For Dr. Ed Grant.
Another proud year
To be part of your
Team To move this
Dept. forward.

Farhood
Jan 2014

Cardiac CT and MR for Adult Congenital Heart Disease

Farhood Saremi
Editor

Cardiac CT and MR for Adult Congenital Heart Disease

Springer

Editor
Farhood Saremi, MD
Department of Radiology
Cardiothoracic Section
University of Southern California
USC Keck Hospital
Los Angeles, CA
USA

ISBN 978-1-4614-8874-3 ISBN 978-1-4614-8875-0 (eBook)
DOI 10.1007/978-1-4614-8875-0
Springer New York Heidelberg Dordrecht London

Library of Congress Control Number: 2013955011

Printed on acid-free paper

Springer is part of Springer Science+Business Media (www.springer.com)

Preface

Different classifications for congenital heart diseases (CHD) have been introduced. These classifications have been mainly based on data obtained from cadaveric and surgical specimens and are designed to simplify the understanding of complexity of this group of abnormalities. However, until recently no single imaging modality has been capable of demonstrating the full spectrum of abnormalities in complex cardiac malformations. In the past years, although plain radiographs, angiography, and echocardiography have been able to answer many questions and guide clinicians and surgeons to treat the patients, in complex cases the shortcomings of these techniques are quite sensible. New generations of MR and CT have facilitated understanding of these complex cases before and after surgical corrections. In fact, the clinical application of CT and MRI has grown dramatically, and cardiologists and cardiothoracic surgeons are ordering these diagnostic modalities more than before.

Along with the advances in diagnostic techniques, the number of adults with CHD has increased over the past decades thanks to parallel advances in surgical techniques and perioperative care. This group of patients comprises important referral cases to hospitals for diagnosis of residual or recurrent lesions requiring serial imaging studies to select candidates for reoperation. In many cases, particularly in immigrants, physicians frequently face complicated CHDs while no clear past history of the disease or the type of surgical treatment can be found. In these cases, a good diagnostic image speaks a thousand words. Images provided by CT and MR can bring a great amount of diagnostic data in these patients with complicated malformations. The element that binds these two modalities in the diagnosis and imaging workup of CHD is their systematic approach to evaluating cardiac anatomy and function. When it comes to the assessment of anatomy, there is no imaging modality that can compete with the speed, accuracy, and spatial resolution of new CT scanners in demonstration of the complex structure of the heart and related vasculature. New generation CT scans can cover the entire anatomic span of the heart and major vessels in a few seconds with spatial resolution of less than 0.5 mm^3. The availability of new low-radiation techniques has made CT an even more attractive choice in many studies. MR is complementary to CT and provides high-resolution anatomic detail in any plane as well as physiologic data that would otherwise be difficult to obtain or unobtainable by either echo or catheterization. Recent technological improvements in MRI hardware and imaging techniques have resulted in dramatic changes to overcome previous limitations of cardiac MR. This is particularly true for imaging of patients with CHD, who are often younger and frequently require continued, lifelong imaging follow-up. Routine availability of high-field magnets, parallel imaging techniques, 2D and 3D steady-state free precession sequences, and high-speed time-resolved MR angiography have opened new gates for cardiac research and improved the evaluation of cardiac pathologies. Time-resolved contrast-enhanced MR angiography with sub-second temporal resolution provides additional dynamic information on blood flow that is less apparent or absent on static MR angiography acquisitions. Newer techniques such as 3D and 4D volumetric flow analyses have facilitated the analysis of shunt flow and post-Fontan hemodynamics. In addition to quantifying the velocity or volume of blood flow through any number of structures of interest, the three-directional flow information acquired with 4D flow MR can be used to qualitatively assess changes in the complex flow patterns within the heart or vasculature.

This book is prepared to serve students, clinicians, and surgeons in the skillful implementation of cardiac MR and CT techniques, coupled with offering a substantial fraction of the existing literature that can be used as a comprehensive resource for CT and MR imaging of CHD. The basics of CT and MR techniques are discussed in the first few chapters in this book. Other chapters focus on common congenital heart problems in adults. The book contains many intriguing cross-sectional and post-processed images that provide an elegant outfit to the content of the book and assist the reader in quickly and easily recognizing various pathologies. Finally, the job would have remained incomplete without the unreserved assistance of Margaret Burns, Developmental Editor; Andy Moyer, Editor; and Wendy Vetter and Wieslawa Langenfeld, the illustrators.

Los Angeles, CA Farhood Saremi, MD

Contents

Contributors

Sonya V. Babu-Narayan, MBBS, BSc, MRCP, PhD NIHR Cardiovascular Biomedical Research Unit, Royal Brompton Hospital and National Heart and Lung Institute, Imperial College London, London, UK

Roy Beinart, MD Division of Cardiology, Johns Hopkins University School of Medicine, Baltimore, MD, USA

William M. Bradlow, BMBS, MRCP, PhD Department of Cardiology, Queen Elizabeth Hospital Birmingham NHS Foundation Trust, Queen Elizabeth Medical Centre, Edgbaston, Birmingham, UK

Stefan Buchner, MD Klinik und Poliklinik für Innere Medizin II, Universitätsklinikum Regensburg, Regensburg, Germany

Harold M. Burkhart, MD Division of Cardiovascular Surgery, Mayo Clinic, Rochester, MN, USA

Michael J. Campbell, MD Division of Pediatric Cardiology, Department of Pediatrics, Duke University Medical Center, Durham, NC, USA

Philip Cascade, MD Division of Cardiothoracic Radiology, Department of Radiology, University of Michigan Health System, Cardiovascular Center, Ann Arbor, MI, USA

Raymond H. M. Chan, MD, MPH, FRCP(C), BScPhm Division of Cardiology, Beth Israel Deaconess Medical Center, PERFUSE Study Group, Boston, MA, USA

Philip Chang, MD Division of Cardiovascular Medicine, Department of Medicine, University of Southern California, Keck School of Medicine, Keck Medical Center of USC and Children's Hospital Los Angeles, Los Angeles, CA, USA

Andrew M. Crean, BSc, BM, MRCP, MSc, FRCR Department of Medicine and Medical Imaging, Toronto Congenital Cardiac Centre for Adults, Peter Munk Cardiac Centre, University Health Network, University of Toronto, Toronto, ON, Canada

Joseph A. Dearani, MD Division of Cardiovascular Surgery, Mayo Clinic, Rochester, MN, USA

Kurt Debl, MD Klinik und Poliklinik für Innere Medizin II, Universitätsklinikum Regensburg, Regensburg, Germany

Scott DeRoo, MD Division of Cardiothoracic Surgery, Columbia University, New York, NY, USA

Jon Detterich, MD Division of Pediatric Cardiology, Department of Pediatrics, University of Southern California, Keck School of Medicine, Children's Hospital Los Angeles, Los Angeles, CA, USA

Jonathan R. Dillman, MD Department of Radiology, University of Michigan Health System, Ann Arbor, MI, USA

Nilda Espinola-Zavaleta, MD, PhD Department of Echocardiography, ABC Medical Center, National Institute of Cardiology Ignacio Chavez, Mexico City, Mexico

Christopher J. François, MD Department of Radiology, School of Medicine and Public Health, University of Wisconsin-Madison, Madison, WI, USA

Julia Geiger, MD Department of Radiology, Medical Physics, University Hospital Freiburg, Freiburg, Germany

Gerald F. Greil, MD, PhD Division of Imaging Sciences and Biomedical Engineering, Department of Pediatric Cardioloy, Guy's and St. Thomas' Hospital/Evelina Children's Hospital, The Rayne Institute, King's College London, London, UK

Matthias Greutmann, MD Congenital Heart Disease Program, Department of Cardiology, Cardiovascular Center, University Hospital Zurich, Zurich, Switzerland

Nobuhisa Hagiwara, MD Department of Cardiology, Tokyo Women's Medical University, Shinjuku, Tokyo, Japan

Linda B. Haramati, MD, MS Cardiothoracic Imaging, Department of Radiology and Medicine, Albert Einstein College of Medicine, Montefiore Medical Center, Bronx, NY, USA

Ee Ling Heng, BSc, MRCP NIHR Biomedical Research Unit, Cardiology Specialty Registrar, Royal Brompton and Harefield NHS Foundation Trust, London, UK

John Hibbeln, MD, FACR Department of Radiology, Rush University Medical Center, Chicago, IL, USA

Ziyad M. Hijazi, MD, MPH, FSCAI Rush Center for Congenital and Structural Heart Disease, Rush University Medical Center, Chicago, IL, USA

Siew Yen Ho, PhD, FRCPath, FESC, FHEA Cardiac Morphology Unit, Royal Brompton Hospital, London, UK

Tiffanie R. Johnson, MD, FAAP, FACC Section of Pediatric Cardiology, Riley Hospital for Children, Indiana University, Indianapolis, IN, USA

Laura Jimenez Juan, MD Department of Radiology, Sunnybrook Health Sciences Centre, University of Toronto, Toronto, ON, Canada

Damien Kenny, MD, MRCPCH Rush Center for Congenital and Structural Heart Disease, Rush University Medical Center, Chicago, IL, USA

Paul Khairy, MD, PhD Electrophysiology Service and Adult Congenital Heart Disease Center, Montreal Heart Institute, Montreal, QC, Canada

Fumiko Kimura, MD, PhD Department of Diagnostic Radiology, Saitama Medical University International Medical Center, Hidaka-shi, Saitama, Japan

Stefan Kislinskiy, MSc Division of Medical and Biological Informatics, German Cancer Research Center (DKFZ), Heidelberg, Germany

Marinos Kontzialis, MD Department of Radiology and Radiological Science, The Johns Hopkins Hospital, Baltimore, MD, USA

Sebastian Leschka, MD Department of Radiology, Institute of Radiology, Kantonsspital St. Gallen, St. Gallen, Switzerland

François Marcotte, MD, FRCPC Non-Invasive Cardiology Service and Adult Congenital Heart Disease Center, Montreal Heart Institute, Montreal, QC, Canada

Michael Markl, PhD Departments of Radiology and Biomedical Engineering, Northwestern University, Chicago, IL, USA

Martin S. Maron, MD Cardiac CT and MRI, Division of Cardiology, Hypertrophic Cardiomyopathy Center, Tufts University School of Medicine, Tufts Medical Center, Boston, MA, USA

Derek Mason, MD Department of Radiology, NYU School of Medicine, New York, NY, USA

Aloha Meave-Gonzalez, MD Cardiovascular Magnetic Resonance Unit, National Institute of Cardiology Ignacio Chavez, Mexico City, Mexico

Raad H. Mohiaddin, MD, FRCR, FRCP, FESC, PhD NIHR Cardiovascular Biomedical Research Unit, Royal Brompton Hospital and National Heart and Lung Institute, Imperial College London, London, UK

François-Pierre Mongeon, MD, SM Non-Invasive Cardiology Service and Adult Congenital Heart Disease Center, Montreal Heart Institute, Montreal, QC, Canada

Jesper Mosegaard, PhD Computer Graphics Lab, The Alexandra Institute Ltd., Århus, Denmark

Luis Muñoz-Castellanos, MD Department of Embryology, National Institute of Cardiology Ignacio Chavez, Mexico City, Mexico

Horia Muresian, MD, PhD Department of Cardiovascular Surgery, University Hospital of Bucharest, Bucharest, Romania

Saman Nazarian, MD, PhD Ventricular Arrhythmia Ablation Service, Cardiac Electrophysiology, Johns Hopkins Hospital, Baltimore, MD, USA

Richard G. Ohye, MD Department of Cardiac Surgery, University of Michigan Health System, Ann Arbor, MI, USA

Sameh M. Said, MD Division of Cardiovascular Surgery, Mayo Clinic, Rochester, MN, USA

Margaret M. Samyn, MD, FAAP, FACC Pediatric Cardiology, The Herma Heart Center, Medical College of Wisconsin, Children's Hospital of Wisconsin, Milwaukee, WI, USA

Damián Sánchez-Quintana, MD, PhD Departamento de Anatomía Humana, Facultad de Medicina de Badajoz, Badajoz, Spain

Farhood Saremi, MD Department of Radiology, Cardiothoracic Section, University of Southern California, USC Keck Hospital, Los Angeles, CA, USA

Laureen Sena, MD Department of Radiology, Boston Children's Hospital, Harvard Medical School, Boston, MA, USA

Thomas Sangild Sørensen, PhD Department of Clinical Medicine and Department of Computer Science, Aarhus University, Aarhus, Denmark

Hugo Spindola-Franco, MD Department of Radiology, Albert Einstein College of Medicine, Montefiore Medical Center, Bronx, NY, USA

Monvadi B. Srichai, MD, FAHA, FACC Department of Radiology and Medicine, NYU School of Medicine, New York, NY, USA

Baskaran Sundaram, MBBS, MRCP, FRCR Division of Cardiothoracic Radiology, Department of Radiology, University of Michigan Health System, Cardiovascular Center 5481, Ann Arbor, MI, USA

Daniel Tobler, MD Congenital Heart Disease Program, Department of Cardiology, University Hospital Basel, Basel, Switzerland

Stephan Waelti, MD Department of Radiology, Institute of Radiology, Kantonsspital St. Gallen, St. Gallen, Switzerland

Rachel M. Wald, MD, FRCPC Departments of Pediatrics, Medicine, Obstetrics/Gynecology and Medical Imaging, Toronto Congenital Cardiac Centre for Adults, Peter Munk Cardiac Centre, University Health Network, University of Toronto, Toronto, ON, Canada

Simon Wildermuth, MD Department of Radiology, Institute of Radiology, Kantonsspital St. Gallen, St. Gallen, Switzerland

Hyun Woo Goo, MD Department of Radiology and Research Institute of Radiology, Asan Medical Center, University of Ulsan College of Medicine, Seoul, South Korea

Chihiro Yamagishi, MD, PhD Department of Pediatrics, Keio University School of Medicine, Tokyo, Japan

Hiroyuki Yamagishi, MD, PhD Division of Pediatric Cardiology, Department of Pediatrics, Keio University School of Medicine, Tokyo, Japan

Andrew Yoon, MD Division of Cardiovascular Medicine, Department of Medicine, University of Southern California, Keck School of Medicine, Keck Medical Center of USC, Los Angeles, CA, USA

Classification and Epidemiology

1

Matthias Greutmann and Daniel Tobler

The advent of open heart surgery has dramatically improved survival in children born with congenital heart disease (CHD). Over the last few decades, mortality has shifted almost entirely to adulthood [1]. This has led to a growing number of adult survivors, particularly to a growing number of adults with complex congenital heart disease. Most patients are however not cured, and many remain at risk for cardiovascular complications and premature death. As most surgical repair techniques were invented only a few decades ago, the cohorts of adult survivors are still emerging and will continue to change in number and age distribution over the upcoming decades.

Historical Perspective

Without intervention, the majority of patients born with complex CHD die in early childhood and survival to adult age is rare [2]. Simple defects, such as isolated ventricular septal defects or a patent ductus arteriosus, have a better natural history and even patients with large defects often reach adulthood without intervention. However, these patients with a large left-to-right shunt are at high risk of developing irreversible pulmonary vascular disease and Eisenmenger syndrome [3]. As a consequence, these patients with Eisenmenger syndrome are at high risk of major morbidity and increased mortality as young adults [4].

In the 1930s and 1940s, techniques to repair or palliate certain forms of congenital heart defects were developed, but only with the introduction of the heart-lung machine into routine clinical practice in the early 1950s, intracardiac repair of CHD became feasible. Over the subsequent decades, pioneer surgeons and cardiologists developed repair techniques for almost all forms of complex CHD. This changed the fate of CHD dramatically. Once highly deadly congenital cardiac lesions, such as tetralogy of Fallot, complete transposition of the great arteries or hearts with univentricular physiology became treatable conditions [5–8]. With improved cardiology care and increasing experience in perioperative management, outcomes rapidly improved.

Classification

Congenital cardiac defects can be classified by a variety of systems. These include classifications based on the type of malformation during the embryologic evolution of the heart (i.e., conotruncal abnormalities, endocardial cushion defects),

M. Greutmann, MD (✉)
Congenital Heart Disease Program,
Department of Cardiology, Cardiovascular Center,
University Hospital Zurich, Raemistrasse 100,
CH-8091 Zurich, Switzerland
e-mail: matthias.greutmann@usz.ch

D. Tobler, MD
Congenital Heart Disease Program,
Department of Cardiology, University Hospital Basel,
Petersgraben 4, CH-4031 Basel, Switzerland
e-mail: daniel.tobler@usb.ch

F. Saremi (ed.), *Cardiac CT and MR for Adult Congenital Heart Disease*,
DOI 10.1007/978-1-4614-8875-0_1, © Springer Science+Business Media New York 2014

classification based on the predominant pathophysiologic or hemodynamic characteristics (cyanotic versus non-cyanotic defects, shunt lesions, etc.), or classification based on clinical severity.

The latter classification based on disease severity is commonly used (Table 1.1). Its intention is to give the clinician a guideline on which adults with CHD can be managed mainly in the general medical community (simple lesions), which adults should be periodically seen in a tertiary care center (lesions of moderate complexity), and which patients should be regularly followed by a multidisciplinary team at a specialized tertiary care center for adults with CHD [2, 9]. It is however important to recognize that even patients with simple lesions at times may also require specialized care and follow-up must be individualized [10].

Table 1.1 Classification of adult congenital heart disease according to disease severity

Simple congenital heart disease
Native disease
Isolated congenital aortic valve disease
Isolated congenital mitral valve disease (e.g., except parachute valve, cleft leaflet)
Small atrial septal defect
Isolated small ventricular septal defect (no associated lesions)
Mild pulmonary stenosis
Small patent ductus arteriosus
Repaired conditions
Previously ligated or occluded ductus arteriosus
Repaired secundum or sinus venosus atrial septal defect without residua
Repaired ventricular septal defect without residua
Congenital heart disease of moderate complexity
Aorto-left ventricular fistulas
Anomalous pulmonary venous drainage, partial or total
Atrioventricular septal defects (partial or complete)
Coarctation of the aorta
Ebstein's anomaly
Infundibular right ventricular outflow obstruction of significance
Ostium primum atrial septal defect
Patent ductus arteriosus (not closed)
Pulmonary valve regurgitation (moderate to severe)
Pulmonary valve stenosis (moderate to severe)
Sinus of Valsalva fistula/aneurysm
Sinus venosus atrial septal defect
Sub- or supravalvular aortic stenosis (except hypertrophic obstructive cardiomyopathy)
Tetralogy of Fallot
Ventricular septal defect with:
Absent valve or valves
Aortic regurgitation
Coarctation of the aorta
Mitral disease
Right ventricular outflow tract obstruction
Straddling tricuspid/mitral valve
Subaortic stenosis
Congenital heart disease of great complexity
Conduits, valved or nonvalved
Cyanotic congenital heart disease (all forms)
Double outlet ventricle
Eisenmenger syndrome
Fontan procedure
Mitral atresia
Single ventricle (also called double inlet or outlet, common or primitive)
Pulmonary atresia (all forms)
Pulmonary vascular obstructive disease
Transposition of the great arteries
Tricuspid atresia
Truncus arteriosus/hemitruncus
Other abnormalities of atrioventricular or ventriculoarterial connection not included above (i.e., crisscross heart, isomerism, heterotaxy syndromes, ventricular inversion)

Modified from Warnes et al. [2]

Incidence and Prevalence

Congenital heart defects are common [2, 11–13]. Their reported incidence varies among different studies depending on the type and setting of the study [13]. The number of patients with lesions of moderate to severe complexity seems to be relatively stable at around 6/1,000 live births with little variation between different countries and little changes over time [13]. Figure 1.1 depicts estimates of the incidence of various congenital heart defects at time of birth, derived from 44 studies of the incidence of congenital heart disease. Among all patients with CHD, ventricular septal defects are the most common defects by far, while among those with lesions of moderate

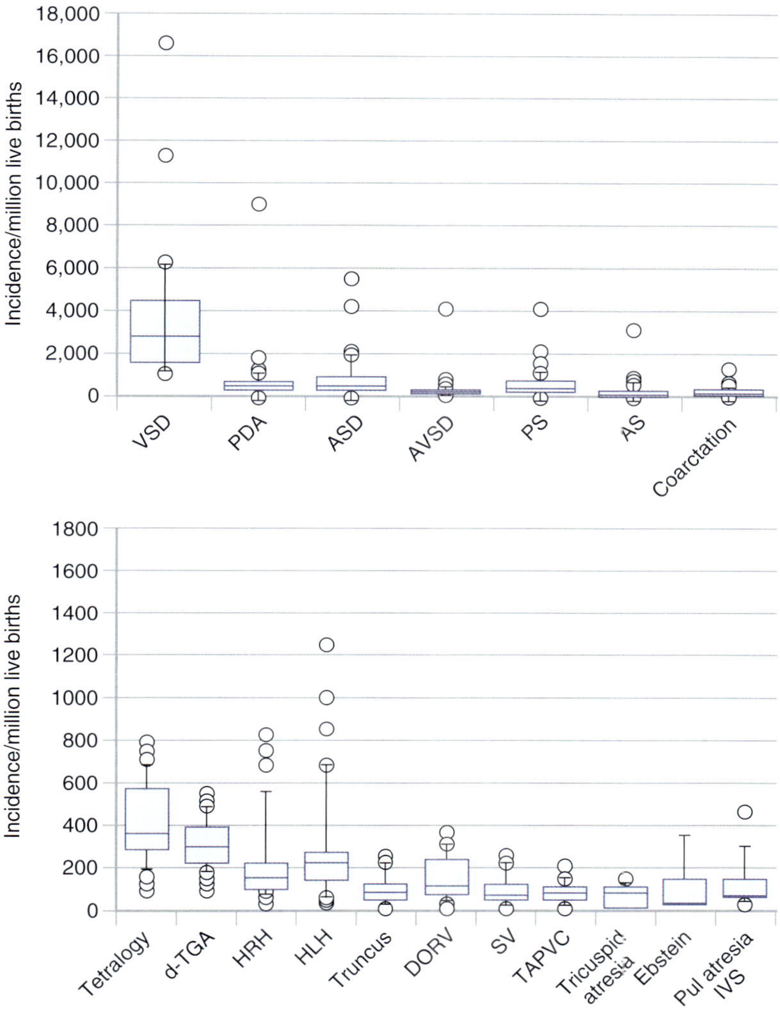

Fig. 1.1 Estimates on incidence of various types of congenital heart defects among live births. Modified *box plots* to show variability of the incidence per million live births of various forms of congenital heart disease. The *rectangle* shows the upper and lower quartiles, and the horizontal line in the middle is the median. The two short horizontal lines connected to the rectangle by thin vertical lines indicate the 90th and 10th percentiles, and data points outside these limits are shown individually. Each panel has a different vertical scale that on the top panel being ten times larger than that on the *bottom panel*. (*Top*) The four major left-to-right shunts (ventricular septal defect *VSD*, patent ductus arteriosus *PDA*, atrial septal defect *ASD*, atrioventricular septal defect *AVSD*) and the three major obstructive lesions (pulmonic stenosis *PS*, aortic stenosis *AS*, coarctation of the aorta *coarctation*). (*Bottom*) Tetralogy of Fallot (tetralogy); complete transposition of the great arteries (*d-TGA*); hypoplastic right heart *HRH*, which includes tricuspid atresia, Ebstein's anomaly, and pulmonary atresia with an intact ventricular septum (pulmonary atresia *IVS*), hypoplastic left heart *HLH*, truncus arteriosus *truncus*, double outlet right ventricle *DORV*, single ventricle *SV*, total anomalous pulmonary venous connection *TAPVC*. The three components of the HRH syndrome do not add up to the total, because not all reports included all three (From Hoffman and Kaplan [13] with permission)

or great complexity (bottom part of the Fig. 1.1), tetralogy of Fallot, complete transposition of the great arteries, and lesions with univentricular physiology have the highest incidence.

In the future, the increasing use of fetal echocardiography and subsequent therapeutic abortion for certain forms of complex CHD may affect their future incidence [14–16]. On the

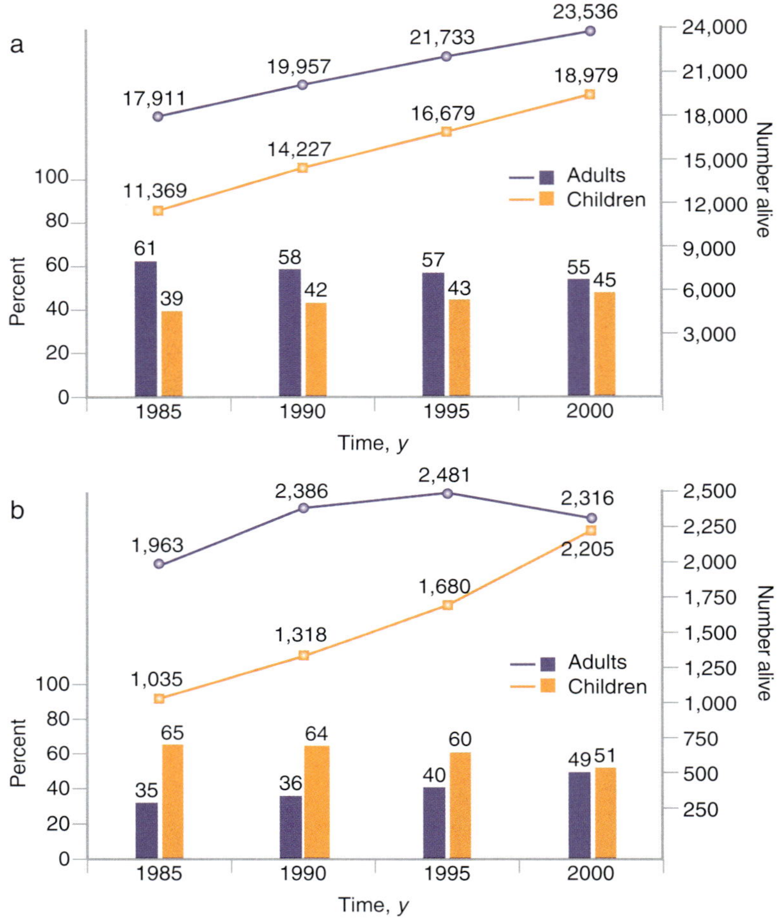

Fig. 1.2 Numbers and proportion of adults and children with all CHD (**a**) and severe CHD (**b**) in 1985, 1990, 1995, and 2000 (From Marelli et al. [24]. Copyright, American Heart Association with permission)

other hand, patients affected by CHD have an increased risk of transmission of a congenital heart defect to their offspring [17, 18]. Most patients born with CHD now reach adulthood and thus childbearing age. Once they have children, the increased incidence of CHD among their offspring may increase the total incidence of babies born with congenital heart disease [19].

While the incidence of CHD has remained relatively stable over time, its prevalence has changed substantially because of improved survival. Nowadays, it is expected that the majority of babies born with complex CHD will survive to adulthood and within the last two decades mortality has shifted almost entirely to adult life [1, 19, 20]. This has led to a growing population of adults with CHD and particularly to a rapid increase of adult survivors with complex CHD as illustrated in Fig. 1.2. Currently, the best available evidence suggests that the overall prevalence of CHD in the adult population is about 3,000 per million [21]. Given that adult patient populations with complex CHD are still emerging, we expect a further increase in the prevalence of adult survivors with complex disease over the next few decades.

Evolution of Current Patient Populations and Future Challenges

Most surgical repair techniques for complex congenital heart lesions have been introduced only a few decades ago and have undergone continuous modification from their invention up to the current era. Thus, the cohorts of adult survivors

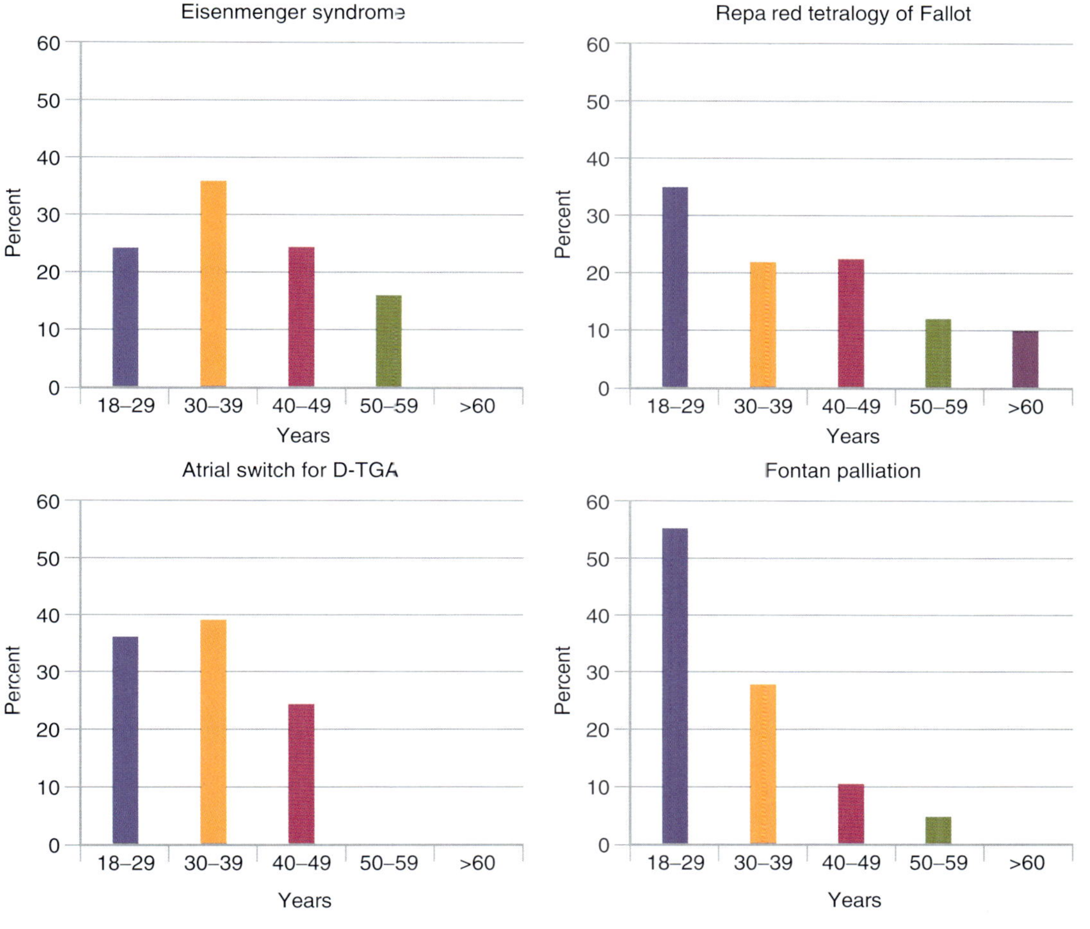

Fig. 1.3 Proportional age distribution among adults with Eisenmenger syndrome, repaired tetralogy of Fallot, atrial switch operation for complete transposition of the great arteries, and Fontan palliation for univentricular physiology followed at the University Hospital Zurich, Switzerland (Abbreviation: *d-TGA* dextro-transposition of the great arteries)

particularly of survivors with complex congenital heart lesions are just emerging, and the number and demographic characteristics of these survivors will change over the next few decades. Most patients are still young adults, but given the historical evolution of repair techniques, there are substantial differences in age distribution among patient cohorts with different congenital cardiac disease entities as illustrated in Fig. 1.3.

Despite dramatic improvements in life expectancy, most survivors of infant heart surgery for congenital heart disease are not cured, and many remain at a substantial risk for cardiovascular complications and premature death. This is particularly true for adult survivors with complex lesions, such as cyanotic heart defects, patients with transposition complexes with systemic right ventricles, patients with repaired tetralogy of Fallot, and those with Fontan palliation for univentricular hearts [4, 22, 23]. With further ageing of these cohorts, complication rates and mortality risk will likely substantially change over the next few decades. In addition, novel patient cohorts, such as adult survivors after the Norwood procedure for palliation of hypoplastic left heart syndrome will emerge and add to the complexity of care for this novel group of young adults with chronic disease.

References

1. Khairy P, Ionescu-Ittu R, Mackie AS, Abrahamowicz M, Pilote L, Marelli AJ. Changing mortality in congenital heart disease. J Am Coll Cardiol. 2010;56:1149–57.
2. Warnes CA, Liberthson R, Danielson GK, et al. Task force 1: the changing profile of congenital heart disease in adult life. J Am Coll Cardiol. 2001;37:1170–5.
3. Wood P. The Eisenmenger syndrome or pulmonary hypertension with reversed central shunt. Br Med J. 1958;2:755–62.
4. Daliento L, Somerville J, Presbitero P, et al. Eisenmenger syndrome. Factors relating to deterioration and death. Eur Heart J. 1998;19:1845–55.
5. Lillehei CW, Cohen M, Warden HE, et al. Direct vision intracardiac surgical correction of the tetralogy of Fallot, pentalogy of Fallot, and pulmonary atresia defects; report of first ten cases. Ann Surg. 1955;142:418–42.
6. Senning A. Surgical correction of transposition of the great vessels. Surgery. 1959;45:966–80.
7. Mustard WT. Successful two-stage correction of transposition of the great vessels. Surgery. 1964;55:469–72.
8. Fontan F, Baudet E. Surgical repair of tricuspid atresia. Thorax. 1971;26:240–8.
9. Warnes CA, Williams RG, Bashore TM, et al. ACC/AHA 2008 guidelines for the management of adults with congenital heart disease: executive summary: a report of the American College of Cardiology/American Heart Association Task Force on Practice Guidelines (writing committee to develop guidelines for the management of adults with congenital heart disease). Circulation. 2008;118:2395–451.
10. Baumgartner H, Bonhoeffer P, De Groot NM, et al. ESC guidelines for the management of grown-up congenital heart disease (new version 2010). Eur Heart J. 2010;31:2915–57.
11. Botto LD, Correa A, Erickson JD. Racial and temporal variations in the prevalence of heart defects. Pediatrics. 2001;107:E32.
12. Ferencz C, Rubin JD, McCarter RJ, et al. Congenital heart disease: prevalence at livebirth. The Baltimore-Washington Infant Study. Am J Epidemiol. 1985;121:31–6.
13. Hoffman JI, Kaplan S. The incidence of congenital heart disease. J Am Coll Cardiol. 2002;39:1890–900.
14. Allan LD, Sharland GK, Milburn A, et al. Prospective diagnosis of 1,006 consecutive cases of congenital heart disease in the fetus. J Am Coll Cardiol. 1994;23:1452–8.
15. Daubeney PE, Sharland GK, Cook AC, Keeton BR, Anderson RH, Webber SA. Pulmonary atresia with intact ventricular septum: impact of fetal echocardiography on incidence at birth and postnatal outcome. UK and Eire Collaborative Study of Pulmonary Atresia with Intact Ventricular Septum. Circulation. 1998;98:562–6.
16. Allan LD, Cook A, Sullivan I, Sharland GK. Hypoplastic left heart syndrome: effects of fetal echocardiography on birth prevalence. Lancet. 1991;337:959–61.
17. Calcagni G, Digilio MC, Sarkozy A, Dallapiccola B, Marino B. Familial recurrence of congenital heart disease: an overview and review of the literature. Eur J Pediatr. 2007;166:111–6.
18. Pierpont ME, Basson CT, Benson Jr DW, et al. Genetic basis for congenital heart defects: current knowledge: a scientific statement from the American Heart Association Congenital Cardiac Defects Committee, Council on Cardiovascular Disease in the Young: endorsed by the American Academy of Pediatrics. Circulation. 2007;115:3015–38.
19. Moons P, Bovijn L, Budts W, Belmans A, Gewillig M. Temporal trends in survival to adulthood among patients born with congenital heart disease from 1970 to 1992 in Belgium. Circulation. 2010;122:2264–72.
20. Gilboa SM, Salemi JL, Nembhard WN, Fixler DE, Correa A. Mortality resulting from congenital heart disease among children and adults in the United States, 1999 to 2006. Circulation. 2010;122:2254–63.
21. van der Bom T, Bouma BJ, Meijboom FJ, Zwinderman AH, Mulder BJ. The prevalence of adult congenital heart disease, results from a systematic review and evidence based calculation. Am Heart J. 2012;164:568–75.
22. Oechslin EN, Harrison DA, Connelly MS, Webb GD, Siu SC. Mode of death in adults with congenital heart disease. Am J Cardiol. 2000;86:1111–6.
23. Verheugt CL, Uiterwaal CS, van der Velde ET, et al. Mortality in adult congenital heart disease. Eur Heart J. 2010;31:1220–9.
24. Marelli AJ, Mackie AS, Ionescu-Ittu R, Rahme E, Pilote L. Congenital heart disease in the general population: changing prevalence and age distribution. Circulation. 2007;115:163–72.

Embryology

2

Hiroyuki Yamagishi and Chihiro Yamagishi

Morphogenesis of the Cardiovascular System

The heart is the first organ that is formed and becomes functional in the human embryo [1, 2]. It bears the circulatory system from the early embryonic period and alters its morphology to each stage of an embryonic growth according to its demand. The early morphogenesis of the heart and great vessels is conserved across species of living things. In the mammals, the complicated process of morphogenesis results in the separable systemic and pulmonary circulation after birth by which oxygen is efficiently supplied to different internal organs in order to maintain their function.

The morphogenesis of the cardiovascular system is started around 3 weeks of gestation and mostly completed by 8 weeks of gestation in human. First, immediately after gastrulation, the cardiac-fated cells of anterior lateral plate mesoderm origin form a crescent-shaped cardiac precursor in front of a notochord (Fig. 2.1a). The cardiac crescent constructs bilateral endocardial tubes that fuse to form the primitive heart tube in the midline of embryo (Fig. 2.1b). The primitive heart tube is a beating tubular structure that maintains blood flow from caudal to rostral direction of the embryo. Along with rightward looping of the primitive heart tube, the right and left ventricles and atria become morphologically apparent (Fig. 2.1c). Endocardial cushions are formed in extracellular matrix (also known as cardiac jelly) of the atrioventricular canal region from the mesenchymal cells which were separated from the endocardium and transformed. An atrioventricular canal is divided by the coalescence of the superior and inferior endocardial cushions. Endocardial cushions also participate in the formation of interatrial septum (closing of ostium primum), atrioventricular valves (mitral and tricuspid valve), and the membranous portion of the interventricular septum. Formation of interatrial septum, interventricular septum, and atrioventricular valves results in the 2-atrium and 2-ventricle heart (Fig. 2.1d).

In the cardiac outflow tract, the conotruncal swellings or cushions form the conotruncal septum that divides a tubular structure into two great vessels, namely, the aorta and the pulmonary trunk, in a spiral fashion (Fig. 2.1e). At the bases of great vessels, semilunar valves are formed. A proper connection of the left ventricle to the aorta and the right ventricle to the pulmonary trunk is indispensable for establishment and separation of the systemic and pulmonary circulation after birth.

The great vessel system arises from six pairs of pharyngeal arch arteries which run through pharyngeal arches symmetrically (Fig. 2.1f).

H. Yamagishi, MD, PhD (✉)
Division of Pediatric Cardiology,
Department of Pediatrics,
Keio University School of Medicine, Tokyo, Japan
e-mail: hyamag@z6.keio.jp

C. Yamagishi, MD, PhD
Department of Pediatrics,
Keio University School of Medicine, Tokyo, Japan

F. Saremi (ed.), *Cardiac CT and MR for Adult Congenital Heart Disease*,
DOI 10.1007/978-1-4614-8875-0_2, © Springer Science+Business Media New York 2014

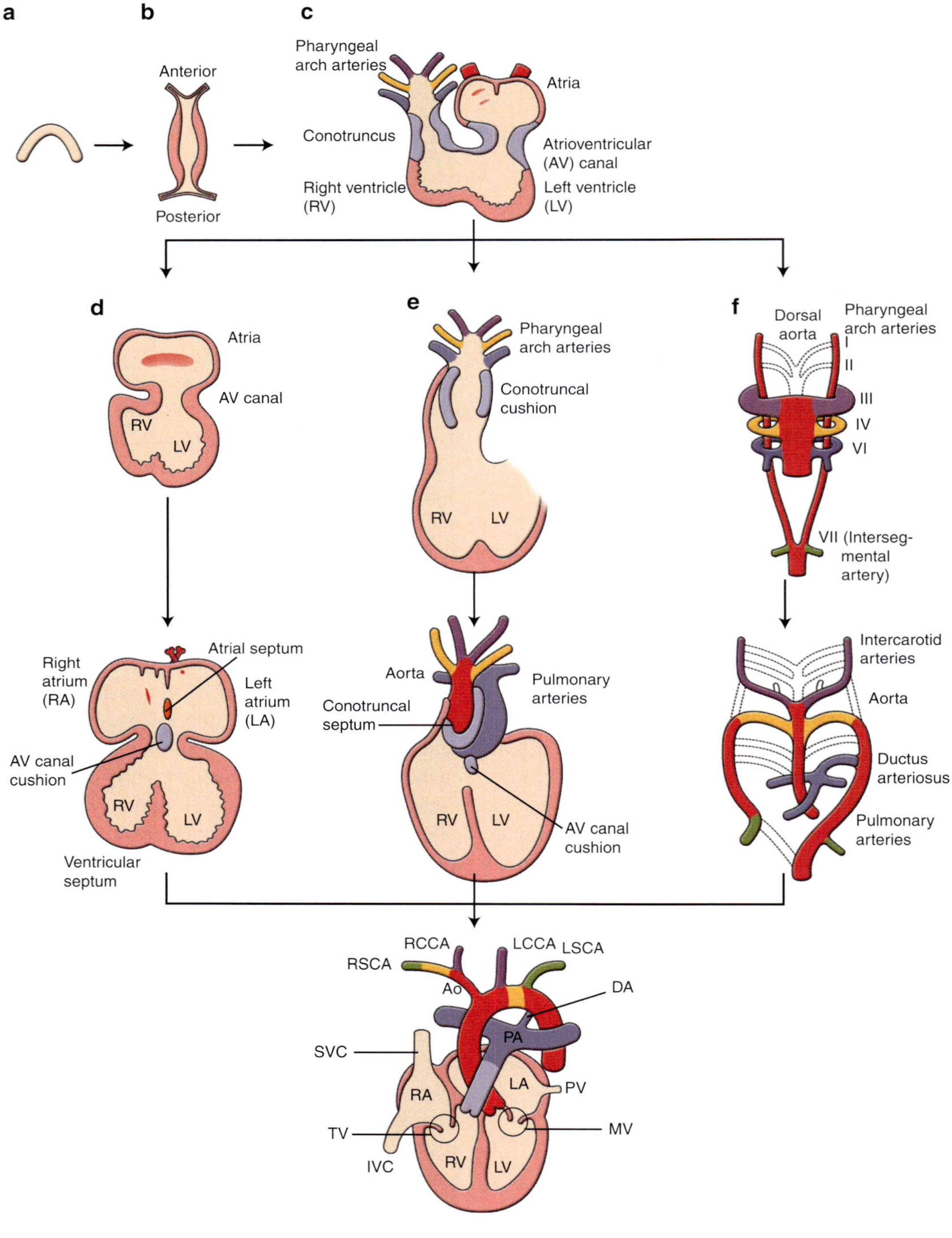

Fig. 2.1 Morphogenesis of the cardiovascular system. (**a**) Cardiac crescent. (**b**) Primitive heart tube. (**c**) Looping. (**d**) Atrioventricle. (**e**) Outflow tract. (**f**) Great vessels. See detail in text. *Ao* aorta, *DA* ductus arteriosus, *IVC* inferior vena cava, *LCCA* left common carotid artery, *LSCA* left subclavian artery, *MV* mitral valve, *PA* pulmonary arteries, *PV* pulmonary veins, *RCCA* right common carotid artery, *RSCA* right subclavian artery, *SVC* superior vena cava, *TV* tricuspid valve

The third, fourth, and sixth pharyngeal arch arteries will remodel and transform to a portion of the aortic arch, arch branches, ductus arteriosus, and a part of branch pulmonary arteries.

Developmental Origins of the Heart

Decades of descriptive embryology, including cell lineage tracings have improved our understandings of developmental origins [1–5]. Cells derived from the anterior lateral plate mesoderm form a crescent shape at approximately 2 weeks of gestation, and by 3 weeks of gestation, these cells coalesce along the ventral midline to form a primitive heart tube, consisting of an interior layer of endocardial cells and an exterior layer of myocardial cells, separated by extracellular matrix, or cardiac jelly, for reciprocal signaling between the two layers. The crescent-shaped pool of cardiogenic progenitor cells is now termed "first heart field" (Fig. 2.2a). The first heart field that forms the heart tube eventually contributes to specific chambers of the future heart, exclusively to the left ventricle and all other parts of the heart, except the cardiac outflow tract.

In addition to the first heart field, it was reported 10 years ago that there was a second source of myocardial cells. In mammalian embryos, this source is lying medially to the cardiac crescent (Fig. 2.2a) and then behind the forming heart tube (Fig. 2.2b), extending into the mesodermal layer of the pharyngeal arches (Fig. 2.2c). This second source is termed "second heart field." The heart tube derived from the first heart field may predominantly provide a scaffold upon which cells from the second heart field migrate into both arterial and venous poles of the heart tube, where they subsequently construct the requisite cardiac components. The contribution of the second heart field to both myocardium and smooth muscle of the arterial pole has been well studied. When the heart tube forms, the second heart field cells migrate into the midline and position themselves dorsal to the heart tube in the pharyngeal mesoderm (Fig. 2.2b). Upon rightward looping of the heart tube, the second heart field cells cross the pharyngeal mesoderm into the anterior and posterior portions, populating a large portion of the outflow tract including future right ventricle and atria (Fig. 2.2c). The addition of the second heart field-derived myocardium to the outflow tract results in its elongation. This elongation is necessary to allow the outflow tract to rotate and shorten sufficiently for correct alignment of the pulmonary and aortic trunks with their respective ventricles.

The third lineage represents cardiac neural crest cells originating from the dorsal neural tube between the mid-otic placode and the caudal boundary of the third somite. After they delaminate from the dorsal neural tube, cardiac neural crest cells migrate into the caudal pharyngeal arches, and the outflow tract where they contribute to the conotruncal cushions that give rise to the outflow tract septum (Fig. 2.2c, d). Migration of the cardiac neural crest cells is also targeted to

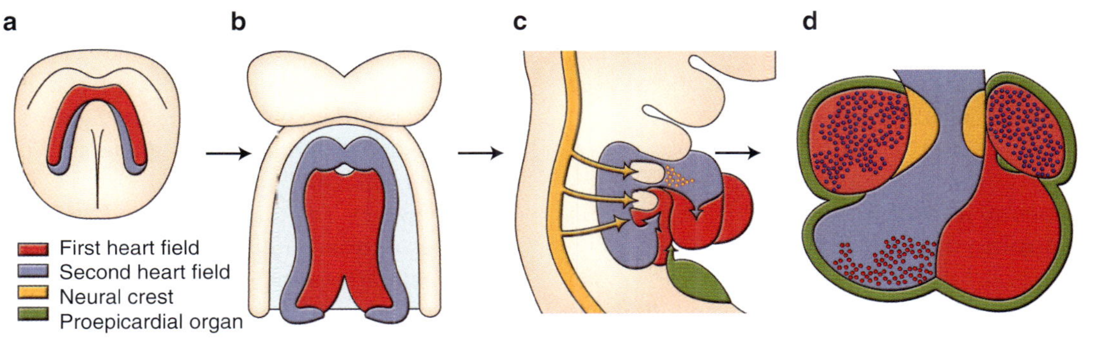

Fig. 2.2 Developmental origins of the heart. (**a**) Cardiac crescent. (**b**) Primitive heart tube. (**c**) Looping heart tube. (**d**) Four chambered heart. See detail in text

pharyngeal arches 3, 4, and 6 which give rise to the future great vessels (Fig. 2.2c). Many signaling pathways are involved in the migration and condensation of cardiac neural crest cells, including reciprocal signaling between the cardiac neural crest cells and the second heart field, which are essential for the development of the outflow tract and the aortic arch system.

The fourth lineage of cardiac precursor cells is the proepicardium. The proepicardium develops from the coelomic mesothelium which overlays the liver bud, and the expression of proepicardium-specific genes is induced in naïve mesothelial cells in response to a localized liver-derived signal. Almost all cells of the epicardium and the coronary vessels arise from the proepicardium, which develops as multiple epithelial villi protruding from the pericardial mesothelium immediately posterior to sinoatrium of the looping stage embryonic heart. The proepicardium extends toward the primitive heart and attaches and spreads over the myocardial surface to form the epicardium (Fig. 2.2c, d). During proepicardium growth and epicardial formation, some proepicardial/epicardial cells undergo an epithelial–mesenchymal transformation (EMT) and give rise to the precursors of the coronary vessels and connective tissue cells.

Embryology of the Heart and Congenital Heart Diseases

Congenital heart diseases are considered to occur as a result of the abnormalities of each step in the morphogenesis of the heart and the great vessels. Current embryological concepts for the genesis of congenital heart diseases are discussed below although not all are proved.

Normal and Abnormal Looping of the Heart [6, 7]

The normal left–right development results in situs solitus with all the asymmetric internal organs placed on the body where they should be, and the looping of the primitive heart tube happens to a rightward convex direction (Fig. 2.3b: dextro-loop; d-loop). When left–right specification does not process normally, the direction of looping will be altered and a range of visceroatrial heterotaxia occurs that is usually associated with complex congenital heart diseases. In case of complete mirror-image reversal of all organs, the looping becomes a leftward convex direction (Fig. 2.3a: levo-loop; l-loop), resulting in a benign dextrocardia without significant cardiac malformations and untoward clinical consequences.

Corrected Transposition of Great Arteries (l-TGA)[8]

This phenotype occurs when the primitive heart tube becomes l-loop; at the same time, an arterial trunk is linearly divided into an anteriorly located left-sided aorta and a posteriorly located right-sided pulmonary arterial trunk (Fig. 2.3c). As a result, there is atrioventricular discordance and ventriculoarterial discordance where the right atrium is connected to the left ventricle contiguous to the pulmonary artery and the left atrium is connected to the right ventricle contiguous to the aorta.

Abnormality of Rightward Shift of the Atrioventricular Canal (Inflow Tract): Tricuspid Atresia (TA) [6, 9, 10]

Around 4 weeks of gestation, the heart looping results in a series circulation from the right atrium, to the left atrium, the left ventricle, and the right ventricle that resembles a hemodynamics of tricuspid atresia (Fig. 2.4). Soon later, the atrioventricular canal shifts rightward and the final relation of the right atrium to the right ventricle and the left atrium to the left ventricle is established, resulting in a parallel circulation (Fig. 2.4 lower). The tricuspid atresia is considered to result from an obstacle of the rightward shift of the atrioventricular canal that leads to complete absence of the tricuspid valve with no direct communication between the right atrium

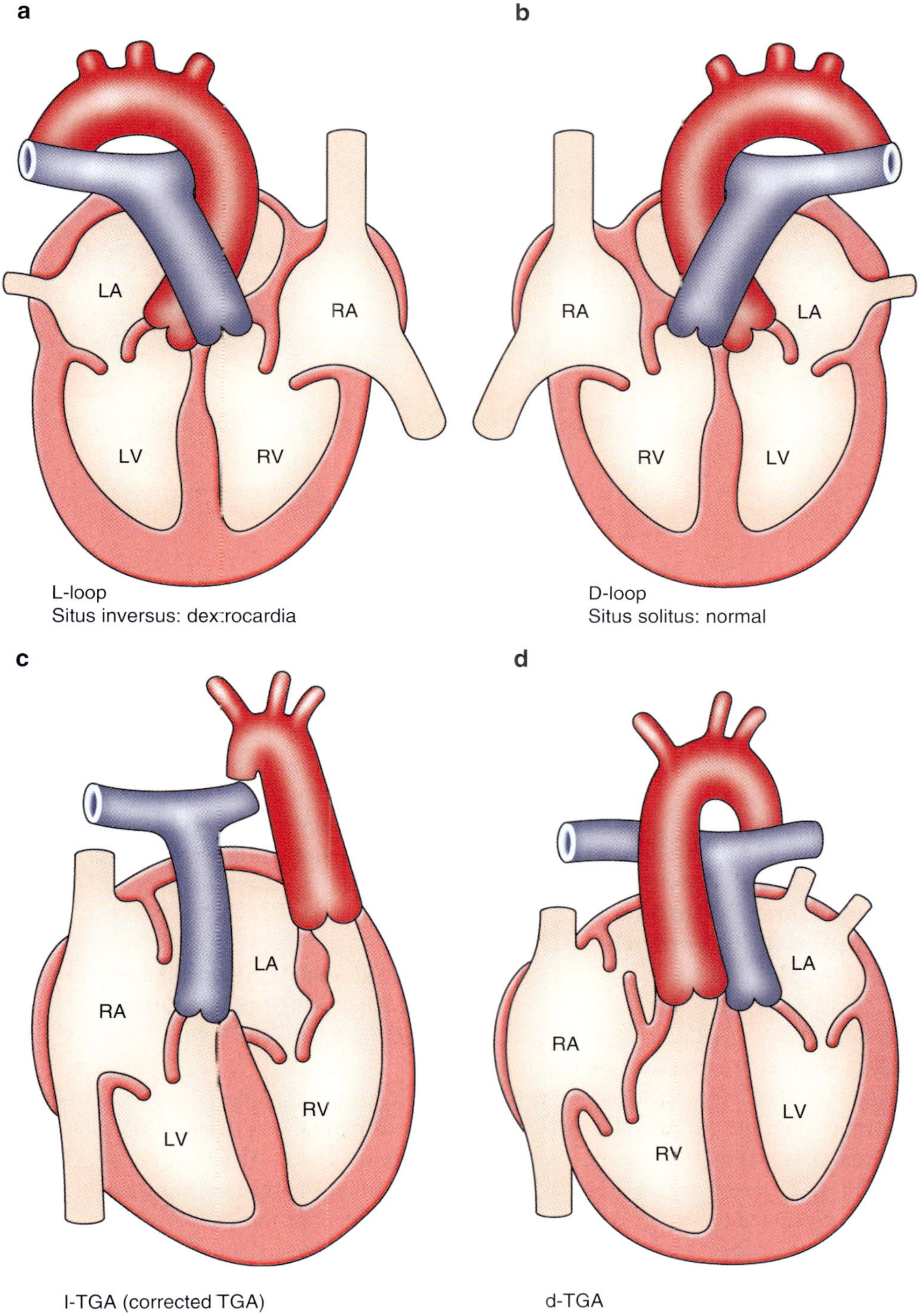

Fig. 2.3 Normal and abnormal looping of the heart. (**a**) Leftward looping. (**b**) Rightward looping. (**c**) L-loop + transposition. (**d**) D-loop + transposition. See detail in text

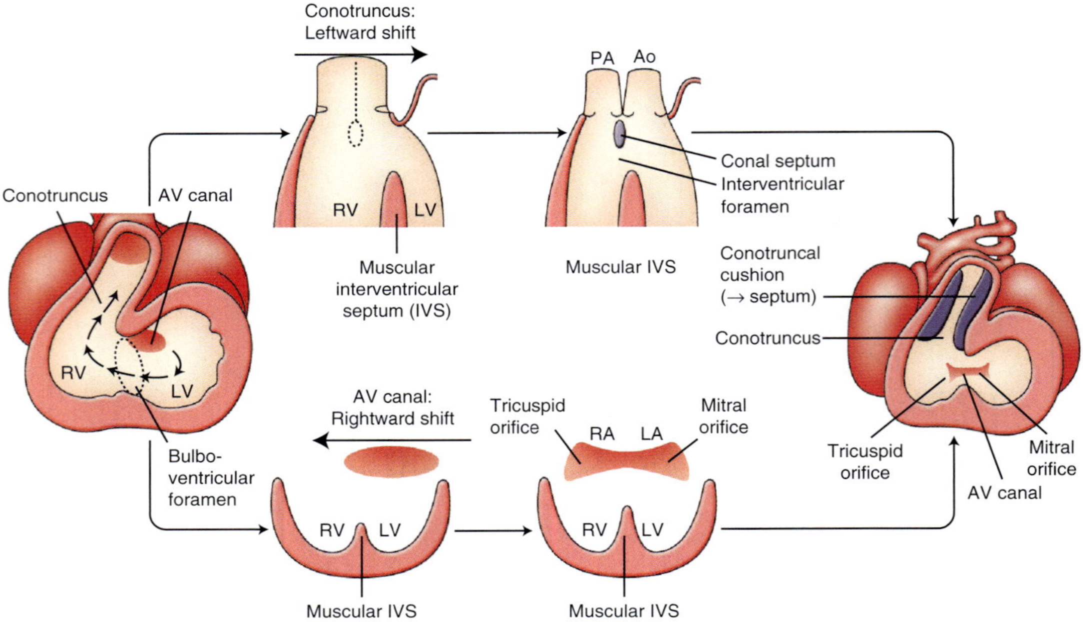

Fig. 2.4 Early development of the inflow tract and the outflow tract. See detail in text. *AV* atrioventricular, *Ao* aorta, *IVS* interventricular septum, *LA* left atrium, *LV* left ventricle, *PA* pulmonary artery, *RA* right atrium, *RV* right ventricle

and the right ventricle. The atretic tricuspid valve is represented by a dimple in the floor of the right atrium. The resulting membrane is usually muscular, but may be fibrous.

Abnormality of Leftward Shift of the Conotruncus (Outflow Tract): Double Outlet Right Ventricle (DORV) [11–13]

Around 4 weeks of gestation, in a process of the looping, the conotruncus shifts leftward, and the relation of the left ventricle to the aorta and the right ventricle to the pulmonary trunk will be established (Fig. 2.4 upper). DORV, in which both great vessels arise from the right ventricle, is presumed to result from an obstacle to leftward shift of the conotruncus. DORV is also implicated in abnormalities of conotruncal rotation, conus formation, and septal formation. It seems reasonable to accept these abnormalities as a spectrum representing a relatively primitive embryologic condition with the origin of both great arteries from the morphologic right ventricle (Fig. 2.5b). The subaortic conus is normally absorbed during the leftward shift of the conotruncus, and fibrous continuation between mitral and aortic valves can be observed. In DORV, bilateral subarterial conus and discontinuity of both semilunar valves with their respective atrioventricular valve are common.

Normal and Abnormal Septation and Alignment of the Outflow Tract [1, 2, 11–14]

The embryonic outflow tract (conotruncus) consists of a distal part, the truncus, and a proximal part or the conus. At 4–5 weeks of gestation, two big swellings in the truncal region (right superior and left inferior truncal cushions) and two small swellings in the conal region (right dorsal and left ventral conal cushions) develop in the outflow tract (Fig. 2.5a). The coalescence of these four cushions is carried out in a spiral fashion that accounts for the adult gross anatomical relationship between the aorta (to the left ventricle) and the pulmonary arterial trunk (to the right ventricle) (Fig. 2.5a).

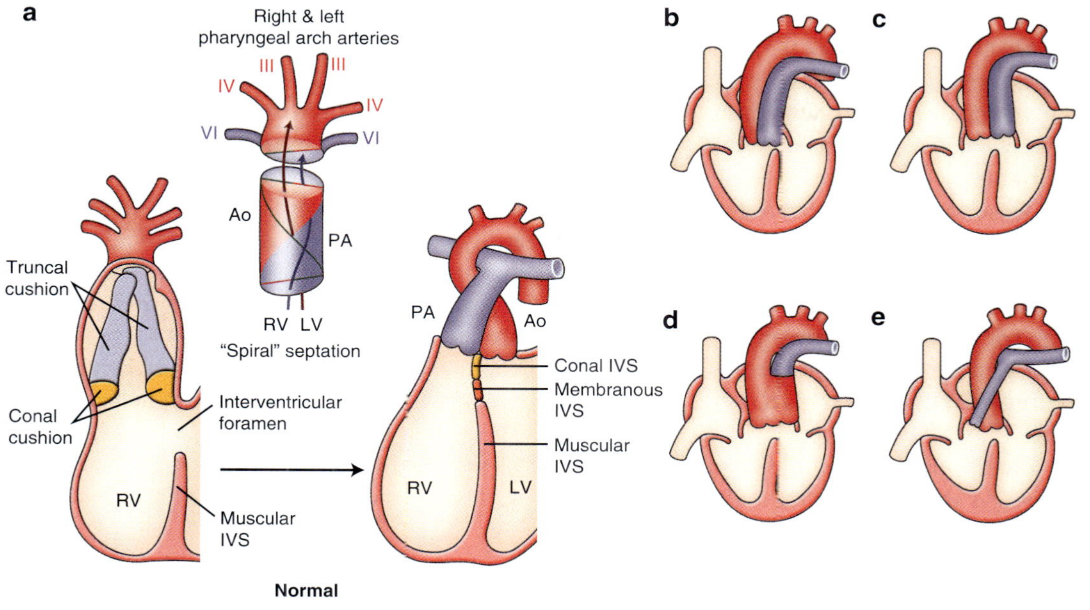

Fig. 2.5 (**a**) Normal and (**b–e**) abnormal septation and alignment of the outflow tract. (**b**) Double outlet right ventricle (DORV). (**c**) Transposition of the great arteries (TGA). (**d**) Persistent truncus arteriosus (PTA). (**e**) Tetralogy of Fallot (TOF). See detail in text. *Ao* aorta, *IVS* interventricular septum, *LV* left ventricle, *PA* pulmonary artery, *RV* right ventricle

There are a variety of clinically important congenital heart diseases associated with abnormalities of the outflow tract. Although they are commonly explained by the developmental abnormalities of cardiac neural crest cells, recently, the involvement of the second heart field for outflow tract defects has been extensively investigated. 22q11.2 deletion syndrome is well known to be highly associated with outflow tract defects.

Transposition of the Great Arteries (TGA) [15]

TGA results from a failure of the outflow tract septation to develop in a spiral fashion, instead it develops in a parallel fashion (Figs. 2.3d and 2.5c). The detailed developmental aspects of the outflow tract septation in a parallel fashion remain largely uncertain. Abnormal development, growth, and absorption of subarterial conus are presumed to be a major factor. Although the normal conus is subpulmonary, left-sided, and anterior, there usually is a subaortic, right-sided, and anterior conus in patients with TGA.

Persistent Truncus Arteriosus (PTA) [1, 2, 12, 14, 16]

PTA results from incomplete formation of the conotruncal septum (Fig. 2.5d). The pathogenesis of PTA is suggested by a key experimental model in which ablation of the cardiac neural cells in chick lead to failure of partitioning of the embryonic truncus arteriosus and disrupted the conotruncal development by interfering with the addition of the myocardium derived from the second heart field. If vestiges of distal truncal septation develop, a short pulmonary arterial trunk can be formed from which the pulmonary arteries arise (Fig. 2.5d). A partial developmental failure of distal truncal septum may result in aorticopulmonary window (AP window). In contrast to PTA, in AP window, semilunar valves are completely divided by the conal septum.

Tetralogy of Fallot (TOF) [1, 2, 12, 14, 17]

TOF refers to the tetrad of overriding aorta, pulmonary stenosis, ventricular septal defect, and right ventricular hypertrophy (Fig. 2.5e). It results from aortic overriding and subpulmonary stenosis created by the deviation of the conal septum, leading to a malalignment between the aorta and the left ventricle with a malalignment-type ventricular septal defect. The anatomic spectrum of TOF is diverse, including cases with pulmonary atresia and those with absent pulmonary valve.

Normal and Abnormal Growth of Ventricles and Alignment of Atrial and Ventricular Septum: Univentricular Heart [18, 19]

At 4 weeks of gestation, right and left ventricles grow and the muscular interventricular septum carries out normal alignment at interatrial septum by looping, and the normal four-chambered heart can be formed (Fig. 2.6c, d). Abnormal growth of the primitive right or left ventricle may result in hypoplasia of the right or left ventricle. Malalignment between the interventricular septum and the interatrial septum could result in unilateral atresia of the atrioventricular valve (tricuspid or mitral atresia) or double inlet ventricle (double inlet right, left or indetermined ventricle) (Fig. 2.6c). These abnormalities consist of a wide spectrum of functional univentricular heart.

Normal and Abnormal Development of Atrial Septum: Atrial Septal Defects (ASD) [20]

At 4–5 weeks of gestation, the crescent-shaped septum primum forms in the roof of the primitive atrium and grows toward to and fuses with the atrioventricular cushions in the atrioventricular canal where the foramen primum between the free edge of the septum primum and the atrioventricular cushions is closed (Fig. 2.6a, d). Meanwhile, the foramen secundum is created in the center of septum primum which is later covered by the septum secundum arising from the atrial roof on the right of the septum primum. The foramen ovale remains patent to maintain blood flow from the right to the left atrium during fetal life.

ASDs are classified according to their location relative to the foramen ovale (Fig. 2.6b). The secundum type is the most common and is considered to result from excessive resorption of the septum primum or secundum. The primum type is probably caused by abnormal development of the atrioventricular cushions and/or dorsal mesenchymal protrusion that arises from the posterior part of second heart field, contributes to the venous pole of the heart tube, and gives rise to the myocardial base of the primary atrial septum. The sinus venosus type is usually associated with anomalous return of the right pulmonary veins. The coronary sinus type is often associated with an unroofed coronary sinus and left atrial connection of a persistent left superior vena cava.

Normal and Abnormal Development of Ventricular Septum: Ventricular Septal Defects (VSD) [21]

At 4 weeks of gestation, the muscular interventricular septum develops in midline on the floor of the primitive ventricles and grows toward the atrioventricular canal (Fig. 2.6d). By 7 weeks of gestation, muscular interventricular septum connects with the bottom edge of conal septum through the atrioventricular cushions, and the interventricular foramen is ultimately closed by the membranous interventricular septum that is formed by the proliferation and fusion of tissues from three sources, partly from the right and left conal cushions and mostly from the atrioventricular cushions (Fig. 2.6e).

The conal type of ventricular septal defect occurs as a result of failure to fuse of the conal cushions (Fig. 2.6f). The muscular type occurs by simple single or multiple perforations in the muscular septum (Fig. 2.6f). The inlet type results from abnormal development of atrioventricular cushions (Fig. 2.6f). The membranous-type ventricular septal defect is the most common congenital heart defect. It can be caused simply by failure of the membranous interventricular septum to develop, but also by malalignment between the conal septum and the muscular septum (Fig. 2.6f–h). The malalignment type is usually associated with complex heart malformations.

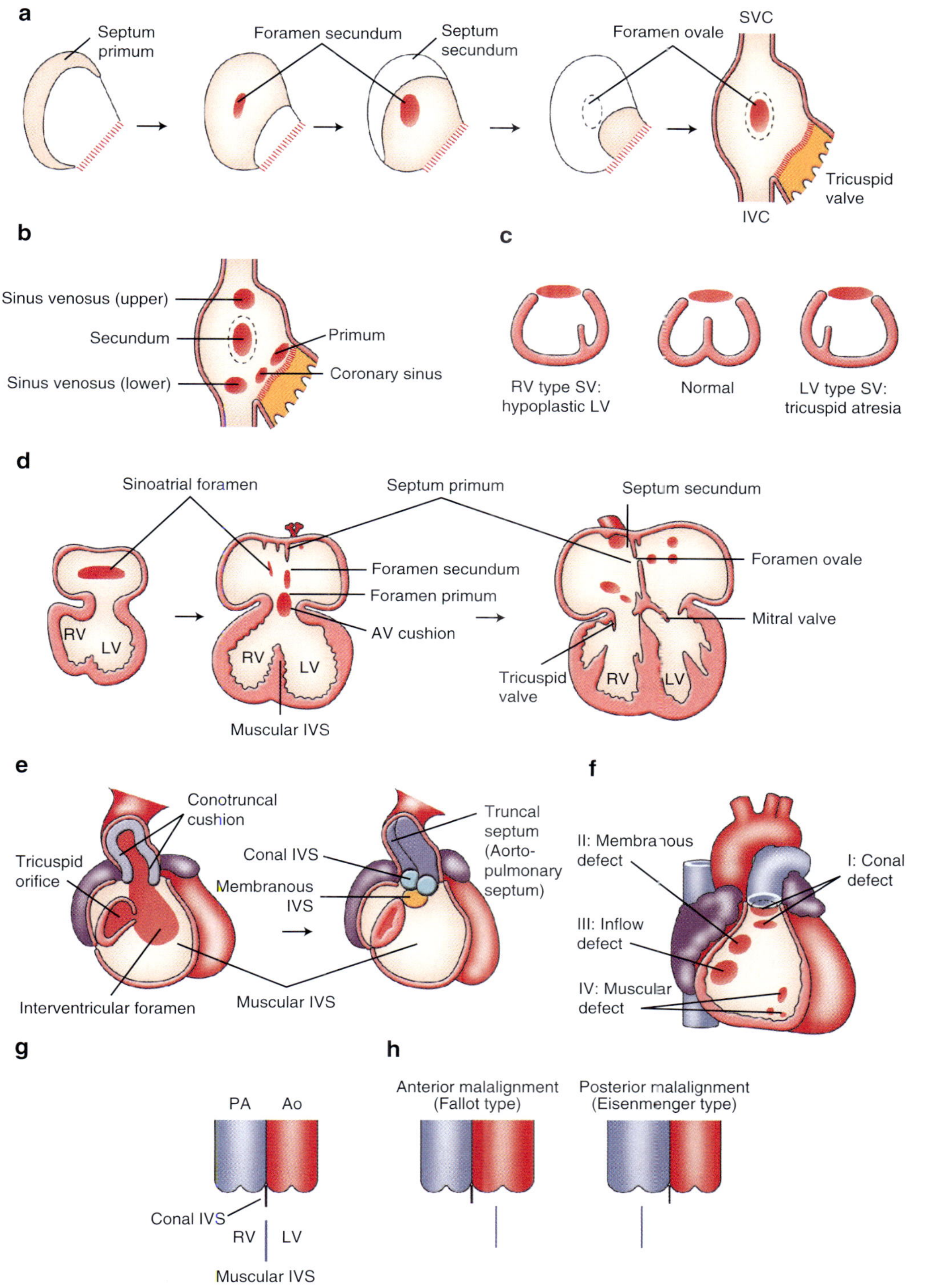

Fig. 2.6 Normal and abnormal development of atrial septum, ventricular septum, and ventricles. (**a**) Atrial septum from right atrium view. (**b**) Atrial septal defect. (**c**) Alignment of AV valves & IVS. (**d**) Atrial and ventricular septum from four chamber view. (**e**) Ventricular and outflow tract septation from right ventricle view. (**f**) Ventricular septal defects. (**g**) Simple perforation. (**h**) Malalignment (of conal septum). See detail in text. *Ao* aorta, *AV* atrioventricular, *IVC* inferior vena cava, *IVS* interventricular septum, *LV* left ventricle, *PA* pulmonary artery, *RV* right ventricle, *SVC* superior vena cava

Usually, anterior malalignment of the conal septum is associated with TOF, while posterior malalignment of the conal septum is associated with coarctation or interruption of the aorta.

Normal and Abnormal Development of Atrioventricular Cushions: Atrioventricular Septal Defects (AVSD) [22]

At 4 weeks of the gestation, an endocardial cushion is formed in the atrioventricular canal by a process called "epithelial–mesenchymal transformation" where the mesenchymal cells are separated from the endocardium and transformed in the extracellular matrix. At 5 weeks of the gestation, the atrioventricular canal is divided by the coalescence of the superior and inferior endocardial cushions into the right-sided tricuspid and the left-sided mitral orifices (Fig. 2.7a). Endocardial cushions also participate in formation of the interatrial septum (closing of the ostium primum), atrioventricular valves (mitral and tricuspid valve), and membranous interventricular septum.

A complete failure of development of atrioventricular endocardial cushions results in complete atrioventricular septal defect which comprises common atrioventricular valve with variable degree of insufficiency (Fig. 2.7a), primum type of ASD (cf. Fig. 2.6b) and membranous/inlet type of VSD (cf. Fig. 2.6f). Partial type of AVSD manifests by a primum ASD with insufficiency of the tricuspid and/or mitral valves.

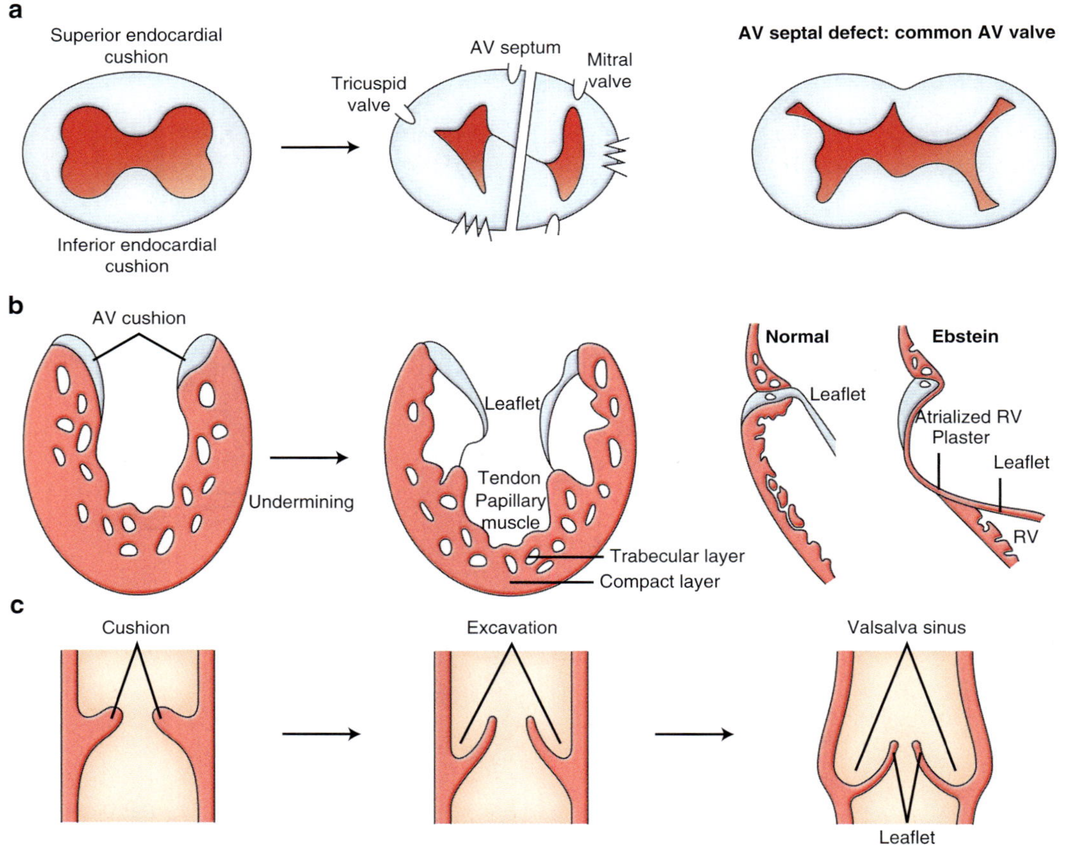

Fig. 2.7 Normal and abnormal development of atrioventricular (*AV*) septum and cardiac valves. (**a**) Development of AV septum. (**b**) Development of AV valve. (**c**) Development of semilunar valve. See detail in text. *RV* right ventricle

Normal and Abnormal Development of Cardiac Valves [9, 23]

Ebstein's Anomaly

The leaflets of atrioventricular valves are derived from the atrioventricular cushions. The leaflets and tendon apparatus which consist of the chordae tendineae and their myotendinous junctions with the papillary muscles are formed mostly by a process called "undermining" (Fig. 2.7b). This process is probably involved by myocardial cell death which delaminates the inner layers of the ventricular inlet and frees the fibrous leaflets.

Ebstein's anomaly of the tricuspid valve includes displacement of the septal and posterior leaflets of the valve into the right ventricle to varying degrees. The portion of the right ventricle between the true valve annulus and the downwardly displaced valve leaflets forms an "atriarized" portion of the right ventricle that is continuous with the true right atrium. It is supposed to result from a defect in undermining that leads to plastering of the valve leaflets to the myocardial layer (Fig. 2.7b).

Abnormalities of Semilunar Valves [9, 24–26]

After division of the outflow tract, the mesenchyme that forms the truncal cushions is remodeled into the aortic and pulmonary valves (Fig. 2.7c). Each valve has three cusps and leaflets. The cushion mesenchyme is derived from epithelial–mesenchymal transformation and from cardiac neural crest cells. The early cusps consist of a core of cushion tissue covered by the endocardium. Excavation of the arterial face of the cusps results in thinning to the final shape that consist of the valve leaflets and Valsalva sinuses (Fig. 2.7c).

A defective process of excavation in the pulmonary valve region results in thick, fused, and/or dysplastic pulmonary valve with stenosis (PS). Pulmonary atresia with intact ventricular septum (PA-IVS) probably occurs after cardiac septation is completed, whereas a diminutive right ventricle and ventriculo-coronary artery connections represent an earlier insult than a well-formed right ventricle and tricuspid valve with fused imperforated pulmonary valve. Aortic valve stenosis (AS) is associated with thickening and increased rigidity of the valve tissue like pulmonary valve stenosis. The aortic valve is often bicuspid with a single, fused commissure and an eccentrically placed orifice which may lead to aortic stenosis and/or insufficiency.

Normal and Abnormal Development of the Arterial System [1, 2, 12, 27]

The great arterial system arises from six pairs of pharyngeal arch arteries that run through pharyngeal arches symmetrically. During 4–5weeks of gestation, the bilaterally symmetric pharyngeal arch arteries and the right and left dorsal aortae undergo remodeling (Fig. 2.8). The first and second pharyngeal arch arteries almost completely regress except to form the maxillary and stapedial arteries, respectively. The third, fourth, and sixth pharyngeal arch arteries result in a portion of the aortic arch and its branches, the ductus arteriosus, and part of branch pulmonary arteries through their remodeling, while the fifth pharyngeal arch arteries completely regress before fully develop.

Interrupted Aortic Arch Type B (IAA-B) [2, 12, 27]

Most anomalies of the aortic arch system result from persistence of parts of the pharyngeal arch arteries and dorsal aortae that normally regress and regression of parts that normally persist. Interrupted aortic arch type B results from abnormal regression of the left fourth pharyngeal arch artery (Fig. 2.8a).

Aberrant Right Subclavian Artery [2, 12, 27]

Aberrant right subclavian artery occurs when the right fourth pharyngeal arch artery abnormally regresses and the right dorsal aorta cranial to the seventh intersegmental artery abnormally persists and forms the retroesophageal portion of the right subclavian artery (Fig. 2.8b).

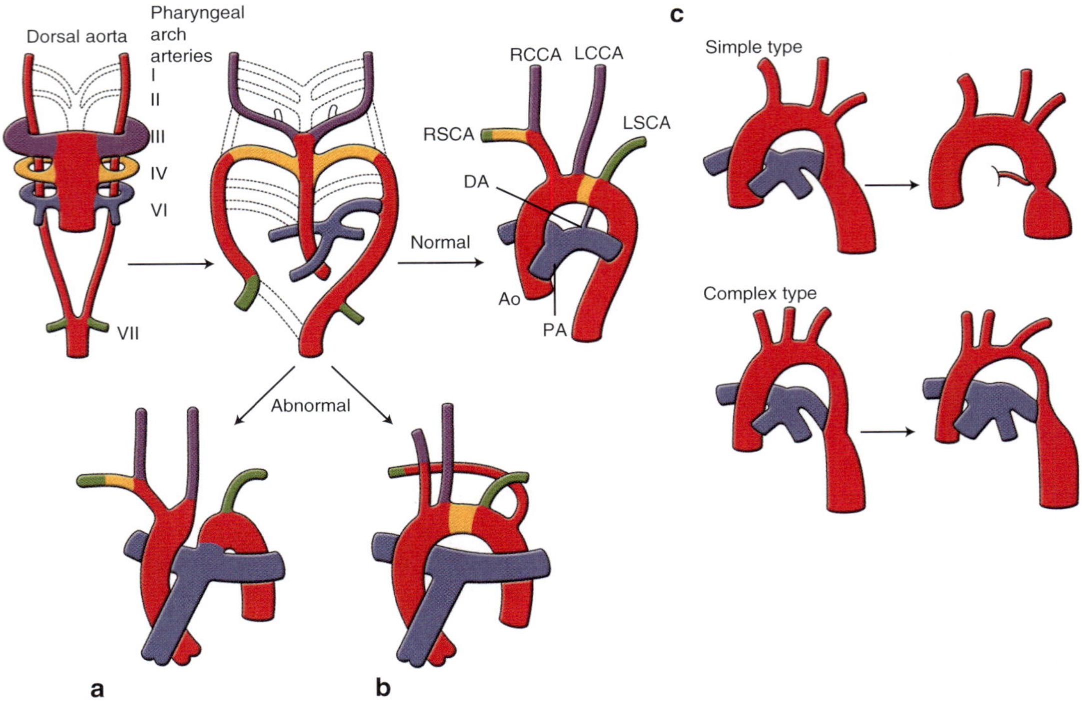

Fig. 2.8 Normal and abnormal development of the arterial system. (**a**) Interrupted aortic arch type B. (**b**) Aberrant right subclavian artery. (**c**) Coarctation of the aorta. See detail in text. *Ao* aorta, *DA* ductus arteriosus, *LCCA* left common carotid artery, *LSCA* left subclavian artery, *PA* pulmonary arteries, *RCCA* right common carotid artery, *RSCA* right subclavian artery

Coarctation of Aorta (CoA) [27]

The simple, or post-ductal, type of coarctation of the aorta may result from abnormal constriction of the aorta together with the ductus arteriosus (Fig. 2.8c). The complex, or preductal, type of coarctation of the aorta may result from a decreased blood flow through preductal aortic arch due to a posterior malalignment of the conal septum, bicuspid aortic valve with aortic stenosis, or other causes (Fig. 2.8c).

Patent Ductus Arteriosus (PDA) [28]

The ductus arteriosus normally develops from the distal portion of the left sixth pharyngeal arch artery and connects the pulmonary trunk to the descending aorta (Fig. 2.8). With a right aortic arch, the ductus arteriosus is commonly on the left, joining the left pulmonary artery and the proximal portion of the left subclavian artery. The exact mechanisms underlying postnatal closure of the ductus arteriosus are not fully understood. An increase in partial pressure of oxygen and release of vasoactive substances, such as acetylcholine, bradykinin, or catecholamines, may contribute to closure of the ductus arteriosus under physiologic conditions. On the other hand, prostaglandins play an active role in maintaining the ductus arteriosus in an open state during normal fetal life. Patency or closure of the ductus arteriosus may represent a balance between the constrictive and relaxing effects by multiple factors.

Normal and Abnormal Development of Pulmonary Veins [29]

At 4 weeks of gestation, the primordial lung buds are enmeshed by the vascular plexus, called the splanchnic and pulmonary venous plexus, that connects to the systemic veins, but not to the heart (Fig. 2.9). By the end of 4 weeks of gestation, the common pulmonary vein derived from pulmonary venous plexus connects to the sinoatrial

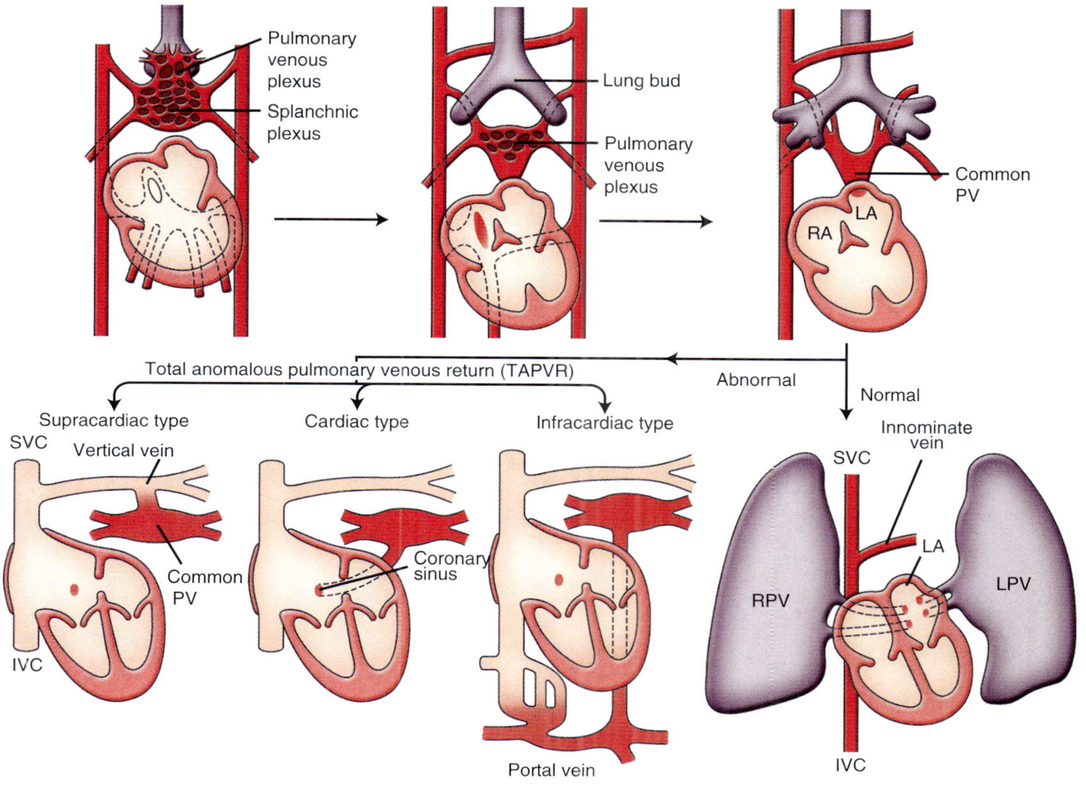

Fig. 2.9 Normal and abnormal development of pulmonary veins. See detail in text. *IVC* inferior vena cava, *LA* left atrium, *LPV* left pulmonary veins, *PV* pulmonary vein, *RA* right atrium, *RPV* right pulmonary veins, *SVC* superior vena cava

portion of the heart. Later, the connections between the pulmonary venous plexus and the systemic veins involute, and finally, the common pulmonary vein is absorbed into the left atrium so that the two right and the two left pulmonary veins connect separately and directly to the left atrium (Fig. 2.9).

Total Anomalous of Pulmonary Venous Return (TAPVR) [29]

TAPVR occurs as a result of developmental failure or early atresia of common pulmonary vein when collateral channels for pulmonary venous return are available in the form of primitive connections between the pulmonary venous plexus and the systemic veins. The type of TAPVR is classified according to the persistent collateral channels from pulmonary to systemic veins as follows: Supracardiac type includes connections to the left innominate vein, the superior vena cava, or the azygos vein; cardiac type includes connections to the coronary sinus or directly to the right atrium; and infracardiac type includes connections below the diaphragm to the inferior vena cava, the portal vein, the hepatic veins, or the ductus venosus (Fig. 2.9).

Normal and Abnormal Development of Coronary Arteries [30–32]

During the early development of the heart, the epicardial precursor cells derived from proepicardial organ contribute to form epicardium spread over the heart (Fig. 2.2c, d). Epithelial–mesenchymal transition provides cells that delaminate and migrate into the myocardium to transform into the vasculogenic mesenchymal cells (Fig. 2.10a). These vasculogenic cells

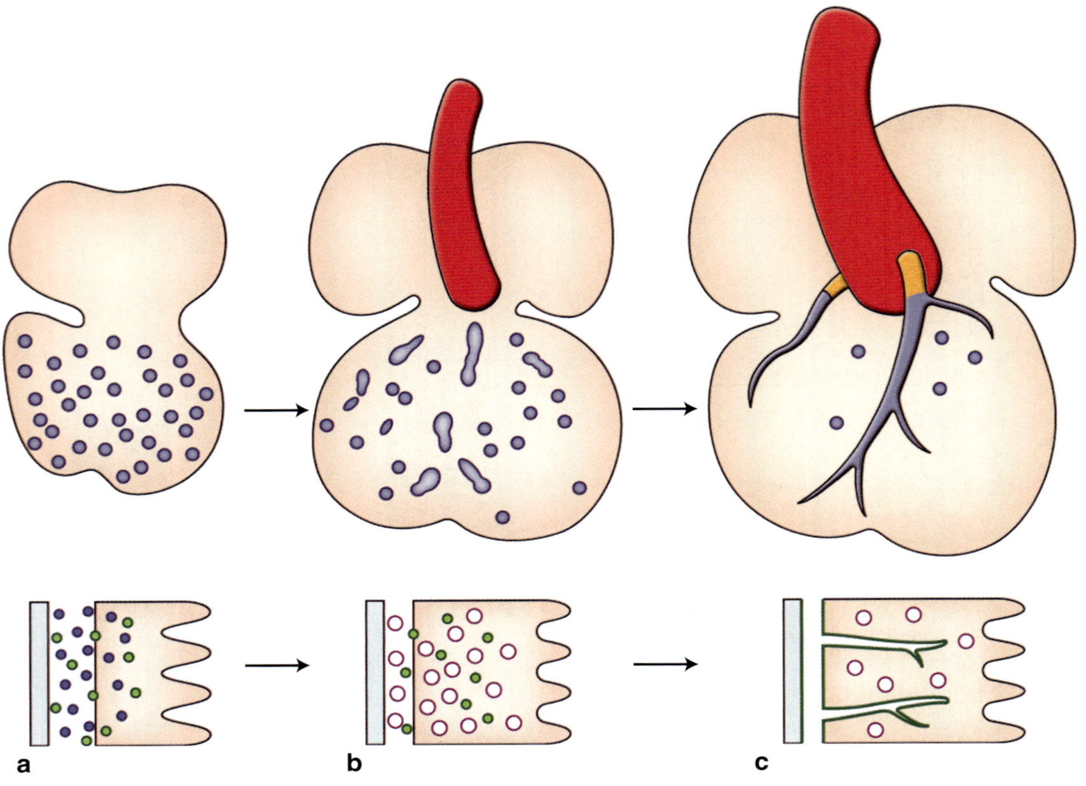

Fig. 2.10 Development of coronary arteries. (**a**) Mesenchymal cells. (**b**) Vascular plexus. (**c**) Coronaries connecting to the aorta. See detail in text. *Small blue circles* represent vasculogenic mesenchymal cells that are derived from epicardium by epithelial–mesenchymal transformation and migrate into the myocardium. A *red* vessel represents the aorta. *Orange* area represents the connection of coronary artery to the aorta

differentiate and link locally to form vascular plexus that induce other mesenchymal cells to become smooth muscle (Fig. 2.10b). Later, these vascular plexi are remodeled into sprouting definitive arteries. Finally, the vascular plexus in the most proximal region links up and gives rise to the major coronaries that eventually connect to the aorta (Fig. 2.10c).

Congenital anomalies of the coronary artery may occur alone or in association with structural heart defects, such as TGA and TOF. There are numerous types of anomalous origin of coronary arteries, including anomalous origin of left coronary arterial branches from the right coronary sinus, anomalous origin of right coronary arterial branches from the left coronary sinus, and anomalous origin of left main coronary artery from the pulmonary artery (Bland–White–Garland syndrome).

References

1. Yamagishi H, Maeda J, Uchida K, et al. Molecular embryology for an understanding of congenital heart diseases. Anat Sci Int. 2009;84:88–94.
2. Kodo K, Yamagishi H. A decade of advances in the molecular embryology and genetics underlying congenital heart defects. Circ J. 2011;75:2296–304.
3. Srivastava D. Making or breaking the heart: from lineage determination to morphogenesis. Cell. 2006;126:1037–48.
4. Vincent SD, Buckingham ME. How to make a heart: the origin and regulation of cardiac progenitor cells. Curr Top Dev Biol. 2010;90:1–41.
5. Snarr BS, Kern CB, Wessels A. Origin and fate of cardiac mesenchyme. Dev Dyn. 2008;237:2804–19.
6. Kirby ML. Molecular control of looping. In: Kirby ML, editor. Cardiac development. New York: Oxford University Press; 2007. p. 87–102.
7. Hagler DJ, O'Leary PW. Cardiac malpositions and abnormalities of atrial and visceral situs. In: Allen HD et al., editors. Moss and Adams' heart disease in infants, children, and adolescents including the fetus

and young adult. Philadelphia: Lippincott Williams & Wilkins; 2001. p. 1151–66.
8. Freedom RM, Dyck JD. Congenitally corrected transposition of the great arteries. In: Allen HD et al., editors. Moss and Adams' heart disease in infants, children, and adolescents including the fetus and young adult. Philadelphia: Lippincott Williams & Wilkins; 2001. p. 1085–101.
9. Kirby ML. Endocardium, cardiac cushions, and valve development. In: Kirby ML, editor. Cardiac development. New York: Oxford University Press; 2007. p. 119–32.
10. Epstein ML. Tricuspid atresia. In: Allen HD et al., editors. Moss and Adams' heart disease in infants, children, and adolescents including the fetus and young adult. Philadelphia: Lippincott Williams & Wilkins; 2001. p. 799–809.
11. Kirby ML. Development of the pole of the heart. In: Kirby ML, editor. Cardiac development. New York: Oxford University Press; 2007. p. 69–86.
12. Kirby ML. Neural crest, great arteries, and outflow septation. In: Kirby ML, editor. Cardiac development. New York: Oxford University Press; 2007. p. 143–60.
13. Hagler DJ. Double-outlet right ventricle and double-outlet left ventricle. In: Allen HD et al., editors. Moss and Adams' heart disease in infants, children, and adolescents including the fetus and young adult. Philadelphia: Lippincott Williams & Wilkins; 2001. p. 1102–28.
14. Yamagishi H, Srivastava D. Unraveling the genetic and developmental mysteries of 22q11 deletion syndrome. Trends Mol Med. 2003;9:383–9.
15. Wernovsky G. Transposition of the great arteries. In: Allen HD et al., editors. Moss and Adams' heart disease in infants, children, and adolescents including the fetus and young adult. Philadelphia: Lippincott Williams & Wilkins; 2001. p. 1027–84.
16. Mair DD, Edwards WD, Julsrud PR, Seward JB, Danielson GK. Truncus arteriosus. In: Allen HD et al., editors. Moss and Adams' heart disease in infants, children, and adolescents including the fetus and young adult. Philadelphia: Lippincott Williams & Wilkins; 2001. p. 910–23.
17. Siwik ES, Patel CR, Zahka KG. Tetralogy of Fallot. In: Allen HD et al., editors. Moss and Adams' heart disease in infants, children, and adolescents including the fetus and young adult. Philadelphia: Lippincott Williams & Wilkins; 2001. p. 880–902.
18. Kirby ML. Chamber specification and ventricular septation. In: Kirby ML, editor. Cardiac development. New York: Oxford University Press; 2007. p. 103–18.
19. Hagler DJ, Edwards WD. Univentricular atrioventricular connection. In: Allen HD et al., editors. Moss and Adams' heart disease in infants, children, and adolescents including the fetus and young adult. Philadelphia: Lippincott Williams & Wilkins; 2001. p. 1129–50.
20. Porter CJ, Feldt RH, Edwards WD, Seward JB, Schaff JV. Atrial septal defects. In: Allen HD et al., editors. Moss and Adams' heart disease in infants, children, and adolescents including the fetus and young adult. Philadelphia: Lippincott Williams & Wilkins; 2001. p. 603–17.
21. McDaniel NL, Gutgesell HP. Ventricular septal defects. In: Allen HD et al., editors. Moss and Adams' heart disease in infants, children, and adolescents including the fetus and young adult. Philadelphia: Lippincott Williams & Wilkins; 2001. p. 636–51.
22. Feldt RH, Edwards WD, Porter CJ, Dearani JA, Seward JB, Puga FJ. Atrioventricular septal defects. In: Allen HD et al., editors. Moss and Adams' heart disease in infants, children, and adolescents including the fetus and young adult. Philadelphia: Lippincott Williams & Wilkins; 2001. p. 618–35.
23. Epstein ML. Congenital stenosis and insufficiency of the tricuspid valve. In: Allen HD et al., editors. Moss and Adams' heart disease in infants, children, and adolescents including the fetus and young adult. Philadelphia: Lippincott Williams & Wilkins; 2001. p. 810–9.
24. Latson LA, Prieto LR. Pulmonary stenosis. In: Allen HD et al., editors. Moss and Adams' heart disease in infants, children, and adolescents including the fetus and young adult. Philadelphia: Lippincott Williams & Wilkins; 2001. p. 820–44.
25. Freedom RM, Nykanen DG. Pulmonary atresia and intact ventricular septum. In: Allen HD et al., editors. Moss and Adams' heart disease in infants, children, and adolescents including the fetus and young adult. Philadelphia: Lippincott Williams & Wilkins; 2001. p. 845–63.
26. Freed MD. Aortic stenosis. In: Allen HD et al., editors. Moss and Adams' heart disease in infants, children, and adolescents including the fetus and young adult. Philadelphia: Lippincott Williams & Wilkins; 2001. p. 970–87.
27. Weinberg PM. Aortic arch anomalies. In: Allen HD et al., editors. Moss and Adams' heart disease in infants, children, and adolescents including the fetus and young adult. Philadelphia: Lippincott Williams & Wilkins; 2001. p. 707–35.
28. Moore P, Brook MM, Heymann MA. Patent ductus arteriosus. In: Allen HD et al., editors. Moss and Adams' heart disease in infants, children, and adolescents including the fetus and young adult. Philadelphia: Lippincott Williams & Wilkins; 2001. p. 652–69.
29. Geva T, Van Praagh S. Anomalies of the pulmonary veins. In: Allen HD et al., editors. Moss and Adams' heart disease in infants, children, and adolescents including the fetus and young adult. Philadelphia: Lippincott Williams & Wilkins; 2001. p. 736–72.
30. Kirby ML. Epicardium and coronary vessel development. In: Kirby ML, editor. Cardiac development. New York: Oxford University Press; 2007. p. 133–42.
31. Reese DE, Mikawa T, Bader DM. Development of the coronary vessel system. Circ Res. 2002;91:761–8.
32. Paul Matherne G. Congenital anomalies of the coronary vessels and the aortic root. In: Allen HD et al., editors. Moss and Adams' heart disease in infants, children, and adolescents including the fetus and young adult. Philadelphia: Lippincott Williams & Wilkins; 2001. p. 675–88.

3 Cardiac MRI Examination: An Overview

Michael J. Campbell

Congenital heart disease is the most common birth defect occurring in 4.8/1,000 births [1]. Previously, many patients with complex congenital heart disease did not survive to adulthood, confining the field of congenital heart disease to pediatric specialists. With improved medical, diagnostic, and interventional techniques, many patients with congenital heart disease are surviving to adulthood [2, 3]. This has created a need for adult providers who are familiar with congenital heart disease and therapies. The increase in the number of congenital heart disease patients has also highlighted a need for further investigation and research with a goal of improved mortality and quality of life.

The first imaging modality used in the imaging of congenital heart disease patients was radiography [4]. Taussig used radiography and fluoroscopy to image the thorax of patients and compared her finding to the clinical presentation and physical examination. As a result, she characterized the radiographic appearance of the thorax to particular congenital heart defects [4]. The field of angiography and cardiac catheterization arose from this technology and experience. Angiography was the mainstay of congenital heart disease imaging until the late 1970s and early 1980s. The emergence of echocardiography in the late 1980s led to its replacement of cardiac catheterization as the leading diagnostic modality. Echocardiography's ability to provide morphologic, hemodynamic, and functional assessment in a safe and noninvasive manner was the primary reason. However, echocardiography has limitations, particularly in patients with adult congenital heart disease (ACHD). As patients age and grow larger, their echocardiographic windows become less ideal, therefore limiting echocardiography's diagnostic utility. This has created the need for an alternative imaging modality to provide comprehensive noninvasive imaging of the patient with congenital heart disease.

Cardiac MRI (CMR) is ideally positioned to fill this need in the imaging of the patient with ACHD. CMRI can overcome the limitations of poor echocardiographic images to provide excellent images in a noninvasive manner. The typical CMR examination consists of multiple imaging sequences which can be used to provide a comprehensive assessment. Traditionally, in adult patients without congenital heart disease, cardiac MRI has been used primarily for assessment of valvular function, coronary artery disease, cardiomyopathy, and other tissue characterization. Many of the MRI sequences used in these patients can be adapted to ACHD.

In this chapter, we will review a typical cardiac MR examination in an ACHD patient. We will review the individual components of the examination in more detail. It is important to note that this meant to serve as a general guide. Often, the examination will need to be adjusted and individualized to the patient's anatomy and history.

M.J. Campbell, MD
Division of Pediatric Cardiology,
Department of Pediatrics, Duke University Medical Center,
7506 Hospital North, 3090, Durham, NC 27710, USA
e-mail: michael.campbell2@duke.edu

F. Saremi (ed.), *Cardiac CT and MR for Adult Congenital Heart Disease*,
DOI 10.1007/978-1-4614-8875-0_3,

Typical Examination

The cardiac MR examination of the patient with ACHD begins with a thorough review of the patient's history. It is imperative that the technologist and interpreting physician understand the basic concepts of the underlying anatomy and interventional history prior to beginning the examination. This allows for proper planning of sequences and helps ensure that accurate and appropriate information is obtained. The typical cardiac MRI in an ACHD patient can last 45–90 min. Preparing prior to the exam allows for efficient use of scanner time and minimizes patient discomfort. Reviewing a patient's history also helps identify possible contraindications to cardiac MRI. ACHD patients have often undergone procedures which can result in metal devices (pacemakers, stents, embolization devices, septal occluders) being placed in the patient. Those performing the examination are responsible for identifying the presence and safety of these devices prior to placing the patient in the scanner. One can refer to one of many references regarding MRI safety [5]. If the presence of metal devices cannot be excluded based on the patient's history, then a chest radiograph can be obtained to rule out the presence of these devices.

There are many approaches to performing a cardiac MRI in ACHD. Most basic studies include morphology imaging, cine imaging, flow analysis, angiography, and post-processing. There are additional sequences which can be added based on the clinical question to be answered. We will describe a typical examination for a new patient at our institution (Fig. 3.1). Patients who have repeat studies often have a more abbreviated examination to evaluate more specific questions. As noted previously, this is meant to serve as a

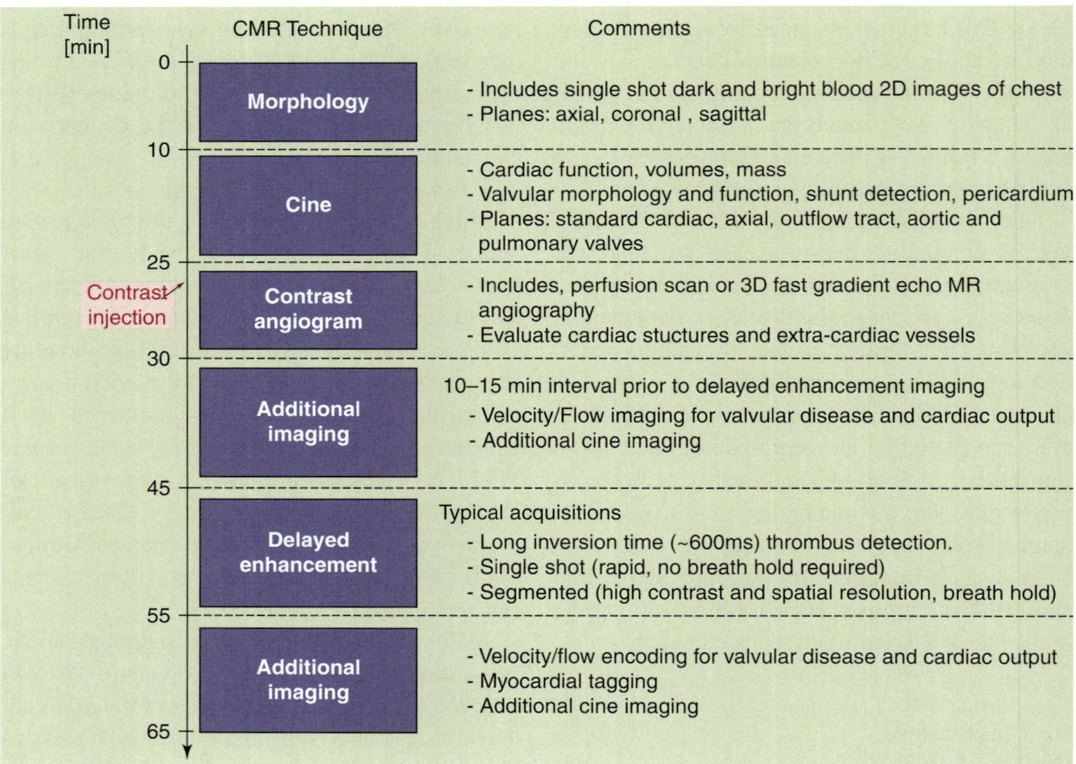

Fig. 3.1 Typical CMR examination in adult congenital heart disease (Image courtesy of Han Kim, MD, Duke University Medical Center)

guide and the study should be changed as appropriate to individualize to the patient.

Our institution's protocol begins with localizer images to center the patient in the magnet and to obtain basic views on which follow-up imaging can be planned. We then perform electrocardiogram (ECG)-gated cine imaging and start by obtaining a short axis stack of images from the apex through the atria. We image through the atria rather than stopping at the base of the ventricles in order to look for atrial septal defects, venous connection anomalies, or baffle leaks/obstructions (i.e., post-atrial switch, post-Fontan). A cine four-chamber view of the heart is obtained next, and a stack of the images from the posterior surface of the heart through the great arteries is performed (alternatively, a series of images in a true axial plane, rather than oriented to the axis of the heart, can be performed). Two- and three-chamber cine images of the left ventricle and a two-chamber image of the right ventricle from an anterior perspective allowing visualization of inflow through the tricuspid valve and outflow out the pulmonary valve are performed next. En face views of the aortic and pulmonary valves are planned off double orthogonal images of the left and right ventricular outflow tracts, respectively. These images are later used for planning flow analysis. Cine imaging is then followed by morphology imaging. Stacks of non-gated black blood and bright blood images (preferably single shot) are obtained through the heart and associated vessels in the axial, sagittal, and coronal planes for both sequences. A gated contrast angiogram of the appropriate anatomy may be performed with gadolinium-based contrast. Contrast-enhanced and non-contrast angiograms will be discussed in much more detail in a subsequent chapter.

Following the administration of gadolinium contrast, delayed enhancement imaging can be performed. Following the contrast-enhanced angiogram, single-shot balanced steady-state free precession (bSSFP) delayed enhancement imaging with a long inversion time (inversion time = 600 ms) is performed in the short and long axis to evaluate for thrombus. During the waiting time to perform delayed enhancement imaging with a null myocardium, velocity-encoded flow analysis can be performed at appropriate locations. Single-shot SSFP delayed enhancement imaging in the short and long axis is then performed with the inversion time set to null normal myocardium. If there is a high index of suspicion for coronary artery disease (CAD) or concern for CAD on the single-shot SSFP delayed enhancement imaging, then segmented gradient echo delayed enhancement images are obtained by taking a stack of images through the ventricles. Whole-heart coronary artery angiography can also be performed as indicated.

Morphology Imaging

Multi-slice morphology imaging is an essential component of the CMR evaluation of ACHD. Our institution typically performs morphology imaging following cine imaging; however, in circumstances where the diagnosis is unknown or scanning time may be limited, it is often advisable to begin the examination with morphology imaging. In patients with complex congenital heart disease, initial localization of the heart and associated structures within the chest is essential. Morphology imaging sequences allow for the single-shot acquisition of large amounts of anatomical information in a relatively short period of time without the need for breath holds. Multi-slice morphology imaging provides contiguous images through the chest which is essential for defining relationships of cardiac structures to one another. Multi-slice image sequences in the axial, sagittal, and coronal planes are generally recommended.

Morphology imaging can be performed with black blood or bright blood imaging (Fig. 3.2). Both modalities can be performed or the modality which produces the best image in that particular patient can be used. Black blood imaging consists of pulse sequences designed to null the blood pool to improve visualization of surrounding structures [6]. Conventional spin echo, fast (turbo) spin echo, and half-Fourier single-shot turbo spin echo (HASTE) are common black blood imaging sequences. All black blood imaging sequences are ECG gated. Fast spin echo is

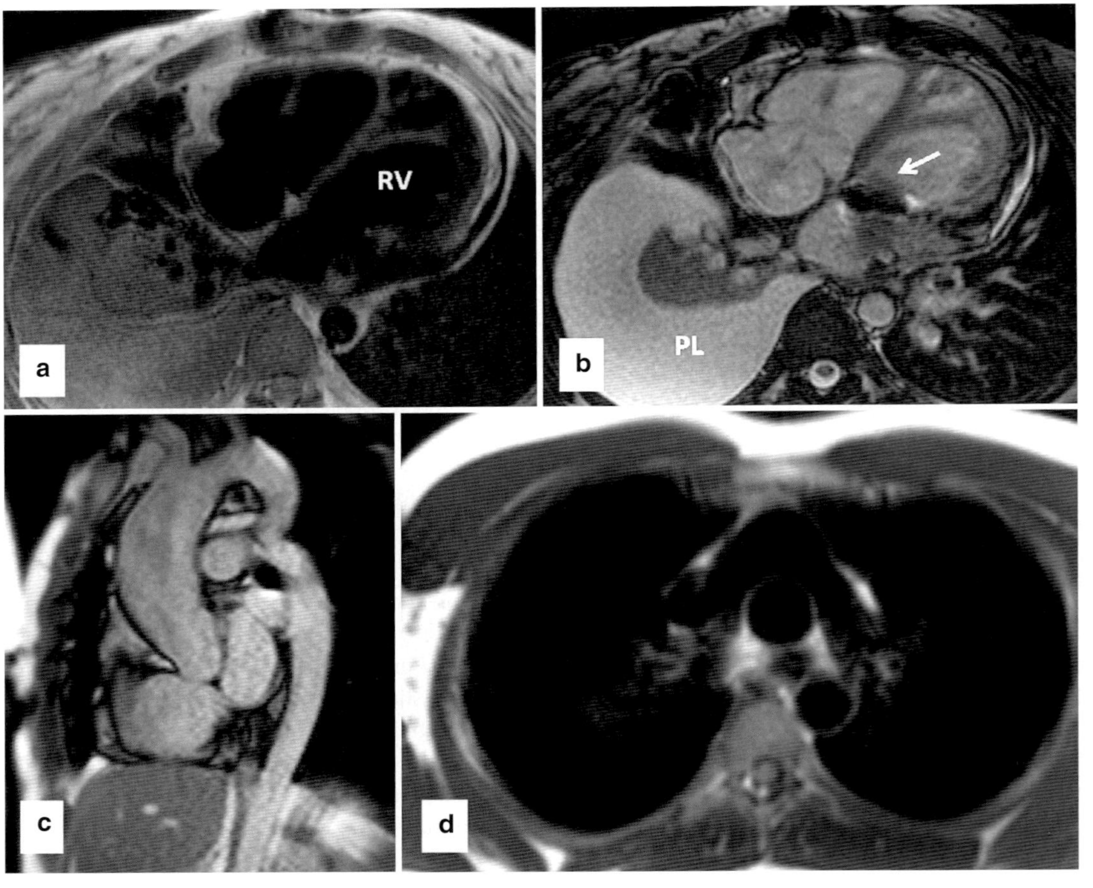

Fig. 3.2 Examples of clinical use of single-shot black blood (double IR-HASTE) and bright blood (bSSFP) sequences in standard body projections. These sequences can provide great amount of anatomical and pathological information in congenital heart malformation which can be used for better implementation of subsequent sequences for a comprehensive MR examination. (**a**) Axial black blood and (**b**) corresponding bright blood views in a patient with congenitally corrected transposition of the great arteries. Note the L-looped morphologic (systemic) right ventricle which is characterized by thickened moderator band. The two sequences are complementary and together can provide added information. In this example the prosthetic tricuspid valve (*arrow*) and left pleural effusion (*PL*) are easier to appreciate on bright blood image. (**c**) Bright blood sagittal image of a patient with coarctation of the aorta. (**d**) Black blood axial image of patient with complete transposition of great arteries following arterial switch operation. Typical appearance of main pulmonary artery anterior to the ascending aorta is shown. *IR-HASTE* inversion recovery half-Fourier single-shot turbo spin echo, *bSSFP* balanced steady-state free precession

most commonly used to obtain high-resolution, single-slice images using a breath hold. HASTE imaging, on the other hand, is used to obtain multi-slice images of the chest in a relatively short period of time and without a breath hold. These images are acquired in a short amount of time; however, the resulting images have less spatial resolution and signal-to-noise ratio. Conversely, because of the short imaging time, respiratory and cardiac motion artifacts are minimized. Black blood imaging should be performed prior to the administration of gadolinium contrast because the shortened T1(and TI) that results from contrast impairs complete suppression of the blood signal [7]. These characteristics make HASTE imaging an ideal modality for a rapid survey of the chest and cardiovascular structures.

Multi-slice bSSFP is usually used for "bright blood" imaging of cardiovascular structures. bSSFP morphology sequences use an imaging engine similar to cine MR SSFP that has been altered to produce a stack of images that progresses through space. This is different from cine MRI images that produce a moving image in a single plane [7]. bSSFP morphology sequences result in a bright blood pool. Artifacts with this sequence can be problematic in ACHD patients with flow or metal artifacts. Multi-slice bSSFP images can be performed before or after the administration of contrast. These images do not require a breath hold and allow for the rapid acquisition of images of the chest (non-ECG gated) in multiple planes.

When interpreting morphology images in ACHD, it is important to first define cardiac position and situs. Congenital heart disease patients with heterotaxy syndromes have abnormalities of organ positioning, including abnormal cardiac position and looping. Morphology imaging is essential in these patients to begin to describe the positions of organs within the chest and abdomen. Next, systemic and pulmonary venous anatomy should be defined. This allows for the identification of patients with systemic venous abnormalities such as a persistent left superior vena cava, interrupted inferior vena cava with azygous continuation, retroaortic innominate vein, and abnormal drainage of the right superior vena cava. Morphology imaging also allows for an evaluation of the patency of these vessels, which is important in a patient population which often requires procedures involving venous cannulation. Assessment of the pulmonary venous anatomy can allow for the identification of anomalous pulmonary venous return and an initial screening for pulmonary vein stenosis.

Morphology imaging also allows for an initial assessment of atrial, ventricular, and great artery morphology (Fig. 3.2a, b). Once this is defined, atrioventricular and ventriculo-arterial relationships can be described. The aorta can be evaluated for abnormalities of sidedness and branching. An initial assessment of the aorta can be performed for aneurysm, dissection, and coarctation (Fig. 3.2c). Many ACHD patients have main and/or branch pulmonary artery stenosis. Morphology imaging allows for the initial assessment of pulmonary artery anatomy (Fig. 3.2d).

Morphology imaging also allows for visualization of noncardiac findings within the chest. It is important to evaluate the mediastinum and lung fields for abnormalities such as pulmonary abnormalities, masses, and infiltrates. The thorax and spine can also be evaluated for bone and soft tissue abnormalities.

In summary, morphology image provides a large amount of anatomical information in multiple planes. This can be performed quickly and without a breath hold. This can allow for rapid diagnosis and it can be used for planning more detailed subsequent imaging during the CMR examination.

Cine Imaging/Functional Assessment

Cine MRI produces a movie of the beating heart in a single prescribed plane. The movie of the beating heart allows for the evaluation of valvular and ventricular function and shunt detection. Cine MRI images can also be obtained in contiguous slices to understand anatomical interrelationships and details. All of these components are critical to the evaluation of ACHD patients. As a result cine MRI is a workhorse of the CMR examination of ACHD patients.

The most common imaging engine used for Cine MRI is ECG-gated bSSFP. ECG-gated bSSFP produces an image at a defined slice position by acquiring data at particular frames of the cardiac cycle over several heartbeats [7]. This produces a cinematic movie of the beating heart at the slice position [6]. bSSFP imaging sequences are relatively short and can be performed with a breath hold to minimize respiratory motion artifacts. Parallel imaging with SENSE (sensitivity encoding) can result in even shorter imaging times [8]. bSSFP images have excellent contrast between the myocardium and blood pool which makes them ideal for ventricular functional assessment. The bSSFP blood-myocardium contrast is mainly secondary to a large difference in T2/T1 relaxation ratio. This ratio is generally high for blood pool and fat (bright) and low for the myocardium (relatively dark) [9].

Cine MRI can also be performed with a fast gradient-recalled echo (GRE) imaging engine. Prior to the emergence of bSSFP, GRE was the primary cine MRI sequence. ECG-gated GRE also produces a moving image by acquiring data at particular frames in the cardiac cycle. GRE relies on the inflow enhancement of blood (time-of-flight effect) to produce contrast between the blood pool and myocardium [6]. Compared to SSFP, GRE has inferior signal-to-noise ratio, less adaptability to parallel imaging resulting in longer acquisition times, and lower temporal resolution.

In ACHD patients, bSSFP is often the preferred cine MRI imaging modality. The high signal-to-noise ratio results in improved blood-endocardial interface and allows for more accurate volumetric measurements and functional assessment. The adaptability of parallel imaging leads to faster imaging and shorter breath holds. The superior temporal resolution leads to a smoother or "less jerky" reproduction of cardiac motion. On the other hand, bSSFP cine imaging is susceptible to dark band flow artifacts. This can often be overcome by frequency shifts or shim adjustment [6] (Fig. 3.3). ACHD patients can be especially susceptible to bSSFP-off resonance artifacts because of flow disturbances (i.e., post-Fontan operation). Sometimes these artifacts cannot be reduced by the usual trouble-shooting. Alternatively in these cases, cine GRE can be used to overcome these limitations.

Anatomic Definition and Valvular Assessment

Cine MRI is very useful for anatomic definition in the ACHD patient. Cine MRI can be obtained in any prescribed plane which is helpful in imaging patients with challenging anatomy. The unlimited nature of imaging planes is one of the main advantages of cine MRI over echocardiography. Cine MR images can be obtained in contiguous slices or "stacks" of images. This is analogous to a "sweep" in an echocardiography plane. This allows for the improved understanding of the relationships of cardiac structures in patients with complex anatomy.

Short axis images of the heart can be obtained by planning a cross section of the heart perpendicular to the long axis of the left ventricle. A "stack" of these short axis images can be created from the cardiac apex through the base of the ventricles (Fig. 3.4). In ACHD patients, it may be prudent to continue this stack through the atria to look for atrial septal defects (ASD) or to assess

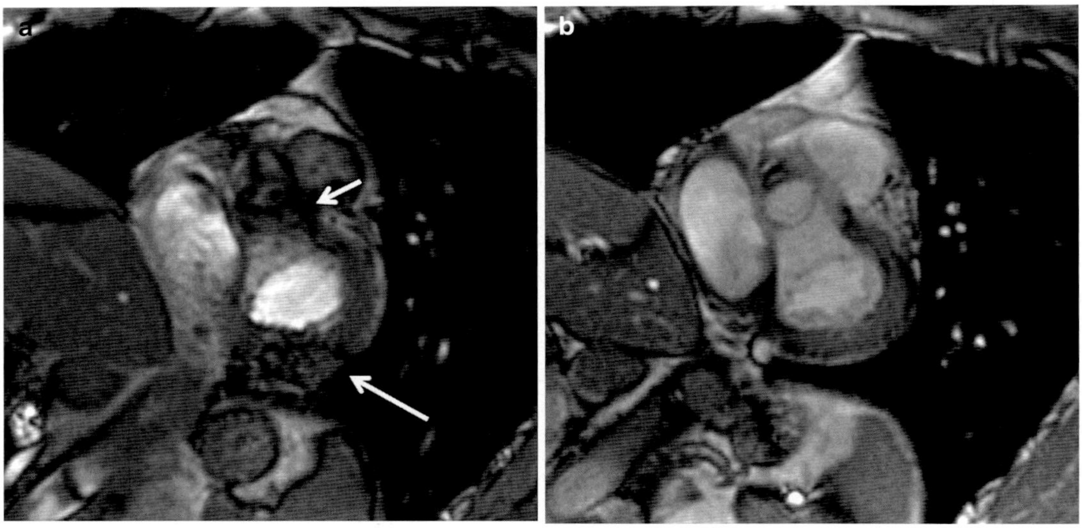

Fig. 3.3 Artifacts in balanced steady-state free precession (bSSFP). (**a**) Dark band and off-resonance artifacts (*arrows*) are corrected by frequency shift adjustment. Note clear view of the aortic valve and posterior wall of the left ventricle after corrections (**b**)

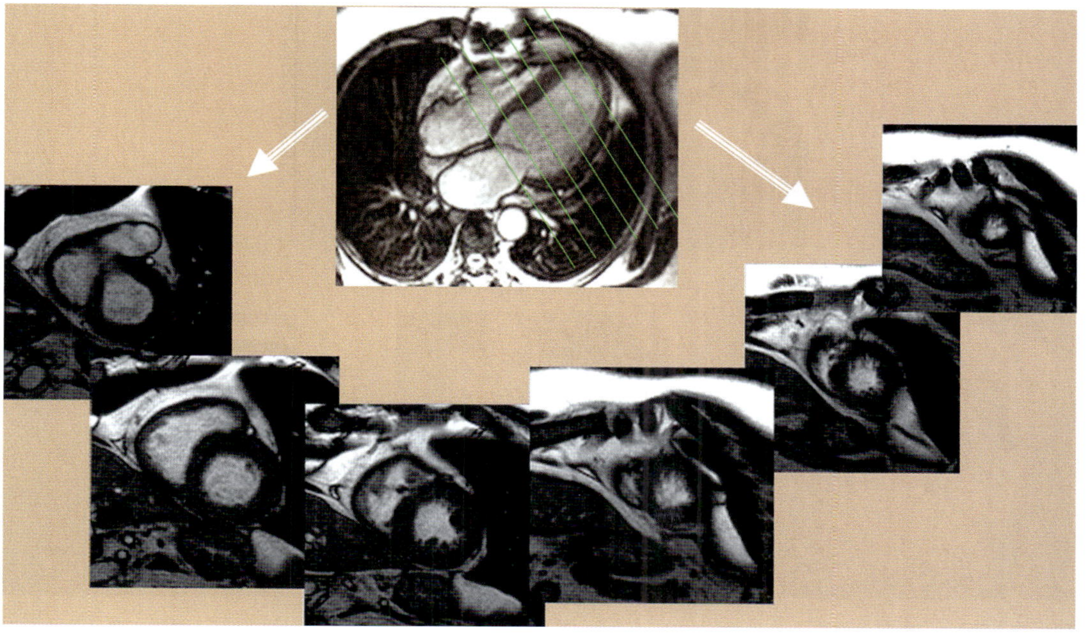

Fig. 3.4 Balanced steady-state free precession (bSSFP). Stack of short axis cine series will be obtained from long axis single-shot scanograms

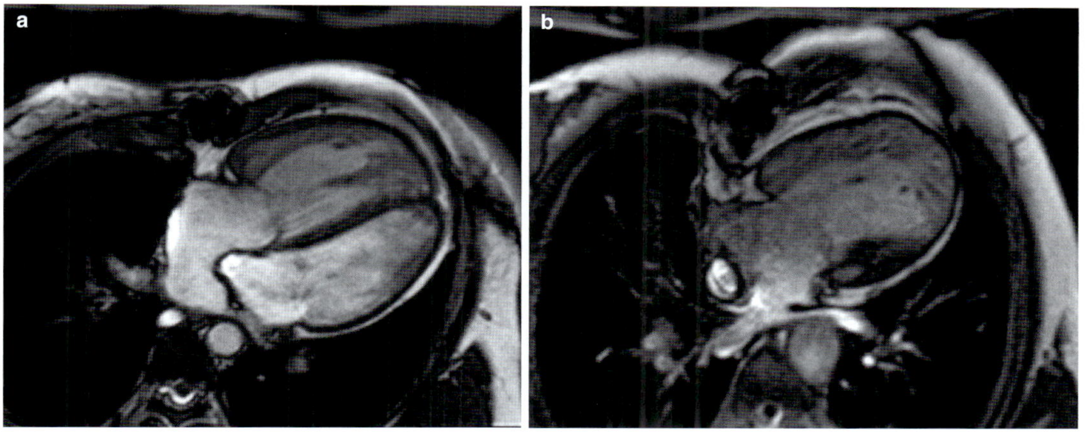

Fig. 3.5 Axial balanced steady-state free precession (bSSFP) provides a four-chamber view of the heart. (**a**) A patient with complete transposition of the great arteries following an atrial switch operation. (**b**) A patient with hypoplastic left heart syndrome following a Fontan operation

atrial baffles in patients who have had atrial switch operations. Short axis images of the ventricles are used predominantly to assess for ventricular wall motion abnormalities and to quantify ventricular volumes, mass, and ventricular function (see section "Functional Assessment" below). Short axis cine images can also be used to define ventricular morphology, assess for ventricular or atrial septal defects, and evaluate atrioventricular valve morphology and function.

Axial or axial oblique images of the heart can be obtained to produce a "four-chamber" view of the heart (Fig. 3.5). Most commonly, this image is obtained at the level of the atrioventricular valves.

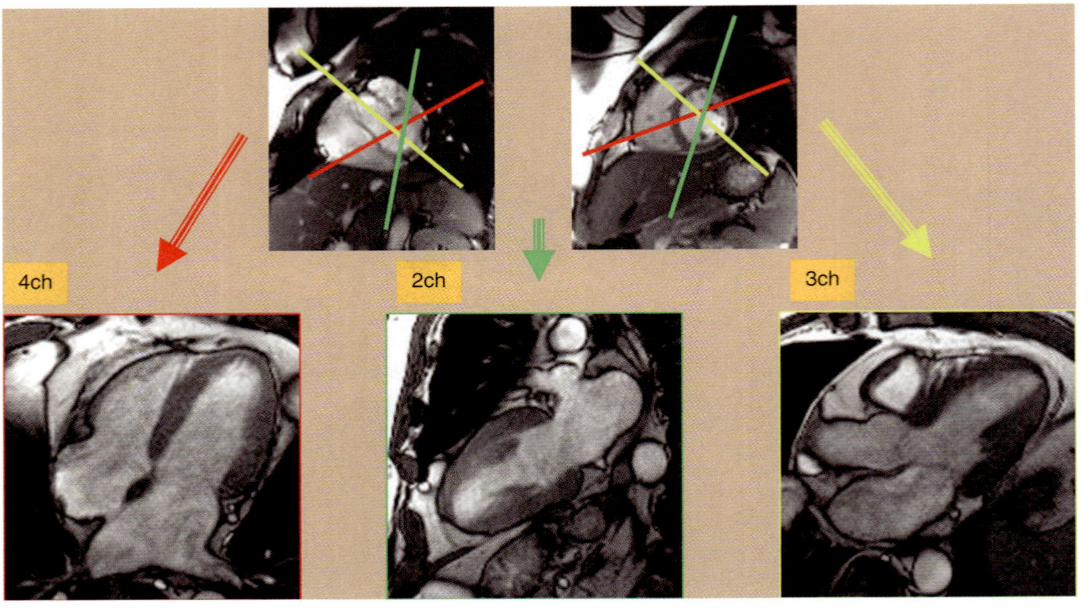

Fig. 3.6 Balanced steady-state free precession (bSSFP). Cardiac long axis views including four-chamber (*4ch*), two-chamber (*2ch*), and three-chamber (*3ch*) can be obtained from the stack of short axis images. Angles are shown in this image. Axial images can be obtained as a reference to facilitate plane adjustment

This allows for definition of cardiac sidedness, atrioventricular relationships, ventricular morphology and function, and atrioventricular valve morphology and function. A stack of these images can be obtained from the inferior surface of the heart superiorly through the great arteries. This facilitates understanding the interrelationships of cardiac structures. These axial or axial oblique images can also be used for volumetric measurements and ventricular functional assessment.

Long axis cine images of the ventricles can also be obtained. A "two-chamber long axis view" of the left ventricle and left atrium is planned off the previously obtained short axis and four-chamber views. This allows for visualization of the left ventricular and mitral valve function. A "three-chamber long axis view" of the left ventricle, left atrium, and left ventricular outflow tract is also obtained (Fig. 3.6). This image is planned from the short axis and "four-chamber" views. This is analogous to a parasternal long axis view in echocardiography and allows for visualization of left ventricular, mitral valve and aortic valve function. An image prescribed parallel to the left ventricular outflow tract (and the aortic root) in the three-chamber view produces an image of the left ventricular outflow tract viewed from an anterior perspective (coronal plane). Using this view and the three-chamber view, an "en face" image (through plane) of the aortic valve can be planned by prescribing double orthogonal planes of the aortic valve. This allows for visualization of aortic valve morphology and function and allows for planning future flow assessment (Fig. 3.7).

Assessment of the right heart structures is particularly important in congenital heart disease patients who often have right ventricular pathology [10]. A long axis cine image of the right ventricle can be obtained by prescribing an imaging plane which bisects the tricuspid valve, right ventricle, and right ventricular outflow tract. This produces an image showing the inflow and outflow of the right ventricle. This allows visualization of the tricuspid valve, right ventricular outflow tract, pulmonary valve, and right ventricular morphology and function (Fig. 3.8). This image can then be used to prescribe and create a sagittal oblique image of the right ventricular outflow tract and pulmonary valve (Fig. 3.8).

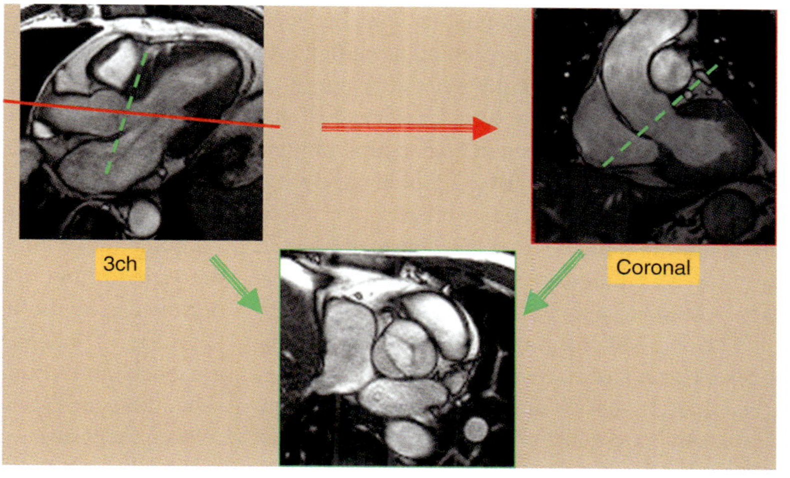

Fig. 3.7 Cine balanced steady-state free precession (bSSFP) technique for en face image of a bicuspid aortic valve. Using a three-chamber (*3ch*) reference image, an image is prescribed parallel to the left ventricular outflow tract (*red line plane*) to obtain a coronal view of the aortic root. From these two reference images, transaxial view of the aortic valve will be obtained (*green planes*)

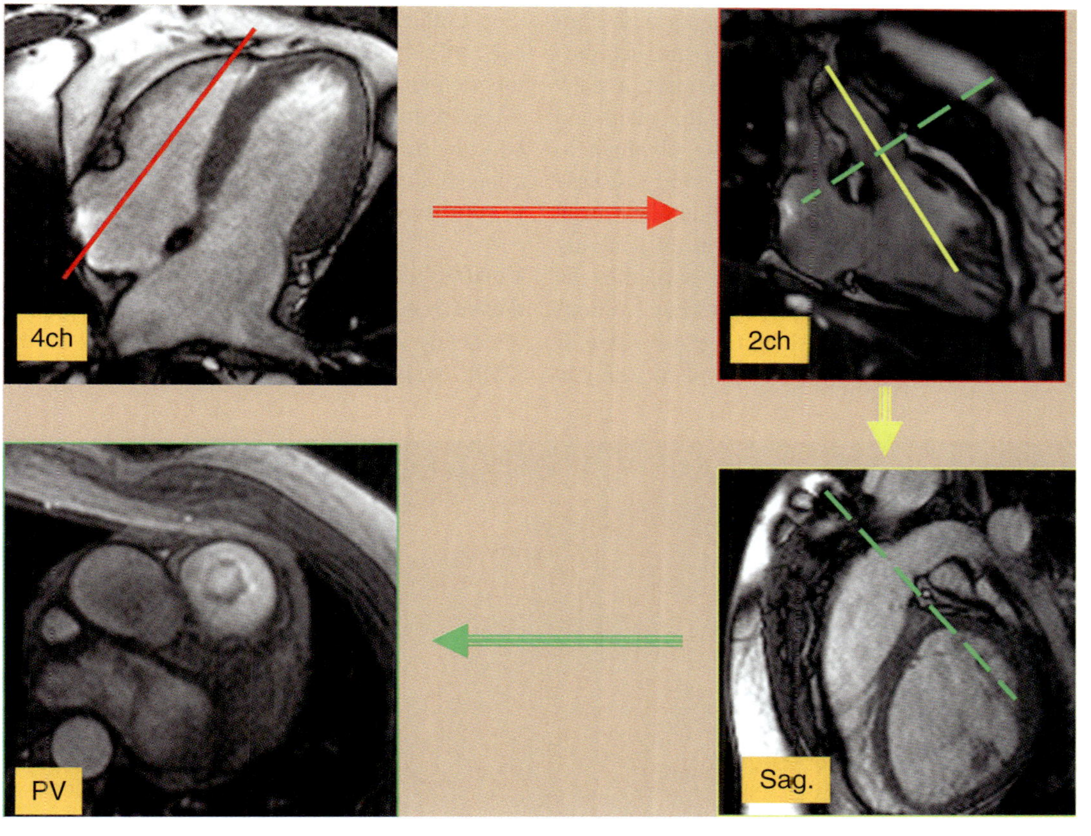

Fig. 3.8 Cine balanced steady-state free precession (bSSFP) technique for the right ventricle views. Using a four-chamber (*4ch*) view and two-chamber (*2ch*) view of the right ventricle will be obtained (*red plane*) which shows the inflow/outflow tracts of the right ventricle. This image can then be used to prescribe (*yellow plane*) and create a sagittal (*sag.*) oblique image of the right ventricular outflow tract and pulmonary valve. Using these two right ventricular views cross-sectional images of the pulmonary valve (*PV*) can easily be prescribed

This is particularly important in patients with pulmonary stenosis or regurgitation, particularly in patients with a transannular patch repair of tetralogy of Fallot. The long axis view of the right ventricle and perpendicular sagittal oblique can then be used to prescribe a double orthogonal image of the pulmonary valve creating an en face image of the pulmonary valve. This can be used to evaluate pulmonary valve function and morphology and to plan for future flow assessment.

The cine MR imaging described above constitutes the standard cine imaging used in adult congenital heart disease patients at our institution. Circumstances occasionally require the expanded use of cine images. Patients with atrioventricular valve disease such as Ebstein's anomaly often require en face imaging of the atrioventricular valves. This provides anatomic definition and functional assessment. Many patients with congenital heart disease will often have branch pulmonary artery disease. In these patients, a stack of axial oblique images through the main and branch pulmonary arteries can be obtained to better identify branch pulmonary artery disease (Fig. 3.9a). Patients who have undergone atrial switch operations have complex atrial anatomy with the pulmonary venous return baffled to the right-sided mitral valve and the systemic venous return baffled to the left-sided tricuspid valve. It can be challenging to image the atrial anatomy in these patients. A stack of coronal oblique images through the atria can allow for evaluation of baffle leaks and obstruction. A sagittal oblique image visualizing the superior and inferior limbs of the systemic venous baffle can also be helpful. Sinus venosus atrial septal defects can be difficult to visualize by standard cine MRI. A bicaval or sagittal oblique view showing the relationship of the superior and inferior vena cava to the atrial septum can be useful in visualizing these defects [11] (Fig. 3.9b). Secundum atrial septal defects are much more common than sinus venosus atrial septal defects. Our institution performs imaging of secundum atrial septal defects by visualizing the atrial septal defect in a four-chamber view of the heart. A perpendicular image of the defect is then obtained producing a short axis view. Both of these images are then used to create an en face view of the atrial septal defect. This image can be used to visualize the size, location, and rims of the defect. A velocity-encoded through plane image of the atrial septal defect can be obtained by copying this image position and then used to quantify the left-to-right shunt (discussed further in velocity-encoded imaging) [12] (Fig. 3.10).

Ventricular Volumes/Functional Assessment

Assessing ventricular function is crucial to the CMR evaluation of the patient with ACHD.

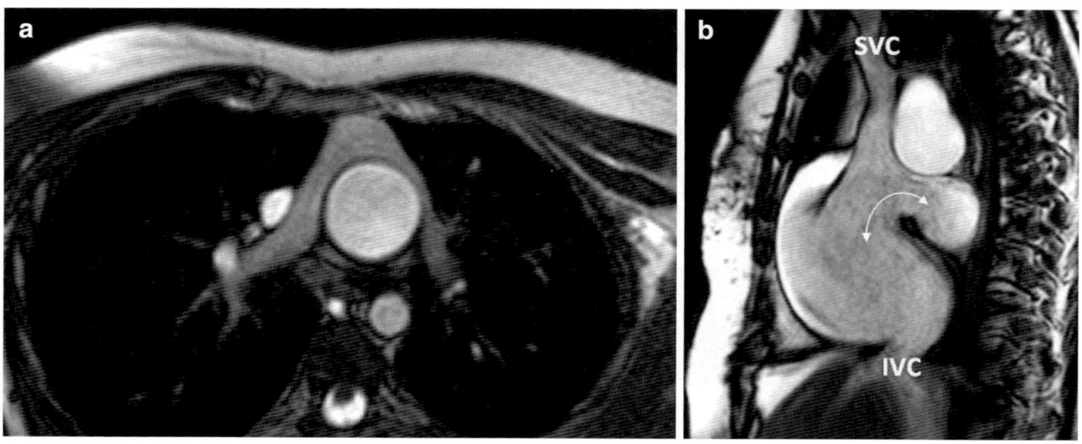

Fig. 3.9 Cine balanced steady-state free precession (bSSFP) technique. (**a**) Axial image of patient with complete transposition of great arteries following arterial switch operation. (**b**) bSSFP sagittal (bicaval) view of the atrial septum in a patient with a sinus venosus atrial septal defect (*arrow*). *SVC* superior vena cava, *IVC* inferior vena cava

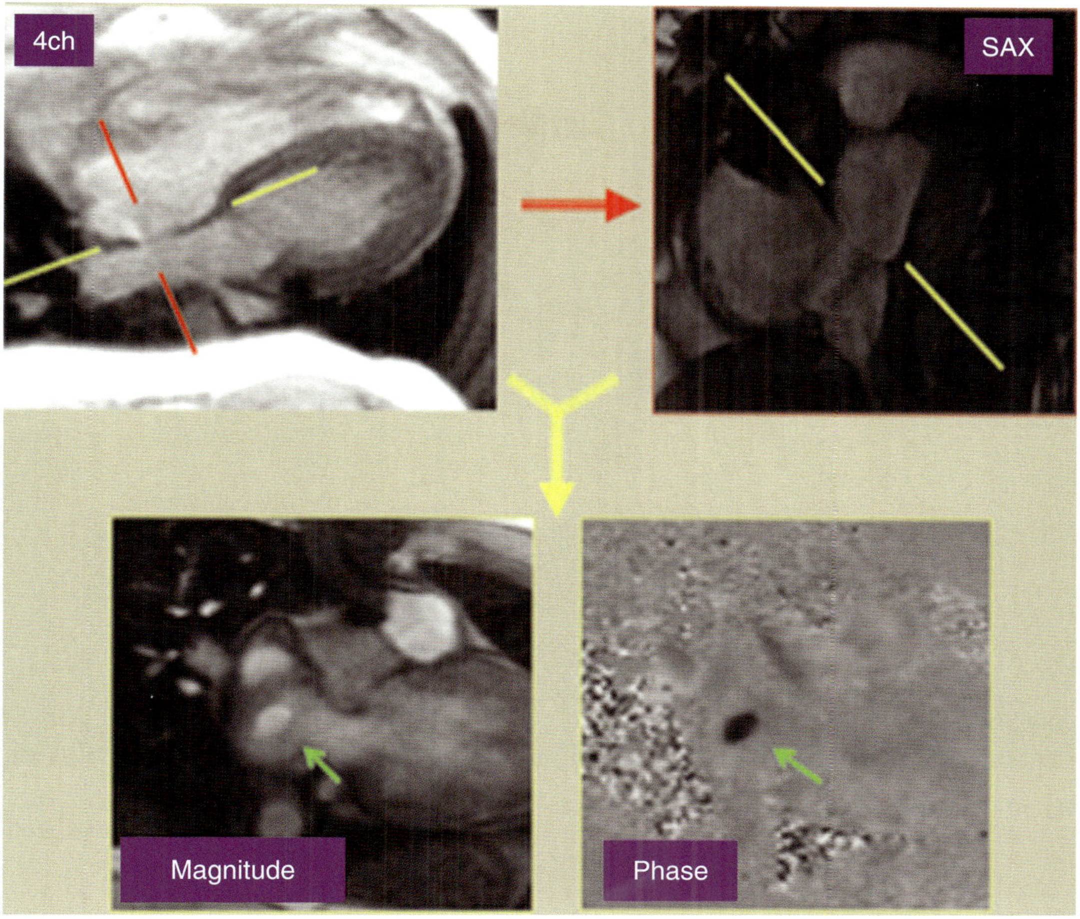

Fig. 3.10 Phase-contrast MRI through plane image looking at the atrial septum from the right atrium in a patient with a secundum atrial septal defect

There are numerous reasons for ventricular dysfunction in these patients. Patients with single-ventricle hearts present one extreme of this spectrum. Those with two functional ventricles can have unique loading conditions, both from pressure and volume loading. ACHD patients have often undergone multiple interventions, placing them at risk for ventricular dysfunction. As these patients continue to age, their incidence of coronary artery disease increases, therefore elevating their risk of ventricular dysfunction.

Multiple measurements have been used to assess global ventricular systolic function. These assessments of systolic function, however, do not necessarily equate to measurements of contractility. They are dependent on ventricular loading conditions (preload and afterload) and often heart rate. One of the most widespread measurements of systolic ventricular function is ejection fraction. Volumetric measurements of the ventricle in diastole and systole are made and used to calculate the stroke volume and ejection fraction: ejection fraction % = (end-diastolic volume − end-systolic volume)/end-diastolic volume. In echocardiography, this is performed by obtaining double orthogonal views of the left ventricular long axis. Most commonly, the modified Simpson's rule or method of disks is used to calculate ventricular volumes [13]. This requires an adequate imaging window with good contrast between the blood pool and myocardium. In ACHD patients who have often had many prior interventions, these conditions often

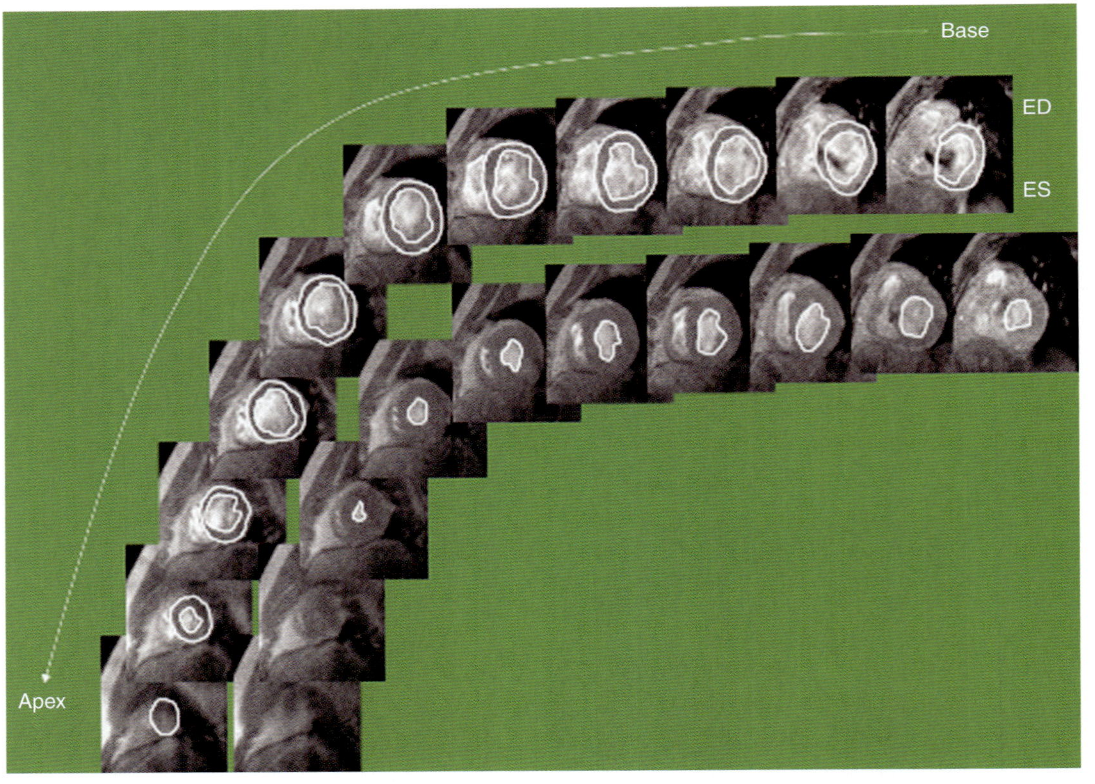

Fig. 3.11 Tracing of cine balanced steady-state free precession (bSSFP) images for ventricular function analysis. Cardiac MR allows for precise and reproducible quantification of wall thickness, ventricular mass, volumes (Courtesy of WJ Manning MD, Harvard Medical School). *ED* end diastole, *ES* end systole

do not exist. bSSFP cine MRI can often overcome these limitations. Echocardiography also provides limited echocardiographic windows of the right ventricle, making volumetric measurements difficult. bSSFP cine MRI can overcome this limitation by allowing for complete visualization of the right ventricular cavity, measurement of ventricular volumes, and the calculation of ejection fraction (Fig. 3.11).

Ventricular volumes and ejection fraction can be measured from a stack of cine MR images in a short axis or axial plane [8, 14]. The ventricular volumes are traced in end diastole and end systole through the entire ventricle (Fig. 3.11). One must be careful to outline only the ventricular cavity. At the level of the atrioventricular valve, the base of the ventricle can move in and out of the plane of the image as the heart moves with the cardiac cycle. This can result in portions of the atria being included in the most basal slice. Ventricular cavity is distinguished from atrial by the shortening of ventricular myocardium during systole. It is also imperative that one be consistent in the inclusion or exclusion of papillary muscles and trabeculations in diastolic and systolic measurements. The ventricular volumes are calculated from the product of the cross-sectional area of the cavity and the thickness of the image slice (prescribed by the user). Volumes are summated to calculate ventricular end-diastolic and end-systolic volumes. An ejection fraction is then calculated from the ventricular volumes. Myocardial mass can be measured by tracing the epicardial border in diastole, subtracting the endocardial volume, and multiplying by the specific gravity of myocardium, 1.05 g/mm^3 [8]. Ventricular volumes and ejection fraction have been validated in animal models and patients [15–17]. Several studies have compared cine MRI measurements of ventricular volumes and ejection fraction to echocardiography and SPECT and have found that cine MRI has greater reproducibility and accuracy [18–20].

Ventricular volumes, mass, and ejection fraction can be compared to published normal values [21, 22]. One group of ACHD patients which have received a great deal of attention in this regard are patients with repaired tetralogy of Fallot [14, 23–27]. Historically, repair of tetralogy of Fallot has involved transannular patch relief of pulmonary stenosis [28–30]. This relieves right ventricular outflow tract obstruction, but results in pulmonary insufficiency. Pulmonary insufficiency can lead to right ventricular dilation and failure. Pulmonary valve replacement is the treatment of choice; however, the timing of replacement is controversial [31]. bSSFP cine MRI measurement of right ventricular volumes and ejection fraction has been proposed and used as one of many criteria in determining timing of pulmonary valve replacement [25, 26, 31].

Cine MRI can also be used for the evaluation of segmental wall motion abnormalities. This is analogous to the evaluation of the left ventricle in the parasternal short axis by echocardiography. The 17-segment model of the left ventricle can be applied and used to classify segmental wall motion abnormalities [32]. Wall motion is classified as normal, hypokinetic, dyskinetic, or akinetic. Areas of abnormal wall motion can be consistent with infarcted myocardium. Combining cine MRI with stress testing can allow for the identification of inducible ischemia (see section "Stress Imaging). ACHD patients can also have abnormal segmental wall motion as a result of patch material and injury from prior interventions, bundle branch block, and a pressure- or volume-loaded right ventricle.

Diastolic function describes the compliance of the ventricles. The gold standard for diastolic function is invasive measurement of ventricular end-diastolic pressure. Cardiac imaging modalities, including CMR, have used indirect data such as atrioventricular valve inflow and pulmonary vein flow patterns, atrial size, and myocardial velocities to assess diastolic function. Phase-contrast analysis of tricuspid and mitral valve inflow and pulmonary venous flow can be performed and used in the assessment of ventricular diastolic function [33, 34]. One group of particular interest in ACHD is repaired tetralogy of Fallot and restrictive right ventricular filling. This is diagnosed by the presence of end-diastolic forward flow on phase-contrast analysis of flow in the main pulmonary artery (Fig. 3.12). This finding has been correlated with worse pulmonary

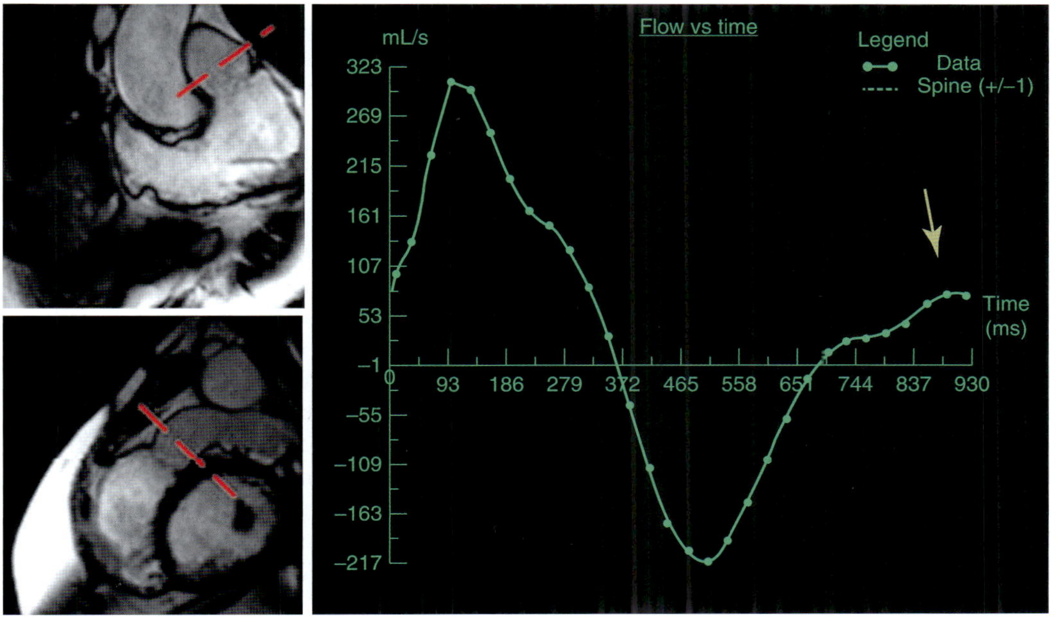

Fig. 3.12 Repaired tetralogy of Fallot and pulmonary regurgitation. Phase-contrast MRI flow diagram of the pulmonary valve is obtained using two orthogonal cine views of the right ventricle outflow tract (marked by *red planes*). There is end-diastolic forward flow (*yellow arrow*) which is indicative of restrictive right ventricular physiology

regurgitation and quality of life [35, 36]. Analysis of myocardial deformation by myocardial tagging or velocity vector imaging (VVI) can also be used to assess regional and global diastolic function. These modalities are discussed further below.

Myocardial Deformation

Within the field of cardiac imaging, there have been a number of recent developments in ventricular mechanics and myocardial deformation. Indices such as strain and strain rate can be evaluated. Myocardial strain is defined as a change in myocardial tissue length. Myocardial strain rate is defined as the rate of change in the length of myocardial tissue over time [37, 38]. These indices allow for assessment of global and regional myocardial function in longitudinal, circumferential, and radial directions. Echocardiographic modalities such as speckle tracking and VVI have been used for these measurements. CMR can also be used for assessment of myocardial deformation and offers some advantages over echocardiography. CMR is not limited by poor echocardiographic windows, and CMR allows for a superior blood pool to endocardium interface which aids in making these measurements.

Myocardial tagging is the gold standard for myocardial deformation evaluation by CMR. This involves superimposing lines or grids on the myocardium and following the subsequent deformation of these lines through the cardiac cycle on a cine MR image [39–43]. This is usually performed before the administration of contrast and requires a unique sequence which applies a prepulse to apply lines and grids [39]. Image acquisition is performed by using a cine MR imaging engine. Post-processing is then performed using an automated harmonic phase analysis (HARP) [39, 42, 43]. Myocardial tagging does have disadvantages in that it requires sequences which are not part of the standard CMR examination and the post-processing is time consuming.

More recently, VVI has emerged as an alternative modality for evaluating myocardial deformation by CMR. This modality involves loading a cine MRI image into vendor-specific software (TomTec™) and tracing the epicardial and endocardial borders of the ventricle and following these locations throughout the cardiac cycle (Fig. 3.13). VVI then uses a hierarchical algorithm to generate values of regional and global myocardial performance [44]. An advantageous feature of VVI, when compared to myocardial tagging, is that VVI does not require specific sequences. Following the CMR examination, DICOM data of cine MR images can be loaded into the software and analysis performed. A disadvantage of CMR VVI is that the mid-myocardium is not evaluated.

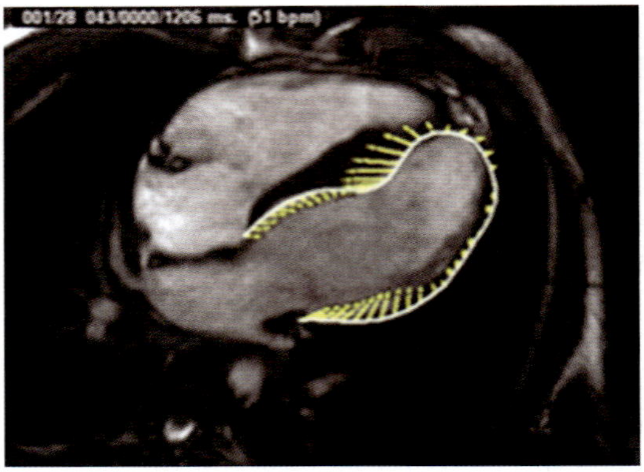

Fig. 3.13 VVI analysis of a cine balanced steady-state free precession (bSSFP) four-chambered view. *Yellow lines* shows ventricular deformity

The application of these myocardial tagging and VVI to ACHD patients is in its infancy. ACHD patients could benefit from this type of imaging because they frequently have regional myocardial dysfunction. Further study in this area could eventually lead to improved understanding of ventricular function in these patients.

Phase Contrast MRI

Hemodynamic assessment is an essential component of imaging patients with ACHD. These patients are at risk for valvular regurgitation and stenosis, arterial and venous stenosis, and intracardiac and extracardiac shunting. One of the strengths of echocardiography has been the use of Doppler technology in this role. CMR can provide excellent image quality with cine and morphology imaging, but, to match the comprehensive utility of echocardiography, a modality for hemodynamic assessment is essential. Phase-contrast CMR (PC-CMR) fills this role [45].

PC-CMR is based on the principle that moving protons, as compared to stationary protons, will experience a phase shift when exposed to a gradient in the direction of flow [7]. A gradient echo imaging engine is used to produce an image in which signal intensity is proportional to flow velocity. The flow in the direction of the applied gradient is white and the flow in the opposite direction is black (Fig. 3.10). Stationary tissue appears null or gray. A retrospective ECG-gated GRE cine imaging engine is used to apply phase contrast throughout the cardiac cycle. Velocity can then be graphed as a function of time [46]. Most commonly, PC-CMR is performed in the through plane, or perpendicular to the direction of flow (Fig. 3.12). The integrated product of the velocities and cross-sectional area of the flow column determines the flow rate. Integration of the area under the curve allows for measurement of forward and reverse volume [46]. In plane phase contrast imaging, which is parallel to the direction of the gradient field can also be used. This is not ideal for quantification of flow but can allow for visualization of the location of maximal flow acceleration (Fig. 3.14).

PC-CMR is applied in the through plane by first setting the imaging plane perpendicular to the vessel or valve to be assessed. A cine MRI image is first obtained perpendicular to the area of interest by using double orthogonal views (Fig. 3.13). The location of the cine image is copied as the image location to be used for phase-contrast CMR. The velocity encoding threshold (VENC) is then set. If the velocity of flow in the image exceeds the VENC, then aliasing of flow will occur, and the protons which exceeded the VENC will then be assigned a negative signal, thereby compromising the accuracy of the measurement [47]. It is also essential to set the VENC close or slightly above to the true maximal velocity. The greater the VENC exceeds the true maximal velocity of the image, the less accurate the measurement [6]. Determining the correct VENC can be time consuming and difficult for a breath-holding patient. When the maximal velocity is unknown, the VENC will be set at what is thought to be an appropriate level and the sequence will be run without a breath hold. If aliasing occurs, sequences will be run without a breath hold until the correct VENC is determined. A breath-hold sequence with the appropriate VENC is then

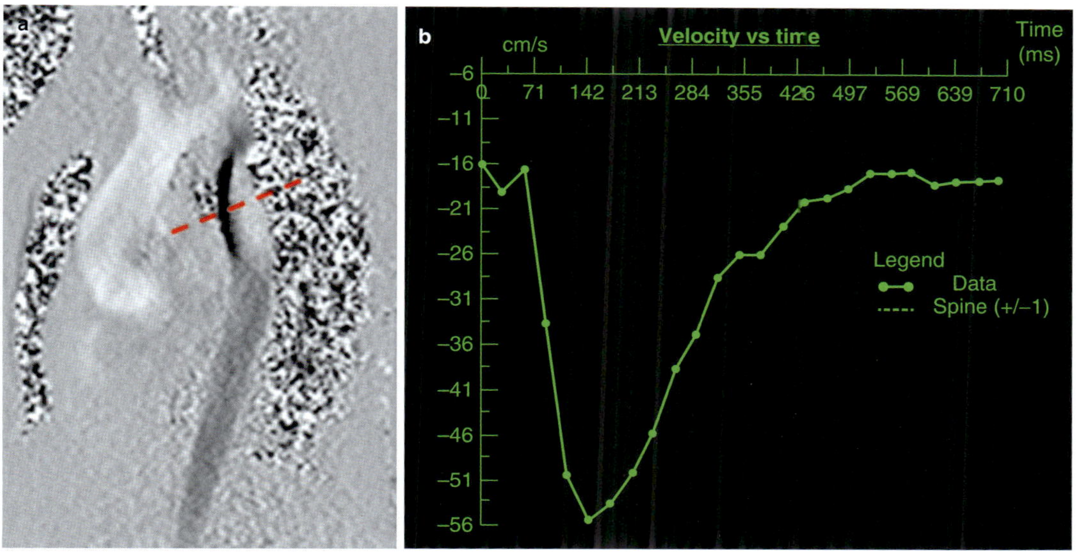

Fig. 3.14 (**a**) In plane phase image of the aortic arch in a patient with coarctation of the aorta. Note the dephasing (*dashed red line*) in the area of the coarctation of the aorta. (**b**) Time velocity diagram of a through plane image of the descending aorta distal to the area of stenosis (*dark line*) showing increased velocity

performed and this is used for measurements. Alternatively, a sequence with multiple averages can be used in free-breathing patients. The finished sequence is then evaluated at a separate workstation using a vendor-specific clinical work station.

Shunting

Many ACHD patients, both repaired and unrepaired, have intracardiac or extracardiac shunting. This shunting can be left to right, right to left, or mixed. When discussing cardiac shunting, the relationship of pulmonary and systemic flow is usually expressed as a Qp/Qs (Qp = pulmonary flow, Qs = systemic flow). When Qp/Qs exceeds 1, pulmonary flow exceeds systemic flow and systemic-to-pulmonary or left-to-right shunting exists. On the contrary when Qp/Qs is less than 1, pulmonary flow is less than systemic flow and pulmonary-to-systemic flow or right-to-left shunting exists. Left-to-right shunting results in normal oxygen content, symptoms of pulmonary overcirculation, and, ultimately, Eisenmenger's physiology. Right-to-left shunting results in diminished oxygen content.

In clinical practice, the gold standard for the measurement of Qp/Qs and intracardiac shunting has been the Fick equation determined by invasive oximetry. Qp/Qs can also be determined by echocardiography; however, this method is dependent on good echocardiographic windows [13]. Echocardiographic determination of Qp/Qs does not directly measure flow but assumes that the flow is equal throughout the flow column. Echocardiography also is limited in that the measurement of the diameter of the vessel is obtained at a different time than the Doppler evaluation of flow velocity [7]. PC-CMR can overcome these limitations in that CMR is not limited by echocardiographic windows, flow across a vessel is directly measured, and the cross-sectional area and velocity measurement are obtained simultaneously [7]. PC-CMR determination of Qp/Qs has compared well with Doppler echocardiography and volumetric assessment of right and left ventricular stroke volume [48–51]. PC-CMR has also been found to agree with the Fick equation in patients with left-to-right shunt who underwent simultaneous PC-CMR and cardiac catheterization [52–56].

With PC-CMR, Qp is usually measured at the main pulmonary artery or pulmonary valve. This is especially useful in the setting of an atrial septal defect, ventricular septal defect, or partial anomalous pulmonary venous return. In the setting of additional sources of pulmonary blood flow such as a patent ductus arteriosus, aortico-pulmonary collaterals, and surgical aorticopulmonary shunt, alternative strategies are required. Flow in the patent ductus arteriosus or surgical aorticopulmonary shunt can be measured directly and added to the main pulmonary artery flow to calculate Qp. Flow in both branch pulmonary arteries distal to the patent ductus arteriosus or surgical shunt can be measured and added to calculate Qp (assuming that the measurement is made proximal to any branch points of the right and left pulmonary arteries) [56]. Flow in all pulmonary veins can also be measured and added to measure Qp.

Qs is usually measured at the ascending aorta or aortic valve. Qs can also be obtained by measuring flow in the superior vena cava and inferior vena cava and adding the two. In patients with patent ductus arteriosus, aorticopulmonary surgical shunts, or aorticopulmonary collaterals, Qs can be obtained by performing PC-MRI in the descending aorta distal to the area of left-to-right shunting and in the superior vena cava before the entrance of the azygous and adding the two [57, 58].

There has been increased interest in the assessment of left-to-right shunting from aorticopulmonary collaterals in the setting of single-ventricle physiology and tetralogy of Fallot [57, 59–61]. Whitehead et al. and Glatz et al. have quantified aorticopulmonary flow in single-ventricle patients with one of two methods: in one method, aorticopulmonary flow = aorta − (SVC + IVC) and in the other method aorticopulmonary flow = (LPV − LPA) + (RPV − RPA) [57, 59, 60]. Tetralogy of Fallot patients with pulmonary atresia and aorticopulmonary collaterals also present a unique approach to PC-MRI. The clinical course and surgical timing are often determined by the amount and distribution of pulmonary blood flow. Historically, many of the most complex patients with this disease were not offered surgical repair, and some of these patients have survived to adulthood with profound cyanosis [62]. Grosse-Wortmann et al. described a method of quantifying pulmonary blood flow with PC-CMR in these patients which would predict postoperative right ventricular systolic pressure. They determined Qs by measuring flow in the descending aorta distal to all collateral vessels and added this to the SVC flow. They calculated Qp by direct measurement or by subtracting descending aortic flow from ascending aortic flow [61].

There are also multiple methods for calculating Qp/Qs in patients with atrial septal defects [12, 54, 63]. A widely used method is to measure pulmonary blood flow at the level of the pulmonary valve or main pulmonary artery and Qs at the aortic valve or ascending aorta. Our institution has described an alternative method which had better correlation with Qp/Qs calculated by the Fisk equation. This method involves obtaining an en face view of the atrial septal defect by planning from double orthogonal views. A PC-CMR through plane image is performed in this position. This allows for visualization of the size of the defect, additional defects, and determination of defect rims (Fig. 3.10). Quantification of flow through the defect can then be performed. Qp is calculated by adding Q_{ASD} to Qs. Qs is measured in the ascending aorta [12].

Regurgitation

Valvular dysfunction and regurgitation is a frequent finding in ACHD. Some common diagnoses in which regurgitation can be seen are bicuspid aortic valve, Ebstein's anomaly, and repaired tetralogy of Fallot. One of the more widespread uses of CMR in the evaluation of ACHD has been the assessment of pulmonary valve regurgitation and right ventricular dilation in repaired tetralogy of Fallot [64, 65]. PC-CMR, in addition to cine MRI, is essential to the assessment of the severity of regurgitation. In plane PC-MRI can be used to visualize regurgitant jets. This can allow for subjective assessment of regurgitation severity and assist with determination of the mechanism of regurgitation. Semilunar valve regurgitation can be assessed by through plane PC-CMR at the level of the valve or great artery proximal to the first branch. Forward and reverse volumes are measured. A regurgitant fraction is then calculated by using the equation: Regurgitant fraction = reverse volume/total forward volume. When performing PC-CMR at the level of the valve, inaccuracies can occur when the plane of the regurgitant jet is eccentric and at an angle to the imaging plane. Because of this our institution frequently performs PC-CMR within the associated great artery: ascending aorta proximal to the innominate artery for the aortic valve and main pulmonary artery for the pulmonary valve (Fig. 3.12). When assessing aortic insufficiency, it can be beneficial to perform PC-CMR in the descending aorta. The presence of flow reversal can be used to help assess severity.

Quantification of atrioventricular valve regurgitation is also an important component of the PC-CMR assessment of the ACHD patient. Atrioventricular valve regurgitation can be measured directly by aligning a through plane PC-CMR image at the level of the plane of the valve. The forward and reverse volume can be measured and regurgitant fraction calculated: Regurgitant fraction = reverse volume/forward volume. This method can be problematic as it can often be difficult to align the PC-CMR with the plane of the valve and regurgitant jet. In the absence of semilunar valve regurgitation, atrioventricular valve regurgitant fraction can be calculated by dividing the reverse volume (directly measured) by the ventricular stroke volume. This can also be done by measuring the forward volume in the associated semilunar valve or great artery and the ventricular stroke volume. Regurgitant fraction of the atrioventricular valve can then be calculated by using the following equation: Regurgitant fraction = (ventricular stroke volume − forward volume of semilunar valve)/ventricular stroke volume.

Stenosis

Valvular stenosis is a frequent finding in ACHD. Pulmonary stenosis, tetralogy of Fallot, bicuspid aortic valve, and repaired atrioventricular septal defects are common diagnosis with valvular stenosis. PC-CMR semilunar valve assessment is accomplished by performing a through plane image at the level of the valve leaflet tips. To ensure accuracy, it is imperative to set the VENC at the minimum value above which aliasing occurs. On the phase-contrasted image, the semilunar valve outflow should be traced to include all of the pixels in the outflow column, but no others. The peak velocity of the flow can then be measured. The modified Bernoulli equation, pressure gradient $=4v^2$, can then be applied to calculate a gradient across the valve. Previous studies have revealed correlation with spectral Doppler echocardiography and cardiac catheterization [66, 67].

Evaluation of atrioventricular valve stenosis can also be performed by PC-CMR [68]. Mitral and tricuspid valve stenoses are frequent findings in a number of ACHD constellations. PC-MRI of the atrioventricular valve is accomplished with a PC-CMR image at the level of the atrioventricular valve leaflet tips [68]. The VENC should again be set properly to the minimum value above which no aliasing occurs. The inflow of the phase-contrast image can be traced, the peak velocity measured, and a mean velocity calculated from the area under the curve. Atrioventricular valve stenosis is commonly reported as a mean gradient, and the modified Bernoulli equation can be used to calculate this gradient [13].

Evaluation of arterial stenosis is critical in patients with branch pulmonary artery stenosis and coarctation of the aorta. ACHD patients, especially those with tetralogy of Fallot and transposition of the great arteries following arterial switch, frequently have branch pulmonary artery stenosis. Branch pulmonary artery stenosis can be measured directly with PC-CMR. A PC-MRI image perpendicular to the long axis of the vessel can be done at the level of the stenosis and a peak velocity and gradient calculated. Flow evaluation of the proximal branch pulmonary arteries can be performed. The flow and forward volume into each branch pulmonary artery can be measured. These values can be compared to each other and to the main pulmonary artery. The percentage of flow to each lung can be calculated. This is analogous to a nuclear lung perfusion scan and studies have confirmed that this modality correlates well with nuclear lung perfusion measurements [69, 70]. Patients with coarctation of the aorta, both repaired and unrepaired, require PC-CMR appraisal of stenosis. It is often advisable to perform in plane PC-CMR in a plane visualizing the aortic arch in an orthogonal sagittal plane with a relatively low VENC. This can allow for visualization of the area of most severe stenosis as identified by the area of maximal aliasing (Fig. 3.14a). A through plane image can be planned at this location and a peak velocity calculated [71]. Through plane PC-CMR can also be performed in the descending aorta. A patient with more severe stenosis can have a flow pattern with diminished amplitude and antegrade flow in diastole (Fig. 3.14b). Collateral volume can be quantified by measuring forward volume in the descending aorta below the level of obstruction and collaterals and proximal to the area of the stenosis. The proximal value is then subtracted from the distal value and the collateral volume calculated [72–76].

Venous stenosis can also be assessed with PC-CMR. Stenosis of the superior vena cava (SVC) can be a complication of surgical repair of superior sinus venosus atrial septal defects. A PC-CMR perpendicular to the long axis of the SVC can allow for measuring the peak and mean velocity across the vessel. Stenosis of the superior systemic limb of the atrial baffle in a transposition of the great arteries patient can also occur and can be evaluated in this manner [77]. Pulmonary venous stenosis can also be a complication of ACHD. Double orthogonal PC-CMR at the orifice of the pulmonary veins can allow for detection of stenosis [78, 79]. This imaging plane is often best planned by using an angiogram. The area under the flow curve can be integrated and mean velocity and gradient calculated.

Patients with single-ventricle physiology who have undergone Fontan completion can also be evaluated for areas of stenosis and flow quantification. Measurements can be performed in the superior vena cava, inferior vena cava, Fontan baffle or conduit, and both branch pulmonary arteries. This allows for the detection of areas of stenosis or disturbed flow and also allows for the evaluation of distribution of flow [80–83].

New Techniques

New techniques involving 3D or 4D flow have been developed [84–89]. These techniques hold promise for the evaluation of flow hemodynamics in ACHD. Studies have begun to evaluate the utility of these modalities in the evaluation of aortic stenosis, coarctation of the aorta, and Fontan patients. Single-ventricle patients with Fontan circulation hold particular promise. These modalities allow for the study and assessment of flow patterns within the Fontan circuit. This can hopefully allow for optimizing the surgical techniques of the Fontan allowing for improved hemodynamics [90]. These modalities are not widely used in clinical practice at this time, but hold great promise for the future.

Delayed Enhancement Imaging

Delayed enhancement CMR (DE-CMR) is used extensively to evaluate infarction, cardiomyopathy, and infiltrative disease in adults with structurally normal hearts [91–97]. The adaptation of this imaging modality to ACHD patients has not been as proliferative. Nevertheless, ACHD patients are at risk for myocardial fibrosis and scar. Abnormal loading conditions, both pressure and volume overloading, can lead to an increased risk of myocardial fibrosis. An example is the systemic right ventricle in patients with transposition of the great arteries (TGA) following an atrial switch operation [98]. ACHD patients also often have a history of multiple prior cardiac interventions. This can lead to hyperenhancement of repaired or patched areas such as a VSD patch or transannular patch in repaired tetralogy of Fallot (TOF). Many ACHD patients have congenital coronary artery abnormalities or undergo surgeries involving reimplantation of the coronary arteries. These patients are at increased risk of myocardial infarction in the perioperative period or later in life. Finally, as ACHD patients age, they will begin to develop coronary artery disease from traditional risk factors. This is an area that will need to be better studied and characterized as these patients continue to age.

DE-CMR is based on differences in signal intensity of abnormal and normal myocardium following the administration of gadolinium contrast. Infarcted or fibrotic myocardium has increased interstitial volume compared to normal myocardium. When gadolinium is administered, the volume of distribution in the abnormal myocardium is increased, resulting in greater signal intensity. Imaging is performed 10–15 min following the administration of a gadolinium-based contrast [91, 99]. This is most commonly performed with a gradient echo imaging engine with an inversion recovery prepulse to provide increased T1 weighting. Image readout occurs in mid-diastole to minimize cardiac motion. Imaging occurs every other heartbeat in order for longitudinal relaxation to recover prior to the next prepulse [7, 91]. The TI is selected so that normal myocardium will appear black or "null" and areas of infarction or fibrosis will hyperenhance and appear bright [99]. Abnormal myocardium appears bright because it will have a more rapid decay of longitudinal magnetization than normal myocardium (Fig. 3.15a, b). These images require a breath hold to minimize respiratory motion.

An ultrafast real-time DE-CMR technique using a single-shot SSFP imaging engine has also been developed [100, 101]. This allows for rapid imaging of the myocardium without breath holding. These images have lower spatial resolution than segmented gradient echo imaging (Fig. 3.15b). A study by Sievers et al. has demonstrated that these images can be rapidly obtained and are highly accurate, although with a reduced sensitivity when compared to segmented gradient echo imaging [101]. This sequence can be especially useful in patients who cannot perform breath holding, are uncooperative, or have arrhythmias [101].

Five minutes following the administration of contrast, single-shot SSFP delayed enhancement images can be performed with the TI set to 500–600 ms. This results in all tissues except thrombus and calcification having equal signal intensity and appearing gray. This sequence can be used to screen for thrombus, and thrombus will appear black in these images (Fig. 3.15c). In the setting

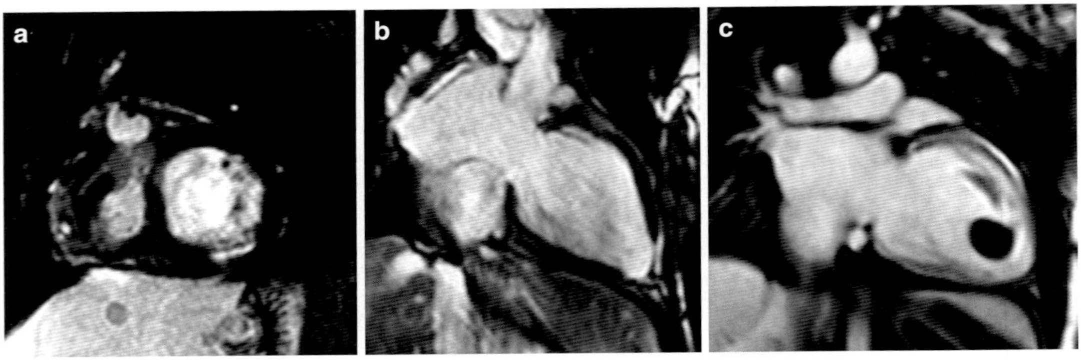

Fig. 3.15 (**a**) Segmented delayed enhancement short axis image of a patient with tricuspid atresia. Note the subendocardial hyperenhancement in the inferior wall which would be consistent with an infarction. (**b**) Two-chambered single-shot delayed enhancement image. Note the apical transmural hyperenhancement which likely represents operative injury at the site left ventriculostomy. (**c**) "High TI" (600 ms) single-shot delayed enhancement two-chambered long axis view of the left ventricle. Note the large thrombus in the left ventricular apex. Note gray signal of the normal myocardium in high TI sequence

of ischemic heart disease, this method has been shown to be superior to transthoracic echocardiography and cine MRI [102, 103]. This imaging modality can be useful in ACHD patients at risk for thrombus. Single-ventricle patients who have undergone the Fontan operation and have low velocity flow within the Fontan are a particularly high-risk group [104].

The use of DE-CMR in patients with ACHD is still very much in its infancy. In 2004, Prakash et al. first reported the feasibility of DE-CMR in congenital heart disease [105]. Harris et al. demonstrated that DE-CMR could detect fibrosis both in unrepaired congenital heart disease and associated with surgical repair [106]. Repaired tetralogy of Fallot is one of the more common diagnosis studied with DE-CMR [107–110]. These patients are at risk for fibrosis because of volume and/or pressure loading from pulmonary regurgitation or residual right ventricular outflow tract obstruction. Transannular patch repair can lead to an aneurysmal right ventricular outflow tract with thinned, scarred myocardium. VSD patches can distort the interventricular septum. Oosterhof et al. demonstrated abnormal DE within the right ventricular outflow tract and correlated an increased amount of hyperenhancement with increased right ventricular volumes [107]. Babu-Narayan performed DE-CMR in patients with repaired TOF and found abnormal DE within the right and left ventricles. Increased abnormal DE was associated with multiple adverse clinical outcomes such as ventricular failure, arrhythmia, exercise tolerance, and neurohumoral activation [108]. Wald et al. used DE-CMR, among other modalities, to evaluate areas of regional right ventricular dysfunction in repaired TOF. They found that a greater extent of regional dysfunction led to reduced global right ventricular function and exercise tolerance [109]. Patients with repaired TOF often have fragmented QRS morphology. Park et al. found that a fragmented QRS was associated with more extensive abnormal DE and dysfunction of the right ventricle [110].

Patients with two-ventricle physiology and a systemic right ventricle, such as TGA following an atrial switch operation and congenitally corrected TGA, have been evaluated for right ventricular fibrosis. Several studies have evaluated for the presence of fibrosis by DE-CMR [98, 111–114]. Fratz et al. and Preim et al. evaluated patients with systemic right ventricles and found that abnormal DE was a rare finding [111, 112]. On the other hand, other groups have demonstrated that this is a common finding [98, 113, 114]. Babu-Narayan et al. demonstrated that the extent of abnormal DE in TGA following atrial switch operation correlates with adverse clinical parameters [98].

Single-ventricle patients have unique hemodynamic demand placed on the ventricular myocardium. Rathod et al. studied DE-CMR patterns in single-ventricle patients with a history of a Fontan operation. They found increased ventricular fibrosis, and this fibrosis was associated with ventricular dysfunction and nonsustained ventricular tachycardia [115]. Harris et al. evaluated six patients with hypoplastic left heart syndrome with DE-CMR and found abnormal delayed enhancement at the site of the Norwood reconstruction [106].

Patients with congenital aortic stenosis have also been found to have abnormal DE-CMR of the left ventricle [116, 117]. Robinson et al. noted left ventricular subendocardial delayed enhancement in several patients who had undergone aortic balloon valvuloplasty [116]. Lasalvia et al. also found left ventricular subendocardial hyperenhancement in a patient with severe congenital aortic stenosis who eventually had ventricular failure and orthotopic heart transplant. The histological specimens of the explanted heart were compared to the DE-CMR images and were found to correlate [117].

There are many more ACHD patient populations which have yet to be studied by DE-CMR. A thorough evaluation of many ACHD patient populations is limited by heterogeneous patient populations and small patient numbers. Studies evaluating DE-CMR patterns in ACHD need to be validated by histology. There are many potential roles for DE-CMR in ACHD which could lead to improved diagnosis, prognostic information, and treatment.

Stress Imaging

Assessment of the heart during exercise can be invaluable for diagnosis and clinical management. Imaging the heart during exercise or stress can allow for assessment of global ventricular function, wall motion abnormalities, inducible ischemia, and intracavitary gradients. Historically, imaging modalities such as nuclear perfusion imaging and echocardiography have been used to image the heart during exercise/stress [118, 119]. CMR also has an important role in diagnostic stress imaging.

Stress CMR imaging is predominantly used in adults with structurally normal hearts for the assessment of coronary artery disease. However, there are uses for stress CMR in ACHD. ACHD patients can have an increased risk of coronary artery disease as a result of congenital coronary artery anomalies, history of coronary artery reimplantation, coronary artery injury associated with prior surgical repair, or standard risk factors. Stress CMR can also be used to assess responses to exercise/stress in ACHD patients without suspected coronary artery disease.

CMR stress testing can be performed by two methods: (1) cine MRI with exercise or pharmacologic stress and (2) stress perfusion CMR with pharmacologic stress. Cine MR images of the ventricle can be obtained with exercise or pharmacologic stress to assess ventricular function and wall motion abnormalities. Exercise testing can be performed using an MRI safe, supine, or upright bicycle ergometer. The patient can exercise while in the bore of the magnet or outside of the bore and then moved in immediately following exercise [120–123]. In theory, exercise should be preferred to pharmacologic stress because pharmacologic stress mimics exercise but does not reproduce all physiological variables [120]. However, motion artifacts and gating issues associated with exercise and hyperventilation can make imaging difficult. Because of these limitations, pharmacologic stress is often used to mimic exercise. Dobutamine is the most commonly used agent. Dobutamine increases myocardial oxygen demand. It acts as an inotropic agent and at higher doses acts as a chronotropic agent as well. Dobutamine has a short half-life (2 min); therefore, it is administered as a continuous infusion. The dose is usually started at 2.5–5 ug/kg/min and increased every 3–5 min until the target heart rate of 85 % of predicted is reached or the maximum dose of 40 ug/kg/min is reached [120]. Contraindications to a dobutamine infusion include an obstruction to systemic inflow or outflow, heart block, or ventricular tachycardia [120]. A stack of cine short axis images can be obtained at rest and with exercise/

stress. Ventricular volumes and ejection fractions can be measured at rest and with exercise/stress and compared. The ventricles can also be assessed for wall motion abnormalities. Abnormalities observed with exercise/stress, but not rest, are consistent with inducible ischemia.

Stress perfusion imaging can also be used in the CMR assessment of coronary artery disease. The patient is given a pharmacologic agent which acts as a coronary vasodilator. Adenosine is most commonly used. Adenosine dilates unobstructed coronary arteries. A patient with a fixed coronary stenosis who is given an adenosine infusion will have a perfusion mismatch between the area of distribution of the affected coronary artery and other areas of myocardium. Adenosine has a very short half-life so it must be given as a continuous infusion (0.14 mg/kg/min). At our institution adenosine is given for 2 min or until the patient experiences typical symptoms of flushing, tachycardia, chest discomfort, shortness of breath, dizziness, and headache [7]. Once the patient is felt to have an adequate physiological response to adenosine, gadolinium is administered and the imaging sequence is initiated. Adenosine is contraindicated in patients with reactive airway disease, second- or third-degree heart block, and in patients taking dipyridamole [120]. Caffeine and theophylline should also be avoided as they act as an adenosine receptor antagonists. Dipyridamole can also be used for CMR stress testing. Dipyridamole inhibits the reuptake of adenosine by endothelial cells, therefore indirectly causing coronary vasodilation by increasing adenosine levels [120]. Regadenoson can also be used for CMR stress testing [124]. It indirectly causes coronary vasodilation because of its action as a selective adenosine A_{2A} receptor antagonist. Regadenoson can be given as a single bolus, eliminating the need for a second IV, and it also has a reduced side effect profile because of its action as a selective adenosine A_{2A} antagonist [125, 126].

CMR stress perfusion imaging is designed to produce a movie of the first-pass perfusion of gadolinium contrast through the myocardium [7]. This allows for the identification of perfusion defects representing areas of distribution of obstructed coronary arteries. Perfusion imaging is performed at stress and at rest, separated by 15 min to allow for contrast washout (Fig. 3.16). Defects which are matched on stress and rest imaging may represent an artifact or an area of infarction which can be confirmed with DE-CMR. Defects which occur at stress, but not rest, represent inducible ischemia and coronary artery disease. Imaging is performed with a gradient echo imaging engine or gradient echo-echo planar hybrid imaging engine with a parallel imaging modifier in a single-shot mode. Four to five short axis slices are obtained with ECG gating every cardiac cycle during the first pass of perfusion [7]. CMR vasodilator myocardial stress perfusion is sensitive and specific for diagnosing coronary artery disease [127–135]. The American College of Cardiology Foundation Appropriateness Criteria Working Group has concluded that stress perfusion CMR is "appropriate" for chest pain syndromes in patients who have intermediate risk of coronary artery disease and for determining the physiological significance of indeterminate coronary artery lesions [7, 136].

Rest perfusion imaging is also frequently used to evaluate a cardiac mass for vascularity [137, 138]. A gradient echo imaging engine is used and image position is planned to best visualize the mass.

The adaptation and use of stress CMR in congenital heart disease has been increasing. The majority of this experience has been with cine MRI. Several studies have performed stress cine MRI in patients with transposition of the great arteries who have undergone an atrial switch operation [139–143]. These studies reveal that these patients do not increase right ventricular stroke volume in response to exercise/stress, and this is felt to be secondary to impaired ventricular filling with exercise as a result of atrial baffles [139–143]. The majority of stress cine MRI studies in this population were performed with dobutamine [140–143]. Roest et al. performed stress cine MRI using a supine bicycle ergometer [139]. Oosterhoff et al. performed exercise and dobutamine stress cine MRI and found that the tests were not interchangeable in this patient population. With dobutamine stress testing, ejection fraction, end-diastolic volume, and end-systolic

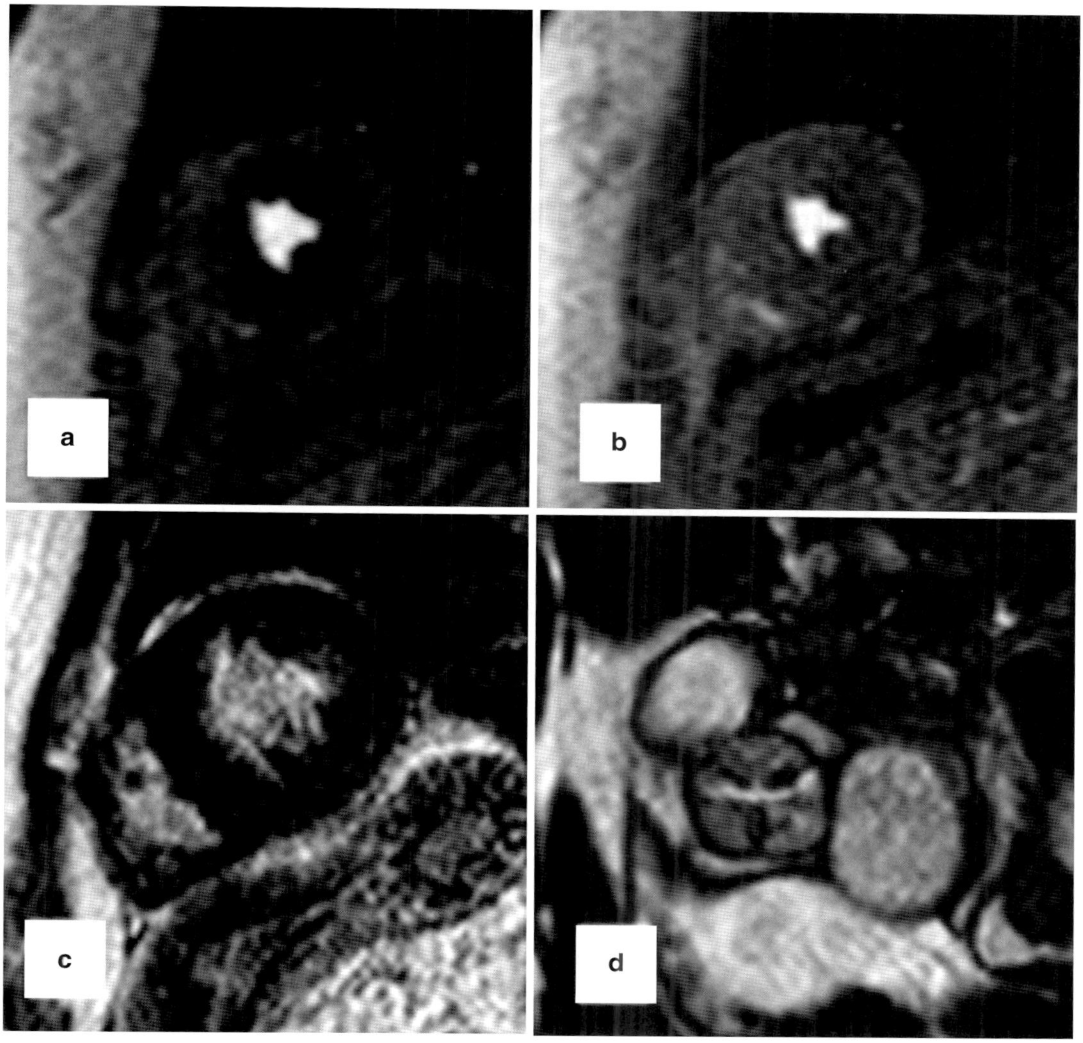

Fig. 3.16 Adenosine stress/rest perfusion and delayed post-contrast images in a patient left ventricular hypertrophy due to stenotic bicuspid aortic valve are shown. (**a**) Stress perfusion shows diffuse subendocardial hypoperfusion. (**b**) Rest perfusion shows normal myocardium. (**c**) Delayed post-contrast image shows no abnormal myocardial enhancement. (**d**) Cine frame shows severe aortic stenosis

volume were increased, but stroke volume was unchanged. With exercise stress testing, ejection fraction decreased while ventricular volumes and stroke volume were unchanged [142].

Patients with congenitally corrected TGA (CC-TGA) also have a systemic morphologic right ventricle. There have been several studies assessing the right ventricle with stress cine MRI and comparing to the systemic right ventricle of patients with complete transposition of the great arteries that have undergone an atrial switch operation [141, 143, 144]. Fratz et al. and Dodge-Khatami et al. performed dobutamine stress cine MRI and found that these patients have a normal response of the right ventricle to exercise with an increase in right ventricular stroke volume [143, 144]. Tulveski et al. also performed dobutamine stress cine MRI and found that right ventricular ejection fraction increased but stroke volume was unchanged [141].

Another ACHD population which has been studied with stress cine MRI is repaired tetralogy of Fallot [35, 122, 145–147]. Roest et al. performed exercise cine MRI (supine bicycle ergometer) and found that pulmonary valve regurgitation was reduced and that there was an abnormal right ventricular response to exercise. There was no change in right ventricular end-systolic volume (indexed) or ejection fraction with exercise. Left ventricular response to exercise was normal [122]. Roest et al. also assessed ascending aortic flow measurements during exercise and concluded that there was an abnormal recovery of left ventricular stroke volume following exercise [145]. Van den Berg et al. performed dobutamine cine MRI and measured pulmonary and tricuspid flow curves at rest and with stress to assess right ventricular filling. They concluded that patients with forward flow in end diastole had an abnormal response to stress with worsening of ventricular filling [35]. In another study, van den Berg et al. also used dobutamine stress cine MRI to assess right ventricular systolic function. In contrast to Roest et al., they found that patients with repaired tetralogy of Fallot have a normal right ventricular response to exercise with a decrease in right ventricular end-systolic volume and an increase in stroke volume [146]. Tulveski et al. performed dobutamine stress CMR in patients with pulmonary stenosis (repaired tetralogy of Fallot, pulmonary stenosis, pulmonary hypertension) and in patients with pulmonary stenosis and regurgitation. With stress, they found that, in both groups, patients had reduced stroke volume, impaired relaxation, and no change in ejection fraction [147].

ACHD patients with single-ventricle physiology and a history of a Fontan operation have been studied during stress with cine MRI and CMR flow assessment [123, 148–152]. Hjortdal et al. performed exercise stress with a bicycle ergometer in patients with a history of a Fontan operation. Velocity flow measurements of the inferior vena cava and aorta were performed and increased flow in the inferior vena cava and aorta was noted, but not the superior vena cava [148, 149]. Pederson et al. also performed bicycle ergometer exercise stress CMR in this group of patients. Velocity flow measurements of the inferior vena cava and branch pulmonary arteries revealed a doubling of inferior vena cava flow and equal distribution to both pulmonary arteries [123]. Ventricular functional response to exercise in Fontan patients has been assessed with dobutamine stress CMR. Robbers-Visser et al. and Schmitt et al. have demonstrated that stroke volume does not increase with exercise and that cardiac output is increased with exercise predominantly with an increase in heart rate [151, 152].

ACHD patients can be at risk for coronary artery disease as a result of congenital coronary artery anomalies, coronary artery reimplantation, perioperative injury, and standard risk factors. Stress CMR can be used for the evaluation of ACHD patients at risk for coronary artery disease. Experience in this field has been limited, but is growing as these modalities are applied to more ACHD patients. Taylor et al. performed adenosine cine MRI in patients with aortic stenosis and transposition of the great arteries following arterial switch operation. They measured volumes and flows and noted increased cardiac output during adenosine infusion. They also concluded that adenosine could be safely administered to patients with congenital heart disease [153]. Strigl et al. reported their experience performing dobutamine stress cine MRI in pediatric congenital heart disease patients with suspected coronary artery disease. They found that the incidence of positive findings was low, but that performing dobutamine stress cine MRI is feasible [154]. Cook et al. performed adenosine stress perfusion in a group of adult patients with a history of repaired coarctation of the aorta. They did not identify inducible ischemia, but did note decreased myocardial perfusion reserve [155]. Buechel et al. reported they experience performing adenosine stress perfusion CMR in pediatric patients with suspected congenital heart disease. They compared adenosine stress perfusion CMR to coronary angiography in some of their patients. They concluded that adenosine stress perfusion CMR is feasible and accurate in pediatric patients with suspected coronary artery disease and congenital heart disease [156].

The use of stress CMR is very much in its early stages. There is much more experience with these modalities in adults with structurally normal hearts and coronary artery disease. As the ACHD population ages, the use of these modalities to identify coronary artery disease will increase. Currently, there are select ACHD patients at high risk for coronary artery disease that can benefit from these modalities. Further research is needed to understand the physiological responses to exercise/stress in patients with congenital heart disease. A better understanding will lay the foundation for improved clinical utility in these patients.

References

1. Ferencz C, Loffredo CA, Rubin JD, et al. Epidemiology of congenital heart disease: the Baltimore Washington Infant Study 1981–1989. Mount Kisco: Futura Publishing; 1993.
2. Marelli AJ, Mackie AS, Ionescu-Ittu R, Rahme E, Pilote L. Congenital heart disease in the general population: changing prevalence and age distribution. Circulation. 2007;115(2):163–72.
3. Williams RG, Pearson GD, Barst RJ, Child JS, del Nido P, Gersony WM, Kuehl KS, Landzberg MJ, Myerson M, Neish SR, Sahn DJ, Verstappen A, Warnes CA, Webb CL, National Heart, Lung, and Blood Institute Working Group on Research in Adult Congenital Heart Disease. Report of the National Heart, Lung, and Blood Institute Working Group on research in adult congenital heart disease. J Am Coll Cardiol. 2006;47(4):701–7.
4. Taussig HB. Congenital malformations of the heart. New York: The Commonwealth Fund; 1947.
5. Ahmed S, Shellock FG. Magnetic resonance imaging safety: implications for cardiovascular patients. J Cardiovasc Magn Reson. 2001;3(3):171–82.
6. Lee V. Cardiovascular MR imaging. Physical principles to practical protocols. Philadelphia: Lippincott Williams & Wilkins; 2006.
7. Kim HW, Crowley AL, Kim RJ. A clinical cardiovascular magnetic resonance service: operational considerations and the basic examination. Cardiol Clin. 2007;25(1):1–13, v.
8. Geva T, Powell AJ. Chapter 7: magnetic resonance imaging. In: Allen HD, Driscoll DJ, Shaddy RE, Feltes TF, editors. Moss and Adams' heart disease in infants, children and adolescents. 7th ed. Philadelphia: Lippincott Williams and Wilkins; 2008. p. 163–99.
9. Carr JC, Simonetti O, Bundy J, Li D, Pereles S, Finn JP. Cine MR angiography of the heart with segmented true fast imaging with steady-state precession. Radiology. 2001;219(3):828–34.
10. Warnes CA. Adult congenital heart disease importance of the right ventricle. J Am Coll Cardiol. 2009; 54:1903–10.
11. Valente AM, Sena L, Powell AJ, Del Nido PJ, Geva T. Cardiac magnetic resonance imaging evaluation of sinus venosus defects: comparison to surgical findings. Pediatr Cardiol. 2007;28(1):51–6.
12. Thomson LE, Crowley AL, Heitner JF, Cawley PJ, Weinsaft JW, Kim HW, Parker M, Judd RM, Harrison JK, Kim RJ. Direct en face imaging of secundum atrial septal defects by velocity-encoded cardiovascular magnetic resonance in patients evaluated for possible transcatheter closure. Circ Cardiovasc Imaging. 2008;1(1):31–40.
13. Snider AR, Serwer GA, Ritter SB. Echocardiography in pediatric heart disease. 2nd ed. St. Louis: Mosby-Year Book Inc; 1997.
14. Fratz S, Schuhbaeck A, Buchner C, Busch R, Meierhofer C, Martinoff S, Hess J, Stern H. Comparison of accuracy of axial slices versus short-axis slices for measuring ventricular volumes by cardiac magnetic resonance in patients with corrected tetralogy of Fallot. Am J Cardiol. 2009;103(12):1764–9. doi:10.1016/j.amjcard.2009.02.030. Epub 2009 May 4.
15. Sechtem U, Pflugfelder PW, Gould RG, Cassidy MM, Higgins CB. Measurement of right and left ventricular volumes in healthy individuals with cine MR imaging. Radiology. 1987;163(3):697–702.
16. Grothues F, Moon JC, Bellenger NG, Smith GS, Klein HU, Pennell DJ. Interstudy reproducibility of right ventricular volumes, function, and mass with cardiovascular magnetic resonance. Am Heart J. 2004;147(2):218–23.
17. Koch JA, Poll LW, Godehardt E, Korbmacher B, Jung G, Mödder U. In vitro determination of cardiac ventricular volumes using MRI at 1.0 T in a porcine heart model. Int J Cardiovasc Imaging. 2001;17(3):237–42.
18. Buser PT, Auffermann W, Holt WW, Wagner S, Kircher B, Wolfe C, Higgins CB. Noninvasive evaluation of global left ventricular function with use of cine nuclear magnetic resonance. J Am Coll Cardiol. 1989;13(6):1294–300.
19. Grothues F, Smith GC, Moon JC, Bellenger NG, Collins P, Klein HU, Pennell DJ. Comparison of interstudy reproducibility of cardiovascular magnetic resonance with two-dimensional echocardiography in normal subjects and in patients with heart failure or left ventricular hypertrophy. Am J Cardiol. 2002; 90(1):29–34.
20. Mogelvang J, Stokholm KH, Stubgaard M. Assessment of right ventricular volumes by magnetic resonance imaging and by radionuclide angiography. Am J Noninvasive Cardiol. 1991;5:321–7.
21. Maceira AM, Prasad SK, Khan M, Pennell DJ. Normalized left ventricular systolic and diastolic function by steady state free precession cardiovascular magnetic resonance. J Cardiovasc Magn Reson. 2006;8(3):417–26.
22. Maceira AM, Prasad SK, Khan M, Pennell DJ. Reference right ventricular systolic and diastolic

function normalized to age, gender and body surface area from steady-state free precession cardiovascular magnetic resonance. Eur Heart J. 2006;27(23):2879–88. Epub 2006 Nov 6.
23. Samyn MM, Powell AJ, Garg R, Sena L, Geva T. Range of ventricular dimensions and function by steady-state free precession cine MRI in repaired tetralogy of Fallot: right ventricular outflow tract patch vs. conduit repair. J Magn Reson Imaging. 2007;26(4):934–40.
24. Geva T, Sandweiss BM, Gauvreau K, Lock JE, Powell AJ. Factors associated with impaired clinical status in long-term survivors of tetralogy of Fallot repair evaluated by magnetic resonance imaging. J Am Coll Cardiol. 2004;43(6):1068–74.
25. Oosterhof T, van Straten A, Vliegen HW, Meijboom FJ, van Dijk AP, Spijkerboer AM, Bouma BJ, Zwinderman AH, Hazekamp MG, de Roos A, Mulder BJ. Preoperative thresholds for pulmonary valve replacement in patients with corrected tetralogy of Fallot using cardiovascular magnetic resonance. Circulation. 2007;116(5):545–51. Epub 2007 Jul 9.
26. Henkens IR, van Straten A, Schalij MJ, Hazekamp MG, de Roos A, van der Wall EE, Vliegen HW. Predicting outcome of pulmonary valve replacement in adult tetralogy of Fallot patients. Ann Thorac Surg. 2007;83(3):907–11.
27. Knauth AL, Gauvreau K, Powell AJ, Landzberg MJ, Walsh EP, Lock JE, del Nido PJ, Geva T. Ventricular size and function assessed by cardiac MRI predict major adverse clinical outcomes late after tetralogy of Fallot repair. Heart. 2008;94(2):211–6. Epub 2006 Nov 29.
28. Blackstone EH, Kirklin JW, Pacifico AD. Decision-making in repair of tetralogy of Fallot based on intra-operative measurements of pulmonary arterial outflow tract. J Thorac Cardiovasc Surg. 1979;77(4):526–32.
29. Naito Y, Fujita T, Manabe H, Kawashima Y. The criteria for reconstruction of right ventricular outflow tract in total correction of tetralogy of Fallot. J Thorac Cardiovasc Surg. 1980;80(4):574–81.
30. Pacifico AD, Kirklin JW, Blackstone EH. Surgical management of pulmonary stenosis in tetralogy of Fallot. J Thorac Cardiovasc Surg. 1977;74(3):382–95.
31. Geva T. Repaired tetralogy of Fallot: the roles of cardiovascular magnetic resonance in evaluating pathophysiology and for pulmonary valve replacement decision support. J Cardiovasc Magn Reson. 2011;13:9. doi:10.1186/1532-429X-13-9.
32. Cerqueira MD, Weissman NJ, Dilsizian V, Jacobs AK, Kaul S, Laskey WK, Pennell DJ, Rumberger JA, Ryan T, Verani MS, American Heart Association Writing Group on Myocardial Segmentation and Registration for Cardiac Imaging. Standardized myocardial segmentation and nomenclature for tomographic imaging of the heart. A statement for healthcare professionals from the Cardiac Imaging Committee of the Council on Clinical Cardiology of the American Heart Association. Circulation. 2002; 105(4):539–42.
33. Lu JC, Cotts TB, Agarwal PP, Attili AK, Dorfman AL. Relation of right ventricular dilation, age of repair, and restrictive right ventricular physiology with patient-reported quality of life in adolescents and adults with repaired tetralogy of Fallot. Am J Cardiol. 2010;106(12):1798–802. doi:10.1016/j.amjcard.2010.08.021. Epub 2010 Nov 2.
34. Rathi VK, Doyle M, Yamrozik J, Williams RB, Caruppannan K, Truman C, Vido D, Biederman RW. Routine evaluation of left ventricular diastolic function by cardiovascular magnetic resonance: a practical approach. J Cardiovasc Magn Reson. 2008;10:36. doi:10.1186/1532-429X-10-36.
35. van den Berg J, Wielopolski PA, Meijboom FJ, Witsenburg M, Bogers AJ, Pattynama PM, Helbing WA. Diastolic function in repaired tetralogy of Fallot at rest and during stress: assessment with MR imaging. Radiology. 2007;243:212–9.
36. Helbing WA, Niezen RA, Le Cessie S, van der Geest RJ, Ottenkamp J, de Roos A. Right ventricular diastolic function in children with pulmonary regurgitation after repair of tetralogy of Fallot: volumetric evaluation by magnetic resonance velocity mapping. J Am Coll Cardiol. 1996;28:1827–35.
37. Mirsky I, Parmley WW. Assessment of passive elastic stiffness for isolated heart muscle and the intact heart. Circ Res. 1973;33(2):233–43.
38. Heimdal A, Stoylen A, Torp H, Skjaerpe T. Real-time strain rate imaging of the left ventricle by ultrasound. J Am Soc Echocardiogr. 1998;11(11):1013–9.
39. Jeung MY, Germain P, Croisille P, El Ghanuddi S, Roy C, Gangi A. Myocardial tagging with MR imaging: overview of normal and pathologic findings. Radiographics. 2012;32(5):1381–98.
40. Zerhouni EA, Parish DM, Rogers WJ, Yang A, Shapiro EP. Human heart: tagging with MR imaging—a method for noninvasive assessment of myocardial motion. Radiology. 1988;169(1):59–63.
41. Axel L, Dougherty L. MR imaging of motion with spatial modulation of magnetization. Radiology. 1989;171(3):841–5.
42. Osman NF, Kerwin WS, McVeigh ER, Prince JL. Cardiac motion tracking using CINE harmonic phase (HARP) magnetic resonance imaging. Magn Reson Med. 1999;42:1048–60.
43. Osman NF, Prince JL. Visualizing myocardial function using HARP MRI. Phys Med Biol. 2000;45: 1665–82.
44. Hor KN, Gottliebson WM, Carson C. Comparison of magnetic resonance feature tracking for strain calculation with harmonic phase imaging analysis. JACC Cardiovasc Imaging. 2010;3(2):144–51.
45. Powell AJ, Geva T. Blood flow measurement by magnetic resonance imaging in congenital heart disease. Pediatr Cardiol. 2000;21(1):47–58.
46. Goldberg A, Jha S. Phase-contrast MRI and applications in congenital heart disease. Clin Radiol. 2012;67(5):399–410.
47. Hosten N, Gutberlet M, Kühne T, Oellinger H, Vogel M, Böckel T, Böck J, Frank J. Cardiac MR flowmetry:

experimental validation and results in patients with operated heart defects. Rofo. 1998;168(5):480–7.
48. Didier D, Ratib O, Lerch R, Friedli B. Detection and quantification of valvular heart disease with dynamic cardiac MR imaging. Radiographics. 2000;20(5):1279–99; discussion 1299–301.
49. Glockner JF, Johnston DL, McGee KP. Evaluation of cardiac valvular disease with MR imaging: qualitative and quantitative techniques. Radiographics. 2003; 23(1):e9.
50. Nishimura T, Yamada N, Itoh A, Miyatake K. Cine MR imaging in mitral regurgitation: comparison with color Doppler flow imaging. AJR Am J Roentgenol. 1989;153(4):721–4.
51. Fujita N, Chazouilleres AF, Hartiala JJ, O'Sullivan M, Heidenreich P, Kaplan JD, Sakuma H, Foster E, Caputo GR, Higgins CB. Quantification of mitral regurgitation by velocity-encoded cine nuclear magnetic resonance imaging. J Am Coll Cardiol. 1994;23(4):951–8.
52. Debl K, Djavidani B, Buchner S, Heinicke N, Poschenrieder F, Feuerbach S, Riegger G, Luchner A. Quantification of left-to-right shunting in adult congenital heart disease: phase-contrast cine MRI compared with invasive oximetry. Br J Radiol. 2009;82(977):386–91.
53. Esmaeili A, Höhn R, Koch A, Vogl TJ, Hofstetter R, Abolmaali N. Assessment of shunt volumes in children with ventricular septal defects: comparative quantification of MR flow measurements and invasive oximetry. Clin Res Cardiol. 2006;95(10):523–30.
54. Petersen SE, Voigtländer T, Kreitner KF, Kalden P, Wittlinger T, Scharhag J, Horstick G, Becker D, Hommel G, Thelen M, Meyer J. Quantification of shunt volumes in congenital heart diseases using a breath-hold MR phase contrast technique – comparison with oximetry. Int J Cardiovasc Imaging. 2002;18(1):53–60.
55. Beerbaum P, Körperich H, Barth P, Esdorn H, Gieseke J, Meyer H. Noninvasive quantification of left-to-right shunt in pediatric patients: phase-contrast cine magnetic resonance imaging compared with invasive oximetry. Circulation. 2001;103(20):2476–82.
56. Hundley WG, Li HF, Lange RA, Pfeifer DP, Meshack BM, Willard JE, Landau C, Willett D, Hillis LD, Peshock RM. Assessment of left-to-right intracardiac shunting by velocity-encoded, phase-difference magnetic resonance imaging. A comparison with oximetric and indicator dilution techniques. Circulation. 1995;91(12):2955–60.
57. Grosse-Wortmann L, Al-Otay A, Yoo SJ. Aortopulmonary collaterals after bidirectional cavopulmonary connection or Fontan completion: quantification with MRI. Circ Cardiovasc Imaging. 2009;2:219–25.
58. Broadhouse KM, Price AN, Durighel G, Cox DJ, Finnemore AE, Edwards AD, Hajnal JV, Groves AM. Assessment of PDA shunt and systemic blood flow in newborns using cardiac MRI. NMR Biomed. 2013;26(9):1135–41.
59. Whitehead KK, Gillespie MJ, Harris MA, Fogel MA, Rome JJ. Noninvasive quantification of systemic-to-pulmonary collateral flow: a major source of inefficiency in patients with superior cavopulmonary connections. Circ Cardiovasc Imaging. 2009;2(5):405–11.
60. Glatz AC, Rome JJ, Small AJ, Gillespie MJ, Dori Y, Harris MA, Keller MS, Fogel MA, Whitehead KK. Systemic-to-pulmonary collateral flow, as measured by cardiac magnetic resonance imaging, is associated with acute post-Fontan clinical outcomes. Circ Cardiovasc Imaging. 2012;5(2):218–25.
61. Grosse-Wortmann L, Yoo SJ, van Arsdell G, Chetan D, Macdonald C, Benson L, Honjo O. Preoperative total pulmonary blood flow predicts right ventricular pressure in patients early after complete repair of tetralogy of Fallot and pulmonary atresia with major aortopulmonary collateral arteries. J Thorac Cardiovasc Surg. 2013.
62. Spaziani G, Favilli S, Fonda C, Chiappa E. Giant aorto-pulmonary collaterals in pulmonary atresia and ventricular septal defect: long-term survival in unoperated adults. J Cardiovasc Med (Hagerstown). 2013;14:613–5.
63. Beerbaum P, Körperich H, Esdorn H, Blanz U, Barth P, Hartmann J, Gieseke J, Meyer H. Atrial septal defects in pediatric patients: noninvasive sizing with cardiovascular MR imaging. Radiology. 2003;228(2):361–9.
64. Helbing WA, de Roos A. Clinical applications of cardiac magnetic resonance imaging after repair of tetralogy of Fallot. Pediatr Cardiol. 2000;21(1):70–9.
65. Johansson B, Babu-Narayan SV, Kilner PJ. The effects of breath-holding on pulmonary regurgitation measured by cardiovascular magnetic resonance velocity mapping. J Cardiovasc Magn Reson. 2009;11:1.
66. Kilner PJ, Firmin DN, Rees RS, Martinez J, Pennell DJ, Mohiaddin RH, Underwood SR, Longmore DB. Valve and great vessel stenosis: assessment with MR jet velocity mapping. Radiology. 1991;178(1):229–35.
67. Eichenberger AC, Jenni R, von Schulthess GK. Aortic valve pressure gradients in patients with aortic valve stenosis: quantification with velocity-encoded cine MR imaging. AJR Am J Roentgenol. 1993;160(5):971–7.
68. Heidenreich PA, Steffens J, Fujita N, O'Sullivan M, Caputo GR, Foster E, Higgins CB. Evaluation of mitral stenosis with velocity-encoded cine-magnetic resonance imaging. Am J Cardiol. 1995;75(5):365–9.
69. Roman KS, Kellenberger CJ, Farooq S, MacGowan CK, Gilday DL, Yoo SJ. Comparative imaging of differential pulmonary blood flow in patients with congenital heart disease: magnetic resonance imaging versus lung perfusion scintigraphy. Pediatr Radiol. 2005;35(3):295–301.
70. Sridharan S, Derrick G, Deanfield J, Taylor AM. Assessment of differential branch pulmonary blood flow: a comparative study of phase contrast magnetic resonance imaging and radionuclide lung perfusion imaging. Heart. 2006;92(7):963–8.
71. Rupprecht T, Nitz W, Wagner M, Kreissler P, Rascher W, Hofbeck M. Determination of the pressure gradient in children with coarctation of the

aorta by low-field magnetic resonance imaging. Pediatr Cardiol. 2002;23(2):127–31.
72. Chernoff DM, Derugin N, Rajasinghe HA, Hanley FL, Higgins CB, Gooding CA. Measurement of collateral blood flow in a porcine model of aortic coarctation by velocity-encoded cine MRI. J Magn Reson Imaging. 1997;7:557–63.
73. Holmqvist C, Ståhlberg F, Hanséus K, Hochbergs P, Sandström S, Larsson EM, Laurin S. Collateral flow in coarctation of the aorta with magnetic resonance velocity mapping: correlation to morphological imaging of collateral vessels. J Magn Reson Imaging. 2002;15(1):39–46.
74. Steffens JC, Bourne MW, Sakuma H, O'Sullivan M, Higgins CB. Quantification of collateral blood flow in coarctation of the aorta by velocity encoded cine magnetic resonance imaging. Circulation. 1994;90(2):937–43.
75. Mohiaddin RH, Kilner PJ, Rees S, Longmore DB. Magnetic resonance volume flow and jet velocity mapping in aortic coarctation. J Am Coll Cardiol. 1993;22:1515–21.
76. Julsrud PR, Breen JF, Felmlee JP, Warnes CA, Connolly HM, Schaff HV. Coarctation of the aorta: collateral flow assessment with phase-contrast MR angiography. AJR Am J Roentgenol. 1997;169:1735–42.
77. Bottega NA, Silversides CK, Oechslin EN, Dissanayake K, Harrison JL, Provost Y, Harris L. Stenosis of the superior limb of the systemic venous baffle following a mustard procedure: an under-recognized problem. Int J Cardiol. 2012;154(1):32–7.
78. Greenway SC, Yoo SJ, Baliulis G, Caldarone C, Coles J, Grosse-Wortmann L. Assessment of pulmonary veins after atrio-pericardial anastomosis by cardiovascular magnetic resonance. J Cardiovasc Magn Reson. 2011;13:72.
79. Grosse-Wortmann L, Al-Otay A, Goo HW, Macgowan CK, Coles JG, Benson LN, Redington AN, Yoo SJ. Anatomical and functional evaluation of pulmonary veins in children by magnetic resonance imaging. J Am Coll Cardiol. 2007;49(9):993–1002.
80. Voges I, Jerosch-Herold M, Hart C, Scheewe J, Gabbert DD, Pardun E, Kramer HH, Rickers C. Anatomical and functional assessment of the intra-atrial lateral tunnel in the Fontan circulation. Eur J Cardiothorac Surg. 2013;44(3):462–7.
81. Hager A, Fratz S, Schwaiger M, Lange R, Hess J, Stern H. Pulmonary blood flow patterns in patients with Fontan circulation. Ann Thorac Surg. 2008;85(1):186–91.
82. Whitehead KK, Sundareswaran KS, Parks WJ, Harris MA, Yoganathan AP, Fogel MA. Blood flow distribution in a large series of patients having the Fontan operation: a cardiac magnetic resonance velocity mapping study. J Thorac Cardiovasc Surg. 2009;138(1):96–102.
83. Klimes K, Abdul-Khaliq H, Ovroutski S, Hui W, Alexi-Meskishvili V, Spors B, Hetzer R, Felix R, Lange PE, Berger F, Gutberlet M. Pulmonary and caval blood flow patterns in patients with intracardiac and extracardiac Fontan: a magnetic resonance study. Clin Res Cardiol. 2007;96(3):160–7.
84. Frydrychowicz A, Bley TA, Dittrich S, Hennig J, Langer M, Markl M. Visualization of vascular hemodynamics in a case of a large patent ductus arteriosus using flow sensitive 3D CMR at 3T. J Cardiovasc Magn Reson. 2007;9(3):585–7.
85. Nett EJ, Johnson KM, Frydrychowicz A, Del Rio AM, Schrauben E, Francois CJ, Wieben O. Four-dimensional phase contrast MRI with accelerated dual velocity encoding. J Magn Reson Imaging. 2012;35(6):1462–71.
86. Hope MD, Hope TA, Crook SE, Ordovas KG, Urbania TH, Alley MT, Higgins CB. 4D flow CMR in assessment of valve-related ascending aortic disease. JACC Cardiovasc Imaging. 2011;4(7):781–7.
87. Hope MD, Meadows AK, Hope TA, Ordovas KG, Saloner D, Reddy GP, Alley MT, Higgins CB. Clinical evaluation of aortic coarctation with 4D flow MR imaging. J Magn Reson Imaging. 2010;31(3):711–8.
88. Brix L, Ringgaard S, Rasmusson A, Sørensen TS, Kim WY. Three dimensional three component whole heart cardiovascular magnetic resonance velocity mapping: comparison of flow measurements from 3D and 2D acquisitions. J Cardiovasc Magn Reson. 2009;11:3.
89. Hussain T, Lossnitzer D, Bellsham-Revell H, Valverde I, Beerbaum P, Razavi R, Bell AJ, Schaeffter T, Botnar RM, Uribe SA, Greil GF. Three-dimensional dual-phase whole-heart MR imaging: clinical implications for congenital heart disease. Radiology. 2012;263(2):547–54.
90. Sundareswaran KS, Haggerty CM, de Zélicourt D, Dasi LP, Pekkan K, Frakes DH, Powell AJ, Kanter KR, Fogel MA, Yoganathan AP. Visualization of flow structures in Fontan patients using 3-dimensional phase contrast magnetic resonance imaging. J Thorac Cardiovasc Surg. 2012;143(5):1108–16.
91. Simonetti OP, Kim RJ, Fieno DS, Hillenbrand HB, Wu E, Bundy JM, Finn JP, Judd RM. An improved MR imaging technique for the visualization of myocardial infarction. Radiology. 2001;218(1):215–23.
92. Kim RJ, Chen EL, Lima JA, Judd RM. Myocardial Gd-DTPA kinetics determine MRI contrast enhancement and reflect the extent and severity of myocardial injury after acute reperfused infarction. Circulation. 1996;94(12):3318–26.
93. Kim RJ, Fieno DS, Parrish TB, Harris K, Chen EL, Simonetti O, Bundy J, Finn JP, Klocke FJ, Judd RM. Relationship of MRI delayed contrast enhancement to irreversible injury, infarct age, and contractile function. Circulation. 1999;100(19):1992–2002.
94. Choudhury L, Mahrholdt H, Wagner A, Choi KM, Elliott MD, Klocke FJ, Bonow RO, Judd RM, Kim RJ. Myocardial scarring in asymptomatic or mildly symptomatic patients with hypertrophic cardiomyopathy. J Am Coll Cardiol. 2002;40(12):2156–64.
95. Moon JC, Mogensen J, Elliott PM, Smith GC, Elkington AG, Prasad SK, Pennell DJ, McKenna WJ. Myocardial late gadolinium enhancement cardiovascular magnetic resonance in hypertrophic cardiomyopathy caused by mutations in troponin I. Heart. 2005;91(8):1036–40.

96. McCrohon JA, Moon JC, Prasad SK, McKenna WJ, Lorenz CH, Coats AJ, Pennell DJ. Differentiation of heart failure related to dilated cardiomyopathy and coronary artery disease using gadolinium-enhanced cardiovascular magnetic resonance. Circulation. 2003;108(1):54–9.
97. Patel MR, Cawley PJ, Heitner JF, Klem I, Parker MA, Jaroudi WA, Meine TJ, White JB, Elliott MD, Kim HW, Judd RM, Kim RJ. Detection of myocardial damage in patients with sarcoidosis. Circulation. 2009;120(20):1969–77.
98. Babu-Narayan SV, Goktekin O, Moon JC, Broberg CS, Pantely GA, Pennell DJ, Gatzoulis MA, Kilner PJ. Late gadolinium enhancement cardiovascular magnetic resonance of the systemic right ventricle in adults with previous atrial redirection surgery for transposition of the great arteries. Circulation. 2005;111(16):2091–8.
99. Kim RJ, Shah DJ, Judd RM. How we perform delayed enhancement imaging. J Cardiovasc Magn Reson. 2003;5:505–14.
100. Li W, Li BS, Polzin JA, Mai VM, Prasad PV, Edelman RR. Myocardial delayed enhancement imaging using inversion recovery single-shot steady-state free precession: initial experience. J Magn Reson Imaging. 2004;20(2):327–30.
101. Sievers B, Elliott MD, Hurwitz LM, Albert TS, Klem I, Rehwald WG, Parker MA, Judd RM, Kim RJ. Rapid detection of myocardial infarction by subsecond, free-breathing delayed contrast-enhancement cardiovascular magnetic resonance. Circulation. 2007;115(2):236–44.
102. Weinsaft JW, Kim HW, Shah DJ, Klem I, Crowley AL, Brosnan R, James OG, Patel MR, Heitner J, Parker M, Velazquez EJ, Steenbergen C, Judd RM, Kim RJ. Detection of left ventricular thrombus by delayed-enhancement cardiovascular magnetic resonance prevalence and markers in patients with systolic dysfunction. J Am Coll Cardiol. 2008;52(2):148–57.
103. Mollet NR, Dymarkowski S, Volders W, Wathiong J, Herbots L, Rademakers FE, Bogaert J. Visualization of ventricular thrombi with contrast-enhanced magnetic resonance imaging in patients with ischemic heart disease. Circulation. 2002;106(23):2873–6.
104. Coon PD, Rychik J, Novello RT, Ro PS, Gaynor JW, Spray TL. Thrombus formation after the Fontan operation. Ann Thorac Surg. 2001;71(6):1990–4.
105. Prakash A, Powell AJ, Krishnamurthy R, Geva T. Magnetic resonance imaging evaluation of myocardial perfusion and viability in congenital and acquired pediatric heart disease. Am J Cardiol. 2004;93(5):657–61.
106. Harris MA, Johnson TR, Weinberg PM, Fogel MA. Delayed-enhancement cardiovascular magnetic resonance identifies fibrous tissue in children after surgery for congenital heart disease. J Thorac Cardiovasc Surg. 2007;133(3):676–81.
107. Oosterhof T, Mulder BJ, Vliegen HW, de Roos A. Corrected tetralogy of Fallot: delayed enhancement in right ventricular outflow tract. Radiology. 2005;237(3):868–71.
108. Babu-Narayan SV, Kilner PJ, Li W, Moon JC, Goktekin O, Davlouros PA, Khan M, Ho SY, Pennell DJ, Gatzoulis MA. Ventricular fibrosis suggested by cardiovascular magnetic resonance in adults with repaired tetralogy of Fallot and its relationship to adverse markers of clinical outcome. Circulation. 2006;113(3):405–13.
109. Wald RM, Haber I, Wald R, Valente AM, Powell AJ, Geva T. Effects of regional dysfunction and late gadolinium enhancement on global right ventricular function and exercise capacity in patients with repaired tetralogy of Fallot. Circulation. 2009;119(10):1370–7.
110. Park SJ, On YK, Kim JS, Park SW, Yang JH, Jun TG, Kang IS, Lee HJ, Choe YH, Huh J. Relation of fragmented QRS complex to right ventricular fibrosis detected by late gadolinium enhancement cardiac magnetic resonance in adults with repaired tetralogy of Fallot. Am J Cardiol. 2012;109(1):110–5.
111. Fratz S, Hauser M, Bengel FM, Hager A, Kaemmerer H. Myocardial scars determined by delayed-enhancement magnetic resonance imaging and positron emission tomography are not common in right ventricles with systemic function in long-term follow up. Heart. 2006;92(11):1673–7.
112. Preim U, Hoffmann J, Lehmkuhl L, Kehrmann J, Riese F, Daehnert I, Kostelka M, Gutberlet M, Grothoff M. Systemic right ventricles rarely show myocardial scars in cardiac magnetic resonance delayed-enhancement imaging. Clin Res Cardiol. 2013;102(5):337–44.
113. Hartke LP, Gilkeson RC, O'Riordan MA, Siwik ES. Evaluation of right ventricular fibrosis in adult congenital heart disease using gadolinium-enhanced magnetic resonance imaging: initial experience in patients with right ventricular loading conditions. Congenit Heart Dis. 2006;1(5):192–201.
114. Giardini A, Lovato L, Donti A, Formigari R, Oppido G, Gargiulo G, Picchio FM, Fattori R. Relation between right ventricular structural alterations and markers of adverse clinical outcome in adults with systemic right ventricle and either congenital complete (after Senning operation) or congenitally corrected transposition of the great arteries. Am J Cardiol. 2006;98(9):1277–82.
115. Rathod RH, Prakash A, Powell AJ, Geva T. Myocardial fibrosis identified by cardiac magnetic resonance late gadolinium enhancement is associated with adverse ventricular mechanics and ventricular tachycardia late after Fontan operation. J Am Coll Cardiol. 2010;55(16):1721–8.
116. Robinson JD, Del Nido PJ, Geggel RL, Perez-Atayde AR, Lock JE, Powell AJ. Left ventricular diastolic heart failure in teenagers who underwent balloon aortic valvuloplasty in early infancy. Am J Cardiol. 2010;106(3):426–9.
117. La Salvia EA, Gilkeson RC, Dahms BB, Siwik E. Delayed contrast enhancement magnetic resonance imaging in congenital aortic stenosis. Pediatr Cardiol. 2006;27(3):388–90.

118. Wann LS, Faris JV, Childress RH, Dillon JC, Weyman AE, Feigenbaum H. Exercise cross-sectional echocardiography in ischemic heart disease. Circulation. 1979;60:1300–8.
119. Beller GA, Zaret BL. Contributions of nuclear cardiology to diagnosis and prognosis of patients with coronary artery disease. Circulation. 2000;101: 1465–78.
120. Robbers-Visser D, Luijnenburg SE, van den Berg J, Moelker A, Helbing WA. Stress imaging in congenital cardiac disease. Cardiol Young. 2009;19(6): 552–62.
121. Roest AA, Kunz P, Lamb HJ, Helbing WA, van der Wall EE, de Roos A. Biventricular response to supine physical exercise in young adults assessed with ultrafast magnetic resonance imaging. Am J Cardiol. 2001;87:601–5.
122. Roest AA, Helbing WA, Kunz P, van den Aardweg JG, Lamb HJ, Vliegen HW, van der Wall EE, de Roos A. Exercise MR imaging in the assessment of pulmonary regurgitation and biventricular function in patients after tetralogy of Fallot repair. Radiology. 2002;223(1):204–11.
123. Pedersen EM, Stenbøg EV, Fründ T, Houlind K, Kromann O, Sørensen KE, Emmertsen K, Hjortdal VE. Flow during exercise in the total cavopulmonary connection measured by magnetic resonance velocity mapping. Heart. 2002;87(6):554–8.
124. Freed BH, Turner KM, Yodwut C, Tarroni G, Estep E, Bhave NM, Narang A, Tanaka S, Corsi C, Gayat E, Czobor P, Cavanaugh K, Lang R, Mor-Avi V, Patel AR. Regadenoson cardiovascular magnetic resonance myocardial perfusion imaging predicts need for future revascularization [abstract]. J Cardiovasc Magn Reson. 2012;14 Suppl 1:P7.
125. Hendel RC, Bateman TM, Cerqueira MD, Iskandrian AE, Leppo JA, Blackburn B, Mahmarian JJ. Initial clinical experience with regadenoson, a novel selective A2A agonist for pharmacologic stress single-photon computed tomography myocardial perfusion imaging. J Am Coll Cardiol. 2005;46:2069–75.
126. Al Jaroudi W, Iskandrian AE. Regadenoson: a new myocardial stress agent. J Am Coll Cardiol. 2009;54:1123–30.
127. Greenwood JP, Younger JF, Brown JM, Everett CC, Bijsterveld P, Ridgway JP, Radjenovic A, Dickinson CJ, Ball SG, Plein S. Cardiovascular magnetic resonance and single-photon emission computed tomography for diagnosis of coronary heart disease (CE-MARC): a prospective trial. Lancet. 2012;379: 453–60.
128. Nandalur KR, Dwamena BA, Choudhri AF, Nandalur MR, Carlos RC. Diagnostic performance of stress cardiac magnetic resonance imaging in the detection of coronary artery disease: a meta-analysis. J Am Coll Cardiol. 2007;50:1343–53.
129. Klem I, Heitner JF, Shah DJ, et al. Improved detection of coronary artery disease by stress perfusion cardiovascular magnetic resonance with the use of delayed enhancement infarction imaging. J Am Coll Cardiol. 2006;47(8):1630–8.
130. Pilz G, Bernhardt P, Klos M, Ali E, Wild M, Hofling B. Clinical implication of adenosine-stress cardiac magnetic resonance imaging as potential gatekeeper to invasive examination in patients with AHA/ACC class II indication for coronary angiography. Clin Res Cardiol. 2006;95:531–8.
131. Plein S, Greenwood JP, Ridgway JP, Cranny G, Ball SG, Sivananthan MU. Assessment of non-ST-segment elevation acute coronary syndromes with cardiac magnetic resonance imaging. J Am Coll Cardiol. 2004;44:2173–81.
132. Plein S, Radjenovic A, Barmby D, Greenwood JP, Ball SG, Sivananthan MU. Coronary artery disease: myocardial perfusion MR imaging with sensitivity encoding versus conventional angiography. Radiology. 2005;235:423–30.
133. Schwitter J, Wacker CM, van Rossum AC, Lombardi M, Al-Saadi N, Ahlstrom H, Dill T, Larsson HBW, Flamm SD, Marquardt M, Johansson L. MR-IMPACT: comparison of perfusion-cardiac magnetic resonance with single-photon emission computed tomography for the detection of coronary artery disease in a multicentre, multivendor, randomized trial. Eur Heart J. 2008;29:480–9.
134. Wong DTL, Leung MCH, Das R, Liew GYH, Dundon BK, Molaee P, Teo KSL, Meredith IT, Worthley MI, Worthley SG. Diagnostic accuracy of adenosine stress cardiovascular magnetic resonance following acute ST-segment elevation myocardial infarction post primary angioplasty. J Cardiovasc Magn Reson. 2011;13:62.
135. Paetsch I, Jahnke C, Wahl A, Gebker R, Neuss M, Fleck E, Nagel E. Comparison of dobutamine stress magnetic resonance, adenosine stress magnetic resonance, and adenosine stress magnetic resonance perfusion. Circulation. 2004;110:835–42.
136. Hendel RC, Patel MR, Kramer CM, Poon M, Hendel RC, Carr JC, Gerstad NA, Gillam LD, Hodgson JM, Kim RJ, Kramer CM, Lesser JR, Martin ET, Messer JV, Redberg RF, Rubin GD, Rumsfeld JS, Taylor AJ, Weigold WG, Woodard PK, Brindis RG, Hendel RC, Douglas PS, Peterson ED, Wolk MJ, Allen JM, Patel MR, American College of Cardiology Foundation Quality Strategic Directions Committee Appropriateness Criteria Working Group; American College of Radiology; Society of Cardiovascular Computed Tomography; Society for Cardiovascular Magnetic Resonance; American Society of Nuclear Cardiology; North American Society for Cardiac Imaging; Society for Cardiovascular Angiography and Interventions; Society of Interventional Radiology. ACCF/ACR/SCCT/SCMR/ASNC/NASCI/SCAI/SIR 2006 appropriateness criteria for cardiac computed tomography and cardiac magnetic resonance imaging: a report of the American College of Cardiology Foundation Quality Strategic Directions Committee Appropriateness Criteria Working Group, American College of Radiology, Society of Cardiovascular Computed Tomography, Society for Cardiovascular Magnetic Resonance, American Society of Nuclear Cardiology, North

American Society for Cardiac Imaging, Society for Cardiovascular Angiography and Interventions, and Society of Interventional Radiology. J Am Coll Cardiol. 2006;48(7):1475–97.
137. Grizzard JD, Ang GB. Magnetic resonance imaging of pericardial disease and cardiac masses. Magn Reson Imaging Clin N Am. 2007;15(4):579–607, vi.
138. Beroukhim RS, Prakash A, Buechel ER, Cava JR, Dorfman AL, Festa P, Hlavacek AM, Johnson TR, Keller MS, Krishnamurthy R, Misra N, Moniotte S, Parks WJ, Powell AJ, Soriano BD, Srichai MB, Yoo SJ, Zhou J, Geva T. Characterization of cardiac tumors in children by cardiovascular magnetic resonance imaging: a multicenter experience. J Am Coll Cardiol. 2011;58(10):1044–54.
139. Roest AA, Lamb HJ, van der Wall EE, Vliegen HW, van den Aardweg JG, Kunz P, de Roos A, Helbing WA. Cardiovascular response to physical exercise in adult patients after atrial correction for transposition of the great arteries assessed with magnetic resonance imaging. Heart. 2004;90(6):678–84.
140. Tulevski II, Lee PL, Groenink M, van der Wall EE, Stoker J, Pieper PG, Romkes H, Hirsch A, Mulder BJ. Dobutamine-induced increase of right ventricular contractility without increased stroke volume in adolescent patients with transposition of the great arteries: evaluation with magnetic resonance imaging. Int J Card Imaging. 2000;16(6):471–8.
141. Tulevski II, van der Wall EE, Groenink M, Dodge-Khatami A, Hirsch A, Stoker J, Mulder BJ. Usefulness of magnetic resonance imaging dobutamine stress in asymptomatic and minimally symptomatic patients with decreased cardiac reserve from congenital heart disease (complete and corrected transposition of the great arteries and subpulmonic obstruction). Am J Cardiol. 2002;89(9):1077–81.
142. Oosterhof T, Tulevski II, Roest AA, Steendijk P, Vliegen HW, van der Wall EE, de Roos A, Tijssen JG, Mulder BJ. Disparity between dobutamine stress and physical exercise magnetic resonance imaging in patients with an intra-atrial correction for transposition of the great arteries. J Cardiovasc Magn Reson. 2005;7(2):383–9.
143. Fratz S, Hager A, Busch R, Kaemmerer H, Schwaiger M, Lange R, Hess J, Stern HC. Patients after atrial switch operation for transposition of the great arteries can not increase stroke volume under dobutamine stress as opposed to patients with congenitally corrected transposition. Circ J. 2008;72(7):1130–5.
144. Dodge-Khatami A, Tulevski II, Bennink GB, Hitchcock JF, de Mol BA, van der Wall EE, Mulder BJ. Comparable systemic ventricular function in healthy adults and patients with unoperated congenitally corrected transposition using MRI dobutamine stress testing. Ann Thorac Surg. 2002;73(6):1759–64.
145. Roest AA, de Roos A, Lamb HJ, Helbing WA, van den Aardweg JG, Doornbos J, van der Wall EE, Kunz P. Tetralogy of Fallot: postoperative delayed recovery of left ventricular stroke volume after physical exercise assessment with fast MR imaging. Radiology. 2003;226(1):278–84.
146. van den Berg J, Strengers JL, Wielopolski PA, Hop WC, Meijboom FJ, de Rijke YB, Boomsma F, Bogers AJ, Pattynama PM, Helbing WA. Assessment of biventricular functional reserve and NT-proBNP levels in patients with RV volume overload after repair of tetralogy of Fallot at young age. Int J Cardiol. 2009;133(3):364–70.
147. Tulevski II, Hirsch A, Dodge-Khatami A, Stoker J, van der Wall EE, Mulder BJ. Effect of pulmonary valve regurgitation on right ventricular function in patients with chronic right ventricular pressure overload. Am J Cardiol. 2003;92(1):113–6.
148. Hjortdal VE, Christensen TD, Larsen SH, Emmertsen K, Pedersen EM. Caval blood flow during supine exercise in normal and Fontan patients. Ann Thorac Surg. 2008;85(2):599–603.
149. Hjortdal VE, Emmertsen K, Stenbøg E, Fründ T, Schmidt MR, Kromann O, Sørensen K, Pedersen EM. Effects of exercise and respiration on blood flow in total cavopulmonary connection: a real-time magnetic resonance flow study. Circulation. 2003;108(10):1227–31.
150. Robbers-Visser D, Helderman F, Strengers JL, van Osch-Gevers L, Kapusta L, Pattynama PM, Bogers AJ, Krams R, Helbing WA. Pulmonary artery size and function after Fontan operation at a young age. J Magn Reson Imaging. 2008;28(5):1101–7.
151. Robbers-Visser D, Jan Ten Harkel D, Kapusta L, Strengers JL, Dalinghaus M, Meijboom FJ, Pattynama PM, Bogers AJ, Helbing WA. Usefulness of cardiac magnetic resonance imaging combined with low-dose dobutamine stress to detect an abnormal ventricular stress response in children and young adults after fontan operation at young age. Am J Cardiol. 2008;101(11):1657–62.
152. Schmitt B, Steendijk P, Ovroutski S, Lunze K, Rahmanzadeh P, Maarouf N, Ewert P, Berger F, Kuehne T. Pulmonary vascular resistance, collateral flow, and ventricular function in patients with a Fontan circulation at rest and during dobutamine stress. Circ Cardiovasc Imaging. 2010;3(5):623–31.
153. Taylor AM, Dymarkowski S, De Meerleer K, Hamaekers P, Gewillig M, Mertens L, Bogaert J. Validation and application of single breath-hold cine cardiac MR for ventricular function assessment in children with congenital heart disease at rest and during adenosine stress. J Cardiovasc Magn Reson. 2005;7(5):743–51.
154. Strigl S, Beroukhim R, Valente AM, Annese D, Harrington JS, Geva T, Powell AJ. Feasibility of dobutamine stress cardiovascular magnetic resonance imaging in children. J Magn Reson Imaging. 2009;29(2):313–9.
155. Cook SC, Ferketich AK, Raman SV. Myocardial ischemia in asymptomatic adults with repaired aortic coarctation. Int J Cardiol. 2009;133(1):95–101.
156. Buechel ER, Balmer C, Bauersfeld U, Kellenberger CJ, Schwitter J. Feasibility of perfusion cardiovascular magnetic resonance in paediatric patients. J Cardiovasc Magn Reson. 2009;11:51.

Magnetic Resonance Angiography

4

Christopher J. François

The clinical use of magnetic resonance angiography (MRA) has rapidly expanded as technological advances in both hardware and imaging techniques overcome previous limitations. This is particularly true for imaging of patients with congenital heart disease (CHD), who are often younger and frequently require continued, lifelong imaging follow-up. In this chapter, we will review recent developments in contrast-enhanced (CE) MRA and non-contrast-enhanced (NCE) MRA techniques applicable to CHD.

Contrast-Enhanced MRA

In general, CE MRA techniques are preferred because they are typically faster with a much larger field of view than NCE MRA techniques. In addition, CE MRA is less susceptible to inflow and pulsatility artifacts. Two complementary approaches to CE MRA are used for imaging the thoracic vasculature: "static" CE MRA and time-resolved CE MRA. Both approaches use gadolinium-based contrast agents (GBCAs) to increase the contrast between the vasculature and surrounding soft tissues. With static CE MRA, the image acquisition is timed to correspond to when there is maximum enhancement of the vessels of interest – either determined a priori with a test bolus injection (Fig. 4.1) or in real time with bolus tracking. Time-resolved CE MRA, on the other hand, does not require any specific timing of image acquisition. Static CE MRA techniques usually have higher spatial resolution and greater volumetric coverage than time-resolved CE MRA sequences, particularly with use of parallel imaging techniques. However, time-resolved CE MRA provides additional dynamic information on blood flow that is less apparent or absent on static CE MRA acquisitions. Further details on these two approaches to CE MRA will be discussed in the following sections.

High-Resolution Static CE MRA

High spatial resolution CE MRA is performed using a 3D spoiled gradient-recalled echo sequence, timed such that the central k-space lines are acquired during peak enhancement of the vessels of interest. Because of the high spatial resolution that can be achieved using modern sequences, typically ≤1.5 mm isotropic, these sequences are used to delineate the complex anatomical structures in patients with CHD (Fig. 4.2). Although previously limited to relatively narrow 3D volumes, improvements in software and hardware design discussed in subsequent paragraphs have enabled substantial accelerations in image acquisition so that it is now possible to obtain high-resolution CE MRA images of the entire thorax (Fig. 4.3) within a short breath hold.

C.J. François, MD
Department of Radiology, School of Medicine and Public Health, University of Wisconsin-Madison, 600 Highland Avenue, Madison, WI 53792-3252, USA
e-mail: cjfrancois@wisc.edu, cfrancois@uwhealth.org

F. Saremi (ed.), *Cardiac CT and MR for Adult Congenital Heart Disease*,
DOI 10.1007/978-1-4614-8875-0_4, © Springer Science+Business Media New York 2014

Contrast Administration

For the majority of CE MRA applications, a single dose of standard, extracellular GBCA (0.1 mmol/kg) is sufficient. Contrast is injected intravenously (IV) through a catheter (preferably through an 18–22 gauge catheter in an antecubital vein) at a variable rate (i.e., 0.5–4.0 mL/s), depending upon the size of the catheter, the quality of the patient's veins, and the length of the acquisition. However, caution should be used

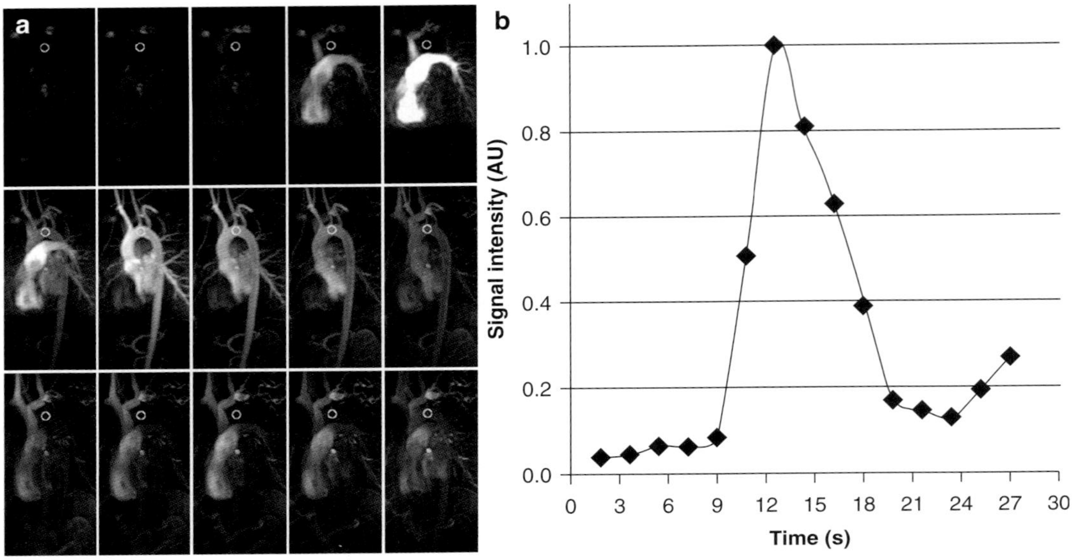

Fig. 4.1 (**a**) Time-resolved CE MRA with fast temporal resolution (≤2 s/image) is used to determine time-to-peak enhancement in the vessel of interest, in this case the aorta. This can be done visually or quantitatively by drawing a region of interest over the aorta (*yellow circle*) and assessing the signal intensity–time curve (**b**) to determine the precise time-to-peak enhancement. Typically, a diagnostic delay (~4–6 s) is added to the time to peak from the test bolus injection due to different amounts of contrast injected between the test bolus and actual 3D CE MRA

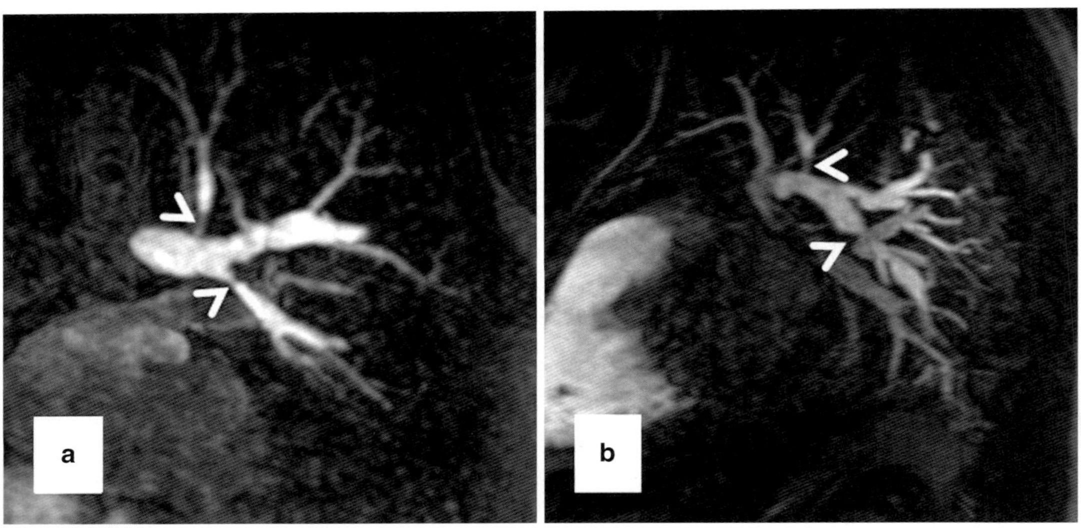

Fig. 4.2 High-resolution 3D CE MRA in 28-year-old male with Alagille syndrome causing multiple branch pulmonary artery stenoses (*arrowheads*). Because of the isotropic spatial resolution, it is possible to generate high-quality (**a**) coronal, (**b**) sagittal, and (**c**) axial multiplanar reformatted and (**d**) volume-rendered images to assess the anatomy and morphology of the cardiovascular system

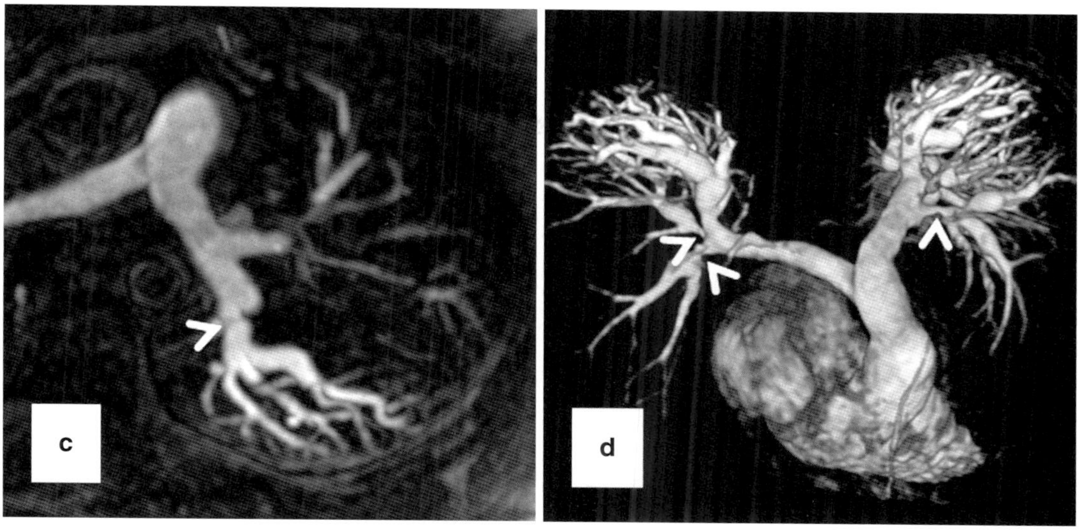

Fig. 4.2 (continued)

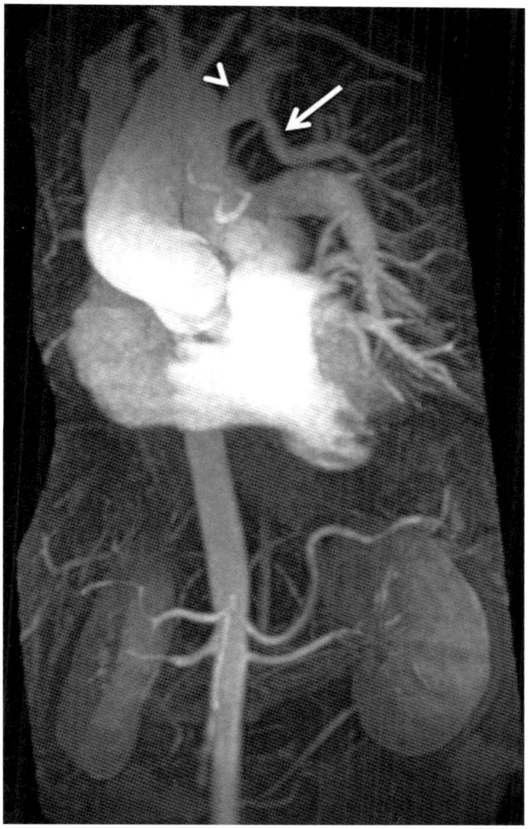

Fig. 4.3 Maximum intensity projection image from 3D CE MRA of the entire thorax in patient with repaired tetralogy of Fallot and partial anomalous venous return from the left upper lobe (*arrow*). The anomalous pulmonary vein drains into the left brachiocephalic vein (*arrowhead*)

when injecting high relaxivity GBCA because when injecting at a high rate, the concentration of GBCA can be high enough to cause T2-star artifact, reducing the overall signal intensity within the vasculature during the first pass (Fig. 4.4). As indicated previously, the image acquisition is timed such that the center of k-space is acquired during maximum enhancement of the vessels of interest, because the center of k-space contributes to the overall signal and enhancement of the image, while the peripheral of k-space contributes to the detail or sharpness of the images (Fig. 4.5). The time-to-peak enhancement of the vessels of interest can be done using a test bolus injection to determine the transit time of a contrast injection from the peripheral IV to the area being imaged [1]. Alternatively, with centric k-space ordering, where the center of k-space is acquired at the beginning of the scan, real-time bolus tracking can be used so that the acquisition can be started precisely when the contrast bolus arrives in the vessels of interest [2]. When the acquisition is not timed appropriately to the passage of the contrast bolus, a variety of different artifacts can occur, including decreased signal-to-noise ratio (SNR), truncation artifact, and edge blurring [3]. Ideally, the contrast bolus injection duration should be equal to the length of acquisition (Fig. 4.6). A benefit of CE MRA, relative to CT angiography (CTA), is that if the

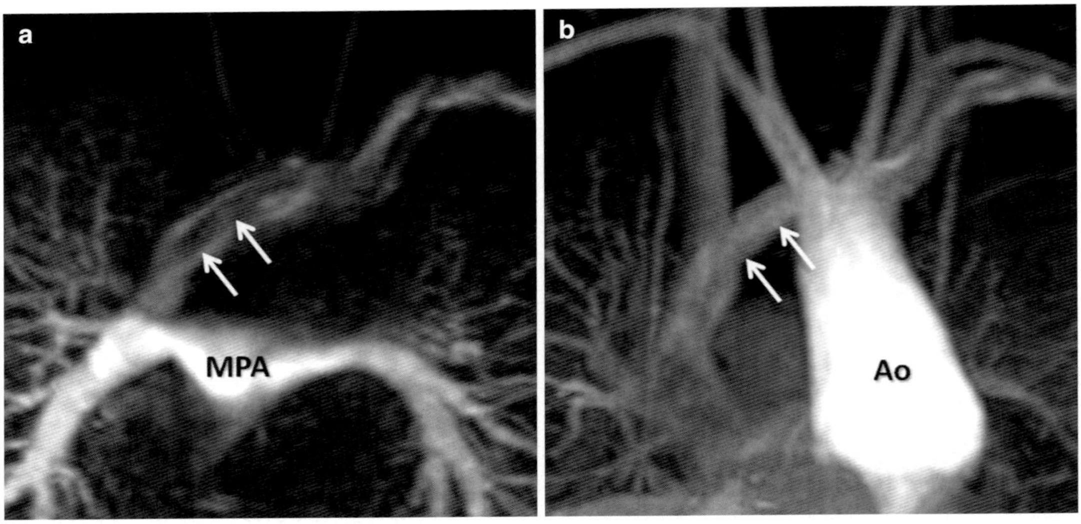

Fig. 4.4 (**a**) T2-star effects of rapid GBCA injection decrease the signal intensity in the left brachiocephalic vein (*arrows*). (**b**) During recirculation, when contrast has been diluted with non-enhanced blood, enhancement of the venous structures is more uniform without any central decrease signal intensity (*arrows*). *MPA* main pulmonary artery, *Ao* aorta

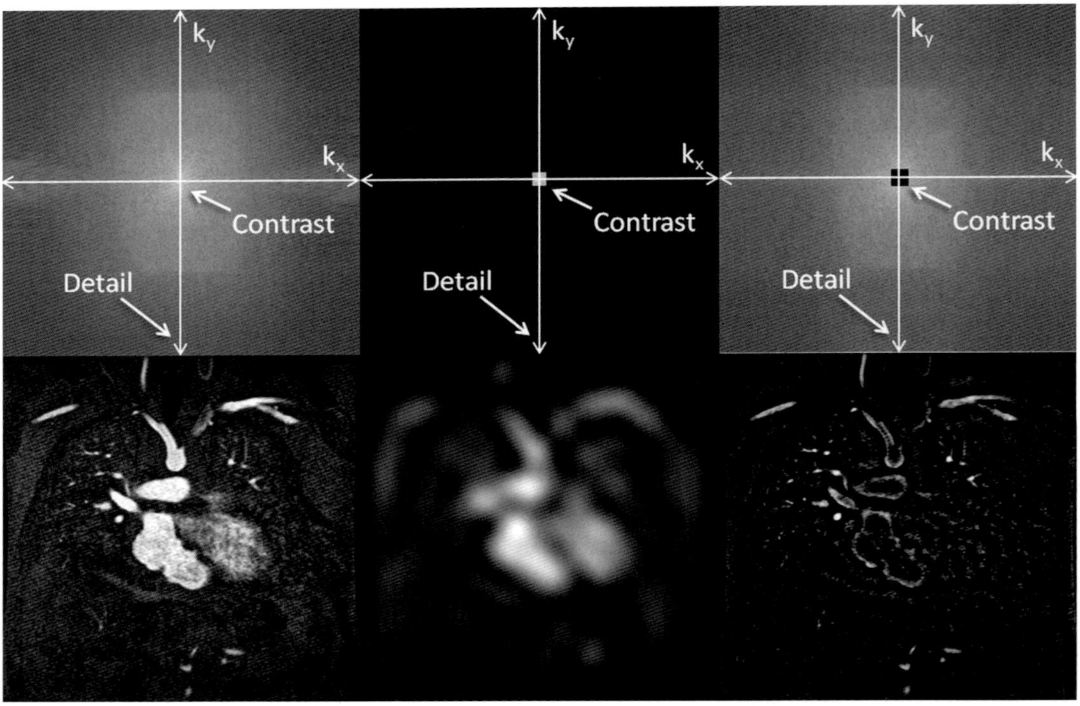

Fig. 4.5 K-space (*top row*) and image space (*bottom row*) images from contrast-enhanced MRA illustrating the differences between fully sampled k-space (*left*), central k-space (*middle*), and outer k-space (*right*) data. The central k-space data contributes to the overall signal of the image, which for contrast-enhanced MRA provides the signal in the vasculature. However, the corresponding image is very blurry. The outer regions of k-space encode for the edges, resulting in images that have sharp vessel definition, but with very little vascular enhancement

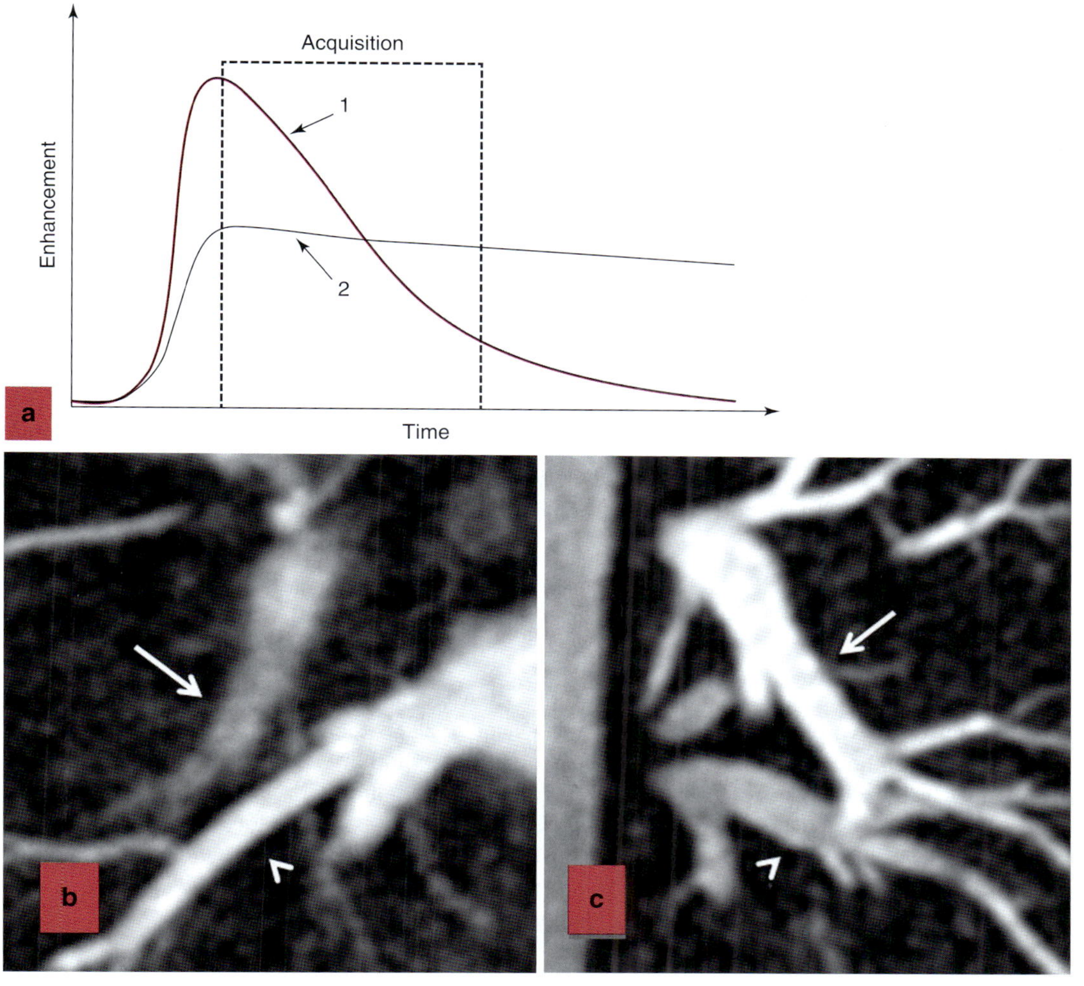

Fig. 4.6 Effects of contrast bolus duration on edge blurring. (**a**) Enhancement time diagram demonstrating two injection strategies. In injection *1*, contrast is injected rapidly, resulting in rapid upslope in enhancement and rapid washout. Although there is bright signal during the early part of the acquisition, resulting in intense contrast enhancement, the later stages of the acquisition occur during diminished enhancement. The loss of signal during the acquisition of the outer regions of k-space results in blurring of the vessels in which the contrast has washed out (**b**). When the contrast is injected more slowly, as in strategy *2*, there is more uniform enhancement throughout the acquisition of k-space. The persistence of enhancement throughout the acquisition, including the higher-order k-space lines, results in improved vascular sharpness (**c**). In (b), the acquisition was 18 s and the bolus duration was 8 s. Although the pulmonary veins (*arrowhead*) are bright and very sharp, the pulmonary arteries (*arrow*) are blurry and poorly enhanced. In (c), the acquisition was 18 s and the bolus duration was 20 s. In this case, pulmonary arteries (*arrow*) and pulmonary veins (*arrowhead*) are very sharp and sufficiently enhanced

image quality is insufficient to make the diagnosis, the acquisition can be repeated with a second injection (Fig. 4.7) with little to no harm to most patients because GBCA is less nephrotoxic and MRA does not require the use of ionizing radiation.

At our institution, we dilute a single dose of GBCA [i.e., 0.1 mmol/kg of gadobenate dimeglumine (Multihance, Bracco Diagnostics Inc. Princeton, NJ, USA) or 0.03 mmol/kg of gadofosveset trisodium (Vasovist, ABLAVAR, EPIX Pharmaceuticals, Inc Cambridge, MA, USA)]

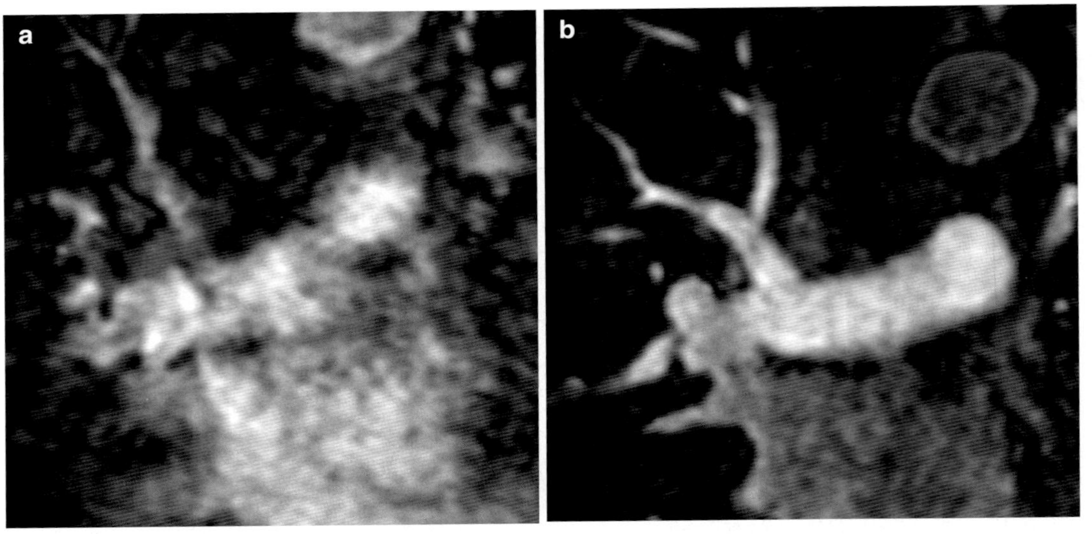

Fig. 4.7 (**a**) Image quality of the initial CE MRA is non-diagnostic due to respiratory motion during the acquisition. (**b**) The CE MRA was repeated after instructing the patient to hold their breath during the entire acquisition, resulting in very high-quality CE MRA with very sharp vessels

with normal saline to achieve a total volume of 30 mL to inject in two phases. We inject 5 mL of diluted contrast at 2 mL/s, resulting in a 2.5 s contrast bolus which we expect to prolong to 3–4 s by the time it gets to the pulmonary circulation, for the time-resolved CE MRA (which has a "temporal resolution" of 3–4 s). We then inject 25 mL at 1.5 mL/s, resulting in a 16–17 s contrast bolus which we expect to prolong to ~20 s by the time it reaches the pulmonary circulation, for the high-resolution 3D CE MRA, which is about 17–20 s long.

ECG Triggering

Conventional three-dimensional (3D) CE MRA can be performed without or with ECG triggering. ECG-triggered CE MRA (Fig. 4.8) is preferred for imaging patients with diseases of the ascending aorta to minimize artifact from cardiac motion [4]. Furthermore, when making measurements of the aorta, or other vessels, it is critical to make double-oblique measurements perpendicular to the vessel long axis (Fig. 4.8b) rather than simply using axial images to avoid overestimating the true size of the vessel [5]. Equally important is to use a consistent method of defining how the measurements are being made, especially when using MRA-derived measurements in comparison with prognostic data obtained using other imaging modalities [6]. A limitation of ECG-triggered CE MRA techniques is that they require more time to acquire and is therefore potentially problematic in patients who have difficulty holding their breath. Acquisition times for ECG-triggered CE MRA can be decreased by limiting the coverage to a thin slab over the aorta or by using parallel imaging.

Parallel Imaging

A major advance in improving the speed of MR image acquisition has been the use of parallel imaging [7–9]. This has been enabled through changes in image reconstruction from undersampled k-space data and use of multichannel receiver coils [10]. With these multichannel receiver coils, each individual coil is used to simultaneously receive the MR signal. The use of parallel imaging to accelerate data acquisition can be used to shorten the scan times to image the same volume [11] or to increase anatomical coverage during the same acquisition time [12]. Using advanced parallel imaging techniques, it is now possible to scan the entire thoracic vasculature within 15–20 s with high, isotropic spatial resolution (Fig. 4.9).

CE MRA at 3.0T

A major motivation for scanning at higher field strengths is that the SNR is proportional to the field strength. Therefore, at 3.0T SNR is approximately twice that at 1.5T. The advantage in SNR at 3.0T,

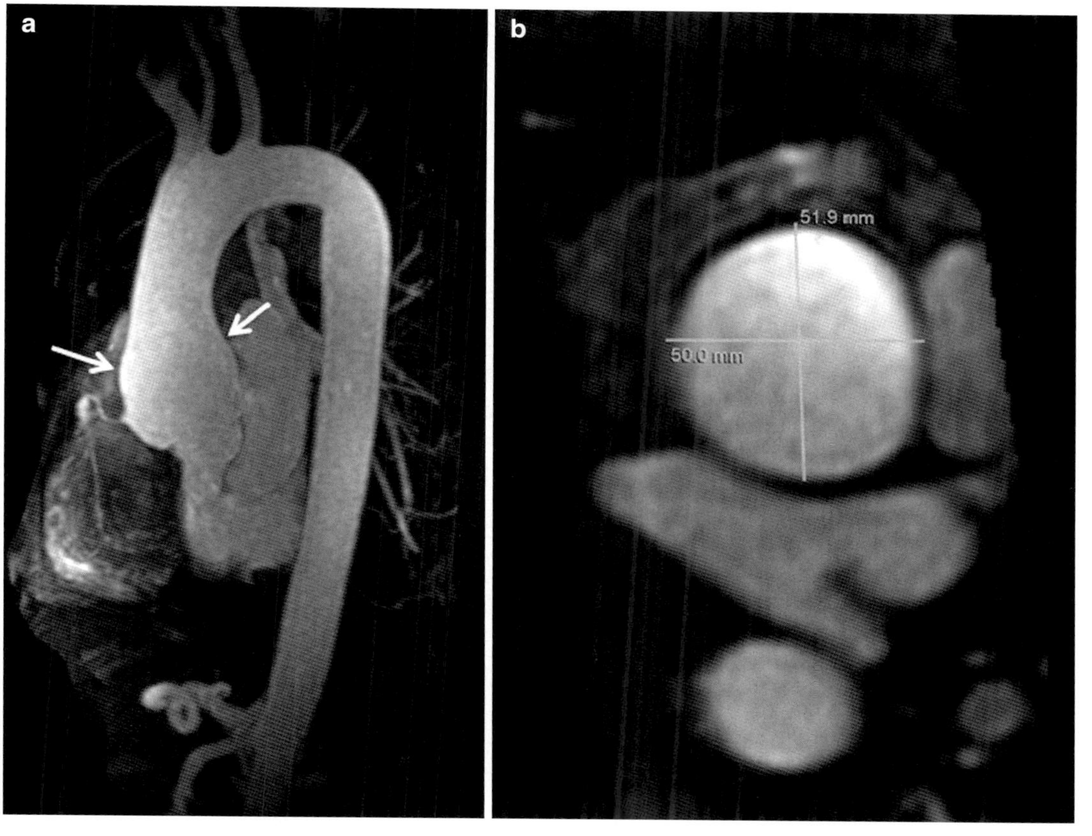

Fig. 4.8 Electrocardiographic (ECG) gated CE MRA in patient with aortic root aneurysm. Use of cardiac gating results in acquisition of images free of cardiac motion artifact. (**a**) On the maximum intensity projection image, the entire ascending aorta, including the aortic root, is well defined with very sharp vessel walls (*arrows*). This is critical when making double-oblique measurements to quantify the maximum dimensions of the aorta (**b**)

relative to 1.5T, can be used to increase spatial resolution, decrease scan time, or a combination of these while obtaining images of relatively similar or better quality as those at 1.5T [13]. In addition, because of the differences in T1 effects of GBCA at 3.0T, there is actually greater vascular contrast, relative to surround soft tissues, at 3.0T compared to 1.5T. Therefore, CE MRA at 3.0T can be performed with smaller doses of GBCA [14–17]. In fact, recent data suggests smaller volumes of GBCA result in higher-quality arterial phase MRA than with larger volumes of GBCA [18].

MRI at 3.0T results in significant challenges and limitations due to the stronger magnetic field that have not yet been fully overcome. At 3.0T, the resonance frequency of water protons is double that at 1.5T. Because the frequency and wavelength are inversely related, the radiofrequency (RF) wavelength of water protons at 3.0T is half that at 1.5T. This shortened wavelength can span the dimensions of the field of view for body imaging, especially in those with a large body habitus [19]. When RF waves overlap within the imaging field, destructive or constructive interference results in areas of darkening or brightening, respectively. RF field homogeneity can be improved by (A) using advanced coil designs, such as multi-coil transmit coils, which can help to suppress eddy currents [20] or (B) implementing new pulse sequences, such as 3D RF pulses [21].

Another potential limitation with performing MRA at 3.0T is that the specific absorption rate (SAR) increases at higher field strengths due to constructive and destructive interference due to RF field inhomogeneity. RF pulses transfer energy to protons within the patient and ultimately generate heat as energy is released. To avoid overheating

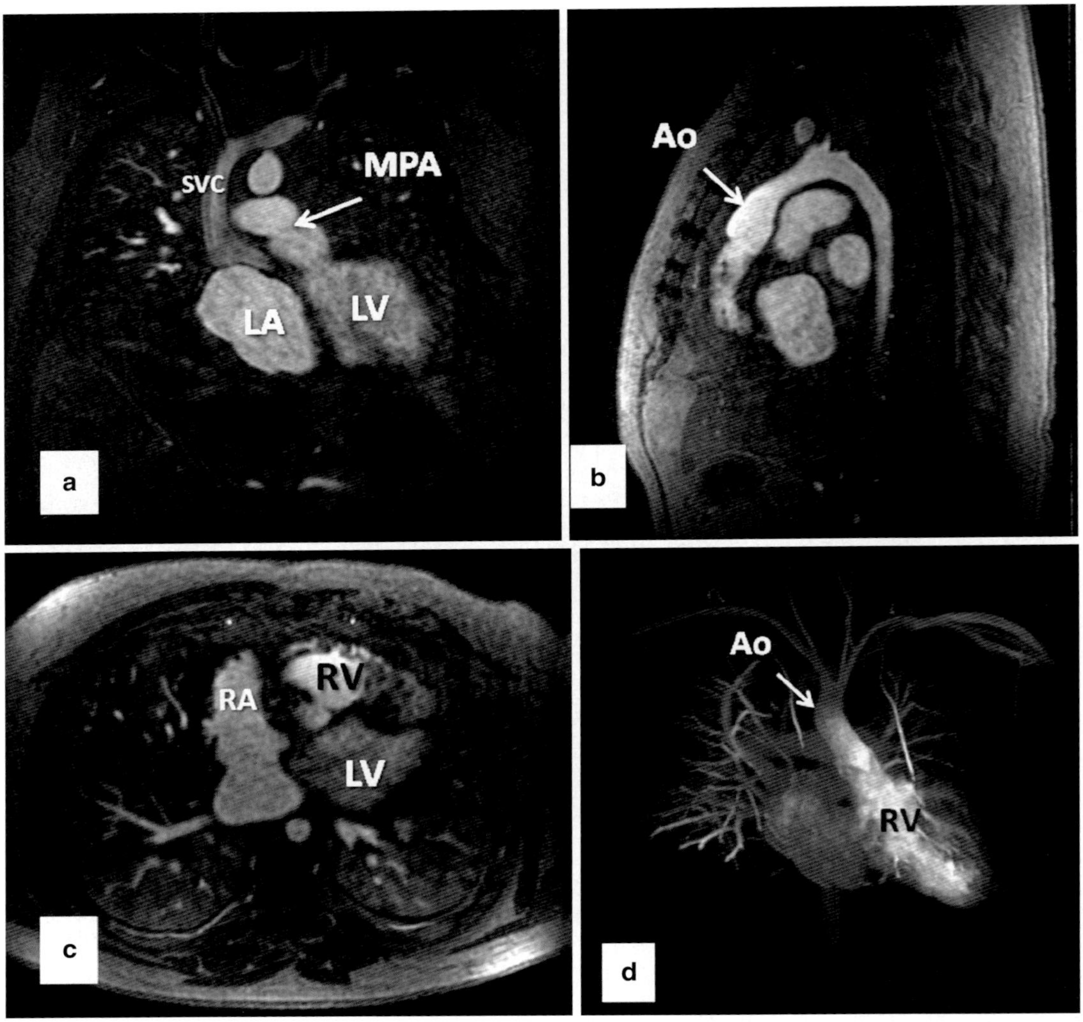

Fig. 4.9 Thirty-two-year-old male with d-TGA status post Mustard procedure. (**a**) Coronal, (**b**) sagittal, and (**c**) axial MPR images from whole chest CE MRA acquired using 2D parallel imaging to accelerate image acquisition ~3.75×. With advanced parallel imaging, acquisition times are decreased sufficiently to acquire images of the entire chest within a short breath hold. Data are isotropic in all three dimensions, enabling high-resolution multiplanar reformation and 3D maximum intensity projection images (**d**) to be generated. *LV* left ventricle, *LA* left atrium, *RV* right ventricle, *RA* right atrium, *SVC* superior vena cava, *MPA* main pulmonary artery, *Ao* aorta

within the patient, which can have detrimental physiologic effects, the SAR is carefully monitored during scanning. The FDA currently limits the total body heating to 4 W/kg during a 15-min period [22, 23]. The SAR estimates the energy transfer to the tissue by the RF pulse and is proportional to the square of the resonance frequency. Therefore, in going from 1.5 to 3.0T, where the resonance frequency is doubled, the SAR increases fourfold for the same sequence, assuming all parameters are equal [24]. As a result, the pulse sequences, acquisition techniques, and hardware designs are modified to work within the allowable constraints of the increased SAR. Parallel imaging helps alleviate this problem by decreasing scan time and the number of RF pulses necessary to acquire an image.

Blood-Pool Contrast Agents

Most CE MRA, as with most CE MRI, is performed with GBCA that are not purely intravascular. Rather, most GBCAs do distribute throughout the extracellular space. For vascular imaging, however, this can be problematic in achieving the greatest contrast between the vessels and their surrounding soft tissues. Intravascular GBCAs are, therefore, another recent advance that has enabled improvement in CE MRA spatial and contrast resolution. Gadofosveset trisodium, the currently only FDA-approved blood-pool GBCA, is a protein-binding intravascular contrast agent that is approved for the evaluation of patients with aortoiliac occlusive disease [25]. Protein binding is what prolongs the intravascular half-life of gadofosveset trisodium relative to other GBCAs. Another factor contributing to its advantage for CE MRA is that gadofosveset trisodium has a higher relaxivity than other GBCAs [26]. Due to its intravascular distribution and greater contrast enhancement, smaller volumes of gadofosveset trisodium are necessary than other GBCAs to achieve the same image quality [27, 28]. Furthermore, the prolonged intravascular half-life extends the amount of time available for scanning during vascular enhancement. Therefore, very high spatial and contrast resolution CE MRA images are feasible during the steady state (Fig. 4.10) which may be

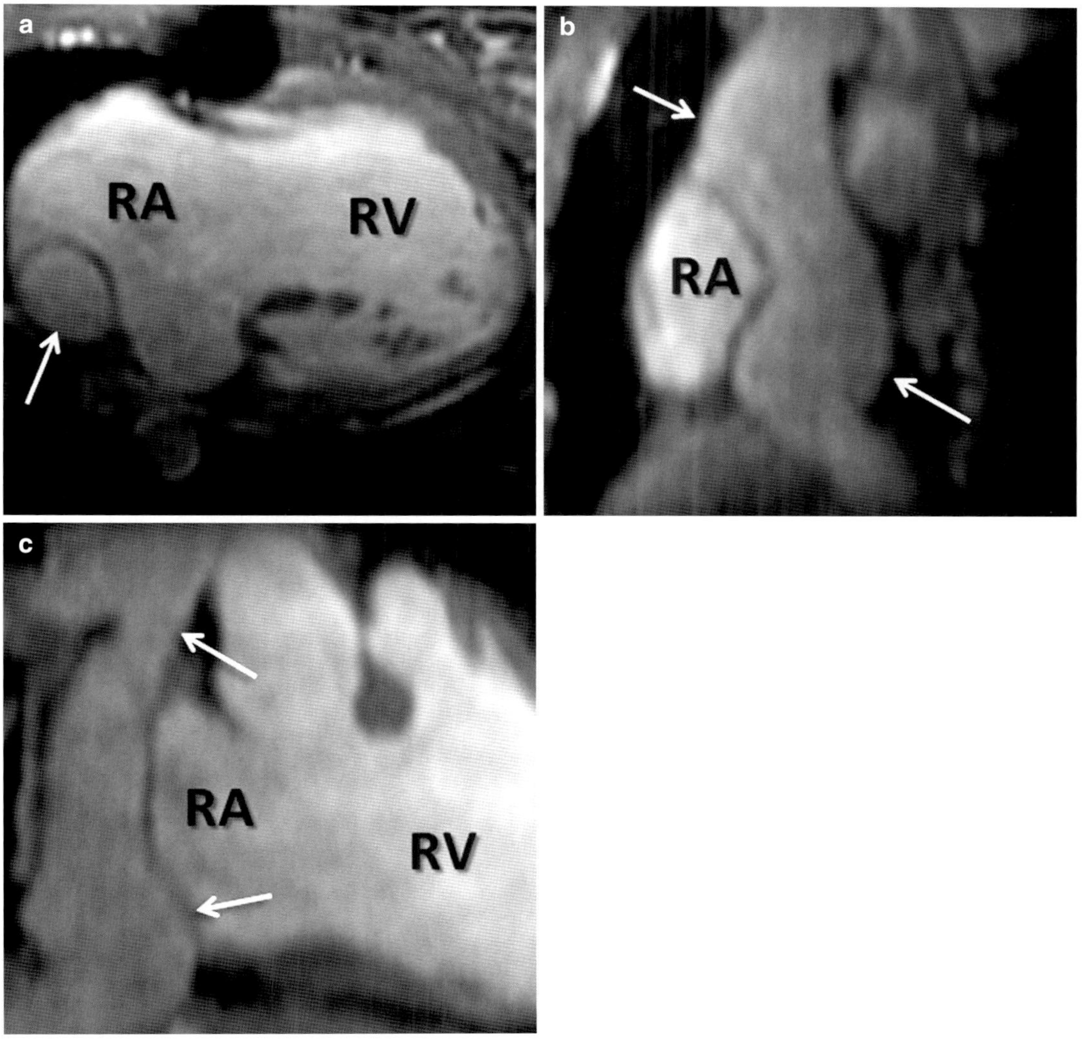

Fig. 4.10 Steady-state CE MRA using navigator respiratory triggering after administration of blood-pool contrast agent. (**a**) Axial, (**b**) sagittal, and (**c**) coronal reformatted images delineate anatomy of extracardiac Fontan (*arrows*) in this patient with double outlet right ventricle (*RV*). *RA* right atrium

beneficial in detecting additional findings not present on first-pass CE MRA [29, 30]. In addition, the prolonged intravascular enhancement with blood-pool contrast agents implies that high-quality imaging can be performed during free breathing using respiratory navigators or bellows for triggering to the same part of the respiratory cycle. This is particularly useful in patients that have difficulty holding their breath [29]. CE MRA during the steady state can also be particularly helpful in patients with cavopulmonary shunts because during the first pass, unenhanced blood from the inferior vena cava will dilute the contrast entering the pulmonary circulation from the superior vena cava.

Time-Resolved CE MRA

Time-resolved CE MRA can help overcome some of the limitations of static 3D CE MRA techniques. A major advantage of time-resolved sequences is the lack of need for precise timing of the acquisition relative to the contrast bolus because data are acquired continuously during the passage of GBCA from the IV catheter throughout the vasculature (Fig. 4.11). There are now multiple methods of accelerating image acquisition to achieve high temporal resolution CE MRA. One method of achieving sub-second temporal resolution is through the use of three-dimensional, asymmetric k-space undersampling combined with thicker slice thickness in the slice-encoding direction [31]. However, because of the relatively thick slice thickness, these acquisitions do not lend themselves to high-quality multiplanar reformations necessary to evaluate the complex anatomy in patients with CHD. To acquire time-resolved data while preserving relatively high spatial information, other approaches are used to accelerate data acquisition based on k-space

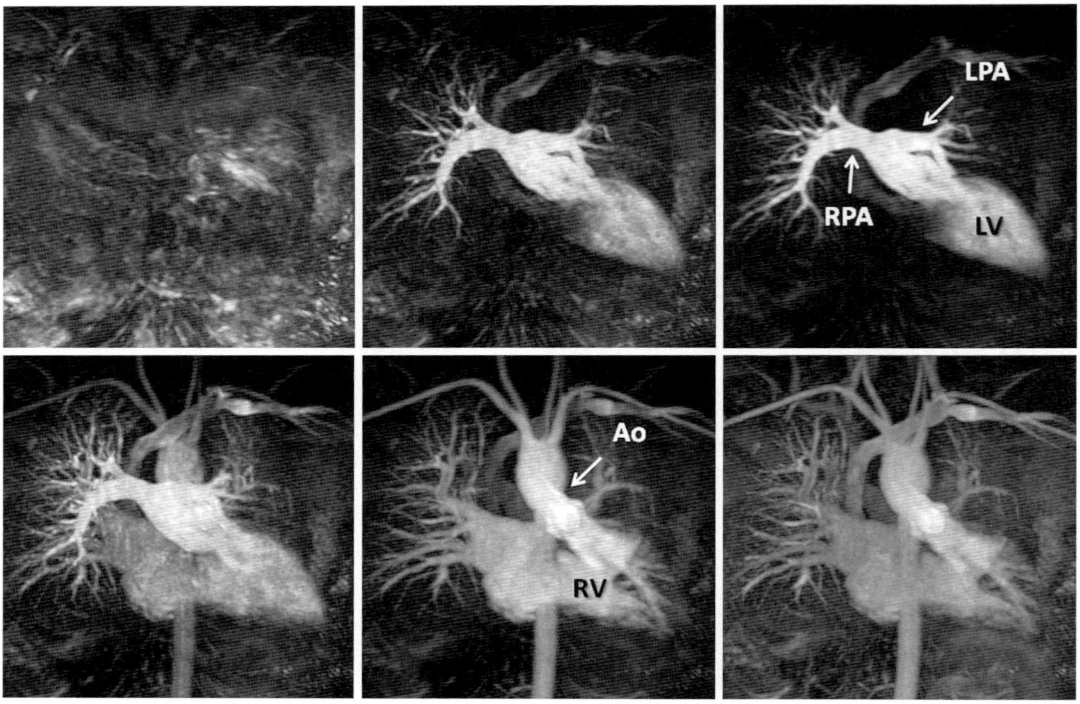

Fig. 4.11 Twenty-year-old male with d-TGA status post Mustard procedure. Maximum intensity images reconstructed from multiple datasets from a time-resolved contrast-enhanced MRA acquisition show asymmetric perfusion of the lungs, with greater perfusion of the right lung than the left lung. *LV* left ventricle, *RV* right ventricle, *RPA* right pulmonary artery, *LPA* left pulmonary artery, *Ao* aorta

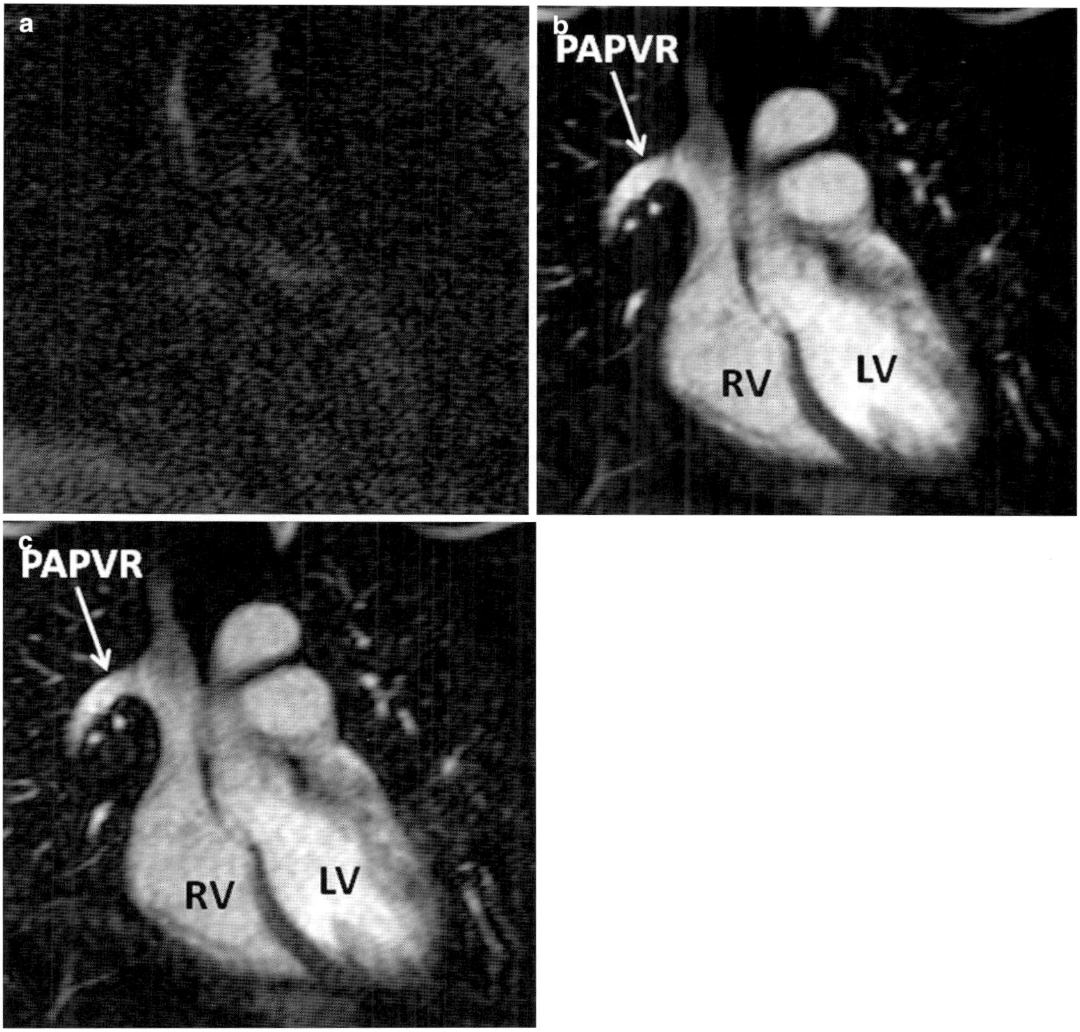

Fig. 4.12 In time-resolved CE MRA, a mask dataset (**a**) is acquired first, prior to the administration of contrast material. Data is then acquired continuously after the injection of contrast to obtain multiple contrast-enhanced MRA datasets (**b**). To remove the background signal, the mask is subtracted from each of the contrast-enhanced dataset to generate images with purely intravascular signal (**c**). *RV* right ventricle, *LV* left ventricle, *PAPVR* partial anomalous pulmonary venous return

undersampling. These are based on acquiring the higher spatial frequencies less frequently [32–35]. As indicated previously, the central k-space data contributes to the high vascular signal, while the outer k-space data contributes to vessel sharpness. Therefore, by updating the center of k-space more frequently and "sharing" the outer regions of k-space between multiple updates of the center of k-space, it is possible to generate images with high contrast, high temporal resolution, and high spatial resolution. To improve the vascular enhancement and SNR of time-resolved CE MRA, a fully k-space sampled non-contrast dataset, or mask, is typically acquired first (Fig. 4.12a). Undersampled k-space images are the acquired during the administration of GBCA (Fig. 4.12b). To generate images with purely vascular signal, the mask images are subtracted from these contrast-enhanced datasets (Fig. 4.12c).

In patients with CHD, time-resolved CE MRA is useful because of the dynamic information that can be obtained from these datasets including transit times through the lungs [36, 37] and relative pulmonary perfusion [38]. This functional information is complementary to the high spatial resolution information obtained from the static 3D CE MRA acquisitions [39]. The relative temporal resolution of time-resolved CE MRA can be adjusted by changing the different parameters to achieve the desired balance between temporal and spatial resolution (Fig. 4.13).

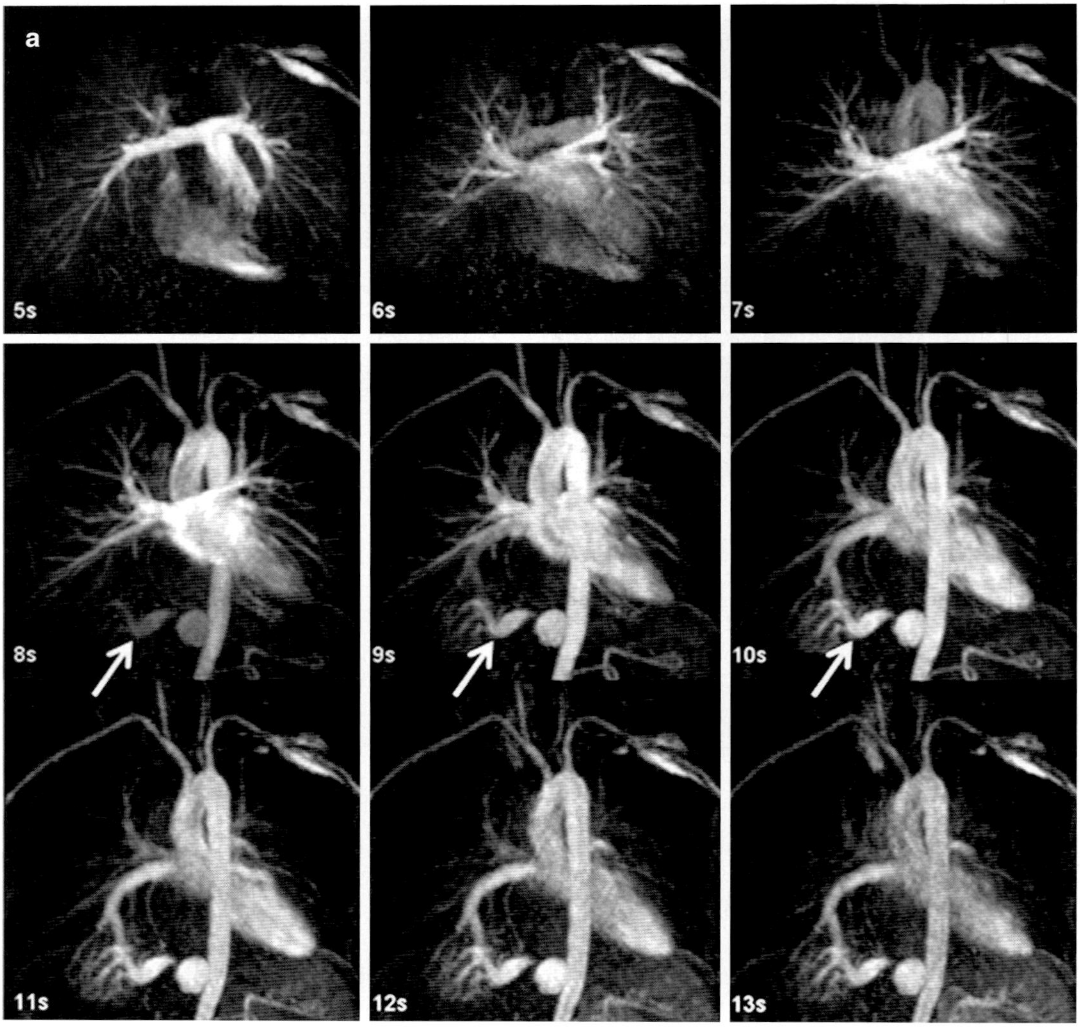

Fig. 4.13 Time-resolved contrast-enhanced MRA (TR CEMRA) with (**a**) 1-s and (**b**) 4-s reconstructed temporal resolution. While the faster temporal resolution TR CEMRA provides greater information on the high flow dynamics through the anomalous artery going to the right lower lobe sequestration (*arrow*), the lower temporal resolution TR CEMRA has higher spatial resolution and can be used to provide more precise measurements of the vessels

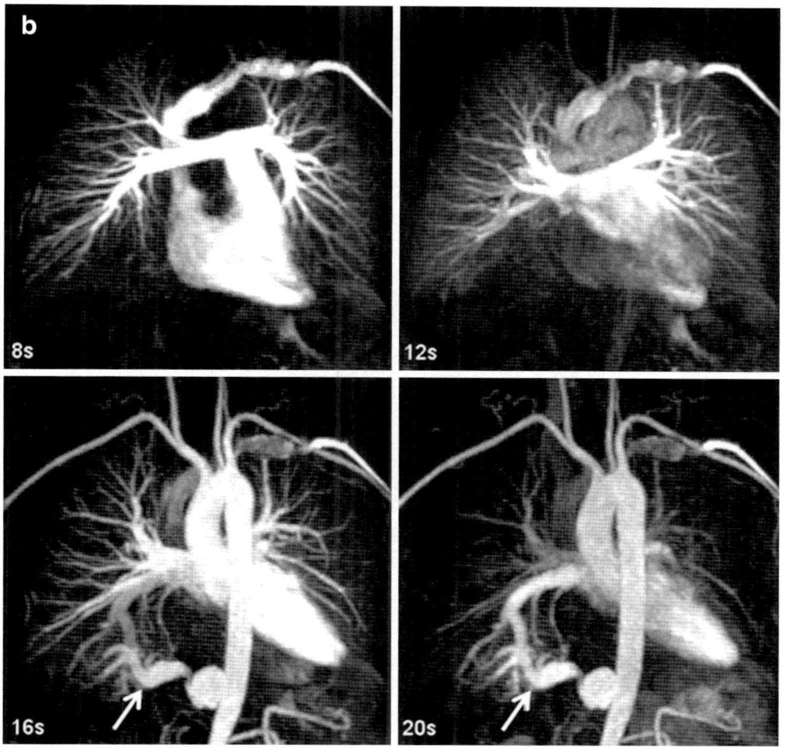

Fig. 4.13 (continued)

Non-Contrast-Enhanced MRA

Long acquisition times and artifacts from cardiac and respiratory motion have traditionally limited the use non-contrast-enhanced (NCE) MRA for cardiothoracic applications. However, improvements in MR software and hardware, as well as concerns over the safety of GBCA in high-risk patient groups, have fostered a renewed interest in NCE MRA. Research linking the administration of GBCA to the development of nephrogenic systemic fibrosis (NSF) in patients with reduced renal function [40–42] has been a primary motivation for expanding the use of NCE MRA for a variety of applications, including thoracic MRA. NCE MRA is also of clinical interest in evaluating patients with other contraindications to GBCA, including poor IV access, pregnancy, or prior allergic reactions to GBCA. Although time-of-flight (TOF) sequences are still used routinely for cervical and intracranial MRA, with diagnostic comparable to CTA and DSA [43, 44], their use in the thorax is markedly limited. In this section, we will review the two main NCE MRA sequences used for cardiothoracic applications, balanced steady-state free precession (bSSFP) and phase-contrast (PC) MRA.

3D bSSFP

For cardiothoracic NCE MRA, 3D bSSFP sequences (Figs. 4.14 and 4.15) are most often used because of (a) inherently high signal of blood compared to surround soft tissues and (b) relative blood flow independence [45]. Image

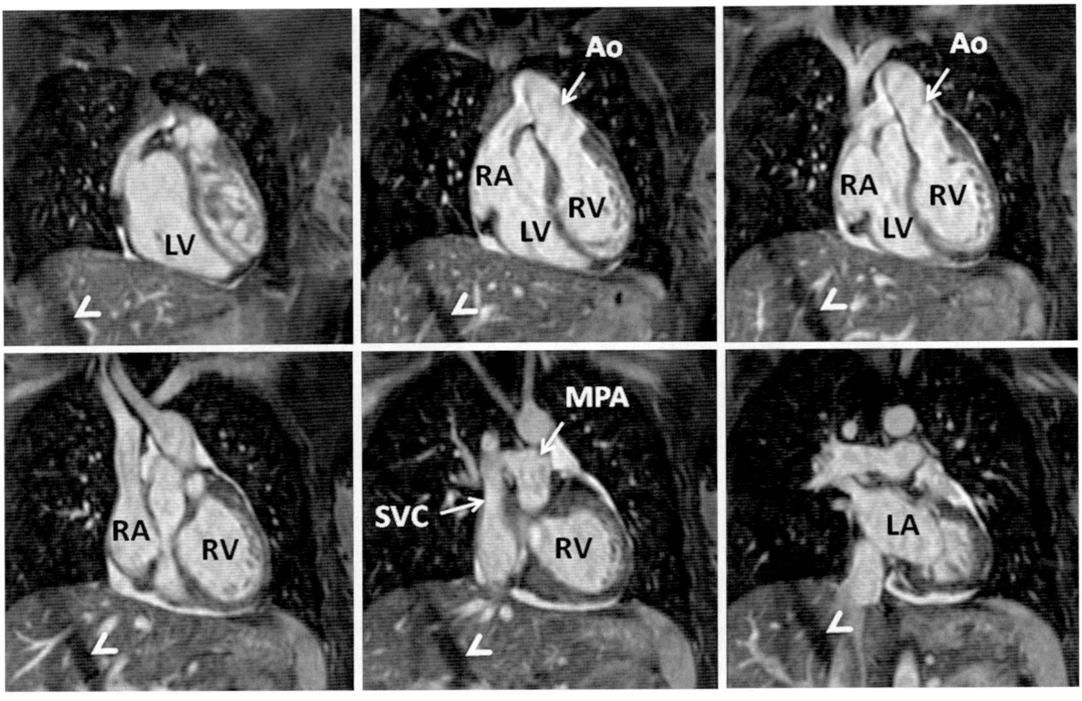

Fig. 4.14 3D balanced SSFP MRA performed without IV contrast and during free breathing using respiratory navigator triggering. High contrast-to-noise and spatial resolution enable accurate assessment of anatomy in this patient with congenitally corrected transposition of the great arteries. The diagonal bands of low signal intensity crossing the right lobe of the liver (*arrowheads*) are related to the navigator. *LV* left ventricle, *LA* left atrium, *RV* right ventricle, *RA* right atrium, *SVC* superior vena cava, *MPA* main pulmonary artery, *Ao* aorta

contrast of bSSFP sequences are determined by the ratio of T2 to T1 of the tissues, which results in the very bright blood-pool signal. Standard 3D bSSFP techniques will produce images that have bright arterial and venous signal, which is typically not a problem for assessment of the larger, central vessels like the aorta, main pulmonary arteries, or pulmonary veins [46–49]. 3D bSSFP MRA is also widely used for coronary MR angiography [50, 51]. These sequences are typically performed using respiratory triggering or navigation to minimize respiratory motion artifacts and ECG triggering to minimize cardiac motion artifacts. However, a limitation of the bSSFP sequence is its susceptibility to field inhomogeneities which occur at the lung–soft tissue interfaces and around metallic implants or devices.

For quantitative measurements of vessel size in the thorax, 3D bSSFP MRA performs very well in comparison with CE MRA. In a comparison of 3D bSSFP and CE MRA, François et al. [46] reported that thoracic aortic measurements were essentially equivalent between the two methods with better delineation of the aortic root with 3D bSSFP. Similar results have been reported for aorta and pulmonary artery measurements in patients with CHD [49].

4D Flow MR

Flow-sensitive, or phase-contrast (PC), MR signal is proportional to the velocity of blood flow and the value set for the velocity encoding (VENC). The VENC is the maximum velocity that can be imaged accurately without aliasing, analogous to aliasing seen with Doppler ultrasound when the maximum Doppler frequency is greater than one half the sampling frequency. Time-resolved, ECG-triggered, two-dimensional

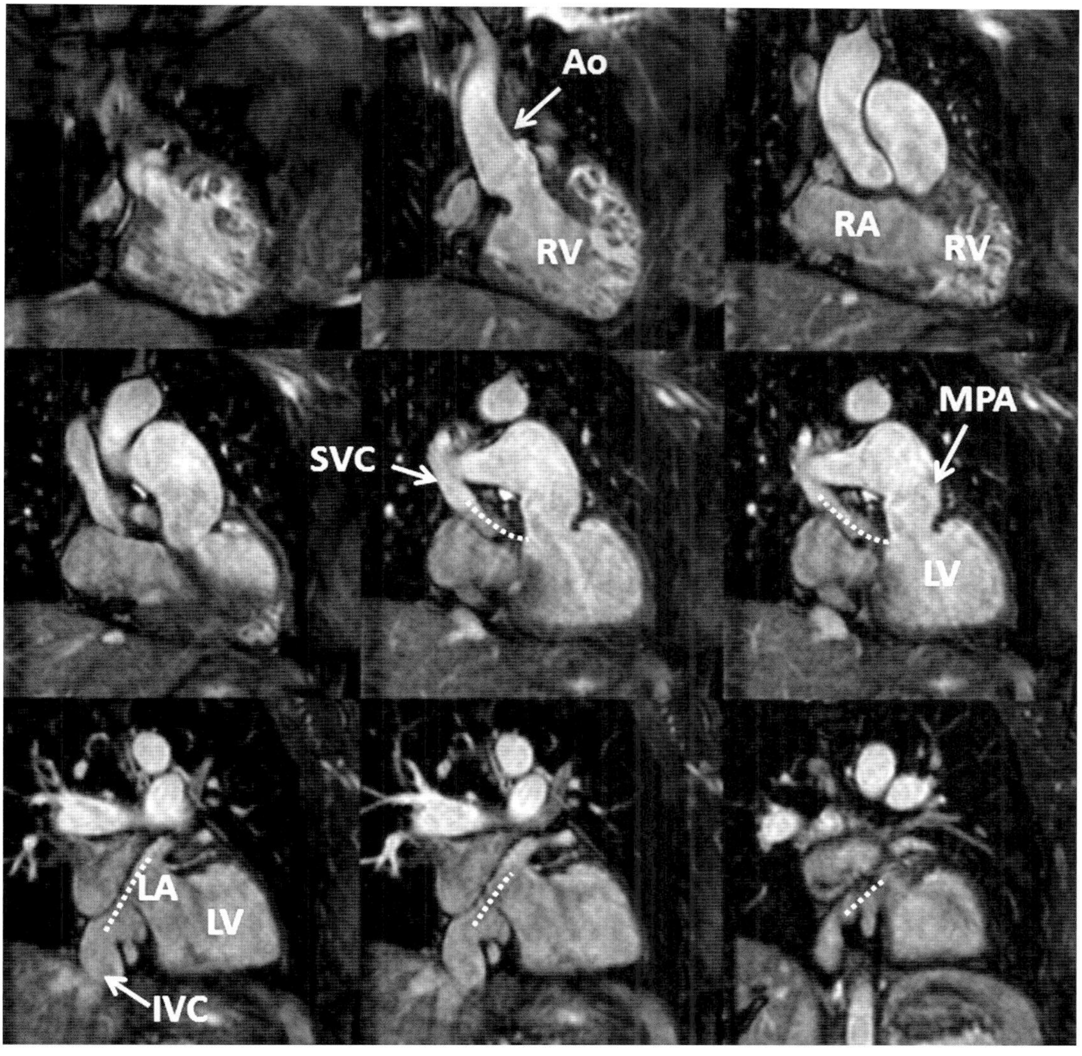

Fig. 4.15 3D balanced SSFP MRA performed without IV contrast and during free breathing using respiratory navigator triggering. High contrast-to-noise and spatial resolution enable accurate assessment of anatomy in this patient with a history of Mustard procedure to repair D-transposition of the great arteries. There is a surgical baffle (*dashed line*) connecting the vena cava (*SVC*, *IVC*) to the left atrium (*LA*), which is connected to the left ventricle (*LV*) and then the main pulmonary artery (*MPA*). Pulmonary venous return is directed to the right atrium (*RA*), right ventricle (*RV*), and into the aorta (*Ao*)

(2D) PC MR is routinely used in cardiac MR to quantify blood flow through the great arteries and cardiac valves [52, 53].

PC NCE MRA is achieved by using a 3D PC sequence with three-directional flow sensitivity [54]. Traditionally, 3D PC MRA was performed without any temporal information to create an angiogram based on the average flow during the acquisition, or a "complex-difference" image [55, 56]. When time-resolved 3D PC MRA data is acquired, based upon binning of the PC data to different phases of the cardiac cycle, it is possible to generate 4D flow-sensitive MR datasets, frequently referred to as "4D flow" [57]. Without the use of any data acquisition acceleration, scan times for 4D flow MRA are very long because of

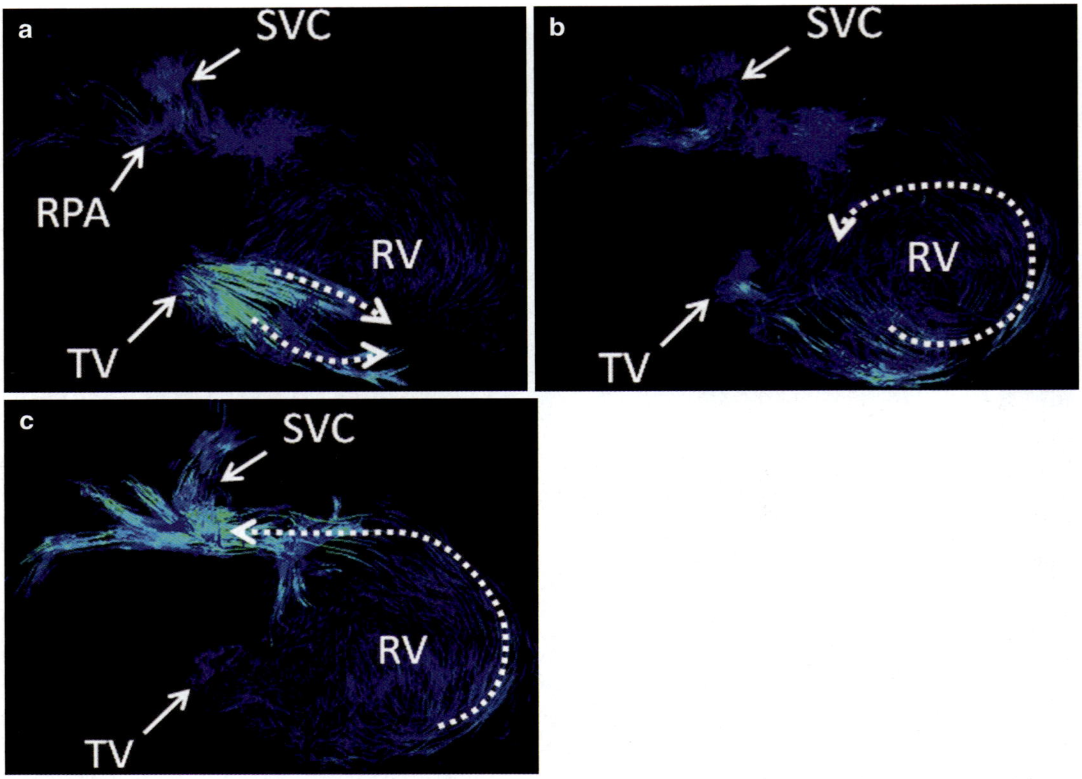

Fig. 4.16 4D flow MRI acquisition in patient with bidirectional Glenn. Particle traces from three phases of the cardiac cycle. In early diastole (**a**), there is brisk flow through the tricuspid valve (*TV*) into the right ventricle (*RV*). During late diastole (**b**), a large vortex forms in the RV (*curved, dashed arrow*). There is also increased flow through the Glenn shunt. During systole (**c**), blood flows from the RV into the pulmonary arteries and retrogrades into the superior vena cava (*SVC*). *RPA* right pulmonary artery

the need to collect data with 3-directional velocity encoding, 3-dimensional spatial encoding, and registration with the cardiac cycle. As a result, currently used 4D flow sequences use a variety of methods to accelerate image acquisition including parallel imaging [58] and 3D radial undersampling [59]. Although these sequences can be used for NCE MRA [60], the greatest potential impact of 4D flow techniques is in their use for quantitative hemodynamic analyses.

Flow quantification with 4D flow is simplified because flow through any number of vessels of interest included in the imaging volume is done post priori [61]. In patients with CHD, this is particularly useful because it is often necessary to quantify flow through multiple vessels and valves [62–69]. In addition to quantifying the velocity or volume of blood flow, the three-directional flow information acquired with 4D flow MR can be used to qualitatively assess changes in the complex flow patterns within the heart or vasculature [58, 69–74]. This is typically performed by viewing these very large datasets in advanced graphics visualization software. The time-resolved 3D velocity data can be displayed in a variety of manners, including velocity vector fields, time-resolved particle traces (Fig. 4.16), or streamlines (Fig. 4.17) [57]. Because 4D flow data are quantitative, additional hemodynamic parameters, beyond velocity and volume, can be quantified. These include pressure gradients (Fig. 4.18) [75–79], wall shear stress [61, 80–85], pulse wave velocity [86, 87], and turbulence [88–91].

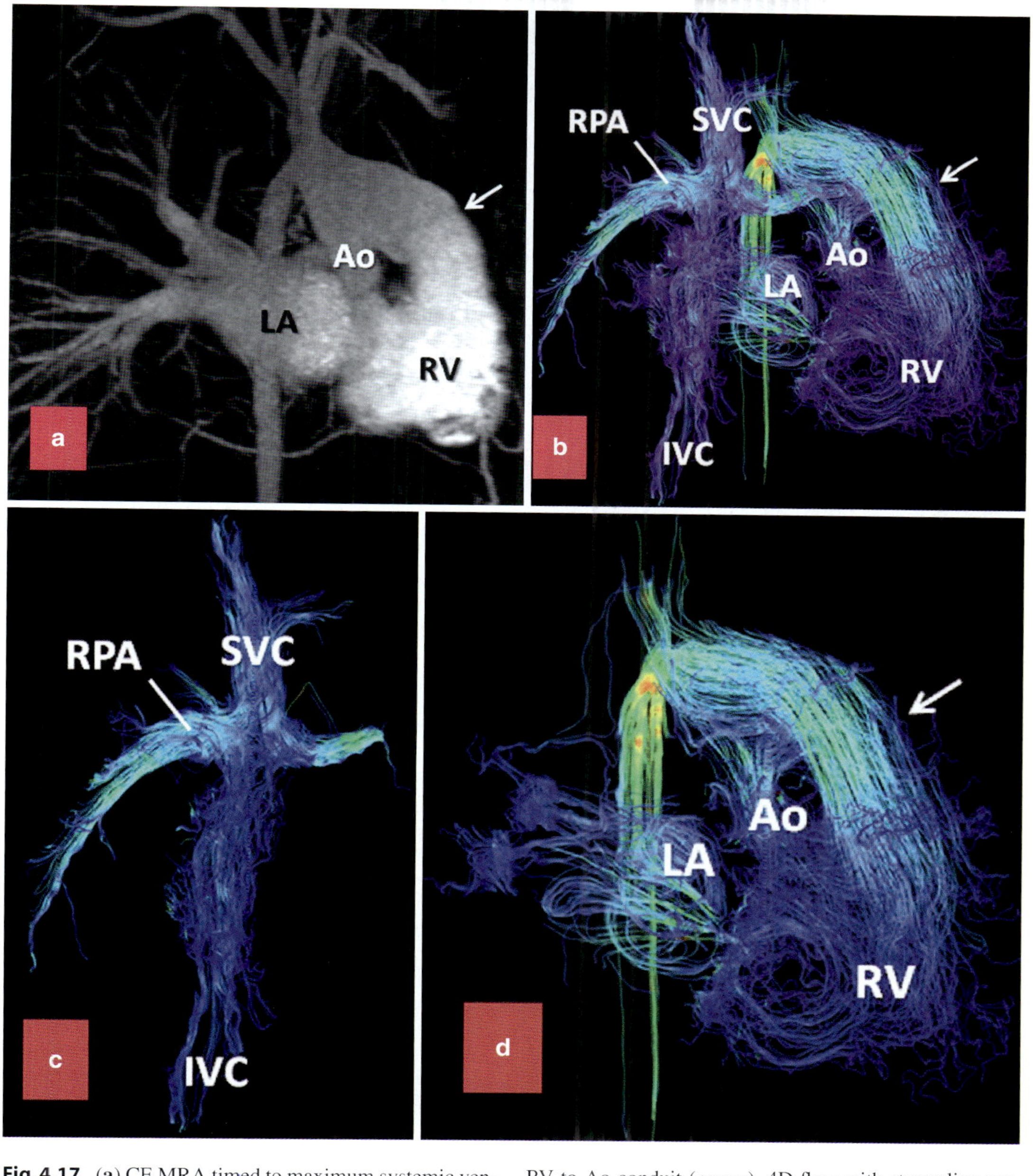

Fig. 4.17 (**a**) CE MRA timed to maximum systemic ventricle enhancement and (**b–d**) 4D flow MRI in a patient with history of Norwood I–III for hypoplastic left ventricle. CE MRA provides excellent detail of the anatomy of the left atrium (*LA*), right ventricle (*RV*), aorta (*Ao*), and RV to Ao conduit (*arrow*). 4D flow with streamline presentation showing the path of blood flow through (**b**) the whole heart, (**c**) the total cavopulmonary shunt, and (**d**) the systemic side of the heart (*arrow*)

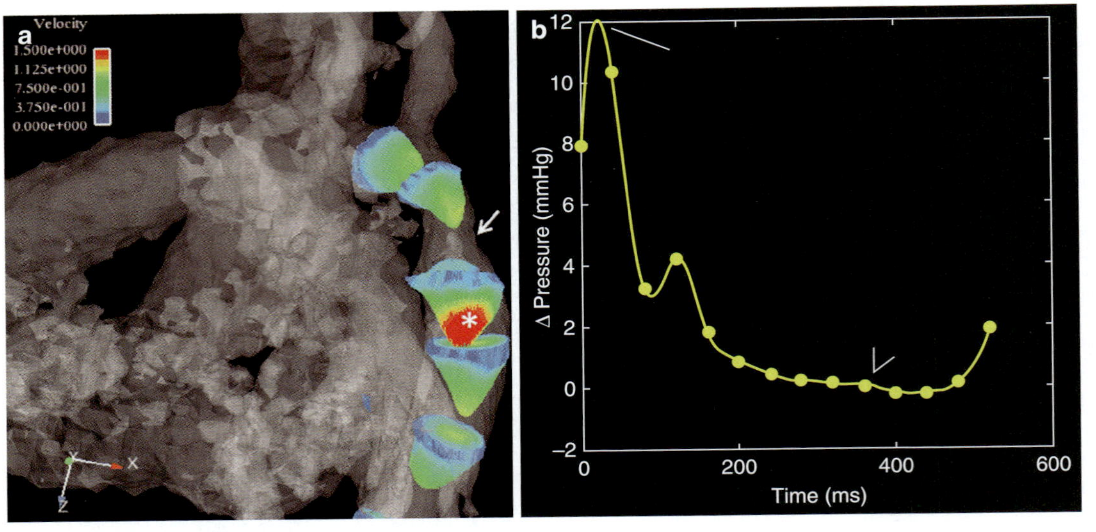

Fig. 4.18 (**a**) Velocity profiles at five locations in the descending thoracic aorta from 4D flow MRI acquisition in patient with aortic coarctation. Elevated velocities (indicated by *red* velocities, *) are present just distal to the coarctation (*arrow*). (**b**) Analysis of the time-resolved velocity profiles can be used to calculate the time-resolved pressure gradient across the stenosis. As expected, the peak pressure gradient across the stenosis occurs during early systole (*arrow*) and decreases during diastole (*arrowhead*)

Summary

Recent improvements in MRI hardware and software have resulted in dramatic changes to how MRA is performed, particularly for thoracic applications. These include the use of 3.0T scanners to achieve higher SNR and CNR to increase spatial resolution or to improve temporal resolution through the use of advanced parallel imaging methods. Intravascular contrast agents have also led to substantial changes in spatial resolution and the ability to perform high-resolution CE MRA during free breathing. NCE MRA methods, especially 3D bSSFP, have also undergone major developments and have had a significant impact on how we analyze the complex anatomy of the heart and thoracic vasculature in patients with CHD. Lastly, 4D flow sequences offer the potential to provide additional hemodynamic information important in the assessment and management of patients with CHD that currently is obtained using only invasive methods.

References

1. Earls JP, Rofsky NM, DeCorato DR, Krinsky GA, Weinreb JC. Breath-hold single-dose gadolinium-enhanced three-dimensional MR aortography: usefulness of a timing examination and MR power injector. Radiology. 1996;201(3):705–10.
2. Wilman AH, Riederer SJ, King BF, Debbins JP, Rossman PJ, Ehman RL. Fluoroscopically triggered contrast-enhanced three-dimensional MR angiography with elliptical centric view order: application to the renal arteries. Radiology. 1997;205(1):137–46.
3. Maki JH, Prince MR, Londy FJ, Chenevert TL. The effects of time varying intravascular signal intensity and k-space acquisition order on three-dimensional MR angiography image quality. J Magn Reson Imaging. 1996;6(4):642–51.
4. Groves EM, Bireley W, Dill K, Carroll TJ, Carr JC. Quantitative analysis of ECG-gated high-resolution contrast-enhanced MR angiography of the thoracic aorta. AJR Am J Roentgenol. 2007;188(2):522–8.
5. Bireley 2nd WR, Diniz LO, Groves EM, Dill K, Carroll TJ, Carr JC. Orthogonal measurement of thoracic aorta luminal diameter using ECG-gated high-resolution contrast-enhanced MR angiography. J Magn Reson Imaging. 2007;26(6):1480–5.
6. Burman ED, Keegan J, Kilner PJ. Aortic root measurement by cardiovascular magnetic resonance:

specification of planes and lines of measurement and corresponding normal values. Circ Cardiovasc Imaging. 2008;1(2):104–13.
7. Griswold MA, Jakob PM, Heidemann RM, et al. Generalized autocalibrating partially parallel acquisitions (GRAPPA). Magn Reson Med. 2002;47(6):1202–10.
8. Sodickson DK, McKenzie CA. A generalized approach to parallel magnetic resonance imaging. Med Phys. 2001;28(8):1629–43.
9. Pruessmann KP, Weiger M, Boesiger P. Sensitivity encoded cardiac MRI. J Cardiovasc Magn Reson. 2001;3(1):1–9.
10. Wilson GJ, Hoogeveen RM, Willinek WA, Muthupillai R, Maki JH. Parallel imaging in MR angiography. Top Magn Reson Imaging. 2004;15(3):169–85.
11. Fenchel M, Doering J, Seeger A, et al. Ultrafast whole-body MR angiography with two-dimensional parallel imaging at 3.0 T: feasibility study. Radiology. 2009;250(1):254–63.
12. Lum DP, Busse RF, Francois CJ, et al. Increased volume of coverage for abdominal contrast-enhanced MR angiography with two-dimensional autocalibrating parallel imaging: initial experience at 3.0 Tesla. J Magn Reson Imaging. 2009;30(5):1093–100.
13. Nael K, Fenchel M, Krishnam M, Finn JP, Laub G, Ruehm SG. 3.0 Tesla high spatial resolution contrast-enhanced magnetic resonance angiography (CE-MRA) of the pulmonary circulation: initial experience with a 32-channel phased array coil using a high relaxivity contrast agent. Invest Radiol. 2007;42(6):392–8.
14. Huang BY, Castillo M. Neurovascular imaging at 1.5 Tesla versus 3.0 Tesla. Magn Reson Imaging Clin N Am. 2009;17(1):29–46.
15. Tomasian A, Salamon N, Lohan DG, Jalili M, Villablanca JP, Finn JP. Supraaortic arteries: contrast material dose reduction at 3.0-T high-spatial-resolution MR angiography–feasibility study. Radiology. 2008;249(3):980–90.
16. Habibi R, Krishnam MS, Lohan DG, et al. High-spatial-resolution lower extremity MR angiography at 3.0 T: contrast agent dose comparison study. Radiology. 2008;248(2):680–92.
17. Attenberger UI, Michaely HJ, Wintersperger BJ, et al. Three-dimensional contrast-enhanced magnetic-resonance angiography of the renal arteries: interindividual comparison of 0.2 mmol/kg gadobutrol at 1.5 T and 0.1 mmol/kg gadobenate dimeglumine at 3.0 T. Eur Radiol. 2008;18(6):1260–8.
18. Rofsky NM, Johnson G, Adelman MA, Rosen RJ, Krinsky GA, Weinreb JC. Peripheral vascular disease evaluated with reduced-dose gadolinium-enhanced MR angiography. Radiology. 1997;205(1):163–9.
19. Collins CM, Liu W, Schreiber W, Yang QX, Smith MB. Central brightening due to constructive interference with, without, and despite dielectric resonance. J Magn Reson Imaging. 2005;21(2):192–6.
20. Vaughan JT, Adriany G, Snyder CJ, et al. Efficient high-frequency body coil for high-field MRI. Magn Reson Med. 2004;52(4):851–9.
21. Saekho S, Yip CY, Noll DC, Boada FE, Stenger VA. Fast-kz three-dimensional tailored radiofrequency pulse for reduced B1 inhomogeneity. Magn Reson Med. 2006;55(4):719–24.
22. Shellock FG, Crues JV. MR procedures: biologic effects, safety, and patient care. Radiology. 2004;232(3):635–52.
23. Shellock FG, Shields Jr CL. Radiofrequency energy-induced heating of bovine articular cartilage using a bipolar radiofrequency electrode. Am J Sports Med. 2000;28(5):720–4.
24. Barth MM, Smith MP, Pedrosa I, Lenkinski RE, Rofsky NM. Body MR imaging at 3.0 T: understanding the opportunities and challenges. Radiographics. 2007;27(5):1445–62.
25. Rapp JH, Wolff SD, Quinn SF, et al. Aortoiliac occlusive disease in patients with known or suspected peripheral vascular disease: safety and efficacy of gadofosveset-enhanced MR angiography–multicenter comparative phase III study. Radiology. 2005;236(1):71–8.
26. Rohrer M, Bauer H, Mintorovitch J, Requardt M, Weinmann HJ. Comparison of magnetic properties of MRI contrast media solutions at different magnetic field strengths. Invest Radiol. 2005;40(11):715–24.
27. Klessen C, Hein PA, Huppertz A, et al. First-pass whole-body magnetic resonance angiography (MRA) using the blood-pool contrast medium gadofosveset trisodium: comparison to gadopentetate dimeglumine. Invest Radiol. 2007;42(9):659–64.
28. Maki JH, Wang M, Wilson GJ, Shutske MG, Leiner T. Highly accelerated first-pass contrast-enhanced magnetic resonance angiography of the peripheral vasculature: comparison of gadofosveset trisodium with gadopentetate dimeglumine contrast agents. J Magn Reson Imaging. 2009;30(5):1085–92.
29. Naehle CP, Kaestner M, Muller A, et al. First-pass and steady-state MR angiography of thoracic vasculature in children and adolescents. JACC Cardiovasc Imaging. 2010;3(5):504–13.
30. Makowski MR, Wiethoff AJ, Uribe S, et al. Congenital heart disease: cardiovascular MR imaging by using an intravascular blood pool contrast agent. Radiology. 2011;260(3):680–8.
31. Finn JP, Baskaran V, Carr JC, et al. Thorax: low-dose contrast-enhanced three-dimensional MR angiography with subsecond temporal resolution – initial results. Radiology. 2002;224(3):896–904.
32. van Vaals JJ, Brummer ME, Dixon WT, et al. "Keyhole" method for accelerating imaging of contrast agent uptake. J Magn Reson Imaging. 1993;3(4):671–5.
33. Korosec FR, Frayne R, Grist TM, Mistretta CA. Time-resolved contrast-enhanced 3D MR angiography. Magn Reson Med. 1996;36(3):345–51.

34. Lim RP, Shapiro M, Wang EY, et al. 3D Time-resolved MR angiography (MRA) of the carotid arteries with time-resolved imaging with stochastic trajectories: comparison with 3D contrast-enhanced Bolus-Chase MRA and 3D time-of-flight MRA. AJNR Am J Neuroradiol. 2008;29(10):1847–54.
35. Haider CR, Hu HH, Campeau NG, Huston 3rd J, Riederer SJ. 3D high temporal and spatial resolution contrast-enhanced MR angiography of the whole brain. Magn Reson Med. 2008;60(3):749–60.
36. Shors SM, Cotts WG, Pavlovic-Surjancev B, Francois CJ, Gheorghiade M, Finn JP. Heart failure: evaluation of cardiopulmonary transit times with time-resolved MR angiography. Radiology. 2003;229(3):743–8.
37. Francois CJ, Shors SM, Bonow RO, Finn JP. Analysis of cardiopulmonary transit times at contrast material-enhanced MR imaging in patients with heart disease. Radiology. 2003;227(2):447–52.
38. Goo HW, Yang DH, Park IS, et al. Time-resolved three-dimensional contrast-enhanced magnetic resonance angiography in patients who have undergone a Fontan operation or bidirectional cavopulmonary connection: initial experience. J Magn Reson Imaging. 2007;25(4):727–36.
39. Wagner M, Nguyen KL, Khan S, et al. Contrast-enhanced MR angiography of cavopulmonary connections in adult patients with congenital heart disease. AJR Am J Roentgenol. 2012;199(5):W565–74.
40. Perazella MA. Advanced kidney disease, gadolinium and nephrogenic systemic fibrosis: the perfect storm. Curr Opin Nephrol Hypertens. 2009;18(6):519–25.
41. Perazella MA, Rodby RA. Gadolinium-induced nephrogenic systemic fibrosis in patients with kidney disease. Am J Med. 2007;120(7):561–2.
42. Sadowski EA, Bennett LK, Chan MR, et al. Nephrogenic systemic fibrosis: risk factors and incidence estimation. Radiology. 2007;243(1):148–57.
43. Provenzale JM, Sarikaya B. Comparison of test performance characteristics of MRI, MR angiography, and CT angiography in the diagnosis of carotid and vertebral artery dissection: a review of the medical literature. AJR Am J Roentgenol. 2009;193(4):1167–74.
44. Buhk JH, Kallenberg K, Mohr A, Dechent P, Knauth M. Evaluation of angiographic computed tomography in the follow-up after endovascular treatment of cerebral aneurysms – a comparative study with DSA and TOF-MRA. Eur Radiol. 2009;19(2):430–6.
45. Miyazaki M, Lee VS. Nonenhanced MR angiography. Radiology. 2008;248(1):20–43.
46. François CJ, Tuite D, Deshpande V, Jerecic R, Weale P, Carr JC. Unenhanced MR angiography of the thoracic aorta: initial clinical evaluation. AJR Am J Roentgenol. 2008;190(4):902–6.
47. Francois CJ, Tuite D, Deshpande V, Jerecic R, Weale P, Carr JC. Pulmonary vein imaging with unenhanced three-dimensional balanced steady-state free precession MR angiography: initial clinical evaluation. Radiology. 2009;250(3):932–9.
48. Krishnam MS, Tomasian A, Malik S, Desphande V, Laub G, Ruehm SG. Image quality and diagnostic accuracy of unenhanced SSFP MR angiography compared with conventional contrast-enhanced MR angiography for the assessment of thoracic aortic diseases. Eur Radiol. 2010;20(6):1311–20.
49. Pasqua AD, Barcudi S, Leonardi B, Clemente D, Colajacomo M, Sanders SP. Comparison of contrast and noncontrast magnetic resonance angiography for quantitative analysis of thoracic arteries in young patients with congenital heart defects. Ann Pediatr Cardiol. 2011;4(1):36–40.
50. Deshpande VS, Li D. Contrast-enhanced coronary artery imaging using 3D trueFISP. Magn Reson Med. 2003;50(3):570–7.
51. Deshpande VS, Shea SM, Laub G, Simonetti OP, Finn JP, Li D. 3D magnetization-prepared true-FISP: a new technique for imaging coronary arteries. Magn Reson Med. 2001;46(3):494–502.
52. Pelc NJ, Herfkens RJ, Shimakawa A, Enzmann DR. Phase contrast cine magnetic resonance imaging. Magn Reson Q. 1991;7(4):229–54.
53. Chai P, Mohiaddin R. How we perform cardiovascular magnetic resonance flow assessment using phase-contrast velocity mapping. J Cardiovasc Magn Reson. 2005;7(4):705–16.
54. Pelc NJ, Bernstein MA, Shimakawa A, Glover GH. Encoding strategies for three-direction phase-contrast MR imaging of flow. J Magn Reson Imaging. 1991;1(4):405–13.
55. De Cobelli F, Mellone R, Salvioni M, et al. Renal artery stenosis: value of screening with three-dimensional phase-contrast MR angiography with a phased-array multicoil. Radiology. 1996;201(3):697–703.
56. Schoenberg SO, Knopp MV, Bock M, et al. Renal artery stenosis: grading of hemodynamic changes with cine phase-contrast MR blood flow measurements. Radiology. 1997;203(1):45–53.
57. Markl M, Frydrychowicz A, Kozerke S, Hope M, Wieben O. 4D flow MRI. J Magn Reson Imaging. 2012;36(5):1015–36.
58. Markl M, Harloff A, Bley TA, et al. Time-resolved 3D MR velocity mapping at 3T: improved navigator-gated assessment of vascular anatomy and blood flow. J Magn Reson Imaging. 2007;25(4):824–31.
59. Gu T, Korosec FR, Block WF, et al. PC VIPR: a high-speed 3D phase-contrast method for flow quantification and high-resolution angiography. AJNR Am J Neuroradiol. 2005;26(4):743–9.
60. Francois CJ, Lum DP, Johnson KM, et al. Renal arteries: isotropic, high-spatial-resolution, unenhanced MR angiography with three-dimensional radial phase contrast. Radiology. 2011;258(1):254–60.
61. Stalder AF, Russe MF, Frydrychowicz A, Bock J, Hennig J, Markl M. Quantitative 2D and 3D phase contrast MRI: optimized analysis of blood flow and vessel wall parameters. Magn Reson Med. 2008;60(5):1218–31.
62. Markl M, Kilner PJ, Ebbers T. Comprehensive 4D velocity mapping of the heart and great vessels by cardiovascular magnetic resonance. J Cardiovasc Magn Reson. 2011;13:7.

63. Nordmeyer S, Berger F, Kuehne T, Riesenkampff E. Flow-sensitive four-dimensional magnetic resonance imaging facilitates and improves the accurate diagnosis of partial anomalous pulmonary venous drainage. Cardiol Young. 2011;21:1–8.
64. Nordmeyer S, Riesenkampff E, Crelier G, et al. Flow-sensitive four-dimensional cine magnetic resonance imaging for offline blood flow quantification in multiple vessels: a validation study. J Magn Reson Imaging. 2010;32(3):677–83.
65. Roes SD, Hammer S, van der Geest RJ, et al. Flow assessment through four heart valves simultaneously using 3-dimensional 3-directional velocity-encoded magnetic resonance imaging with retrospective valve tracking in healthy volunteers and patients with valvular regurgitation. Invest Radiol. 2009;44(10):669–75.
66. Uribe S, Beerbaum P, Sorensen TS, Rasmusson A, Razavi R, Schaeffter T. Four-dimensional (4D) flow of the whole heart and great vessels using real-time respiratory self-gating. Magn Reson Med. 2009;62(4): 984–92.
67. Valverde I, Simpson J, Schaeffter T, Beerbaum P. 4D phase-contrast flow cardiovascular magnetic resonance: comprehensive quantification and visualization of flow dynamics in atrial septal defect and partial anomalous pulmonary venous return. Pediatr Cardiol. 2010;31(8):1244–8.
68. Westenberg JJ, Roes SD, Ajmone Marsan N, et al. Mitral valve and tricuspid valve blood flow: accurate quantification with 3D velocity-encoded MR imaging with retrospective valve tracking. Radiology. 2008; 249(3):792–800.
69. Frydrychowicz A, Landgraf B, Wieben O, Francois CJ. Images in Cardiovascular Medicine. Scimitar syndrome: added value by isotropic flow-sensitive four-dimensional magnetic resonance imaging with PC-VIPR (phase-contrast vastly undersampled isotropic projection reconstruction). Circulation. 2010;121(23):e434–6.
70. Frydrychowicz A, Markl M, Harloff A, et al. Flow-sensitive in-vivo 4D MR imaging at 3T for the analysis of aortic hemodynamics and derived vessel wall parameters. Rofo. 2007;179(5):463–72.
71. Hope TA, Markl M, Wigstrom L, Alley MT, Miller DC, Herfkens RJ. Comparison of flow patterns in ascending aortic aneurysms and volunteers using four-dimensional magnetic resonance velocity mapping. J Magn Reson Imaging. 2007;26(6):1471–9.
72. Markl M, Geiger J, Kilner PJ, et al. Time-resolved three-dimensional magnetic resonance velocity mapping of cardiovascular flow paths in volunteers and patients with Fontan circulation. Eur J Cardiothorac Surg. 2011;39(2):206–12.
73. Geiger J, Markl M, Jung B, et al. 4D-MR flow analysis in patients after repair for tetralogy of Fallot. Eur Radiol. 2011;21(8):1651–7.
74. Francois CJ, Srinivasan S, Schiebler ML, et al. 4D cardiovascular magnetic resonance velocity mapping of alterations of right heart flow patterns and main pulmonary artery hemodynamics in tetralogy of Fallot. J Cardiovasc Magn Reson. 2012;14:16.
75. Lum DP, Johnson KM, Paul RK, et al. Transstenotic pressure gradients: measurement in swine – retrospectively ECG-gated 3D phase-contrast MR angiography versus endovascular pressure-sensing guidewires. Radiology. 2007;245(3):751–60.
76. Turk AS, Johnson KM, Lum D, et al. Physiologic and anatomic assessment of a canine carotid artery stenosis model utilizing phase contrast with vastly undersampled isotropic projection imaging. AJNR Am J Neuroradiol. 2007;28(1):111–5.
77. Bley TA, Johnson KM, Francois CJ, et al. Noninvasive assessment of transstenotic pressure gradients in porcine renal artery stenoses by using vastly undersampled phase-contrast MR angiography. Radiology. 2011;261(1):266–73.
78. Tyszka JM, Laidlaw DH, Asa JW, Silverman JM. Three-dimensional, time-resolved (4D) relative pressure mapping using magnetic resonance imaging. J Magn Reson Imaging. 2000;12(2):321–9.
79. Bock J, Frydrychowicz A, Lorenz R, et al. In vivo noninvasive 4D pressure difference mapping in the human aorta: phantom comparison and application in healthy volunteers and patients. Magn Reson Med. 2011;66(4):1079–88.
80. Barker AJ, Lanning C, Shandas R. Quantification of hemodynamic wall shear stress in patients with bicuspid aortic valve using phase-contrast MRI. Ann Biomed Eng. 2010;38(3):788–800.
81. Boussel L, Rayz V, Martin A, et al. Phase-contrast magnetic resonance imaging measurements in intracranial aneurysms in vivo of flow patterns, velocity fields, and wall shear stress: comparison with computational fluid dynamics. Magn Reson Med. 2009;61(2):409–17.
82. Frydrychowicz A, Stalder AF, Russe MF, et al. Three-dimensional analysis of segmental wall shear stress in the aorta by flow-sensitive four-dimensional-MRI. J Magn Reson Imaging. 2009;30(1):77–84.
83. Oyre S, Pedersen EM, Ringgaard S, Boesiger P, Paaske WP. In vivo wall shear stress measured by magnetic resonance velocity mapping in the normal human abdominal aorta. Eur J Vasc Endovasc Surg. 1997;13(3):263–71.
84. Bieging ET, Frydrychowicz A, Wentland A, et al. In vivo three-dimensional MR wall shear stress estimation in ascending aortic dilatation. J Magn Reson Imaging. 2011;33(3):589–97.
85. Petersson S, Dyverfeldt P, Ebbers T. Assessment of the accuracy of MRI wall shear stress estimation using numerical simulations. J Magn Reson Imaging. 2012;36(1):128–38.
86. Markl M, Wallis W, Strecker C, Gladstone BP, Vach W, Harloff A. Analysis of pulse wave velocity in the thoracic aorta by flow-sensitive four-dimensional MRI: reproducibility and correlation with characteristics in patients with aortic atherosclerosis. J Magn Reson Imaging. 2012;35(5):1162–8.
87. Markl M, Wallis W, Brendecke S, Simon J, Frydrychowicz A, Harloff A. Estimation of global aortic pulse wave velocity by flow-sensitive 4D MRI. Magn Reson Med. 2010;63(6):1575–82.

88. Arzani A, Dyverfeldt P, Ebbers T, Shadden SC. In vivo validation of numerical prediction for turbulence intensity in an aortic coarctation. Ann Biomed Eng. 2012;40(4):860–70.
89. Petersson S, Dyverfeldt P, Gardhagen R, Karlsson M, Ebbers T. Simulation of phase contrast MRI of turbulent flow. Magn Reson Med. 2010;64(4):1039–46.
90. Dyverfeldt P, Gardhagen R, Sigfridsson A, Karlsson M, Ebbers T. On MRI turbulence quantification. Magn Reson Imaging. 2009;27(7):913–22.
91. Dyverfeldt P, Sigfridsson A, Kvitting JP, Ebbers T. Quantification of intravoxel velocity standard deviation and turbulence intensity by generalizing phase-contrast MRI. Magn Reson Med. 2006;56(4):850–8.

Principles of CT Imaging

5

Sebastian Leschka, Stephan Waelti,
and Simon Wildermuth

The traditional imaging modality for the pre- and postoperative evaluation of patients with congenital heart disease (CHD) had been catheter angiography but had been replaced by echocardiography for most conditions [1]. However, several anatomical structures including the pulmonary vasculature, the aortic arch, and the right ventricle are sometimes difficult to evaluate with transthoracic echocardiography. Albeit these structures are better visualized with transesophageal echocardiography, the method is limited in patients with pulmonary enlargement [2]. Moreover, the diagnostic quality and interpretation of echocardiography highly depends on the operator and the presence of an adequate acoustic window. In recent years, magnetic resonance imaging (MRI) has been introduced in the diagnostic armamentarium for patients with CHD because of its noninvasiveness, the accurate morphological and functional information provided, and that neither iodinated contrast agent nor ionizing radiation is required. Therefore, MRI is considered an excellent diagnostic tool particularly for the evaluation of young children with CHD, because they may require several follow-up examinations during their lifetime. As a drawback, the utilization of MRI may be limited in the many patients who have undergone surgical corrections of CHD and those who have implanted pacemakers or cardioverter-defibrillator. In addition, the long examination time of MRI often requires lengthy period of patient sedation.

Since its introduction in the 1970s, computed tomography (CT) has become an important diagnostic tool in medicine with a widespread utilization for imaging of all body regions and an estimated 72 million scans performed in the United States in 2007 [3]. Visualization of the heart has been of great interest for radiologists since the early beginning of CT. In his novel prize lecture in 1979, Sir Godfrey N. Hounsfield has had hypothesized on the future of CT for cardiac imaging:

> [...] Various attempts have been made to achieve useful pictures of the heart. The time available for taking a picture of the heart is obviously longer than one heartbeat. Some experiments were conducted some time ago using conventional CT machines but in which the traverse of the detectors was synchronized to the heart beat via an electrocardiograph, passing over the heart in diastole (when the heart movement is at a minimum). [...] The heart chambers can be discerned by a little intravenous injected contrast media. [...] A further promising field may be the detection of the coronary arteries. It may be possible to detect these under special conditions of scanning. [...] [4].

Another 30 years of technical development were required to achieve the current state of modern CT systems being robust and accurate for cardiac imaging.

S. Leschka, MD (✉) • S. Waelti, MD
S. Wildermuth, MD
Department of Radiology, Institute of Radiology,
Kantonsspital St. Gallen, Rorschacher Strasse 95,
CH-9007 St. Gallen, Switzerland
e-mail: sebastian.leschka@kssg.ch

F. Saremi (ed.), *Cardiac CT and MR for Adult Congenital Heart Disease*,
DOI 10.1007/978-1-4614-8875-0_5, © Springer Science+Business Media New York 2014

Due to improvements in medical management and surgical procedures, it is estimated that 85 % of the children with CHD will survive to adulthood [5] and around 50 % of these children will require follow-up examinations in adult life [6]. Thus, precise follow-up imaging of these patients is important not only for monitoring the lesions and their functional status but also to provide accurate information on the anatomical relationship of the coronary arteries as well as cardiac and extracardiac structures to plan possible surgical reinterventions. Disadvantages of CT are the exposure of the patients to ionizing radiation and the cumulative radiation exposure during lifetime as well as the risks inherent in the application of iodinated contrast agent. Accounting for these drawbacks, patients should be carefully selected for CT imaging, and strategies for the reduction of the radiation exposure need to be applied.

Parameters Defining a CT System's Performance

Visualization of the moving heart and the coronary arteries requires the highest technical demands of any imaged body region because of the small size and tortuous course of the coronary arteries and the continuous motion during the cardiac cycle. Therefore, first, the CT system used needs to provide a high temporal resolution to compensate for the rapid and continuous cardiac movement. Second, a high spatial resolution is required to accurately visualize small cardiac structures of interest (e.g., small atrial septal defects) and the coronary arteries for possibly associated coronary malformations. And third, the CT system should facilitate a high coverage speed in the *z*-axis direction and consequently a short acquisition time which reduces the breath-hold time and may omit the requirement of patient sedation. In addition, CT imaging at very high volume coverage speed using a second-generation 128-slice dual-source CT system with pitch values of 3.2 may avoid the necessity for electrocardiographic (ECG) synchronization as it has been recently reported for CT imaging of the aortic root and the proximal parts of the coronary arteries [7].

Spatial Resolution

The spatial resolution of a CT system depends on the physical width of the detector in the longitudinal direction. Ideally isotropic voxel imaging should be achieved. That means that a voxel has the same size in all dimensions. Isotropic voxels are required to reconstruct images in all planes at the same high quality. Current CT systems provide an isotropic spatial resolution of up to 0.4 mm [8]. Importantly, as CT slice thickness is typically 0.5–0.6 mm, the spatial resolution in the longitudinal *z*-axis may not be completely isotropic with the in-plane resolution resulting in volume averaging of data with the reconstruction of longitudinal structures in a minor degree but usually do not substantially influence the quality of multiplanar reformations (MPR). Further, improved spatial resolution at a level of 0.2 mm had been advocated for a detailed evaluation of small structures or severely calcified arteries [9]. However, a further increase in spatial resolution will require a higher radiation exposure to maintain sufficient signal-to-noise ratio [9].

A good illustration for the effect of spatial resolution is the analogy to the film grain in photography. High-grain films [*CT*: *low spatial resolution*] are usually more sensitive to the incoming light [*CT*: *radiation exposure*] but have lower detail resolution. In contrast, small-grain films [*CT*: *high spatial resolution*] are less sensitive to the light [*CT*: *radiation exposure*] but have a higher resolution. The effects of film grain can be objectionably noticeable in an over-enlarged film photograph (Fig. 5.1a, b). In digital cameras, an image sensor with more elements [*CT*: *smaller detector size*] will result in an image with better resolution like small-grain films.

Temporal Resolution

The temporal resolution depends on the gantry rotation time. For artifact-free imaging of the beating heart and the coronary arteries, a temporal resolution of less than 100 ms is desirable to permit reliable evaluation of these structures even at elevated heart rates [9].

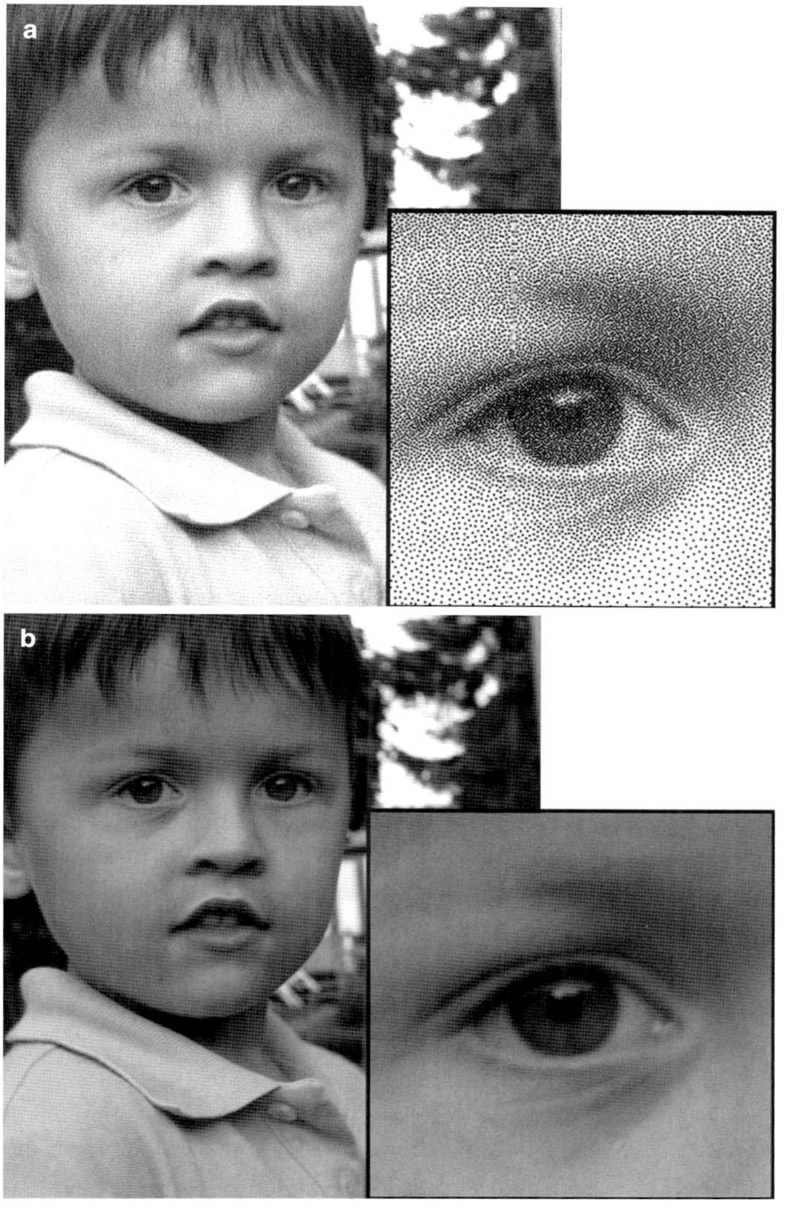

Fig. 5.1 (**a**) Analogy of photography for spatial resolution: High-grain films (low spatial resolution) are more sensitive to incoming light (radiation exposure) but have lower detail resolution. (**b**) Small-grain films (high spatial resolution) are less sensitive to light (radiation exposure) but have higher detail resolution

In order to compensate for motion artifacts of the beating heart, the CT data acquisition is commonly synchronized with the ECG signal. The most commonly used approach for synchronization is retrospective ECG gating in which images are acquired throughout the cardiac cycle, and those time points depicting the coronary arteries without motion artifacts are retrospectively selected for image reconstruction. The projection data of a half gantry rotation is then required for image reconstruction (half-scan reconstruction), and thus, the temporal resolution corresponds to the half of the rotation time. Modern CT systems provide a gantry rotation time of down to 270 ms with a resulting temporal resolution of 135 ms. When using a mono-segment half-scan reconstruction method, further improvements in gantry rotation time are mandatory to achieve a temporal resolution of better than 100 ms. However, the mechanical forces increase with higher gantry rotation times. CT systems with a gantry rotation time of 330 ms are associated with a mechanical force of around 28 g. Therefore, rotation times of less than 200 ms required for a temporal resolution of 100 ms in a mono-segment half-scan reconstruction appear to be beyond today's mechanical limits (i.e., *mechanical forces>75 g*) [9].

The temporal resolution can be improved by using the scan data from more than one heart cycle for reconstruction of the images (multi-segment reconstruction) [10]. The images are then reconstructed using the partial scan data of projection sectors from multiple consecutive heart cycles resulting in a temporal resolution of up to a quarter of the rotation time when using two consecutive heartbeats and up to a sixth of the rotation time when using three heartbeats and so forth. Despite the theoretically improved temporal resolution, multi-segment reconstruction does not necessarily improve image quality as this algorithm is sensitive to changing heart rates. Therefore, the use of partial data from more than two consecutive heartbeats is usually not practical.

Another approach for improving temporal resolution at a given gantry rotation time is the dual-source CT system. A dual-source CT system consists of two X-ray tubes and two detectors mounted on the gantry with an angular offset of 90° working simultaneously. Therefore, only a quarter of rotation of each tube instead of a half of rotation with single-source CT is necessary to acquire the required projection data for image reconstruction. The temporal resolution improves to one quarter of the rotation time using only a single heartbeat for image reconstruction [8].

In photography, the shutter speed is analogous to the temporal resolution of CT. The shutter speed or exposure time is the effective length of time the camera's shutter is open. Images taken at a low shutter speed, meaning a long exposure time [*CT*: *low temporal resolution*], will result in blurred display of moving structures (Fig. 5.2). Using a high shutter speed, meaning a short exposure time [*CT*: *high temporal resolution*], will result in a frozen display of the moving structure [*CT*: *the heart*].

Z-Axis Coverage Speed

The coverage speed in *z*-axis is related to the longitudinal axis covered by the detector array, the gantry rotation speed, and the pitch value used. The higher the coverage speed in the *z*-axis, the shorter is the acquisition time. The scan time becomes important in CT imaging of patients being unable to hold their breath for a longer time or who are unable to cooperate (e.g., toddlers). One important benefit of short acquisition time is the lower occurrence of heart rate variability: A long breath-hold is frequently accompanied with tachycardia at the end of acquisition causing a considerable variability in the length of heart cycles [11]; a shorter breath-hold time reduces heart rate variability and may improve image quality of the images acquired during the end of the scan. In addition, when the scan time is reduced, there is also a shorter period required for the contrast opacification of the cardiac structures and consequently permits a smaller volume of contrast media to be used.

Recent Developments in CT Imaging

CT imaging has undergone a rapid technical improvement – in particular in the last 10 years. Modern CT systems provide high scan speed and high temporal and high spatial resolution. Thus, CT combines the advantages of widespread availability and short acquisition time. When being synchronized to the ECG signal, CT accurately delineates rapid moving cardiac structures and allows the assessment of the anatomical relationship of the coronary arteries to the adjacent structures and associated coronary artery anomalies [12].

Single-Slice Helical CT

The introduction of the single-slice helical CT into clinical practice was an important step toward the widespread utilization of CT in clinical routine improving the image quality

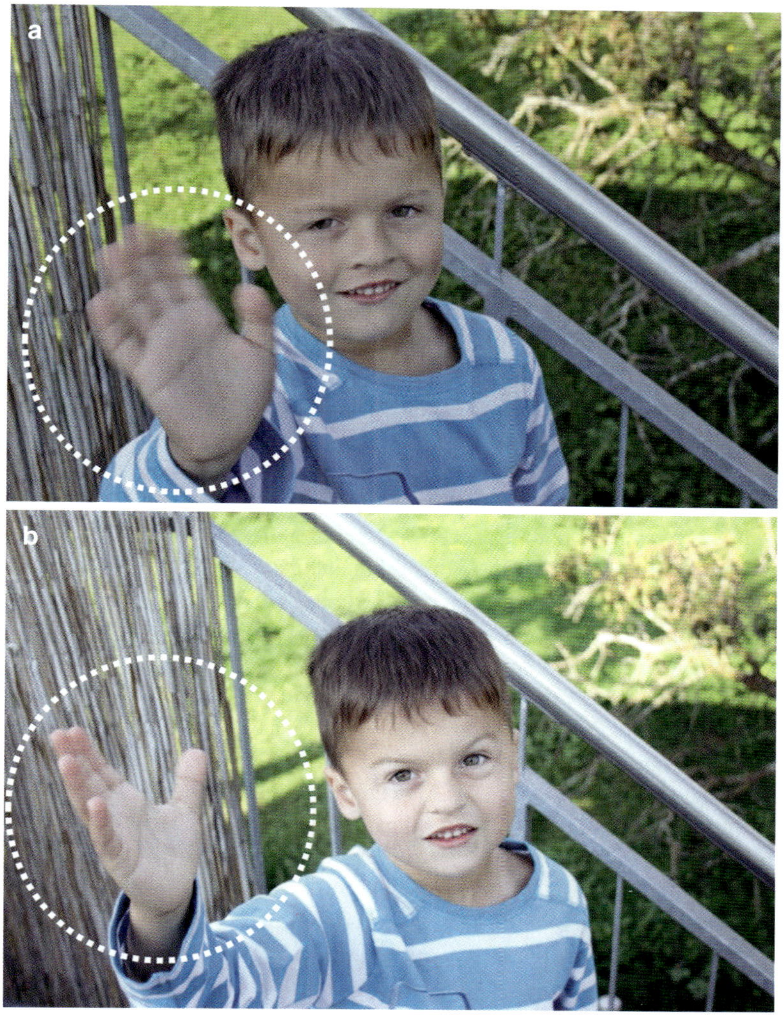

Fig. 5.2 (**a**) Analogy of photography for temporal resolution: Images taken at a low shutter speed (1/25 s), meaning a long exposure time (low temporal resolution), result in blurred moving structures. (**b**) Images taken at a high shutter speed (1/500 s), meaning a short exposure time (high temporal resolution), will result in a sharp moving structures

in general and rendering CT fast enough for daily clinical routine. The gantry rotation time of single-slice helical CT was around 0.8 s which leads to a temporal resolution of 400 ms by using a half-scan reconstruction technique. The reconstructed slice thickness was about 3–5 mm. Although a better temporal resolution of 50–100 ms was available in the early 1980s with electron beam CT, single-slice helical CT established itself for cardiac imaging due to its availability in many institutions worldwide. In addition, newly introduced postprocessing techniques, including segmentation algorithms of the cardiac cycle, allowed to investigate a particular cardiac phase. When using a single-slice helical CT, occasionally the diagnosis of coronary artery stenosis in large proximal vessels [13], cardiac thrombus [14], and congenital heart disease [15] could be established under optimal conditions with very slow heart rates. However, most often the coronary arteries were displayed as "dancing vessels" or "ghosts" due to limitations in temporal resolution. Nevertheless, in consideration of the expected improvements of the temporal and spatial resolution, it became evident that cardiac CT imaging will become a practical and valuable tool despite the limitations present in these days.

Multi-Slice CT

The next step of CT evolution on the way to cardiac imaging was the implementation of multi-slice CT technology – coupled with a decreased size of the single detector element, the faster gantry rotation speed, and the increased volume coverage.

Since 1999 4-slice CT systems became clinically available providing gantry rotation times of 500–800 ms, resulting in a temporal resolution of 250–400 ms. The spatial resolution in *z*-axis was 1.0–1.25 mm and *z*-axis coverage was around 2 cm. The CT examination of the entire heart was feasible within a 40–50 s acquisition time – unfortunately being longer than most patients could hold their breath. Therefore, preoxygenation was often used to reduce breathing artifacts. Despite optimal preparation, only the proximal to mid coronary artery segments could be depicted without artifacts [16–24]. Images of distal segments and side branches suffered from the insufficient quality, and up to 32 % of coronary segments had to be excluded from analysis in the published 4-slice CT studies [22]. Therefore, the 4-slice CT system was still not robust enough to be implemented into daily clinical practice for cardiac CT imaging.

In 2001 16-slice CT systems became available. They provided gantry rotation times of 380–500 ms, resulting in a temporal resolution of 190–250 ms, and images were reconstructed with a slice thickness of 0.5–0.75 mm. The examination of the entire heart could be finished within a single breath-hold of around 20 s omitting the previous requirements of preoxygenation. In contrast to the 4-slice CT systems, even small coronary segments and side branches could be reliably evaluated [11, 25–34]. Nevertheless, 29 % of coronary artery segments remained not evaluative due to insufficient contrast attenuation in 52 %, to coronary artery motion artifacts in 45 %, to small vessel caliber in 31 %, to breathing artifacts in 19 %, and due to severe calcifications in 5 % [35]. Therefore, 16-slice CT systems were still not robust enough for cardiac imaging in all patients.

In 2004 64-slice CT systems became available. They provided gantry rotation times of 330–400 ms, resulting in a temporal resolution of 165–200 ms. The slice thickness was 0.5–0.625 mm, and detector covered 19.2–40 mm. The 64-slice CT systems allowed an examination of the entire heart within less than 10 s. Even detailed evaluation of small-sized branches of less than 1 mm in diameter was possible. The improvements in temporal resolution and the *z*-axis coverage speed allowed a precise characterization of the morphology and function of the aortic [36–40] and the mitral valve [40, 41]. Therefore, the 64-slice CT has been considered the first CT system being robust enough for cardiac CT imaging in daily clinical practice [42–50]. Despite its improved temporal resolution, the 64-slice CT system still needed a low and stable heart rate for optimal image quality [51], making a premedication with beta-blockers prior to coronary CT angiography frequently required. However, a precise morphological and functional evaluation of the heart of CHD patients could be commonly performed without medicamentous heart rate control.

State-of-the-Art CT Systems

The remaining challenges of temporal resolution and detector coverage have led to the development of the latest CT systems: 256-/320-slice CT and dual-source CT.

Large Volume Coverage CT (256-Slice CT/320-Slice CT)

In order to overcome limitations of CT for coronary visualization in patients with irregular heart rhythm, Toshiba introduced in 2006 the first CT system capable of covering the entire heart within a single heartbeat, using a large detector system with a 256-slice detector array and a spatial resolution of 0.5 mm resulting in a *z*-axis coverage of 128 mm. These technical improvements permit coverage of the entire heart in a single gantry rotation. On the other hand, because of increasing weight of the rotating elements, this CT system is

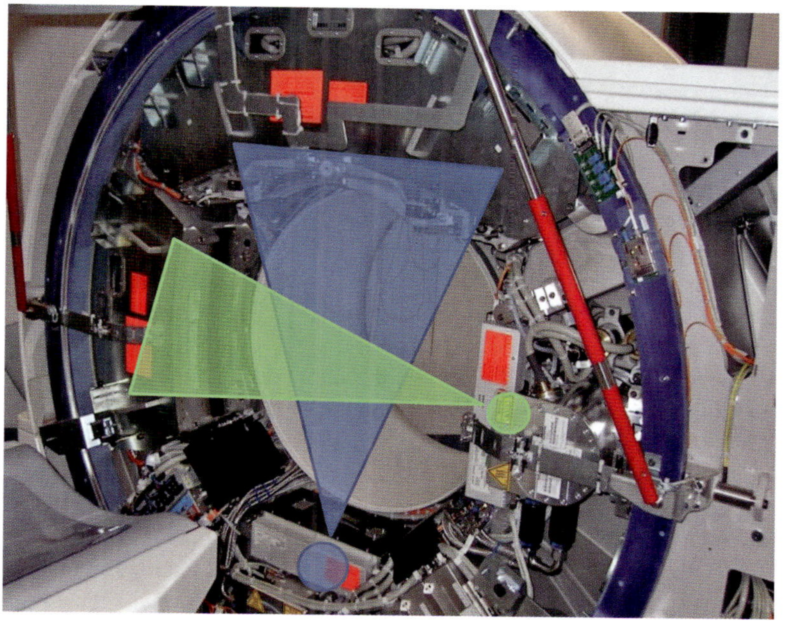

Fig. 5.3 Dual-source CT: Two corresponding detectors are mounted onto the rotating gantry with an angular offset of 90°

limited by its long gantry rotation time of 500 ms. Nevertheless, initial results from small patient cohorts show great promise for assessing coronary artery stenosis with the 256-slice CT system [52, 53]. In 2007 Philips introduced another 256-slice CT system but with a lower gantry rotation time of 270 ms. Later, a 320-slice CT system with a detector coverage of 160 mm and a gantry rotation time of 350 ms was introduced by Toshiba. First results show great promise for imaging the coronary arteries within a single heartbeat [54]. Large volume coverage CT might open the field for new cardiac imaging applications, including observation of evolving processes such as coronary contrast flow and whole heart perfusion.

Dual-Source CT

In 2005 Siemens introduced a CT scanner with two X-ray tubes and two corresponding detectors mounted onto the rotating gantry with an angular offset of 90°, the so-called dual-source CT [8] (Fig. 5.3). Each detector array of the first generation of dual-source CT is capable of acquiring 64 slices. This construction led to a reduction of the rotation needed to acquire the required projection data for image reconstruction from half a rotation in single-source CT to a quarter of a rotation in dual-source CT. Thus, the gantry rotation time of 330 ms results in a temporal resolution of 83 ms in a mono-segment reconstruction mode that is consistent throughout various heart rates owing to individual adaptation of the table pitch. Due to the high temporal resolution, several studies demonstrated a high diagnostic accuracy of dual-source CT for the assessment of coronary artery stenosis combined with a low rate of nonevaluative coronary segments [55–62] and permits coronary imaging even at high heart rates [8, 63, 64]. In addition, by operating both tubes at different tube voltages, dual-energy cardiac CT can be performed, which may help to identify myocardial perfusion defects [65].

Recently, Siemens introduced the second-generation dual-source CT which is capable of acquiring 2 × 128 slices. The gantry rotation time has been reduced to 280 ms, leading to a temporal resolution of 75 ms. In contrast to the other CT systems, where a low pitch is needed for overlapping data acquisition, the second-generation dual-source CT can achieve gapless z-axis sampling even at a pitch value of up to 3.2. Therefore, it enables coverage of the entire heart in a single heartbeat.

Development of Technical Parameters

The development of multi-slice CT scanners led to an enormous improvement of the technical parameters defining the cardiac imaging capabilities.

Development of Spatial Resolution

Compared to 64-slice CT systems, the temporal resolution has not substantially improved with 256-slice/320-slice or dual-source CT systems. Interestingly, blooming artifacts of severely calcified vessels walls are less pronounced in dual-source CTCA than in 64-slice CTCA [55]. Given that the spatial resolution of single-source 64-slice CT and dual-source CT is the same, this difference in calcification dependency could indicate that blooming artifacts may be sometimes superimposed by additional motion artifacts [55] and thus be dependent on the temporal resolution. Therefore, artifacts from clip material and devices might be reduced in CT imaging of CHD patients after surgery when using state-of-the-art CT systems.

Development of Temporal Resolution

A gantry rotation time of less than 100 ms is required to overcome the challenge of motion artifacts at high heart rates. In order to achieve this goal, two different approaches have been developed: the multi-segment reconstruction algorithm and the dual-source concept.

In the multi-segment reconstruction concept, small portions of projection data are selected from two or more heart cycles, and all projections are combined to obtain sufficient data for image reconstruction. The maximal achievable temporal resolution is half of the gantry rotation time and divided by the number of heart cycles averaged for image reconstruction. Although effectively improving the temporal resolution, the multi-segment reconstruction approach may be a cause of additional motion artifacts. The cardiac position in the thoracic cage is not absolutely fixed and depends on the actual ventricular filling and function, even at a steady heart rate. Due to merging of data from two or more consecutive cycles, the resulting image data do not exactly match together, leading to motion artifacts. These motion artifacts are even seen in patients with regular heart rate and more pronounced in patients with variable heart rate and result in an increased vessel blurring [51, 66, 67]. These disadvantages have even been reported for modern CT systems with high temporal resolution [68].

The other approach to improve the temporal resolution is the dual-source CT concept. Because images are obtained in a quarter of the rotation, the temporal resolution is around 75–83 ms using a mono-segment reconstruction from a single heartbeat for the individual image thereby avoiding artifacts from averaging projection data from several consecutive heartbeats. Several studies have shown improved image quality by reducing motion artifacts without administration of beta-blockers for heart rate control [55–57, 61].

Development of *Z*-Axis Coverage

The *z*-axis coverage speed has tremendously increased during the CT development. While acquisition of the entire heart needs more than 40 s with a 4-slice CT and around 20 s with a 16-slice CT, the acquisition with current 64-slice CT systems takes less than 10 s. With the most advanced CT systems (e.g., 320-slice CT and second-generation dual-source CT systems), the entire heart is imaged within a single heartbeat.

The increase in *z*-axis coverage speed led to a concomitant decrease in the amount of contrast media required for cardiac CT. The contrast media amount was reduced from 160 mL in the beginning of cardiac CT with 4-slice CT systems [69] to around 50–80 mL with 320-slice CT and dual-source CT [54, 55, 57, 61, 64, 70]. Therefore, state-of-the-art CT systems have the potential to reduce the risk of contrast-induced nephropathy.

Table 5.1 Relevant CT parameters for imaging adult patients with congenital heart disease using a dual-source CT system

Slice collimation	Thin collimation: 2×64×0.6 mm Thick collimation: 2×24×1.2 mm
Tube voltage/tube current	BMI ≤25 kg/sqm: 100 kVp/150 mAs (ECG-synchronized: 100 kVp/220 mAs) BMI >25 kg/sqm: 120 kVp/180 mAs (ECG-synchronized: 120 kVp/330 mAs)
Gantry rotation time	330 ms
Pitch	1 (non-ECG-synchronized CT) 0.2–0.5 (retrospective ECG-gated CT; pitch depending on the heart rate)

CT Imaging Protocols in CHD Patients

All protocols and recommendations within this section are valid for current dual-source CT systems but might be easily adapted to other CT systems. The CT imaging protocol should be adapted according to the suspected cardiac defect, the type of previous surgical repair, and the patient's compliance. The relevant CT parameters for CHD imaging in adult patients are summarized in Table 5.1.

Patient Preparation

Good image quality is one of the key factors for a good diagnosis and additionally reduces the time needed for interpretation of the cardiac CT study. Therefore, every patient preparation should be optimized for the scan to be successful. Many of the steps that ensure a good image quality take place even before the scanning begins.

Patient preparation includes instruction to the patient, correct positioning of the patient on the CT table, ECG lead placement if ECG synchronization is intended, and placement of a peripheral venous catheter for the contrast agent. The size of the venous access line depends on the CT protocol. For high-quality CT angiographic images, an 18-gauge or larger catheter is the preferred administration route. A right-arm injection is preferable to avoid artifacts from undiluted contrast agent in the left brachiocephalic vein.

Although the rate of not-evaluative coronary segments has been markedly declined when using modern scanner types, a low and particularly regular heart rate is still one of the major determinants for good image quality. Thus the patient should be imaged in a calm and comfortable ambience to avoid influences on the heart rate by anxiety or agitation. We give patients explicit breathing instructions and practice correct breathing without pressuring before the scan. The patient is instructed to suspend respiration at the appropriate time and to hold still during the scan. The patient is also informed about the possible instantaneous effects of contrast material including warmth, pelvic tingling, and a metallic taste in the mouth to minimize worry during the examination.

When to Use ECG Synchronization and When Not?

Data acquisition in cardiac CT can be performed non-ECG-synchronized or synchronized to the ECG signal by retrospectively gated or prospectively triggered techniques. In general, ECG synchronization leads to a reduction of motion artifacts but increases the radiation exposure [71]. For most instances, the non-ECG-synchronized technique is sufficient, while ECG synchronization is mandatory in patients with a complex cardiac abnormality or a small-sized intracardiac abnormality or communication or when the coronary arteries need to be investigated.

Non-ECG-Synchronized CT

Non-ECG-synchronized cardiac CT provides a fast acquisition of the cardiac and extracardiac structures, but due to heart motion artifacts, it is less suited for the detailed visualization of small cardiac and coronary structures. Using a pitch of around 1 is usually a good balance between acquisition time, radiation dose, and image quality. To reduce radiation dose and improve image quality in non-ECG-synchronized CT, thicker detector collimation is preferred, at the expense of reduced visualization of small-sized structures. Furthermore, when using a thicker collimation, the acquisition time is lower, and thereby, the respiratory motion artifacts might be reduced. If possible, non-ECG-synchronized CT in patients with CDH is performed during breath-hold. If this is not possible, the CT examination could be performed in free-breathing technique, avoiding excessive respiratory excursion. In modern CT systems, respiratory artifacts are less pronounced. It has been reported in non-ECG-synchronized CT acquisitions that 82 % of patients with CHD, the origins and proximal segments of the coronary arteries are evaluative [72]. The radiation dose of this scan technique in young children is usually less than 1 mSv [73].

ECG-Synchronized CT

The synchronization of the CT data acquisition with the ECG signal is important for sufficient compensation of cardiac motion artifacts and is of utmost importance for the evaluation of small-sized cardiac structures, intracardiac communications, and the coronary arteries and commonly improves visualization of the aortic root. The ECG synchronization can be performed with three different acquisition modes: retrospectively ECG-gated helical CT (*single- and dual-source CT*), prospectively ECG-triggered sequential CT (*single- and dual-source CT*), and prospectively ECG-triggered high-pitch helical CT (*only dual-source CT*).

Retrospective ECG Gating

For a long time, retrospective ECG gating has been the standard acquisition mode for helical cardiac CT. In retrospective ECG-gated CT, the data acquisition is performed with continuous scanner table motion and spiral acquisition with overlap of the radiation beam on each spiral synchronized to the ECG (Fig. 5.4a). Thus, low pitch values are necessary for gapless data acquisition, and radiation dose are substantial higher than when using non-ECG-synchronized CT as each portion of the heart is imaged more than once, while ECG is recorded. Then, in the retrospective, images are reconstructed in the optimal phase of the cardiac cycle providing the least motion artifacts and used for the interpretation. The surplus of information across different phases of the cardiac cycle can be used for ventricular functional analysis.

Prospective ECG Triggering

If there is a high probability that just a single reconstruction in the diastole is required for a diagnostic image, usually in patients with a low and stable heart rate, prospectively ECG-triggered sequential CT is an alternative acquisition mode. Using this mode, the CT table is stationary during image acquisition and moves in the following heartbeat to the next position for the next sequential scan ("step-and-shoot mode") (Fig. 5.4b). With a 64-slice CT, complete coverage of the heart requires 5–8 heartbeats, with a 128-slice dual-source CT 2–3 heartbeats and with a 320-slice CT only a single heartbeat. The radiation dose of prospectively ECG-triggered sequential CTCA is low with an effective radiation dose of 1–4 mSv because there is little overlap between adjacent sequential scans and X-ray exposure is limited to a small interval in the cardiac cycle [74, 75]. Prospective ECG triggering can be used to reduce radiation dose in other types of cardiac CT studies as well, such as evaluation of coronary artery bypass grafts [76] and triple-rule-out studies in acute chest pain [77]. Several studies have demonstrated a high diagnostic accuracy of prospectively ECG-triggered coronary CT angiography [74, 78, 79]. A heart rate threshold of up to 70 or 65 bpm is used in most of the studies performing ECG-triggered CTCA. Husmann et al. [80] reported that 98.9 % of all coronary artery segments were evaluative at heart rates of up to 63 bpm, while only 85 % were assessable at higher heart rates. Faster CT systems and advanced acquisition techniques may increase the heart rate threshold in prospectively gated CT above the level of 70 bpm, at a similar ability to assess coronary segments as in retrospective ECG gating [81].

In *prospective ECG-triggered CT*, the patient is irradiated only at selectable heart phases, and the table is moved in a sequential manner, remaining stationary while data are acquired. This leads to smaller effective patient dose of

1–3 mSv in adults [82] and 0.2–0.7 mSv in newborns and infants [83]. Limitations of this technique are the missing ability to assess the ventricular function and the impairment of the image quality in case of arrhythmia. Nevertheless, prospective ECG-triggered CT has almost completely replaced the retrospective ECG-gated acquisition in patients with CHD. For patients with heart rates <75 bpm, we predefine the data acquisition in the diastolic phase at 70 % relative to the R-R interval and for patients with a heart rate of more than 75 bpm in the systolic phase at 30 %. We still perform a retrospective ECG-gated CT – if ECG synchronization is required – in patients with arrhythmia and if multiphase functional evaluation is required.

Most recently, an adaptation of the prospective ECG-triggered CT technique to a dual-step mode has been introduced to provide ventricular functional analysis at low radiation dose [84].

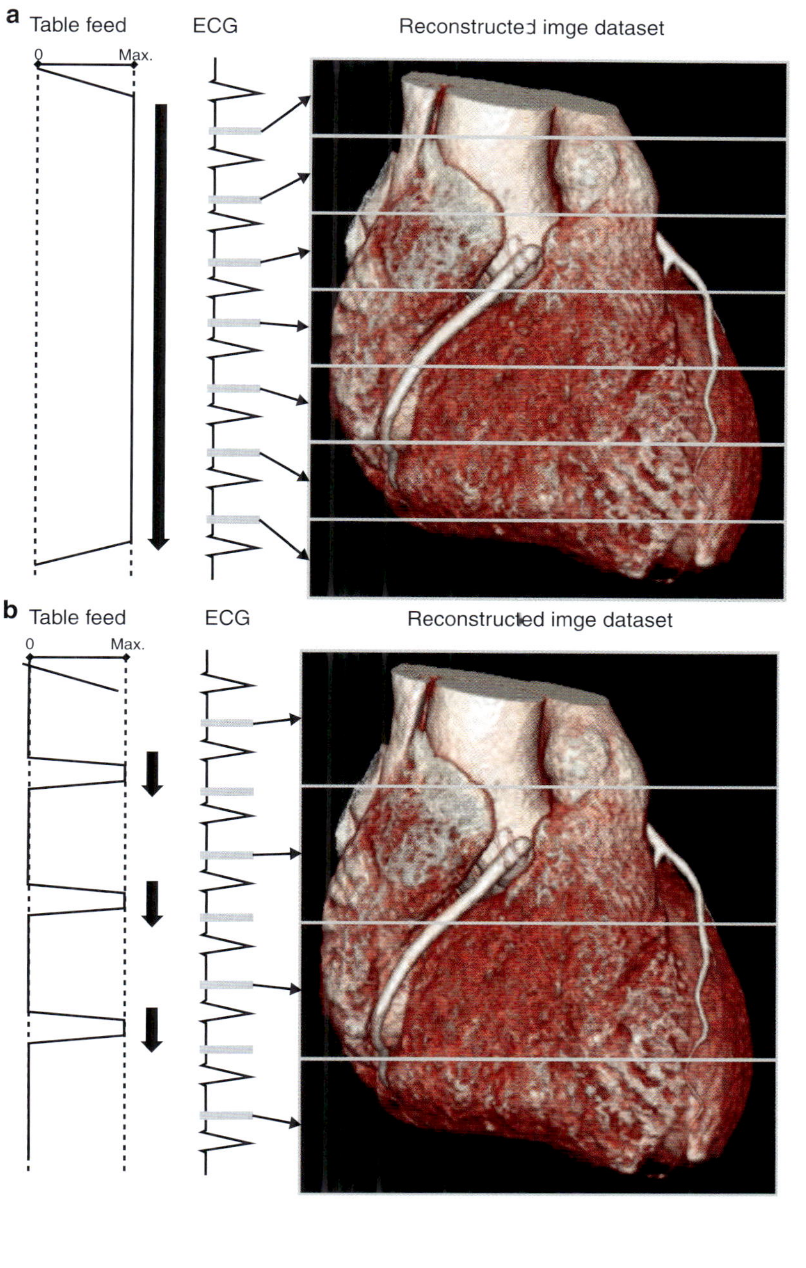

Fig. 5.4 (**a**) Retrospective ECG gating: The data acquisition is performed with continuous scanner table motion and spiral acquisition with overlap of the radiation beam on each spiral synchronized to the ECG. Then, in the retrospective, images are reconstructed in the optimal phase of the cardiac cycle providing the least motion artifacts. (**b**) Prospective ECG-triggered CT: The patient is irradiated only at selectable heart phases, and the table is moved in a sequential manner, remaining stationary while data are acquired. (**c**) High-pitch helical prospectively gated CT: This scanning mode permits cardiac CT to be performed in a small fraction of a single heartbeat. Because the high-pitch scan is limited to the diastole in a single heartbeat, the heart rhythm needs to be prospectively predicted

Fig. 5.4 (continued)

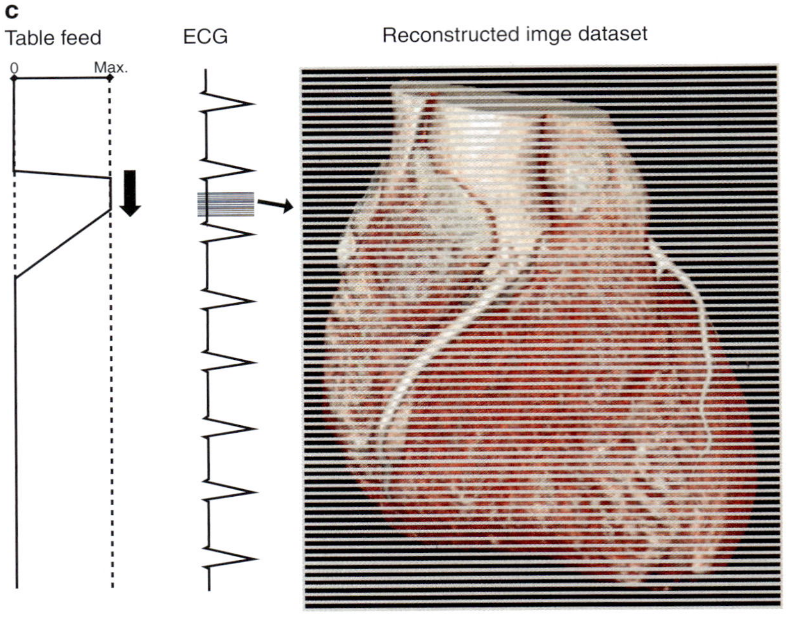

High-Pitch Helical Prospectively Gated CT

In order to gain sufficient projection data from image reconstruction in retrospectively ECG-gated cardiac CT, pitch is usually limited to low values of 0.2–0.5. Higher pitch values would result in less projection overlap. If the pitch is increased to more than 1.5, projection gaps will occur resulting in severe artifacts. In dual-source CT systems, the second tube-detector combination can fill these projection gaps occurring at high pitch values. Pitch values of 3.2–3.4 are feasible using a second-generation 128-slice dual-source CT system, leading to an acquisition time of approximately 250 ms (Fig. 5.4c). This permits cardiac CT to be performed in a small fraction of a single heartbeat. Because the high-pitch scan is limited to the diastole in a single heartbeat, the heart rhythm needs to be prospectively predicted. Therefore, it is essential for high-pitch helical prospectively gated CT to only be performed in patients with low and regular heart rates. Radiation dose is very low due to the short acquisition time and the little overlap between spiral acquisitions. Achenbach et al. [85] evaluated high-pitch helical prospectively gated CT in 50 patients with a body weight of less than 100 kg and a heart rate of 60 bpm or less with a resulting radiation dose of 0.9 mSv. Leschka et al. [86] reported a high diagnostic accuracy of high-pitch coronary CT angiography for the assessment of coronary artery stenosis at a submillisievert radiation dose. Alkadhi and colleagues [78] investigated the diagnostic performance of high-pitch cardiac CT in comparison to prospectively ECG-triggered CT in patients with a heart rate of less than 70 bpm and found similar diagnostic accuracies for the assessment of coronary artery stenosis at a 30 % lower radiation dose at high-pitch CT. In addition, high-pitch helical prospectively gated CT can be used to evaluate the coronary artery bypass graft patency at a low effective radiation dose of approximately 2.3 mSv [87].

Selection of Protocols Depending on the Type of CHD

The scan range and the acquisition mode and whether ECG synchronization is performed depend on the type of CHD to be investigated. Table 5.2 provides recommendations for CT protocols for different CHDs.

Contrast Agent Application

To avoid high-contrast artifacts in the left brachiocephalic vein, a right-arm contrast media

Table 5.2 Recommended scan range and ECG synchronization depending on the congenital heart disease type

Congenital heart disease type	Scan range	ECG synchronization required?	Comment
Aortic coarctation	Aortic arch to diaphragm	No	Thin collimation is recommended for identification of collateral pathways
Anomalous pulmonary venous return	Aortic arch to diaphragm	No	Scan range should be extended to the level of the kidneys in the infracardiac type
Patent ductus arteriosus	Aortic arch to diaphragm	No	Thin collimation is recommended for identification of small ductus arteriosus
Persistent superior left vena cava	Aortic arch to diaphragm	No	
Atrial septal defect	Below tracheal bifurcation to diaphragm	Yes	ECG synchronization may be beneficial for small intracardiac shunts
Ventricular septal defect	Below tracheal bifurcation to diaphragm	Yes	ECG synchronization may be beneficial for small intracardiac shunts
Tetralogy of Fallot	Above the pulmonary bifurcation to diaphragm	No	–
Common aortic-pulmonary trunk	Above the pulmonary bifurcation to diaphragm	No	–
Transposition of the great arteries	Above the pulmonary bifurcation to diaphragm	No	–
Univentricular heart	Below tracheal bifurcation to diaphragm	No	No saline chasing bolus should be used to avoid washout
Double outlet ventricle	Above the pulmonary bifurcation to diaphragm	No	No saline chasing bolus should be used to avoid washout
Isomerism	Below tracheal bifurcation to diaphragm	Yes	ECG synchronization is recommendable for morphological identification of the atrial appendages to determine sideness; the scan range must include the thorax and spleen for identification of extracardiac abnormalities
Coronary artery anomaly	Below tracheal bifurcation to diaphragm	Yes	Thin collimation and ECG synchronization are mandatory

injection is preferable. In neonates and young children, nonionic iodinated contrast agent is injected at a dose of 2 mL per kg body weight to a maximum amount of 100 mL. The injection rate is set at 1 mL/s but might be increased to 2 mL/s in patients with a large intracardiac communication. In adults, 1.5 mL/kg body weight is injected at a rate of 3–4 mL/s. A saline bolus should be applied after the injection of the contrast media to reduce the artifacts from undiluted contrast media and to reduce the total amount of contrast media. To determine the scan delay in ECG-synchronized CT, the bolus-tracking technique is advantageous. For this purpose, the region of interest (ROI) in pediatric patients is placed in the left ventricle, and a threshold attenuation of 200 HU is set. However, when in doubt about the intracardiac connections and the timing of the contrast attenuation of the different cardiac chambers, in the individual patient monitoring the arrival of contrast material in the cardiac chambers and manually starting the CT acquisition is often the safer way for sufficient contrast attenuation of the cardiac cavities and adjacent arteries and veins. In adult patients, the ROI is placed in the ascending or descending aorta, and the attenuation threshold is set at 140–180 HU.

When performing a non-ECG-synchronized CT in pediatric patients, a fixed scan delay is usually sufficient. The start delay is set on 12 s for peripheral injection and on 8 s for central venous injection.

Image Reconstruction and Postprocessing

On the axial images, the oblique orientation of the heart often leads to unfavorable cutting angles and partial volume effects. The image reconstruction technique used depends on the diagnostic task, and usually a combination of different visualization techniques is required. In addition, to facilitate the communication between the radiologist and the referring physician, the presentation of the findings should be adapted to the field of the referring physician. For example, while surgeons will prefer realistic 3D images simulating a surgical view, cardiologists are used to conventional angiographic images. To generate the desired presentation, axial data need to be processed.

Multiplanar Reformation (MPR)

MPR is a 2D postprocessing technique allowing to display one plane inside the original 3D image volume (Fig. 5.5). This plane may be orthogonal to the axial slices of the image volume (i.e., coronal or sagittal MPR), oblique, or replaced by an arbitrary curved surface (i.e., curved MPR). In cardiac CT oblique, MPR is often used to show the four-chamber view and the short-axis view. To display the complete course of a vessel in a single 2D image, curved MPR enables to align a course along the vessel centerline. Current dedicated workstations permit an automatic definition of the vessel centerline after the user has selected one or more seeding point inside the lumen of the vessel. A drawback of the curved MPR technique is that only a single vessel branch may be displayed at any time. MPR is the most popular method of reconstruction in cardiac CT. Due to its easy handling, MPR is least susceptible to wrong operation by the radiologist among all postprocessing techniques.

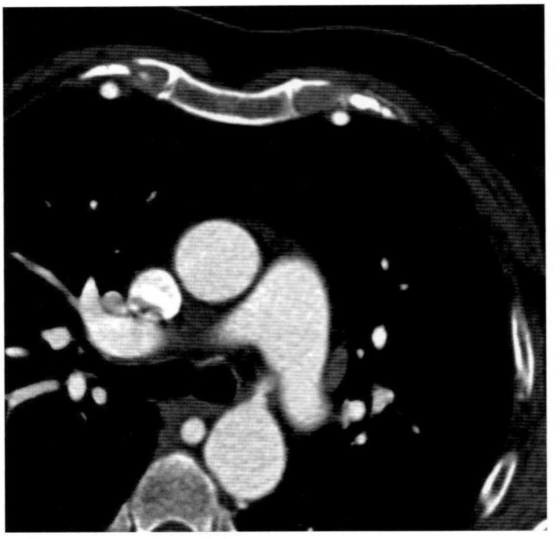

Fig. 5.5 Multiplanar reformation (MPR) technique in a patient with an aortic coarctation displaying one plane inside the original 3D image volume

Nevertheless, continuous adaptation of the reformatted planes is required to avoid improper plane orientation which might introduce false or mask pathological findings.

Maximum Intensity Projection (MIP)

MIP is the simplest 3D postprocessing technique. A virtual camera sends multiple beams through the 3D volume dataset, whereas only the highest-attenuation voxels are retained, allowing a fast display of a part of the total dataset. The parameters that have to be chosen are the window setting and the beam angulation which determine the viewing orientation. MIP is suited to display vascular structures in a single image (Fig. 5.6a). Sometimes, the significant information reduction in MIP proves to be a disadvantage. When applied to the entire image volume, the vascular structures can be overlaid and therefore be obscured with the cardiac cavities filled with contrast agent, high-attenuation pericardial metallic clips, or bones of the chest (Fig. 5.6b). Thin-slab MIP is a technique to remove high-attenuation voxels of surrounding structures from the rendering by cutting planes in front and behind a vessel. In defiance of these shortcomings, MIP has become an important complementary tool for the visualization of thoracic vasculature.

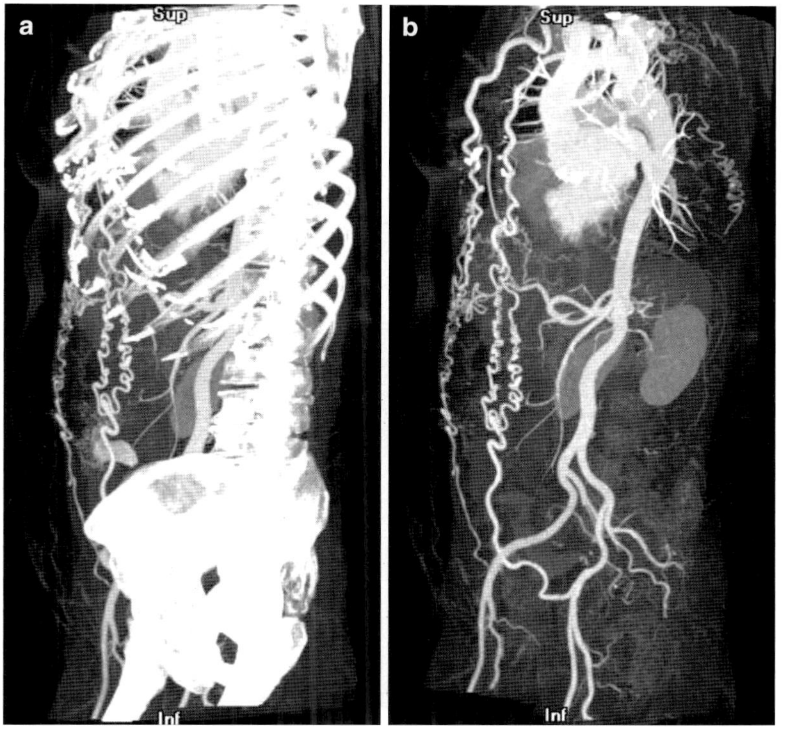

Fig. 5.6 (**a**) Maximum intensity projection (MIP) technique applied to the entire image volume in a patient with aortic coarctation. The bones obscure the vascular structures. (**b**) Thin-slab MIP in the same patient: The high-attenuation voxels of the bones are removed, leading to an improved visualization of the vascular structures and the collateral circulation in aortic coarctation

Direct Volume Rendering (DVR)

As in the MIP technique, a virtual camera sends multiple beams through the 3D volume dataset, but, in contrast to the MIP technique, a physically based model defines the attenuation properties of each voxel density encountered along the beam. A transfer function maps Hounsfield units to colors and opacities that are then integrated along the beam. Therefore, a color defines a distinct structure, and separate tissues can be classified and rendered from completely transparent to completely opaque. To enhance the 3D impression, the image volume usually is illuminated with a virtual external light. Direct volume rendering technique is able to produce realistic images and provides a good overview of the anatomy (Fig. 5.7a, b). In general, the multitude of parameters renders DVR a computationally intensive and time-consuming postprocessing technique. Albeit DVR being an excellent "nature-like" display of the cardiac and extracardiac structures for the referring physician, DVR is very susceptible to wrong operation by the radiologist and inappropriate setting may mask or artificially display a pathological finding.

Radiation Dose Issues

In any CT study, the ALARA principles ("as low as reasonable achievable"), i.e., dose reduction to the lowest value maintaining image quality at a diagnostic level, should be followed. The balance between low radiation dose and diagnostic image quality is the most crucial step in radiation dose reduction. If the CT study loses its diagnostic capability to answer the clinical question of interest due to excessive dose reduction, there is no benefit for the patient [88]. However, the application of more radiation dose than needed to answer the clinical question will unlikely increase the diagnostic capability of the study and may harm the patient [88]. The goal is to acquire at least diagnostic image quality and not best achievable image quality. To achieve this goal, familiarity with more noisy images is a must.

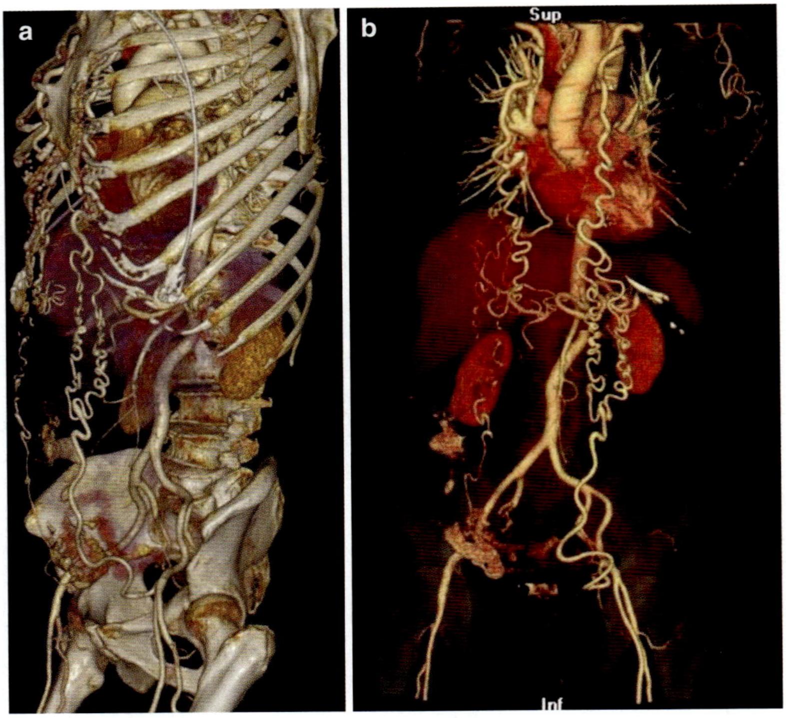

Fig. 5.7 (**a**) Direct volume rendering (DVR) technique in a patient with aortic coarctation clearly providing the anatomical details. (**b**) Direct volume rendering (DVR) technique in a patient with aortic coarctation: The opacity of the bone dense Hounsfield units is reduced displaying them transparent, leading to an excellent visualization of the vascular structures

PROTECTION I, a large international multicenter trial, has identified several predictors of higher radiation exposure in cardiac CT [89]. They included 1965 CT coronary angiography studies from 50 centers and estimated a median effective radiation dose of 12 mSv. Several predictors of higher radiation dose have been identified, such as increased body weight (5 % increase in radiation dose for a 10 kg increase in body weight), larger scan length (5 % increase in radiation dose for each cm scan length), or unstable heart rhythm (10 % increase in dose compared to sinus rhythm) [89]. The radiation dose saving potential of several techniques has been investigated too, ranging from 25 to 78 % of radiation dose reduction [89]. These techniques included the different acquisition modes concerning ECG and supplemental radiation dose reduction strategies. Interestingly, neither the number of performed coronary CT angiography nor the experience of a particular center had any significant effect on the radiation dose [89].

Compared to conventional coronary angiography (CCA), CT coronary angiography (CTCA) caused a higher radiation dose exposure. This was one of the most important obstacles for CTCA to become a standard tool in the cardiac imaging armamentarium. In a 16-slice CT radiation dose of a CTCA has been estimated of about 9 mSv [90]. The radiation dose substantially increased in 64-slice to approximately 15 mSv in men and 20 mSv in women [48]. The radiation dose estimates of CTCA were achieved when using common retrospective ECG triggering for phase synchronization. In CCA, the radiation dose is significantly lower, approximately 2.1–7 mSv [45, 91]. Improvements in CT technique offered a substantial dose reduction. Tube current modulation during the different phases of the cardiac cycle (ECG pulsing) is one possibility. During predefined phases of the cardiac cycle likely to be used for image reconstruction, a maximal tube current is applied. During the remaining phases, tube current is reduced [64]. Using this technique, radiation doses of 6.4 mSv for 16-slice CT [92], 9.4 mSv for 64-slice CT [92], and 8.8 mSv for dual-source CT [93] have been reported. The reduction of the tube voltage is another possibility to reduce radiation dose. A tube voltage of 80 kVp in slim patients with a body weight below 60 kg led to a dose saving potential of 88 % [94]. Tube voltages of 100 kVp have been successfully

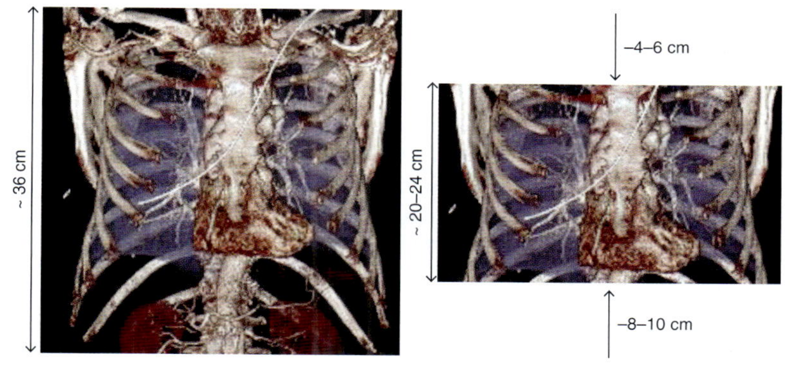

Fig. 5.8 Restriction of z-axis coverage: For patients with CHD CT acquisition from the aortic arch to the bottom of the heart is sufficient. Average reduction in scan length of 12–16 cm leads to a radiation dose saving potential of around 30 %

used in 16-slice CT [92], 64-slice CT [92], and dual-source CT [95, 96], reporting a dose saving potential of up to 40 %. This benefit is independent and incremental from radiation dose savings by using ECG pulsing.

The use of prospective ECG gating, so-called sequential cardiac scanning, is one of the most effective methods of radiation dose reduction in CTCA. This technique was first used in electron beam CTCA in 1995 [97]. X-ray is turned up during a short period of the cardiac cycle and turned down during rest of the cycle. It is recommended for patients with heart rates below 70 bpm. Several studies have reported excellent image quality [82, 98, 99] and diagnostic accuracy [74, 100] of prospectively ECG-gated CTCA at radiation doses of 1–3 mSv [74, 82, 98–100].

General Strategies for Reduction of Radiation Exposure

In most pediatric patients with a congenital heart disease, several follow-up studies will be performed during lifetime. Therefore, radiation dose reduction is of utmost importance in this patient group, even more than in adult patients.

Restriction of *Z*-Axis Coverage

The z-axis coverage is one of the largest contributors to radiation dose in CT imaging. For CHD patients with suspected malformations of the heart and the extracardiac vasculature, the CT acquisition could be frequently limited to a scan from immediately above the aortic arch to the bottom of the heart and does not need to cover the whole chest (Fig. 5.8). One drawback might be the limited ability to identify incidental findings including pulmonary nodules. However, reporting of incidental noncardiac findings in cardiac CT studies have been shown to increase surgical rates, costs, and patient's anxiety, all without proof of improvement in outcomes [101].

When imaging solely of the heart is intended, the scout view is rather inaccurate in determining the required z-axis coverage. Following the frequent recommendations of manufacturers to scan from the tracheal bifurcation to below the diaphragm will result in a large z-axis coverage with unnecessary imaging structures above and below the heart. In a recent study using scan length adjustment methods in retrospective ECG-gated cardiac CT, we demonstrated a dose reduction potential of 0.7 mSv per 1 cm reduction in scan range [102]. There are several options to more precisely define the needed scan range in z-axis than the manufacturers' recommendations. One possibility is to plan the scan range with the scout image but to start the scan from 1 to 2 cm below the tracheal bifurcation and to end the scan 1 cm below the cardiac apex. This will leave sufficient but not excessive margins above and below the cardiac margins to compensate for breathing movement [102, 103]. In CHD patients, depending on type of abnormality, larger scan coverage may be required beyond the heart boundaries to cover the entire anatomy (Table 5.2).

Application of Dedicated Cardiac Bowtie Filters

State-of-the-art CT systems provide implemented beam-shaping filter to limit the scan field of view (FoV) in order to reduce radiation intensity in the scan plane. Using this dedicated cardiac bowtie filter in CT studies focussed on cardiac pathologies permits for lower radiation exposure by limiting the scatter radiation of the X-rays toward the detectors, and it is more efficient to irradiate detectors directly across from the X-ray tube as less photons are required [104]. In cardiac CT, the heart is centered within the chest; consequently, the scan FoV can be limited to around 25 cm. Budoff has reported a dose reduction of 40 % by using a small field bowtie filter rather than a large field filter [104]. Thus, routine use of dedicated cardiac bowtie filter is recommendable for radiation dose reduction purpose and improves image quality. One drawback of limiting the scan FoV by small field bowtie filters might be the reduced image quality outside the scan FoV and though of incidental noncardiac findings. However, in our experience, an adequate diagnosis of associated extracardiac pathologies and malformations remains still feasible.

Protection of Radiosensitive Organs

Bismuth shields have been introduced for chest CT to reduce radiation exposure to superficial radiosensitive organs (i.e., the breast and thyroid glands), and significant radiation dose reductions of 29–57 % have been reported using these shields [105, 106]. For cardiac CT, the available data of using these shields is limited. In calcium scoring a decrease in radiation dose of 37 % to the breast has been reported [107]. However, Geleijns and colleagues [108] demonstrated that the organ dose reduction can more efficiently be obtained by optimizing the tube current. In addition, use of these bismuth shields may interfere with anatomy-based tube current modulation techniques with the risk of totally increased radiation exposure to the children. At current, no valid data exist of the radiation dose reduction potential and potential negative effects on noise and signal-to-noise ratio for dedicated cardiac CT. We therefore do not use this technique in our institution.

Optimization of Tube Voltage

The effects of changing the tube voltage settings are less predictable than those of changing the tube current. Changes in tube voltage affect the peak photon energy and radiation exposure approximately varies with the square of the peak tube voltage. The effect of lower tube voltage on image quality and radiation dose has been investigated by several studies. Abada et al. [94] used an 80-kVp tube voltage setting in 11 slim patients with a body weight of less than 60 kg and reported a radiation dose reduction of 88 % compared to the standard 120-kVp tube voltage. Leschka et al. [95] reported a dose reduction of 25 % in 100 kVp retrospectively ECG-gated cardiac CT in normal-weighted patients (BMI <25 kg/sqm). In the PROTECTION I trial [89], the radiation dose of 100-kVp cardiac CT was associated with a radiation dose reduction of 46 % compared to 120-kVp studies. Interestingly, tube voltage reduction does not only affect the radiation dose but additionally affects the contrast attenuation of iodine and consequently the contrast opacification of the coronary arteries. This effect is caused by an increase in the photoelectric effect and a decrease in Compton scattering. As a consequence, the attenuation of the contrast in the coronary arteries is approximately one quarter to one third higher at 100 kVp than it is at 120 kVp, leading to a higher signal-to-noise ratio (SNR) [95]. The increased contrast opacification offers the possibility to reduce the amount of intravenous contrast medium by around one third. Likewise, the higher SNR in low kVp examinations can be used to additionally reduce the tube current by accepting more image noise because of the higher SNR and thereby further reducing the radiation dose [95].

Optimization of Tube Current

The tube current directly affects the number of generated photons. This leads to a predictable effect on radiation dose and image noise. In fact, the tube current alterations are approximately proportional to the radiation dose and the image noise. Therefore, tube current optimization offers an effective opportunity to reduce the radiation dose. In most CT systems, the vendor's default settings often use too high tube current for best image quality at the expense of the radiation dose [104]. In obese patients, standard tube current

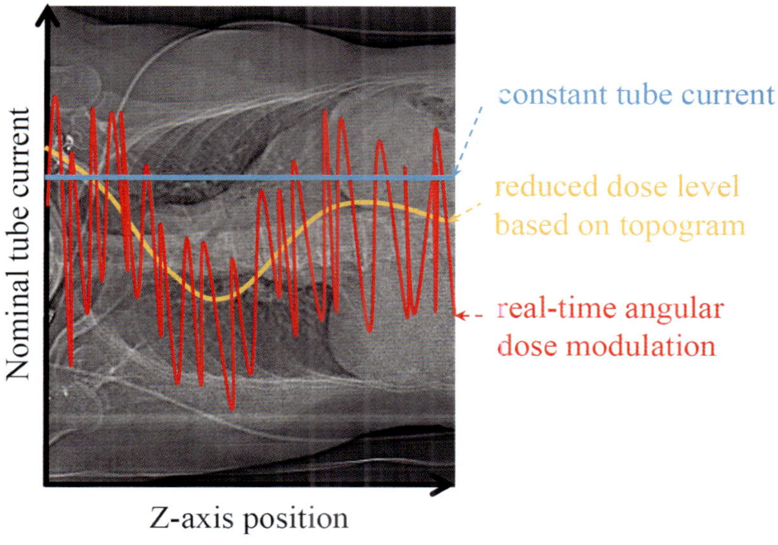

Fig. 5.9 Anatomy-based tube current modulation: The tube current is automatically and real-time adjusted based on the noise of the previous image

needs to be increased in order to compensate for higher photon scatter and higher image noise. In contrast, thinner patients are exposed to an unnecessary high dose if standard tube current settings are used because X-ray attenuation is lower in slim patients.

Anatomy-Based Tube Current Modulation

Anatomy-based tube current modulation has been developed for body CT [109]. It modulates the radiation dose according to the patient's morphology in the scan plane or in the *z*-axis or both (Fig. 5.9) thus aiming to facilitate the optimization of image quality and radiation exposure and thereby eliminating arbitrary selection of tube current by CT technologists and radiologists. The user only selects the reference noise index (i.e., GE), the reference image acquisition (i.e., Philips), the reference tube current-time product (i.e., Siemens), or the reference standard deviation of attenuation (i.e., Toshiba) and then the tube current is adjusted so that all images will have a similar user-selected quantum noise level independent of patient size and anatomy. The tube current modulation for each anatomic region is automatically determined with calculations of patient density, size, and shape (beam attenuation) performed by using a single scout projection acquired before the actual examination and a set of empirically determined noise prediction coefficients. A dose reduction of up to 40 % has been reported in chest CT [110].

ECG-Based Tube Current Modulation

For retrospectively ECG-gated cardiac CT, the full tube current can be restricted to a certain part of the cardiac cycle because data from the high movement periods of the cardiac cycle (ventricular contraction in mid- to end-systole and atrial contraction in end-diastole) are frequently not required for image reconstruction. The ECG-controlled tube current modulation ("ECG pulsing") considers this by limiting the nominal full tube current to a predefined interval within the cardiac cycle while reducing the tube current in the remaining part of the cardiac cycle to 20 % or less of the normal output [111]. The image quality is impaired by noise outside the full tube current window thereby rendering those phases of the cardiac cycle inadequate for detailed morphological evaluation but provide sufficient image quality for ventricular functional analysis. Due to technological advances of CT systems, especially the higher temporal resolution, the ECG-controlled tube current modulation is appropriate for daily use. In the PROTECTION I trial, ECG pulsing was used in 73 % of studies with a dose reduction of 25 % [89]. In another study, ECG pulsing was used in 82 % of patients in daily routine without substantial impairment of image quality [92]. Unfortunately, the anatomy-based tube current modulation is not completely compatible with ECG-synchronized protocols due to interference with the ECG pulsing [104, 112].

Patients with irregular or high heart rate might not benefit from ECG-controlled tube current modulation because optimal reconstruction might not be predefined in the case of premature heartbeat or additional systolic reconstruction might be required in high heart rate. Advanced ECG pulsing algorithms automatically detect heart rhythm irregularities, and then stopping ECG pulsing in real time during acquisition is currently provided by different vendors of CT systems. Otherwise, there needs to be a trade-off between ECG pulsing settings and the heart rate. For patients with higher heart rates, automatic or manual adjustment of the full tube current width of ECG pulsing are available in order to widen the pulsing width in patients at higher heart rates to include the systole [64]. In contrary, at low and stable heart rates pulsing width can be used as narrow as possible in the mid-diastole [64].

The efficiency of ECG-controlled tube current modulation for radiation dose reduction depends on the heart rate and on the number of sources (single- or dual-source CT). In single-source CT, ECG pulsing is most efficient at a low heart rate, while in higher heart rate, the efficiency decreases because of subsequent widening of the full tube current window. In contrast, in dual-source CT higher heart rates are associated with a lower radiation dose because the negative effect of higher pulsing width is compensated by the heart rate-adapted pitch of dual-source CT with a pitch of 0.5 at above 80 bpm compared to a pitch of 0.2 at below 60 bpm [93]. Optimal ECG pulsing window settings for cardiac CT depend on the patient's heart rate and have been recommended as follows [64]: 60–70 % of the R-R interval at heart rates ≤60 bpm, 60–80 % at heart rates of 60–70 bpm, 55–80 % at heart rates of 70–80 bpm, and 30–80 % at heart rates >80 bpm. The ECG pulsing technique has been reported to reduce the radiation dose by up to 64 % [113]. Figure 5.10 provides a schematic demonstration of the tube current application in the different acquisition modes.

Iterative Reconstruction

Recently, iterative image reconstruction algorithms have been introduced into CT imaging by different vendors. The commonly used filtered back projection technique for image reconstruction has limitations regarding image noise and requires a higher amount of photons to achieve adequate signal-to-noise ratios [88]. In contrast, iterative reconstruction algorithms provide higher flexibility for accurate physical noise modeling and geometric system description [114]. Leipsic and colleagues [115] demonstrated an image noise reduction of up to 43 % when using iterative instead of filtered back projection reconstruction. By using iterative reconstruction with lower image noise than filtered back projection, tube current can be reduced by approximately the same rate to keep relative image noise maintained, while radiation dose is reduced. A recent multicenter trial performed in 1,202 consecutive patients demonstrated that iterative reconstruction permits a radiation dose reduction of 44 % in average compared to filtered back projection, while image interpretability and SNR were similar between both reconstruction techniques [116].

Practical Approach to the Use of Radiation Dose Reduction Techniques

Patient-specific parameters such as body habitus and heart rate need to be used in clinical routine for efficient application of radiation dose reduction strategies without sacrificing the diagnostic capability of the cardiac CT study.

Selection of the Acquisition Mode

Non-ECG-synchronized CT is commonly sufficient for CT work-up of most CHD types (Table 5.2). When ECG synchronization is required, the most important parameter for selection of the acquisition mode is the heart rate. If available, high-pitch prospectively ECG-gated helical CT should be performed in patients with a heart rate of 60 bpm or less and when the heart rate is stable (i.e., maximum of 2 bpm changes in heart rate between heartbeats). Prospectively

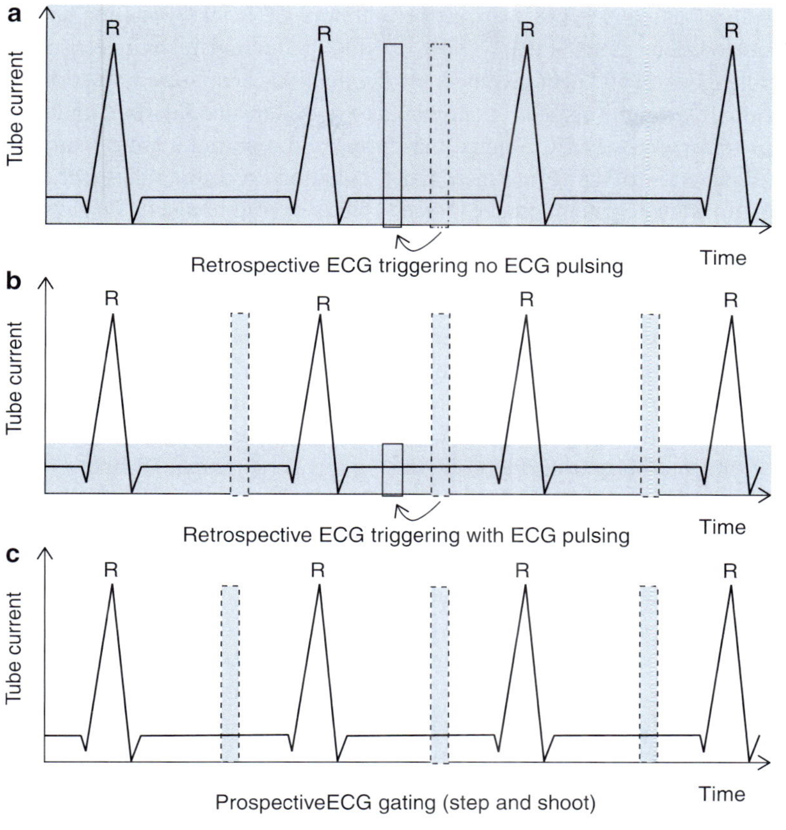

Fig. 5.10 (**a**) Retrospective ECG triggering without ECG pulsing: Full tube current is applied during the entire cardiac cycle. Images can be reconstructed in any phase of the cardiac cycle at the same image noise level. (**b**) Retrospective ECG triggering with ECG pulsing: Full tube current is only applied in predefined parts of the cardiac cycle and reduced in the remainder. Images can be reconstructed at low noise level in the full tube current parts but at higher noise in the cardiac cycle parts with reduced tube current output. (**c**) Prospectively ECG-triggered sequential CT: The CT table is stationary during image acquisition and moves in the following heartbeat to the next position for the next sequential scan ("step-and-shoot mode"). The reconstruction time point within the cardiac cycle has to be defined prior to the image acquisition

ECG-gated sequential CT can be used for all patients with a heart rate of 70 bpm or less and when there is only minor heart rate variability (i.e., maximum of 4 bpm changes in heart rate between heartbeats).

Retrospectively ECG-triggered helical CT remains the alternative CT mode in all patients with a heart rate above 70 bpm or in patients with severe heart rate irregularities. Modern CT systems are capable of compensating heart rate irregularities when ECG pulsing is applied. Therefore, ECG-controlled tube current modulation should be used whenever retrospective ECG-triggered cardiac CT is performed. In addition, retrospectively ECG-triggered helical CT is the preferred acquisition mode when ventricular functional analysis is required.

Individual Adaptation of Tube Current and Tube Voltage Settings

A practical approach for individual adaptation of tube current and tube voltage for radiation dose reduction is to divide patients into three categories (slim, normal weight, and overweight) and define parameters for each category. Manual selection of scanning parameter settings for individual patients might be based on the body weight [117], body mass index (BMI) [96], the anteroposterior chest diameter [118], or on the image noise from previous scans [112].

Jung and colleagues [117] demonstrated by using an individually weight-adapted examination protocol in retrospectively ECG-gated cardiac CT a dose reduction of 18 % for men and 26 % for women, while constant image noise was achieved and diagnostic image quality was preserved.

The chest diameter is a strong indicator of higher radiation dose with a difference of 5 cm in the diameter corresponds to a factor of two or more higher radiation dose required for the same image noise [119]. Rogalla et al. [118] investigated the use of the anteroposterior diameter for selection of tube current in cardiac CT and found a lower interindividual image noise variation when using the diameter instead of the BMI for tube current adaptation. However, there are considerable differences in chest attenuation between men and women, and there are large interindividual differences in fat distribution.

Paul and Abada [112] have introduced a noise-based approach for the adaptation of tube current and tube voltage in cardiac CT. Their principle is to calculate the noise from a low-dose pre-control scan (120 kVp, 20 mAs) at the bottom part of the heart as reference and then adjust tube voltage and tube current in six different settings to acquire cardiac CT with sufficient image quality for interpretation at a low dose level. This approach might be the most practical and dose efficient for adaptation of tube current and tube voltage because individual body morphology at the heart level is directly translated into scanning parameter settings.

Combined Approaches

In general, the highest radiation dose reduction is obtained when the radiation dose reduction techniques are used in a combined approach. LaBounty and colleagues [120] prospectively evaluated patients before and after initiation of different dose reduction techniques including BMI and heart rate-based protocols and scan length reduction and found 20 % reduction in radiation dose for each 100-mA reduction in tube current. Raff et al. [121] evaluated a large cohort of 4,995 patients and applied several dose reduction techniques such as scan length reduction, heart rate reduction, ECG-controlled tube current modulation, and reduced tube voltage and reported a more than 50 % reduction in radiation dose compared with the control period, while overall image quality was maintained. One simple and straightforward approach has been published by Alkadhi and colleagues [96]. The authors used the heart rate and the BMI to select the acquisition mode and the tube current and tube voltage settings. In 150 consecutive patients, the radiation dose potential was up to 88 % in selected patients with low heart rate and low BMI and was more than 50 % in average for the study population compared to an otherwise applied retrospectively ECG-gated standard cardiac CT protocol.

Specific Considerations for CT Imaging in Pediatric Patients with CHD

Imaging of pediatric patients is for some reasons different from imaging adult patients with CHD including the patient preparation procedure, the contrast agent application, and the CT scanning parameters and acquisition mode. Notably, radiation dose reduction is of utmost importance in children because they have greater radiosensitivity, a longer life expectancy, and might require several follow-up studies during lifetime.

Patient Information and Preparation

Preprocedure preparation is the most important step of the examining pediatric CHD patients. Failure and ambiguity in the preparation will prevent a successful CT study. The specific factors that have to be taken into account in preprocedure preparation are:

- The age and developmental stage of the child or young person
- Previous experiences with CT imaging
- Anxiety level and coping styles
- The role and anxiety of the parents

For the children, the CT study can be a situation of high psychological stress, as the examination procedure might be unknown to the children and is performed in an unfamiliar technical environment and in the presence of unknown persons. In addition, painful sensations might occur before and during the CT study including the placing of the IV access line and the contrast agent injection. Therefore, preparation of the children for the CT examination should include a psychological preparation to provide information and reduce anxiety. One of the most important goals in the preprocedure preparation of children is to attain its agreement to perform the CT study, and this could in our experience only be obtained by gaining a confiding relationship to the child.

For the parents, the CT study of their children could be a distressing event as well, because they have to experience their children lying in the CT system, and they may fear the result from the examination. The radiologist should take some time to explain the CT examination to the parents and to answer all questions that may arise. One has to bear in mind that anxiety of the parents is easily transferred to the children. Information to the parents and children should be provided about the imaging procedure itself (i.e., steps that the children must perform and steps that healthcare professionals will perform), and the sensations the children can expect to feel (e.g., pain when placing the IV access, warmness, and taste sensations when the iodinated contrast agent is injected). The information for the parents should also include information of the applied radiation exposure and the potential risk for the children. Parents are frequently informed from press releases about the potential risk of CT imaging and are often concerned about the increased lifetime risk of cancer. Larson and colleagues [122] investigated how parents' understanding and willingness to permit their children to undergo CT imaging change after receiving information regarding radiation exposure and potential risk. Of the 100 parents who have been surveyed, their willingness to have their child undergo the CT examination did not significantly changed, and 62 % of patients reported no change in level of concern after reading the handout [122]. In our experience, a brief informational handout or a one-on-one interview with the radiologist can improve the parental understanding of the potential risk of cancer related to pediatric CT without causing parents to refuse the CT study recommended by the referring physician.

The preparation and information of the children needs to be age-dependent. In our experience, it is often very helpful to simulate the CT examination prior to the image acquisition with the children or his favorite toy in order that the children becomes used to the procedures and the ambience. In addition – especially when imaging young children – the technical environment can be made more appropriate for children by using painted curtains, wall paintings, or placing stuffed animals around the CT machine. In our experience, the children's agreement to perform the CT study is increased when the different steps of the procedure are explained to them by their parents – after detailed instruction of the parents by the radiologist. The presence of one or both of the parents in the CT room will help the children to feel as safe and secure as possible.

Sedation

Sedation of pediatric patients is not recommended on a routine basis but depends on the children's age and anxiety.

Infants (0–12 Months Old)

In this age, CT examination can be frequently done without medical sedation using the "natural sleep" phase, which may be induced by feeding in a serene and comfortable environment beginning 30–40 min prior to the CT study. The presence of familiar objects such as a favorite blanket, toy, or pacifier can help comfort the children.

Sleeping infants will be covered in a prewarmed cotton blanket and placed in a lateral position on the CT table with the head placed on a soft pillow. Additional cotton blankets will be positioned close to the front and back of the infant to avoid movement. In small infants, in

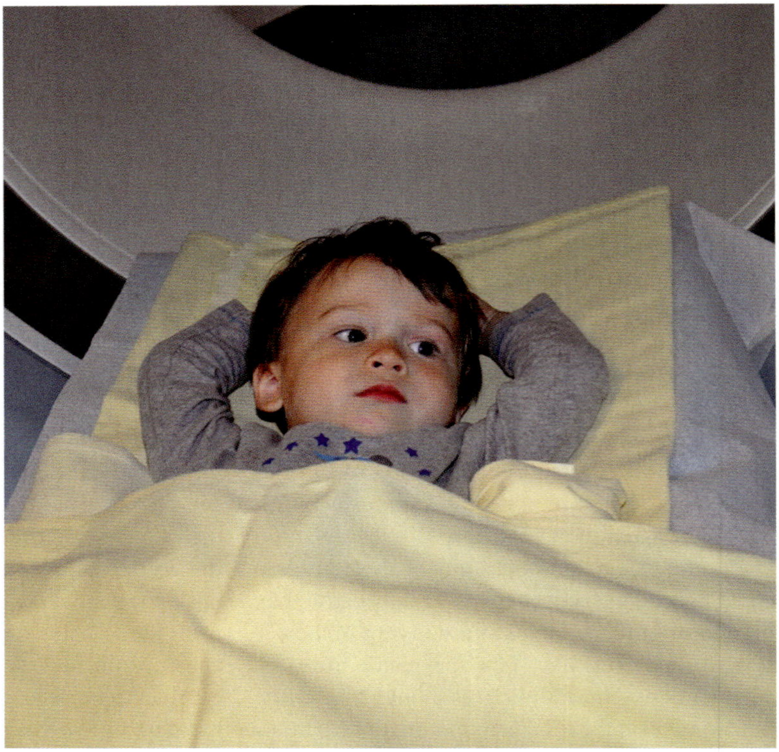

Fig. 5.11 A 2-year-old preschool child is placed in a comfortable position and "fixed" in warm blankets for the CT acquisition. In this case, no medicamentous sedation was required

whom the feeding-induced natural sleep failed, the need of medical sedation could be frequently prevented by short-time fixation using a vacuum pillow. This pillow is composed of an airtight flexible cover filled with small solid polystyrene balls which can easily be wrapped around the baby and provides firm but soft fixation [123]. However, the medicolegal and ethical aspects of short-time fixation versus medical sedation being different among countries need to be addressed. In addition, the advantages and disadvantages of a short-time fixation versus medical sedation need to be discussed with the parents.

Toddlers and Preschool Children (1–5 Years Old)

Toddlers and older children are placed in a supine position on the CT table. Warm blankets on the side will help to attain the children in a comfortable position and thereby reduce the ability to move during the data acquisition often without the children is being aware of this 'fixation' (Fig. 5.11). In this age, the parents have commonly the best access to their children, and the preprocedure information talk with the parents should help the parents to assure the children to perform the CT study. Nevertheless, in this age group, there is the largest need of sedation. If sedation is necessary, we prefer a short-term bodyweight-adapted sedation with midazolam hydrochloride via the rectal route (Table 5.3).

School Age and Older (6+ Years)

One of the most important steps in preparing children of this age is to attain its agreement to perform the CT study. In common, this agreement is not obtained *via* the parents like in younger children but by the performing radiologist directly convincing the children. In this age group, there are also more gender-specific differences in the information talk: While girls are more likely convinced with the consideration of *looking inside their body*, boys are usually more interested to learn about the *secrets of the technique* of the CT system. In general, sedation could be most often avoided in this age group.

Table 5.3 Scheme for rectal application of midazolam depending on the children's body weight

Body weight (kg)	Dose (mg)
<5	No application of midazolam
5–6	2.5
6–8	3
8–10	4
10–12	5
12–14	6
14–16	7
16–18	8
18–20	9
20–30	10

Table 5.4 Relevant CT parameters for imaging pediatric patients with congenital heart disease using a dual-source CT system

Slice collimation	Thin collimation: 2×64×0.6 mm Thick collimation: 2×24×1.2 mm
Tube voltage/ tube current	<20 kg: 80 kVp/50 mAs 20–30 kg: 80 kVp/80 mAs 30–50 kg: 80 kVp/150 mAs 50–60 kg: 80 kVp/250 mAs
Gantry rotation time	330 ms
Pitch	1 (non-ECG-synchronized CT) 0.2–0.5 (retrospective ECG-gated CT; pitch depending on the heart rate)

Radiation Dose Issues

In common, ECG-synchronized CT is not used in the pediatric work-up due to its higher radiation dose. The larger cardiac structures are affected by motion only to a minor degree; therefore, ECG synchronization does not significantly improve the image quality. Moreover, ECG-synchronized CT is associated with a longer scan time, and therefore, motion artifacts due to respiration or body motion might be more crucial than the beneficial effects of cardiac motion suppression in pediatric patients.

CT imaging for CHD in neonates and children should always be performed at an 80-kVp setting. Cardiac CT with a tube voltage of 80 kVp has been successfully performed in adults with a body weight below 60 kg [94]. In children, CT with 80 kVp provides sufficient image quality when the tube current output is adapted to the patient's body weight (Table 5.4). Besides the advantage of saving radiation dose, the 80-kVp setting provides to reduce the total amount of contrast agent because iodine has a higher attenuation at lower energy. In addition, non-ECG-synchronized CT is the preferred CT technique in neonates and children because of the higher heart rates in those patients and the shorter acquisition times of non-ECG-synchronized CT which results in fewer respiratory artifacts. If an ECG synchronization technique is required, the CT protocol should be performed with very narrow ECG pulsing window width to limit the radiation exposure.

References

1. Goo HW, Park IS, Ko JK, et al. CT of congenital heart disease: normal anatomy and typical pathologic conditions. Radiographics. 2003;23(Spec No):S147–65.
2. Goo HW. State-of-the-art CT, imaging techniques for congenital heart disease. Korean J Radiol. 2010; 11(1):4–18.
3. Berrington de Gonzalez A, Mahesh M, Kim KP, et al. Projected cancer risks from computed tomographic scans performed in the United States in 2007. Arch Intern Med. 2009;169(22):2071–7.
4. Lindsten J. Nobel lectures, physiology or medicine 1971–1980. Singapore: World Scientific Publishing Co.; 1992.
5. Moller JH, Taubert KA, Allen HD, Clark EB, Lauer RM. Cardiovascular health and disease in children: current status. A Special Writing Group from the Task Force on Children and Youth, American Heart Association. Circulation. 1994;89(2):923–30.
6. Wren C, O'Sullivan JJ. Survival with congenital heart disease and need for follow up in adult life. Heart. 2001;85(4):438–43.
7. Karlo C, Leschka S, Goetti RP, et al. High-pitch dual-source CT angiography of the aortic valve-aortic root complex without ECG-synchronization. Eur Radiol. 2011;21(1):205–12.
8. Flohr TG, McCollough CH, Bruder H, et al. First performance evaluation of a dual-source CT (DSCT) system. Eur Radiol. 2006;16(2):256–68.
9. Flohr TG, Schoepf UJ, Ohnesorge BM. Chasing the heart: new developments for cardiac CT. J Thorac Imaging. 2007;22(1):4–16.
10. Kachelriess M, Ulzheimer S, Kalender WA. ECG-correlated image reconstruction from subsecond multi-slice spiral CT scans of the heart. Med Phys. 2000;27(8):1881–902.
11. Nieman K, Rensing BJ, van Geuns RJ, et al. Non-invasive coronary angiography with multislice spiral computed tomography: impact of heart rate. Heart. 2002;88(5):470–4.

12. Kacmaz F, Ozbulbul NI, Alyan O, et al. Imaging of coronary artery anomalies: the role of multidetector computed tomography. Coron Artery Dis. 2008;19(3):203–9.
13. Mochizuki T, Murase K, Koyama Y, Higashino H, Ikezoe J. LAD stenosis detected by subsecond spiral CT. Circulation. 1999;99(11):1523.
14. Mochizuki T, Koyama Y, Tanaka H, Ikezoe J, Shen Y, Azemoto S. Images in cardiovascular medicine. Left ventricular thrombus detected by two- and three-dimensional computed tomographic ventriculography: a new application of helical CT. Circulation. 1998;98(9):933–4.
15. Mochizuki T, Murase K, Higashino H, Koyama Y, Azemoto S, Ikezoe J. Images in cardiovascular medicine. Demonstration of acute myocardial infarction by subsecond spiral computed tomography: early defect and delayed enhancement. Circulation. 1999; 99(15):2058–9.
16. Becker CR, Knez A, Leber A, et al. Detection of coronary artery stenoses with multislice helical CT angiography. J Comput Assist Tomogr. 2002; 26(5):750–5.
17. Dirksen MS, Jukema JW, Bax JJ, et al. Cardiac multidetector-row computed tomography in patients with unstable angina. Am J Cardiol. 2005; 95(4):457–61.
18. Gaudio C, Mirabelli F, Alessandra L, et al. Noninvasive assessment of coronary artery stenoses by multidetector-row spiral computed tomography: comparison with conventional angiography. Eur Rev Med Pharmacol Sci. 2005;9(1):13–21.
19. Herzog C, Ay M, Engelmann K, et al. Visualization techniques in multislice CT-coronary angiography of the heart. Correlations of axial, multiplanar, three-dimensional and virtual endoscopic imaging with the invasive diagnosis. Rofo. 2001;173(4):341–9.
20. Kopp AF, Schroeder S, Kuettner A, et al. Non-invasive coronary angiography with high resolution multidetector-row computed tomography. Results in 102 patients. Eur Heart J. 2002;23(21):1714–25.
21. Leber AW, Knez A, Becker C, et al. Non-invasive intravenous coronary angiography using electron beam tomography and multislice computed tomography. Heart. 2003;89(6):633–9.
22. Morgan-Hughes GJ, Marshall AJ, Roobottom CA. Multislice computed tomographic coronary angiography: experience in a UK centre. Clin Radiol. 2003;58(5):378–83.
23. Nieman K, Oudkerk M, Rensing BJ, et al. Coronary angiography with multi-slice computed tomography. Lancet. 2001;357(9256):599–603.
24. Nieman K, Rensing BJ, van Geuns RJ, et al. Usefulness of multislice computed tomography for detecting obstructive coronary artery disease. Am J Cardiol. 2002;89(8):913–8.
25. Cademartiri F, Runza G, Marano R, et al. Diagnostic accuracy of 16-row multislice CT angiography in the evaluation of coronary segments. Radiol Med. 2005; 109(1–2):91–7.
26. Hoffmann MH, Shi H, Schmitz BL, et al. Noninvasive coronary angiography with multislice computed tomography. JAMA. 2005;293(20):2471–8.
27. Hoffmann U, Moselewski F, Cury RC, et al. Predictive value of 16-slice multidetector spiral computed tomography to detect significant obstructive coronary artery disease in patients at high risk for coronary artery disease: patient-versus segment-based analysis. Circulation. 2004;110(17):2638–43.
28. Kuettner A, Beck T, Drosch T, et al. Diagnostic accuracy of noninvasive coronary imaging using 16-detector slice spiral computed tomography with 188 ms temporal resolution. J Am Coll Cardiol. 2005;45(1):123–7.
29. Kuettner A, Trabold T, Schroeder S, et al. Noninvasive detection of coronary lesions using 16-detector multislice spiral computed tomography technology: initial clinical results. J Am Coll Cardiol. 2004;44(6):1230–7.
30. Martuscelli E, Romagnoli A, D'Eliseo A, et al. Accuracy of thin-slice computed tomography in the detection of coronary stenoses. Eur Heart J. 2004;25(12):1043–8.
31. Mollet NR, Cademartiri F, Krestin GP, et al. Improved diagnostic accuracy with 16-row multi-slice computed tomography coronary angiography. J Am Coll Cardiol. 2005;45(1):128–32.
32. Mollet NR, Cademartiri F, Nieman K, et al. Multislice spiral computed tomography coronary angiography in patients with stable angina pectoris. J Am Coll Cardiol. 2004;43(12):2265–70.
33. Paul JF, Ohanessian A, Caussin C, et al. Visualization of coronary tree and detection of coronary artery stenosis using 16-slice, sub-millimeter computed tomography: preliminary experience. Arch Mal Coeur Vaiss. 2004;97(1):31–6.
34. Schuijf JD, Bax JJ, Salm LP, et al. Noninvasive coronary imaging and assessment of left ventricular function using 16-slice computed tomography. Am J Cardiol. 2005;95(5):571–4.
35. Garcia MJ, Lessick J, Hoffmann MH. Accuracy of 16-row multidetector computed tomography for the assessment of coronary artery stenosis. JAMA. 2006;296(4):403–11.
36. Stolzmann P, Knight J, Desbiolles L, et al. Remodelling of the aortic root in severe tricuspid aortic stenosis: implications for transcatheter aortic valve implantation. Eur Radiol. 2009;19(6):1316–23.
37. Halpern EJ, Mallya R, Sewell M, Shulman M, Zwas DR. Differences in aortic valve area measured with CT planimetry and echocardiography (continuity equation) are related to divergent estimates of left ventricular outflow tract area. AJR Am J Roentgenol. 2009;192(6):1668–73.
38. Shah RG, Novaro GM, Blandon RJ, Whiteman MS, Asher CR, Kirsch J. Aortic valve area: meta-analysis of diagnostic performance of multi-detector computed tomography for aortic valve area measurements as compared to transthoracic echocardiography. Int J Cardiovasc Imaging. 2009;25(6):601–9.

39. Alkadhi H, Desbiolles L, Husmann L, et al. Aortic regurgitation: assessment with 64-section CT. Radiology. 2007;245(1):111–21.
40. Boehm T, Husmann L, Leschka S, Desbiolles L, Marincek B, Alkadhi H. Image quality of the aortic and mitral valve with CT: relative versus absolute delay reconstruction. Acad Radiol. 2007;14(5):613–24.
41. Alkadhi H, Desbiolles L, Stolzmann P, et al. Mitral annular shape, size, and motion in normals and in patients with cardiomyopathy: evaluation with computed tomography. Invest Radiol. 2009;44(4):218–25.
42. Ehara M, Surmely JF, Kawai M, et al. Diagnostic accuracy of 64-slice computed tomography for detecting angiographically significant coronary artery stenosis in an unselected consecutive patient population: comparison with conventional invasive angiography. Circ J. 2006;70(5):564–71.
43. Leber AW, Knez A, von Ziegler F, et al. Quantification of obstructive and nonobstructive coronary lesions by 64-slice computed tomography: a comparative study with quantitative coronary angiography and intravascular ultrasound. J Am Coll Cardiol. 2005;46(1):147–54.
44. Leschka S, Alkadhi H, Plass A, et al. Accuracy of MSCT coronary angiography with 64-slice technology: first experience. Eur Heart J. 2005;26(15):1482–7.
45. Mollet NR, Cademartiri F, van Mieghem CA, et al. High-resolution spiral computed tomography coronary angiography in patients referred for diagnostic conventional coronary angiography. Circulation. 2005;112(15):2318–23.
46. Nikolaou K, Knez A, Rist C, et al. Accuracy of 64-MDCT in the diagnosis of ischemic heart disease. AJR Am J Roentgenol. 2006;187(1):111–7.
47. Ong AT, Serruys PW, Mohr FW, et al. The SYNergy between percutaneous coronary intervention with TAXus and cardiac surgery (SYNTAX) study: design, rationale, and run-in phase. Am Heart J. 2006;151(6):1194–204.
48. Pugliese F, Mollet NR, Runza G, et al. Diagnostic accuracy of non-invasive 64-slice CT coronary angiography in patients with stable angina pectoris. Eur Radiol. 2006;16(3):575–82.
49. Raff GL, Gallagher MJ, O'Neill WW, Goldstein JA. Diagnostic accuracy of noninvasive coronary angiography using 64-slice spiral computed tomography. J Am Coll Cardiol. 2005;46(3):552–7.
50. Ropers D, Rixe J, Anders K, et al. Usefulness of multidetector row spiral computed tomography with 64- × 0.6-mm collimation and 330-ms rotation for the noninvasive detection of significant coronary artery stenoses. Am J Cardiol. 2006;97(3):343–8.
51. Leschka S, Wildermuth S, Boehm T, et al. Noninvasive coronary angiography with 64-section CT: effect of average heart rate and heart rate variability on image quality. Radiology. 2006;241(2):378–85.
52. Kido T, Kurata A, Higashino H, et al. Cardiac imaging using 256-detector row four-dimensional CT: preliminary clinical report. Radiat Med. 2007;25(1):38–44.
53. Motoyama S, Anno H Sarai M, et al. Noninvasive coronary angiography with a prototype 256-row area detector computed tomography system: comparison with conventional invasive coronary angiography. J Am Coll Cardiol. 2008;51(7):773–5.
54. Rybicki FJ, Otero HJ, Steigner ML, et al. Initial evaluation of coronary images from 320-detector row computed tomography. Int J Cardiovasc Imaging. 2008;24(5):535–46.
55. Scheffel H, Alkadhi H, Plass A, et al. Accuracy of dual-source CT coronary angiography: first experience in a high pre-test probability population without heart rate control. Eur Radiol. 2006;16(12):2739–47.
56. Leber AW, Johnson T Becker A, et al. Diagnostic accuracy of dual-source multi-slice CT-coronary angiography in patients with an intermediate pretest likelihood for coronary artery disease. Eur Heart J. 2007;28(19):2354–60.
57. Johnson TR, Nikolaou K, Busch S, et al. Diagnostic accuracy of dual-source computed tomography in the diagnosis of coronary artery disease. Invest Radiol. 2007;42(10):684–91.
58. Ropers U, Ropers D, Pflederer T, et al. Influence of heart rate on the diagnostic accuracy of dual-source computed tomography coronary angiography. J Am Coll Cardiol. 2007;50(25):2393–8.
59. Brodoefel H, Burgstahler C, Tsiflikas I, et al. Dual-source CT: effect of heart rate, heart rate variability, and calcification on image quality and diagnostic accuracy. Radiology. 2008;247(2):346–55.
60. Leschka S, Scheffel H, Desbiolles L, et al. Combining dual-source computed tomography coronary angiography and calcium scoring: added value for the assessment of coronary artery disease. Heart. 2008;94(9):1154–61.
61. Alkadhi H, Scheffel H, Desbiolles L, et al. Dual-source computed tomography coronary angiography: influence of obesity, calcium load, and heart rate on diagnostic accuracy. Eur Heart J. 2008;29(6):766–76.
62. Tsiflikas I, Brodoefel H, Reimann AJ, et al. Coronary CT angiography with dual source computed tomography in 170 patients. Eur J Radiol. 2010;74(1):161–5.
63. Matt D, Scheffel H, Leschka S, et al. Dual-source CT coronary angiography: image quality, mean heart rate, and heart rate variability. AJR Am J Roentgenol. 2007;189(3):567–73.
64. Leschka S, Scheffel H, Desbiolles L, et al. Image quality and reconstruction intervals of dual-source CT coronary angiography: recommendations for ECG-pulsing windowing. Invest Radiol. 2007;42(8):543–9.
65. Ruzsics B, Lee H, Zwerner PL, Gebregziabher M, Costello P, Schoepf UJ. Dual-energy CT of the heart for diagnosing coronary artery stenosis and myocardial ischemia-initial experience. Eur Radiol. 2008;18(11):2414–24
66. Flohr T, Ohnesorge B. Heart rate adaptive optimization of spatial and temporal resolution for electrocardiogram-gated multislice spiral CT of the heart. J Comput Assist Tomogr. 2001;25(6):907–23.
67. Wintersperger BJ, Nikolaou K, von Ziegler F, et al. Image quality, motion artifacts, and reconstruction

timing of 64-slice coronary computed tomography angiography with 0.33-second rotation speed. Invest Radiol. 2006;41(5):436–42.
68. Leschka S, Alkadhi H, Stolzmann P, et al. Mono- versus bisegment reconstruction algorithms for dual-source computed tomography coronary angiography. Invest Radiol. 2008;43(10):703–11.
69. Achenbach S, Ulzheimer S, Baum U, et al. Noninvasive coronary angiography by retrospectively ECG-gated multislice spiral CT. Circulation. 2000;102(23):2823–8.
70. Rist C, Johnson TR, Muller-Starck J, et al. Noninvasive coronary angiography using dual-source computed tomography in patients with atrial fibrillation. Invest Radiol. 2009;44(3):159–67.
71. Leschka S, Oechslin E, Husmann L, et al. Pre- and postoperative evaluation of congenital heart disease in children and adults with 64-section CT. Radiographics. 2007;27(3):829–46.
72. Goo HW, Yang DH. Coronary artery visibility in free-breathing young children with congenital heart disease on cardiac 64-slice CT: dual-source ECG-triggered sequential scan vs. single-source non-ECG-synchronized spiral scan. Pediatr Radiol. 2010;40(10):1670–80.
73. Yang DH, Goo HW, Seo DM, et al. Multislice CT angiography of interrupted aortic arch. Pediatr Radiol. 2008;38(1):89–100.
74. Scheffel H, Alkadhi H, Leschka S, et al. Low-dose CT coronary angiography in the step-and-shoot mode: diagnostic performance. Heart. 2008;94(9):1132–7.
75. Earls JP, Berman EL, Urban BA, et al. Prospectively gated transverse coronary CT angiography versus retrospectively gated helical technique: improved image quality and reduced radiation dose. Radiology. 2008;246(3):742–53.
76. Lee JH, Chun EJ, Choi SI, et al. Prospective versus retrospective ECG-gated 64-detector coronary CT angiography for evaluation of coronary artery bypass graft patency: comparison of image quality, radiation dose and diagnostic accuracy. Int J Cardiovasc Imaging. 2011;27(5):657–67.
77. Shuman WP, Branch KR, May JM, et al. Prospective versus retrospective ECG gating for 64-detector CT of the coronary arteries: comparison of image quality and patient radiation dose. Radiology. 2008;248(2):431–7.
78. Alkadhi H, Stolzmann P, Desbiolles L, et al. Low-dose, 128-slice, dual-source CT coronary angiography: accuracy and radiation dose of the high-pitch and the step-and-shoot mode. Heart. 2010;96(12):933–8.
79. Dewey M, Zimmermann E, Deissenrieder F, et al. Noninvasive coronary angiography by 320-row computed tomography with lower radiation exposure and maintained diagnostic accuracy: comparison of results with cardiac catheterization in a head-to-head pilot investigation. Circulation. 2009;120(10):867–75.
80. Husmann L, Valenta I, Gaemperli O, et al. Feasibility of low-dose coronary CT angiography: first experience with prospective ECG-gating. Eur Heart J. 2008;29(2):191–7.
81. Xu L, Yang L, Zhang Z, et al. Low-dose adaptive sequential scan for dual-source CT coronary angiography in patients with high heart rate: comparison with retrospective ECG gating. Eur J Radiol. 2010;76(2):183–7.
82. Stolzmann P, Leschka S, Scheffel H, et al. Dual-source CT in step-and-shoot mode: noninvasive coronary angiography with low radiation dose. Radiology. 2008;249(1):71–80.
83. Goo HW, Seo DM, Yun TJ, et al. Coronary artery anomalies and clinically important anatomy in patients with congenital heart disease: multislice CT findings. Pediatr Radiol. 2009;39(3):265–73.
84. Feuchtner G, Gotti R, Plass A, et al. Dual-step prospective ECG-triggered 128-slice dual-source CT for evaluation of coronary arteries and cardiac function without heart rate control: a technical note. Eur Radiol. 2010;20(9):2092–9.
85. Achenbach S, Marwan M, Ropers D, et al. Coronary computed tomography angiography with a consistent dose below 1 mSv using prospectively electrocardiogram-triggered high-pitch spiral acquisition. Eur Heart J. 2010;31(3):340–6.
86. Leschka S, Stolzmann P, Desbiolles L, et al. Diagnostic accuracy of high-pitch dual-source CT for the assessment of coronary stenoses: first experience. Eur Radiol. 2009;19(12):2896–903.
87. Goetti R, Leschka S, Baumuller S, et al. Low dose high-pitch spiral acquisition 128-slice dual-source computed tomography for the evaluation of coronary artery bypass graft patency. Invest Radiol. 2010;45(6):324–30.
88. Earls JP, Leipsic J. Cardiac computed tomography technology and dose-reduction strategies. Radiol Clin North Am. 2010;48(4):657–74.
89. Hausleiter J, Meyer T, Hermann F, et al. Estimated radiation dose associated with cardiac CT angiography. JAMA. 2009;301(5):500–7.
90. Bae KT, Hong C, Whiting BR. Radiation dose in multidetector row computed tomography cardiac imaging. J Magn Reson Imaging. 2004;19(6):859–63.
91. Kocinaj D, Cioppa A, Ambrosini G, et al. Radiation dose exposure during cardiac and peripheral arteries catheterisation. Int J Cardiol. 2006;113(2):283–4.
92. Hausleiter J, Meyer T, Hadamitzky M, et al. Radiation dose estimates from cardiac multislice computed tomography in daily practice: impact of different scanning protocols on effective dose estimates. Circulation. 2006;113(10):1305–10.
93. Stolzmann P, Scheffel H, Schertler T, et al. Radiation dose estimates in dual-source computed tomography coronary angiography. Eur Radiol. 2008;18(3):592–9.
94. Abada HT, Larchez C, Daoud B, Sigal-Cinqualbre A, Paul JF. MDCT of the coronary arteries: feasibility of low-dose CT with ECG-pulsed tube current modulation to reduce radiation dose. AJR Am J Roentgenol. 2006;186(6 Suppl 2):S387–90.
95. Leschka S, Stolzmann P, Schmid FT, et al. Low kilovoltage cardiac dual-source CT: attenuation, noise, and radiation dose. Eur Radiol. 2008;18(9):1809–17.

96. Alkadhi H, Stolzmann P, Scheffel H, et al. Radiation dose of cardiac dual-source CT: the effect of tailoring the protocol to patient-specific parameters. Eur J Radiol. 2008;68(3):385–91.
97. McCollough CH. Maximizing dose reductions with cardiac CT. Int J Cardiovasc Imaging. 2009;25(6):647.
98. Gopal A, Mao SS, Karlsberg D, et al. Radiation reduction with prospective ECG-triggering acquisition using 64-multidetector computed tomographic angiography. Int J Cardiovasc Imaging. 2009;25(4):405–16.
99. Earls JP. How to use a prospective gated technique for cardiac CT. J Cardiovasc Comput Tomogr. 2009;3(1):45–51.
100. Stolzmann P, Scheffel H, Leschka S, et al. Influence of calcifications on diagnostic accuracy of coronary CT angiography using prospective ECG triggering. AJR Am J Roentgenol. 2008;191(6):1684–9.
101. Budoff MJ, Gopal A. Incidental findings on cardiac computed tomography. Should we look? J Cardiovasc Comput Tomogr. 2007;1(2):97–105.
102. Leschka S, Kim CH, Baumueller S, et al. Scan length adjustment of CT coronary angiography using the calcium scoring scan: effect on radiation dose. AJR Am J Roentgenol. 2010;194(3):W272–7.
103. Gopal A, Budoff MJ. A new method to reduce radiation exposure during multi-row detector cardiac computed tomographic angiography. Int J Cardiol. 2009;132(3):435–6.
104. McCollough CH, Primak AN, Braun N, Kofler J, Yu L, Christner J. Strategies for reducing radiation dose in CT. Radiol Clin North Am. 2009;47(1):27–40.
105. Fricke BL, Donnelly LF, Frush DP, et al. In-plane bismuth breast shields for pediatric CT: effects on radiation dose and image quality using experimental and clinical data. AJR Am J Roentgenol. 2003;180(2):407–11.
106. Hopper KD, King SH, Lobell ME, TenHave TR, Weaver JS. The breast: in-plane x-ray protection during diagnostic thoracic CT – shielding with bismuth radioprotective garments. Radiology. 1997;205(3):853–8.
107. Yilmaz MH, Yasar D, Albayram S, et al. Coronary calcium scoring with MDCT: the radiation dose to the breast and the effectiveness of bismuth breast shield. Eur J Radiol. 2007;61(1):139–43.
108. Geleijns J, Salvado Artells M, Veldkamp WJ, Lopez Tortosa M, Calzado Cantera A. Quantitative assessment of selective in-plane shielding of tissues in computed tomography through evaluation of absorbed dose and image quality. Eur Radiol. 2006;16(10):2334–40.
109. Kalender WA, Wolf H, Suess C, Gies M, Greess H, Bautz WA. Dose reduction in CT by on-line tube current control: principles and validation on phantoms and cadavers. Eur Radiol. 1999;9(2):323–8.
110. Das M, Mahnken AH, Muhlenbruch G, et al. Individually adapted examination protocols for reduction of radiation exposure for 16-MDCT chest examinations. AJR Am J Roentgenol. 2005;184(5):1437–43.
111. Fuchs TO, Kachelriess M, Kalender WA. System performance of multislice spiral computed tomography. IEEE Eng Med Biol Mag. 2000;19(5):63–70.
112. Paul JF, Abada HT. Strategies for reduction of radiation dose in cardiac multislice CT. Eur Radiol. 2007;17(8):2028–37.
113. Weustink AC, Mollet NR, Pugliese F, et al. Optimal electrocardiographic pulsing windows and heart rate: effect on image quality and radiation exposure at dual-source coronary CT angiography. Radiology. 2008;248(3):792–8.
114. Thibault JB, Sauer KD, Bouman CA, Hsieh J. A three-dimensional statistical approach to improved image quality for multislice helical CT. Med Phys. 2007;34(11):4526–44.
115. Leipsic J, Labounty TM, Heilbron B, et al. Adaptive statistical iterative reconstruction: assessment of image noise and image quality in coronary CT angiography. AJR Am J Roentgenol. 2010;195(3):649–54.
116. Leipsic J, Labounty TM, Heilbron B, et al. Estimated radiation dose reduction using adaptive statistical iterative reconstruction in coronary CT angiography: the ERASIR study. AJR Am J Roentgenol. 2010;195(3):655–60.
117. Jung B, Mahnken AH, Stargardt A, et al. Individually weight-adapted examination protocol in retrospectively ECG-gated MSCT of the heart. Eur Radiol. 2003;13(12):2560–6.
118. Rogalla P, Blobel J, Kandel S, et al. Radiation dose optimisation in dynamic volume CT of the heart: tube current adaptation based on anterior-posterior chest diameter. Int J Cardiovasc Imaging. 2010;26(8):933–40.
119. Starck G, Lonn L, Cederblad A, Forssell-Aronsson E, Sjostrom L, Alpsten M. A method to obtain the same levels of CT image noise for patients of various sizes, to minimize radiation dose. Br J Radiol. 2002;75(890):140–50.
120. LaBounty TM, Earls JP, Leipsic J, et al. Effect of a standardized quality-improvement protocol on radiation dose in coronary computed tomographic angiography. Am J Cardiol. 2010;106(11):1663–7.
121. Raff GL, Chinnaiyan KM, Share DA, et al. Radiation dose from cardiac computed tomography before and after implementation of radiation dose-reduction techniques. JAMA. 2009;301(22):2340–8.
122. Larson DB, Rader SB, Forman HP, Fenton LZ. Informing parents about CT radiation exposure in children: it's OK to tell them. AJR Am J Roentgenol. 2007;189(2):271–5.
123. Nievelstein RA, van Dam IM, van der Molen AJ. Multidetector CT in children: current concepts and dose reduction strategies. Pediatr Radiol. 2010;40(8):1324–44.

Echocardiographic Imaging in Adult Congenital Heart Disease

6

Jon Detterich, Andrew Yoon, and Philip Chang

Echocardiography (echo) remains the primary imaging modality for the anatomical and basic functional assessment of the heart with congenital defects. As with many techniques shared between adult and pediatric cardiology, echo imaging has been adapted to imaging pediatric subjects and concentrates heavily on the structural delineation of cardiac anatomy, both normal and abnormal. Adult echo imaging, alternatively, concentrates primarily on the functional characterization of cardiac structures owing largely to the fact that the majority of adult hearts are structurally normal to begin with. The application of echo imaging to adult congenital heart disease (ACHD) patients requires a strong integration of both approaches to and applications of echo imaging.

In this chapter, the basic application of echo will be discussed as it relates to imaging congenital heart disease (CHD). This discussion will begin with a review of the general application of transthoracic echo imaging in ACHD and expand to include additional imaging tools including color Doppler imaging, tissue Doppler imaging (TDI), transesophageal echo (TEE), 3-dimensional (3D) imaging, and intracardiac and intravascular echo (ICE and IVUS). Finally, the limitations of echo will be discussed within the context of combining the echo and advanced imaging modalities to comprehensively evaluate structural and functional features of hearts with newly diagnosed, unrepaired, and repaired forms of CHD.

J. Detterich, MD
Division of Pediatric Cardiology, Department of Pediatrics, University of Southern California, Keck School of Medicine, Children's Hospital Los Angeles, Los Angeles, CA, USA

A. Yoon, MD
Division of Cardiovascular Medicine, Department of Medicine, University of Southern California, Keck School of Medicine, Keck Medical Center of USC, Los Angeles, CA, USA

P. Chang, MD (✉)
Division of Cardiovascular Medicine, Department of Medicine, University of Southern California, Keck School of Medicine, Keck Medical Center of USC and Children's Hospital Los Angeles, Los Angeles, CA, USA
e-mail: philip.chang@med.usc.edu

History of Ultrasound

The use of sound waves to determine location and movement of sound-generating objects in 3D space has existed in nature but has only been integrated into man-made technology within the last century. The use of ultrasonic sound waves as well as the development of the piezoelectric crystal resulted in the ability to use this science in a broad array of applications. The first use of ultrasound (US) in medical imaging occurred in 1941, when Karl Dussik of Austria performed US imaging of the brain ventricles [1]. Dr. Helmet Hertz and Dr. Inge Edler of Sweden were the first physicians to use the pulse-reflect US method to

F. Saremi (ed.), *Cardiac CT and MR for Adult Congenital Heart Disease*,
DOI 10.1007/978-1-4614-8875-0_6,

examine cardiac structures in 1953 [2]. This method progressively developed into echo or the application of US imaging techniques to the evaluation of cardiac structure and function. Today, echo has become a vital and necessary component to the clinical practice of modern cardiology. Certainly, echo has become integral to the detection and serial evaluation of patients with CHD. Thus far, no other noninvasive imaging modality is capable of matching the quickness, versatility, and cost-effectiveness of echo in imaging cardiac structures and function with both high spatial and temporal resolution and minimal risk to the patient.

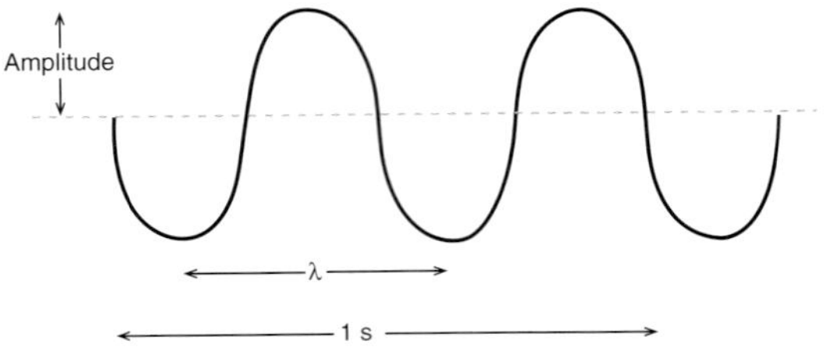

Fig. 6.1 Representation of sound waves. Amplitude is the maximum extent of an acoustic oscillation, measured from a position of equilibrium. Wavelength (λ) is the distance between successive sound wave crests and represents one sound wave cycle. Frequency is the number of cycles per 1 s (in this example, 2) and is measured in Hertz (Hz). Propagation velocity (not depicted above) is the speed at which an acoustic signal travels through a medium

Basic Principles of Ultrasound

A brief and necessarily simplified review of US principles is presented here both as an introduction and to provide a framework for understanding various echo capabilities.

Echo image acquisition involves placement of a transducer on the patient's chest wall. US waves are generated and directed from the transducer as focused beams through the patient. As with any wave, sound waves are characterized by their frequency, propagation velocity, wavelength, and amplitude (Fig. 6.1). In clinical echo, sound waves with a frequency of 2–8 MHz are used. As the US wave propagates through the patient's tissue, the tissue particles vibrate longitudinally, with alternating regions of compression and rarefaction. The velocity of the propagation is approximately 1,540 m/s in blood. Diagnostic US utilizes wavelengths of 0.15–1.5 mm, which determines image resolution (1–2 wavelengths). Sound waves with short wavelengths have high image resolution but poorer penetration compared to longer wavelengths. Conversely, longer wavelengths have better tissue penetration but poorer image resolution. Amplitude is a measure of the strength of the sound wave and is measured in decibels.

US waves interact with internal tissue structures via reflection, refraction, and attenuation. Reflection consists of specular and scattered varieties. Specular reflection occurs when US waves interact with anatomic structures with a lateral dimension larger than the wavelength of US, such as tissue interfaces or valve leaflets. The US reflects off of these tissue boundaries and returns to the transducer. The amount of sound wave that returns to the transducer (i.e., the signal strength) depends on the angle of reflection between the tissue interface and the transducer. The optimal angle with the maximal amount of reflected US occurs when the tissue interface is perpendicular to the transducer. When the tissue interface is parallel in alignment to the transducer, no US wave returns to the transducer and signal dropout occurs. Scattered reflection results in the characteristic speckle pattern of tissues seen on US images. These speckles are the result of constructive and destructive US interference backscattered from Rayleigh scatterers, which are anatomic structures with a lateral dimension smaller than the wavelength of US. Signals produced by scattered echoes are considerably lower in comparison to specular echoes, because the overall percentage of energy reflected back to the US transducer is much lower due to their considerably smaller size.

Refraction occurs when US waves travel from one tissue to another tissue with different acoustic impedances. Acoustic impedance (Z) is an inherent characteristic of tissues and depends on the density of the tissue (p) and the propagation velocity of US within that tissue (c):

$$Z = pc$$

This difference in acoustic impedances encountered by the US wave as it crosses from one tissue interface to another causes the beam to deviate at an angle away from its original straight line path. As impedance increases, more US will be reflected, and this deviation can lead to "double image" artifacts.

Attenuation occurs when signal strength is lost, either due to reflection, scattering, or absorption. Absorption is the conversion of US to heat, which is consequently absorbed by the body tissues. Air is a significant source of signal attenuation given its high acoustic impedance. Any air between the transducer and cardiac structures results in significant signal attenuation. For this reason, a water-soluble gel is used to form an airless contact between the transducer and the patient's skin, greatly facilitating the transfer of sound waves into and out of the body. The lungs are also filled with air, and careful manual positioning of the transducer is required to obtain adequate imaging of cardiac structures while avoiding the lung fields, especially in patients with hyperinflated lung conditions such as COPD, mechanically assisted ventilation, and pneumothorax.

Piezoelectricity

The piezoelectric crystal within the US transducer acts as both a signal transmitter and signal receiver. Most current commercial transducers use ceramics for the piezoelectric material. When an alternating electric current is applied to the piezoelectric crystal, it rapidly vibrates, emitting a high-frequency US as it expands and contracts. The transducer emits a short burst of US, lasting 1–6 μs, called the pulse length. The transducer then enters into a receiver mode referred to as "dead time," waiting for reflected US waves to return. The combined duration of a single pulse length time and dead time is known as the pulse repetition frequency. When a reflected US wave returns to the crystal, it induces the crystalline generation of an electric current that is detected. This transmit-receive cycle is repeated temporally and spatially, and the differences in time delay of the reflected sound waves received by the transducer are used to generate the US image. To create a 2-dimensional echocardiogram sector image, the transducer must emit and receive at repetition rates of 3,000–5,000 times/s.

Ultrasound Imaging

The simplest type of US imaging is based on the alternating pulsed transmission and reception along a single US beam. This is used in M-mode imaging, when the image obtained along a single US beam is recorded over time in what is sometimes referred to as the "ice pick" view (Fig. 6.2a). A phased array sector scanner must be used to obtain the familiar 2-dimensional (2D) echo images. In phased array scanners, numerous small piezoelectric crystals are interconnected electrically and arranged in an array. Each crystal is connected to an electrode, which enables each crystal to transmit and receive US signals. The electrical excitation of each crystal within the array is timed such that excitation for every crystal does not occur simultaneously but rather in a timed sequential excitation pattern, allowing the US beams to be "steered" through a sector arc to generate a 2D image (Fig. 6.2b).

During the transmission of US waves, the frequency of the original wave may be altered by nonlinear tissue interactions. These interactions result in the generation of new frequencies that were not present in the original transmitted US beam. These new frequencies are integer multiples of the original signal and are known as harmonic frequencies. If the original sound wave has a frequency of f, the harmonic frequencies are 2f, 3f, etc. The original US beam undergoes significant attenuation as it propagates through the patient's tissue but generates new harmonic waves with higher-frequency oscillations than the original US beam. These higher-frequency waves have higher spatial resolution and increase in strength as the US wave penetrates the body. Harmonic frequencies are optimal at depths of 4–8 cm which is ideal for imaging cardiac structures. Additionally, strong

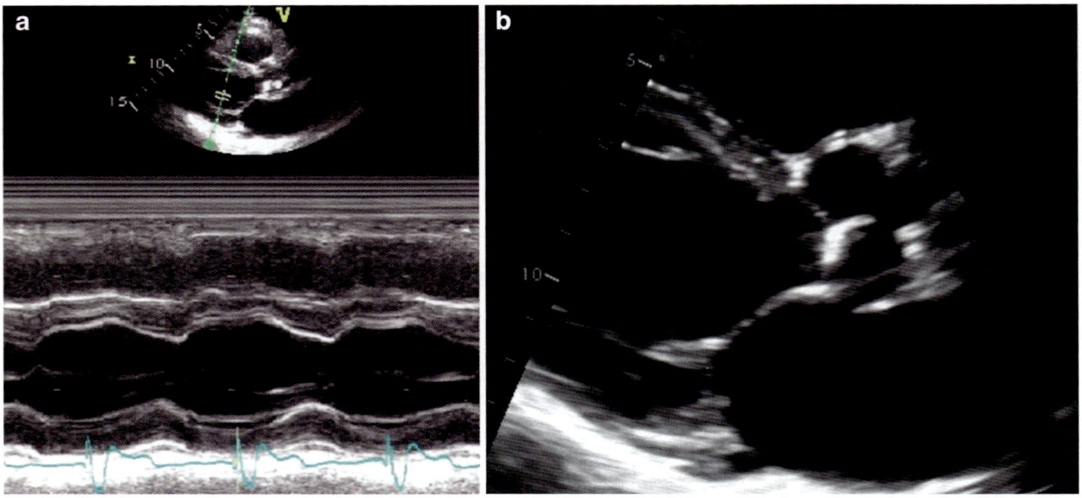

Fig. 6.2 M-mode and 2-dimensional echo imaging. (**a**) Demonstrates an M-mode (motion mode) tracing of the left ventricle. M-mode is an ultrasound representation of the depth of echo-producing interfaces in a single sampling line, displayed as a function of time. (**b**) Demonstrates a 2-dimensional ultrasound image of the same left ventricle through combining of images acquired from multiple ultrasound beams in a phased array

US waves create strong harmonic frequencies, while weak US waves produce almost no harmonic frequencies. In tissue harmonic imaging, the reflected signal from the original US beam is suppressed, and the harmonic frequencies are used to construct the image. The development of tissue harmonic imaging has been instrumental in significantly improving echo image quality, particularly in the visual assessment of endocardial borders.

Doppler Echocardiography

Doppler echo is the detection of signals from anatomic structures with a lateral dimension smaller than the wavelength of US. Doppler echo is integral in the echocardiographic measurement of blood velocities, tissue velocities, and in newer techniques measuring ventricular torsion and strains. For a stationary anatomic structure, any US waves that strike the anatomic structure and reflect back to the transducer will have the same frequency as the originally transmitted US beam. If the anatomic structure is in motion in a direction away from the transducer, the frequency of the reflected beams will be lower than the originally transmitted frequency. If the anatomic structure is moving toward the transducer, the frequency of the reflected beams will be faster than the originally transmitted signal frequency. This is the same sound wave phenomenon observed when a train moving toward an observer has a high-pitched whistle, which then changes to a low-pitched whistle as the train travels away from the observer. The difference in frequencies between the originally transmitted frequency and the reflected, returning frequency is known as the Doppler shift. In echo, it is possible to calculate the velocity of blood as it travels through cardiac structures by detecting the Doppler shift from the scattered echo's reflected from the thousands of blood cells located within the US beam. The velocity of the moving blood cells can be calculated using the equation:

$$V = c(F_s - F\tau)/\ (2F\tau\ \text{-}\cos\theta)$$

$F\tau$ is the transmitted frequency, F_s is the frequency of the signal returning from the blood, c is the velocity of sound waves in blood (1,540 m/s), and $\cos\theta$ is the intercept angle

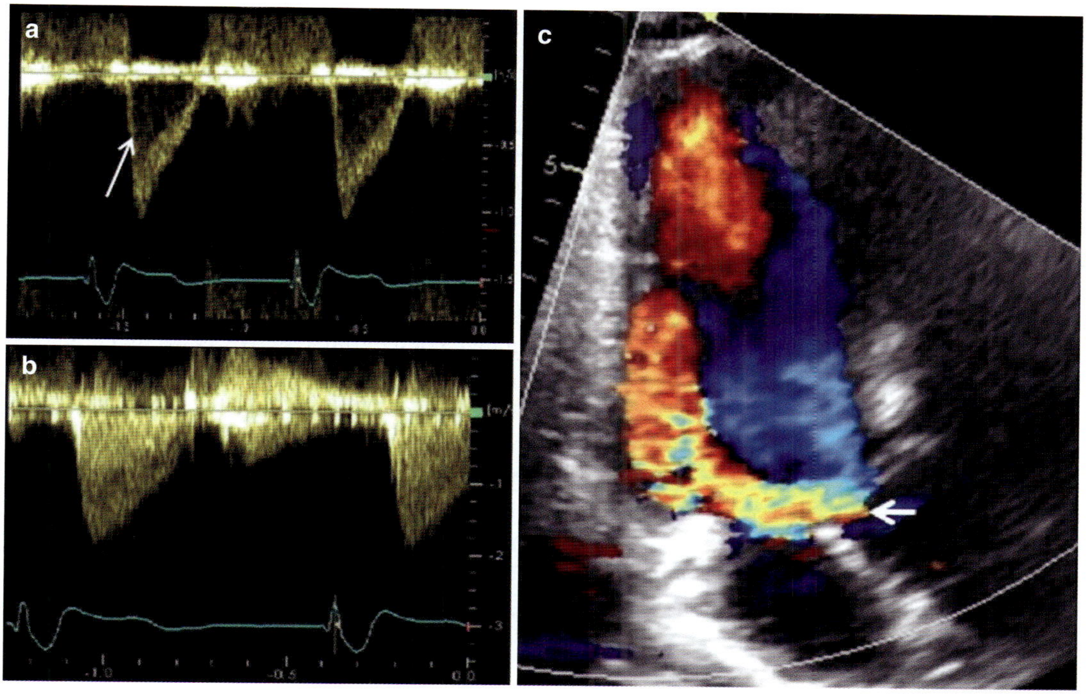

Fig. 6.3 Examples of Doppler echo imaging. (**a**) Shows pulse wave Doppler of a sample site within the left ventricular outflow tract in a normal heart, demonstrating a narrow band of laminar spectral output (*arrow*). (**b**) Shows the continuous wave Doppler of the same left ventricular outflow tract demonstrating all of the various velocities encountered by the ultrasound beam, including the narrow band noted in the pulse wave Doppler example in (**a**). (**c**) Shows color Doppler over the left ventricular outflow tract demonstrating a large, diastolic, regurgitant jet (*arrow*) in a patient with severe aortic regurgitation

between the US beam and the direction of blood flow. In cardiac applications, care must be taken to align the transducer parallel to the direction of blood flow so that $\cos\theta = 1$. Although small angle deviations typically result in minor underestimations of blood velocity, an angle deviation of 60° between the US beam and the direction of blood flow can result in a 50 % underestimation of blood velocity.

There are three types of Doppler interrogations performed during a typical echocardiogram study: continuous wave (CW) Doppler, pulse wave (PW) Doppler, and color Doppler (Fig. 6.3). In CW Doppler, two crystals are used. One crystal is set to continuously transmit an US signal, and the other crystal is set to continuously receive return signals. Along the single US beam, every Doppler shift is recorded simultaneously and displayed in graph format as velocity versus time. The advantage of this method is that high velocities can be measured accurately due to the continuous US signal transmission and data reception. In contrast to CW Doppler which samples all velocities along the beam length, PW Doppler allows for the measurement of velocity at a prespecified sample depth. A pulse of US frequency is transmitted to the sample site, and after a specific time period, the receiver detects the reflected signal. The specified time interval is determined by the time it takes the US to reach the sample depth and return and is called the pulse repetition frequency. Color flow imaging is conceptually analogous to PW Doppler, but instead of a single sample point, numerous sample points along multiple sampling lines are obtained. By combining data points among the different sample sites, mean blood flow velocities are calculated and a 2D image of blood flow is constructed. By convention, flow toward the transducer is depicted in red, and flow away from the transducer is depicted in blue. A third color, typically yellow or green, may be used to indicate "variance" or excessive variation in velocity within the sample points to represent nonlaminar or high-velocity blood flow.

Echo Application in Congenital Heart Disease

The incorporation of echo into the evaluation of CHD has changed the course of management for patients born with heart defects [3–5]. Prior to widespread use of 2D echo, diagnosis and follow-up evaluation of CHD was done primarily by history, physical exam, chest X-ray, electrocardiogram, and cardiac catheterization. There is still no replacement for a detailed history and physical exam, but a detailed anatomic and hemodynamic evaluation is necessary upon initial diagnosis to properly plan for both initial intervention and subsequent follow-up care. Cardiac catheterization historically had been the only diagnostic tool to acquire anatomic, functional, and hemodynamic data to guide management. While the information derived from catheterization was incredibly valuable, its invasive nature and lack of portability remained its biggest disadvantages [6, 7]. Technological advances have allowed the incorporation of US imaging as a noninvasive method of evaluating patients with CHD. The high temporal and spatial resolution of echo enables it to provide accurate and comprehensive anatomic and functional diagnostic assessments that, in turn, guide the management and follow-up of patients. For a large proportion of patients, a high-quality echo study provides sufficient information to recommend specific surgical or percutaneous therapies without the need for more invasive diagnostics [8, 9]. Today, it is rare for patients with even the most complex cardiac defects to require catheterization prior to initial surgery.

2-Dimensional Echocardiographic Imaging in Congenital Heart Disease

Cardiac pathological studies have resulted in the development of a structured framework for describing and communicating CHD lesions. The heart is a complex 4-dimensional (4D) structure that moves in both time and space. Since most imaging modalities are displayed on a 2D screen, the 3D and 4D reconstruction must occur in the human mind to fully appreciate the pathophysiology. In fact, the development and application of 3D echo in CHD is largely founded on how sonographers and echocardiographers are already mentally interpreting image slices and formulating these 3D and 4D images. In order to establish a clear and consistent way of describing the myriad of CHD lesions and the immense intralesion variability, pathologists in the past developed the segmental approach for the description of CHD [10, 11]. The Van Praagh's developed the three-level cardiac segmentation approach, which includes:

1. Visceroatrial situs
2. Ventricular looping
3. Great artery relationship

Each segment is designated by a letter, which delineates their position in space (Fig. 6.4). The segmental approach provides a uniform method of describing basic cardiac anatomy. Once segmentation has been established, additional attention is then paid to describing the individual connections between respective segments and describing the specific features within each segment (i.e., chamber size, valve architecture, great vessel caliber, and course). The end result is a consistent way of describing all aspects of the cardiac anatomy, providing a way for individuals to piece together any defect even before performing or reviewing any imaging study.

Given the superior temporal and spatial resolution of echo, the 2D "sweep" of the anatomy begins the process of combining anatomic evaluation and connection. The use of short clips in single planes to evaluate a single valve or structure is of limited utility in the CHD population given the lack of ability to create a 3D mental

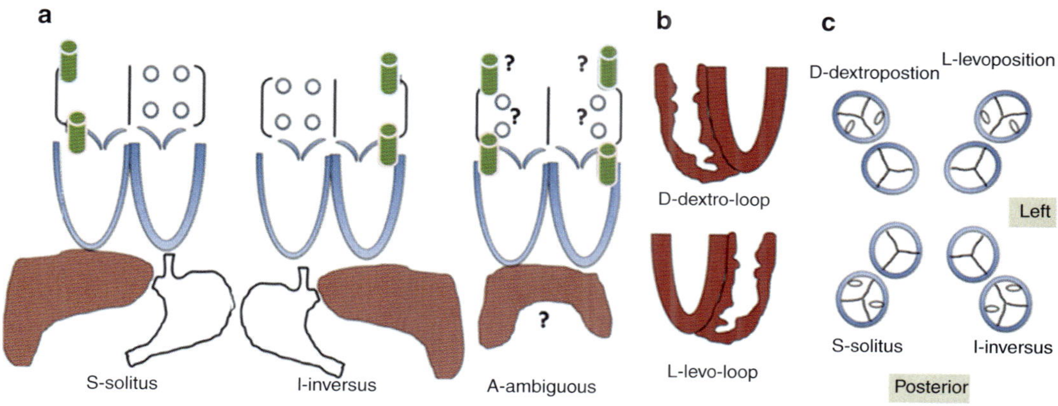

Fig. 6.4 Schematic illustration of the segmental approach to describing cardiac anatomy. Analysis begins with evaluation of visceroatrial situs (**a**) with consideration of the anatomic positioning of the abdominal viscera (liver, spleen, stomach), inferior systemic venous drainage (i.e., IVC or azygous or hemiazygous continuation), and atrial anatomy (including which chambers receive systemic and pulmonary venous drainage). Segmental description continues with delineation of ventricular looping (**b**; D- vs. L-looping) and ends with description of the anatomic relationship of the great arteries to each other (**c**). Each segment is labeled with a letter designation as listed in each panel

picture of the heart. The incorporation of "sweeps" to the evaluation of cardiac anatomy applies to standard transthoracic and transesophageal approaches in CHD echo.

Echo "sweeps" for the imaging of CHD involve pivoting the transducer in standard views to obtain a series of imaging slices that provide left-to-right, superior-to-inferior, and superficial-to-deep contour. The combination of sweeps in all standard views can then be used to generate mental or computer-processed 3D depictions of cardiac structures. Sonographers utilize typical subcostal, parasternal, apical, and suprasternal notch windows to acquire these sweeps. Occasionally, alternate windows and modified views need to be utilized, particularly in cases of unusual cardiac positioning, dextrocardia, or anomalous, aberrant, or hypoplastic vascular structures.

In TEE, sweeps are obtained by rotating the transducer along its axis, raising or lowering the probe tip to various levels within the upper gastrointestinal tract, and flexing the transducer tip along its fulcrum, thereby acquiring image slices at a certain level and orientation of the transducer within the chest (Fig. 6.5). Similar to transthoracic imaging, these slices are then integrated mentally or through image processing to yield 3D depictions of structures.

Transthoracic Echocardiography in Congenital Heart Disease

Transthoracic echo (TTE) remains the primary diagnostic tool complementing history and physical examination in the evaluation of CHD, owing largely to its portability and high spatial and temporal resolution. Infant and child heart disease is often easily imaged with few limitations. However, as the patient grows, so do the soft tissues and lungs, which will limit resolution of imaging and the ability to find adequate echo windows. US does not travel through air, so any lung that overlies cardiovascular structures will obscure the image, rendering the structure indecipherable. Furthermore, disorganized scar tissue, for example, following cardiac surgery, and bone will obscure imaging and limit the reader's ability to accurately comment on the cardiovascular structural details.

As with standard adult echo, CHD echo incorporates views from the parasternal, apical, and suprasternal notch locations on the chest. Orthogonal views are obtained by rotating the transducer 90°. In addition, CHD echo incorporates a greater emphasis on the subcostal or subxyphoid views obtained by placing the transducer just below the xyphoid process, in the epigastric space, utilizing the liver to improve image quality.

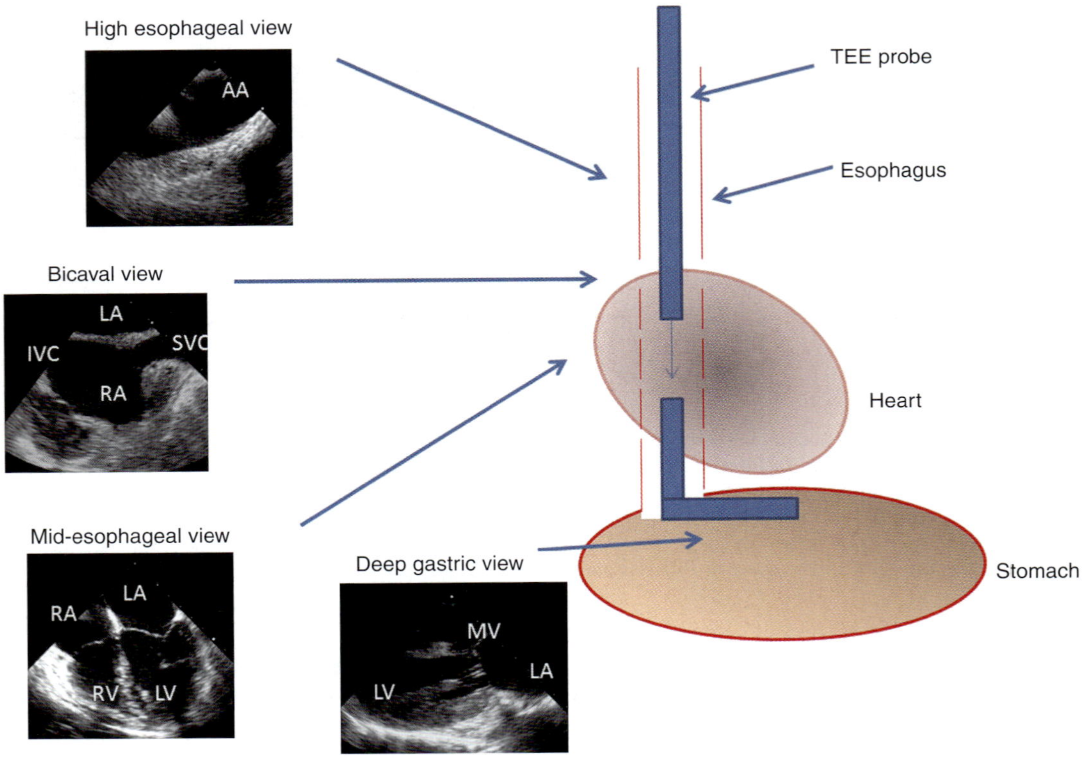

Fig. 6.5 Schematic of transesophageal echo (TEE) imaging. During TEE imaging, the imaging probe is placed down the esophagus and oriented to obtain 2- and 3-dimensional images along with color and spectral Doppler tracings. The transducer tip can be rotated to obtain orthogonal views from a single location within the esophagus. The probe is also advanced or withdrawn to acquire images at varying depths within the esophagus. The probe tip can also be flexed and placed into the stomach for deep gastric imaging. *AA* aortic arch, *SVC* superior vena cava, *IVC* inferior vena cava, *LA* left atrium, *RA* right atrium, *LV* left ventricle, *RV* right ventricle, *MV* mitral valve

Sweeps are performed by pivoting the transducer at each site and in each orthogonal projection. The following paragraphs review the standard TTE views with accompanying TTE images of CHD lesions to provide the reader with examples of what is best seen and imaged from various positions along the chest and epigastrium.

The subcostal view provides excellent imaging of the heart with CHD. Combined orthogonal views from this location give the echocardiographer a comprehensive overview of the entire heart (Figs. 6.6 and 6.7). Caval and pulmonary venous return, visceral and atrial situs, ventricular looping, and outflow tract arrangement are all demonstrable from this position. The presence of an interrupted inferior vena cava and either azygous or hemiazygous venous continuation is best viewed from the subcostal location. Additionally, the atrial septum is best profiled by virtue of the more perpendicular imaging plane relative to the septum's spatial lie. The ventricular sizes and intraventricular septum are well profiled, and all four valves and the outflow tracts are seen, permitting one to determine ventricular looping and great arterial relationship, along with a basic description of the intersegmental connections. The subcostal short-axis view is valuable in assessing vena caval size and flow characteristics, descending aortic flow, and inferiorly draining anomalous pulmonary veins. In palliated single-ventricle patients, the subcostal short-axis view also provides an excellent way to assess the IVC flow through the Fontan connection (Fig. 6.8).

The parasternal view provides excellent imaging of the ventricles and, in particular, the left ven-

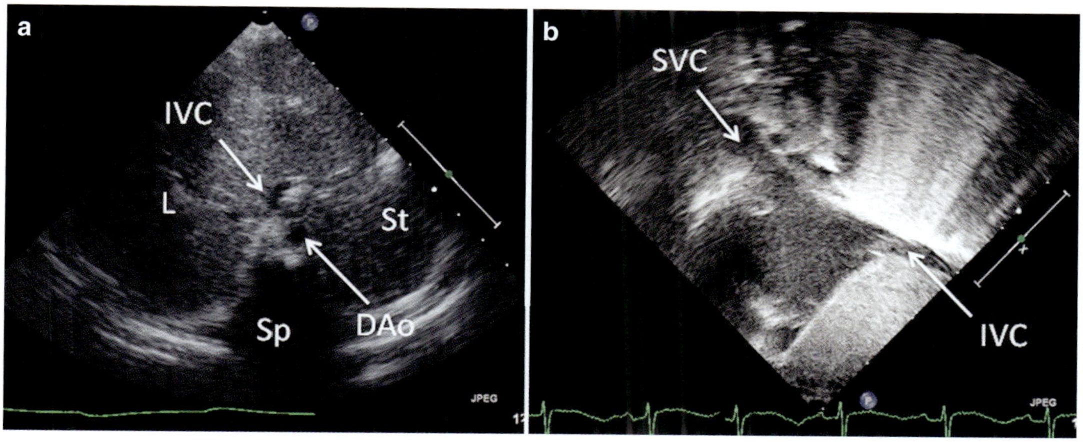

Fig. 6.6 Transthoracic imaging from the subcostal view. (**a**) Depicts a sweep at the subxyphoid process from caudal, posterior, and deep in the abdomen up to the heart which is cranial, anterior, and superficial. The sweep shows visceral situs with the descending aorta (*DAo*) leftward of the spine (*Sp*), the inferior vena cava (*IVC*) anterior and rightward to the aorta, the liver (*L*) positioned to the patient's right, and the stomach (*St*) on the patient's left. Collectively, these structures define visceral situs solitus. (**b**) Depicts additional subcostal imaging in an orthogonal plane to demonstrate superior and inferior vena caval (*SVC, IVC*) return to the morphologic right atrium, helping to confirm atrial situs solitus

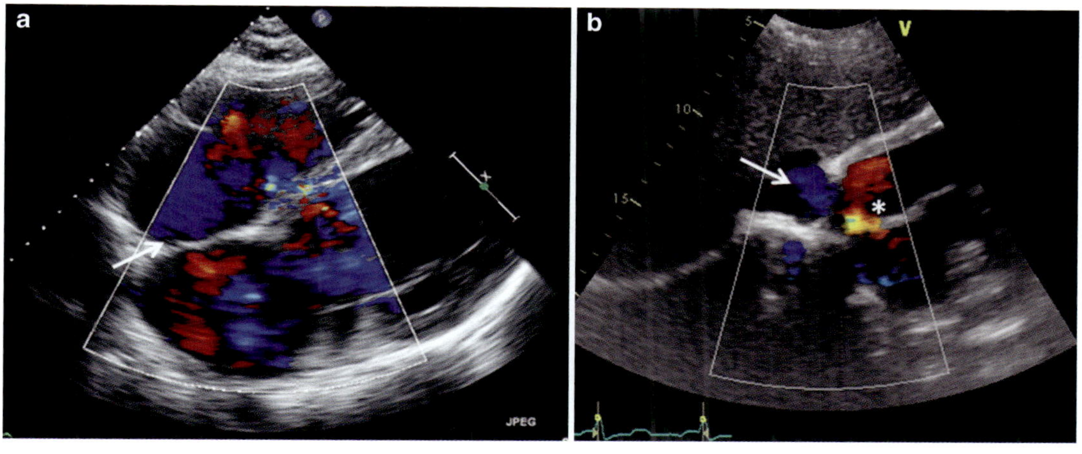

Fig. 6.7 Transthoracic echo imaging from the subcostal view. (**a**) Demonstrates a subcostal long-axis slice in an adult with an unrepaired ventricular septal defect. Comprehensive imaging was necessary to ensure lack of other associated defects prior to performing surgical defect closure. Subcostal views offer the best plane for imaging the atrial septum as the plane of imaging is nearly perpendicular to the septum, resulting in the clearest delineation of its structure. In this example, 2-dimensional and color Doppler imaging demonstrate an intact atrial septum (*arrow*). (**b**) Demonstrates subcostal long-axis imaging in an adult patient with palliated single-ventricle congenital heart disease (pulmonary atresia, intact ventricular septum, hypoplastic right ventricle). Two-dimensional and color Doppler imaging show low-velocity flow from the IVC to an extracardiac Fontan conduit (*arrow*). In addition, an atrial level defect from prior atrial septectomy is noted with bidirectional shunting on color Doppler imaging (*). Left-to-right shunting is noted in the image above

tricle. Tricuspid and mitral valve architecture are well delineated. The ventricular septum is profiled extremely well given the perpendicular relationship between the imaging plane and septal lie (Fig. 6.9). Depending on body habitus, the right ventricle may be imaged to varying degrees, and one can appreciate

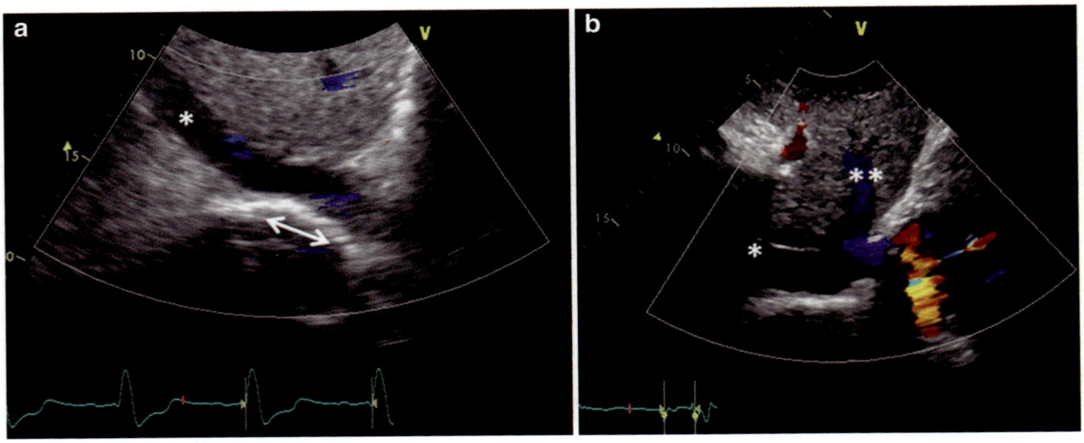

Fig. 6.8 Transthoracic echo imaging from the subcostal view in Fontan patients. (**a**) Demonstrates a subcostal short-axis slice showing a normal-sized inferior vena cava (*) that is anastomosed directly to an extracardiac Fontan conduit (*bidirectional arrow*). Color Doppler demonstrates low-velocity flow through the cava and conduit. The conduit appears more echo-bright on 2-dimensional imaging compared to normal vascular or cardiac tissue. (**b**) Demonstrates a similar subcostal slice in a Fontan patient palliated with a variant of an atriopulmonary Fontan. Marked dilation of the inferior vena cava (*) and hepatic veins (**) is noted. Low-velocity color flow is again noted consistent with passive venous return to the pulmonary arteries

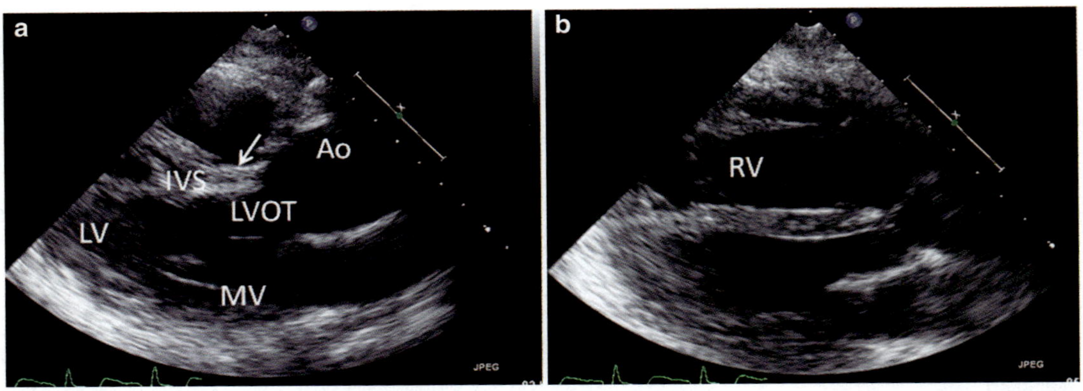

Fig. 6.9 Transthoracic echo imaging of a young adult with repaired tetralogy of Fallot. Images from the parasternal long-axis view are shown. (**a**) Shows a more posterior angled imaging plane, profiling the left ventricle (*LV*), mitral valve (*MV*), ventricular septum (*IVS*), and left ventricular outflow tract (*LVOT*) to the ascending aorta (*AAo*). The patch used to close the ventricular septal defect can be seen (*arrow*) without gross 2-dimensional evidence of a residual defect. The ascending aorta is severely dilated. (**b**) Shows a more anterior imaging plane in the same transthoracic view by "sweeping" the ultrasound probe from deep to superficial along the chest wall. In this view, the right ventricle (*RV*) is well profiled and noted to be significantly dilated with a chamber size that is nearly twice that of the left ventricle, frequently the consequence of right ventricular outflow tract and pulmonary valve pathology

chamber size, wall thickness, and systolic function. The ventricular outflows and semilunar valves are imaged well, providing the sonographer with excellent opportunities to assess for congenital and postoperative status of these structures. The parasternal short-axis views allow for imaging of the atrial septum and pulmonary veins when sweeping near the base of the heart; however, this can be limited. The right ventricular outflow, main pulmonary artery, and proximal branch pulmonary vessels are well profiled from the short-axis view. Finally, the right ventricular size is better visualized from the short-axis view, and septal motion is easily assessed in this imaging plane (Fig. 6.10).

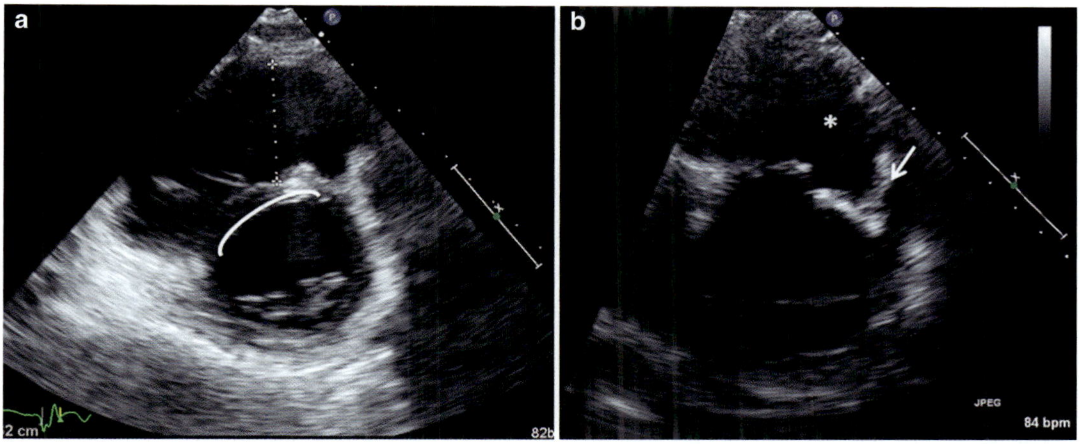

Fig. 6.10 Transthoracic imaging using the parasternal short-axis sweep in a patient with repaired tetralogy of Fallot. (**a**) Shows a slice upon sweeping from apex to base at the level of the mitral valve leaflets. The right ventricular chamber is noted to be severely dilated (measuring 3.62 cm from septum to free wall). The ventricular septal curvature remains rounded and bowing into the right ventricular cavity (*curved line*) suggesting that right ventricular pressures are less than those in the left ventricle. (**b**) Shows a short-axis slice toward the basal aspect of the heart highlighting the right ventricular outflow tract. The outflow tract is open without evidence of subvalvular obstruction (*). A bioprosthetic valve, implanted previously to address pulmonary insufficiency, is noted in the pulmonary position (*arrow*)

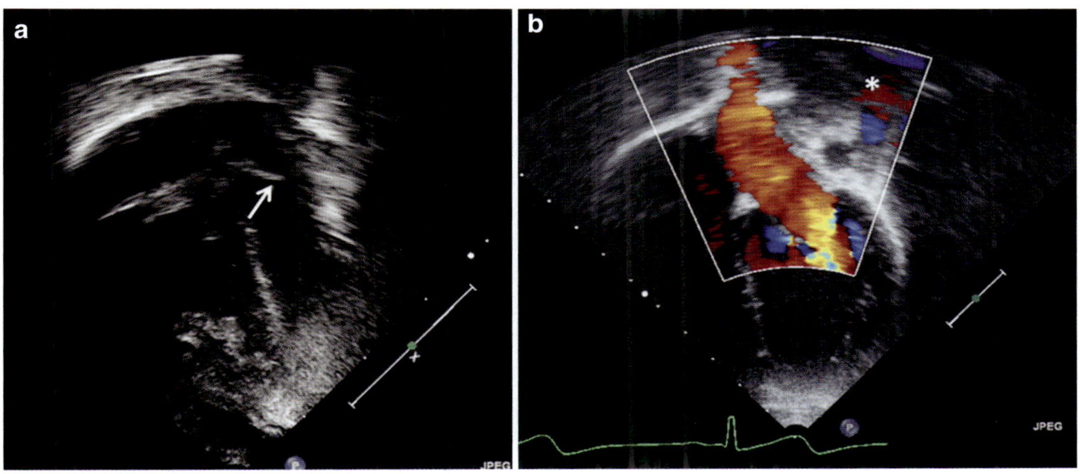

Fig. 6.11 Transthoracic echo imaging in the apical four-chamber view. (**a**) Demonstrates a 2-dimensional view showing an example of dropout in the ventricular septum (*arrow tip*), which gives the impression of the presence of a ventricular septal defect. Dropout can occur when the beam of imaging is parallel the structure being imaged. (**b**) Demonstrates color Doppler assessment in the left atrium in the 4-chamber view. From this view, pulmonary venous return can be partially evaluated, as depicted in this example where the right upper pulmonary vein is seen draining correctly into the left atrium (*)

The apical views are most intuitive to understand as all four chambers are typically displayed with the atrioventricular valves and outflow tracts seen reasonably well with deep to superficial sweeping of the transducer (Fig. 6.11). Atrial and ventricular septal defects can sometimes be seen with color flow, but 2D imaging may project a false finding of a defect as the septa are more parallel to the imaging plane, resulting in dropout. The apical view provides excellent views to evaluate

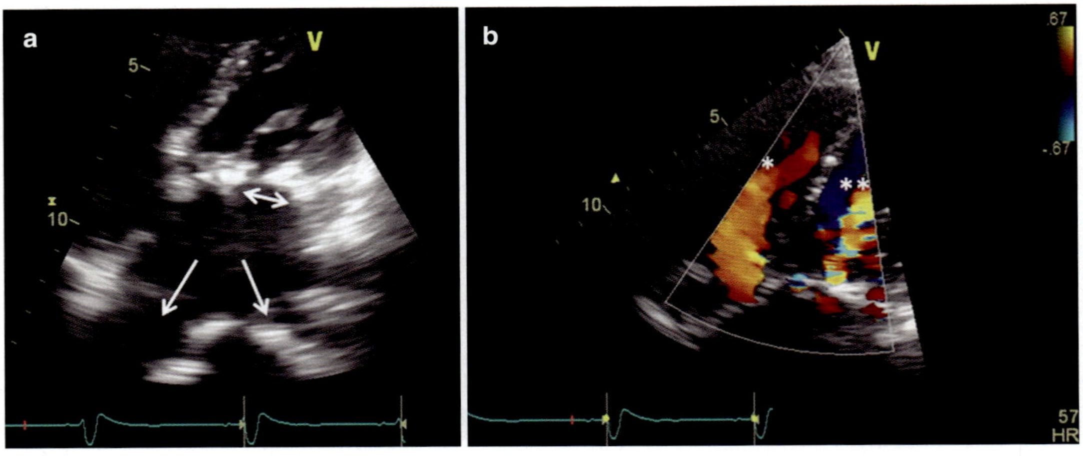

Fig. 6.12 Apical four-chamber view of a young adult with previously repaired complete atrioventricular canal defect. (**a**) Demonstrates a 2-dimensional view highlighting the repaired/constructed left-sided atrioventricular valve. The functional valve orifice is narrowed (*bidirectional arrow*) resulting in mitral inflow stenosis. The left atrium and pulmonary veins are visibly dilated (*arrows*), consistent with elevated left atrial and pulmonary venous pressures in the context of valve stenosis. (**b**) Demonstrates color flow across the left and right atrioventricular valves (repaired/constructed tricuspid and mitral valves) in the same patient. Note that both valves sit at the same plane within the heart, consistent with a prior atrioventricular canal defect. Tricuspid inflow is unobstructed (*), while mitral inflow demonstrates significant color aliasing (**), consistent with stenosis and an elevated left atrium-left ventricular pressure gradient

ventricular and atrial chamber sizes. Pulmonary venous return, mitral and tricuspid valve morphology and function, and surgically created baffles within the atria can be imaged reasonably well from this site, provided the body habitus and cardiac size are permitting (Figs. 6.12 and 6.13).

Suprasternal views allow evaluation of the aortic arch, superior pulmonary veins, superior caval return, and branch pulmonary vessels (Figs. 6.14 and 6.15). From this view, the echocardiographer can obtain views of a bidirectional Glenn anastomosis, evaluate for aortic coarctation, and demonstrate anomalous pulmonary venous return, especially superiorly to the superior systemic veins. Aortic root and arch size are generally seen as well. While the findings that can be seen from this view are important, imaging windows are frequently limited due to body habitus, lung interference, and postoperative changes in the CHD patient.

Limitations of TTE multiply as the patient's size increases and following multiple cardiac surgeries. Bone, fat, scar, and air do not transmit US, so the imaging is easily shadowed in a large postoperative patient. The superiority of echo's spatial resolution over MRI is readily apparent in an infant or young child; however, that quickly changes when the imaging windows are limited. Depth of penetration is dependent on transducer frequency, with lower-frequency transducers penetrating further into the chest. Despite better penetration, spatial resolution quickly degrades, and the ability to see posterior structures declines rapidly as body habitus increases.

Transesophageal Echocardiography in Congenital Heart Disease

TEE provides additional echo views of cardiac structures in a more invasive fashion (Figs. 6.16 and 6.17). Younger patients often require sedation before performance of a transesophageal study, and there is a small but non-ignorable risk of complications, namely, irritation or damage to the esophagus. While TEE is widely applied in

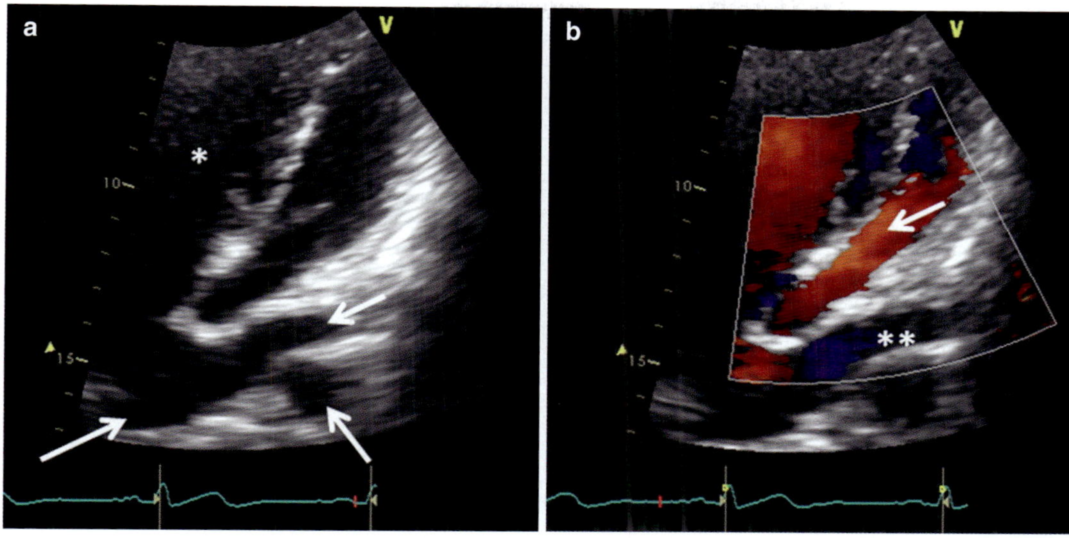

Fig. 6.13 Apical four-chamber view of a young adult with physiologically repaired D-transposition of the great arteries. An atrial level switch operation (Senning procedure) was previously performed. (**a**) Demonstrates pulmonary venous return (*arrows*) to the pulmonary venous baffle with channeling of flow to the tricuspid valve and systemic right ventricle (*). (**b**) Shows color Doppler flow over the systemic venous baffle and mitral valve (*arrow*). Color flow suggests no obstruction to systemic venous baffle flow to the mitral valve. Far-field color imaging (**) demonstrates low-velocity flow within the pulmonary venous baffle, also suggesting no obstruction in this other surgically created atrial chamber

adult patients without limitation due to size, the smallest of pediatric patients may be precluded from this imaging approach owing to the proportionate large caliber of the transducer probe relative to the esophagus.

When combined, TTE and TEE provide a near 360° depiction of cardiac structures. Structures closer to the chest wall are better imaged using transthoracic means, while deeper structures are seen better when approached from a posterior and intrathoracic origin within the chest.

Color and Spectral Doppler in Congenital Heart Disease

In addition to detailed assessment of cardiac anatomy, basic physiological and functional parameters can be evaluated with the use of color flow mapping and spectral Doppler. Color flow mapping is used to evaluate flow disruptions, abnormal flow patterns, and directionality of blood flow. Spectral Doppler allows estimates of peak instantaneous velocity at a single point using pulse wave Doppler or over a distance along an US beam using continuous wave Doppler. The modified Bernoulli equation can be used to convert velocity into an estimate of pressure gradient by the equation:

$$\Delta P = 4v2$$

The modified Bernoulli equation and spectral Doppler velocity measurement provide a noninvasive method for serial measurement of stenotic vessels or valves. Evaluation of flow on top of a 2D image provides an added layer of assurance that 2D anatomy corresponds with the suspected pathophysiology.

The velocity scale used for color flow mapping can be adjusted for low- or high-velocity blood flow. Venous flow mapping should be performed at low velocity to ensure visualization of slow venous blood flow. Arterial flow should be evaluated at higher velocities. Using the correct velocity scale for the vascular structure of interest will allow the sonographer to visualize

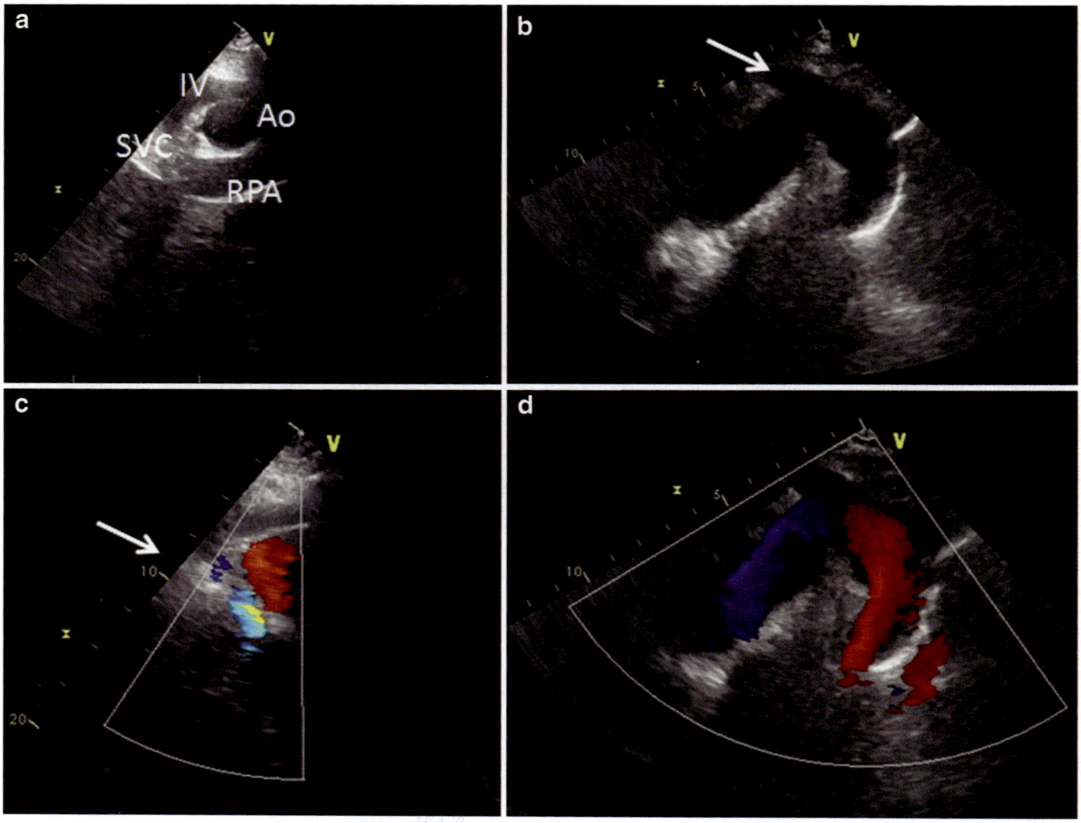

Fig. 6.14 Transthoracic echo imaging from the suprasternal notch. (**a**, **c**) Demonstrate imaging of an adult following repair of a sinus venosus atrial septal defect and partial anomalous pulmonary venous connection. Two-dimensional imaging demonstrates the course of the innominate vein (*IV*) and right superior vena cava (*SVC*). The right pulmonary artery (*RPA*) and aortic arch (*Ao*) are also noted and are both dilated. Color imaging demonstrates turbulent flow (*blue jet*, *arrow*) from the right upper pulmonary venous flow baffled through the repaired atrial septal defect into the left atrium. (**b**, **d**) Demonstrate similar suprasternal image slices in a patient with severe neoaortic insufficiency and aortic arch aneurysm diagnosed decades after an arterial switch operation and arch augmentation to address transposition of the great arteries with arch hypoplasia. Two-dimensional imaging demonstrates the severely dilated and tortuous arch in its entirety. The right innominate artery is also noted to be dilated (*arrow*). Color Doppler during diastole shows retrograde flow from the descending thoracic aorta coursing back to the aortic root (*red to blue color jet*), consistent with severe aortic insufficiency

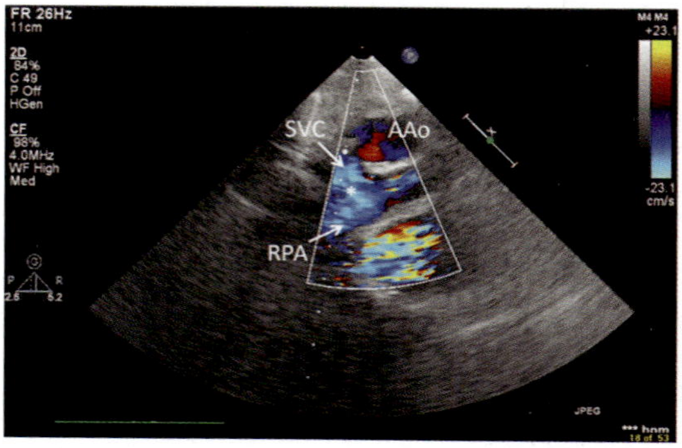

Fig. 6.15 Transthoracic echo imaging from the suprasternal notch in a single-ventricle congenital heart disease patient. An orthogonal plane of imaging creates a short-axis view from the suprasternal notch, allowing one to see a cross-sectional view through the ascending aorta (*AAo*). The superior vena cava (*SVC*) is noted to drain to the right of the aorta with a direct connection to the right pulmonary artery (*RPA*) in a bidirectional Glenn connection (*). A bidirectional Glenn anastomosis is performed during a second palliative operation to manage patients with single-ventricle lesions

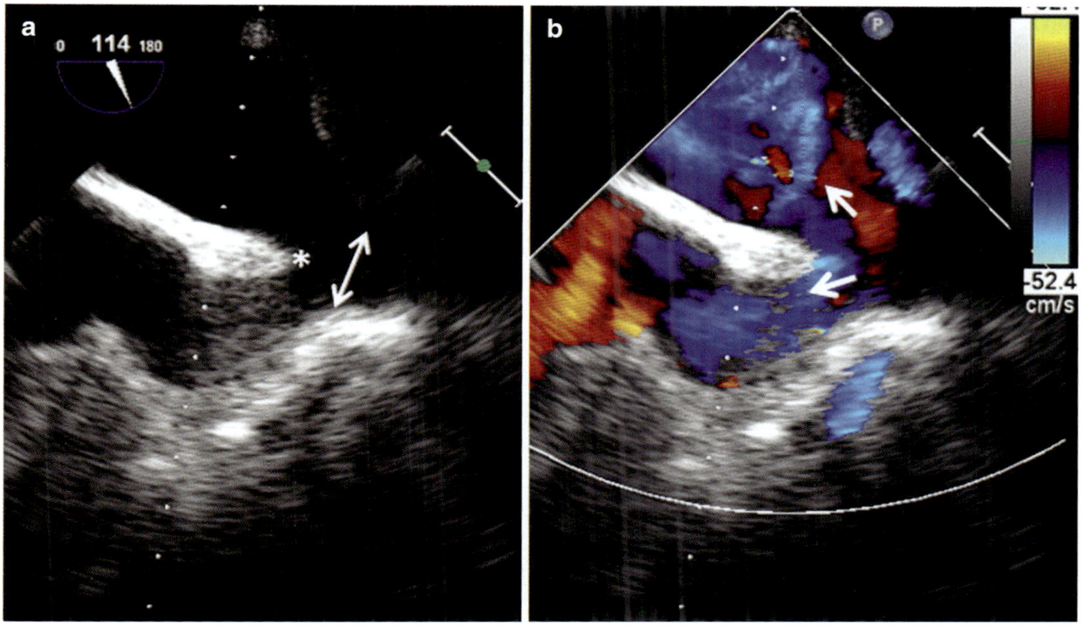

Fig. 6.16 Transesophageal echo imaging, bicaval view, of a 52-year-old patient with previously unrepaired congenital heart disease consisting of a sinus venosus-type atrial septal defect and partial anomalous pulmonary venous connections. (**a**) Two-dimensional imaging shows the defect involving the crest of the atrial septum (*) and an abnormally medial insertion of the superior vena cava overriding the septum (*bidirectional arrow*), as is frequently the case with this defect. (**b**) Color Doppler flow shows streaming of caval flow to both the left and right atria (*arrows*). The patient exhibited hypoxemia with a room air pulse oximetry value of 92 %

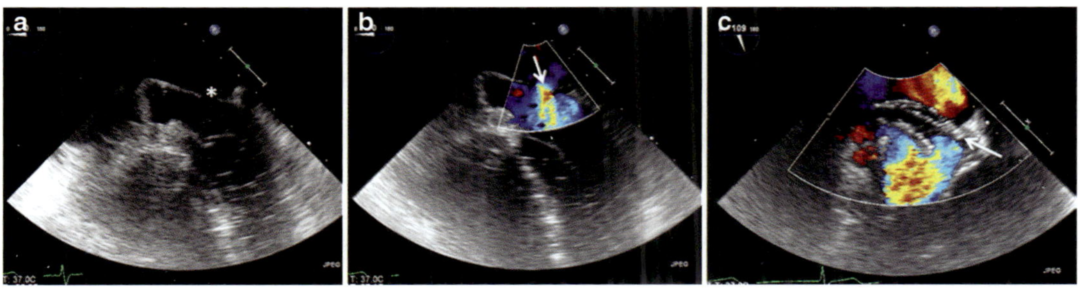

Fig. 6.17 Transesophageal imaging in a young adult with physiologically repaired D-transposition of the great arteries. A prior atrial level switch procedure (Mustard's procedure) was performed. A baffle leak was suspected on transthoracic echo imaging and confirmed with transesophageal echo prior to transvenous dual chamber pacemaker implantation for a history of sick sinus syndrome. (**a**, **b**) Demonstrate the location of the baffle leak (*) within the lateral aspect of the baffle wall overlying the mitral valve. Color Doppler flow demonstrates shunting across the leak (*arrow*) from the pulmonary venous to systemic venous atrial limbs, consistent with a physiologic left-to-right shunt. (**c**) Demonstrates the appearance of the baffle wall following deployment of an Amplatzer septal occluder device (*arrow*). The device is seated with the discs spanning the leak with color flow demonstrating no significant residual shunting

transitions between laminar flow and turbulent flow, indicating areas of acute angle change or stenosis. In patients with CHD, this is a crucial link between the anatomy as seen on 2D imaging and the physiology of stenosis, regurgitation or simply directionality of flow. For instance, complex heterotaxy syndrome can manifest as interruption of the IVC with azygous continuation to the SVC or infracardiac total anomalous pulmonary venous drainage below the diaphragm. On the initial 2D US examination, the vascular anatomy can be confusing as these draining vessels can appear in a similar region, but the direction of blood flow will clue the sonographer into which structure is more likely. An azygous continuation of the IVC will drain superiorly causing the low-velocity color signal to be blue (away from the transducer) in the subcostal imaging planes, whereas an inferiorly draining pulmonary venous confluence will appear red (toward the transducer) in the subcostal imaging planes. Also, if the correct velocity is used for the color scale, regions of narrowing or dilation can be seen as turbulent flow as described in the prior section, "Doppler Echocardiography."

In addition, color flow mapping augments 2D imaging when spatial limitation or imaging artifact obscures structures such as small vessel connections. An important example of this is in the case of anomalous left coronary artery off the pulmonary artery (ALCAPA). 2D imaging of anomalous coronary arteries may be limited in terms of concise determination of ostial origin and vessel course. Color Doppler permits direct evaluation of the directionality of blood flow within an imaged vessel, thereby providing further confirmatory evidence of an anomalous origin.

Evaluation of obstructed blood flow utilizes both color flow mapping and spectral Doppler. Color flow mapping allows the sonographer to visualize the specific region of obstruction and the region of highest velocity. Spectral Doppler, either PW or CW, is then used to estimate the peak and/or mean velocity, which correlate with the peak-to-peak gradient measured by catheterization. Pre- and postsurgical valvular stenoses and vascular stenoses are also followed in this manner.

Limitations of color and spectral Doppler include incident angle of interrogation, imaging through bone and air, probe frequency, and choice of CW or PW. The incident angle of interrogation is the angle at which a Doppler beam contacts the vessel or region of interest. The beam must be parallel with the blood flow to gain maximal accuracy of velocity estimation. The greater the difference in angle between the interrogation beam and blood flow, the greater the error will be when estimating the velocity. Newer systems and probes can adjust for angle differences but if the beam is perpendicular to flow, both color flow mapping and spectral Doppler analysis will be difficult and may lead to incorrect diagnosis. Imaging difficulties through air and bone are similar to standard 2D echo imaging; however, where 2D imaging can fail due to air and bone, color flow mapping and spectral Doppler can function well enough to be diagnostic. Spectral Doppler by itself does not require a 2D image and can be performed "blindly" as was historically the case in the early era of echo. Probe frequency will affect the ability for spectral and color Doppler to evaluate blood flow of varying velocities as described in the previous section. Lower-frequency US probes offer a more robust assessment over a larger range of velocities compared to higher-frequency probes. Finally, PW is limited in its capacity to evaluate high-velocity blood flow compared to CW Doppler, and this is related to the pulse frequency of US transmission as described previously.

Tissue Doppler in Congenital Heart Disease

TDI is employed in echo imaging for a more direct assessment of myocardial function. Whereas color and spectral Doppler assess blood flow that results from myocardial contraction, TDI filters out the high-frequency blood flow signal, allowing the lower-frequency motion of the myocardium to be measured as a myocardial velocity. This can be displayed in 2D color imaging similar to color Doppler blood flow, where red color indicates myocardial motion toward the transducer and blue color indicates motion away from the transducer. TDI can also be displayed using PW Doppler at a specific point along the ventricular chamber, which will display the resultant velocity change over time at that particular region. Further expanded applications of TDI include color Doppler myocardial imaging

(CDMI) which tracks a region of myocardium in space, similar to tracking two adjacent points in the myocardium during myocardial strain analysis. The MRI equivalent to this technique is the use of magnetic myocardial tagging to track myocardial change in space over time. The benefit of TDI is direct assessment of myocardial motion rather than extrapolating functional assessment from measures of blood flow and change in cavity size (i.e., ejection fraction measurement). While blood flow and change in chamber size during the cardiac cycle are important metrics for assessing overall cardiovascular function, direct myocardial measurement as described above using TDI improves our understanding of the system's component parts.

Since TDI measures the myocardium throughout the cardiac cycle, it is used to assess diastolic function simultaneously with systolic function in the same beat. An example of this is the myocardial performance index (MPI), which can be determined using both spectral Doppler and TDI. Utilizing spectral Doppler analysis of blood flow during systole and diastole requires a change in position of the acquisition cursor while imaging. Therefore, two separate images must be acquired and attention paid to heart rate consistency between the two images. LV myocardial performance index (MPI), a metric that includes the isovolumic relaxation time (IVRT), isovolumic contraction time (IVCT), and LV ejection time (LVET), is measured by acquiring a spectral Doppler tracing at the LV outflow tract to obtain LVET and at the mitral valve to obtain the interval between A-wave completion and onset of the E-wave (Fig. 6.18). By subtracting the LVET from the inter-mitral interval, one can then derive a combined IVCT and IVRT. Using the spectral Doppler approach for MPI assessment introduces potential for inaccurate measurements by virtue of the fact that multiple measurements have to be made during different cardiac cycles. In contrast, TDI allows the same measurements to be made in a single beat, without adjusting the cursor position, and with superior accuracy of each component. The IVCT and IVRT can be measured directly using TDI rather than extrapolating these intervals from spectral Doppler measurements.

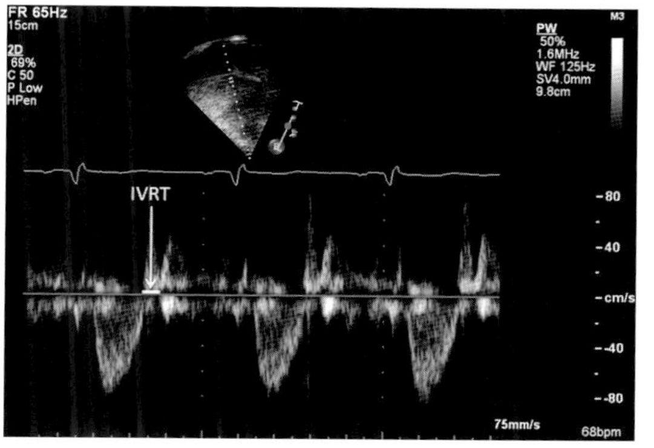

Fig. 6.18 Example of measuring isovolumic relaxation time (*IVRT*) of the left ventricle with spectral Doppler. Several cardiac cycles are recorded using spectral Doppler at the left ventricular outflow tract. Additional spectral Doppler evaluation at the mitral valve inflow is necessary to acquire additional measurements as part of determining the myocardial performance index (MPI)

TDI provides additional utility in echo imaging in the evaluation of global myocardial function given that it is less dependent on geometric constraints compared to methods employed for ejection or shortening fraction calculations.

TDI techniques vary in spatial resolution; however, they all share the advantage of high temporal resolution with frame rates as high as 300 frames per second. The spatial resolution is dependent on the TDI technique being employed. PW Doppler examination of myocardial velocity suffers from a lack of myocardial tracking. Newer myocardial tracking of ventricular wall segments by CDMI provides better regional characterization through improved spatial resolution while maintaining excellent temporal resolution. In this case the tag remains on the myocardium, similar to MRI tissue tagging. However, where MRI tags move in plane and out of plane, the echo-based technique only moves in 2 dimensions and, thus, can only provide motion characteristics in either a longitudinal direction or radial direction.

Individual TDI-derived velocities have been correlated with various components of myocardial function. For instance, the *E*/*E′* ratio is the ratio between peak E-wave velocity measured from spectral Doppler-derived mitral inflow (*E*) and peak E-wave from TDI-derived mitral annular motion (*E′*). This has been correlated with the pulmonary capillary wedge pressure as determined by right heart catheterization. The peak S-wave on TDI at the lateral tricuspid valve annulus has been correlated with pulmonary vascular resistance. CDMI is being utilized to measure myocardial strain and strain rate on a regional basis, providing more detailed wall motion analysis.

Intracardiac and Intravascular Echocardiography in Congenital Heart Disease

ICE and IVUS have extended the US imaging modality further into the endocardial and endovascular spaces, expanding its application in cardiac imaging. Both imaging approaches are progressively incorporating other avenues of utility in cardiac imaging. However, they both remain relatively limited for the evaluation of CHD.

IVUS imaging is frequently incorporated in the evaluation of vessel lumen patency during coronary arterial catheterization and is an important tool to help assess coronary arterial stenoses, atherosclerotic plaque burden and distribution, vascular wall characterization, and patency of previously implanted stents during percutaneous intervention [12–16]. It has also become an important adjunct tool during percutaneous coronary interventions, providing an additional level of assessment at the time of vessel dilation or stent deployment [14]. In addition to coronary arterial imaging, it has also been incorporated into diagnostic imaging of the pulmonary arterial vasculature in patients with pulmonary arterial hypertension [17]. Finally, this imaging approach has also been incorporated for pulmonary vein imaging and endovascular procedures such as IVC filter deployment [18–20].

IVUS imaging is performed at the time of cardiac catheterization, which requires venous or arterial access with long outer, introducing sheath support. The high-frequency (20–40 MHz) imaging catheter is passed over a guide wire to the distal most part of the vessel of interest and is then slowly withdrawn (usually at a rate of 0.5 mm/s) while acquiring images of the vessel wall and lumen. Due to its close proximity to the structures being imaged as well as use of high-frequency ultrasonic waves, imaging resolution and clarity are excellent for imaging epicardial coronary and smaller branch pulmonary arterial and venous vessels.

While the modality provides excellent imaging in the small vessel space, this is rarely required for general diagnostic or therapeutic purposes in patients with CHD. What is imaged by IVUS is typically seen during an initial survey and characterization of CHD lesions by standard transthoracic and possibly transesophageal imaging approaches first. In addition, small vessel structures such as anomalous coronary arterial origins and courses and anomalous pulmonary venous drainage or stenoses typically require angiography or advanced imaging with cardiac MRI or CT, further limiting IVUS to more of a therapeutic adjunct tool.

With regard to its specific application in CHD, IVUS has been incorporated into the late assessment of patients who have undergone previous arterial switch operation (ASO) for transposition of the great arteries (TGA). In this operation, the great vessels are switched and the coronary arteries are also transferred from their native sites to join the aorta and left ventricle at the neoaortic root. IVUS was incorporated into the follow-up care of 22 TGA patients who had undergone ASO repair [21]. The youngest patient evaluated with IVUS in the study was 5 years old (range 5–21.6 years). A high percentage (89 %) of vessels imaged demonstrated intimal proliferation to varying degrees with nearly half of the patients having moderate-to-severe coronary arterial intimal thickening based on IVUS imaging, demonstrating its utility in follow-up for this unique and growing population as well as the concerning degree of small vessel disease that remains worrisome but otherwise difficult to quantify.

Our institution has incorporated IVUS in the anatomic and hemodynamic evaluation of cavopulmonary connections in single-ventricle patients (Fig. 6.19). In select patients with atriopulmonary Fontan connection variants, IVUS has been utilized during diagnostic catheterization for formal assessment of pulmonary arterial, Fontan, and caval pressures in the context of right heart failure and failing Fontan symptomatology. IVUS imaging of the anastomotic sites between the atrium and pulmonary artery has offered adjunctive assessments while limiting the amount of contrast and angiographic radiation that may have been otherwise required.

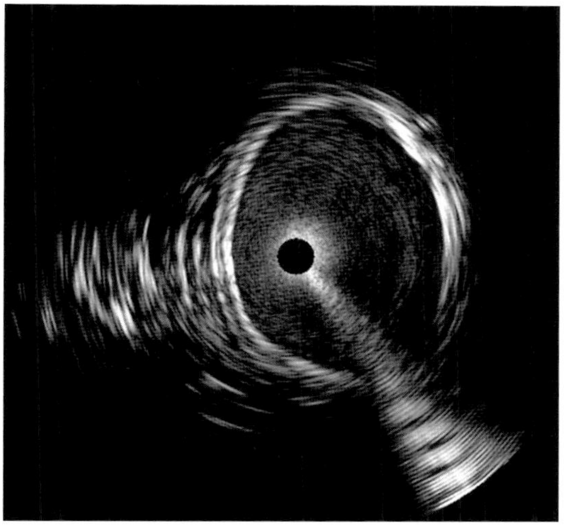

Fig. 6.19 Intravascular ultrasound (IVUS) imaging in a 43-year-old patient with palliated single-ventricle congenital heart disease consisting of tricuspid atresia and hypoplastic right ventricle. The patient had previously undergone Fontan palliation with a Kreutzer connection, incorporating a conduit between the right atrium and hypoplastic right ventricle, thereby bypassing the atretic tricuspid valve. During diagnostic catheterization, IVUS was used to evaluate the intraluminal characteristics of the Kreutzer conduit. The image above demonstrates complete patency of the conduit lumen without evidence of pannus ingrowth or luminal kinking

Similar to IVUS, ICE imaging is also performed at the time of cardiac catheterization. ICE catheters are comprised of high-frequency (greater than 20 MHz) transducers with either phased array or single crystal designs mounted at the tip of the catheter. Typically, venous access with at least a 9-French sheath is required to accommodate the catheter. The catheter is steerable and therefore has some degree of maneuverability to position the transducer to image left and right heart structures. ICE imaging is generally applied in the interventional and therapeutic arenas for procedures such as noncoronary cardiac interventions and electrophysiologic studies involving catheter ablation. This imaging modality provides excellent visualization of the atrial septum, making it a valuable tool for transseptal puncture for right atrial-to-left atrial access as well as percutaneous device closure of a patent foramen ovale or secundum-type atrial septal defects [22–25] (Fig. 6.20). ICE has also been used in the diagnostic and therapeutic aspects of prosthetic valve management. It provides a valuable extension to standard TTE and TEE imaging of prosthetic valves to evaluate for perivalvular leaks and valve vegetations and to further expand the assessment of prosthetic valve stenosis or regurgitation [26]. ICE is also being

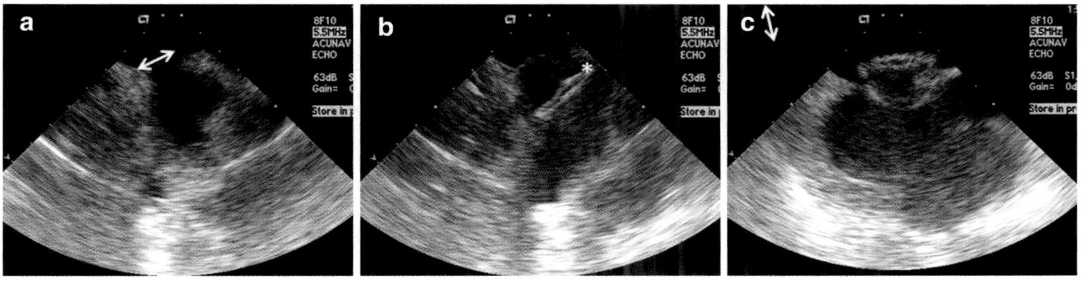

Fig. 6.20 Intracardiac echo (ICE) imaging during percutaneous ASD closure. (**a**) Demonstrates ICE imaging with the probe tip located in the right atrium. In this imaging plane, the atrial septum and associated defect (*bidirectional arrow*) are clearly seen. (**b**) Demonstrates imaging during occlusion device (*) deployment. The left atrial disc of the device has been released on the left atrial side of the defect. A floppy and aneurysmal septum primum (*arrow*) is noted in conjunction with the atrial septal defect. (**c**) Shows the occlusion device seated across the atrial septal defect (*bidirectional arrow*). Both discs have been deployed and released with complete defect occlusion. The septal rims are noted in this view as well

incorporated for percutaneous valve replacement procedures such as transcatheter aortic valve implantation [27, 28].

In patients with CHD, ICE imaging has occasionally been utilized for interventional and electrophysiologic procedures [29–32]. ICE provides an additional measure of real-time imaging for navigating within baffle limbs, performing transbaffle punctures, and positioning catheters through preexisting leaks (as in the case of fenestrated Fontan conduits or atrial baffle leaks). It also provides a way to directly image catheter position and contact during catheter ablation and to monitor for the development of pericardial effusions during interventional procedures. In addition to atrial defect closure, the use of ICE in Fontan fenestration closure has been anecdotally described, and its incorporation during percutaneous closure of atrial baffle leaks in adults with TGA has been reported [33]. Its superiority relative to TEE for these applications remains debated [24, 25], and its incorporation in such applications will likely remain the individual decision of the practicing physician utilizing these imaging tools. Furthermore, the applications noted above in CHD are extensions to how ICE is already incorporated for atrial septal access and defect closure in patients with structurally normal hearts. As with IVUS, ICE is generally not incorporated for the initial diagnosis and characterization of CHD lesions. From a diagnostic standpoint, it can provide adjunct information when standard TTE and TEE imaging are limited.

The application of IVUS and ICE in the echocardiographic assessment of CHD is limited for several reasons. First, the invasive vascular requirement for ICE and IVUS, coupled with adequate TTE and TEE imaging quality for the majority of CHD-related structures, limits the regular use of IVUS and ICE for pure diagnostic purposes. Advanced imaging techniques often supplant IVUS and ICE as well given their less invasive approaches and ability to acquire far more information than these two expanded echo modalities can provide. Second, vascular access may be limited in adult patients with CHD due either to small patient and/or small vessel sizes or obstructed vessels from prior instrumentation and procedures. Lack of access precludes use of either IVUS or ICE. Third, the relatively narrow range of structures that these approaches are capable of imaging largely limits their use to interventional and therapeutic applications such as imaging catheter location and contact, assessing device seating and stability, and surveying the endocardial wall and pericardial space during interventional procedures in the event of hemodynamic instability (i.e., to rule out pericardial effusion).

Integration of Echocardiography with Advanced Cardiac Imaging

Advanced cardiac imaging using computed tomography (CT) and magnetic resonance imaging (MRI) has become an extremely useful adjunct to standard echo and catheterization in the evaluation of CHD. In certain arenas, advanced imaging has served as an alternative to more invasive testing in the planning and recommendation for therapeutic interventions as is the case with the application of cardiac MRI in place of diagnostic catheterization with angiography for second-stage palliative surgical planning for hypoplastic left heart syndrome [34]. These imaging modalities continue to have limitations though, namely, their lack of portability, costly maintenance, and staffing requirements. CT has the additional disadvantage of radiation exposure concerns. MRI is limited due to longer scan times and the need for sedation or possibly general anesthesia for younger patients or those with developmental impairments that may limit their ability to cooperate during the scan. However, where echo and catheterization fall short, advanced imaging can fill in the gap. In fact, the application of CT and MRI is growing dramatically in their ability to provide high-resolution anatomic detail in any plane as well as physiologic data that would otherwise be difficult to obtain or unobtainable by either echo or catheterization. The ultimate tie that binds all of these modalities in the diagnosis and management of CHD is the systematic approach to evaluating cardiac anatomy, connections, and physiology.

The quality of anatomical assessment of CHD by either echo or MRI is difficult to compare. On the one hand, echo is, by far, more available but generally requires the interpreting physician to generate a mental 3D picture of the heart being imaged. Additionally, the quality of imaging declines with larger or obese body habitus or following cumulative cardiac surgeries. Imaging using MRI may be viewed as more intuitive given a more holistic image set that is generated, and high-quality imaging can be obtained in patients with severely limited echo windows. However, interpreting the images acquired from MRI still requires an intimate knowledge of CHD and the systematic approach to CHD description and classification.

Cardiac function can be assessed in many ways using echo and MRI modalities, from global measures such as ejection fraction and cardiac output to more specific measures such as regional wall motion or isovolumic interval assessment. Intrinsic myocardial fiber function is not assessed using echo at this time. The ideal assessment of function is a load-independent description of myocardial contractility, and the ideal diastolic assessment is re-creation of a diastolic compliance curve. However, there is no single measure at our disposal that can fully assess both systolic and diastolic function. Cardiac functional assessment by echo or MRI is quite different, but both aim to describe similar features of myocardial mechanics. A comparison between the tools of functional assessment using either modality is mentioned below:

1. Echocardiographic global LV systolic function is measured by using either a shortening fraction on M-mode or by measuring ejection fraction in the apical four-chamber view by modified Simpson's model. Both methods are incomplete because they make geometric assumptions that may not apply to the disease condition.

   MRI provides a true ejection fraction based on LV end-diastolic volume and LV end-systolic volume that is measured using 3D reconstruction of the LV. Wall motion abnormalities can be documented, and true volume assessments can be made regardless of the geometry and regardless of imaging windows.

2. Isovolumic relaxation, passive LV filling, and active/atrial systolic LV filling are specific portions of diastole that serve different functions during ventricular diastole. Pulmonary vein spectral Doppler, mitral inflow Doppler, TDI, and left atrial size/volume are examples of different assessments performed using echo to assess ventricular diastolic function. Each metric provides one aspect of diastole; therefore, they are utilized in combination to give a broader view of diastolic function as a whole.

   MRI can provide similar metrics for diastolic functional assessment. While echo can assess beat-to-beat changes due to higher temporal resolution, MRI is an average over multiple cardiac cycles.

3. TDI analysis on echo provides a highly reproducible measure of strain and wall motion analysis similar to tissue characterization by tagged MRI scanning. The ability to track wall motion has gained more attention over the last decade with the goal of direct myocardial assessment versus surrogate measures by blood flow characterization or geometric chamber changes.

Conclusions

In summary, echo continues to be the primary modality for cardiac imaging in CHD due to its portability and excellent temporal and spatial resolution. However, in the older patient where US windows are limited and for adults with repaired or palliated CHD, MRI is playing an increasing role in defining both anatomy and function in a safe manner with improved spatial resolution. Furthermore, direct and very accurate measurements of both RV and LV volumes can be made using MRI along with flow quantification in any of the extracardiac vessels or across the cardiac valves with the ability to quantify both forward flow and regurgitant flow. Both imaging modalities have their strengths and limitations, but when combined in the appropriate settings, they provide an incredible wealth of information that is vital to the management of ACHD patients.

References

1. Dussik KT. Uber die Moglichkeit Hochfrequente Mechanische schwingungen als Diagnostiches Hilfsmittel zu Verwerten. Z Neurol. 1941;174:153.
2. Edler I, Hertz CH. Use of ultrasonic reflectoscope for the continuous recording of movements of heart walls. Kungl Fysiogr Sallsk Lung Forth. 1954;24:40.
3. Gutgesell HP, Huhta JC, Latson LA, Huffines D, McNamara DG. Accuracy of two-dimensional echocardiography in the diagnosis of congenital heart disease. Am J Cardiol. 1985;55:514–8.
4. Bash SE, Huhta JC, Vick III GW, Gutgesell HP, Ott DA. Hypoplastic left heart syndrome: is echocardiography accurate enough to guide surgical palliation? J Am Coll Cardiol. 1986;7:610–6.
5. Krabill KA, Ring WS, Foker JE, Braunlin EA, Einzig S, Berry JM, et al. Echocardiographic versus cardiac catheterization diagnosis of infants with congenital heart disease requiring surgery. Am J Cardiol. 1987;60:351–4.
6. Lipshultz SE, Sanders SP, Mayer JE, Colan SD, Lock JE. Are routine preoperative cardiac catheterization and angiography necessary before repair of ostium primum atrial septal defect? J Am Coll Cardiol. 1988;11:373–8.
7. Davis JT, Allen HD, Cohen DM, Teske DW, Cassidy SC, Craenen JM, et al. Use of cardiac catheterization in pediatric cardiac surgical decisions. Thorac Cardiovasc Surg. 1994;42:148–51.
8. Currie PJ, Seward JB, Hagler DJ, Tajik AJ. Two-dimensional/Doppler echocardiography and its relationship to cardiac catheterization for diagnosis and management of congenital heart disease. Cardiovasc Clin. 1986;17:301–22.
9. Tworetzky W, McElhinney DB, Brook MM, Reddy VM, Hanley FL, Silverman NH. Echocardiographic diagnosis alone for the complete repair of major congenital heart defects. J Am Coll Cardiol. 1999;33:229–33.
10. Van Praagh R. Terminology of congenital heart disease. Glossary and commentary. Circulation. 1977;56:139–43.
11. Van Praagh R. Diagnosis of complex congenital heart disease: morphologic-anatomic method and terminology. Cardiovasc Intervent Radiol. 1984;7:115–20.
12. Tobis JM, Mallery J, Mahon D, Lehmann K, Zalesky P, Griffith J, Gessert J, Moriuchi M, McRae M, Dwyer ML. Intravascular ultrasound imaging of human coronary arteries in vivo. Analysis of tissue characterizations with comparison to in vitro histological specimens. Circulation. 1991;83:913–26.
13. Golinvaux N, Maehara A, Mintz GS, Lansky AJ, McPherson J, Farhat N, Marso S, de Bruyne B, Serruys PW, Templin B, Cheong W-F, Aaskar R, Fahy M, Mehran R, Leon M, Stone GW. An intravascular ultrasound appraisal of atherosclerotic plaque distribution in diseased coronary arteries. Am Heart J. 2012;163:624–31.
14. Mantziari A, Ziakas A, Stavropoulos G, Styliadis IH. Clinical applications of intravascular ultrasound (IVUS): experience from an academic high volume centre in Northern Greece. Hippokratia. 2011;15(1):60–3.
15. Maehara A, Mintz GS, Weissman NJ. Advances in intravascular imaging. Circ Cardiovasc Interv. 2009;2:482–90.
16. Nicholls SJ, Hsu A, Wolski K, Hu B, Bayturan O, Lavoie A, Uno K, Tuzcu EM, Nissen SE. Intravascular ultrasound-derived measures of coronary atherosclerotic plaque burden and clinical outcome. J Am Coll Cardiol. 2010;55:2399–407.
17. Bressollette E, Dupuis J, Bonan R, Doucet S, Cernacek P, Tardif J-C. Intravascular ultrasound assessment of pulmonary vascular disease in patients with pulmonary hypertension. Chest. 2001;120:809–15.
18. Cabrera JA, Sánchez-Quintana D, Farré J, Navarro F, Rubio JM, Cabestrero F, Anderson RH, Ho SY. Ultrasonic characterization of the pulmonary venous wall: echocardiographic and histological correlation. Circulation. 2002;106:968–73.
19. Guerra PG, Thibault B, Dubuc M, Talajic M, Roy D, Crépeau J, Nattel S, Tardif J-C. Identification of atrial tissue in pulmonary veins using intravascular ultrasound. J Am Soc Echocardiogr. 2003;16:982–7.
20. Oppat WF, Chiou AC, Matsumura JS. Intravascular ultrasound-guided vena cava filter placement. J Endovasc Surg. 1999;6:285–7.
21. Pedra SRFF, Pedra CAC, Abizaid AA, Braga SLN, Staico R, Arrieta R, Costa Jr JR, Vaz VD, Fontes VF, Sousa JER. Intracoronary ultrasound assessment late after the arterial switch operation for transposition of the great arteries. J Am Coll Cardiol. 2005;45:2061–8.
22. Daoud EG, Kalbfleisch SJ, Hummel JD. Intracardiac echocardiography to guide transseptal left heart catheterization for radiofrequency catheter ablation. J Cardiovasc Electrophysiol. 1999;10:358–63.
23. Earing MG, Cabalka AK, Seward JB, Bruce CJ, Reeder GS, Hagler DJ. Intracardiac echocardiographic guidance during transcatheter device closure of atrial septal defect and patent foramen ovale. Mayo Clin Proc. 2004;79:24–34.
24. Boccalandro F, Baptista E, Muench A, Carter C, Smalling RW. Comparison of intracardiac echocardiography versus transesophageal echocardiography guidance for percutaneous transcatheter closure of atrial septal defect. Am J Cardiol. 2004;93:437–40.
25. Rigatelli G, Dell'Avvocata F, Cardaioli P, Giordan M, Braggion G, Aggio S, Roncon L, Chen-Scarabelli C, Scarabelli TM, Faggian G. Five-year follow-up of transcatheter intracardiac echocardiography-assisted closure of interatrial shunts. Cardiovasc Revasc Med. 2011;12:355–61.
26. Kolodner DQ, Shimbo D, Magnano AR. Intracardiac echocardiography in the diagnosis of prosthetic valve endocarditis. Heart. 2007;93:1120.
27. Ussia GP, Barbanti M, Sarkar K, Cumbo M, Aruta P, Scarabelli M, Cammalleri V, Immè S, Pistritto AM, Gulino S, Deste W, Zingali G, Garretto V, Mulè M, Scandura S, Tamburino C. Accuracy of intracardiac echocardiography for aortic root assessment in

patients undergoing transcatheter aortic valve implantation. Am Heart J. 2012;163:684–9.
28. Bartel T, Bonaros N, Müller L, Friedrich G, Grimm M, Velik-Salchner C, Feuchtner G, Pedross F. Intracardiac echocardiography: a new guiding tool for transcatheter aortic valve replacement. J Am Soc Echocardiogr. 2011;24:966–75.
29. Barker PCA. Intracardiac echocardiography in congenital heart disease. J Cardiovasc Transl Res. 2009; 2:19–23.
30. den Uijl DW, Blom NA, Wijnmaalen AP, Bax JJ, Schalij MJ, Zeppenfeld K. Real-time integration of intracardiac echocardiography to facilitate atrial tachycardia ablation in a patient with a Senning baffle. Circ Arrhythm Electrophysiol. 2009;2: e28–30.
31. Peichl P, Kautzner J, Gebauer R. Ablation of atrial tachycardias after correction of complex congenital heart diseases: utility of intracardiac echocardiography. Europace. 2009;11:48–53.
32. Traykov VB, Pap R, Bencsik G, Makai A, Forster T. Ventricular location of a part of the right atrial isthmus after tricuspid valve replacement for Ebstein's anomaly: a challenge for atrial flutter ablation. J Interv Card Electrophysiol. 2009;25:199–201.
33. Kuppahally SS, Litwin SE, Green LS, Ishihara SM, Freedman RA, Michaels AD. Utility of intracardiac echocardiography for atrial baffle leak closure in repaired transposition of the great arteries. Echocardiography. 2010;27:E90–3.
34. Brown DW, Gauvreau K, Powell AJ, Lang P, Colan SD, Del Nido PJ, Odegard KC, Geva T. Cardiac magnetic resonance versus routine cardiac catheterization before bidirectional glenn anastomosis in infants with functional single ventricle: a prospective randomized trial. Circulation. 2007;116:2718–25.

Right Ventricle Outflow Tract

7

Farhood Saremi, Siew Yen Ho, and Damián Sánchez-Quintana

With rapid development in imaging technology, cardiac CT and MR have become the ideal methods for the assessment of complex morphology and function of the conotruncal region including the right ventricle out flow tract (RVOT). Detailed information about the embryology and anatomy of RVOT provides a better understanding of the spectrum of diseases of this region and helps to narrow differential diagnosis of pathologies involving this important structure. This will be discussed first in this chapter. Following to that, the role of CT and MR to evaluate morphology and function in relation to developmental malformation of the RVOT will be reviewed. A spectrum of conotruncal anomalies with abnormally positioned great arteries may arise from a perturbation of RVOT formation. Complications after RVOT surgery in congenital heart disease are common, and many need follow-up imaging for diagnosis and surgical planning. In this regard, the spectrum of diseases, differential diagnosis, and postoperative findings will be described.

Developmental Considerations

The two fields of cardiac progenitors are now recognized as the primary, and secondary or anterior, heart fields [1–4] It is the primary heart field that produces the straight heart tube. In mouse, there is firm evidence that the primary heart field gives rise to the left ventricle (LV), with the secondary field forming both the RV and the outflow tract (OFT) [4]. With looping of the heart tube, the ventricular trabeculations start to form at the outer curvature, permitting identification of the cranial part of the tube as OFT or conotruncus.

The initial OFT extends proximally from the distal ventricular groove to the pericardial reflections and demonstrates a characteristic dogleg bend which divides it into two myocardial subsegments, a proximal subsegment or the conus and a distal subsegment or the truncus [5]. The truncus arteriosus is a short segment interposed between the conus and the aortic sac. The latter transforms into the ascending aorta and pulmonary trunks.

The initial OFT is mainly myocardial and increases almost 6-fold in length between HH12 (Hamburger–Hamilton stages) and 24 (Fig. 7.1) [6]. Subsequently the initial musculature of the walls of the truncus and distal conus disappears by apoptosis, transdifferentiation, absorption into the developing RV, or a combination of

F. Saremi, MD (✉)
Department of Radiology, Cardiothoracic Section, University of Southern California, USC Keck Hospital, 1500 San Pablo St., Los Angeles, CA 90033, USA
e-mail: fsaremi@usc.edu

S.Y. Ho, PhD, FRCPath, FESC, FHEA
Cardiac Morphology Unit, Royal Brompton Hospital, London, SW3 6LY, UK

D. Sánchez-Quintana, MD, PhD
Departamento de Anatomía Humana, Facultad de Medicina de Badajoz, Badajoz, 06071, Spain
e-mail: damians@unex.es, dasaqui55@yahoo.com

F. Saremi (ed.), *Cardiac CT and MR for Adult Congenital Heart Disease*,
DOI 10.1007/978-1-4614-8875-0_7, © Springer Science+Business Media New York 2014

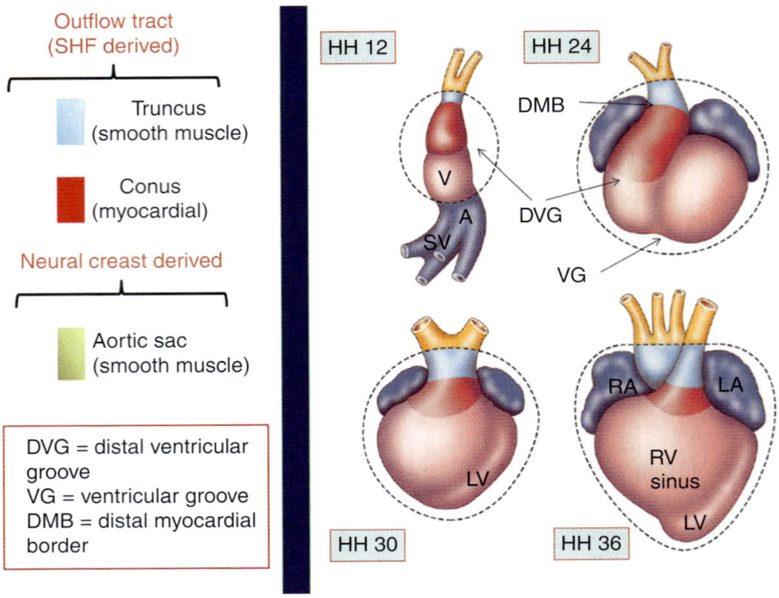

Fig. 7.1 The developing outflow tract in embryonic chicken hearts at stages 12, 24, 30, and 36 H/H. The area of the outflow tract (OFT) extends between distal ventricular groove (*DVG*) of the right ventricle and the junction with aortic sac at pericardial reflections and divided into the conus (proximal OFT shown in red) and the truncus (distal OFT in *light blue*). The OFT is divided into two parts, conus and truncus, and the junction between the two will be distal myocardial border (*DMB*). The images show that the OFT is initially mainly myocardial (*red part*) in its entirety, increasing in length up to HH24. The OFT myocardium, subsequently, shortens as a result of ventricularization, contributing to the trabeculated free wall, as well as the infundibulum, of the right ventricle (*RV*). Note the absolute reduction in the length of the OFT between 30 and 36 H/H stages, as well as the relative reduction in relation to the ventricles, which have increased in size by cardiomyocyte proliferation. The OFT has also been divided by septation into pulmonic and systemic outflows, and the aortic root has rotated to a posterior position, where it connects with the left ventricle (*LV*). The dotted line around the heart indicates the pericardium. *A* primitive atrium, *LA* left atrium, *RA* right atrium, *SV* sinus venosus, *V* primitive ventricle

these processes [7]. With further development, these new portions will be remodeled into the intrapericardial portions of the aorta and pulmonary trunk and arterial valves and their supporting sinuses. In contrast, myocardial tissue is being added to the proximal portion of the conus. As development proceeds, the single OFT undergoes remodeling into separate pulmonary and aortic arteries. The aorticopulmonary septation involves interactions between diverse cell types, including myocardium, endocardium, and neural crest cells [8]. The distal portion of aortic sac is also being considered as an entirely neural crest derivative.

OFT undergoes rotation during its remodeling. Rotation of the myocardium at the base of the OFT is probably essential to achieve normal positioning of the great arteries with respect to each other at the ventriculoarterial junction [9, 10]. In addition to abnormal OFT septation caused by neural crest cell defects, a spectrum of conotruncal anomalies with abnormally positioned great arteries may arise from a perturbation of myocardial rotation including tetralogy of Fallot (TOF), persistent truncus arteriosus, double outlet right ventricle (DORV), and transposition of the great arteries (TGA) [10, 11]. A short outflow tract as obtained experimentally through secondary heart field ablation may not allow a normal conotruncal rotation [4]. Although in conotruncal anomalies including TOF, the infundibular septum is not always short. It is believed that any time the RV shows a short outflow tract, a total or partial lack of conotruncal rotation and remodeling is inevitably present [9] (Fig. 7.2).

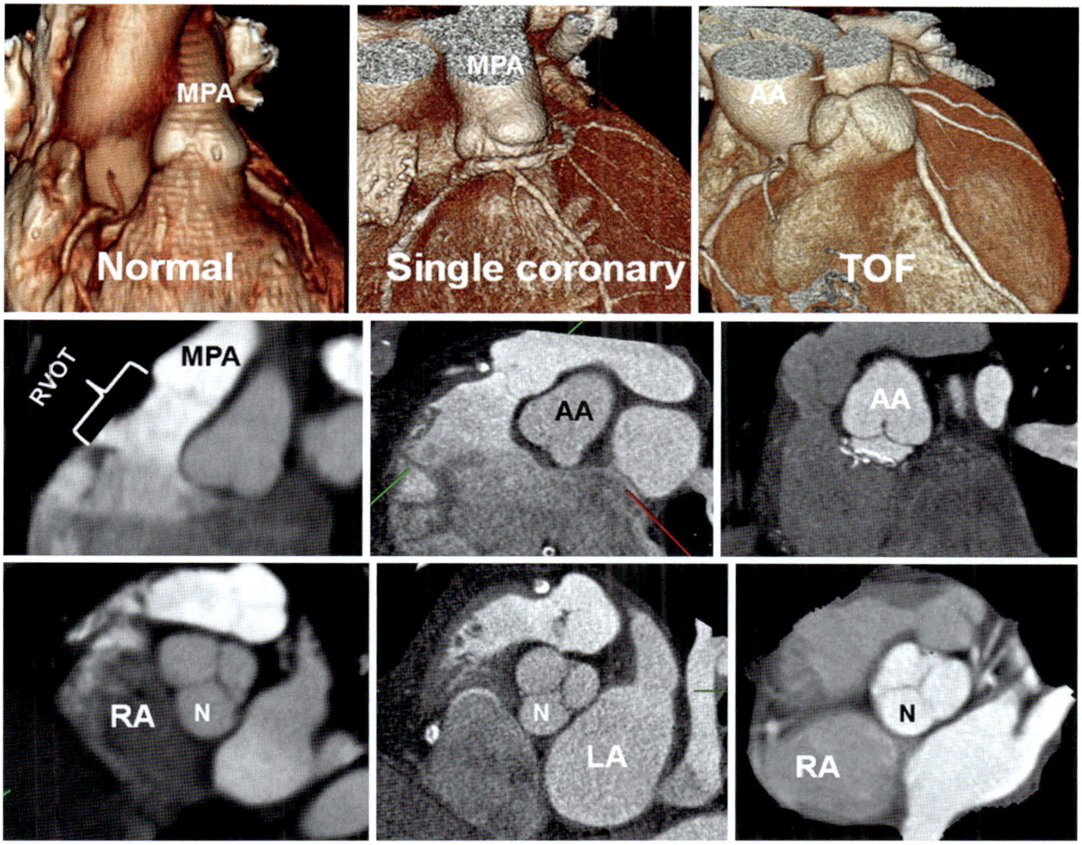

Fig. 7.2 Variations in right ventricle outflow tract (*RVOT*) length. In normal example the pulmonary valve extends well above the coronary sinuses of the ascending aorta (*AA*). The RVOT has a vertical course, and the middle of noncoronary (*N*) sinus overlays the interatrial septum. In patients with single coronary artery arising from the right coronary sinus and tetralogy of Fallot (*TOF*), the RVOT is short, and the aortic root is rotated clockwise facing the right atrium (*RA*). The RVOT is thickened and narrowed in TOF. Although in conotruncal anomalies including TOF the infundibular septum is not always short, it is believed that any time the RV shows a short outflow tract, a total or partial lack of conotruncal rotation is present. *LA* left atrium, *MPA* main pulmonary artery

Anatomical Evaluation of RVOT

Imaging Techniques

Cardiac CT and MR allow comprehensive morphological and functional assessment of the heart within a single examination. Higher spatial resolution and availability of isotropic multiplanar data acquisition of cardiac CT angiography make it the preferred technique over current routine MR techniques for detailed anatomical study of the RVOT. Using new CT scanners, entire heart acquisition can be obtained in a short breath hold combined with thin slices (0.5–0.75 mm). This greatly reduces motion artifacts, and the thin collimation improves the depiction of small structures. Anatomical analysis of the RV can be performed with a dedicated ECG-gated right heart study or as part of CT coronary angiography [12, 13]. In the latter, most of the time sufficient attenuation for visualization of the right heart can be obtained by split-bolus injection in which an initial bolus of contrast medium (50–75 mL) is followed by 50 mL of a 70 %:30 % saline-to-contrast medium mixture and a 30-mL saline chaser at a rate of 4–5 mL/s [13]. A dedicated right heart examination with CT requires ECG gating/triggering and homogeneous enhancement of the right atrium and ventricle to an optimum Hounsfield unit of 350–400. Scan can be started early (i.e., main pulmonary artery triggering) to include the right heart only. For certain cases with congenital heart disease, a modified injection protocol using dual extremity contrast injections into the antecubital and femoral veins is described which provides homogeneous images of the right atrium and ventricle [14] (Chap. 10 for detail). Different sequences can be used to evaluate the RVOT morphology with MRI including MR angiography, dark/bright blood sequences, and cine images. In addition to routine short- and long-axis cine [ECG-gated cine balanced steady-state free precession (SSFP)] views, transaxial and sagittal images may help to show the abnormality. ECG-triggered, double inversion recovery fast (segmented or single shot) spin-echo sequence with blood suppression is a great technique for anatomical imaging of the outflow tracts and major vessels especially in patients with metallic implant artifacts or those with compromised renal function and contraindication to gadolinium-enhanced MRI.

Anatomical Landmarks

The RV in the normal heart is the most anteriorly situated cardiac chamber and marks the inferior border of the cardiac silhouette. In contrast to the near conical shape of the LV, the RV appears triangular when viewed from the side and crescent shaped when viewed in cross section [15–18]. The curvature of the ventricular septum places the RVOT antero-cephalad to that of the LV's resulting in a characteristic "crossover" relationship between right and left ventricular outflows. This important spatial relationship can be lost in congenital heart malformations such as TGA. The overlap between left ventricular inlets and outlets puts the aortic outflow tract immediately behind the septum that separates it from the RV inlet, giving the "wedged" position of the aortic root.

Traditionally, the RV is divided into the sinus and conus parts, but in more recent decades, both the right and left ventricles have been described as having three components: the inlet, apical trabecular, and outlet portions (Fig. 7.3) [15–17]. In the analysis of congenitally malformed hearts, this tripartite concept is more useful than the traditional bipartite division. The inlet portion of the RV surrounds the leaflets of the tricuspid valve and supports its papillary muscles and tension apparatus. A distinguishing feature of the tricuspid valve is the direct attachment of its septal leaflet to the ventricular septum. The apical portion of the RV is characterized typically by heavy trabeculations. Distinguishing features of the outlet portion of the RV include:

Pulmonary Infundibulum

The pulmonary infundibulum (conus) is a tubular muscular structure that supports the leaflets of the pulmonary valve. Its length, size, and angle vary. The size of the infundibulum is independent of the general size of the RV.

Supraventricular Crest

The posterior (paraseptal) wall of the infundibulum is formed by a prominent muscular ridge, known as the supraventricular crest (crista supraventricularis or ventriculoinfundibular fold) which separates the inlet and outlet components of the RV (Figs. 7.3, 7.4, and 7.5). This is in contrast to the LV where the aortic and mitral valves are in fibrous continuity. Although it looks like a ridge from the perspective of the RV cavity, the supraventricular crest is in fact an infolding of the ventricular wall (the ventriculoinfundibular fold) inserting into the ventricular septum. It is separated from the aorta by the epicardial fat, and any incision through it will lead outside the heart into the vicinity of the right coronary artery (Figs. 7.3 and 7.4). Only the central portion of its inferior most part between the limbs of the septomarginal trabeculation contributes to the interventricular septum (muscular outlet septum or conal septum) [17] (Figs. 7.4 and 7.5). In the normal heart, however, this area is exceedingly small and can hardly be distinguished from the septomarginal trabeculation by CT.

Septomarginal Trabeculation

The septomarginal trabeculation is a prominent Y-shaped muscular strap reinforcing the septal surface. It bifurcates into anterosuperior and

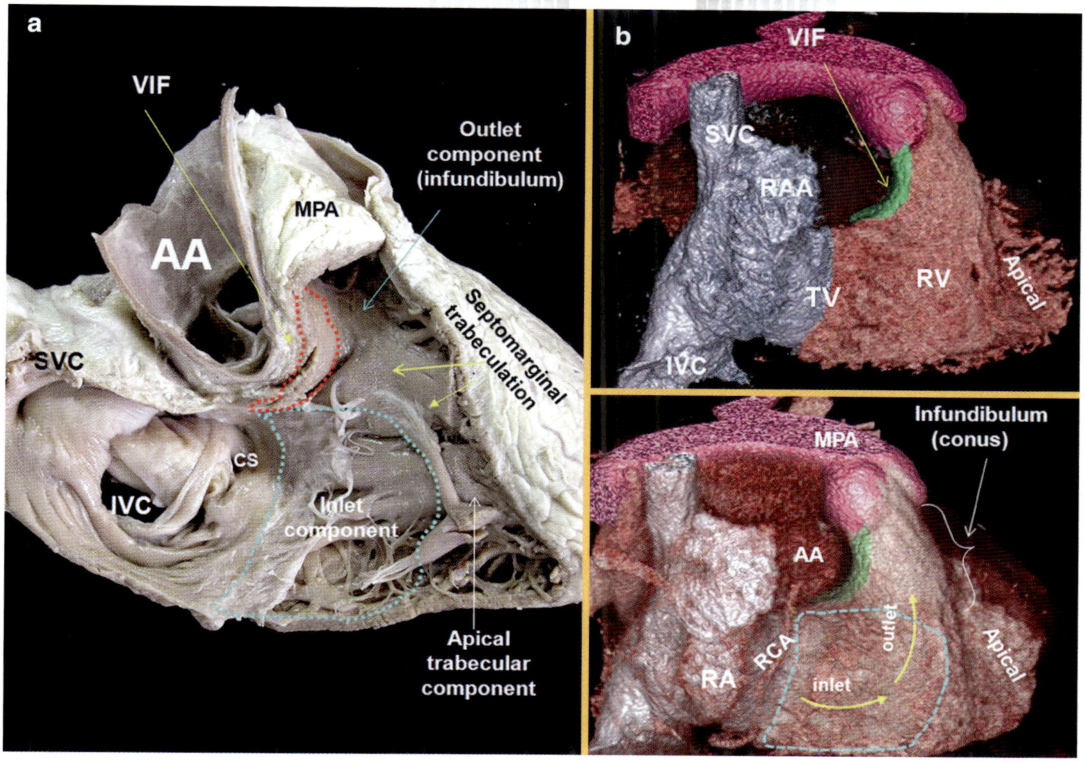

Fig. 7.3 Right anterior oblique views (two chambers) of the right heart are shown. (**a**) Cadaveric specimen. (**b**) Volume-rendered images of a right heart CT. The right ventricle comprises of three components: the inlet, apical trabecular, and outlet portions. The outflow tract, the infundibulum or conus, separates the tricuspid and pulmonary valves. The axis of the orifices of the inlet and outlet roughly forms an angle of 60°. The supraventricular crest is composite of the ventriculoinfundibular fold (*VIF*) cradled between the limbs of septomarginal trabeculation. It is separated from the right aortic sinus by the epicardial fat. *AA* ascending aorta, *MPA* main pulmonary artery, *RA* right atrium, *RAA* right atrial appendage, *SVC* superior vena cava, *IVC* inferior vena cava, *CS* coronary sinus

inferoposterior limbs (Fig. 7.6) which clasp the supraventricular crest. The anterosuperior limb extends along the infundibulum to the leaflets of the pulmonary valve. The posterior limb runs onto and overlays the ventricular septum, toward the right ventricular inlet, giving rise to the medial papillary muscle complex. The body of septomarginal trabeculation extends to the apex of the ventricle, where it gives rise to the moderator band and anterior papillary muscle before breaking up into the general apical trabeculations. The body of the septomarginal trabeculation is interventricular rather than supraventricular and when enlarged can appear as a bump on the septum on cross-sectional imaging. When hypertrophied, the septomarginal band can divide the RV into two chambers (double-chambered RV) [19].

Moderator Band

It is considered as part of the septomarginal trabeculation, supporting the anterior papillary muscle of the tricuspid valve and, from this point, crossing to the free wall of the ventricle. The moderator band incorporates the right atrioventricular bundle, as conduction tissue fibers move toward the apex of the ventricle before entering the anterior papillary muscle. It is usually located equidistant from the tricuspid valve and the apex and can be identified in 90 % of hearts. In 40 % the band is a short and thick trabeculation. The average thickness of the band is 4.5 mm, and its length is 16 mm, ranging from 11 to 24 mm [20]. The moderator band is supplied by branches of the left anterior descending (LAD) artery named the artery of the moderator band. The artery

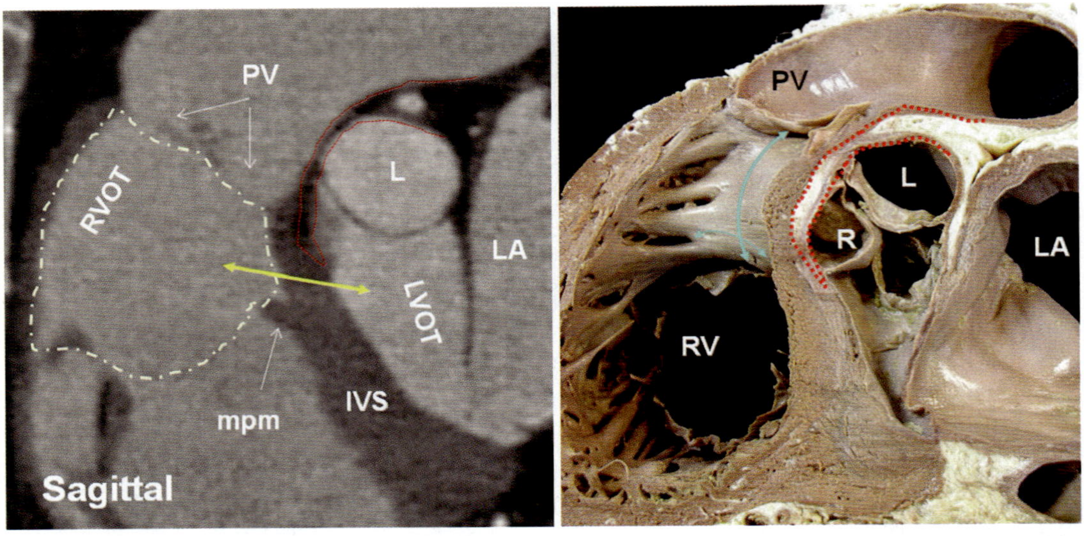

Fig. 7.4 Sagittal views of CT and cadaveric specimen at the right ventricle outflow tract (RVOT). Note fat plane (*dotted red line*) extending between the posterior wall of the RV infundibulum (supraventricular crest) (*blue arrows*) and the anterior wall of ascending aorta making surgical resection of the infundibulum possible. The height of supraventricular crest varies from patient to patient; however, most of it is separated from the aorta by epicardial fat and can be surgically removed without entering the left ventricular cavity. Only the central portion of its inferiormost part may form part of the interventricular septum. The term supraventricular crest is replaced by ventriculoinfundibular fold, representing any muscular structure interposed between the attachments of the leaflets of the atrioventricular and arterial valves. The inferior central part of it is called outlet septum which is part of septomarginal trabeculation. The outlet septum above the level of medial papillary (*double headed yellow arrow*) muscle (mpm) is shown by yellow arrow. However, its true existence is questionable given the limited spatial resolution of CT compared with histological slices. *PV* pulmonary valve, *L* left aortic sinus, *R* right aortic sinus, *RV* right ventricle, *LA* left atrium, *IVS* interventricular septum, *LVOT* left ventricle outflow tract

supplying the band makes anastomotic connections at the base of the anterior papillary muscle with branches of the right coronary artery.

Medial Papillary Muscle of the Conus

The medial (septal) papillary muscle of the conus presents in 82 % of the hearts, while in the rest, it is replaced by tendinous chords [21] (Figs. 7.4 and 7.6). It is a single papilla in 50 % and double in 30 %. It connects with the septal and anterior leaflets of the tricuspid valve. It represents an important surgical landmark for the location of the right bundle branch to avoid injury to the bundle during surgical correction of certain types of ventricular septal defects.

Pulmonary Valve

The pulmonary root is the part of RVOT that supports the leaflets of the pulmonary valve. It consists of three sinuses of Valsalva confined proximally by the semilunar attachments of the valvular leaflets and distally by the sinotubular junction. Different nomenclatures have been used to define the anatomical location of the pulmonary valve sinuses base on their spatial location in relation to the body of the heart itself (Fig. 7.7). Because of the semilunar shape of the pulmonary leaflets (similar to the aortic valve), this valve does not have a ringlike annulus. The sinotubular junction of the pulmonary trunk marks the level of the commissures between the annuli (Fig. 7.7). Compared to the aortic root, the pulmonary sinotubular junction is less obvious on CT images. A second junction exists at the ventriculoarterial junction. The bases of the sinuses within the ventricle cross the anatomical ventriculoarterial junction. The anatomical ventriculoarterial junction forms the annulus. The semilunar attachment of the valvular leaflets which forms the hemodynamic ventriculoarterial

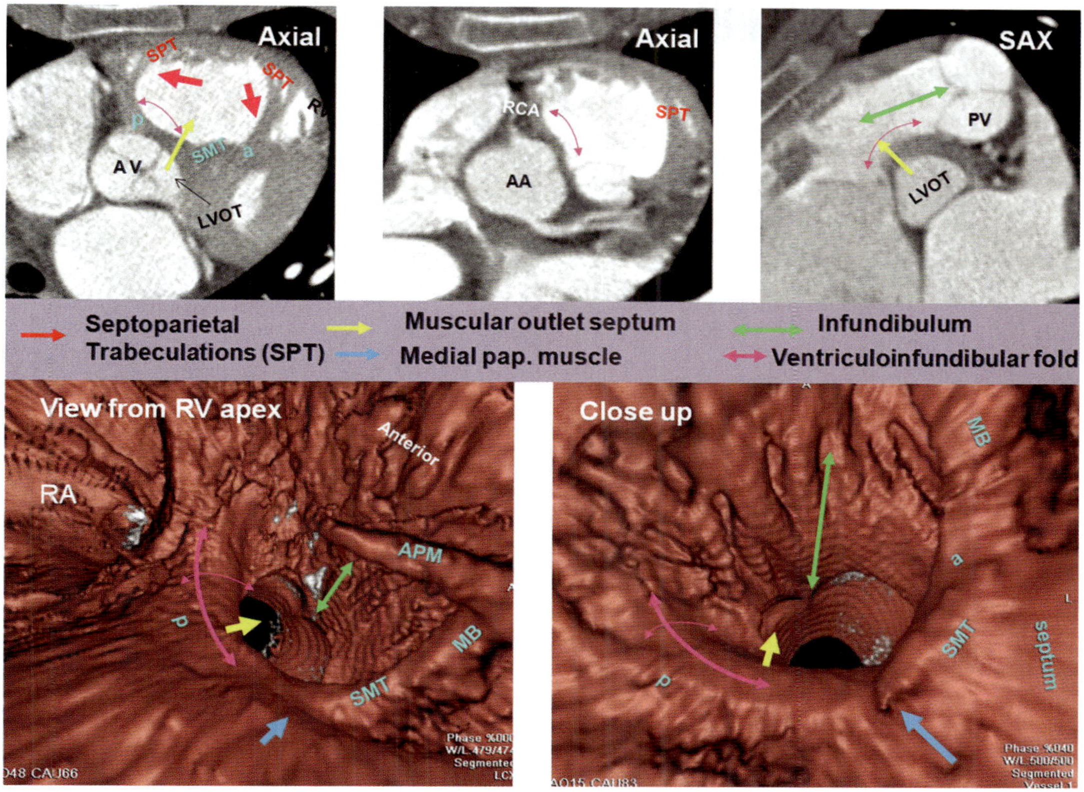

Fig. 7.5 Right ventricle (*RV*) infundibulum. The posterior wall of RV infundibulum is the continuation of the infundibulum into the ventriculoinfundibular fold (supraventricular crest). It is a free-standing wall except its mid-inferiormost part which contributes to the interventricular septum also known as the outlet septum (*yellow arrows*). One slice above it (second axial cut) at the orifice of the right coronary artery (*RCA*) demonstrates extension of fat plane between the ascending aorta and RVOT. The RCA can be injured at the time of pulmonary valve surgery. The ventriculoinfundibular fold is located between the antero-cephalad (septal band) (*a*) and postero-caudal (parietal band) (*p*) limbs of the septomarginal trabeculations (*SMT*), and its width is shown by double-headed purple arrows. The cradle between the SMT limbs and the ventriculoinfundibular fold forms the supraventricular crest. Note smooth surface of ventriculoinfundibular fold compared to the rest of RV infundibulum which is trabeculated. The anterior limb runs superiorly into the infundibulum and supports the leaflets of the pulmonary valve (*PV*). Multiple muscular bundles that extend from the cephalad margin of the septomarginal trabeculation and run onto the parietal wall of the outflow tract are designated as the septoparietal trabeculations (SPT) (*red arrows*). *AA* ascending aorta, *AV* aortic valve, *PUV* pulmonary valve, *MB* moderator band, *RA* right atrium

junction crosses the anatomical ventriculoarterial junction. The leaflets are thickened along their semilunar line of attachment. The fibrous interleaflet trigones are the areas of arterial wall proximal to the semilunar attachments of the leaflets and therefore are incorporated within the ventricular cavity. Their tips point toward the commissures. The musculature of the subpulmonary infundibulum raises the pulmonary valve above the ventricular septum to position the pulmonary valve as the most superiorly situated of the cardiac valves. This anatomical feature makes possible the safe resection of the pulmonary valve, including its basal attachments within the infundibulum from the rest of the RVOT.

Arterial Supply and Anatomical Variants

The conotruncal structures are normally vascularized by anterior and posterior arterial branches

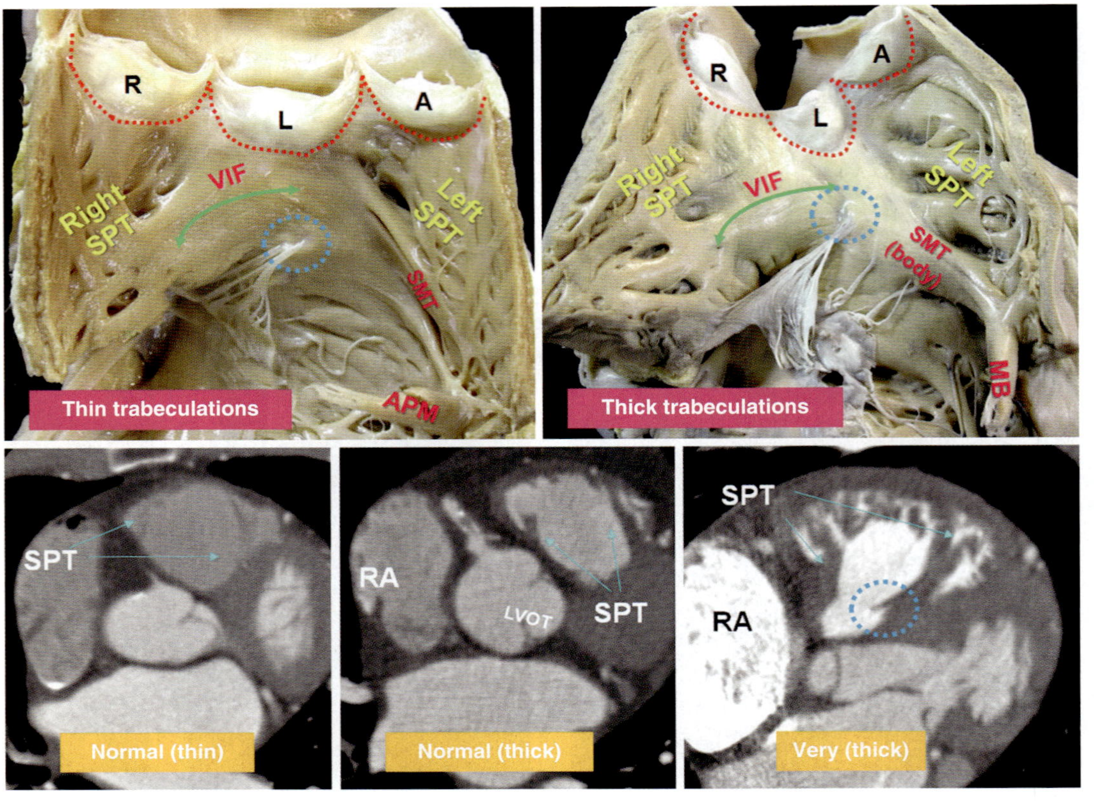

Fig. 7.6 Variation of trabeculations in RVOT. Upper panel: RVOT open-book dissection views. The septomarginal trabeculation (*SMT*) is a muscle strap plastered onto the septal part. The ventriculoinfundibular fold (*VIF*) extends between SMT and the pulmonary valve and forms the paraseptal wall of the RVOT. The septoparietal trabeculations (*SPT*) originate from the anterior margin of the SMT and run round the parietal quadrant of the endocardial infundibulum along the right and left septoparietal walls of the RVOT. These trabeculations vary in number (5–22 trabeculations) and thickness (2–10 mm). The SPTs can be flat or prominent and may be hypertrophied as in pulmonary hypertension or tetralogy of Fallot, contributing to muscular subpulmonary stenosis. The SMT continues to apex and turns into the moderator band (*MB*) and anterior papillary muscle. *Blue circles* demarcate medial papillary muscle. Lower panel demonstrates variable thickness of the SMT and its SPTs. Note marked thickening of the RVOT in the last image in a patient with pulmonary valve stenosis. The right atrium (*RA*) is markedly enlarged. *A* anterior, *R* right posterior, and *L* left posterior are pulmonary sinuses, *LVOT* left ventricle outflow tract, *RA* right atrium, *red dotted line* denotes margin of the pulmonary valve leaflets

from the right and left coronary arteries [22]. On the right side, the branches arise from the conal branch of the right coronary artery or directly from the aorta. On the left side, they arise from the LAD, the left main, or directly from the aorta. The right anterior conal branch is the most constant and conspicuous branch participating in the preconal circulation, also known as Vieussens' arterial ring [22] (Fig. 7.8). This collateral intercoronary connection extends between the conus artery and first right ventricular branch (left anterior conus branch) of the LAD artery. The Vieussens' arterial ring will become dilated when there is proximal LAD artery occlusion or, less frequently, RCA occlusion. Generally, three major collateral pathways at conotruncal level provide circulation between right and left coronary system in all congenital or acquired forms of one-sided coronary occlusion and are used as the basis for different classifications [23]. These three collateral circulation pathways include preconal (precardiac), retroconal (interarterial), and retroaortic. In coronary ostial atresia, because intercoronary collaterals develop very early in

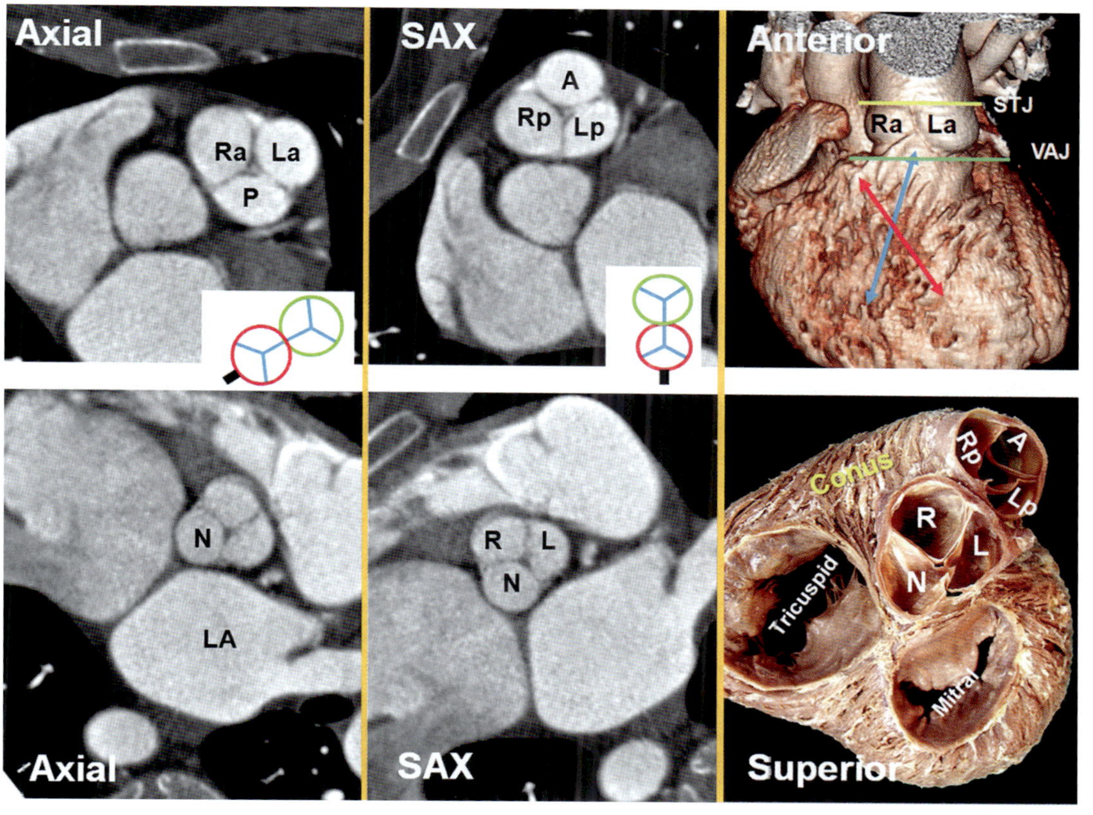

Fig. 7.7 Pulmonary valve sinuses. When heart is viewed in attitudinal anatomical position as sitting in the thorax (i.e., axial views), the pulmonary leaflets and sinuses are seen to be posterior (*P*), right anterolateral (*Ra*), and left anterolateral (*La*). However, in relation to the heart (i.e., short-axis views), the pulmonary sinuses can be named anterior (*A*), left posterior (*Lp*), and right posterior (*Rp*). According to their relation to the aorta, sinuses will be left-facing, right-facing, and nonfacing. Same rule can be applied to the aortic valve as seen in the above examples. The relationship of the pulmonary and aortic valve (*green and red circles*) as well as their orientation in relation to the body (axial) and the heart (short axis, SAX) are drawn; the *black line* shows the location of the interatrial septum. Crossover arrangement between left and right ventricular outflow tracts (*red and blue arrows* respectively) is also shown. The term "pulmonary annulus" denotes the semilunar fibrous attachment of each of the pulmonary leaflets. They are much less sturdy than the aortic annuli. *LA* left atrium, *N* noncoronary sinus, *STJ* sinotubular junction (*yellow line*), *VAJ* ventriculoarterial junction (*green line*)

life, they can be large and overall angiographic appearance of the anomaly can be difficult to differentiate from congenital single coronary artery malformation. In congenital single coronary artery, the blood flow is always centrifugal from larger caliber arteries proximally to smaller ones distally. In ostial atresia the blood flows from the intact right or left coronary artery to the abnormal side via one or more collateral arteries whose caliber is smaller than that of the target vessels (Fig. 7.9). The incidence of a major coronary artery crossing the RVOT in TOF is between 5 and 12 % [24]. Preoperative recognition of such arteries may be important in reconstructive surgery of the RVOT (Fig. 7.10). Infundibular and preventricular branches should not be mistaken for a major coronary artery arising crossing the RVOT.

Morphological Changes in Adult CHD

Major advances in cardiac surgery over the past 50 years have resulted in a marked increase in the number of patients with congenital heart disease

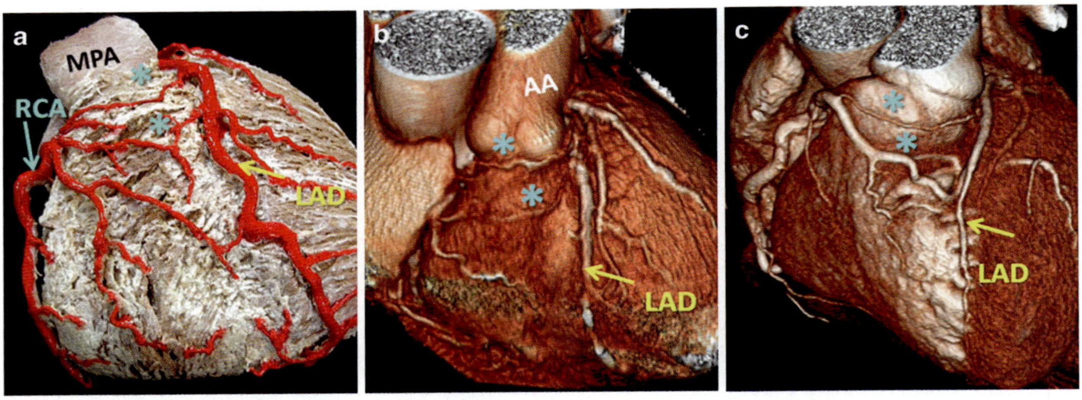

Fig. 7.8 Vieussens' arterial ring; preconal arterial anastomotic rings (*) between pulmonary conus branches arising from the RCA and the LAD artery are shown (**a**) participating in vascular supply to infundibulum as well as the anterior right ventricle. These collaterals may be enlarged in acquired obstructive (**b**) or congenital (**c**) coronary disease. *AA* ascending aorta, *MPA* main pulmonary artery, *RCA* right coronary artery, *LAD* left anterior descending artery

reaching adulthood. In many cases initial surgery is indicated on the basis of echo, with catheterization for physiological assessment if required. CT and MR have a prominent role in follow-up, either to monitor changes during staged surgical repair or to look for complications which are common and many need imaging for diagnosis and surgical planning. However, it is not unusual to discover an RVOT malformation for the first time and without a history of past surgery.

RVOT Stenosis: Pre- and Postoperative Findings

RVOT stenosis is usually secondary to pulmonary valve diseases, but stenotic lesions at subvalvular or supravalvular levels are not uncommon. Causes of RVOT stenosis are listed in Fig. 7.11.

Pulmonary Valve Stenosis

Isolated pulmonary stenosis (PS) is almost always congenital and many can be asymptomatic when first diagnosed. It is not unusual to suspect PS in a young patient on routine chest x-ray or CT by noticing enlarged main and left pulmonary arteries. With severe PS, symptoms of dyspnea, fatigue, chest pain, palpitations, and decreased exercise tolerance may occur. Three morphological types are described [18, 25–28] (Table 7.1). The most common type of congenital PS (40–60 %) is a dome-shaped pulmonary valve, which is characterized by a mobile valve and 2–4 raphes and incomplete separation of valve cusps due to commissural fusion resulting in funnel with a small circular orifice (Fig. 7.12a). The line of basal attachment of the domed valve is not semilunar; instead, the sinuses are shallow and the line attachment appears somewhat circular. A waist-like narrowing of the sinotubular junction may be seen is some cases. Dysplastic pulmonary valve is the second most common PS (20–30 %) and is associated with immobile thickened cusps and in some cases a hypoplastic ventriculoarterial junction [26] (Fig. 7.12b). Cauliflower-like myxomatous thickening is limited to the free margin of the leaflets, and the proximal part of leaflets is intact. The commissures are not fused, the sinuses are deep, and the lines of attachment are semilunar, all as seen in normal hearts. The semilunar attachment of the pulmonary valve leaflets is an essential feature for normal function of the valve. Shallow attachment and lack of "height" of the overall valvular apparatus can cause pulmonary stenosis due to limiting mobility of the free edge of the leaflets even in the absence of commissural fusion. Of those cases with PS who require active treatment whether interventional or surgical, dysplastic

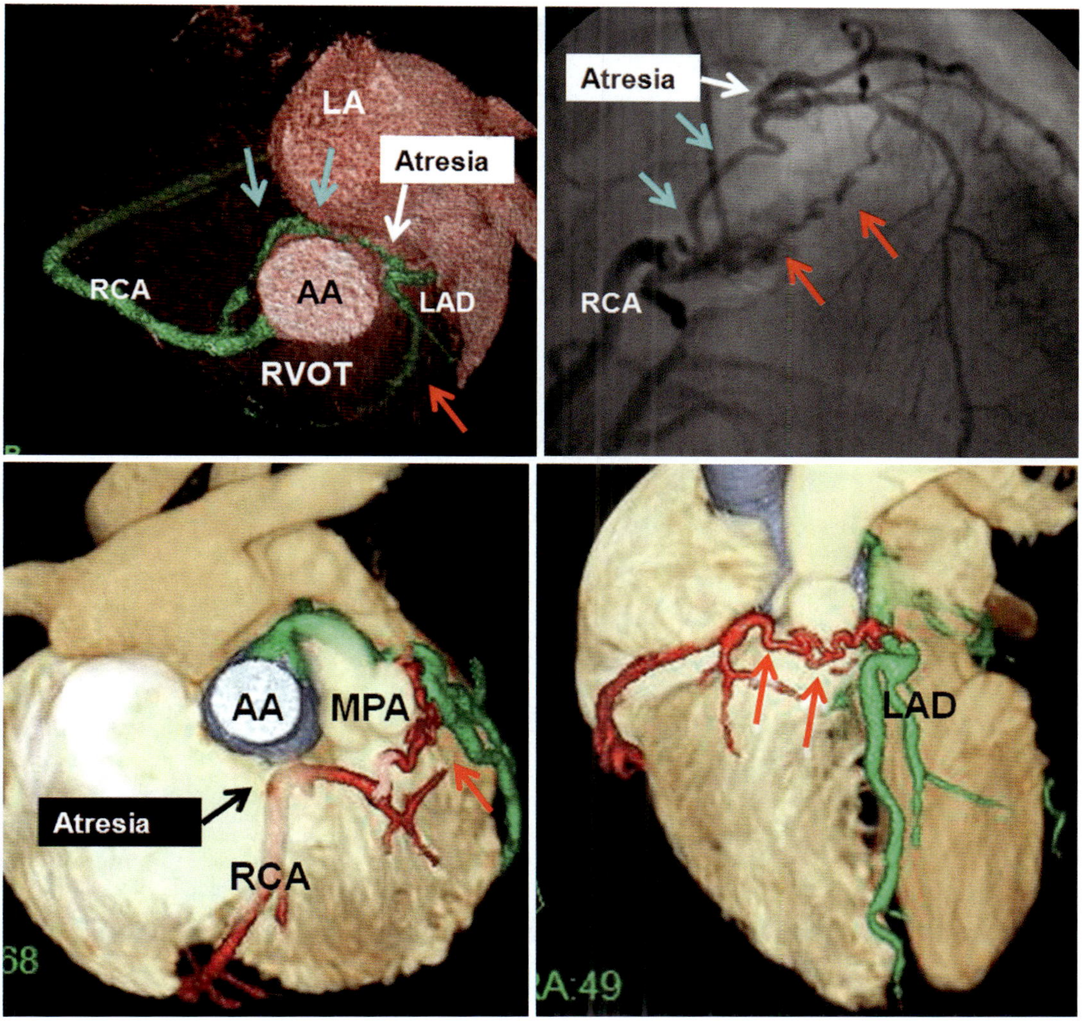

Fig. 7.9 *Upper row* shows left coronary ostial atresia with retroaortic (*blue arrows*) and preconal (*red arrows*) collaterals between the right and left coronary systems. *Lower row* shows right coronary ostial atresia with preconal (*red arrows*) collaterals between the right and left coronary systems in a patient with congenital pulmonary valve stenosis. *AA* ascending aorta, *LA* left atrium, *LAD* left anterior descending artery, *MPA* main pulmonary artery, *RVOT* right ventricle outflow tract, *RCA* right coronary artery

valves would be far more common. Milo et al. [25] described a third morphology of PS with deep "bottle-shaped" sinuses and an hourglass deformity due to supravalvular narrowing at the sinotubular junction (Fig. 7.12c). Although the later morphology is reported in 16 % of patients with congenital PS, it is not accepted as a separate variant by every investigator [26]. Dome-shaped valve with dysplastic leaflets is another uncommon variant. Different morphologies can be equally distinguished with cardiac MR and CT angiography. Bicuspid or multicuspid valve is rare [27] (Fig. 7.13). In bicuspid valve, one leaflet can be larger containing a shallow raphe or both leaflets may be equal in size. Stenosis and post-stenostic dilatation are common. Compared to bicuspid valve, quadricuspid pulmonary valve is usually asymptomatic. Mild pulmonary regurgitation (PR) is not uncommon. Congenital variations can be isolated but are often associated with

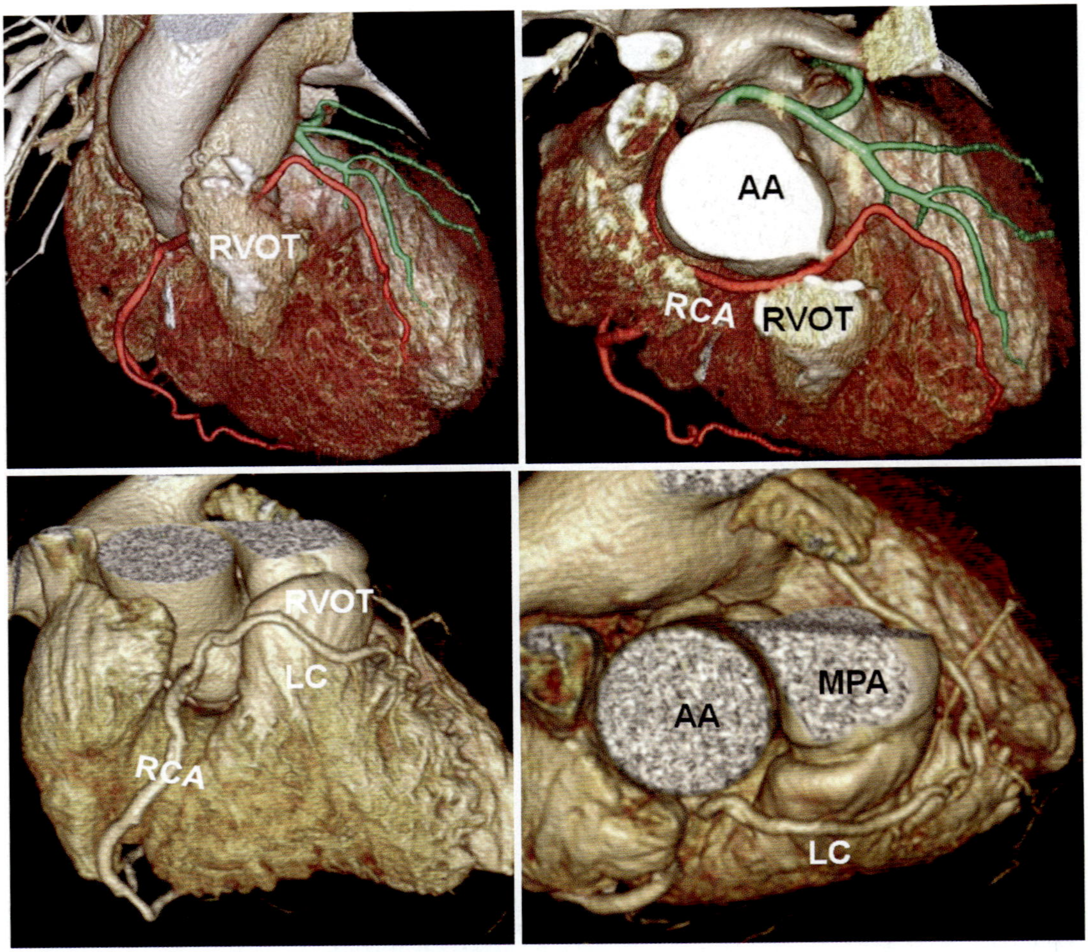

Fig. 7.10 Anomalous course of the coronary arteries next to the right ventricle outflow tract (*RVOT*). *Upper row* shows repaired RVOT in tetralogy. Anomalous course of the right coronary artery (*RCA*) behind the RVOT conduit is seen. *Lower row* shows a single RCA with preconal course of the left coronary (*LC*) artery. *AA* ascending aorta, *MPA* main pulmonary artery

other congenital heart anomalies. For example, tetralogy of Fallot can be associated with a bicuspid pulmonary valve. Congenital pulmonary valve anomalies can also be associated with extracardiac anomalies as in Noonan syndrome and LEOPARD syndrome, which is often associated with a dysplastic pulmonary valve.

Chronic PS results in RV hypertrophy, especially at the RVOT. When prominent, RVOT hypertrophy can lead to secondary dynamic subvalvular stenosis. Distinguishing between valvular stenosis and subvalvular dynamic stenosis secondary to infundibular hypertrophy can become challenging. Subvalvular dynamic obstruction (late systolic stenosis), in fact, often accompanies severe valvular PS and is characterized by a late-peaking jet in MRI similar to that of dynamic LV outflow obstruction. PS can also result in post-stenotic dilatation of the pulmonary trunk and left pulmonary artery. For symptomatic patients with dome-shaped pulmonary valve, balloon valvuloplasty is indicated when a peak instantaneous gradient >50 mmHg is present [28]. A successful procedure is defined by final peak gradient of <30 mmHg and is obtained in >90 % [29]. If the valve is dysplastic, surgery is

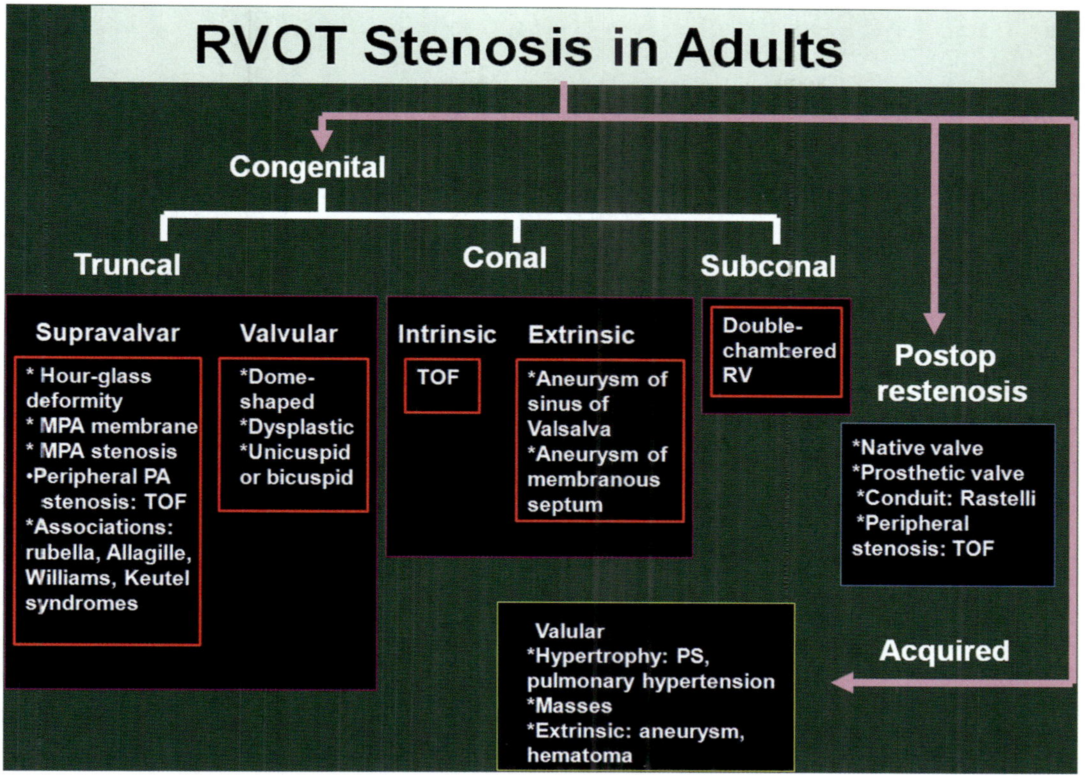

Fig. 7.11 Causes of RVOT stenosis in adults. *TOF* tetralogy of Fallot, *MPA* main pulmonary artery, *PA* pulmonary artery, *PS* pulmonary stenosis, *RV* right ventricle

Table 7.1 Congenital pulmonary valve stenosis

A. Dome-shaped
Very common: 80–90 % of all congenital right ventricle outflow tract lesions
Low familial inheritance
2–4 raphes but no separation into valve cusps
Treatment: balloon valvotomy
B. Dysplastic
10–20 %
Trileaflet with markedly thickened leaflets
Associations: hypoplastic ventriculoarterial junction. Noonan's syndrome
Treatment: partial or total valvotomy, a transannular patch
C. Bicuspid/quadricuspid
Rare
Usually asymptomatic
Common with other congenital heart diseases

more likely to be required; if there is annular or pulmonary trunk hypoplasia, a transannular patch may become necessary. In patients with PS and significant pulmonary regurgitation, valve replacement is required. Mechanical valve replacement is used rarely because of thrombosis issues. Bioprosthetic valves and pulmonary homografts are preferred [30].

Tetralogy of Fallot

TOF consists of a large nonrestrictive subaortic ventricular septal defect (VSD), dextroposed aorta riding up over the septal defect, and RVOT obstruction (Fig. 7.14). TOF without PS is called Eisenmenger complex (Fig. 7.15). Subpulmonary stenosis, which is an essential part of TOF, is mainly due to anterosuperior malalignment of the muscular outlet septum relative to the limbs of the septomarginal trabeculation, coupled with thickened septoparietal trabeculations

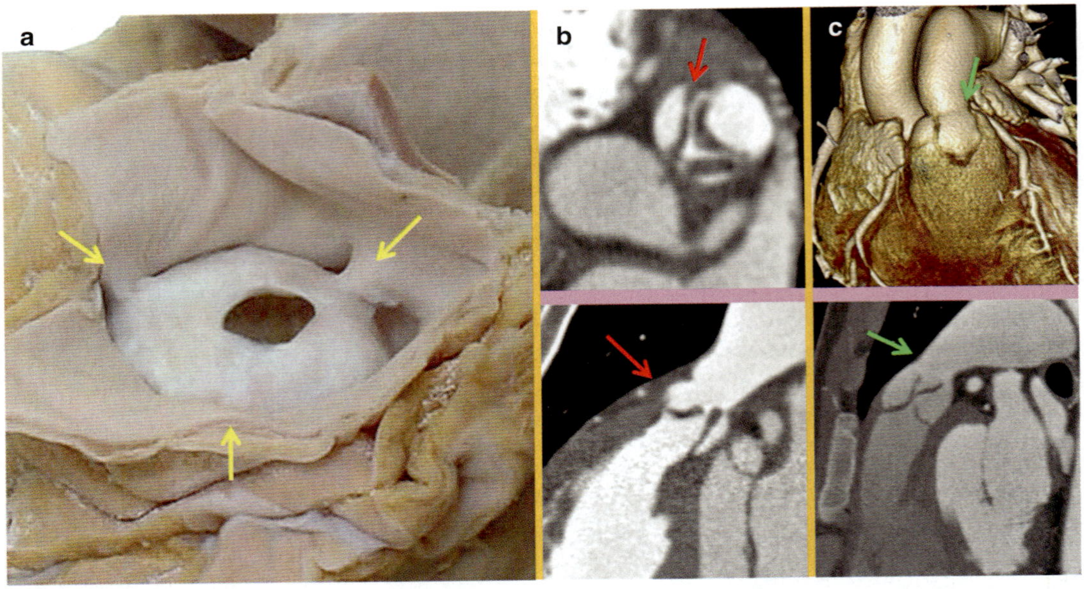

Fig. 7.12 (**a**). Dome-shaped pulmonary valve viewed from the arterial aspect. It is characterized by narrow opening and incomplete separation of the valve cusps. The fused commissures (*yellow arrows*) pull the sinotubular junction toward the central circular orifice. (**b**) Axial and sagittal CT appearance of a dysplastic pulmonary stenosis. Club-shaped myxomatous thickening (*red arrows*) is limited to the free margin of the leaflets, and the proximal part of leaflets appears intact. Note the trileaflet thickened valve and no commissural fusion with hypoplastic ventriculoarterial junction. In dysplastic pulmonary valve, there are three distinct cusps and no commissural fusion. (**c**) Volume-rendered and sagittal CT images in a patient with LEOPARD syndrome and pulmonary stenosis (*arrows*). Note mild thickening of the valve leaflets and narrowing at sinotubular junction giving an hourglass appearance

[17, 31, 32] (Fig. 7.14). Stenosis can also occur at subpulmonic level by hypertrophy of the septomarginal trabeculation or the moderator band. This gives the arrangement often described as "two-chambered right ventricle." The subpulmonary infundibulum itself varies markedly in length and can sometimes be short especially in Eisenmenger complex (Fig. 7.2). In most other instances of TOF, the narrowed infundibular chamber is normal in length but sometimes has considerable length. Absent pulmonary valve syndrome occurs in less than 3–6 % of TOF patients [17]. This syndrome is associated with significant pulmonary artery dilatation and airway compression. Pulmonary atresia in TOF is also due to severe deviation of the outlet septum. However, isolated pulmonary atresia can rarely occur as a result of valve imperforation rather than severe stenosis. In pulmonary atresia blood supply to the right and left pulmonary arteries (if not atretic) will be provided by a large patent ductus arteriosus or multiple aortopulmonary collateral arteries. Extensive reconstructive surgery is required in extreme cases.

Patients with TOF have remarkable intrinsic histological abnormalities and reduced elasticity in both ascending aorta and pulmonary artery, and it appears that TOF repair does not improve these abnormalities [33, 34]. Aortic root dilation with or without aortic regurgitation is common [33]. Cardiac MRI or CT can address these major clinical implications (Fig. 7.14). The concept of aortic overriding is shown in Fig. 7.16. Note that mild overriding above the ventricular septum can be seen in normal instances. Greater than 50 % overriding falls into definition of DORV subgroup. However, in TOF there is always fibrous continuity between the anterior mitral leaflet, while in DORV this may not be the case (Fig. 7.16). The concept of dextroposition is shown in Fig. 7.17.

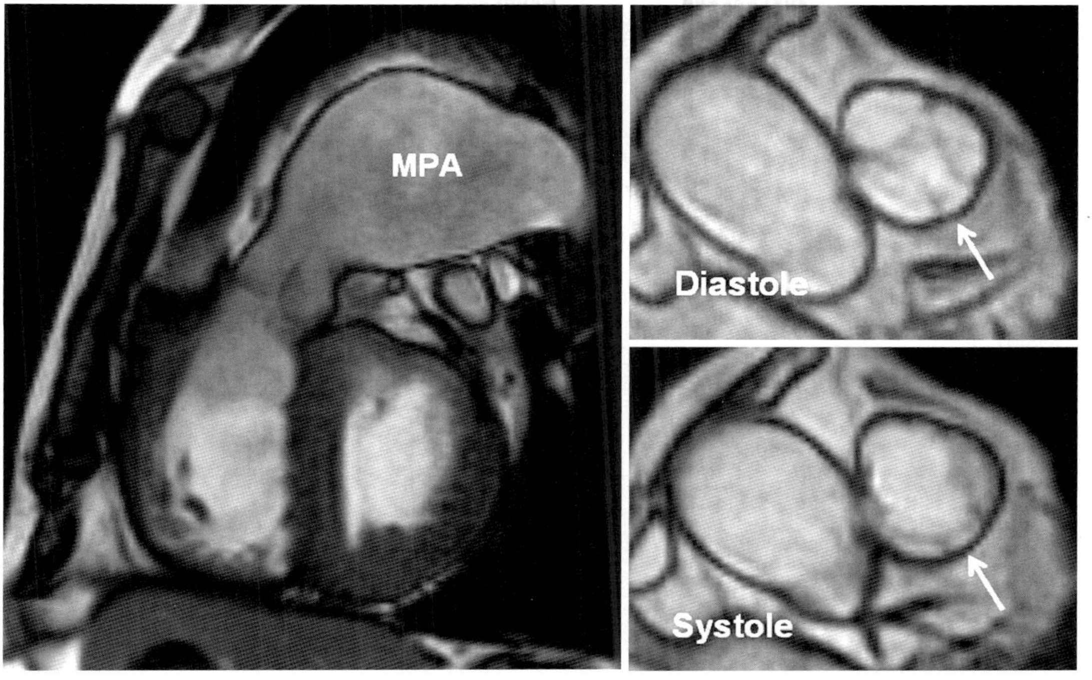

Fig. 7.13 A 51-year-old male with mild pulmonary regurgitation and pulmonary hypertension. Long-axis and short-axis MR images of a quadricuspid valve are shown. The valve is shown at two different phases of cardiac cycle. One rudimentary extra cusp between the left posterior and anterior (nonfacing) cusps (*arrows*) is seen. The right ventricle is hypertrophied and the main pulmonary artery (*MPA*) is dilated

Double-Chambered Right Ventricle

Double-chambered RV (DCRV) is characterized by subinfundibular stenosis due to aberrant hypertrophied septomarginal trabeculations or abnormal moderator band that divides the RV cavity into a proximal high-pressure and a distal low-pressure chamber [19, 35, 36] (Fig. 7.18). The severity of the DCRV stenosis tends to increase with time [36]. DCRV is usually associated with a perimembranous VSD. MRI and CT are usually diagnostic, identifying the degree and location of the obstruction and the presence of a VSD. The degree of stenosis can be best quantified with MR phase-contrast techniques. The indications for surgery in DCRV are similar to those for pulmonary valve stenosis (peak gradients >50 mmHg). Muscular resection and correction of VSD have excellent long-term results and low rates of recurrence [37].

Post-RVOT Repair Changes

Most TOF patients in adult life have undergone either palliative or total repair early in life. Total repair involves a patch closure of the VSD and relief of the RVOT obstruction. In TOF more than one-third of patients receive a transannular RVOT patch using pericardium, Dacron, or polytetrafluoroethylene, and 10 % of TOF patients receive valved conduits, Hancock, homograft, or bovine jugular vein [38]. An extracardiac conduit interposition between the RVOT and main pulmonary artery or individual pulmonary branches may be necessary in the presence of pulmonary atresia or an anomalous left coronary artery crossing the RVOT [39] (Fig. 7.19). Cryopreserved valved aortic homografts are more popular than pulmonary homografts, but accelerated aortic homograft fibrocalcifications have been described [40]. The Contegra valved bovine jugular vein has been used as a better alternative to homografts in

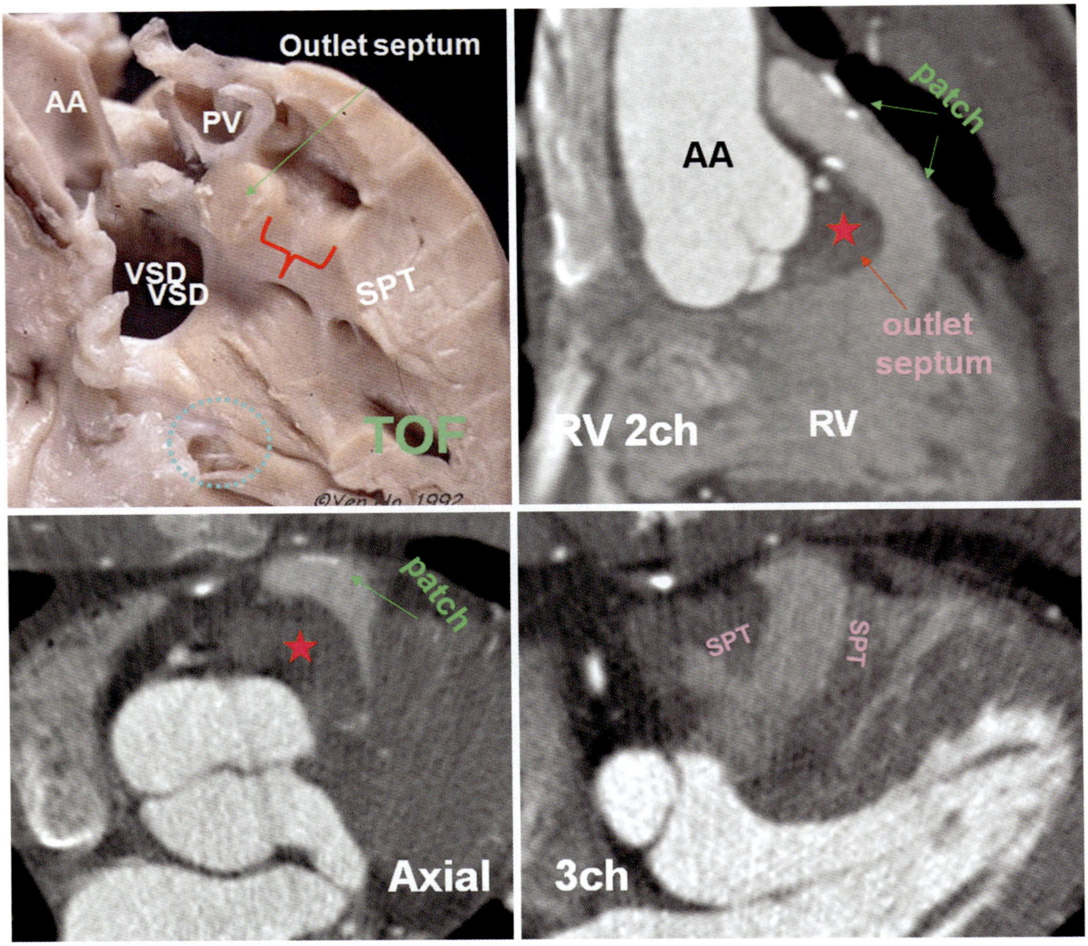

Fig. 7.14 Cadaveric specimen demonstrates phenotypic features of tetralogy of Fallot (*TOF*) including a large nonrestrictive subaortic perimembranous ventricular septal defect (*VSD*) with the aorta overriding the septal defect. The muscular outlet septum is displaced anterocephalad to the limbs of the septomarginal trabeculation, and there is hypertrophy of the septoparietal trabeculations (*SPT*). Subpulmonary obstruction (*red bracket*) is generally produced between the muscular outlet septum and the hypertrophied SPTs. There is continuity between the leaflets of the aortic and tricuspid valves in the postero-inferior margin of the VSD. Note the VSD is located anterior to the medial papillary muscle (*blue circle*). CT images show repaired TOF with markedly thickened outlet septum (*red stars*) and the SPT. Status post transpulmonary patch surgery covering the anterior wall of the RVOT. In this patient the RVOT is long. The ascending aorta (*AA*) is dilated. The muscular outlet septum is located cephalad to the SPTs. *PV* pulmonary valve, *RV 2ch* right ventricle two chamber, *3ch* three chamber

RVOT reconstruction [41]. The diameter of the grafts ranges from 12 to 22 mm and length is 10–12 cm. High pressure in the conduit may lead to aneurysmal dilatation (one-third of the conduits) and valve regurgitation. Dacron conduits are least popular for extensive fibrous sheathing and calcifications (Fig. 7.19). Conduit narrowing at the pulmonary anastomosis (distal suture line) is relatively common which may be associated with conduit dilatation. A complete assessment of pulmonary arterial system with CT or MR may be necessary before RVOT reoperation to find associated complications [42] (Fig. 7.20). Residual branch pulmonary artery stenosis is common after repair. Demonstration of substantial branch pulmonary artery stenosis, especially in the setting of free pulmonary regurgitation, should be treated by balloon dilation with or

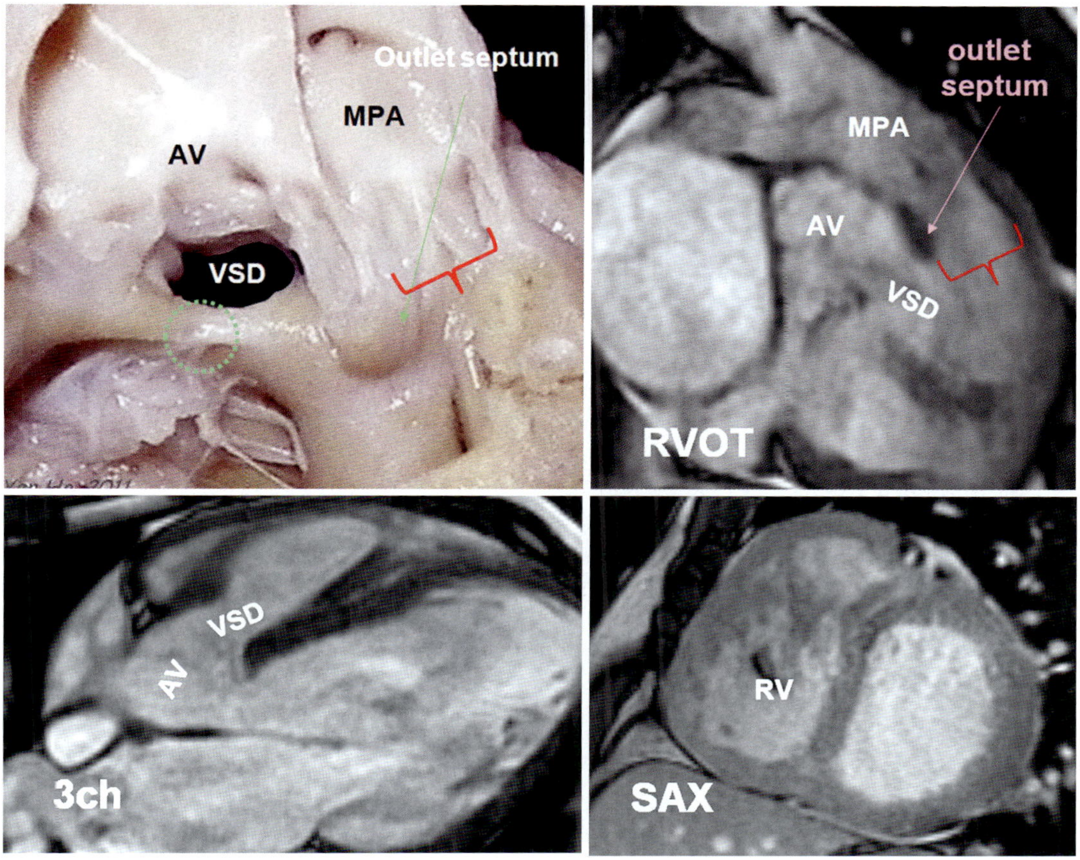

Fig. 7.15 Cadaveric specimen demonstrates phenotypic features of Eisenmenger complex. A subaortic ventricular septal defect (*VSD*) is shown. The outlet septum is mildly displaced superiorly but without causing subpulmonary obstruction (*red bracket*). Note the VSD is located anterior to the medial papillary muscle (*green circle*). MR images are obtained in a 35-year-old male with unrepaired tetralogy. Subaortic VSD and aortic overriding are shown. Outlet septum is superiorly displaced. There is no subpulmonary stenosis (*red bracket*). The right ventricle (*RV*) is thickened wall and appears mildly dilated. *AV* aortic valve, *MPA* main pulmonary artery, *RVOT* right ventricle outflow tract, *SAX* short axis, *3ch* three chamber

without implantation of an endoluminal stent (Fig. 7.21). Repeat sternotomy should be performed with special care in post-OFT surgery cases because of the risk of conduit adherence to the sternum. CT scanning of the chest is helpful in these complex patients (Fig. 7.19).

Recently, percutaneous valve replacement has been performed successfully in RVOT inside a failing bioprosthetic valve or conduit and has now been extended to include patients with native PS [43–45]. Morphology of the RVOT is a major determinant of suitability for percutaneous pulmonary valve replacement. This can easily be done by CT or MRI. Different RVOT morphologies exist (Fig. 7.22). An aneurysmal (pyramidal) [45] morphology is the most common (50 %) and related to the presence of a transannular patch. This morphology is not suitable for percutaneous pulmonary valve implantation. In patients with conduits, other morphologies are more common. The current device for pulmonary valve implantation, made of a platinum–iridium alloy, performs best in cylindrical, rigid (to avoid fracture) RVOTs that measure 14–22 mm diameter. These requirements make the device unsuitable in most of the patients.

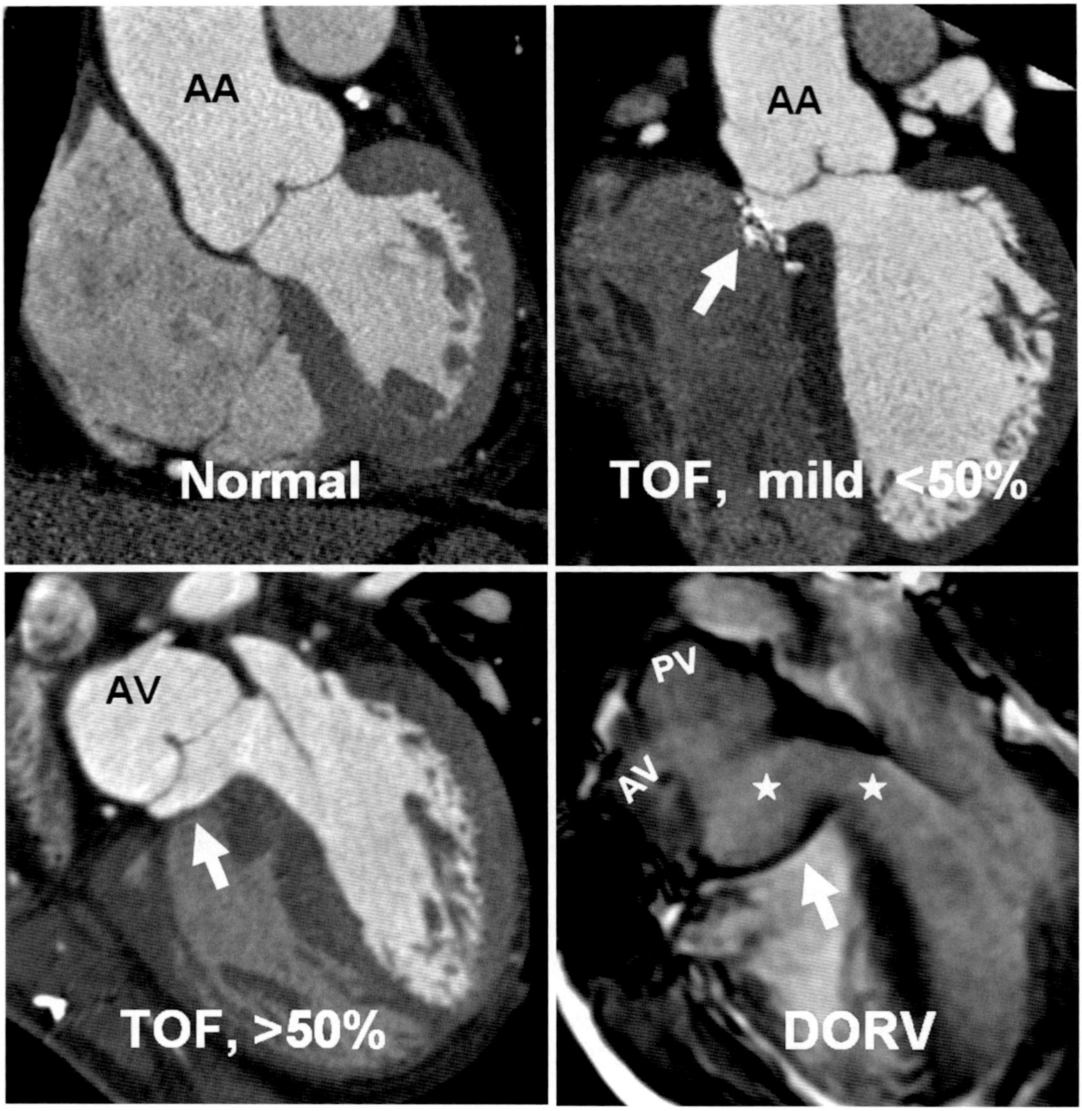

Fig. 7.16 The concept of aortic overriding. Coronal views of the heart at the level of the aortic root demonstrate the relationship of the aorta to interventricular septum. Mild dextroposition of the aorta is normal. When it overrides the septum greater than 50 %, it falls in definition of DORV. However, in this example aortic–mitral fibrous continuity which is essential for diagnosis of TOF still exists. In DORV both aortic valve (*AV*) and pulmonary valve (*PV*) arise from the right ventricle, and the pulmonary valve is usually located on the left side of the aorta. This will result in lack of fibrous continuity between the mitral and aortic valves as shown in this image. *Arrows* point to patch repaired VSDs. *Stars* denote left ventricle baffle. *AA* ascending aorta

Double Outlet Right Ventricle (DORV)

DORV is a type of abnormal ventriculoarterial connection in which both great vessels arise entirely or predominantly (>50 % circumference) from the RV [46]. New classification defines four types of DORV based on the clinical presentation and surgical treatment approach: VSD type (24 %), Fallot type (36 %), TGA type (Taussig–Bing) (18 %), and DORV noncommitted VSD (22 %) [47–49]. The VSD is typically large and has four potential locations: subaortic, subpulmonic, doubly committed, or remote

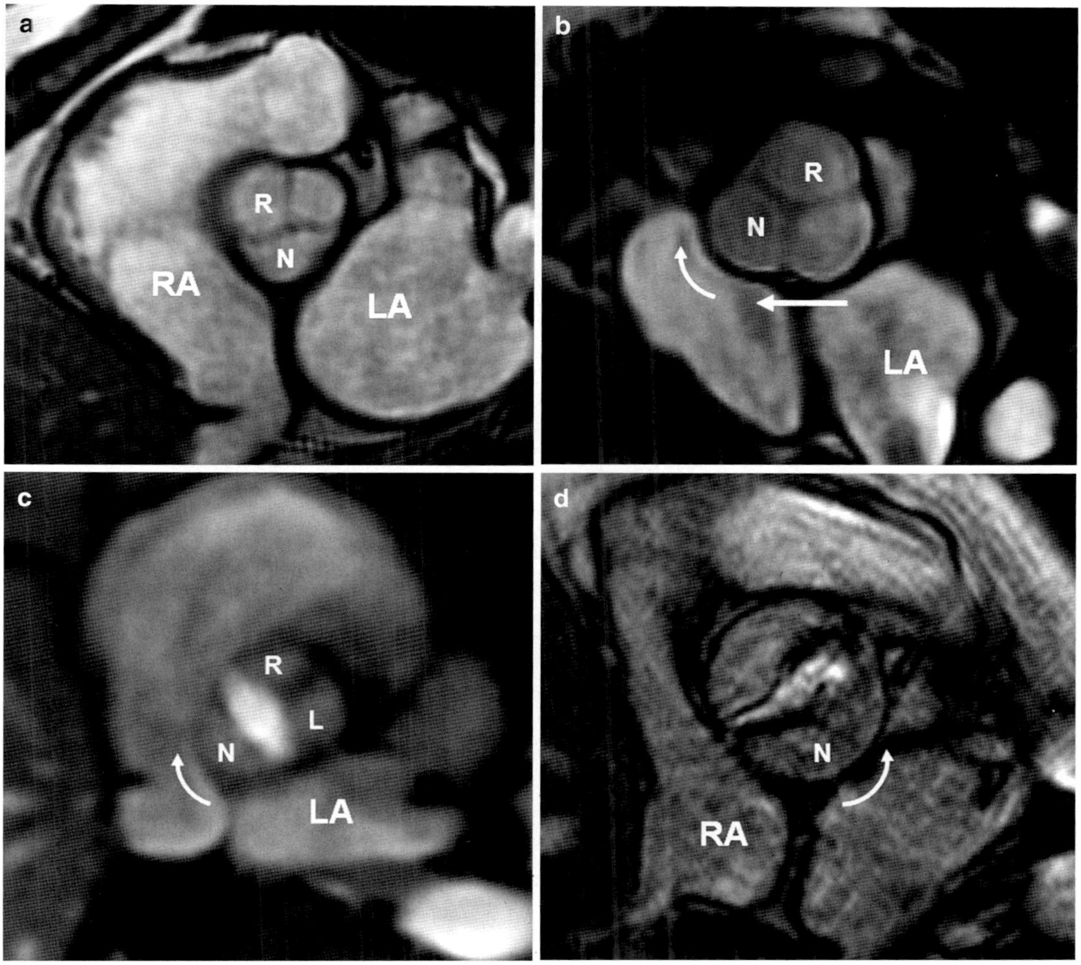

Fig. 7.17 The concept of dextroposition. The term dextroposition indicates that there is specific anatomical evidence that the aortic root is rotated in a clockwise direction (looking from below) and is partially transposed to the right. (**a**) Normal heart with normal aortic root showing the noncoronary aortic sinus (*N*) facing the interatrial septum. In normal patients mild clockwise rotation of the aortic root toward the right atrium (*RA*) is not unusual. (**b**) Typical changes of the aortic root in tetralogy of Fallot (TOF) including clockwise rotation (*curved arrow*) and rightward translation (*straight arrow*). The root is also dilated causing aortic regurgitation in many adult TOF cases. Aortic root rotation is not limited to TOF and is seen in many conotruncal anomalies. (**c**, **d**) Demonstrate changes of the aortic root in two patients with bicuspid aortic valve, one with a raphe between the right (*R*) and the left (*L*) sinuses (**c**) and second without the raphe (**d**). Clockwise rotation is seen in **c** and counterclockwise rotation in (d). (**d**) Shows aortic stenosis. *LA* left atrium

noncommitted [47]. MR is accurate in pre- and postoperative assessment of DORV patients [50]. The spatial relationship between semilunar valves, great arteries, outlet septum, and VSD can be accurately assessed by MRI [50, 51]. The data for the role of CT in DORV is limited. In one study using electron beam CT, the range of diagnostic accuracy for all VSD types in DORV was 88–100 % for 3D CT and 71–94 % for echocardiography [52]. CT also provides clear delineation of the outlet septum which defines the location of the VSD. The outlet septum attaches to the anterior or posterior limbs of septomarginal trabeculations in subaortic or subpulmonic VSDs respectively. In the doubly committed VSD, the muscular outlet septum is

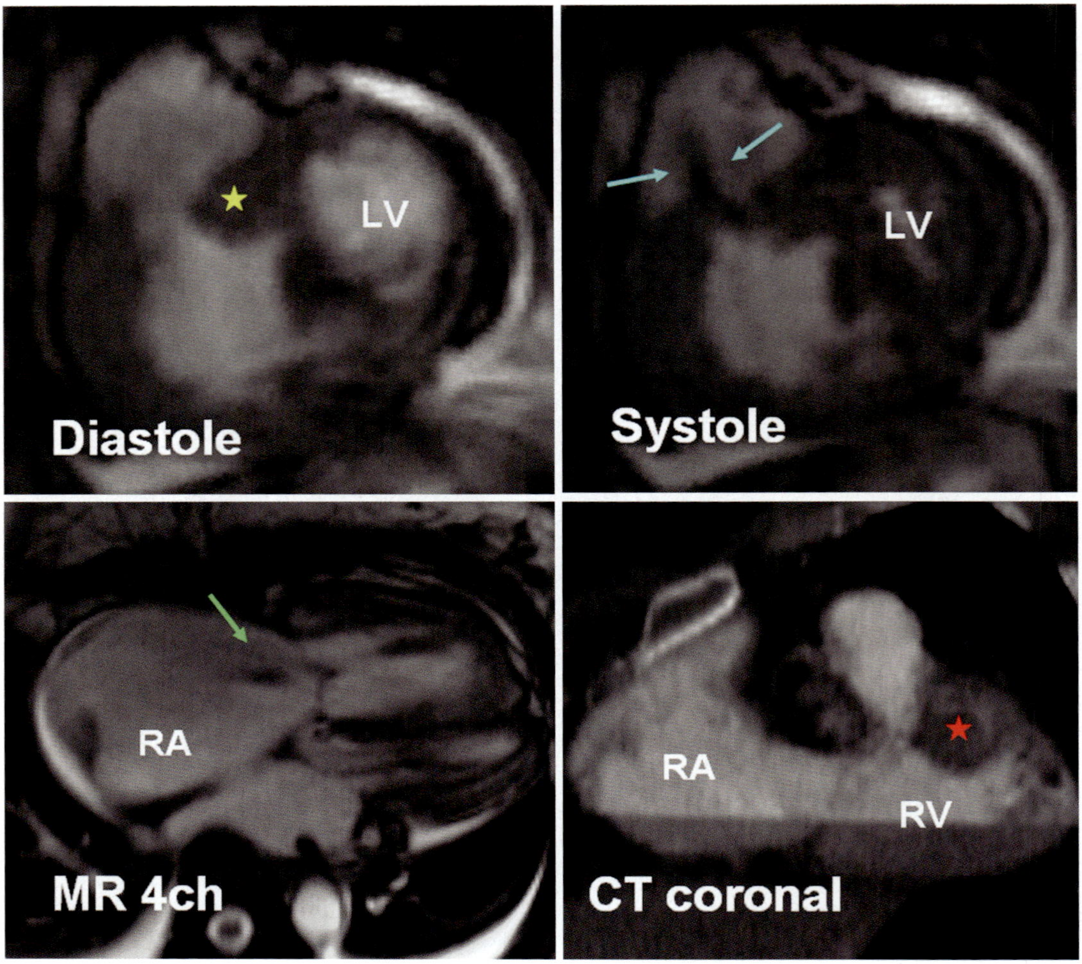

Fig. 7.18 A 48-year-old female with double-chambered right ventricle (*RV*). Severe RVOT stenosis is seen as a result of thickened septomarginal (*yellow star*) and septoparietal (*red star*) trabeculations. Jet flow is seen in systole (*blue arrows*). Thickened wall RV inlet is shown. The right atrium (*RA*) and the RV are enlarged, and there is mild to moderate tricuspid regurgitation (*green arrow*). *LV* left ventricle

absent [48]. The arterial trunks may vary in location, with the aorta generally to the right of the pulmonary trunk (Fig. 7.23). If the trunks spiral as they leave the base of the heart, the VSD is usually subaortic. If the trunks are parallel with the aorta anterior and rightward, the VSD is usually subpulmonic. When the VSD is only under the pulmonary trunk, the configuration is called the Taussig–Bing heart [18, 48]. Usually, there is no fibrous continuity between the semilunar and atrioventricular valves with both great arteries arising predominantly from the RV.

Postoperative DORV

Depending on the anomaly, different surgical methods are used in DORV. In unrestrictive subaortic VSD type, the VSD is closed to include the aortic valve as part of the LV, creating a tunnel that excludes the RV from the systemic circulation. An intraventricular tunnel made of a Gore-Tex patch can baffle blood from the LV through the VSD to the aorta [53, 54]. In Fallot type there is usually a subaortic VSD with pulmonary stenosis. A Rastelli repair is performed, with creation of an intraventricular tunnel to baffle LV to the aorta and placement

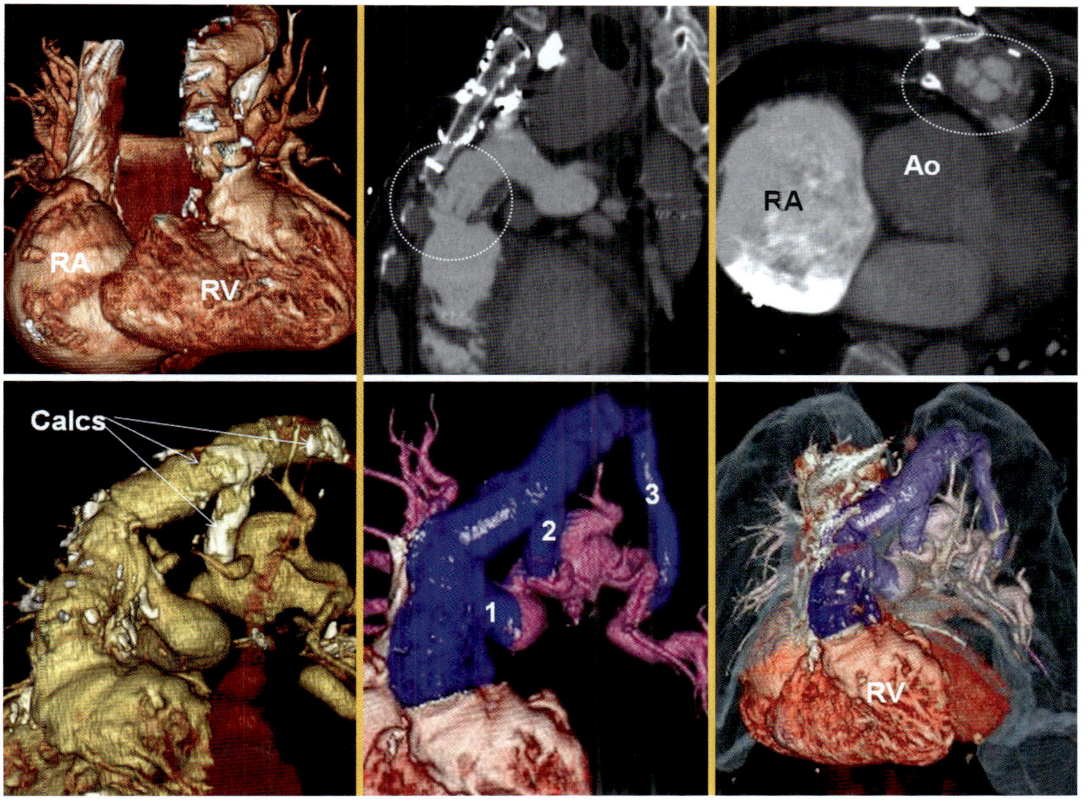

Fig. 7.19 A 48-year-old with history of tetralogy of Fallot (TOF) and pulmonary atresia. Long conduit is shown (*blue colored*) extending between the right ventricle outflow tract and left pulmonary artery branched with three separate connections (*1–3*) to the left pulmonary artery branches. The right atrium (*RA*) and right ventricle (*RV*) are markedly dilated. The aorta is also enlarged (*Ao*). Note close approximation of the pulmonary valve conduit to the sternum (*white circles*). Extensive calcifications (calcs) are shown

of a RV-to-pulmonary artery conduit (valved homograft) (Fig. 7.23). TGA type usually has a subpulmonary VSD without pulmonary stenosis. Complete repair with an arterial switch operation and a VSD to pulmonary artery baffle is required in the neonatal period. Repair of DORV with a remote noncommitted VSD can be very complex [53]. In postoperative cases MRI or CT can easily shows the morphology and patency of both outflow tracts. In postoperative patient, issues that should be assessed with imaging include the status of both ventricles, any evidence for subaortic or subpulmonary obstruction if a tunnel-type operation has been performed, the presence of a residual VSD, and evidence for conduit stenosis or regurgitation.

Complete Transposition of the Great Arteries

In this anomaly ventriculoarterial discordance exists, meaning the aorta arises from the morphological RV and the pulmonary artery arises from the morphological LV [55, 56] (Fig. 7.24a, b). In TGA the aorta and main pulmonary artery are parallel rather than crossing, and in most cases the aorta is located right anterior to the pulmonary artery (Fig. 7.24). It is not uncommon to see the aorta directly anterior to the pulmonary artery [57]. Rarely, the arrangement is side-by-side, with the aorta on the right and in front of the tricuspid valve [58]. RV dysfunction and pulmonary hypertension are recognized late outcome after the Mustard or Senning procedures [59, 60]. In arterial switch

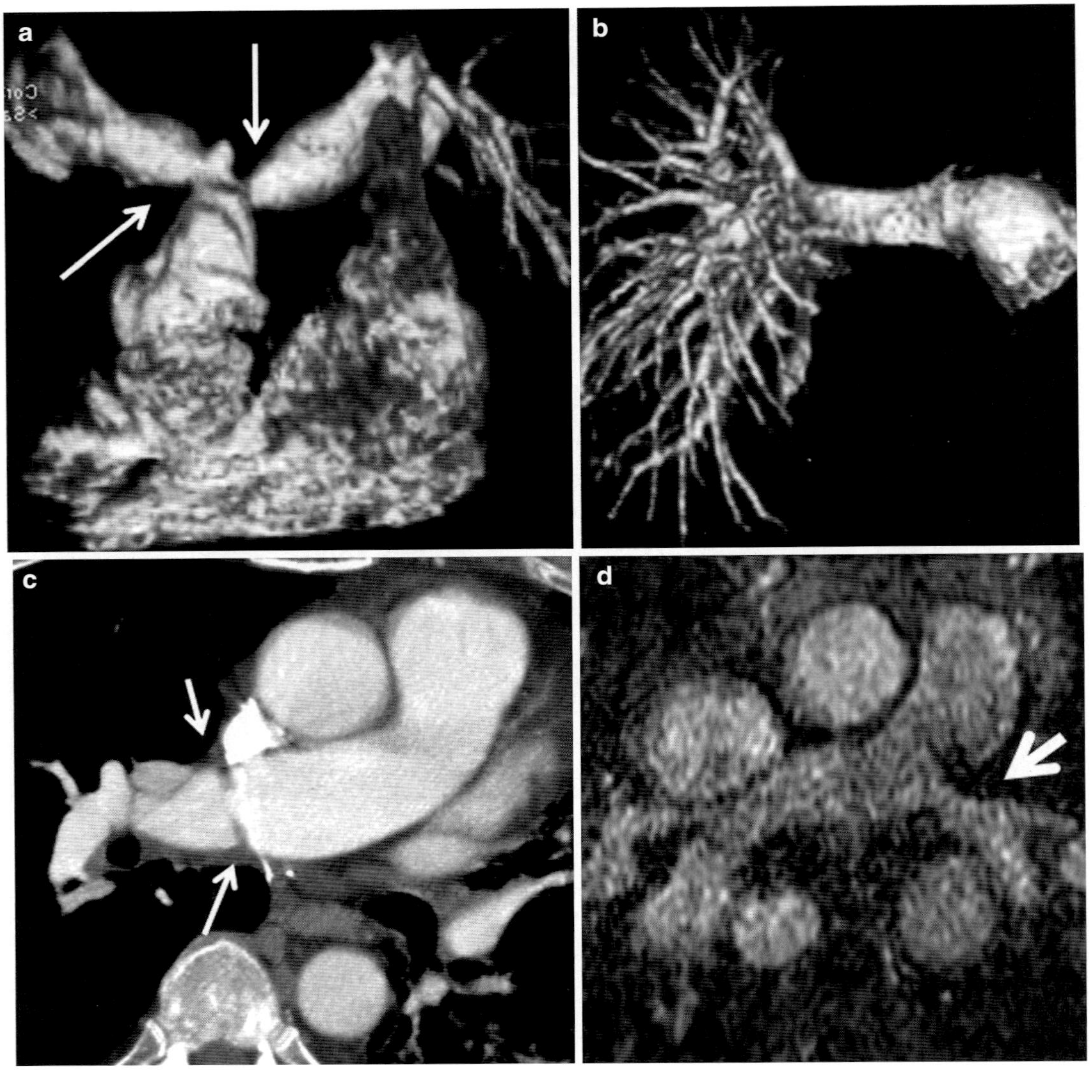

Fig. 7.20 Associated findings in pulmonary branches of different adult patients with repaired TOF represented with RVOT regurgitation. A comprehensive assessment of pulmonary branches is necessary before pulmonary valve implantations. (**a**) Severe right and left pulmonary arteries stenosis (*arrows*). (**b**) Absence of left pulmonary artery. (**c**) Annular stenosis of distal right pulmonary artery (*arrows*). (**d**) Mild narrowing of left pulmonary artery (*arrow*)

Fig. 7.22 Morphology of the RVOT in repaired TOF is a major determinant of suitability for percutaneous pulmonary valve replacement. Untreated TOF is shown for comparison (female 54 years old). Type I is aneurysmal (pyramidal) shape and the most common (50 %) and not a good candidate for valve replacement. Type II is cylindric with a constant diameter (14 %). Type III has an inverted pyramidal appearance (3 %), Type IV is fusiform (17 %), and Type V is narrow and tubular (13 %). Note stenosis at distal end of homograft in the fusiform RVOT. MR or CT is necessary for 3-dimensional analysis and appropriate measurements. MR assessment of right and left pulmonary arteries is necessary for hemodynamic analysis in each candidate

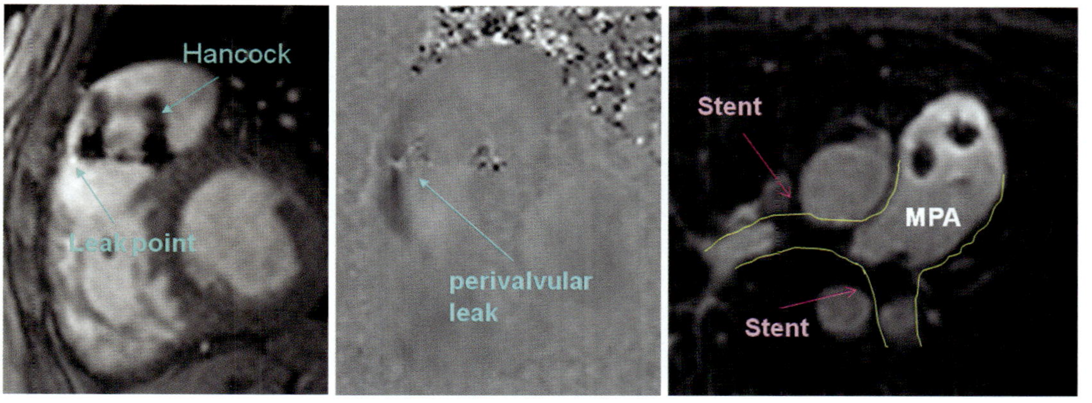

Fig. 7.21 Tetralogy of Fallot (TOF) with anterior perivalvular leak (*blue arrows*). Status post Hancock pulmonary valve replacement and stenting of right and left pulmonary arteries (*pink arrows*). The metallic struts of the bioprosthetic valve cause artifacts that compromised a full evaluation of the pulmonary valve. The measured regurgitant fraction from the perivalvular insufficiency was approximately 15 %. The proximal portion of the main pulmonary artery (*MPA*) was aneurysmal measuring 4.8 × 3.8 cm. Substantial branch pulmonary artery stenosis was treated by balloon dilation and endoluminal stent before valve replacement

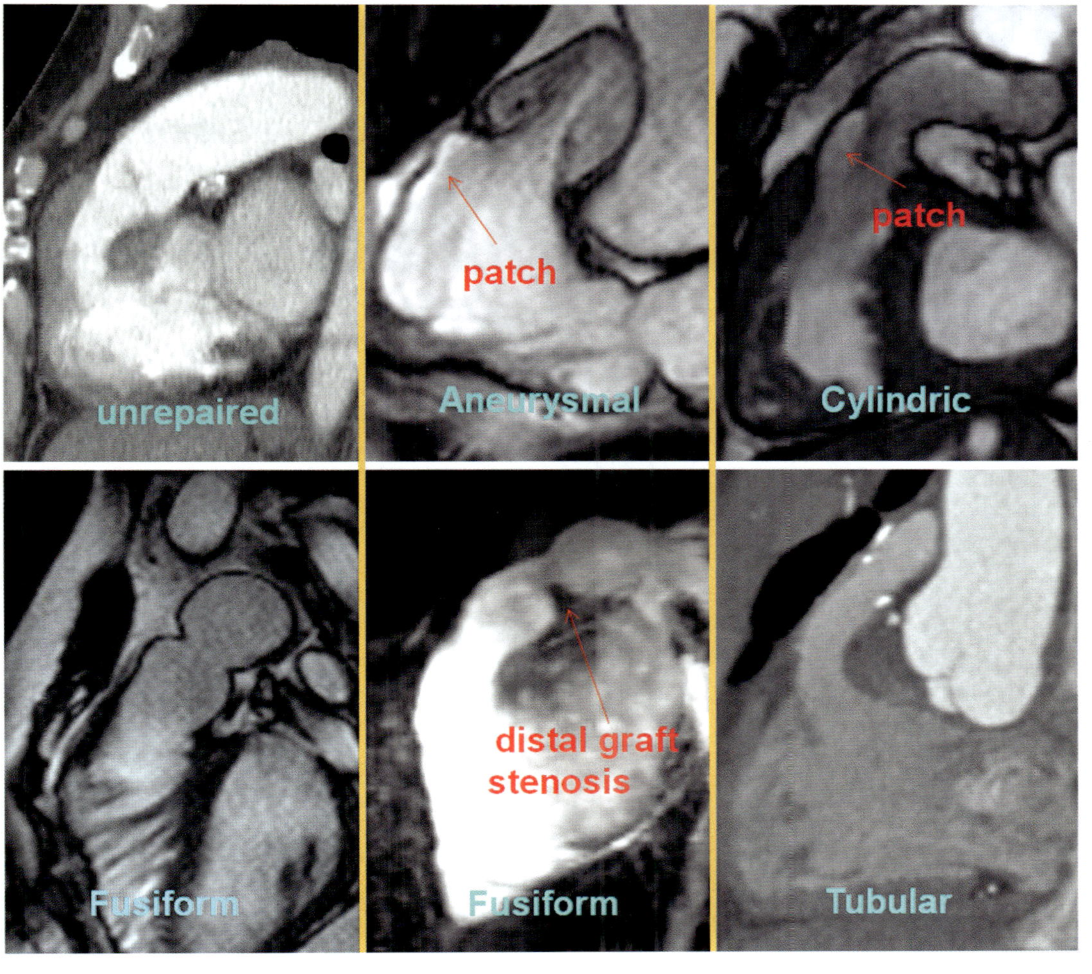

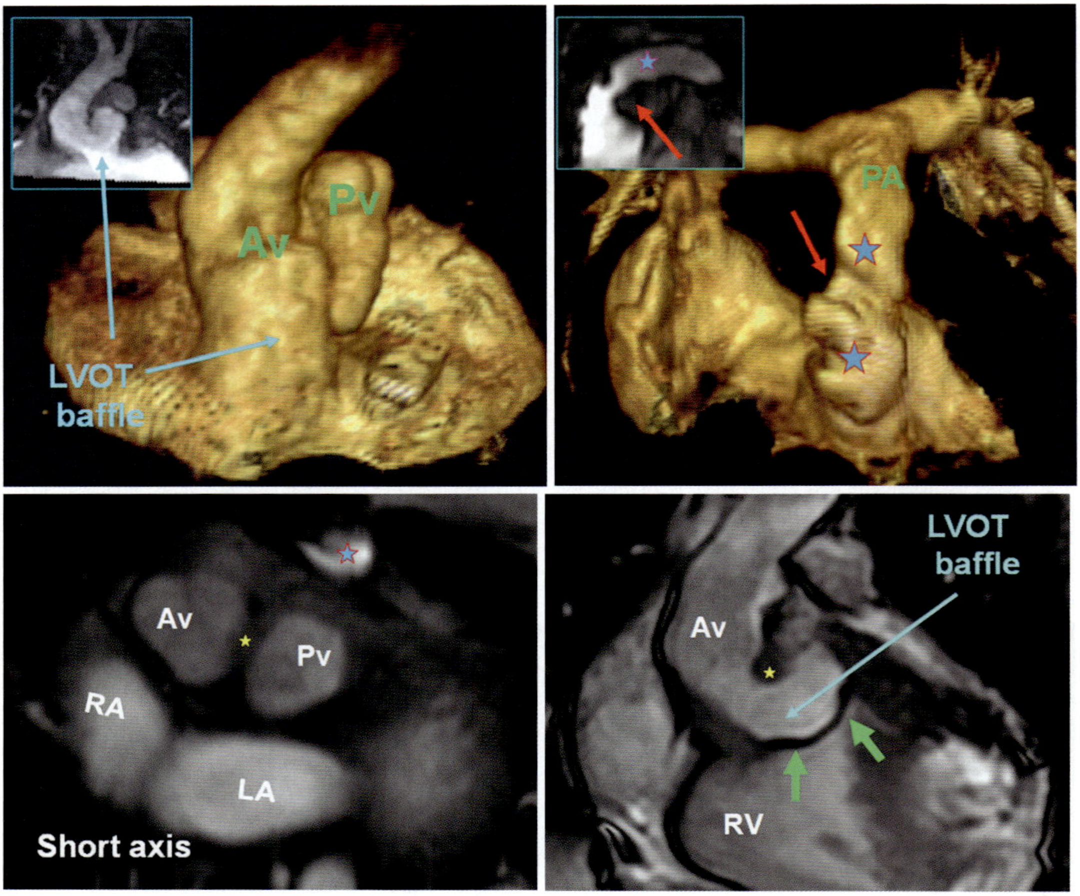

Fig. 7.23 Spectrum of findings in repaired DORV. A 22-year-old male status post Rastelli repair for double outlet right ventricle (DORV). Rastelli repair is performed by an intraventricular tunnel made of a Gore-Tex patch (*green arrows*) to baffle left ventricular blood to the aorta (*blue stars*) and placement of a right ventricular-to-pulmonary artery (*PA*) conduit. RV-to-PA conduit shows mild narrowing (*red arrows*). Note side-by-side position of the aortic (A) and pulmonary (P) valves and the outlet septum between them (*yellow stars*). *RV* right ventricle, *RA* right atrium, *LA* left atrium, *LVOT* left ventricle outflow tract

procedure the pulmonary artery is brought forward anterior to the aorta and the coronary buttons are sutured into the "neoaorta" [61]. Complications can be shown by CT or MRI. These include distortion of the RVOT and pulmonary arteries, neoaortic root dilatation with aortic regurgitation, and rarely coronary artery stenosis [61].

Congenitally Corrected TGA

In congenitally corrected TGA (ccTGA), blood flows in the normal direction but through the "wrong" ventricle (Fig. 7.24c, d). The morphological LV and mitral valve supply the pulmonary circulation, and the morphological RV and tricuspid valve supply the systemic circulation [62, 63]. The most common anatomical arrangement is situs solitus with L-looping of the ventricles and the aorta anterior and leftward of the pulmonary artery [62]. At the earliest sign of deterioration in systemic ventricular function, systemic atrioventricular valve regurgitation should be suspected [64, 65]. Most centers would not recommend a prophylactic double switch procedure for patients without associated abnormalities in whom RV and tricuspid valve function is normal. Regular assessment of ventricular function using cardiac MRI every few years is suggested [64].

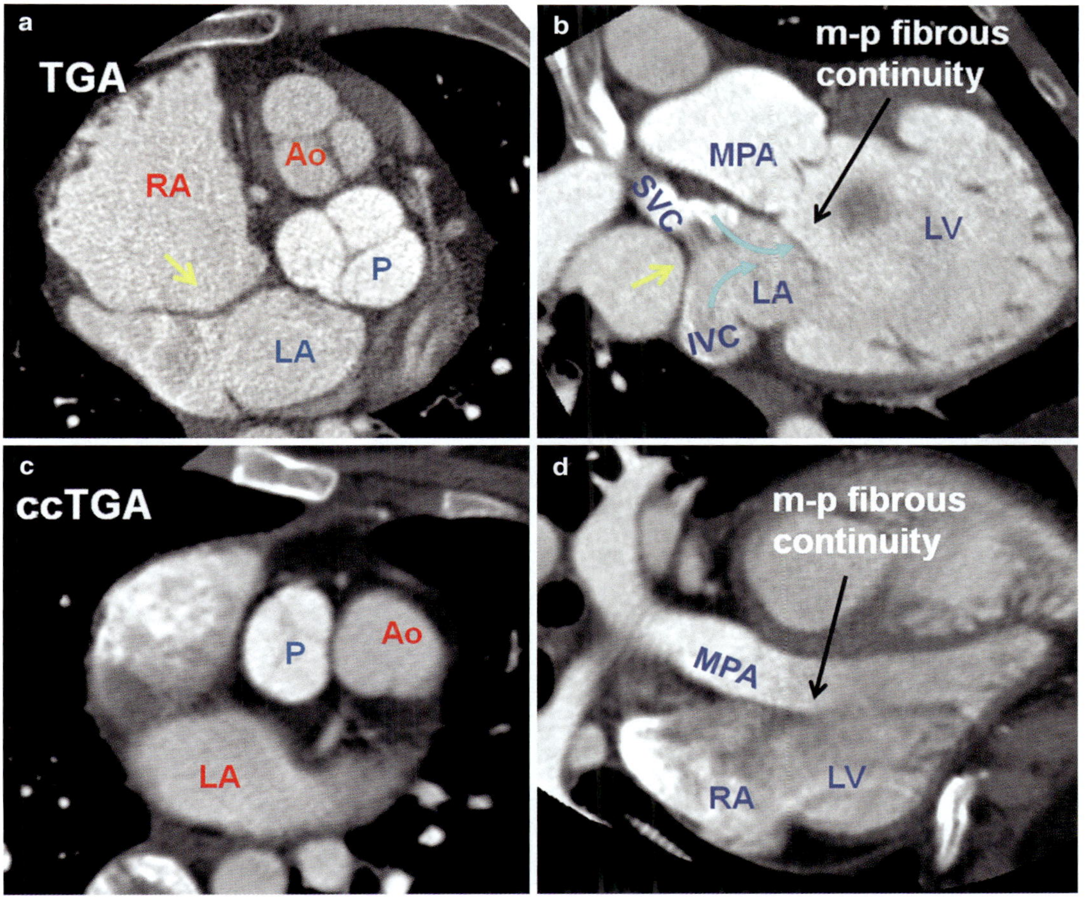

Fig. 7.24 Anatomical features of the outflow tract in transposition of great arteries (TGA) and congenitally corrected malposition of great arteries (ccTGA). (**a**, **b**) TGA status post atrial switch. In TGA the aortic valve (*Ao*) is located anterior to the pulmonary valve (*P*) in most cases, and the great arteries are parallel rather than crossing as they do in the normal heart. The second most common arrangement is with the aorta just anterior to the pulmonary artery. There is fibrous continuity of the mitral and pulmonary valves (m–p continuity). Intra-atrial baffle (*yellow arrows*) shifts deoxygenated blood of the SVC and IVC into the left atrium (*LA*) vestibule, left ventricle (*LV*), and main pulmonary artery (*MPA*). The right ventricle is the systemic ventricle and will be hypertrophied. (**c**, **d**) In ccTGA the ventricles are congenitally inverted with the LV located behind the sternum. The pulmonary (*P*) and aortic (*Ao*) valves are usually side-by-side with the aorta on the left. This anatomical arrangement of great arteries can be rarely seen in TGA (<10 %). The pulmonary artery in ccTGA arises directly from the LV with direct fibrous continuity between the mitral and pulmonary valves. *IVC* inferior vena cava, *RA* right atrium, *SVC* superior vena cava

Truncus Arteriosus

Truncus arteriosus consists of a single arterial trunk giving origin to the pulmonary arteries, the coronary arteries, and the systemic circulation [66]. Several classifications of the common trunk have been proposed on the basis of the origins of the pulmonary arteries [66, 67]. Progressive dilatation of the common trunk as a result of cystic medial necrosis is common. The common trunk usually overrides a large, nonrestrictive VSD resulting from absence of the infundibular septum [18]. It lies between the 2 limbs of the septomarginal trabeculation. The truncal valve is usually tricuspid but can vary between 1 to 6 cusps [18]. The basic repair involves closing the VSD and separating the PAs and attaching them to a valved conduit arising from RVOT [68] (Fig. 7.25). Most patients have reoperation by 10–12 years for conduit replacement (usually because of the small size of the original conduit)

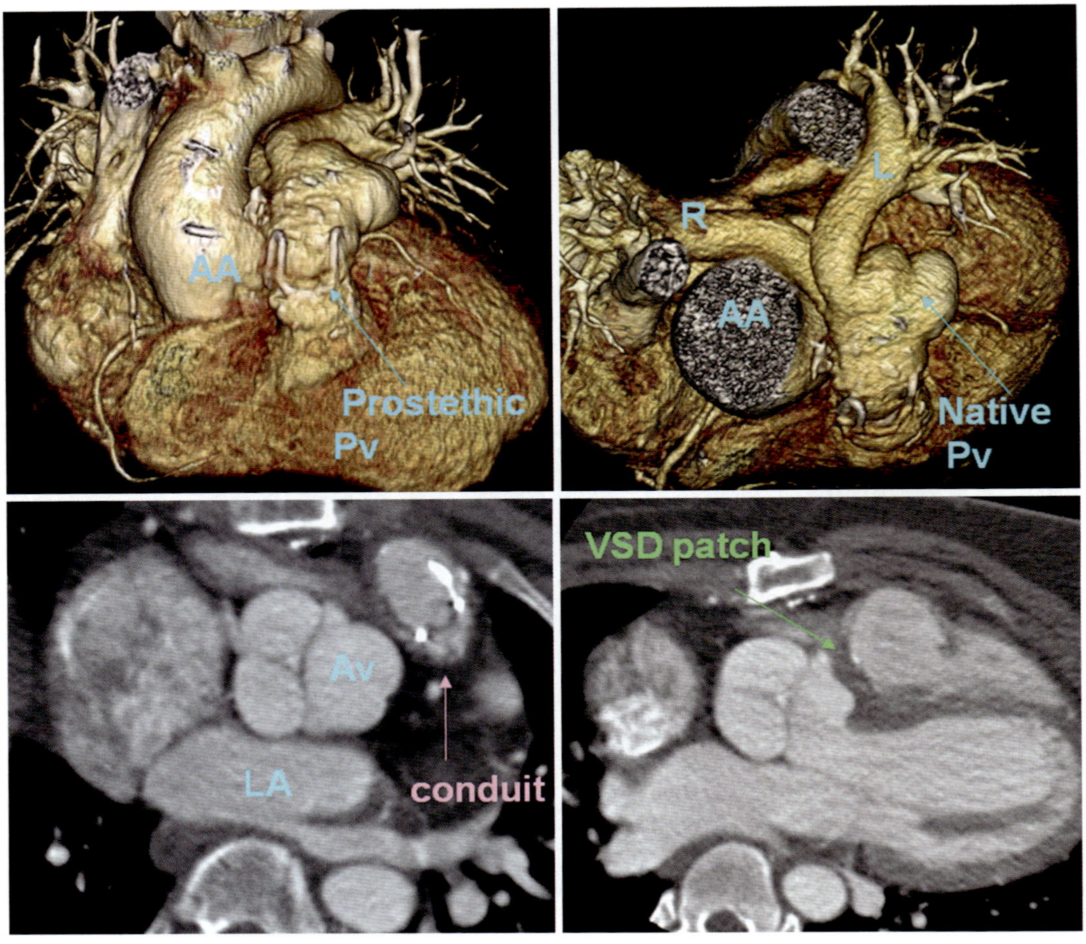

Fig. 7.25 Repaired truncus arteriosus. A prosthetic valve is placed in right ventricle pulmonary artery conduit. Conduit homograft is partially calcified. Sub-truncal VSD patch is shown (*green arrow*). *AA* ascending aorta, *AV* aortic valve, *VSD* ventricular septal defect, *PV* pulmonary valve, *R* right pulmonary artery, *L* left pulmonary artery

or truncal valve replacement because of valvular insufficiency. Truncus arteriosus should not be mistaken with hemitruncus [69]. Hemitruncus is best defined as a condition in which one branch of the pulmonary artery (usually the right) originates from the ascending aorta and the other branch has a normal course arising from a normal main pulmonary artery (Fig. 7.26).

Functional Analysis of the RVOT

Accurate quantification of the RV volume and function has remained clinically challenging despite advances in cardiac imaging. The three-dimensional nature and complex anatomy of the RV make CT and MR ideal tools for assessing its size and function.

Imaging Techniques

Cardiac MRI is an excellent noninvasive imaging modality for RV function analysis and when serial monitoring is necessary (i.e., systemic RV) can be repeated. Unfortunately, in presence of a cardiac pacer, MRI is relatively contraindicated, although this circumstance is changing. In patients with a pacemaker, CT may be a better choice for functional assessment of RVOT

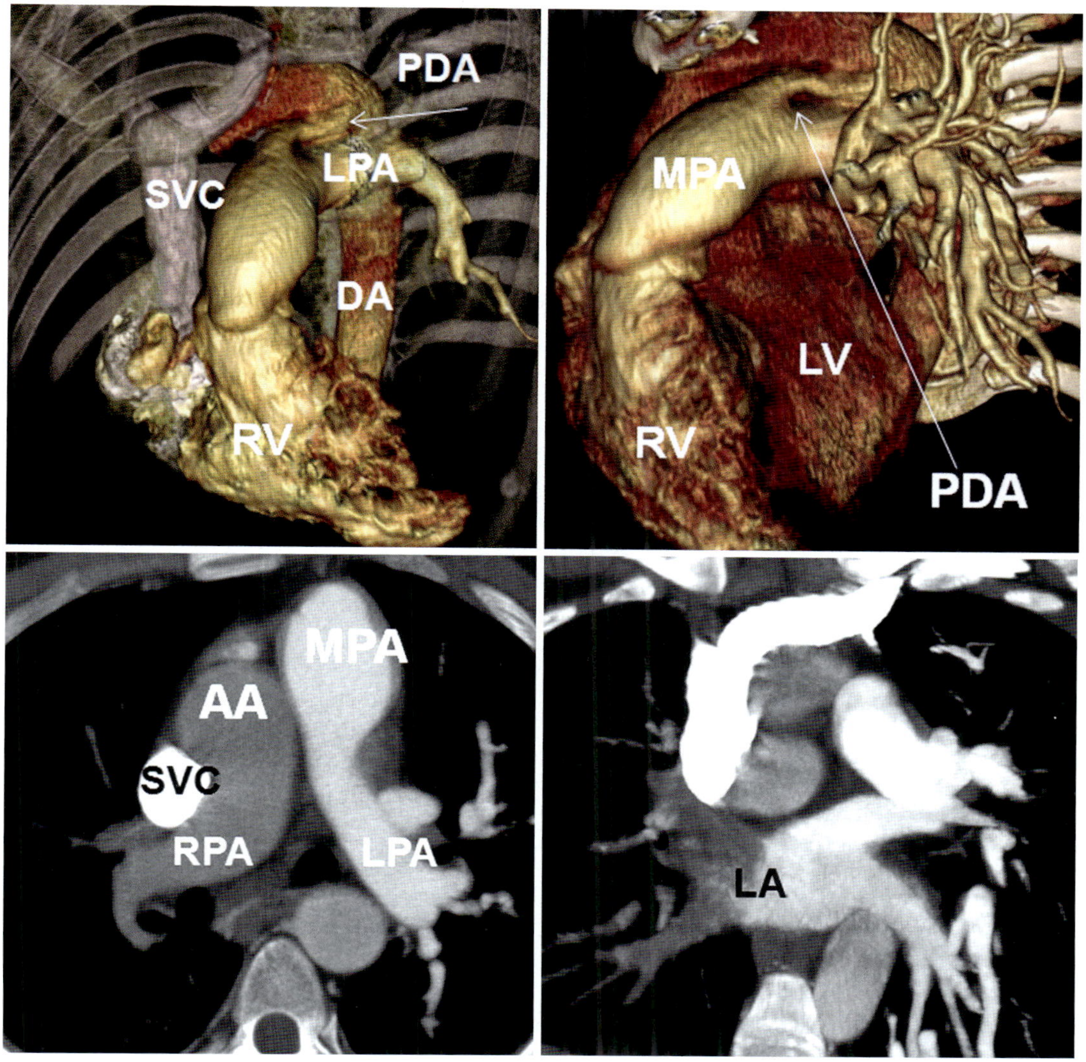

Fig. 7.26 Hemitruncus with anomalous origin of the right pulmonary artery (*RPA*) from the ascending aorta (*AA*). A patent ductus arteriosus (*PDA*) also exists. The CT data is obtained at pulmonary phase and only the right heart is opacified. The left pulmonary artery (*LPA*) originates normally from the main pulmonary artery (*MPA*). Delayed opacification of the RPA as a result of its origin from the aorta has given a double contrast to the left atrium (*LA*) with incomplete filling of the right pulmonary veins. *RV* right ventricle, *LV* left ventricle

especially when evaluation of anatomy and complications related to surgery is also desired and limitations exist for performing echocardiography. Functional MR analysis of the RV and RVOT can be obtained using balanced SSFP cine images [70]. Manual or automated tracing of the endocardial borders of the RV will be performed at end-systolic and end-diastolic phases. The RV volume is then automatically calculated by summation of slice volumes. The process is then repeated by tracing the endocardial borders of the RV inlet or outlet according to the described anatomical landmarks earlier. Using long-axis cross-reference images will help to correctly localize the level of atrioventricular and ventriculoarterial valves as well as the border between the inlet and outlet on short-axis images. Because of RV conduction delay in repaired TOF, the end-diastolic and end-systolic phases of the RV lag the LV. Therefore, images at these phases selected for the

LV volume measurement on short-axis images may not be the same phase for the RV.

Functional analysis can be performed using retrospective ECG-gated cardiac CT. Temporal resolution of CT is not as fast as MRI. With dual source scanners and new reconstruction algorithm, faster temporal resolution (i.e., 83 ms) can be obtained; this way the image quality can be improved by reducing motion artifact [71]. A comprehensive functional assessment of the RV may necessitate MR flow quantification at the level of valves or when RVOT stenosis is suspected on cine images (i.e., double-chambered RV). With new MR phase-contrast techniques, volumetric evaluation of hemodynamics is possible [72]. Care should be taken to avoid sternal wires and surgical clips when localizing the image plane to obtain routine phase-contrast measurements. Both breath hold and free breathing techniques have been used during phase-contrast data collection. It is claimed that pulmonary regurgitant fraction is artificially low in expiratory breath hold technique compared to free breathing or inspiratory breath hold data acquisitions [73].

Arrangement of Muscle Bundles

Architecture of the myocardial strands in the left and right ventricles is fundamentally different (Fig. 7.27). In the relatively thin wall RV circumferential and longitudinal orientations predominate [46, 74, 75]. Subepicardial myofibers retain the circumferential arrangement, and deeper subendocardial myofibers are arranged longitudinally. The hypertrophied RV in TOF can change in architecture to resemble the sandwich pattern (prominent circumferential middle layer) seen in the normal left ventricle (LV) [74]. In the RV, the fibers' orientation can be different in the infundibulum. Myocardial strands are mainly aligned in circular fashion in the subepicardium of the RVOT and form the bulk of the wall [75] (Fig. 7.2). At the subendocardium of the infundibulum, there are longitudinally aligned myofibers, these forming the series of septoparietal trabeculations that branch laterally from the septomarginal trabeculation and may form parallel or crossed strands (Figs. 7.6 and 7.27). These septoparietal trabeculations can be flat or prominent and may be hypertrophied as in pulmonary hypertension, TOF, or pulmonary valve stenosis, contributing to muscular pulmonary subvalvular stenosis (Fig. 7.6).

Regional Differences in Right Ventricular Systolic Function

Global assessment of the RV function is difficult owing to the underlying complex anatomy with the inlet and outlet contracting almost perpendicular to each other. When the overall RV function is taken into account, it is important to mention that the inlet part of the RV has a greater contribution compared with the outlet. The outlet (infundibulum) comprises 20 % of the RV volume and contributes 15 % of the total RV ejection fraction [70]. The conduction in the RV is provided by a single long fascicle and takes time resulting in a peristaltic-like motion with the outlet following the RV inlet by >15 % of the cardiac cycle delay [70]. This pattern can be lost in pulmonary hypertension patients, and all RV components may reach minimum volume simultaneously [76, 77]. Furthermore, RVOT fractional shortening will be reduced early in patients with pulmonary hypertension, while their right ventricular systolic long-axis excursion may remain stable [76] (Fig. 7.28). RVOT fractional shortening is simply calculated as the percentage shortening in RVOT anteroposterior diameter in systole with respect to that in diastole using a three-chamber or axial view. The right ventricular systolic long-axis excursion is the difference between diastolic and systolic lengths of RV measured from the lateral margin of tricuspid ring to the RV apex on a four-chamber view. Using CT data, it is seen that RVOT diameter and cross-sectional area measured during systole are larger in patients with pulmonary hypertension compared with normal subjects, whereas diastolic values are not significantly different [12].

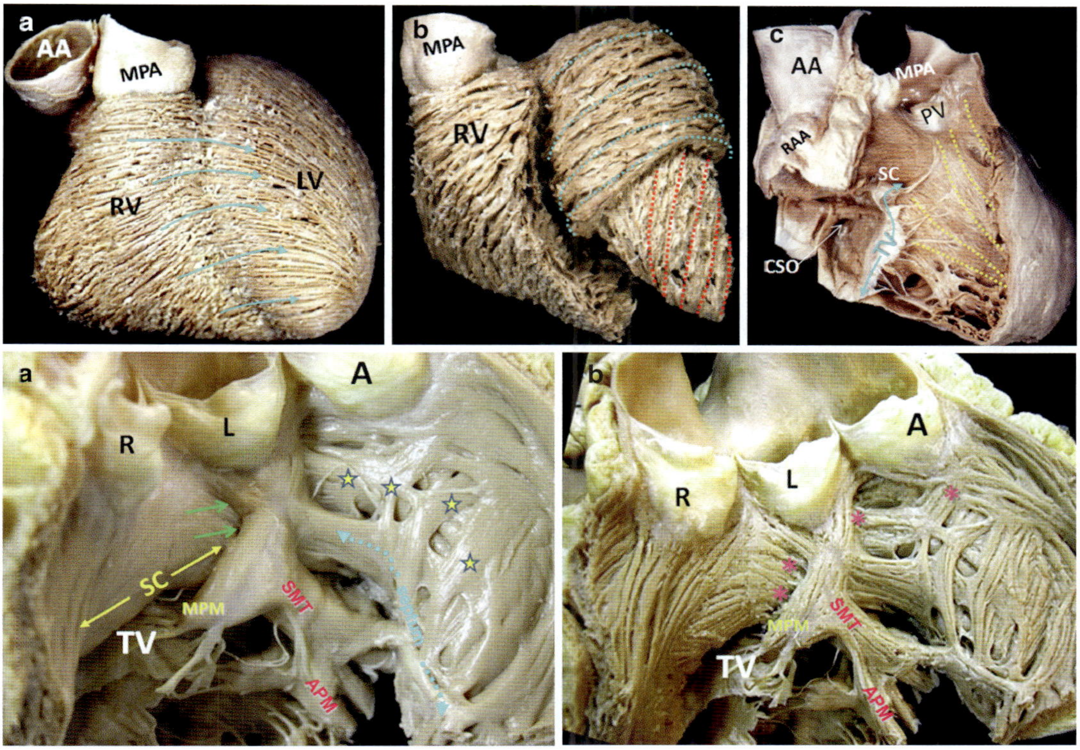

Fig. 7.27 *Upper panel*: (**a**–**c**) These dissections show the change in the myocardial grain, representing the overall oblique or circumferential orientation of the myocardial strands in the epicardial or superficial region (**a**) of the right ventricular walls. Note that there is continuity between the superficial fibers of the right and left ventricle (*arrows*). (**b**) Demonstrates prominent circumferential middle of the left ventricle (*blue dotted lines*) which is absent within the normal right ventricle. (**c**) Demonstrates the deep or subendocardial region in an opened right ventricle (*yellow dotted lines*). This deep region can also be seen in the left ventricle (*red dots*) in image **b**. Note subendocardial myocardial strands are longitudinally or obliquely arranged at right angles with respect to epicardial strands. *RV* Right ventricle, *LV* Left ventricle, *AA* Aorta, *CSO* Coronary sinus orifice, *RAA* Right atrial appendage, *TV* Tricuspid valve (*blue line*), *PV* Pulmonary valve, *MPA* Main pulmonary artery. *Lower panel*: (**a**) Endocardial view of the RVOT. Note that endocardial infundibular sleeve consists of septoparietal trabeculations (*stars*) arising from the septomarginal trabeculation (*SMT*), the medial papillary muscle (*MPM*) and the junction (*green arrows*) between the supraventricular crest (*SC*) shown by (*yellow arrows*), and SMT. The interventricular septum is shown by dotted (*blue line*). (**b**) Same specimen showing the RVOT subendocardial myofibers arrangements. Note the crossing architecture pattern of the myocardial strands between the SMT with the septoparietal trabeculations and supraventricular crest below the pulmonary valve (*asterisks*). *L* left, *A* anterior, *R* right, *TV* tricuspid valve, *APM* anterior papillary muscle

Right Ventricle Outflow Tract Stenosis

RVOT hypertrophy is common in chronic pulmonary valve stenosis and may lead to a fixed or dynamic subvalvular stenosis (Fig. 7.3). RVOT stenosis, which can be due to extrinsic or intrinsic causes, can result in hemodynamic instability and defined as "significant" when the peak right ventricular-to-pulmonary artery systolic gradient exceeds 25 mmHg. Furthermore, significant RVOT stenosis is defined as "fixed" if there is no change in RVOT dimensions during the cardiac cycle and as "dynamic" if RVOT dimensions increase appreciably in diastole [78]. A hypertrophied RV can maintain its function for years, even when RV pressures are near systemic. Symptoms occur at a variable level of valve gradient but usually much later than an RV pressure exceeding 50 % of systemic pressure. Echocardiography is the best modality for diagnosis and grading of stenosis. MR and CT can

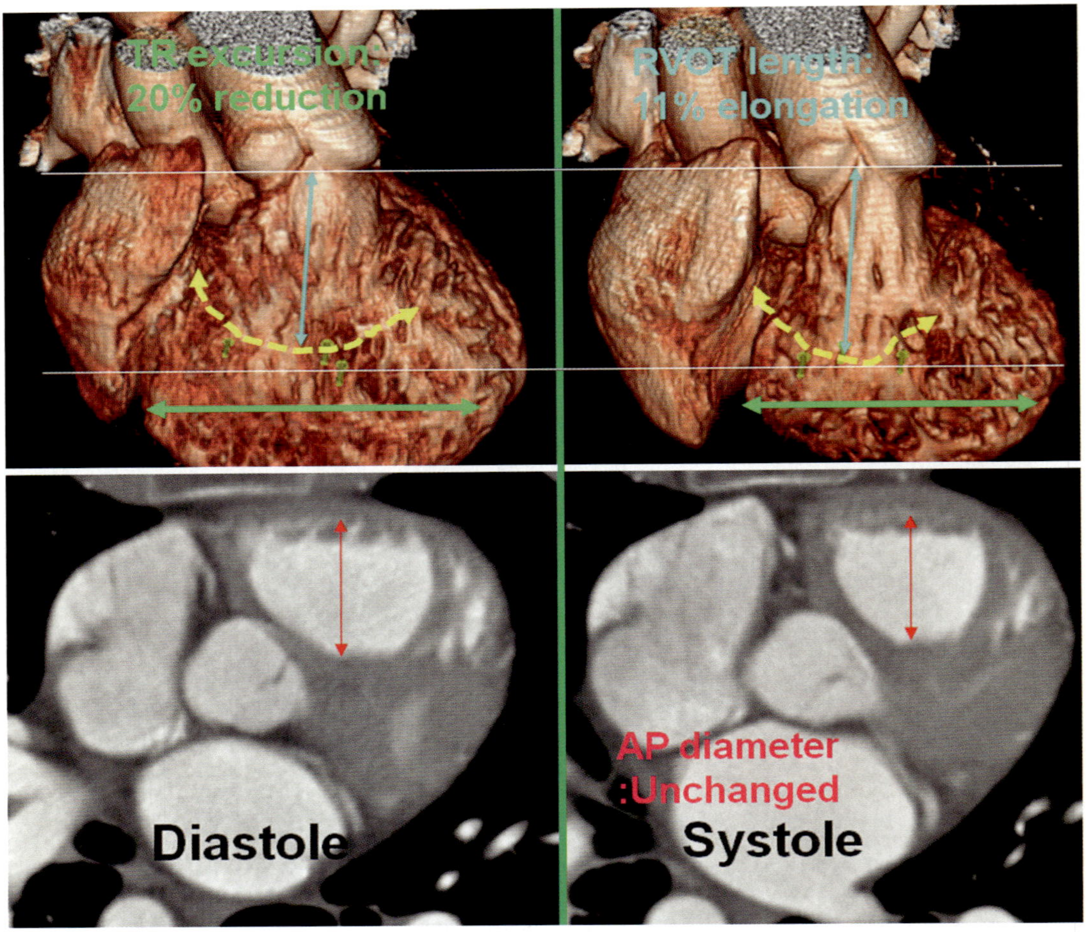

Fig. 7.28 Right ventricle outflow tract (*RVOT*) function in pulmonary hypertension. In pulmonary hypertension, compared to normal, tricuspid ring (*TR*) excursion (*green arrows*) only mildly decreases, but the RVOT anteroposterior diameter (*AP*) remains unchanged or mildly contracted in systole compared to diastole (*red arrows*). AP shortening fraction is used as one of the early parameters that will change in pulmonary hypertension. Note the length of RVOT (*blue arrows*) is not only changed but mildly increased in systole compared to diastole. *Yellow curve* shows the beginning of the RVOT

also provide valuable information on valve mobility, RV size and function, the presence of post-stenotic dilatation, locating a pulmonary subvalvular stenosis, and associated pathologies [79] (Fig. 7.29).

RVOT and RV Function in Repaired TOF

Evaluation of the regional adaptation of three components of the morphological RV to different conditions of loading by imaging techniques can be important especially in repaired congenital heart disease. The apical trabecular component provides the major ejectile momentum of the ventricle, and its function is maintained in patients with slight-to-moderate ventricular dysfunction. The outlet part, in contrast, shows a consistently and markedly decreased ejection fraction irrespective of the nature of the overload. In post-repair TOF, although the surgical subjects have lower RVOT ejection fraction and higher indexed volumes, most show reserved inlet ejection fraction [80]. The pulmonary infundibulum may be essential for right ventricular ejection and for maintaining pulmonary valve competence.

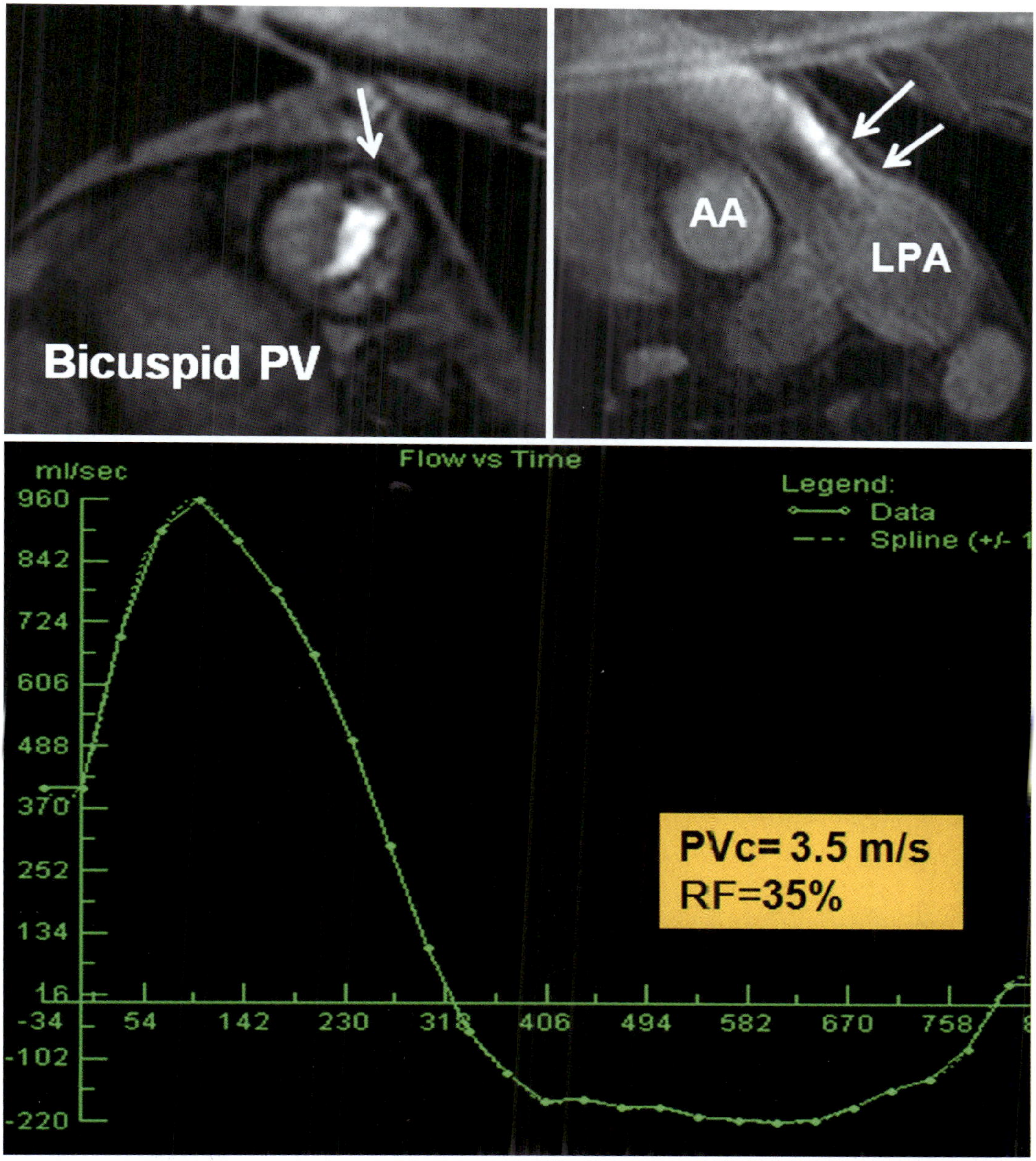

Fig. 7.29 Transaxial and long-axis MRI of a stenotic bicuspid pulmonary valve (PV) (*arrow*) with jet flow (*double arrows*) and post-stenotic dilatation of the left pulmonary artery (*LPA*) are shown in upper row. Systolic flow turbulence and increased peak velocity (*PVc*) of 3.5 m/s by phase velocity mapping were seen. Flow profile, mL/s versus time (ms), is shown. There was moderate (free) pulmonary valve insufficiency with regurgitant fraction (*RF*) 35 %. The regurgitant fraction is defined as regurgitant volume divided by the stroke volume. *AA* ascending aorta

Transannular patching gives excellent relief of the RVOT obstruction but invariably causes pulmonary insufficiency, hypokinesis and aneurysm of the RVOT, and fibrosis (Fig. 7.30). Surgical attempts to preserve pulmonary valve competence by limiting the patching to the ventricular area below the pulmonary valve may not protect patients from the late deleterious consequences

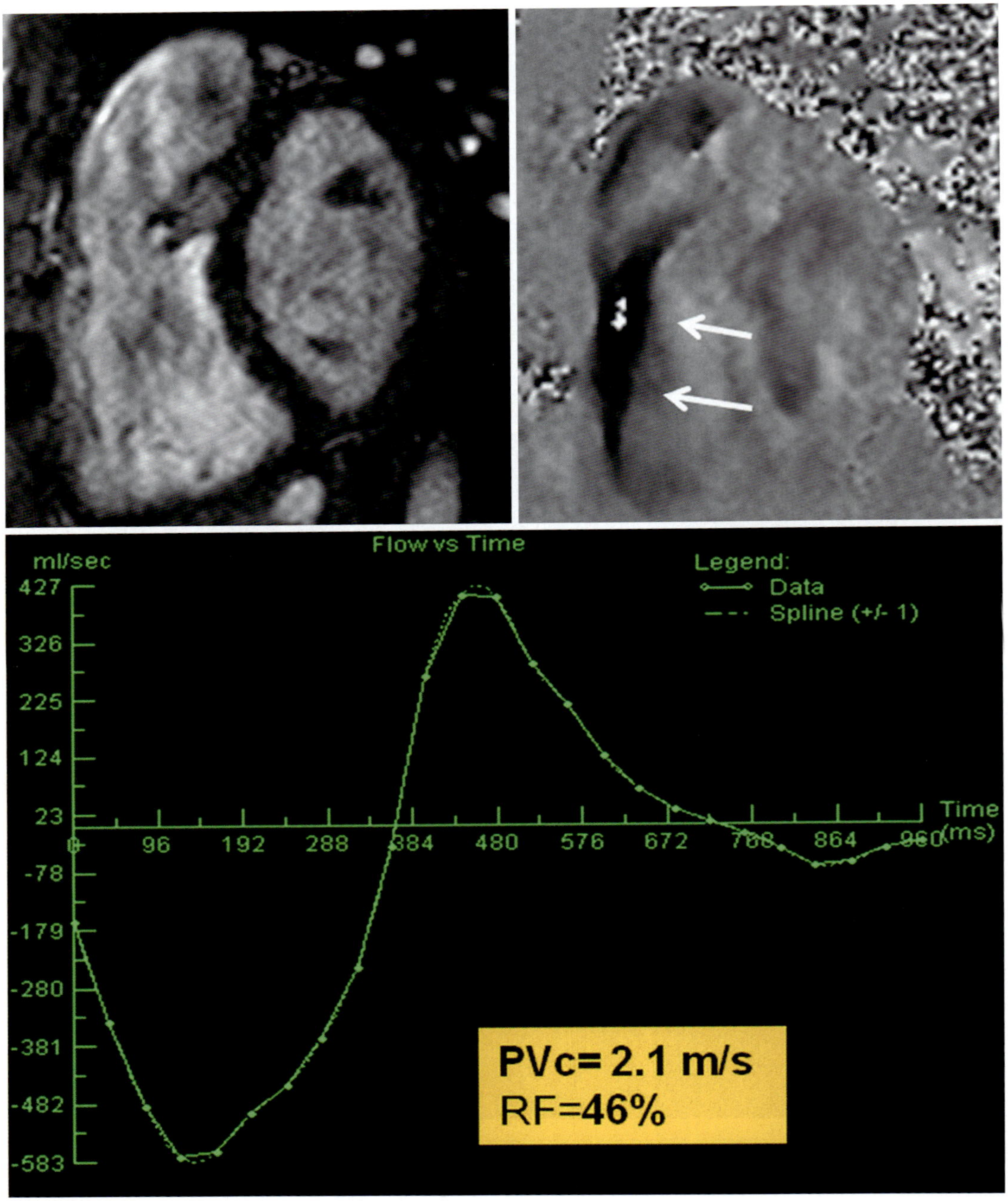

Fig. 7.30 Post-repaired tetralogy of Fallot showing free flow regurgitation at pulmonary valve level best shown on phase image (*arrows*). Flow profile, mL/s versus time (ms), shows moderate to severe pulmonary valve insufficiency with a regurgitant fraction (*RF*) of 46 %. Peak velocity (*PVc*) was 2.1 m per second (m/s). Time-flow volume curve is recorded reverse with forward flow shown in negative direction. Note mild late diastolic forward flow due to forced atrial contraction related to impaired relaxation of the right ventricle. Documentation of severe pulmonary regurgitation, exercise limitation, and excessive right ventricular dilatation, defined by a RV/LV ratio of 2:1 by MRI, has been used as criteria for valve replacement

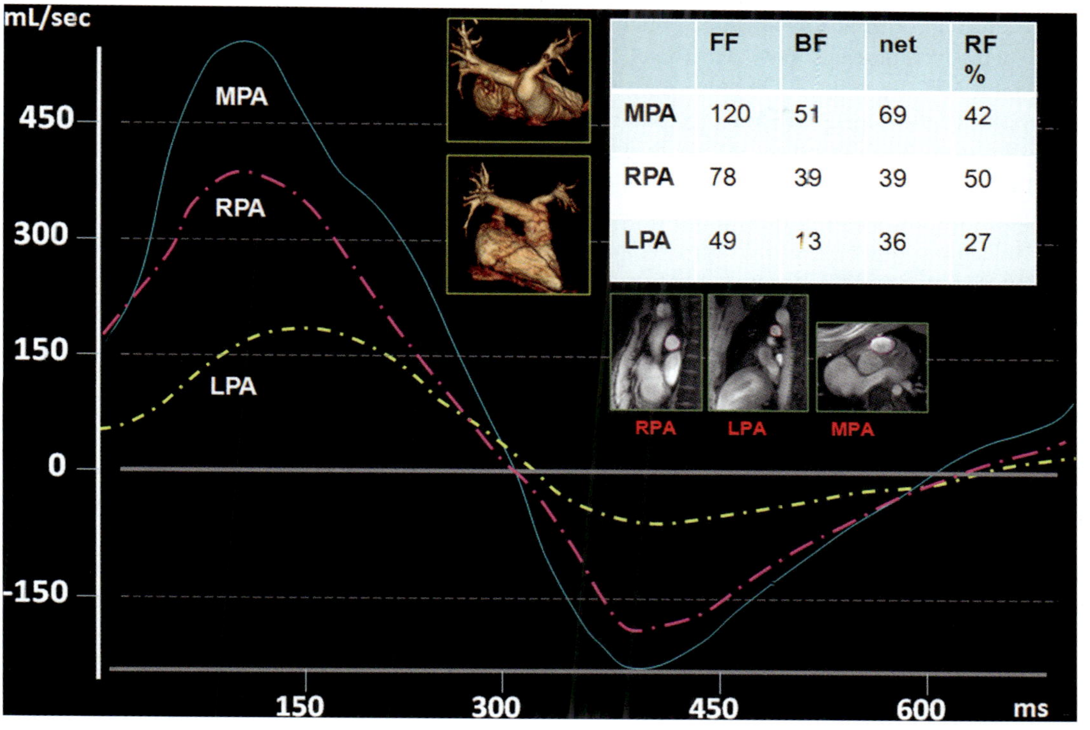

Fig. 7.31 Time-flow curves, phase-contrast magnitude views, and volume-rendered MR angiography of pulmonary arteries are shown. Status after tetralogy of Fallot repair with larger right pulmonary artery (*RPA*) compared to the left pulmonary artery (*LPA*). Differential regurgitant fraction (*RF*) of the RPA and LPA is shown. Despite larger size of RPA, the net flow to both RPA and LPA is almost equal due to larger RF of the RPA. The elevated RPA–RF may be related to elevated right-sided pulmonary vascular resistance. *BF* backward flow, *MPA* main pulmonary artery, *FF* forward flow

of RV dilatation [81]. It is possible that the source of global RV dysfunction in repaired TOF is because of the dyskinesis of the infundibulum and dyssynchrony of RV contraction [82]. There is a close relationship between the degree of pulmonary insufficiency and RV diastolic dimensions and stroke volume. Adverse ventricular–ventricular interaction could be an important mechanism in which RV dilatation and dysfunction lead to LV dysfunction. In phase-contrast analysis of the outflow tract regurgitation, both regurgitant volume and fraction values are equally important and should be reported [83]. Regurgitant fraction (regurgitant volume x 100/forward flow volume, in %) can be artificially high in the presence of low RV systolic function but modest amount of regurgitant volume. It is also important to measure differential regurgitant fraction of the left and right pulmonary artery branches. In the absence of stenosis or marked dilatation of one vessel, regurgitant fraction is usually higher on the left side and may be related to increased peripheral vascular resistance [84] (Fig. 7.31). Indications of pulmonary valve replacement include in moderate to severe insufficiency, RV/LV diameter or end-diastolic volume ratio >2, RV end-diastolic volume index >150–160 mL/m^2, RV and/or LV dysfunction, and large RVOT aneurysm. Cardiac MR is the ideal method for longitudinal follow-up in patients with repaired TOF. Following percutaneous valve replacement, end-diastolic and end-systolic volumes decrease by 30–40 %, and tricuspid regurgitation improves, although global RV systolic function (measured as ejection fraction) remains unchanged. The RV size may not return to normal in preoperative end-diastolic volume index >170 mL/m^2 [79].

Detailed information about three-dimensional (3D) hemodynamics and flow alterations occurring in the RVOT and the entire pulmonary vascular system in post-repair TOF are important before valve surgery. Time-resolved 3D phase-contrast MRI with three-directional velocity encoding, also known as flow-sensitive 4D-MRI, has introduced as a valuable method for comprehensive analysis of RVOT function [72]. Routine phase-contrast methods can be used to quantify differential pulmonary flow in order to assess the significance of a branch pulmonary stenosis. A severe discrepancy in pulmonary blood flow (>35 %) requires treatment of the branch pulmonary stenosis before repair of the RVOT [79]. Identification of residual intracardiac shunt with cardiac MR is also important before percutaneous pulmonary valve replacement. For example, in the presence of a moderate pulmonary regurgitation (35 % regurgitant fraction) and RV dilatation, even a small shunt (i.e., <1.3 pulmonary-to-systemic flow ratio) can be problematic and should be treated.

RVOT Function in Systemic RV

In patients with ccTGA and post-atrial switch TGA, the RV functions as the systemic pumping chamber. In these condition the infundibulum is very short and underdeveloped, and RV dysfunction and tricuspid regurgitation are common (Fig. 7.24). A shift in the systemic RV myostructure from longitudinal to circumferential shortening is seen as an adaptive response to the systemic load when compared with the normal RV. However, in contrast to the normal LV, ventricular torsion is essentially absent and strain rate is reduced [85–87]. It seems that ventricular hypertrophy, the design of the respective atrioventricular valve, the lack of torsion, reduced strain rate, and possibly myocardial ischemia might be factors responsible for accelerated failure of the systemic RV [86–89]. Generally, the goals of MRI after an atrial switch procedure include evaluations of the function and size of the ventricles, careful assessment of the intra-atrial baffle for leak and stenosis, atrioventricular valves for regurgitation, and outflow tracts for obstruction. The number of adult patients with ccTGA who need CT or MRI for early detection of complications has been increasing, due to better imaging techniques as well as increasing life expectancy of these patients. A small percentage of patients with ccTGA have no intracardiac defect and may remain asymptomatic until age 40–50. The role of MRI or CT in these cases is mainly in the assessment of systemic RV function and associated tricuspid regurgitation. CT may be advantageous over MRI in delineation of the coronary anatomy origin before surgery or in patients with an endocardial pacer.

RVOT Myocardial Scar

Detection of myocardial scar in MR or CT exam of adult congenital heart malformations is not uncommon and most of the time is located at areas of patch repairs or ventriculostomy (Fig. 7.32). Scar tissue and/or patch material in the RVOT can adversely affect RV mechanics after TOF repair. In post-repair TOF, regional functional abnormalities and hyperenhancement are most common in the RVOT [90]. Hyperenhancement frequently extends to the anterior RV free wall and neighboring segments. Typical sites of hyperenhancement include anterior wall of RVOT (99 %), VSD patch area (98 %), moderator band (24 %), site of apical vent insertion in the LV (48 %), and inferior (80 %) and superior (24 %) insertion points [90]. Delayed myocardial enhancement in the systemic RV (TGA with atrial switch and ccTGA) is not uncommon and has direct correlation with patient age, myocardial wall thickness, and end-systolic volume of the RV and may be associated with cardiac arrhythmia and sudden death [85]. Enhancement patterns include localized full-thickness RV anterior wall enhancement, small patchy areas of enhancement, and VSD closure site. It is important to remember that in the presence of subendocardial or transmural enhancement in a vascular territory, coronary artery disease should be excluded. Enhancement at RV free-wall insertion to interventricular septum is a common finding and seems more characteristic of continuous pressure overload [85]. RVOT wall enhancement in arrhythmogenic right ventricular cardiomyopathy/dysplasia (ARVD/C) is not uncommon [91].

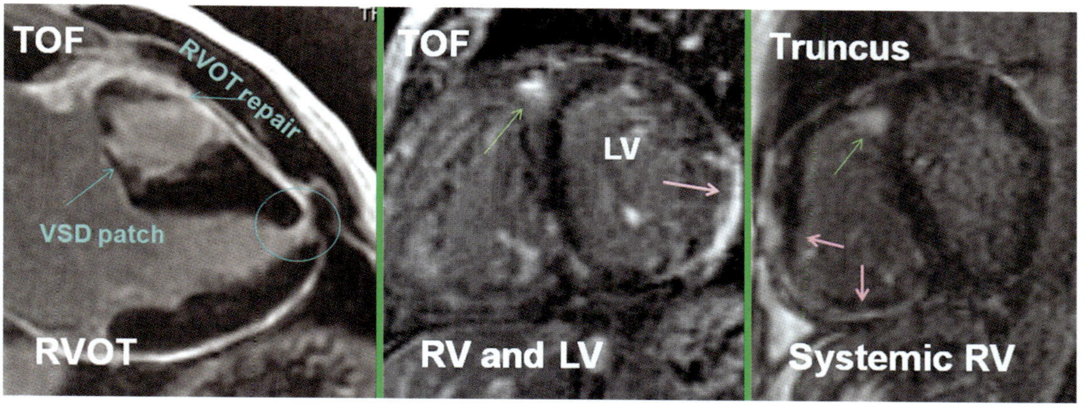

Fig. 7.32 Common locations of RVOT myocardial scars. In tetralogy of Fallot (*TOF*), scars at surgical repair site, around VSD patch, and ventriculostomy site are the most common locations. The right ventricle (*RV*) free wall can easily be involved in systemic RV (*red arrows*) as shown in this 41-year-old patient with truncus arteriosus and single ventricle. Enhancing sites at the RV free-wall insertion sites to the septum are benign findings (*green arrows*). The left ventricle wall is involved in middle image (*red arrow*). Scars in RVOT may predispose to cardiac arrhythmias. *LV* left ventricle, *VSD* ventricular septal defect

RVOT and Cardiac Arrhythmias

The RVOT is generally a common source of cardiac arrhythmias. The embryonic OFT consists of slowly conducting tissue until it is incorporated into the ventricles and develops rapid conducting properties. It is suggested [92] that remnants of the embryonic OFT phenotype and expression profile in the adult RVOT determine the electrophysiological and structural characteristics that make the RV more vulnerable for arrhythmias. Patients with TOF have higher rate of atrial and ventricular arrhythmias [93]. Potential risk factors for ventricular tachycardia (VT) include aneurysmal dilation of the RVOT, RV dilatation, and pulmonary regurgitation. Ventricular arrhythmias are usually localized to the RVOT act, and the scars at infundibulotomy, VSD patch repair, or ventriculostomy may increase the risk [93].

Morphological changes of the RV free wall are described in patients with idiopathic RVOT tachycardia using MRI including fat deposition, wall thinning, saccular aneurysm, and dyskinesis in up to 60–65 % of cases [94, 95]. VT is also a common complication in patients with arrhythmogenic right ventricular cardiomyopathy/dysplasia (ARVD/C) and may arise from the RVOT [96]. Currently, RVOT ventricular tachycardia ablation is guided by traditional electrophysiologic and electroanatomic methods. CT and MR can help in demonstrating myocardial scar, vascular integrity of the RVOT, and better localizing the source of arrhythmia by image fusion techniques. The relationship of coronaries with RVOT can nicely be depicted with CT scan. When distance between the coronary arteries and the ablation sites is found to be less than 5 mm, cryoablation or 4-mm-tip catheters may be considered to avoid short- and long-term damage to the coronary arteries [97]. Fat deposition in the RV and RVOT wall is not limited to idiopathic VT or ARVD [98]. It is seen in 25 % asymptomatic general population and increases with age [99, 100]. Fat can develop at the site of any myocardial scar including the site of surgery (i.e., Ross procedure). The relation of RV fat with RV function or OFT arrhythmias is not clear.

Rare Causes of RVOT Obstruction

Extrinsic RVOT obstruction has been recognized as a possible cause of hemodynamic instability after cardiac surgery and should be reported in postoperative chest CT scans [81]. Extrinsic compression can occur from an aortic or pulmonary artery aneurysm or postoperative mediastinal hematoma [101]. Intrinsic obstruction is mainly related to congenital heart disease. Hypertrophic cardiomyopathy and ventricular non-compaction may rarely cause RVOT obstruction [102, 103].

Post-Ross Outflow Tract

The Ross procedure is aortic valve replacement with the autologous pulmonary valve which eliminates problems with aortic prosthetic valve or allograft replacements especially in children [104]. It is a procedure of choice in children with severe anomaly of the aortic valve and/or left ventricular outflow tract obstruction [105]. The main concern after surgery is dilatation of the neoaortic root leading to progression of aortic regurgitation, especially in the settings of geometric mismatch of the aortic and pulmonary roots and regurgitant valve (Fig. 7.33).

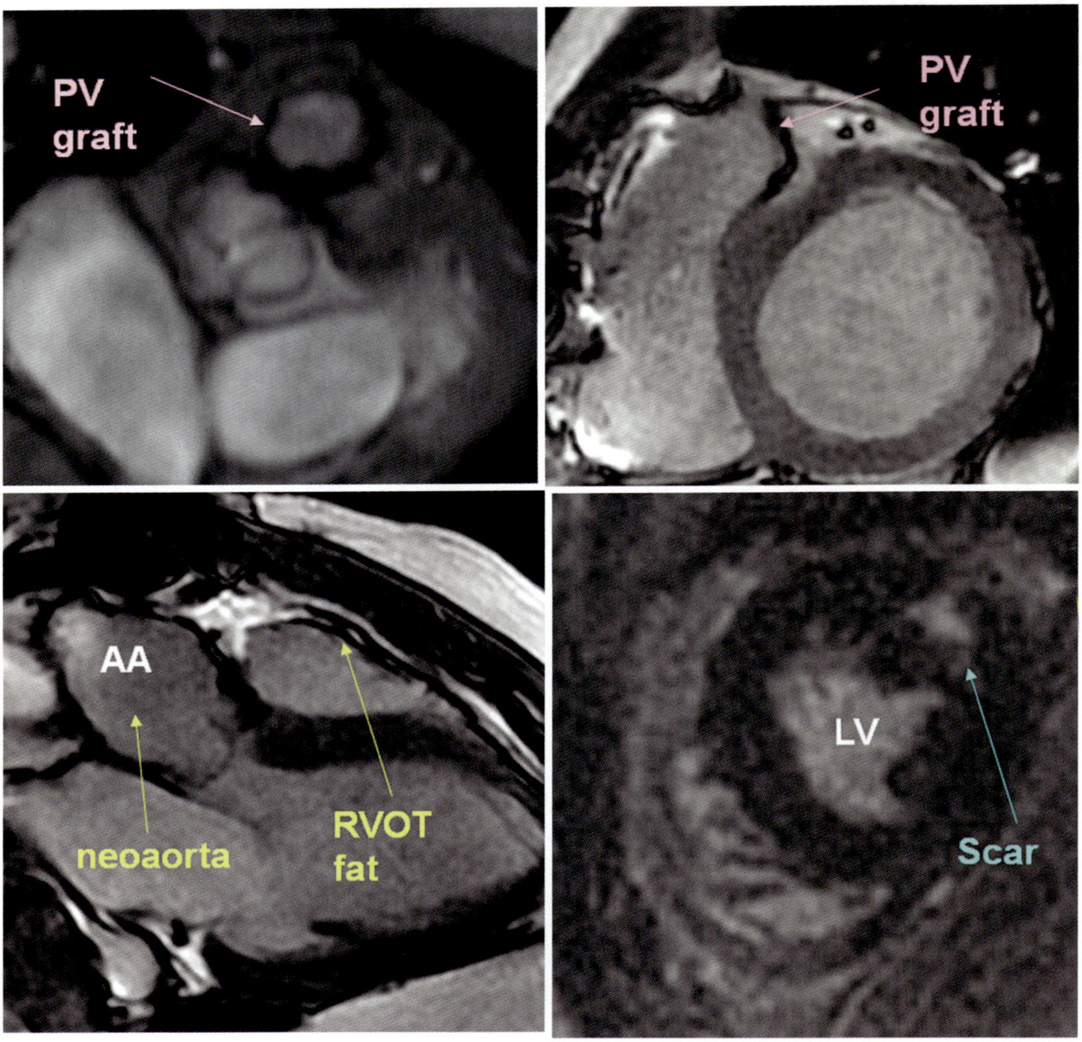

Fig. 7.33 A 29-year-old male with congenital heart disease, status post Ross procedure, and pulmonary homograft revision. MR images show dilated aortic root (pulmonary autograft) and severe aortic regurgitation with regurgitant fraction of 45 %. The bioprosthetic pulmonary valve (*PV*) showed mild stenosis and regurgitation. Note fatty degeneration of right ventricle outflow tract (*RVOT*) and intramyocardial scar of the left ventricle (*LV*). *AA* ascending aorta

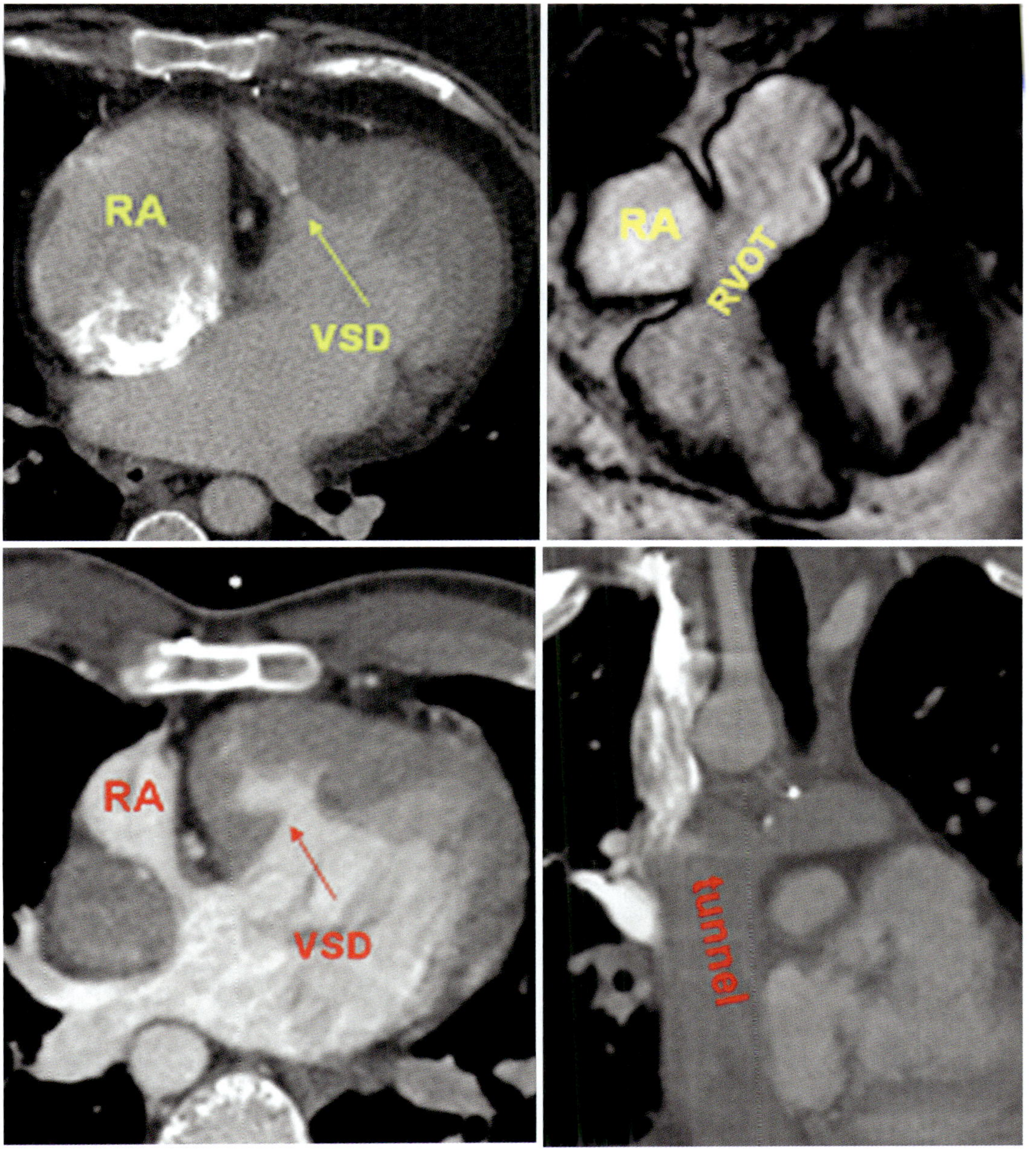

Fig. 7.34 Axial and coronal CT images. Bjork surgery showing right atrium (*RA*) to RVOT (*upper row*) versus total cavopulmonary connection with extracardiac lateral Fontan tunnel (*bottom*) for tricuspid atresia. Note markedly dilated right RA in Bjork. *RV* right ventricle, *RVOT* right ventricle outflow tract. *VSD* ventricular septal defect

Problems with the homograft used in reconstruction of the RVOT are not usually significant, although mild regurgitation is common and up to about 20 % of patients tend to have mild gradients which can be relieved with balloon dilatation [105].

Bjork Surgery

The procedure involves right atrium to RV connection and has been done in the past for tricuspid atresia (Fig. 7.34). The usual surgical approach for tricuspid atresia is Blalock–Taussig shunt or pulmonary artery band soon after birth, followed by Glenn surgery (bidirectional cavo-pulmonary shunt) at 3–6 months of age, and finally Fontan surgery at 2–3 years of age [106].

Conclusion

Detailed information about the embryology and anatomy of RVOT provides a better understanding of the spectrum of diseases involving this important area and helps to narrow differential diagnosis of malformations involving this important structure. CT and MR can provide most of the data regarding anatomical, functional, and pathological changes of the RVOT.

References

1. Waldo KL, Kumiski DH, Wallis KT, et al. Conotruncal myocardium arises from a secondary heart field. Development. 2001;128:3179–88.
2. Kirby ML. Cardiogenic fields and heart tube formation. In: Kirby ML, editor. Cardiac development. 1st ed. Oxford/New York: Oxford University Press; 2007. p. 21–35.
3. Kelly RG, Brown NA, Buckingham ME. The arterial pole of the mouse heart forms from Fgf10-expressing cells in pharyngeal mesoderm. Dev Cell. 2001;1: 435–40.
4. Waldo KL, Hutson MR, Ward CC, et al. Secondary heart field contributes myocardium and smooth muscle to the arterial pole of the developing heart. Dev Biol. 2005;281:78–90.
5. Webb S, Qayyum SR, Anderson RH, Lamers WH, Richardson MK. Septation and separation within the outflow tract of the developing heart. J Anat. 2003;202(4):327–42.
6. Rana MS, Horsten NCA, Tesink-Taekema S, Lamers WH, Moorman AFM, van den Hoff MJB. The trabeculated right ventricular free wall in the chicken heart forms by ventricularization of the myocardium initially forming the outflow tract. Circ Res. 2007;100:1000–7.
7. van den Hoff MJB, Moorman AFM, Ruijter JM, et al. Myocardialization of the cardiac outflow tract. Dev Biol. 1999;212:477–90.
8. Waldo KL, Hutson MR, Stadt HA, Zdanowicz M, Zdanowicz J, Kirby ML. Cardiac neural crest is necessary for normal addition of the myocardium to the arterial pole from the secondary heart field. Dev Biol. 2005;281:66–77.
9. Restivo A, Piacentini G, Placidi S, Saffirio C, Marino B. Cardiac outflow tract: a review of some embryogenetic aspects of the conotruncal region of the heart. Anat Rec A Discov Mol Cell Evol Biol. 2006;288(9):936–43.
10. Bajolle F, Zaffran S, Kelly RG, et al. Rotation of the myocardial wall of the outflow tract is implicated in the normal positioning of the great arteries. Circ Res. 2006;98(3):421–8.
11. Hoffman JI, Kaplan S. The incidence of congenital heart disease. J Am Coll Cardiol. 2002;39:1890–900.
12. Revel MP, Faivre JB, Remy-Jardin M, Delannoy-Deken V, Duhamel A, Remy J. Pulmonary hypertension: ECG-gated 64-section CT angiographic evaluation of new functional parameters as diagnostic criteria. Radiology. 2009;250(2):558–66.
13. Kerl JM, Ravenel JG, Nguyen SA, et al. Right heart: split-bolus injection of diluted contrast medium for visualization at coronary CT angiography. Radiology. 2008;247(2):356–64, 57.
14. Saremi F, Kang J, Rahmanuddin S, Shavelle D. Assessment of post-atrial switch baffle integrity using a modified dual extremity injection cardiac computed tomography angiography technique. Int J Cardiol. 2013;162(2):e25–7.
15. Ho SY, Nihoyannopoulos P. Anatomy, echocardiography, and normal right ventricular dimensions. Heart. 2006;92 Suppl 1:i2–13.
16. Haddad F, Hunt SA, Rosenthal DN, Murphy DJ. Right ventricular function in cardiovascular disease, part I: anatomy, physiology, aging, and functional assessment of the right ventricle. Circulation. 2008;117(11):1436–48.
17. Anderson RH, Jacobs ML. The anatomy of tetralogy of Fallot with pulmonary stenosis. Cardiol Young. 2008;18 Suppl 3:12–21.
18. Bashore TM. Adult congenital heart disease: right ventricular outflow tract lesions. Circulation. 2007;115(14):1933–47.
19. Alva C, Ho SY, Lincoln CR, Rigby ML, Wright A, Anderson RH. The nature of the obstructive muscular bundles in double-chambered right ventricle. J Thorac Cardiovasc Surg. 1999;117(6):1180–9.
20. Loukas M, Klaassen Z, Tubbs RS, et al. Anatomical observations of the moderator band. Clin Anat. 2010;23(4):443–50.
21. Loukas M, Tubbs RS, Louis Jr RG, et al. An endoscopic and anatomical approach to the septal papillary muscle of the conus. Surg Radiol Anat. 2009;31(9):701–6.
22. Hansen MW, Merchant N. Images in cardiovascular medicine. Vieussens' ring: combining computed tomography coronary angiography and magnetic resonance imaging in assessing collateral pathways. Circulation. 2006;114(16):e545–6.
23. Saremi F, Goodman G, Wilcox A, Salibian R, Vorobiof G. Coronary artery ostial atresia: diagnosis of conotruncal anastomotic collateral rings using CT angiography. JACC Cardiovasc Imaging. 2011;4(12):1320–3.
24. Li J, Soukias ND, Carvalho JS, Ho SY. Coronary arterial anatomy in tetralogy of Fallot: morphological and clinical correlations. Heart. 1998;80(2): 174–83.

25. Milo S, Fiegel A, Shem-Tov A, Neufeld HN, Goor DA. Hour-glass deformity of the pulmonary valve: a third type of pulmonary valve stenosis. Br Heart J. 1988;60(2):128–33.
26. Stamm C, Anderson RH, Ho SY. Clinical anatomy of the normal pulmonary root compared with that in isolated pulmonary valvular stenosis. J Am Coll Cardiol. 1998;31(6):1420–5.
27. Berdajs D, Lajos P, Zund G, Turina M. The quadricuspid pulmonary valve. Its importance in the Ross procedure. J Thorac Cardiovasc Surg. 2003;125:198–9.
28. Warnes CA, Williams RG, Bashore TM, et al. ACC/AHA 2008 guidelines for the management of adults with congenital heart disease: a report of the American college of cardiology/American Heart Association Task Force on Practice Guidelines (writing committee to develop guidelines on the management of adults with congenital heart disease). Circulation. 2008;118:e714–833.
29. Kan JS, White Jr RI, Mitchell SE, Gardner TJ. Percutaneous balloon valvuloplasty: a new method for treating congenital pulmonary valve stenosis. N Engl J Med. 1982;307:510–4.
30. Kanter KR, Budde JM, Parks WJ, et al. One hundred pulmonary valve replacements in children after relief of right ventricular outflow tract obstruction. Ann Thorac Surg. 2002;73:1801–6.
31. Becker AE, Connor M, Anderson RH. Tetralogy of Fallot: a morphometric and geometric study. Am J Cardiol. 1975;35:402–12.
32. Howell CE, Ho SY, Anderson RH, Elliott MJ. Variations within the fibrous skeleton and ventricular outflow tracts in tetralogy of Fallot. Ann Thorac Surg. 1990;50:450–7.
33. Tan JL, Davlouros PA, McCarthy KP, Gatzoulis MA, Ho SY. Intrinsic histological abnormalities of aortic root and ascending aorta in tetralogy of Fallot: evidence of causative mechanism for aortic dilatation and aortopathy. Circulation. 2005;112:961–8.
34. Bédard E, McCarthy KP, Dimopoulos K, Giannakoulas G, Gatzoulis MA, Ho SY. Structural abnormalities of the pulmonary trunk in tetralogy of Fallot and potential clinical implications: a morphological study. J Am Coll Cardiol. 2009;54(20):1883–90.
35. Ibrahim T, Dennig K, Schwaiger M, Schomig A. Images in cardiovascular medicine: assessment of double chamber right ventricle by magnetic resonance imaging. Circulation. 2002;105:2692–3.
36. Oliver JM, Garrido A, Gonzalez A, et al. Rapid progression of midventricular obstruction in adults with double-chambered right ventricle. J Thorac Cardiovasc Surg. 2003;126:711–7.
37. Hachiro Y, Takagi N, Koyanagi T, Morikawa M, Abe T. Repair of double-chambered right ventricle: surgical results and long-term follow-up. Ann Thorac Surg. 2001;72:1520–2.
38. Tirilomis T, Friedrich M, Zenker D, Seipelt RG, Schoendube FA, Ruschewski W. Indications for reoperation late after correction of tetralogy of Fallot. Cardiol Young. 2010;20(4):396–401.
39. Shebani SO, McGuirk S, Baghai M, et al. Right ventricular outflow tract reconstruction using Contegra valved conduit: natural history and conduit performance under pressure. Eur J Cardiothorac Surg. 2006;29(3):397–405.
40. Tweddell JS, Pelech AN, Frommelt PC, et al. Factors affecting longevity of homograft valves used in right ventricular outflow tract reconstruction for congenital heart disease. Circulation. 2000;102 Suppl 3:130–5.
41. Bove T, Demanet H, Wauthy P, et al. Early results of valved bovine jugular vein conduit versus bicuspid homograft for right ventricular outflow tract reconstruction. Ann Thorac Surg. 2002;74:536–41.
42. Oosterhof T, van Straten A, Vliegen HW, et al. Preoperative thresholds for pulmonary valve replacement in patients with corrected tetralogy of Fallot using cardiovascular magnetic resonance. Circulation. 2007;116:545–51.
43. Khambadkone S, Bonhoeffer P. Nonsurgical pulmonary valve replacement: why, when, and how? Catheter Cardiovasc Interv. 2004;62:401–8.
44. Lurz P, Coats L, Khambadkone S, et al. Percutaneous pulmonary valve implantation: impact of evolving technology and learning curve on clinical outcome. Circulation. 2008;117(15):1964–72.
45. Schievano S, Coats L, Migliavacca F, et al. Variations in right ventricular outflow tract morphology following repair of congenital heart disease: implications for percutaneous pulmonary valve implantation. J Cardiovasc Magn Reson. 2007;9(4):687–95.
46. Nielsen E, Smerup M, Agger P, et al. Normal right ventricular three-dimensional architecture, as assessed with diffusion tensor magnetic resonance imaging, is preserved during experimentally induced right ventricular hypertrophy. Anat Rec (Hoboken). 2009;292(5):640–51.
47. Lev M, Bharati S, Meng CCL, Liberthson RR, Paul MH, Idriss F. A concept of double-outlet right ventricle. J Thorac Cardiovasc Surg. 1972;64:271–81.
48. Walters III HL, Mavroudis C, Tchervenkov CI, Jacobs JP, Lacour-Gayet F, Jacobs ML. Congenital heart surgery nomenclature and database project: double outlet right ventricle. Ann Thorac Surg. 2000;69(4 Suppl):S249–63.
49. Lacour-Gayet F, Maruszewski B, Mavroudis C, Jacobs JP, Elliott MJ. Presentation of the international nomenclature for congenital heart surgery. The long way from nomenclature to collection of validated data at the EACTS. Eur J Cardiothorac Surg. 2000;18:128–35.
50. Beekmana RP, Roest AA, Helbing WA, et al. Spin echo MRI in the evaluation of hearts with a double outlet right ventricle: usefulness and limitations. Magn Reson Imaging. 2000;18(3):245–53.
51. Mayo JR, Roberson D, Sommerhoff B, Higgins CB. MR imaging of double outlet right ventricle. J Comput Assist Tomogr. 1990;14(3):336–9.
52. Chen SJ, Lin MT, Liu KL, et al. Usefulness of 3D reconstructed computed tomography imaging for

double outlet right ventricle. J Formos Med Assoc. 2008;107(5):371–80.
53. Artrip JH, Sauer H, Campbell DN, et al. Biventricular repair in double outlet right ventricle: surgical results based on the STS-EACTS International Nomenclature classification. Eur J Cardiothorac Surg. 2006;29(4):545–50.
54. Barbero-Marcial M, Tanamati C, Atik E, Ebaid M. Intraventricular repair of double-outlet right ventricle with noncommitted ventricular septal defect: advantages of multiple patches. J Thorac Cardiovasc Surg. 1999;118:1056–67.
55. Hornung TS, Derrick GP, Deanfield JE, Redington AN. Transposition complexes in the adult: a changing perspective. Cardiol Clin. 2002;20:405–20.
56. Warnes CA. Transposition of the great arteries. Circulation. 2006;114:2699–709.
57. Paladini D, Volpe P, Sglavo G, et al. Transposition of the great arteries in the fetus: assessment of the spatial relationships of the arterial trunks by four-dimensional echocardiography. Ultrasound Obstet Gynecol. 2008;31(3):271–6.
58. Yasui H, Nakazawa M, Morishima M, Miyagawa-Tomita S, Momma K. Morphological observations on the pathogenetic process of transposition of the great arteries induced by retinoic acid in mice. Circulation. 1995;91(9):2478–86.
59. Mee RB. Severe right ventricular failure after Mustard or Senning operation: two-stage repair: pulmonary artery banding and switch. J Thorac Cardiovasc Surg. 1986;92(Pt 1):385–90.
60. Ebenroth ES, Hurwitz RA, Cordes TM. Late onset of pulmonary hypertension after successful Mustard surgery for d-transposition of the great arteries. Am J Cardiol. 2000;85:127–30.
61. Jatene AD, Fontes VF, Paulista PP, et al. Anatomic correction of transposition of the great vessels. J Thorac Cardiovasc Surg. 1976;72:364–70.
62. Blume E, Chung T, Hoffer FA, Geva T. Anatomically corrected malposition of the great arteries {S, D, L}. Circulation. 1998;97:1207.
63. Allwork SP, Bentall HH, Becker AE, et al. Congenitally corrected transposition of the great arteries: morphologic study of 32 cases. Am J Cardiol. 1976;38:910–23.
64. Hornung TS, Calder L. Congenitally corrected transposition of the great arteries. Heart. 2010;96:1154–61.
65. Prieto LR, Hordof AJ, Secic M, Rosenbaum MS, Gersony WM. Progressive tricuspid valve disease in patients with congenitally corrected transposition of the great arteries. Circulation. 1998;98:997–1005.
66. Van Praagh R. Truncus arteriosus: what is it really and how should it be classified? Eur J Cardiothorac Surg. 1987;1:65–70.
67. Calder L, Van Praagh R, Van Praagh S, et al. Truncus arteriosus communis: clinical, angiocardiographic, and pathologic findings in 100 patients. Am Heart J. 1976;92:23–38.
68. McGoon DC, Rastelli GC, Ongley PA. An operation for the correction of truncus arteriosus. JAMA. 1968;205:69–73.
69. Vida VL, Sanders SP, Bottio T, et al. Anomalous origin of one pulmonary artery from the ascending aorta. Cardiol Young. 2005;15:176–81.
70. Geva T, Powell AJ, Crawford EC, Chung T, Colan SD. Evaluation of regional differences in right ventricular systolic function by acoustic quantification echocardiography and cine magnetic resonance imaging. Circulation. 1998;98(4):339–45.
71. Nance Jr JW, Bastarrika G, Kang DK, et al. High-temporal resolution dual-energy computed tomography of the heart using a novel hybrid image reconstruction algorithm: initial experience. J Comput Assist Tomogr. 2011;35(1):119–25.
72. Geiger J, Markl M, Jung B, et al. 4D-MR flow analysis in patients after repair for tetralogy of Fallot. Eur Radiol. 2011;21(8):1651–7.
73. Johansson B, Babu-Narayan SV, Kilner PJ. The effects of breath-holding on pulmonary regurgitation measured by cardiovascular magnetic resonance velocity mapping. J Cardiovasc Magn Reson. 2009;11:1.
74. Sanchez-Quintana D, Anderson RH, Ho SY. Ventricular myoarchitecture in tetralogy of Fallot. Heart. 1996;76:280–6.
75. Anderson RH, Smerup M, Sanchez-Quintana D, Loukas M, Lunkenheimer PP. The three-dimensional arrangement of the myocytes in the ventricular walls. Clin Anat. 2009;22(1):64–76.
76. Lindqvist P, Henein M, Kazzam E. Right ventricular outflow-tract fractional shortening: an applicable measure of right ventricular systolic function. Eur J Echocardiogr. 2003;4(1):29–35.
77. Calcutteea A, Chung R, Lindqvist P, Hodson M, Henein MY. Differential right ventricular regional function and the effect of pulmonary hypertension: three-dimensional echo study. Heart. 2011;97(12):1004–11.
78. Denault AY, Chaput M, Couture P, Hébert Y, Haddad F, Tardif JC. Dynamic right ventricular outflow tract obstruction in cardiac surgery. J Thorac Cardiovasc Surg. 2006;132(1):43–9.
79. Geva T. Repaired tetralogy of Fallot: the roles of cardiovascular magnetic resonance in evaluating pathophysiology and for pulmonary valve replacement decision support. J Cardiovasc Magn Reson. 2011;13:9.
80. Bodhey NK, Beerbaum P, Sarikouch S, et al. Functional analysis of the components of the right ventricle in the setting of tetralogy of Fallot. Circ Cardiovasc Imaging. 2008;1(2):141–7.
81. d'Udekem Y, Ovaert C, Grandjean F, et al. Tetralogy of Fallot: transannular and right ventricular patching equally affect late functional status. Circulation. 2000;102(19 Suppl 3):III116–22.
82. Lytrivi ID, Ko HH, Srivastava S, et al. Regional differences in right ventricular systolic function as determined by cine magnetic resonance imaging after infundibulotomy. Am J Cardiol. 2004;94(7):970–3.
83. Wald RM, Redington AN, Pereira A, et al. Refining the assessment of pulmonary regurgitation in adults after tetralogy of Fallot repair: should we be

measuring regurgitant fraction or regurgitant volume? Eur Heart J. 2009;30(3):356–61.
84. Harris MA, Whitehead KK, Gillespie MJ, et al. Differential branch pulmonary artery regurgitant fraction is a function of differential pulmonary arterial anatomy and pulmonary vascular resistance. JACC Cardiovasc Imaging. 2011;4(5):506–13.
85. Babu-Narayan SV, Goktekin O, Moon JC, et al. Late gadolinium enhancement cardiovascular magnetic resonance of the systemic right ventricle in adults with previous atrial redirection surgery for transposition of the great arteries. Circulation. 2005;111:2091–8.
86. Davlouros PA, Niwa K, Webb G, Gatzoulis MA. The right ventricle in congenital heart disease. Heart. 2006;92(Suppl I):i27–38.
87. Pettersen E, Helle-Valle T, Edvardsen T, et al. Contraction pattern of the systemic right ventricle shift from longitudinal to circumferential shortening and absent global ventricular torsion. J Am Coll Cardiol. 2007;49:2450–6.
88. Graham Jr TP, Bernard YD, Mellen BG, et al. Long-term outcome in congenitally corrected transposition of the great arteries: a multi-institutional study. J Am Coll Cardiol. 2000;36:255–61.
89. Hauser M, Bengel FM, Hager A, et al. Impaired myocardial blood flow and coronary flow reserve of the anatomical right systemic ventricle in patients with congenitally corrected transposition of the great arteries. Heart. 2003;89:1231–5.
90. Wald RM, Haber I, Wald R, Valente AM, Powell AJ, Geva T. Effects of regional dysfunction and late gadolinium enhancement on global right ventricular function and exercise capacity in patients with repaired tetralogy of Fallot. Circulation. 2009;119(10):1370–7.
91. Tandri H, Saranathan M, Rodriguez ER, et al. Noninvasive detection of myocardial fibrosis in arrhythmogenic right ventricular cardiomyopathy using delayed-enhancement magnetic resonance imaging. J Am Coll Cardiol. 2005;45(1):98–103.
92. Boukens BJ, Christoffels VM, Coronel R, Moorman AF. Developmental basis for electrophysiological heterogeneity in the ventricular and outflow tract myocardium as a substrate for life-threatening ventricular arrhythmias. Circ Res. 2009;104(1):19–31.
93. Harrison DA, Harris L, Siu SC, et al. Sustained ventricular tachycardia in adult patients late after repair of tetralogy of Fallot. J Am Coll Cardiol. 1997;30(5):1368–73.
94. Globits S, Kreiner G, Frank H, et al. Significance of morphological abnormalities detected by MRI in patients undergoing successful ablation of right ventricular outflow tract tachycardia. Circulation. 1997;96(8):2633–40.
95. White RD, Trohman RG, Flamm SD, et al. Right ventricular arrhythmia in the absence of arrhythmogenic dysplasia: MR imaging of myocardial abnormalities. Radiology. 1998;207(3):743–51.
96. Miljoen H, State S, de Chillou C, et al. Electroanatomic mapping characteristics of ventricular tachycardia in patients with arrhythmogenic right ventricular cardiomyopathy/dysplasia. Europace. 2005;7(6):516–24.
97. Vaseghi M, Cesario DA, Mahajan A, et al. Catheter ablation of right ventricular outflow tract tachycardia: value of defining coronary anatomy. J Cardiovasc Electrophysiol. 2006;17(6):632–7.
98. Burke AP, Farb A, Tashko G, Virmani R. Arrhythmogenic right ventricular cardiomyopathy and fatty replacement of the right ventricular myocardium: are they different diseases? Circulation. 1998;97:1571–80.
99. Tansey DK, Aly Z, Sheppard MN. Fat in the right ventricle of the normal heart. Histopathology. 2005;46:98–104.
100. Raney AR, Saremi F, Kenchaiah S, et al. Multidetector computed tomography shows intramyocardial fat deposition. J Cardiovasc Comput Tomogr. 2008;2(3):152–63.
101. Tardif JC, Taylor K, Pandian NG, Schwartz S, Rastegar H. Right ventricular outflow tract and pulmonary artery obstruction by postoperative mediastinal hematoma: delineation by multiplane transesophageal echocardiography. J Am Soc Echocardiogr. 1994;7:400–4.
102. Stierle U, Sheikhzadeh A, Shakibi JG, Langbehn AF, Diederich KW. Right ventricular obstruction in various types of hypertrophic cardiomyopathy. Jpn Heart J. 1987;28:115–25.
103. Sirin BH, Kurdal AT, Iskesen I, Cerrahoglu M. Right ventricular outflow obstruction of the patient with biventricular non-compaction. Thorac Cardiovasc Surg. 2010;58(6):364–6.
104. Ross D. Pulmonary valve autotransplantation (the Ross operation). J Card Surg. 1988;3(Suppl):313–9.
105. Hraska V, Krajci M, Haun C, et al. Ross and Ross-Konno procedure in children and adolescents: mid-term results. Eur J Cardiothorac Surg. 2004;25(5):742–7.
106. Bjork VO, Olin CL, Bjarke BB, Thoren CA. Right atrial right ventricular anastomosis for correction of tricuspid atresia. J Thorac Cardiovasc Surg. 1979;77(3):452–8

Left Ventricular Outflow Tract

8

Stefan Buchner and Kurt Debl

Left ventricular outflow tract obstructions (LVOTO) encompass a series of stenotic lesions starting in the left ventricular outflow tract (LVOT), including the aortic valve and extending to the ascending aorta. Depending on definition, also intraventricular obstruction and hypoplastic left heart syndrome are included in the types of LVOTO.

Left ventricular outflow tract obstructions can occur at several levels (Fig. 8.1):

- Valvular LVOTO in the adult patient with congenital heart disease is usually due to bicuspid aortic valve. It usually occurs isolated but can be associated with other abnormalities, the most common being coarctation of the aorta, persistent ductus arteriosus, or aneurysm of the ascending aorta.
- Subvalvular LVOTO is usually either a discrete fibromuscular ridge which partially or completely encircles the LVOT or a long fibromuscular narrowing beneath the base of the aortic valve.
- Supravalvular LVOTO may occur rarely in isolation as an hourglass deformity. It is more often diffuse, however, involving the major arteries to varying degrees and begins at the superior margin of the sinuses of Valsalva.

S. Buchner, MD (✉) • K. Debl, MD
Klinik und Poliklinik für Innere Medizin II,
Universitätsklinikum Regensburg,
Franz-Josef-Strauss-Allee 11,
93053 Regensburg, Germany
e-mail: stefan.buchner@klinik.uni-regensburg.de;
kurt.debl@klinik.uni-regensburg.de

Embryology

Valvulogenesis is a complex process during embryonic development whereby a fragile gelatinous matrix is remodeled into thin fibrous leaflets capable of maintaining unidirectional flow over a lifetime. Defective valvulogenesis can result in impaired cardiac function and lifelong complications [1]. A variety of signaling pathways, transcription factors, and genes are involved during valvulogenesis. In the recent years, a large number of genes that play important roles in heart development have been identified [2].

In the outflow tract, mesenchymal cells originating from migrating cardiac neural crest cells will reach the outflow tract cushions and together with endocardially derived mesenchymal cells will contribute to the formation of the aortic and pulmonary valves. Growth factors signal the process of endocardium-to-mesenchyme transformation (EMT) resulting in formation of prevalvular cushions. EMT is followed by a remodeling process whereby mesenchyme differentiates into collagen secreting interstitial valve fibroblasts. This complex process leads to leaflet compaction, attenuation, and formation of fibrous continuities that are indicative of the mature valve tissue (Fig. 8.2). Subtle perturbations in endocardial cushion development can lead to heart valve diseases, including bicuspid aortic valve (BAV) [1, 3].

The morphology of the BAV usually includes leaflets of unequal size as the result of the fusion of two cusps. The larger leaflet is characterized by a raphe, which is a thin ridge of tissue that represents

F. Saremi (ed.), *Cardiac CT and MR for Adult Congenital Heart Disease*,
DOI 10.1007/978-1-4614-8875-0_8, © Springer Science+Business Media New York 2014

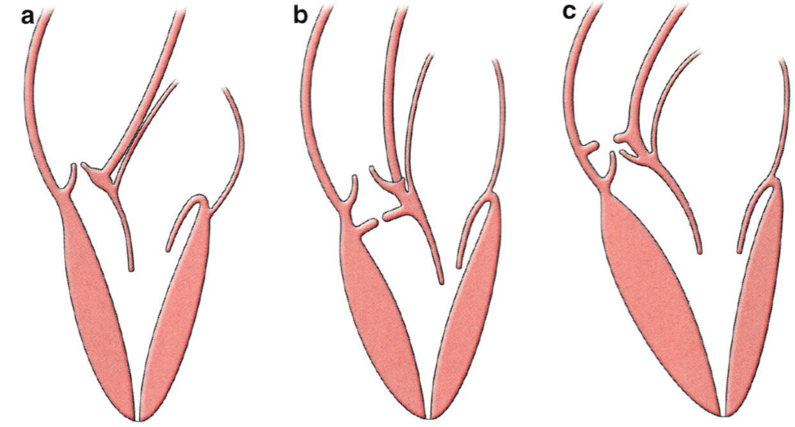

Fig. 8.1 Types of congenital left ventricular outflow tract obstruction. (**a**) Valvular aortic stenosis. (**b**) Subvalvular aortic stenosis. (**c**) Supravalvular aortic stenosis

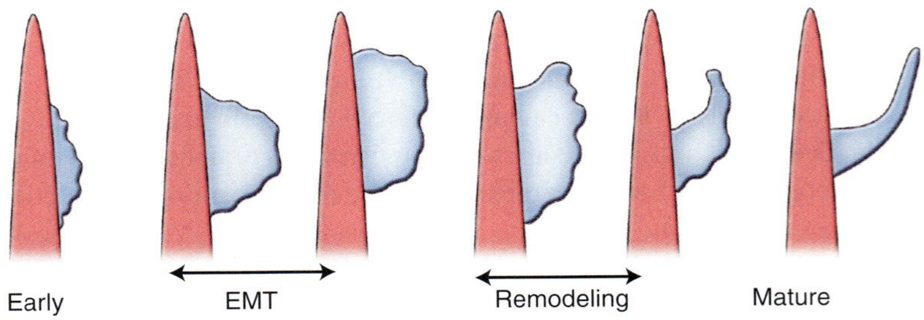

Fig. 8.2 Schematic illustration of valvular morphogenesis. Endothelial-to-mesenchymal transition (*EMT*) is followed by a remodeling process whereby mesenchyme differentiates to fibroblasts. This process leads to leaflet compaction and mature valve tissue

the location where the two cusps fused during valve development. The most frequent BAV subtypes are those with fusion of the right and left (RL) coronary leaflet and those with fusion of the right and noncoronary (RN) leaflet. Insight into the etiology of the RN and RL BAVs was further gained from studies of Nos3 null mice as well as the inbred Syrian hamsters strain which selectively display RN and RL subtypes, respectively. These studies suggested that the BAV-RN is caused by defective formation of the outflow tract cushion, whereas the BAV-RL is likely the result of defective outflow tract septation [4, 5]. Thus, the two BAV subtypes appear to have distinct etiologies.

Imaging Techniques

Cardiac MRI and CT provide highly reproducible and accurate assessments of the structure and function of the left ventricle and valves. They can be used for accurate depiction of complex cardiovascular anatomic and functional features both before and after surgery. The comprehensive evaluation of the LVOT and aortic valve has been expanded. Especially, CT and MRI can be used for accurate morphologic characterization of the aortic valve. MRI can visualize the cardiac structure and function without contrast medium, whereas for CT contrast medium by bolus injection of an iodinated contrast is necessary for adequate analysis of cardiac anatomy.

MRI typically involves ECG gating and breath-hold acquisitions. SSFP (steady-state free precession) sequences allow best functional and anatomic analysis of the cardiac structures and the aortic root. Functional analysis of the left ventricle is usually performed by semiquantitative tracing of myocardial borders by modified Simpson's rule or newer 4D analysis. SSFP sequences are applied in short-axis, long-axis, and orthogonally angulated views to allow morphologic evaluation of the valve and the LVOT. If information about the velocity of flow across the aortic valve/LVOT is specifically requested, velocity-encoded phase-contrast cine images are acquired perpendicular to aortic blood flow. Comprehensive 4D velocity MRI for visualization and quantification of cardiovascular hemodynamics has been recently developed to understand these pathologies. A delayed contrast-enhanced technique (gadolinium) MRI is usually used to visualize the extent of myocardial fibrosis, especially in left ventricular hypertrophy.

CT with a single breath-hold acquisition allows perfect anatomic images of the whole heart including the LVOT, aortic valve, and aortic root. With advances in CT scanners and software, high-quality 2D reformatted and 3D reconstructed images can be generated to understand the complex cardiovascular anatomy. These scanners generate isotropic data sets with voxels measuring less than 1 mm in the *x*-, *y*-, and *z*-planes. A combination of 2D multiplanar and 3D maximum-intensity-projection and volume-rendered images is most commonly used. Two-dimensional multiplanar reformations can be generated in any plane with resolution comparable with that of axial images. Three-dimensional maximum-intensity-projection and volume-rendered images can be used to display a portion of defined cardiac structures which provides high spatial resolution in all 3 dimensions and thus excellent visualization of the LVOT, aortic valve, and aortic root. Functional analysis with CT is also possible, but this is addressed by increased radiation expose.

Anatomy of the LVOT

CT and MRI provide a clear definition of the LVOT (Figs. 8.3 and 8.4). The LVOT is the region of the left ventricle that lies between the anterior cusp of the mitral valve and the ventricular septum. In the anterior wall are both the muscular

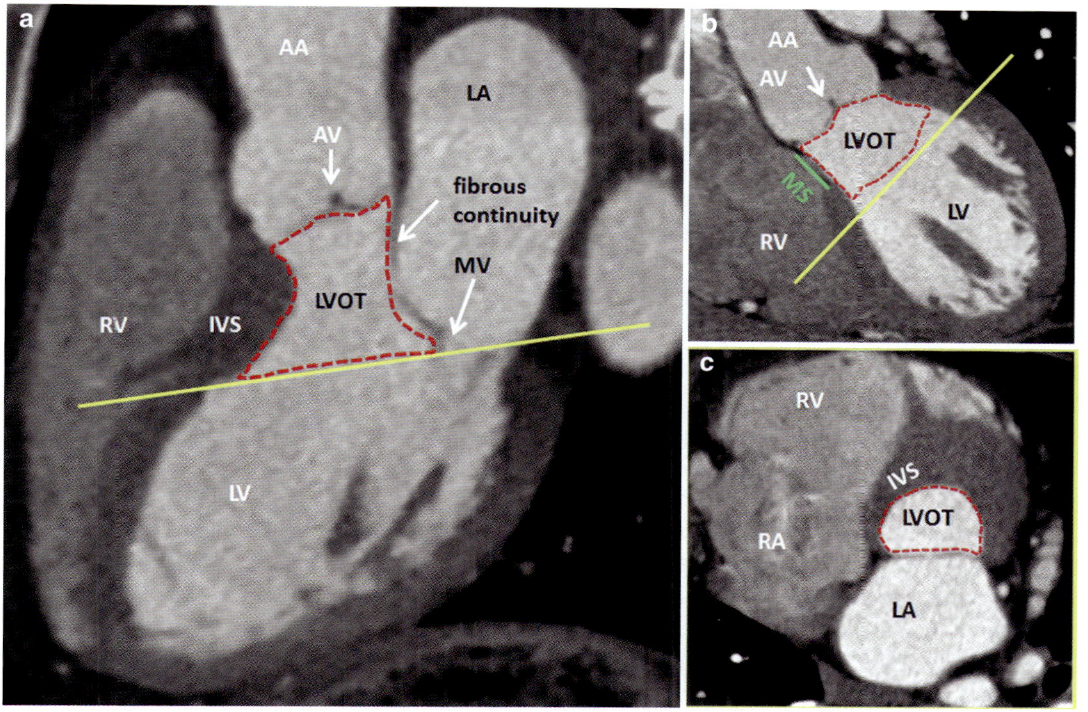

Fig. 8.3 CT of the LVOT and its neighbor structures. (**a**, **b**) Long-axis views. (**c**) Cross-sectional orthogonal view of the basal LVOT (corresponding *yellow lines*) showing the elliptical shape of the bottom of LVOT. *AA* ascending aorta, *AV* aortic valve, *IVS* interventricular septum, *LA* left atrium, *LV* left ventricle, *LVOT* left ventricle outflow tract, *MV* mitral valve, *RA* right atrium, *RV* right ventricle, *MS* membranous septum (*green line*), *Dotted red line* delimits LVOT

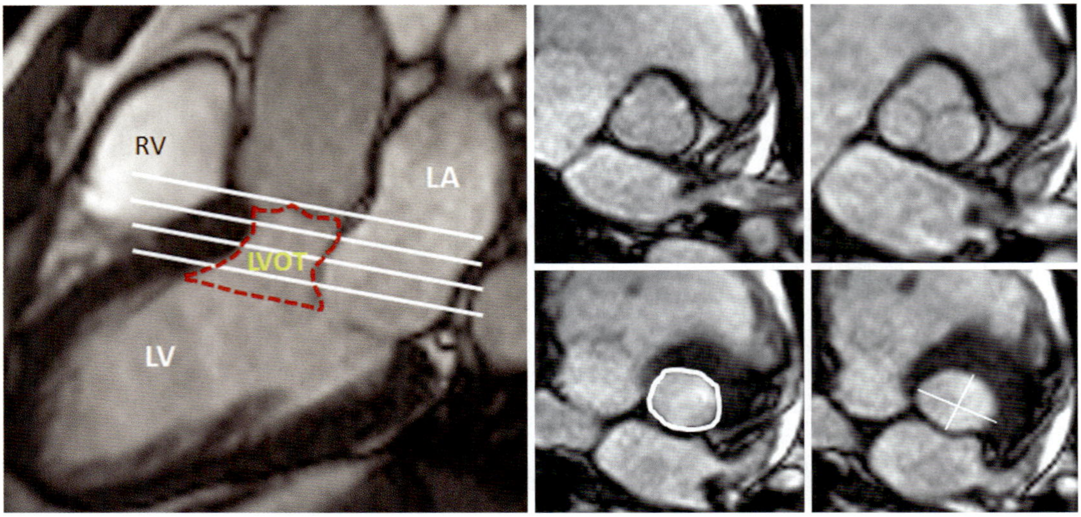

Fig. 8.4 Short-axis MRI of the LVOT at different levels. *LA* left atrium, *LV* left ventricle, *LVOT* left ventricle outflow tract, *RV* right ventricle, *Red dotted line* delimits the LVOT at different levels (*white lines*), LVOT circumference and diameters are shown in white

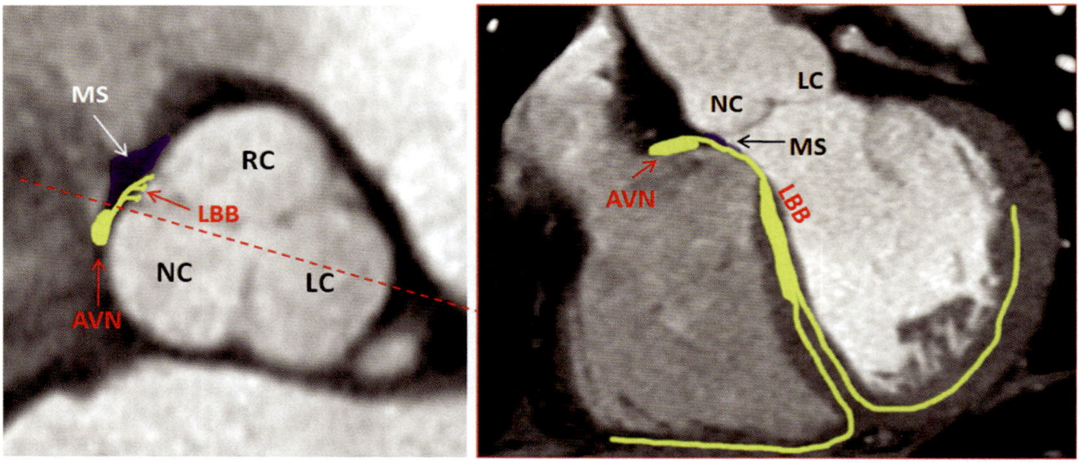

Fig. 8.5 Anatomic landmarks of the cardiac conduction system by CT. *AVN* atrioventricular node, *LBB* left bundle branch, *LC* left cusp, *MS* membranous septum, *NC* noncoronary cusp, *RC* right cusp *dotted red line* in axial view shows the level of coronal plane

and membranous parts of the ventricular septum. The atrioventricular bundle lies at the junction of the muscular and membranous parts of the septum (Fig. 8.5). The posterior wall of the outflow tract is formed not only by the anterior mitral cusp but also by the intervalvular septum and, in its upper part, by a curtain formed by the fusion of the anterior and posterior mitral cusps. The roof of the LVOT is formed by the aortic valve. The LVOT area is not exclusively circular but often assumes a more ellipsoid-like shape. Dynamic changes of the LVOT area during systole are detectable in normal individuals. LVOT is more circular during systole, but the AP diameter remains smaller than the transverse diameter throughout the cardiac cycle. The oval shape of the LVOT has important implications when LVOT area is calculated from LVOT diameters.

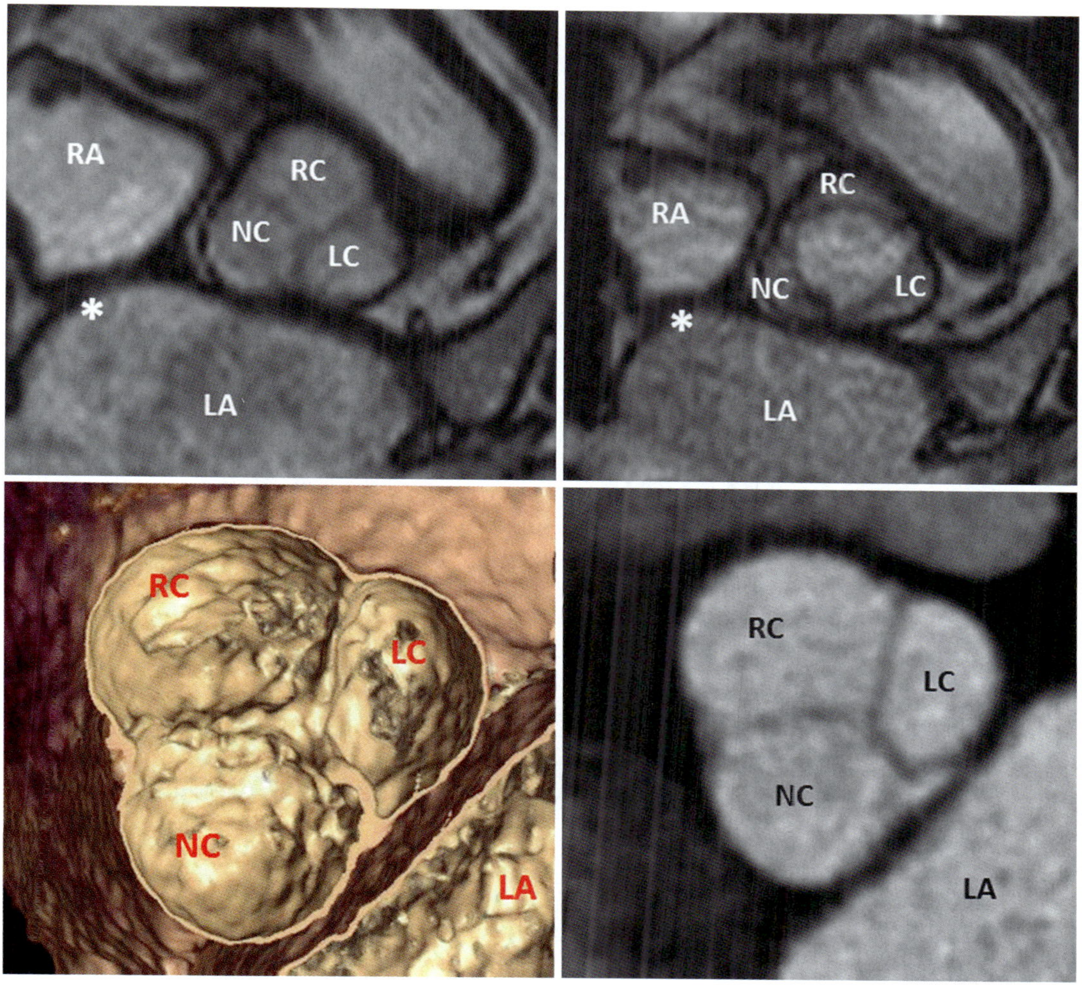

Fig. 8.6 MRI of a tricuspid aortic valve with three cusps during diastole (*left*) and systole (*right*). Interatrial septum (*). Image reconstruction to obtain a cross-sectional multidetector CT image at the level of the aortic leaflet tips. *LA* left atrium, *LAA* left atrial appendage, *LC* left cusp, *NC* noncoronary cusp, *RA* right atrium, *RC* right cusp

Aortic Valve

The normal aortic valve is a trileaflet valve with the left and right cusps giving rise to the left and right coronary arteries, respectively (Fig. 8.6). The noncoronary cusp is in fibrous continuity with the anterior leaflet of the mitral valve. The aortic valve has a semilunar attachment to the junction of the left ventricular outlet and the aortic root. The cusps have a main core of fibrous tissue with endocardial linings on each surface. The cusps are thickened at the midpoint to form a nodule. The area of the aortic orifice in a normal adult is 3.0–4.0 cm^2. The imaging plane of the aortic valve to identify the cusps is defined by obtaining long-axis views of the LVOT and the proximal aorta (3-chamber and 2-chamber views). The valvular plane is then obtained by orthogonal views perpendicular to the annulus (Fig. 8.7).

Anatomy of the Ascending Aorta and Aortic Root

CT and MRI allow a detailed understanding of the complex three-dimensional aortic root

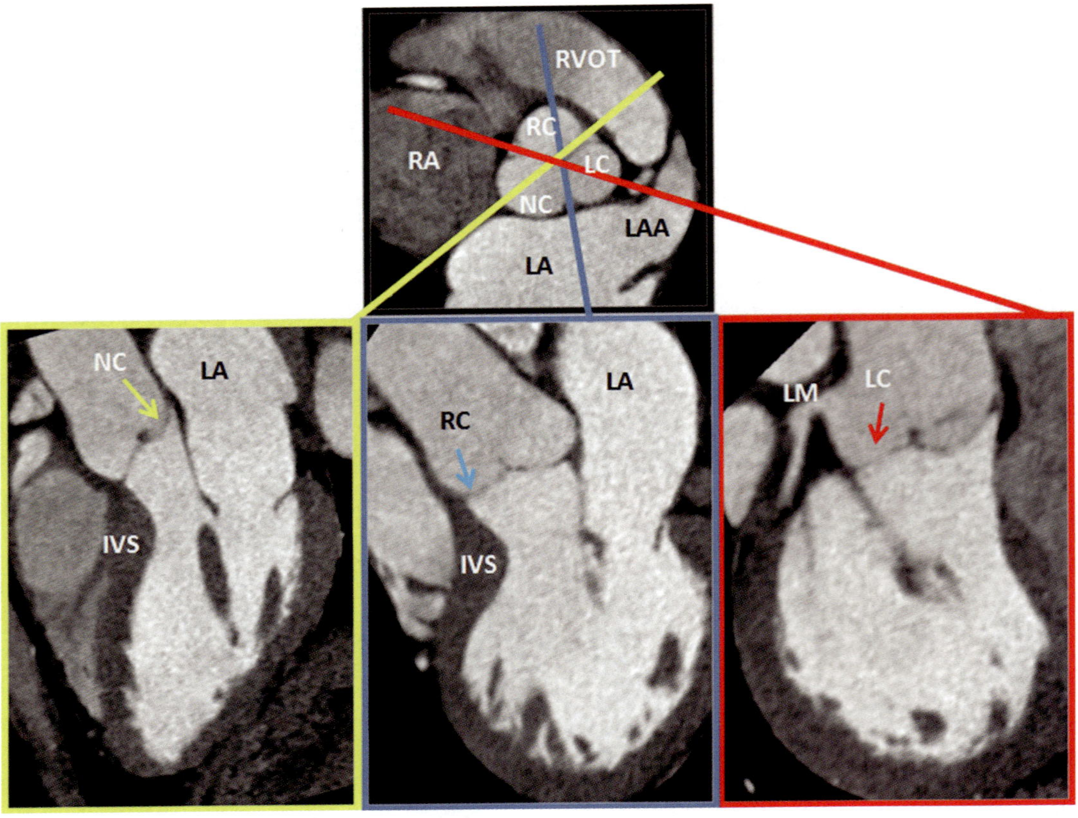

Fig. 8.7 Plane selection by CT. From a short-axis image, imaging planes were planned through each of the three cusps of the aortic valve. *Left* (LC, *red*), *right* (RC, *blue*), and noncoronary (NC, *yellow*) cusps. *IVS* interventricular septum, *LA* left atrium, *LC* left cusp, *LM* left main artery, *NC* noncoronary cusp, *RA* right atrium, *RC* right cusp, *LAA* left atrial appendage, *RVOT* right ventricle outflow tract

anatomy, including the crown-shaped anatomic aortic annulus, the virtual basal ring, the sinuses of Valsalva, the valve leaflets, and the sinotubular junction (Figs. 8.8 and 8.9). The ascending aorta consists of the aortic root and the tubular segment [6]. The border between the two is called the sinotubular junction. The aortic root, representing the outflow tract from the left ventricle, provides the supporting structures for the leaflets of the aortic valve and forms the bridge between the left ventricle and the ascending aorta. The top end of LVOT, the aortic annulus, the commissures, the sinuses of Valsalva, the coronary ostia, and the sinotubular junction are the framework in which the valve leaflets are hanging. The annulus is an oval-shaped, 3-pronged coronet with 3 anchor points at the nadir of each aortic cusp [7]. The attachment of the aortic cusps is semilunar, extending throughout the aortic root from the LV distally to the sinotubular junction. The anatomic boundary between the left ventricle and the aorta, however, is found at the point where the ventricular structures change to the fibroelastic wall of the arterial trunk. This locus is not coincident with the basal attachment of the leaflets of the aortic valve.

The root is much wider at the midpoint of the sinuses than at either the sinotubular junction or the basal attachment of the leaflets [8]. This becomes of significance when considering measurements of the annulus because the hinges of the leaflets extend through all these three levels. The appropriate measuring points are at the bottom of the basal valvular attachments, at the widest point of the sinuses, and at the sinotubular

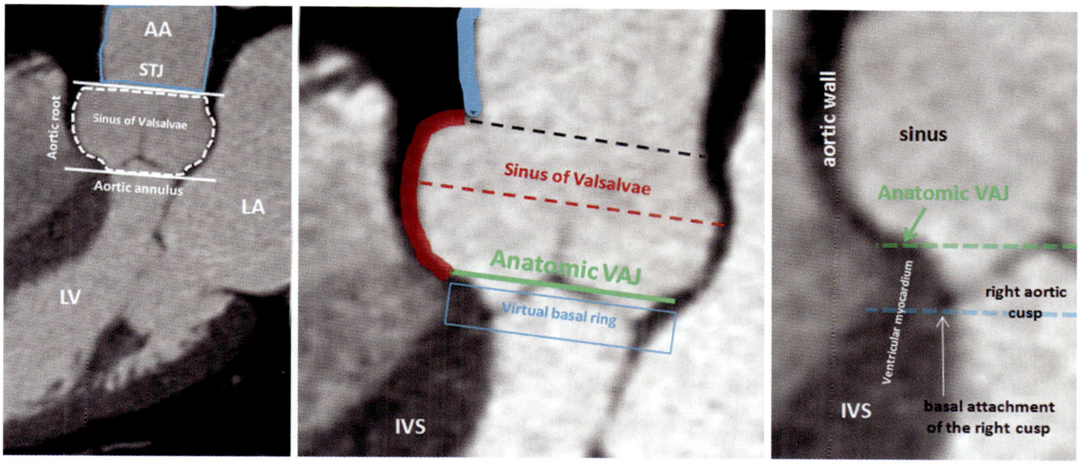

Fig. 8.8 CT of the ascending aorta and the aortic root with its anatomic landmarks of sinotubular junction (*STJ*) and aortic annulus (*delimited by white lines*). The aortic root can further be divided in subsegments: the aortic valve, the sinus of Valsalva, (*dotted red line*) the anatomic ventriculo-aortic junction (*VAJ*), and the virtual basal ring (*blue line*). The virtual basal ring represents the level of the basal insertions of the aortic cusps at the left ventricle. The aortic cusps extend from sinusal level through the anatomic VAJ to the virtual basal ring. As shown, the bottom of the cusps sags through the anatomic VAJ. The entire circumference of the AJ and the basal attachment of the aortic cusps can be accurately identified using CT. The *green line* shows the level of the VAJ with the transformation of the arterial wall into the ventricular wall. The *black line* shows the STJ. *AA* ascending aorta, *IVS* interventricular septum, *LA* left atrium, *LV* left ventricle

junction. Beyond diameter measurements, the perimeter appears especially useful for definition of the exact size in multiplanar CT or MRI. An exact visualization of the aortic root and ascending aorta is important as diseases of these structures are commonly related to bicuspid aortic valve disease and in an interventional and surgical context.

Left Ventricular Systolic Function

Cardiac volumes and ejection fraction have important prognostic and therapeutic implications in cardiology. Systolic left ventricular ejection fraction is a strong predictor for prognosis in valvular heart disease [9]. Left ventricular end-diastolic volume and end-systolic volume measurement by section summation of contiguous MRI short-axis images is the reference standard for left ventricular function. Cine images in short-axis and two long-axis orientations are used for left ventricular function analysis by guide-point modeling ventricular function analysis (Fig. 8.10).

Left Ventricular Mass

LVOTO results in concentric hypertrophy which is characterized by a reduced end-diastolic radius-to-wall thickness ratio or volume-to-mass ratio (Fig. 8.11). The left ventricular response to LVOTO is complex. It consists of a combination of wall thickening and a change in cavity size with associated effects on systolic and diastolic function. Concentric hypertrophy is defined by a combination of left ventricular hypertrophy and increased relative wall thickness. Patients with LVOTO had wide variation in left ventricular geometry and function [10]. Left ventricular hypertrophy is associated with myofibrillar hypertrophy, but also fibrosis, which is the deposition of collagen and fibronectin. Focal scarring can be observed in severe left ventricular hypertrophy caused by aortic stenosis and correlates with the severity of left ventricular remodeling [11] (Fig. 8.11). The amount of myocardial fibrosis by delayed contrast enhancement is associated with the degree of left ventricular functional improvement and all-cause mortality late after aortic valve replacement in patients with severe aortic valve disease [12].

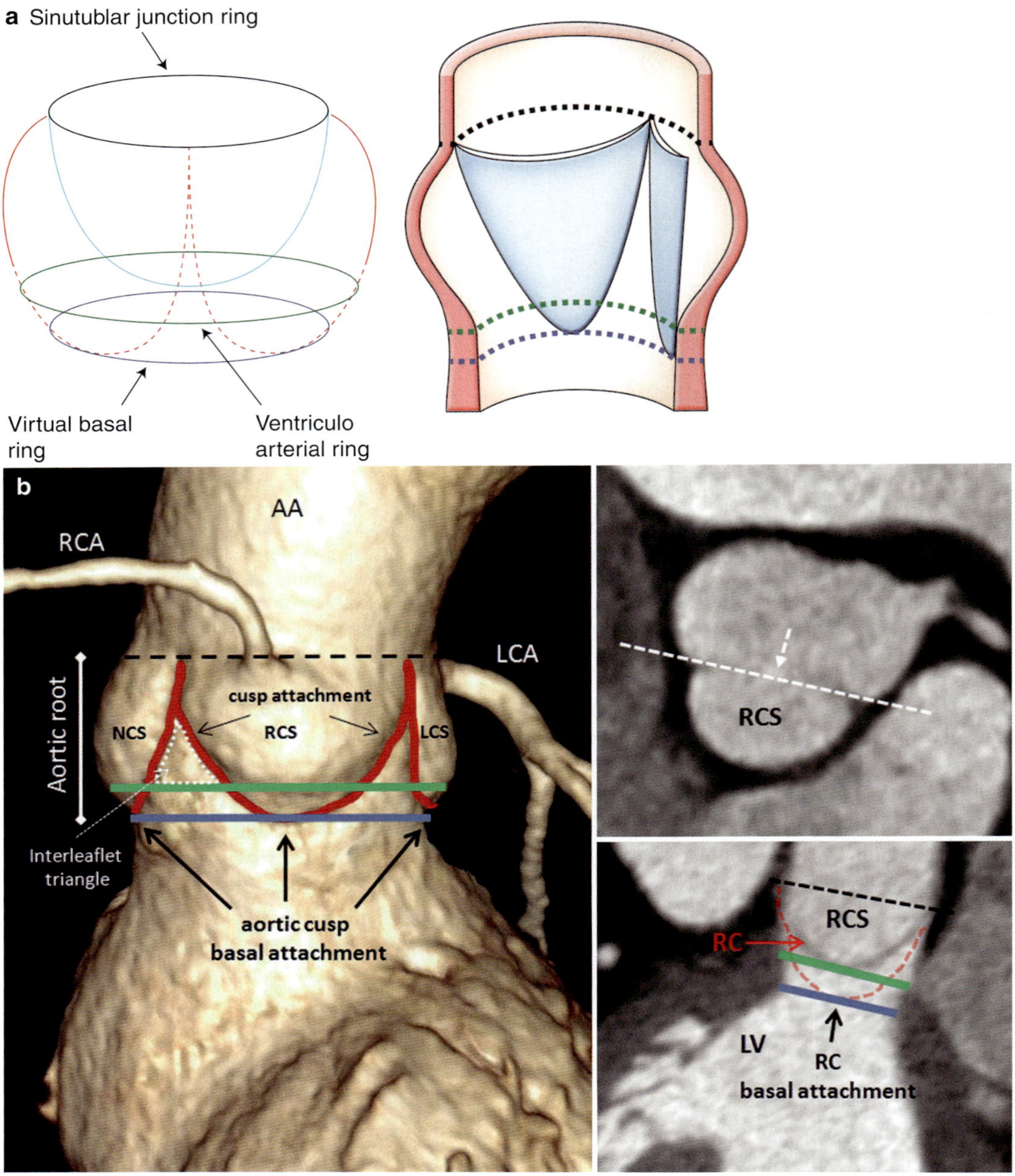

Fig. 8.9 Schematic representation (**a**) and contrast volume-rendering CT (**b**) of the aortic root with its anatomic landmarks. The virtual ring represents the lowest points of attachment of the aortic leaflets into the LV. The semilunar valves extend from the sinotubular junction (*STJ*) (*black line*) across the anatomic ventriculoarterial junction (*VAJ*) (*green line*) to the virtual basal ring (*blue line*). This creates a triangle of artery as part of the ventricle between each leaflet (*dotted white line*). The curved reconstructed CT images show the right coronary sinus (*RCS*) and sinus in relation to the anatomic VAJ and the virtual basal ring. The two top attachments of the right coronary cusp (*RC*) are shown, and an angulated view (*dotted white line*) is reconstructed. This view shows the basal attachment of the right coronary cusp. *AA* ascending aorta, *LA* left atrium, *LCA* left coronary artery, *LCS* left coronary sinus, *LV* left ventricle, *NCS* noncoronary sinus, *RCA* right coronary artery (A adapted from Anderson [8] with permission)

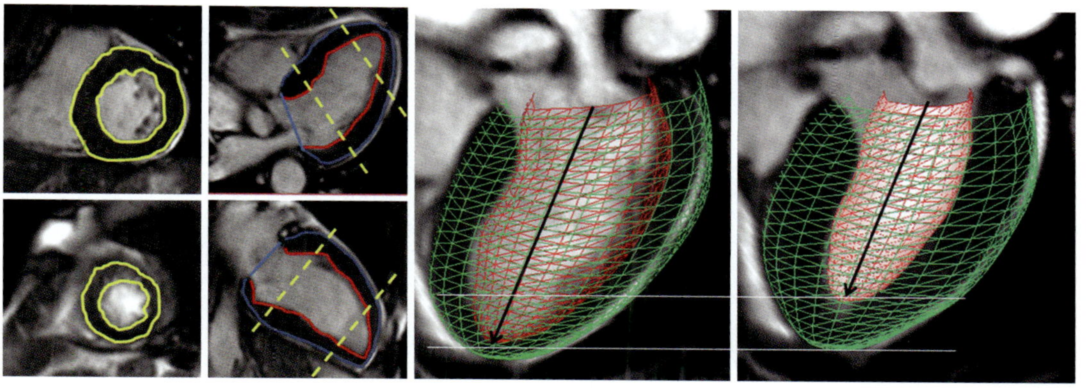

Fig. 8.10 Endocardial and epicardial contours are drawn in short-axis and long-axis views. The contours are drawn in end-diastole and end-systole to calculate left ventricle volumes and ejection fraction. The heart model clearly shows the short-axis contraction compared to the long-axis contraction of the left ventricle

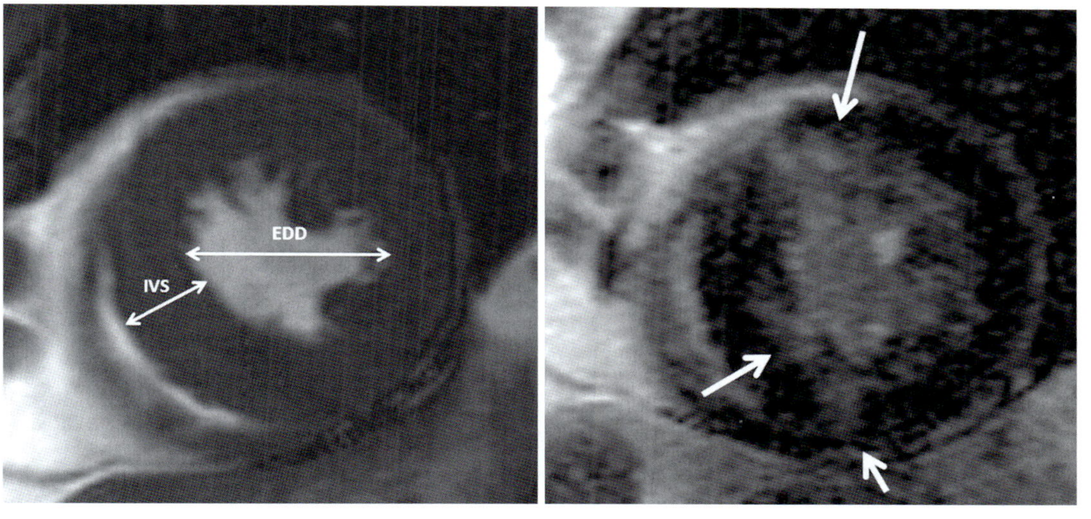

Fig. 8.11 Left ventricular hypertrophy and fibrosis. Short-axis cine and delayed contrast-enhanced cardiovascular MR image show concentric left ventricular hypertrophy and patchy areas of delayed hyperenhancement (*arrows*), corresponding to myocardial fibrosis. The concentric hypertrophy is characterized by a reduced end-diastolic radius-to-wall thickness ratio (EDD/IVS). *EDD* end-diastolic diameter, *IVS* interventricular septum

Valvular LVOTO: Aortic Valve Stenosis

The normal aortic valve is trileaflet. Congenital forms of valve disease are either unicuspid, bicuspid, or quadricuspid. Bicuspid aortic valve is the most common congenital cardiac anomaly occurring in 1–2 % of the population with a male predominance (4:1) [13] (Fig. 8.12). Mutations in the NOTCH-I gene have been related to bicuspid aortic valve. Valve dysfunction in BAV is characterized by an earlier onset and a higher rate of progression in comparison to patients with tricuspid aortic valve disease [14]. Further, BAV has a predisposition to infective endocarditis [15]. Aortic stenosis is the most common complication of patients with BAV [16]. Twenty percent of patients with bicuspid aortic valve have an associated cardiovascular abnormality, such as patent ductus arteriosus or aortic coarctation. Aortic stenosis does not become hemodynamically significant unless the valve area is reduced to approximately 1.0 cm^2.

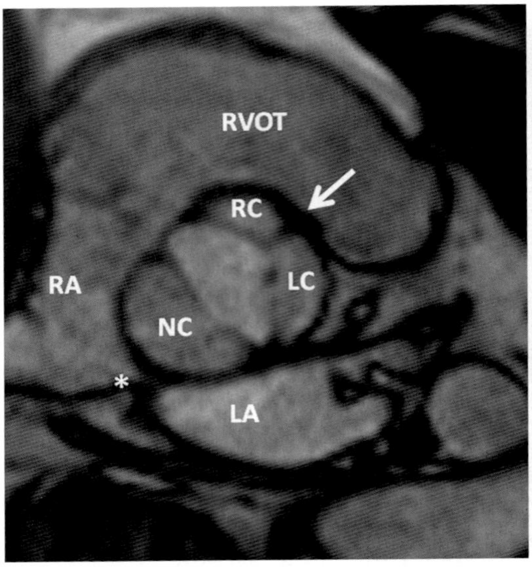

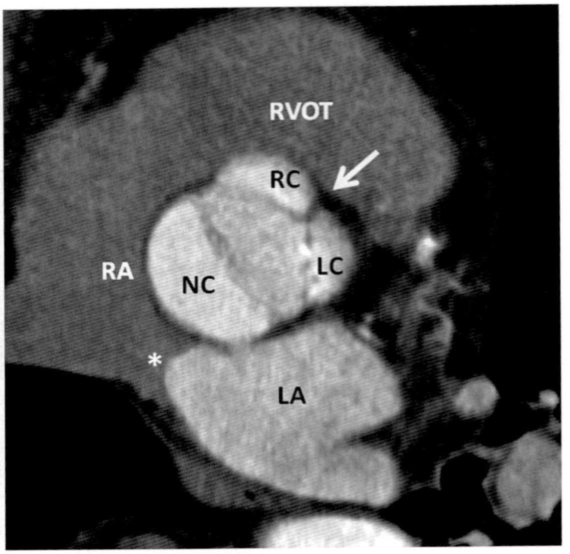

Fig. 8.12 Normal bicuspid aortic valve. MRI and CT of a patient with a bicuspid aortic valve which has three cusps and one raphe (Sievers Type 1 – RL). The fusion of the cusps is between the right (*RC*) and left coronary cusps (*LC*) representing a typical thickened raphe (*white arrow*). The orientation of the atrial septum allows the assignment of the noncoronary cusp. Thus, the noncoronary cusp is always close to the atrial septum. The orifice area is 1.4 cm^2 in MRI and 1.5 cm^2 in CT, respectively. Interatrial septum (*). *LA* left atrium, *LC* left cusp, *NC* noncoronary cusp, *RA* right atrium, *RC* right cusp, *RVOT* right ventricle outflow tract

Anatomy and Classification of Bicuspid Valve

Bicuspid aortic valve stands for a common congenital aortic valve malformation with heterogeneous morphologic phenotypes (Fig. 8.13). In general, a purely bicuspid aortic valve has only two cusps and has a characteristic fish-mouth appearance on short-axis images. Histopathological findings, however, show additional phenotypes of the bicuspid aortic valve regarding to the number of raphes, spatial position of cusps or raphes, and the functional status of the valve [16]. Thus, over the past years, different bicuspid aortic valve classifications were described. These classifications, however, are not uniform and easily applicable. Recently, a systematic classification of BAV with respect to the numbers and spatial position of the cusps and raphes, as well as the functional status, was found reliable and appropriate for a classification system from a surgical point of view (Table 8.1) (Fig. 8.14) [17]. By applying Sievers' classification system, MRI and CT allow excellent characterization of valve phenotype in patients with bicuspid aortic valve for improved management of this entity (Figs. 8.15, 8.16, and 8.17) [18–21].

Calcium Score

The method of the calcium scoring of the coronary arteries is well established as the imaging-based tool to assess cardiovascular risk. A few studies used the method of calcium scoring for assessment of the calcium content in the evaluation of the aortic valve disease [22–25] and demonstrated a good correlation between transaortic gradients on echocardiography and valvular calcium. Between bicuspid and tricuspid aortic valves, the calcium score is equal. Histoarchitectural distribution of calcific deposits is different between bicuspid and tricuspid stenotic aortic valves which can be visualized by CT (Fig. 8.18). Thus, BAV has more diffuse distribution than the more superimposed nodular form of the tricuspid stenotic valve [26]. Further, midline calcifications on raphes were quite commonly observed in BAVs [27].

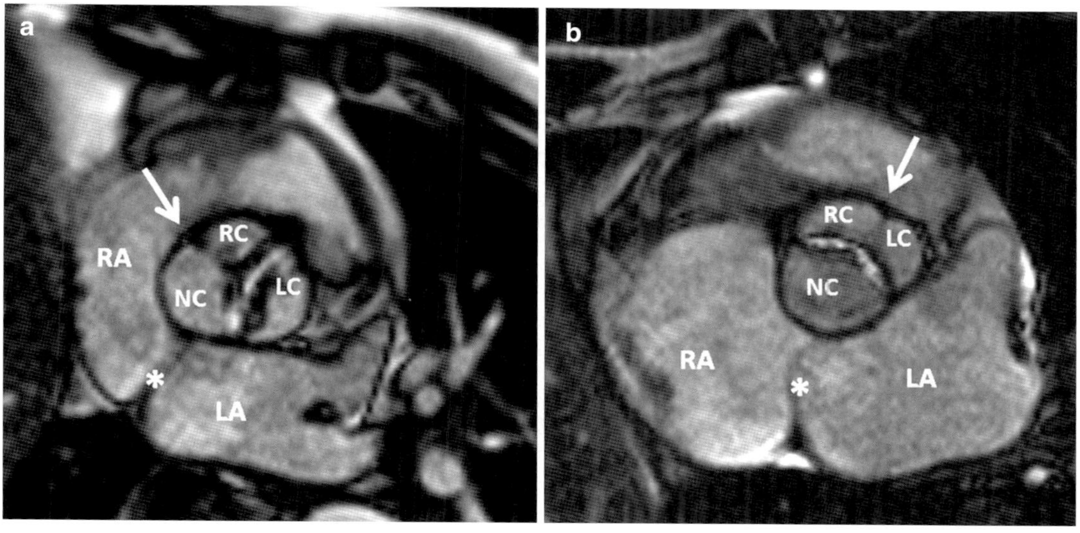

Fig. 8.13 Bicuspid aortic valve. MRI of a stenotic bicuspid aortic valve. (**a**) Fusion of the right and noncoronary cusps (Sievers Type 1 – RN) and (**b**) fusion of the right and left coronary cusps (Sievers Type 1 – RL). *White arrows* indicate the raphe. Note the noncoronary cusp is close to the left atrial septum (*). *LA* left atrium, *LC* left cusp, *NC* noncoronary cusp, *RA* right atrium, *RC* right cusp

Table 8.1 Distribution of BAV phenotype according to Sievers' BAV nomenclature system

			Main category					
	n	Modality	Type 0 (0 raphe)		Type 1 (1 raphe)			Type 2 (2 raphes)
Sievers et al. [17]	304	intraoperative	21 (7 %)		269 (88 %)			14 (5 %)
Buchner, Debl et al. [18, 20]	117	MRI	15 (13 %)		90 (77 %)			12 (10 %)
Kari et al. [21]	127	intraoperative/ CT	28 (22 %)		97 (76 %)			2 (2 %)
			Subcategory					
			Lateral	Anterior/ posterior	RL	RN	LN	RL/RN/LN
			13 (4 %)	7 (2 %)	216 (71 %)	45 (15 %)	3 (1 %)	14 (5 %)
			11 (11 %)	4 (4 %)	76 (72 %)	14 (13 %)	0 (0 %)	12 (10 %)
			18 (14 %)	10 (7 %)	84 (66 %)	11 (9 %)	2 (2 %)	2 (2 %)

Main category is defined by the number of raphes. Subcategory is defined by the orientation of the cusps in Type 0 and the position of the raphes in Types 1 and 2.
Abbreviations: *n* number, *RL* right-left, *RN* right noncoronary, *LN* left noncoronary.

Definition and Quantification of Aortic Stenosis

The main features of the clinical assessment and decision making are symptoms, the grade of stenosis, and LV geometry and function. Additionally, the size of the ascending aorta is important in the management of patients with BAV. Accurate determination of the severity of aortic stenosis is important for timely and appropriate surgical interventions. In addition to the calculation of the effective orifice area using the continuity equation by transthoracic Doppler echocardiography, anatomic determination of aortic valve area can be

Fig. 8.14 Definition of bicuspid aortic valve (*BAV*) phenotypes (MRI and CT imaging view) according to Sievers (modified). *Sievers Type 0*: BAV without raphe, the orientation of the free edge of the cusps defined either lateral (BAV-LA) or anterior-posterior (BAV-AP). *Sievers Type 1*: BAV with 1 raphe, BAV-RL (fusion of the right and left coronary cusps), BAV-RN (fusion of the right and noncoronary cusps), and BAV-LN (fusion of the left and noncoronary cups). *Sievers Type 2*: BAV with 2 raphes. *L* left, *R* right, and *N* noncoronary sinuses

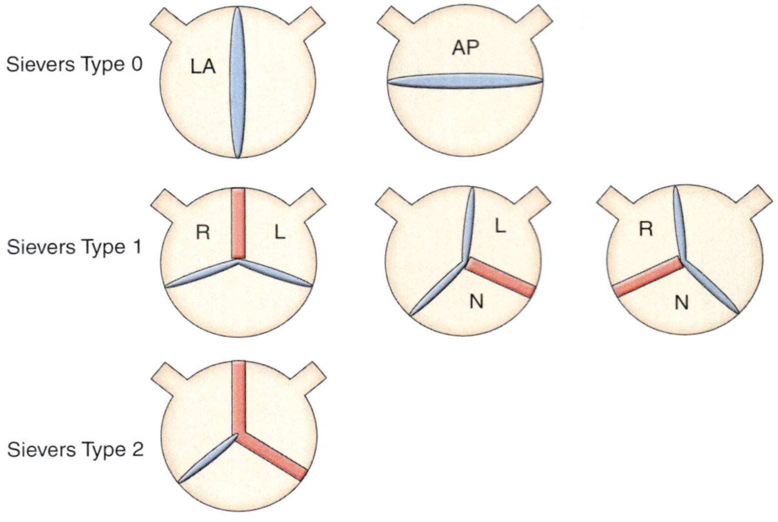

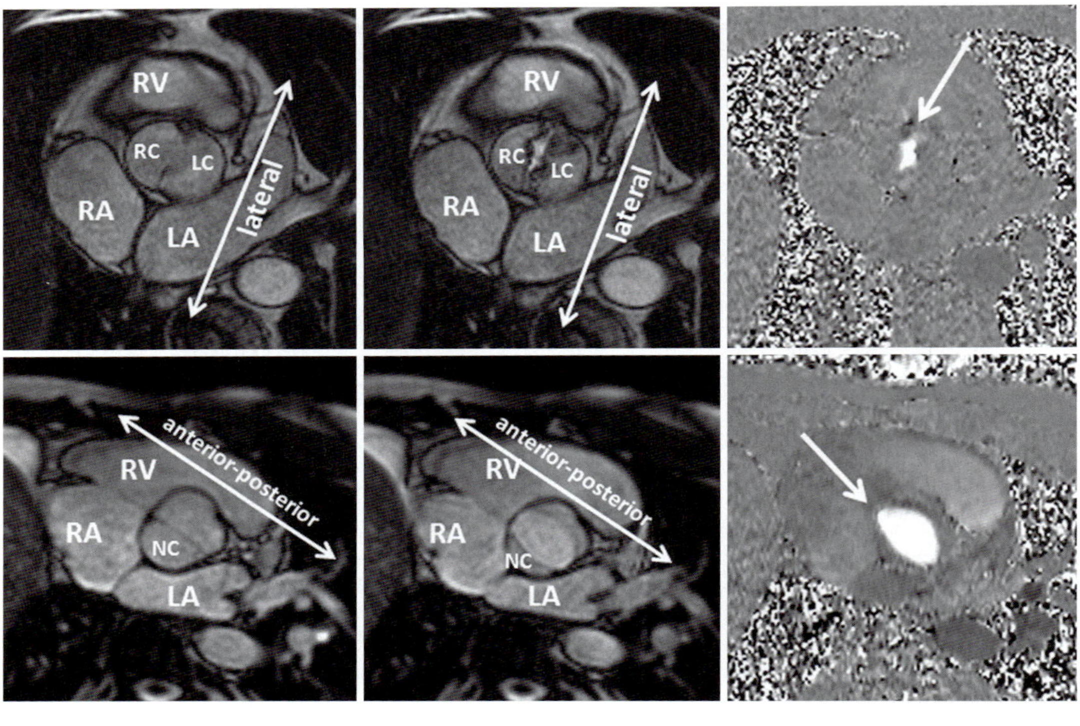

Fig. 8.15 *Bicuspid aortic valve Sievers Type 0*. Two different patients with cine MRI findings of a bicuspid aortic valve with no raphe. One patient had a stenotic bicuspid (*arrow*) aortic valve with the free edge of the cusps in the lateral orientation (*upper row*). The other patient had a bicuspid aortic valve (*arrow*) with the free edge of the cusps in the anteroposterior orientation (*lower row*). Additionally, phase-contrast MRI demonstrates clearly the shape of the stenotic and the normal orifice of a bicuspid valve. *LA* left atrium, *LC* left cusp, *NC* noncoronary cusp, *RA* right atrium, *RC* right cusp, *RV* right ventricle

easily performed by MRI and CT using planimetry [28–30]. Of note, the effective aortic valve orifice is smaller than the anatomic area. The current guidelines do not differentiate between these methods regarding the cutoff values for severity of aortic stenosis. MRI and CT studies for

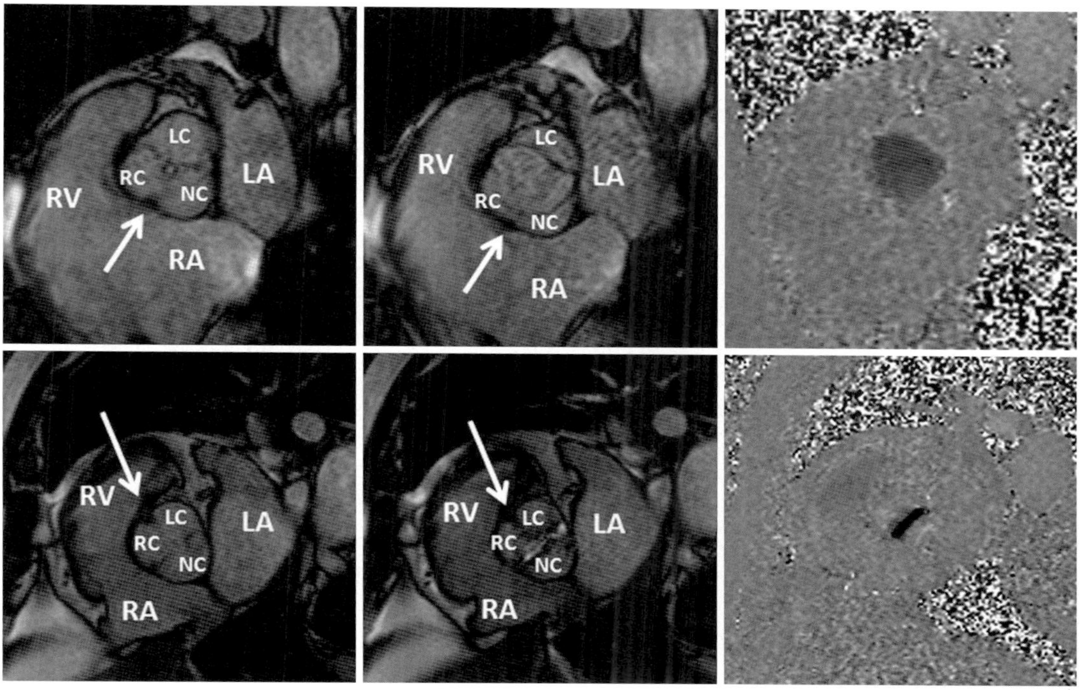

Fig. 8.16 *Bicuspid aortic valve Sievers Type 1*. Two different patients with cine MRI findings of a bicuspid aortic valve with raphe. The first patient (*upper row*) had a bicuspid aortic valve with a raphe between (*arrow*) the right (*RC*) and noncoronary cusps (*NC*). The second patient (*lower row*) had a stenotic bicuspid aortic valve with a raphe between (*arrow*) the right and left coronary cusps. Additionally, phase-contrast MRI demonstrates clearly the shape of the stenotic and the normal orifice. *LA* left atrium, *LC* left cusp, *NC* noncoronary cusp, *RA* right atrium, *RC* right cusp, *RV* right ventricle

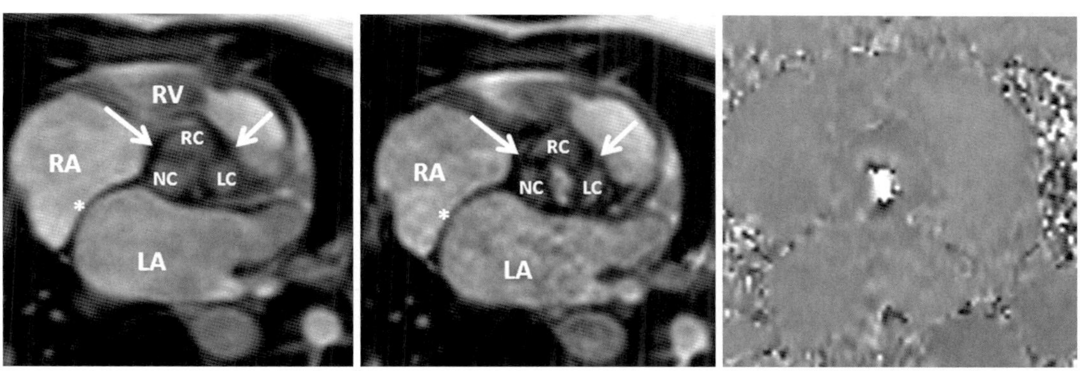

Fig. 8.17 *Bicuspid aortic valve Sievers Type 2*. MRI findings of a bicuspid aortic valve with two raphes. The one fusion (*arrow*) of the right (*RC*) and noncoronary cusps (*NC*) and one fusion of the right (RC) and left coronary cusps (*LC*). Additionally, phase-contrast MRI demonstrates clearly the shape of the stenotic. *LA* left atrium, *LC* left cusp, *NC* noncoronary cusp, *RA* right atrium, *RC* right cusp, *RV* right ventricle

the quantification of stenotic aortic valves have focused on direct planimetry of the stenotic aortic valve or jet area (Fig. 8.19) and have shown promising results compared with other standard methods [28–31]. Calculation of the effective aortic valve area by the continuity equation is also possible by MRI (Fig. 8.20) and has been investigated using velocity-encoded cine magnetic resonance [32, 33]. Accurate planimetry of aortic valve area can be challenging because orthogonal

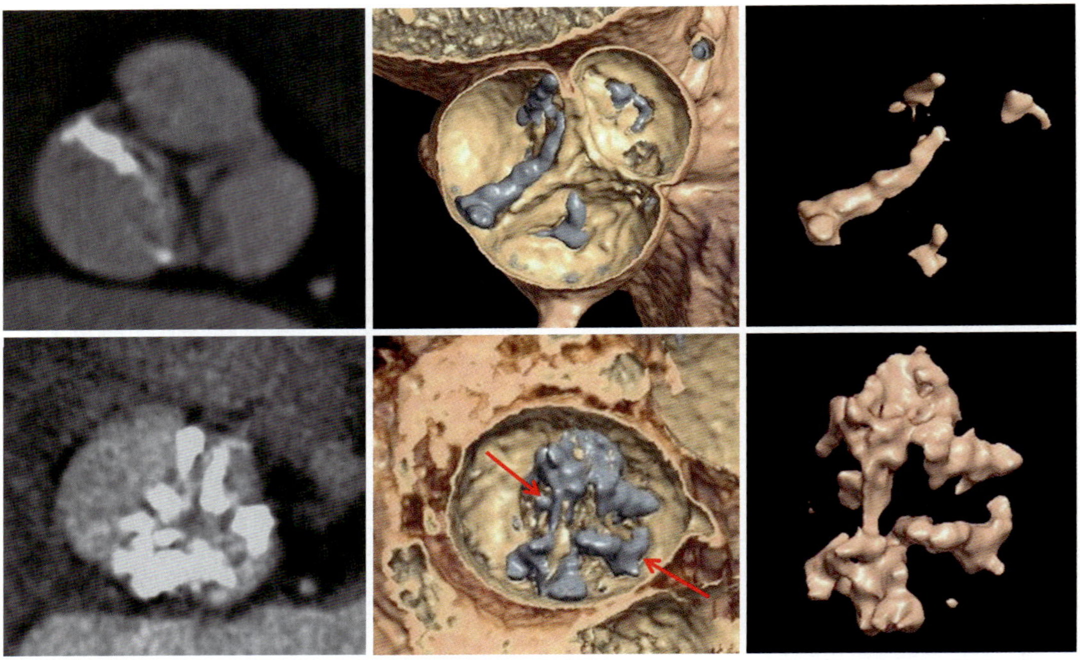

Fig. 8.18 Short-axis two-dimensional and volume-rendered CT images show heavily calcified, thickened, and stenosed tricuspid and bicuspid aortic valves. In tricuspid stenotic aortic valve (*upper row*), the distribution of the calcified deposits is more nodular. In bicuspid stenotic aortic valve (*lower row*), the distribution of the calcified deposits is mainly along the free edges and the raphe (*red arrow*). Volume-rendered CT allows to visualize the chalk skeleton of the valve to analyze the volume

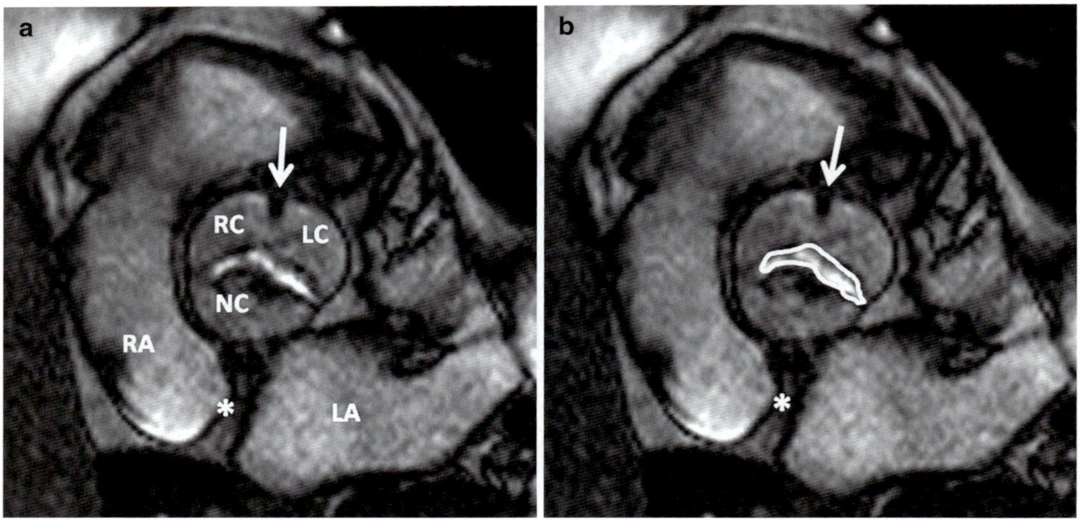

Fig. 8.19 MRI of a stenotic right-left bicuspid aortic valve (Sievers Type 1 – RL). (**a**) The rim of the cusps is clearly shown. Consequently, an exact planimetry of the stenotic anatomic orifice is possible (0.8 cm^2). The location of the raphe is between the right and left coronary cusps (*white arrow*). (**b**) Aortic valve orifice area was measured by precisely delineating the edges of the maximal systolic opening of the leaflets on each scanning plane in systole. Only the smallest of these measurements was retained as the aortic valve orifice (**b**). *RA* right atrium, *LA* left atrium, *NC* noncoronary cusp. Interatrial septum (*). *LC* left cusp, *RC* right cusp

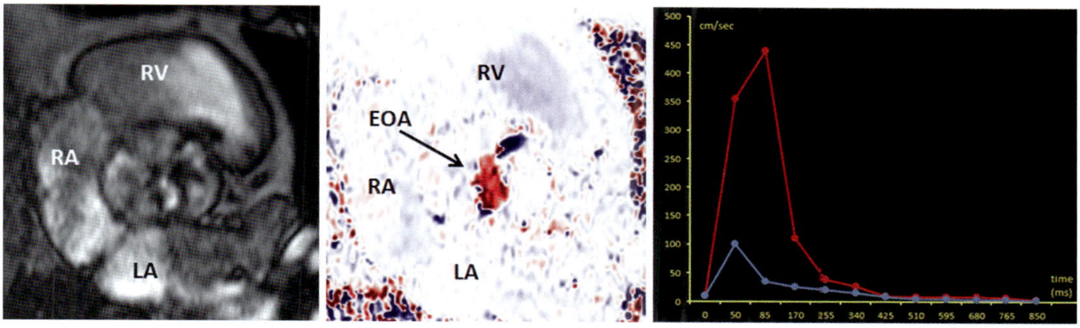

Fig. 8.20 Flow images through the stenotic bicuspid aortic valve. The magnitude image details the anatomy, contour, and shape of the stenotic orifice (*arrow*). On the phase velocity map, flow in the phase-encoding direction represents the effective orifice area (*EOA*; *red* signal). The area graph of the data obtained from the velocity maps demonstrated the areas under the curves of transaortic velocity time integral in the aortic valve (*red line*) and velocity time integral of the left ventricle outflow tract (*blue line*). The calculated velocity ratio is the effective curve expressed as a proportion of the left ventricle outflow tract curve. *LA* left atrium, *RA* right atrium, *RV* right ventricle

angulated short-axis views have to be positioned exactly at the level of the aortic valve cusps, resulting in overestimation of the aortic valve orifice in some patients (Fig. 8.21). In addition to planimetry, MRI allows the determination of functional hemodynamic parameters, such as flow velocities and effective orifice areas. The new approach of a serial systolic planimetry velocity-encoded MRI sequence (VENC-MRI) facilitates the sizing of blood-filled cardiac structures with the registration of changes in magnitude during systole [34]. Additionally, the subvalvular VENC-MRI measurements improve the clinically important exact determination of the LVOT area with respect to its specific eccentric configuration and its systolic deformity. MRI and CT allow assessment of the myocardial morphology and function, morphology of the aortic valve and aortic valve stenosis severity, and an exact measurement and characterization of the aortic root and ascending aorta.

Discrepancies in the Assessment of Aortic Valve Area Using Different Methods

A severe aortic stenosis induces an obstruction of transvalvular blood flow that leads to a subsequent increase in left ventricular afterload. The adult normal aortic valve area is 3.0–4.0 cm^2. In significant aortic stenosis, valve area must be reduced to one-fourth before any significant changes in hemodynamics occur. Severe aortic stenosis is thus defined as a valve area of less than 1.0 cm^2. Aortic valve area can be measured by different techniques to assess stenosis severity. These techniques provide the anatomic orifice area (AOA), the effective orifice area (EOA), and the Gorlin area (GA) [35]. The differences in effective and anatomic aortic valve area are depicted in Fig. 8.22.

Anatomic orifice area (AOA):

- Anatomic area of the stenotic aortic valve orifice assessed by planimetry
- Measured by imaging techniques (echocardiography, MRI, CT)

Effective orifice area (EOA):

- Minimal cross-sectional area of the flow jet downstream of the anatomic stenotic aortic valve.
- EOA represents functional severity.
- Measured by echocardiography and MRI using the continuity equation (measurement of velocities and gradients).
- EOA < AOA because of flow contraction (Cc, coefficient of contraction); Cc is dependent on valve geometry, valve inflow shape, and jet eccentricity.
- For a given AOA, EOA as a measure of functional severity tends to be smaller in bicuspid valve stenosis than in tricuspid valve stenosis. This phenomenon appears to be primarily related to greater jet eccentricity in BAV.

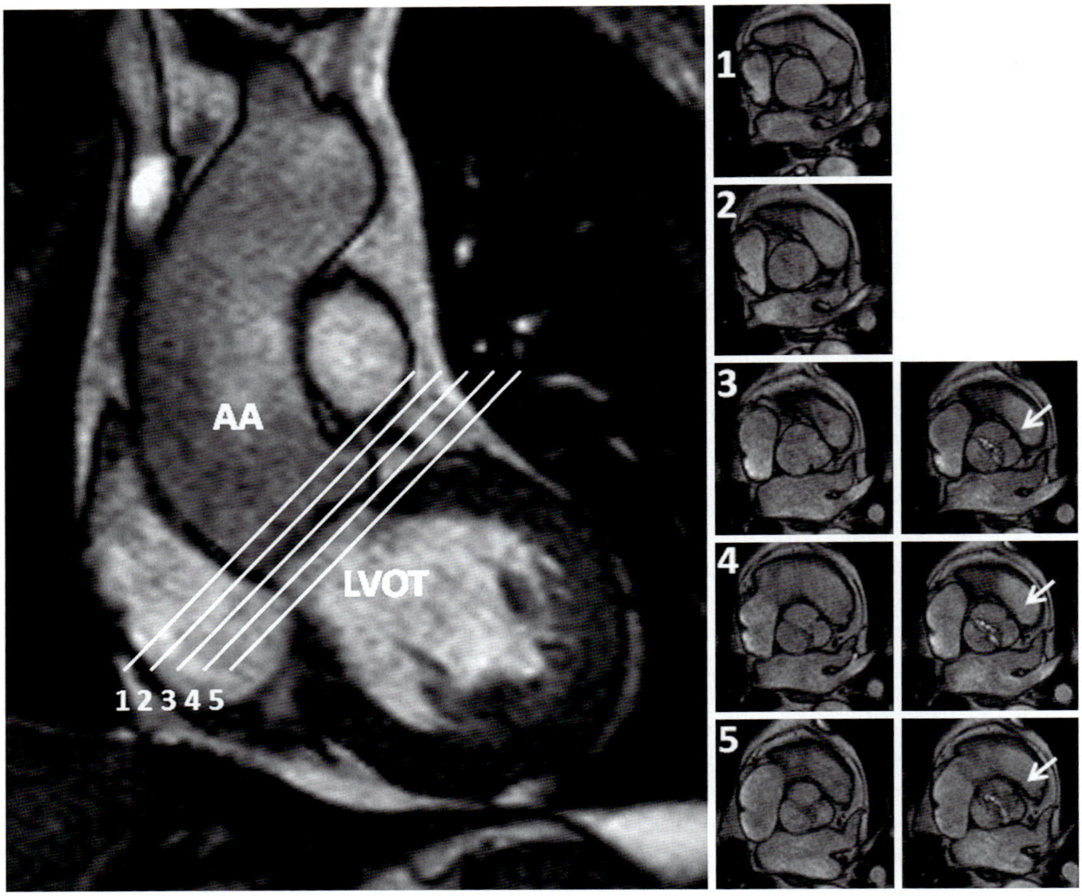

Fig. 8.21 Stepwise positioning of the aortic valve slices using an adjusted long-axis view of the left ventricular outflow tract (*LVOT*). A stenotic right–left bicuspid aortic valve (Sievers Type 1 – RL) at systole and diastole. *White arrows* show the location of the raphe between the right and left coronary cusps at systole. Stepwise positioning is necessary to clearly identify the raphe (1–5). Slice thickness 5 mm, shift wise in 2.5 mm steps. *AA* ascending aorta

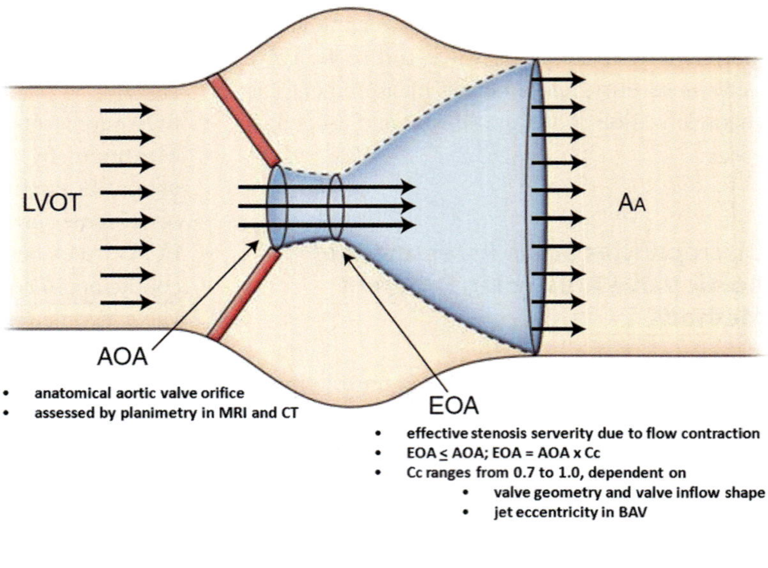

Fig. 8.22 Schema of the systolic flow through a stenotic aortic valve; *LVOT* left ventricular outflow tract, *Ao* area of the ascending aorta, *AOA* anatomic orifice area, *EOA* effective orifice area, *Cc* coefficient of flow contraction, *BAV* bicuspid aortic valve, *AA* ascending aorta

Gorlin area (GA):

- Assessed by the Gorlin formula at catheterization [36].
- GA is usually higher than EOA, especially in small aortas due to the pressure recovery phenomenon.
- Discrepancies between Gorlin area and EOA are mainly dependent on the pressure recovery phenomenon.

AOA, EOA, and GA represent different hemodynamic parameters, and the differences among them are highly dependent on valve inflow geometry and aortic cross-sectional area [35, 37, 38]. Furthermore, the discrepancies of these three aortic valve area parameters are highly patient specific. Especially in BAV, the correct assessment of stenosis severity can be challenging, because AOA seems to underestimate functional stenosis severity systematically due to jet eccentricity [39, 40]. These inaccuracies of the assessment of aortic valve area by different techniques have to be taken into account in the decision making in patients with aortic stenosis. EOA as a measure of functional severity should probably the preferred parameter of stenosis severity in BAV.

Grading Severity

Guidelines by the ACC/AHA and ESC have categorized aortic stenosis severity as mild, moderate, or severe to provide guidance for clinical decision making (Table 8.2). A normal aortic valve area in adults is 3.0–4.0 cm^2. Severe stenosis is present when valve area is reduced to 25 % of the normal size so that a value of 1.0 cm^2 is one reasonable definition of severe aortic stenosis in adults [41].

Table 8.2 Grading aortic stenosis

	Mild	Moderate	Severe
Vmax (cm/s)	250–300	300–400	>400
Mean gradient (mmHg)	<20	20–40	>40
Valve area (cm^2)	>1.5	1.0–1.5	<1.0
Valve area indexed (cm^2/m^2 BSA)	>0.85	0.60–0.85	<0.60
Velocity ratio	>0.50	0.25–0.50	<0.25

Abbreviations: *Vmax* maximum velocity, *BSA* body surface area, *cm/s* centimeter per second

Aortic Root and Ascending Aorta Involvement in Bicuspid Aortic Valve

Bicuspid aortic valve disease is increasingly recognized as a disease of the entire proximal aorta including both valvular and vascular complications [13]. Dilatation of the proximal aorta is a frequent finding in BAV and independent from the severity of valve dysfunction. Intrinsic vascular matrix remodeling of the proximal aorta is the structural basis of aortic dilatation in BAV [42]. Additionally, in a bicuspid aortic valve, the valve anatomy gives rise to altered hemodynamics, independently of valve function, with turbulent eccentric flow acceleration in the ascending aorta (Fig. 8.23) [43]. Furthermore, dilatation of the proximal aorta seems to be independent of coexistent valve dysfunction [44]. Time-resolved 3D phase-contrast magnetic resonance imaging (4D flow) is an effective means of evaluating dynamic multidirectional blood flow in the thoracic aorta (Fig. 8.24) [45, 46]. CT and MRI play an increasing role in imaging of patients with BAV, providing excellent spatial resolution. CT and MRI should be regularly used in patients with bicuspid aortic valves when morphology of the aortic root or ascending aorta cannot be assessed accurately by echocardiography [47].

More accurate quantification of the size of the aortic root and ascending aorta can be obtained with image reconstruction and postprocessing options of MRI or CT (Fig. 8.25). Important clinical consequences of these abnormalities of the proximal aorta are progressive dilatation and dissection. Consequently, patients with BAV should receive a careful assessment of both valve function and dilatation of the ascending aorta [42]. These patients with ascending aorta dilatation should be carefully monitored with respect to progressive dilatation.

Treatment

An accurate preoperative assessment of function and morphology in bicuspid aortic valve disease is essential, thus MRI and CT are complementary tools to echocardiography. Surgical interventions are indicated for patients with severe stenosis who

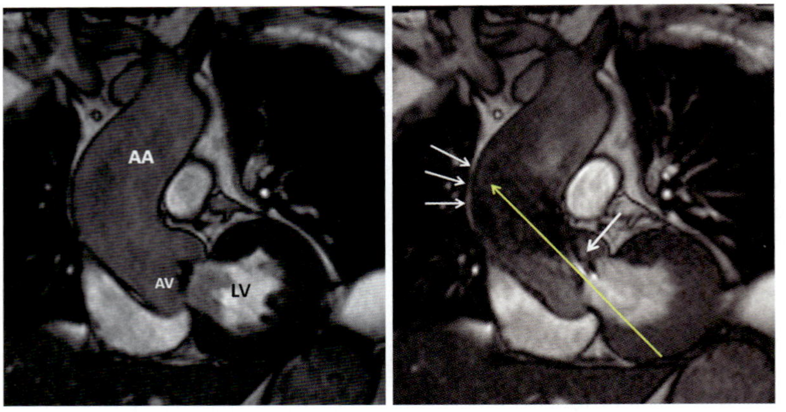

Fig. 8.23 MRI of a stenotic bicuspid aortic valve with dilatation of the ascending aorta (*AA*). (**a**) Long-axis view of the left ventricular outflow tract (*LVOT*). In systole, the *arrow* demonstrates flow turbulence (signal void) that begins at the level of the aortic valve leaflets. The LVOT view shows aortic valve stenosis with a jet (*white arrow*) in the aorta (peak velocity 405 cm/s). The jet direction (*yellow arrow*) is to the lateral wall (*small arrows*) of the dilated ascending aorta. *AV* aortic valve, *LV* left ventricle

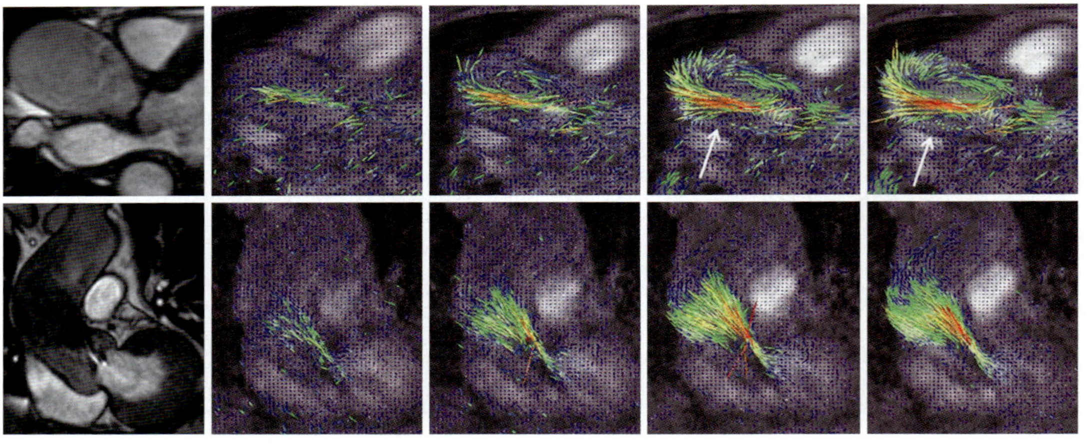

Fig. 8.24 Flow analysis in a patient with a severe stenotic bicuspid aortic valve and an ascending aortic aneurysm. Sequences of flow during systole in two long-axis views. 3-Dimensional streamlines clearly show asymmetric aortic outflow and an accelerated flow channel along the outer aortic curvature (*white arrows*) and the onset of substantial helical flow during peak systole. The complex flow resulted in considerable variation of peak velocities along the aorta, like *fireworks*

are symptomatic or have left ventricular systolic dysfunction [47]. Mechanical prostheses or bioprosthetic valves are generally preferred. Also, the Ross procedure has been used in patients with BAV [48]. This procedure involves excision of the diseased aortic valve and aortic root with subsequent placement of a pulmonary autograft in the aortic position. An aortic homograft is usually placed in the pulmonary position.

Posttreatment

Left ventricular hypertrophy and reduced left ventricular function are largely reversible after successful aortic valve replacement [49]. Left ventricular mass regression after aortic valve replacement is a marker of favorable LV remodeling [50]. MRI and CT allow analyzing the cardiac adaption before and after aortic valve replacement.

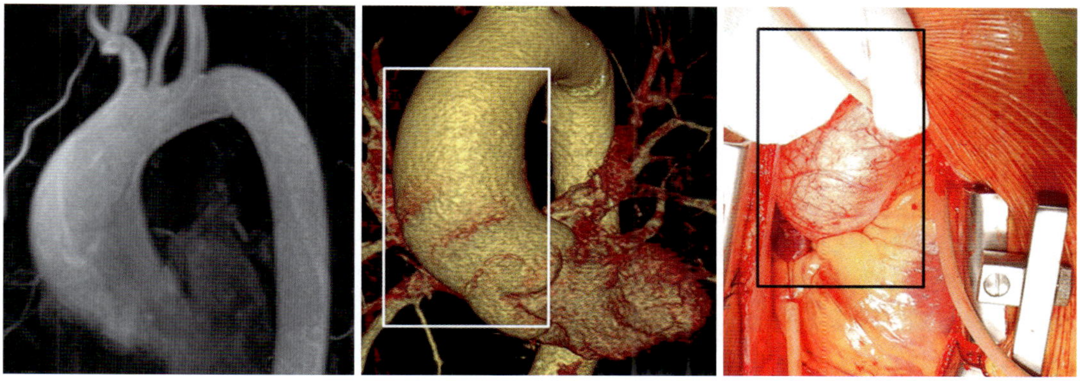

Fig. 8.25 Bicuspid aortic valve Sievers Type 1 – RL – with an aneurysm of ascending aorta. Contrast-enhanced 3-dimensional cardiovascular MRI, volume-rendering CT, and in situ image of the ascending aorta (*delimited by box*) show fusiform aneurysm (5.5 cm)

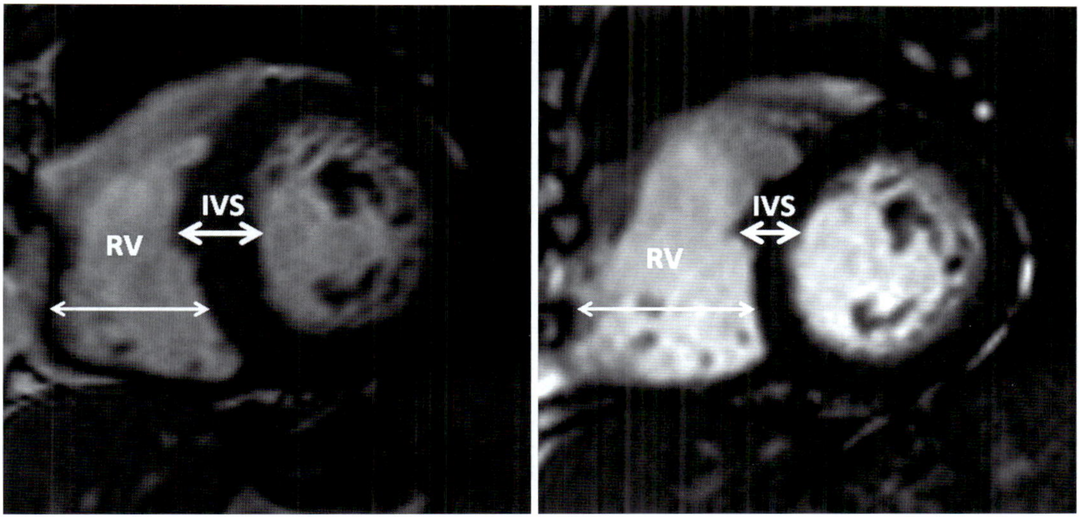

Fig. 8.26 Time changes of left ventricular mass in a 64-year-old man with an initial stenotic bicuspid aortic valve after Ross procedure. Cine MRI images preoperatively and after 5-year follow-up are shown. The calculated left ventricular mass was 341 and 209 g, respectively. Note the increase diameter of the right ventricle. *IVS* interventricular septum, *RV* right ventricle

The exact assessment of the extent of postoperative left ventricular mass regression is possible (Fig. 8.26). Especially, in young adults with severe aortic valve disease, a marked regression in LV hypertrophy has been demonstrated by MRI after Ross procedure [51]. Rarely, RVOT obstruction and aortic regurgitation have been noted after Ross procedure. Thus, in postoperative care, CT and MRI allow exact evaluation and visualization of the RVOT (RVOT obstruction, delayed enhancement) (Figs. 8.27, 8.28, and 8.29). Furthermore, an exact visualization of the reconstructive aortic root and aortic valve as well as detection of aortic valve incompetence is possible (Fig. 8.30).

Subvalvular LVOTO

Subvalvular left ventricular outflow tract obstruction – also often called "subaortic stenosis" – includes a variety of obstructions of the left ventricular outflow tract, ranging from a short

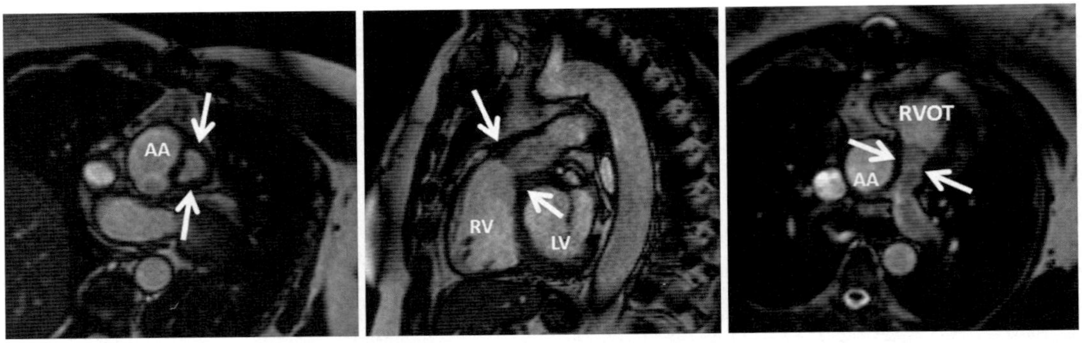

Fig. 8.27 A 58-year-old woman who underwent Ross procedure. There is pulmonary homograft stenosis (*arrows*). Cine images of right ventricular outflow tract (*RVOT*), pulmonary root, and pulmonary trunk in short-axis and sagittal orientation reveal narrowing of the pulmonary homograft conduit. The valve remains competent, with the stenosis appearing in the homograft conduit. *AA* ascending aorta, *LV* left ventricle, *RV* right ventricle

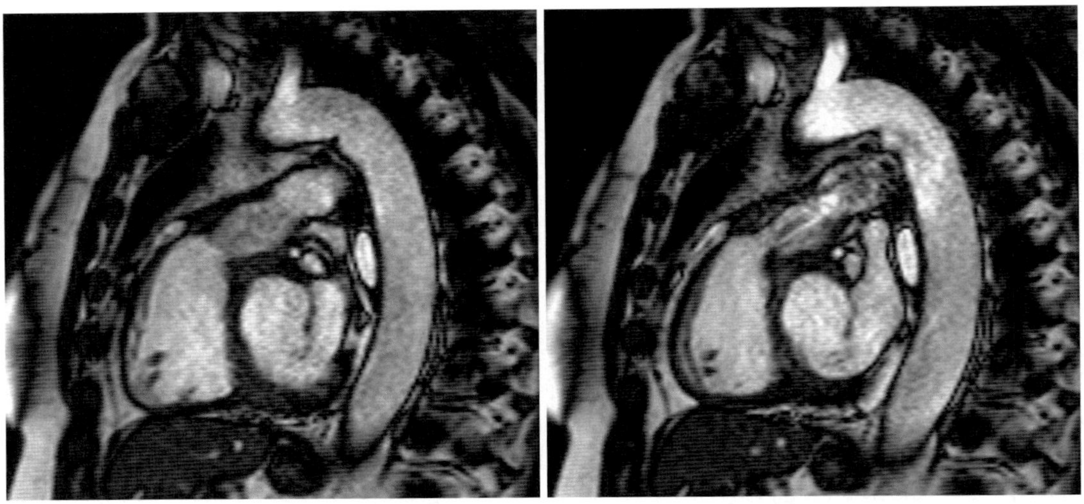

Fig. 8.28 The right ventricular outflow tract after Ross procedure. The bioprosthetic pulmonary valve showed a stenosis in systolic phase with an increase flow of 230 cm/s

(discrete) subvalvular membrane to long, tunnel-like narrowing. Subvalvular LVOTO is a rare condition but remains an important differential diagnosis in hypertrophic cardiomyopathy with LVOT obstruction and in aortic stenosis. Subvalvular LVOTO constitutes 8–20 % of all forms of LVOT obstruction in children [52, 53]. The fibromuscular type and the tunnel type are infrequently seen in adults. Subvalvular stenosis in adults is usually a result of a discrete subaortic membrane or ridge just below the valve. Most commonly, a discrete crescent-shaped ridge or fibroelastic membrane protrudes from the left septal surface into the subaortic region, or a fibromuscular collar encircles the LVOT with attachments to the anterior leaflet of the mitral valve [54]. A genetic predisposition has been suggested as there are reports of a familial incidence [55]. Subvalvular LVOTO has a male predominance (2:1). The underlying genetic predisposition and various geometric and anatomic variations of the LVOT lead to flow turbulence at this level which may damage the endothelium and promote fibrin deposition [56, 57]. Subvalvular LVOTO often

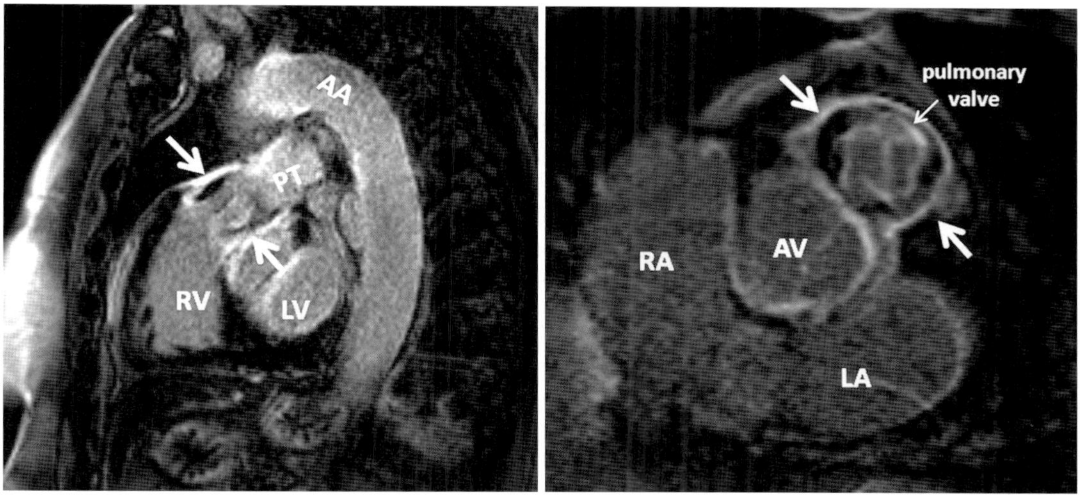

Fig. 8.29 A 52-year-old man who underwent Ross procedure. Delayed enhancement of the pulmonary homograft conduit in sagittal and short-axis view reveals markedly delayed enhancement (*white arrows*) corresponding to inflammatory appearance of the graft. *AA* ascending aorta, *AV* aortic valve, *LV* left ventricle, *PT* pulmonary truncus, *RV* right ventricle

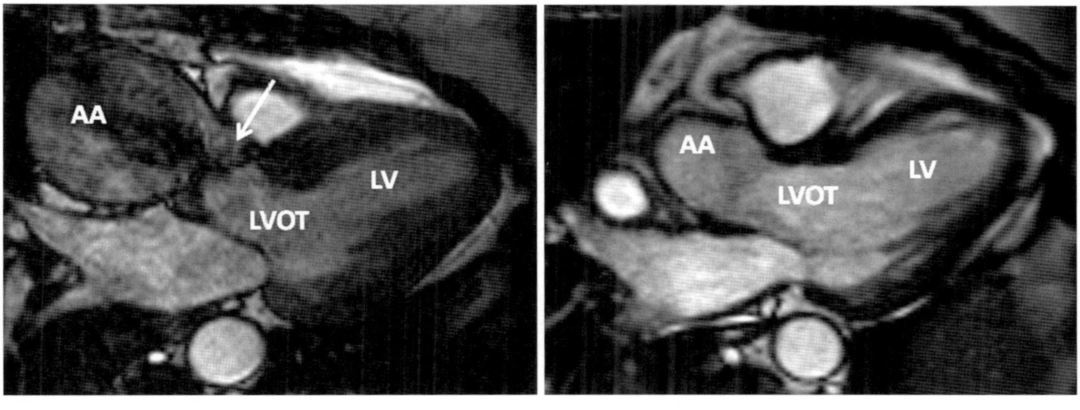

Fig. 8.30 Three-chamber cine image of the left ventricular outflow tract (*LVOT*) with a stenotic bicuspid aortic valve before Ross procedure. In systole, the *arrow* demonstrates flow turbulence (signal void) that begins at the level of the aortic valve leaflets. Six years after Ross procedure, the aortic graft is normal without regurgitation. Note the regression of the left ventricular mass. *AA* ascending aorta, *LV* left ventricle

progresses, but progress rate is variable, and low gradients may remain for many years [57]. It is often associated with aortic regurgitation (up to 60 % of cases) through an otherwise normal valve which has been damaged by the subvalvular jet of blood [58]. An association with other congenital lesions is frequent, e.g., small ventricular septal defects. These patients are particularly prone to endocarditis.

Imaging

Echocardiography including color Doppler is surely the modality of choice to establish the diagnosis and to assess the extent and hemodynamic severity of subvalvular LVOT. In differential diagnosis of hypertrophic obstruction cardiomyopathy and of aortic stenosis, CT and MRI demonstrate the potential of the noninvasive

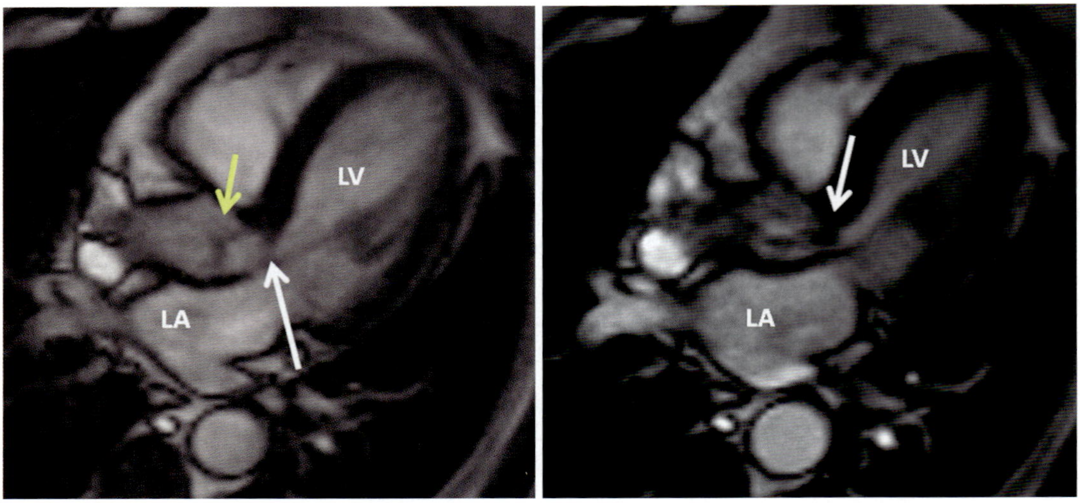

Fig. 8.31 MRI of a subvalvular aortic stenosis with a subvalvular membrane. In the diastolic image, a short membrane (*white arrows*) is just close to the aortic valve (*yellow arrow*). In the systole, a turbulent jet across the membrane is seen. *LA* left atrium, *LV* left ventricle

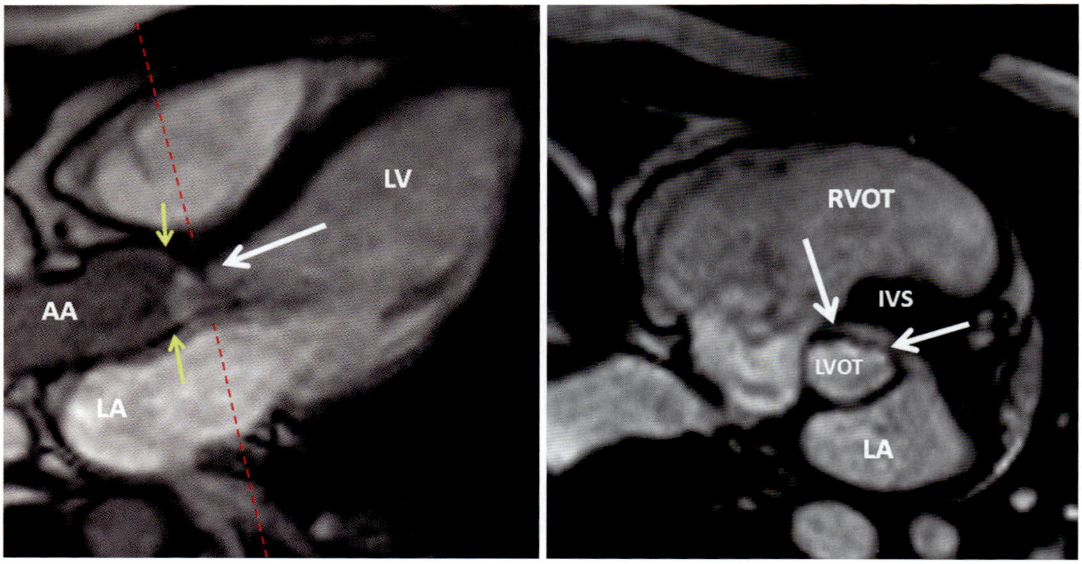

Fig. 8.32 MRI of a left ventricular outflow tract (*LVOT*) view with a subvalvular membrane (*white arrow*) just close to the aortic valve (*yellow arrows*). The LVOT is obstructive by the membrane. In the corresponding short-axis view (at the level of *dotted red line*), the subvalvular membrane (*white arrows*) is markedly shown as a half moon in the LVOT. *AA* ascending aorta, *LA* left atrium, *IVS* interventricular septum, *LV* left ventricle, *RVOT* right ventricle outflow tract

modality for a comprehensive evaluation of patients with the disease (Fig. 8.31). Both imaging methods can be helpful to characterize the complex LVOT anatomy and demonstrate the membrane in these patients (Figs. 8.32 and 8.33). CT is not supposed to provide hemodynamic measures by being a purely excellent morphology-based imaging tool. However, CT also allows the quantification of severity by planimetric measurements of left ventricular obstruction. MRI

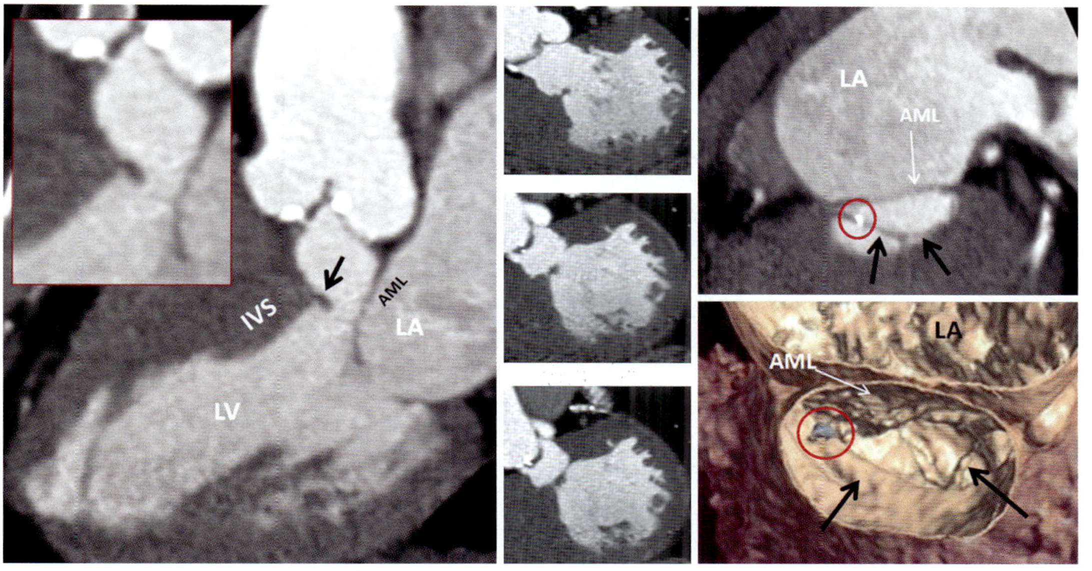

Fig. 8.33 A 71-year-old man with a slightly calcified aortic valve and a subvalvular membrane. CT with oblique reconstruction showing the discrete membrane (*arrow*) originating from the interventricular septum (*IVS*). The anterior mitral valve leaflet (*AML*) constituting the medial border of the left ventricular outflow tract. Volume-rendered image gives an impression of the spatial relationship of the subvalvular membrane with thicker and a thinner part. Note the calcified part of the membrane (*circle*). *LA* left atrium, *LV* left ventricle, rectangle box is an enlarged view of the left ventricle outflow tract

provides excellent morphologic assessment of the subaortic stenosis (Fig. 8.34). The LVOT area at the level of discrete membrane shows often a dynamic change during one cardiac cycle being the smallest in systole. Information from CT and MRI may prove useful for preoperative planning of cardiac surgery.

Grading and Treatment

Symptomatic patients with mean Doppler-derived gradient of >50 mmHg (spontaneous or under exercise test) or severe aortic regurgitation have a poor prognosis [59]. Surgical resection is the intervention of choice for treatment of subvalvular LVOTO. Asymptomatic patients should be considered for surgery when LV ejection fraction is <50 % (gradient may be <50 mmHg due to low flow) or AR is severe and LV end-systolic diameter >50 mm and/or ejection fraction <50 %, mean Doppler gradient is ≥50 mmHg and marked LV hypertrophy, or mean Doppler gradient is ≥50 mmHg and blood pressure response is abnormal on exercise testing. To date, there are no cutoff values for MRI and CT available.

Supravalvular LVOTO

Congenital supravalvular LVOTO is the rarest (<7 %) obstructive lesion of the LVOT affecting both sexes equally. Usually supravalvular LVOTO is part of Williams syndrome. The Williams syndrome occurs in chromosome 7q11.23 microdeletion and is associated with mental retardation, hypercalcemia, and a variety of cardiovascular anomalies [60]. Also, there is a familial variant with normal facies or associated with rubella syndrome. And aortic regurgitation is common. Focal pulmonary arterial stenosis and diffuse hypoplasia of the pulmonary arterial bed are the next most common lesions [50] with this syndrome. The pathology of supravalvular LVOTO is not simple supravalvular; rather, it tends to involve the aortic valve and the ascending aorta of varying severity, which is most pronounced at the sinotubular junction. In most

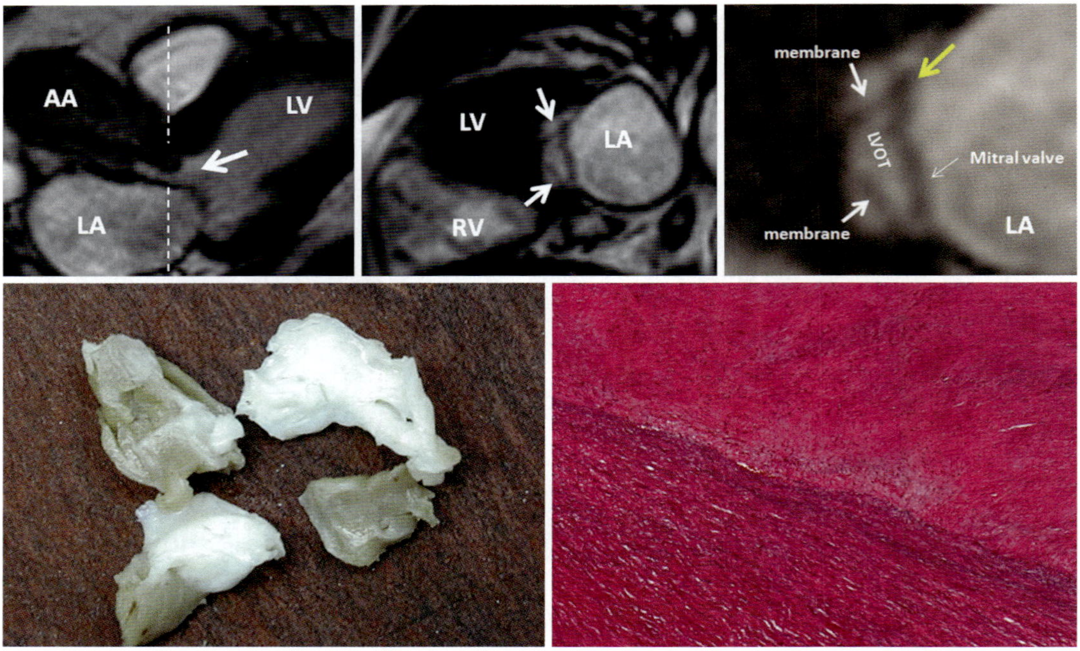

Fig. 8.34 A 63-year-old woman with a symptomatic subvalvular aortic stenosis. Long axis three chamber MRI shows the subaortic membrane that caused obstruction of the LVOT and thickening of the aortic valve leaflets. The angulated cine MRI image the angulated short axis cine MRI image of LVOT (at the level of *dotted white line*) shows a thin subaortic membrane (between *arrows*). The membrane is attached to the anterior leaflet of the mitral valve (*yellow arrow*). Macroscopic examination after resection of the subaortal membrane and myectomy (Morrow procedure) showed multiple fragments of dense fibrous tissue. Histology (elastica van Giesson) revealed layers of fibroelastic tissue (collagen fibers in *pink* and elastic fibers in *blue*) consistent with a subaortic membrane. *AA* ascending aorta, *LA* left atrium, *LV* left ventricle, *RV* right ventricle

cases the aortic valve is abnormal with, e.g., bicuspid. Further, aortic stenosis or regurgitation is seen frequently. Supravalvular LVOTO is usually a progressive disease. MRI and CT provide excellent anatomic visualization of the level and severity of the lesion and the associated cardiovascular anomalies. In asymptomatic young adults, a resting angiographic gradient greater than 50 mmHg or progressive aortic valve dysfunction has been used as criteria for intervention.

References

1. Butcher JT, Markwald RR. Valvulogenesis: the moving target. Philos Trans R Soc Lond B Biol Sci. 2007;362:1489–503.
2. Laforest B, Nemer M. Genetic insights into bicuspid aortic valve formation. Cardiol Res Pract. 2012;2012: 180297.
3. Combs MD, Yutzey KE. Heart valve development: regulatory networks in development and disease. Circ Res. 2009;105:408–21.
4. Fernandez B, Fernandez MC, Duran AC, Lopez D, Martire A, Sans-Coma V. Anatomy and formation of congenital bicuspid and quadricuspid pulmonary valves in Syrian hamsters. Anat Rec. 1998;250:70–9.
5. Fernandez B, Duran AC, Fernandez-Gallego T, et al. Bicuspid aortic valves with different spatial orientations of the leaflets are distinct etiological entities. J Am Coll Cardiol. 2009;54:2312–8.
6. Anderson RH. Clinical anatomy of the aortic root. Heart. 2000;84:670–3.
7. Ho SY. Structure and anatomy of the aortic root. Eur J Echocardiogr. 2009;10:i3–10.
8. Anderson R. The surgical anatomy of the aortic root. Multimed Man Cardiothorac Surg. 2007;2007(102): 1–8. doi:10.1510/mmcts.2006.002527.
9. Otto CM, Burwash IG, Legget ME, et al. Prospective study of asymptomatic valvular aortic stenosis. Clinical, echocardiographic, and exercise predictors of outcome. Circulation. 1997;95:2262–70.
10. Buchner S, Debl K, Haimerl J, et al. Electrocardiographic diagnosis of left ventricular hypertrophy in aortic valve disease: evaluation of

ECG criteria by cardiovascular magnetic resonance. J Cardiovasc Magn Reson. 2009;11:18.
11. Debl K, Djavidani B, Buchner S, et al. Delayed hyper-enhancement in magnetic resonance imaging of left ventricular hypertrophy caused by aortic stenosis and hypertrophic cardiomyopathy: visualisation of focal fibrosis. Heart. 2006;92:1447–51.
12. Azevedo CF, Nigri M, Higuchi ML, et al. Prognostic significance of myocardial fibrosis quantification by histopathology and magnetic resonance imaging in patients with severe aortic valve disease. J Am Coll Cardiol. 2010;56:278–87.
13. Fedak PW, Verma S, David TE, Leask RL, Weisel RD, Butany J. Clinical and pathophysiological implications of a bicuspid aortic valve. Circulation. 2002;106:900–4.
14. Michelena HI, Desjardins VA, Avierinos JF, et al. Natural history of asymptomatic patients with normally functioning or minimally dysfunctional bicuspid aortic valve in the community. Circulation. 2008;117:2776–84.
15. Horstkotte D, Loogen F. The natural history of aortic valve stenosis. Eur Heart J. 1988;9(Suppl E):57–64.
16. Roberts WC. The congenitally bicuspid aortic valve. A study of 85 autopsy cases. Am J Cardiol. 1970;26:72–83.
17. Sievers HH, Schmidtke C. A classification system for the bicuspid aortic valve from 304 surgical specimens. J Thorac Cardiovasc Surg. 2007;133:1226–33.
18. Buchner S, Hulsmann M, Poschenrieder F, et al. Variable phenotypes of bicuspid aortic valve disease: classification by cardiovascular magnetic resonance. Heart. 2010;96:1233–40.
19. Ko SM, Song MG, Hwang HK. Bicuspid aortic valve: spectrum of imaging findings at cardiac MDCT and cardiovascular MRI. AJR Am J Roentgenol. 2012;198:89–97.
20. Debl K, Djavidani B, Buchner S, et al. Unicuspid aortic valve disease: a magnetic resonance imaging study. Rofo. 2008;180:983–7.
21. Kari FA, Fazel SS, Mitchell RS, Fischbein MP, Miller DC. Bicuspid aortic valve configuration and aortopathy pattern might represent different pathophysiologic substrates. J Thorac Cardiovasc Surg. 2012;144: 516–7.
22. Willmann JK, Kobza R, Roos JE, et al. ECG-gated multi-detector row CT for assessment of mitral valve disease: initial experience. Eur Radiol. 2002;12: 2662–9.
23. Koos R, Mahnken AH, Sinha AM, Wildberger JE, Hoffmann R, Kuhl HP. Aortic valve calcification as a marker for aortic stenosis severity: assessment on 16-MDCT. AJR Am J Roentgenol. 2004;183:1813–8.
24. Ferda J, Linhartova K, Kreuzberg B. Comparison of the aortic valve calcium content in the bicuspid and tricuspid stenotic aortic valve using non-enhanced 64-detector-row-computed tomography with prospective ECG-triggering. Eur J Radiol. 2008;68:471–5.
25. Morgan-Hughes GJ, Owens PE, Roobottom CA, Marshall AJ. Three dimensional volume quantification of aortic valve calcification using multislice computed tomography. Heart. 2003;89:1191–4.
26. Isner JM, Chokshi SK, DeFranco A, Braimen J, Slovenkai GA. Contrasting histoarchitecture of calcified leaflets from stenotic bicuspid versus stenotic tricuspid aortic valves. J Am Coll Cardiol. 1990;15:1104–8.
27. Joo I, Park EA, Kim KH, Lee W, Chung JW, Park JH. MDCT differentiation between bicuspid and tricuspid aortic valves in patients with aortic valvular disease: correlation with surgical findings. Int J Cardiovasc Imaging. 2012;28:171–82.
28. Debl K, Djavidani B, Seitz J, et al. Planimetry of aortic valve area in aortic stenosis by magnetic resonance imaging. Invest Radiol. 2005;40:631–6.
29. Kupfahl C, Honold M, Meinhardt G, et al. Evaluation of aortic stenosis by cardiovascular magnetic resonance imaging: comparison with established routine clinical techniques. Heart. 2004;90:893–901.
30. Chun EJ, Choi SI, Lim C, et al. Aortic stenosis: evaluation with multidetector CT angiography and MR imaging. Korean J Radiol. 2008;9:439–48.
31. Feuchtner GM, Muller S, Bonatti J, et al. Sixty-four slice CT evaluation of aortic stenosis using planimetry of the aortic valve area. AJR Am J Roentgenol. 2007;189:197–203.
32. Garcia J, Kadem L, Larose E, Clavel MA, Pibarot P. Comparison between cardiovascular magnetic resonance and transthoracic Doppler echocardiography for the estimation of effective orifice area in aortic stenosis. J Cardiovasc Magn Reson. 2011;13:25.
33. Yap SC, van Geuns RJ, Meijboom FJ, et al. A simplified continuity equation approach to the quantification of stenotic bicuspid aortic valves using velocity-encoded cardiovascular magnetic resonance. J Cardiovasc Magn Reson. 2007;9:899–906.
34. Sagmeister F, Herrmann S, Ritter C, et al. Functional cardiac MRI for assessment of aortic valve disease. Radiologe. 2010;50:541–7.
35. Garcia D, Kadem L. What do you mean by aortic valve area: geometric orifice area, effective orifice area, or gorlin area? J Heart Valve Dis. 2006;15: 601–8.
36. Gorlin R, Gorlin SG. Hydraulic formula for calculation of the area of the stenotic mitral valve, other cardiac valves, and central circulatory shunts. I. Am Heart J. 1951;41:1–29.
37. Richards KE, Deserranno D, Donal E, Greenberg NL, Thomas JD, Garcia MJ. Influence of structural geometry on the severity of bicuspid aortic stenosis. Am J Physiol Heart Circ Physiol. 2004;287:H1410–6.
38. Gilon D, Cape EG, Handschumacher MD, et al. Effect of three-dimensional valve shape on the hemodynamics of aortic stenosis: three-dimensional echocardiographic stereolithography and patient studies. J Am Coll Cardiol. 2002;40:1479–86.
39. Garcia D, Pibarot P, Landry C, et al. Estimation of aortic valve effective orifice area by Doppler echocardiography: effects of valve inflow shape and flow rate. J Am Soc Echocardiogr. 2004;17:756–65.

40. Donal E, Novaro GM, Deserrano D, et al. Planimetric assessment of anatomic valve area overestimates effective orifice area in bicuspid aortic stenosis. J Am Soc Echocardiogr. 2005;18:1392–8.
41. Vahanian A, Alfieri O, Andreotti F, et al. Guidelines on the management of valvular heart disease (version 2012). Eur Heart J. 2012;33:2451–96.
42. Tadros TM, Klein MD, Shapira OM. Ascending aortic dilatation associated with bicuspid aortic valve: pathophysiology, molecular biology, and clinical implications. Circulation. 2009;119:880–90.
43. den Reijer PM, Sallee 3rd D, van der Velden P, et al. Hemodynamic predictors of aortic dilatation in bicuspid aortic valve by velocity-encoded cardiovascular magnetic resonance. J Cardiovasc Magn Reson. 2010;12:4.
44. Fernandes S, Khairy P, Graham DA, et al. Bicuspid aortic valve and associated aortic dilation in the young. Heart. 2012;98:1014–9.
45. Barker AJ, Markl M, Burk J, et al. Bicuspid aortic valve is associated with altered wall shear stress in the ascending aorta. Circ Cardiovasc Imaging. 2012;5:457–66.
46. Hope MD, Hope TA, Crook SE, et al. 4D Flow CMR in assessment of valve-related ascending aortic disease. JACC Cardiovasc Imaging. 2011;4:781–7.
47. Bonow RO, Carabello BA, Kanu C, et al. ACC/AHA 2006 guidelines for the management of patients with valvular heart disease: a report of the American College of Cardiology/American Heart Association Task Force on Practice Guidelines (writing committee to revise the 1998 Guidelines for the Management of Patients with Valvular Heart Disease): developed in collaboration with the Society of Cardiovascular Anesthesiologists: endorsed by the Society for Cardiovascular Angiography and Interventions and the Society of Thoracic Surgeons. Circulation. 2006;114:e84–231.
48. Luciani GB, Favaro A, Casali G, Santini F, Mazzucco A. Ross operation in the young: a ten-year experience. Ann Thorac Surg. 2005;80:2271–7.
49. Monrad ES, Hess OM, Murakami T, Nonogi H, Corin WJ, Krayenbuehl HP. Time course of regression of left ventricular hypertrophy after aortic valve replacement. Circulation. 1988;77:1345–55.
50. Krayenbuehl HP, Hess OM, Monrad ES, Schneider J, Mall G, Turina M. Left ventricular myocardial structure in aortic valve disease before, intermediate, and late after aortic valve replacement. Circulation. 1989;79:744–55.
51. Djavidani B, Schmid FX, Keyser A, et al. Early regression of left ventricular hypertrophy after aortic valve replacement by the Ross procedure detected by cine MRI. J Cardiovasc Magn Reson. 2004;6:1–8.
52. Trinchero R, Demarie D, Orzan F, et al. Fixed subaortic stenosis. Natural history of patients with mild obstruction and follow-up of operated patients. G Ital Cardiol. 1988;18:738–44.
53. Kelly DT, Wulfsberg E, Rowe RD. Discrete subaortic stenosis. Circulation. 1972;46:309–22.
54. Katz NM, Buckley MJ, Liberthson RR. Discrete membranous subaortic stenosis. Report of 31 patients, review of the literature, and delineation of management. Circulation. 1977;56:1034–8.
55. Fatimi SH, Ahmad U, Javed MA, Shamim S, Ahmad R. Familial membranous subaortic stenosis: review of familial inheritance patterns and a case report. J Thorac Cardiovasc Surg. 2006;132:1484–6.
56. Tutar HE, Atalay S, Turkay S, Gumus H, Imamoglu A. Echocardiographic, morphologic, and geometric variations of the left ventricular outflow tract: possible role in the pathogenesis of discrete subaortic stenosis. Angiology. 2000;51:213–21.
57. Oliver JM, Gonzalez A, Gallego P, Sanchez-Recalde A, Benito F, Mesa JM. Discrete subaortic stenosis in adults: increased prevalence and slow rate of progression of the obstruction and aortic regurgitation. J Am Coll Cardiol. 2001;38:835–42.
58. Ibrahim M, Kostolny M, Hsia TY, et al. The surgical history, management, and outcomes of subaortic stenosis in adults. Ann Thorac Surg. 2012;93:1128–33.
59. Baumgartner H, Bonhoeffer P, De Groot NM, et al. ESC guidelines for the management of grown-up congenital heart disease (new version 2010). Eur Heart J. 2010;31:2915–57.
60. Urban Z, Zhang J, Davis EC, et al. Supravalvular aortic stenosis: genetic and molecular dissection of a complex mutation in the elastin gene. Hum Genet. 2001;109:512–20.

Repaired Tetralogy of Fallot

9

Ee Ling Heng and Sonya V. Babu-Narayan

Tetralogy of Fallot: The Lesion

The anatomy of tetralogy of Fallot (TOF), together with the pathophysiological consequences, was first described by Etienne-Louis Fallot in 1888. The tetrad of overriding aorta, right ventricular (RV) outflow tract obstruction, ventricular septal defect (VSD) and consequent RV hypertrophy is all due to antero-cephalad deviation of the outlet septum during fetal development. TOF is the most common cyanotic congenital heart disease (CHD), accounting for 10 % of CHD patients and occurring in 1 in 3,600 births [1]. It carries a recurrence risk of 3 % in siblings. There is genetic microdeletion in 22q11 in 15–25 % of TOF patients in whom TOF is part of DiGeorge syndrome. There is a spectrum of morphology, despite the four features that comprise 'tetralogy', and the severity of the RV outflow tract (RVOT) obstruction is the major determinant of first clinical presentation.

E.L. Heng, BSc, MRCP
NIHR Biomedical Research Unit,
Cardiology Specialty Registrar, Royal Brompton
and Harefield NHS Foundation Trust, London, UK

S.V. Babu-Narayan, MBBS, BSc, MRCP, PhD (✉)
NIHR Cardiovascular Biomedical Research Unit,
Royal Brompton Hospital and National Heart
and Lung Institute, Imperial College London,
Sydney Street, London SW3 6NP, UK
e-mail: s.babu-narayan@imperial.ac.uk

Early Interventions for Tetralogy of Fallot

Surgical palliation was achieved using the Blalock–Taussig shunt (subclavian artery to ipsilateral pulmonary artery connection) in 1944, a landmark event as these patients underwent the first cardiac surgery. Subsequently, surgical repair was described in the 1950s with the advent of cardiopulmonary bypass. Primary surgical repair involves patch closure of the VSD and intervention to the RVOT to relieve obstruction. RV muscle bundles are resected. Depending on the size of the outflow tract, pulmonary valve and pulmonary arteries; an RVOT patch, transannular patch and/or pulmonary artery (PA) patch may be required for RVOT reconstruction. In the variants with anomalous coronary arteries or in pulmonary atresia-type Fallot, an RV to PA conduit may be used.

Contemporary cohorts of TOF patients include older patients that have had generous transannular patching to relieve RVOT obstruction completely but at the expense of loss of integrity of the native pulmonary valve and large akinetic regions in the RVOT. In the modern era, transannular patching is avoided if possible and a degree of RVOT residual obstruction is accepted. Older adult patients will have undergone ventriculotomy and potentially late repair after a preceding shunt as opposed to younger patients that reflect current practice of a transatrial, transpulmonary approach and early repair. Late presentation of TOF in adulthood is possible and repair can be

F. Saremi (ed.), *Cardiac CT and MR for Adult Congenital Heart Disease*,
DOI 10.1007/978-1-4614-8875-0_9,

considered. Since the introduction of surgical repair, there is now a large population of adults with repaired TOF requiring medical care.

Late Complications and Survival

Unrepaired TOF is associated with 20 % mortality within the first year, in stark contrast to 90 % patients surviving beyond 30 years after surgical repair [2]. Although surgical developments have revolutionised survival prospects in this group, there remains a long-term 3.7–6 % risk of sudden cardiac death or ventricular tachycardia [3]. The majority of adult TOF patients are physically unrestricted from a cardiac perspective, but lifelong surveillance is imperative to monitor for late complications of pulmonary regurgitation and RV overload, in addition to arrhythmias, heart failure and sudden cardiac death. There can be concurrent left heart sequelae of left ventricular dysfunction, aortic root dilatation and associated aortic regurgitation. Rare cases of aortic dissection have been reported.

Pulmonary regurgitation is a frequent finding in TOF patients in adulthood. Severe chronic pulmonary regurgitation can be clinically well tolerated for decades. However, it is associated with progressive RV dysfunction, left ventricle (LV) dysfunction, exercise intolerance, arrhythmias, symptomatic heart failure and sudden death. Pulmonary valve replacement (PVR) can lead to reduced RV volume, improved biventricular mechanics and improved symptoms. The optimal timing of pulmonary valve replacement remains controversial, but cardiovascular magnetic resonance (CMR)-measured RV volumes is increasingly valued for aiding decision-making in asymptomatic patients.

General Merits and Limitations of CMR in TOF

CMR has an established role in the management of TOF patients. It provides detailed imaging in any plane, is the gold standard for quantification of pulmonary regurgitation, is especially adept in quantifying degree of obstruction in multilevel right-sided obstruction, can quantify right as well as left ventricular volumes and function as well as provide anatomical and functional data for extracardiac structures such as pulmonary arteries and major aortopulmonary collateral arteries. CMR is exquisitely suited to serial clinical surveillance in patients with TOF as it provides unrestricted and comprehensive access to cardiovascular anatomy and function without exposure to ionising radiation. Exposure to radiation from diagnostic investigation causes genuine harm for adult CHD (ACHD) patients [4]. The reproducibility of measurements facilitates lifelong clinical monitoring with serial imaging, which is often necessary in ACHD patients. CMR can be utilised safely in pregnancy without the use of gadolinium (unless essential). The spatial and anatomical information obtained can aid in planning and directing subsequent transcatheter procedures to minimise procedural time and radiation, for example, coiling of major aortopulmonary collateral arteries or electrophysiology ablation procedures in complex CHD patients [5].

The use of CMR is limited by its cost, availability and lack of portability. It remains operator and equipment dependent and can be time-consuming when compared to other imaging modalities. Implantable pacemakers and defibrillators generally preclude CMR, although recent developments have included MR-compatible devices. MR safety checks should be meticulous in individuals with implantable devices to ensure that only patients with MR-compatible pacing systems in the absence of old pacing leads undergo scanning safely. Cardiovascular CT provides a complementary role and can be invaluable when used selectively, for example, in patients who cannot undergo CMR, for preoperative coronary artery assessment in older patients, for evaluation of major aortopulmonary collateral arteries and in preprocedure planning for percutaneous pulmonary valve insertion. Small residual intracardiac shunts and less than moderate tricuspid regurgitation are often more sensitively assessed by echocardiography.

CMR Acquisition Techniques Helpful in TOF Assessment

Multislice Imaging

Multislice imaging is helpful in TOF as in any CHD to obtain scout images for piloting of subsequent breath-hold cine acquisitions. Coronal, sagittal and transaxial multislice images should be taken using either rapid acquisition by half-Fourier acquisition single-shot turbo spin-echo (HASTE) – dark-blood sequence – or a bright-blood sequence such as balanced steady-state free precession (bSSFP) to obtain contiguous slices covering the heart and mediastinum.

Cine Imaging

Cine imaging with bSSFP is utilised for imaging and measuring ventricular function, mass and valvular pathology due to the preferable blood–myocardial interface contrast. Volume measurements can be obtained by manual contouring of diastolic and systolic frames or derived from semiautomated programmes.

Phase-Shift Velocity Mapping

Phase-shift velocity mapping enables accurate and versatile flow assessment by tracking frequency changes experienced by moving nuclei relative to applied magnetic gradients [6]. Clinical applications of this include the calculation of cardiac output, shunt flow and assessment of severity of aortic or pulmonary regurgitation. Low to high velocity flows can be measured by selecting the appropriate plane, echo time, velocity-encoding direction and velocity sensitivity for a particular flow assessment. Velocities can be encoded in or through an image plane – flow volume can be measured by acquiring images through the plane transecting the vessel (i.e. encoding velocity in direction of slice-selection gradient). The luminal cross-sectional area and mean velocity within the area is measured throughout the phases of the cardiac cycle, which then produces a flow curve. Systolic forward flow and diastolic flow reversal can then be computed by integration of areas.

Velocity mapping also enables shunt quantification by measuring aortic and pulmonary flows. This typically involves two separate acquisitions – the aortic flow is obtained from a plane transecting the aortic root at the level of the sinotubular junction, whereas pulmonary flow is obtained from a plane transecting the pulmonary trunk proximal to its bifurcation. These measurements are particularly relevant in the context of intracardiac shunts.

Throughplane velocity mapping can delineate shunts such as ventricular septal defects and measure velocities and cross-sectional areas through stenotic vessels and valves. Jet velocity mapping can be employed in the assessment of stenotic lesions not readily accessed by echocardiography, such as double-chamber RV, branch PA stenoses or RV–PA conduits.

The recommended acquisition plane for imaging aortic flow is across the aortic sinuses, between the valve and sinotubular junction, just proximal to the origin of the coronary arteries. However, displacement of the aortic root can cause underestimation of the regurgitant flow and volume as the aortic root moves 6–12 mm during the backflow of aortic regurgitation into the left ventricle. This together with the variability of breath-hold positions can cause inaccuracies, which can be minimised by acquiring images at or immediately above the sinotubular junction at end diastole. Motion tracking and heart motion-adapted flow measurements have been proposed as a potential solution but has yet to be incorporated into current commercial CMR systems [7].

It is important to be aware of limitations in current phase velocity mapping given the emphasis on these measurements in ACHD CMR assessments. Velocity images are formed by subtracting the phase image of two acquisitions with differing velocity sensitivity, with phase differences between the two images causing stationary tissue to display an apparent nonzero velocity, known as background offset or baseline errors [7]. The accuracy of measured regurgitant fraction is therefore influenced by the well-recognised problem of velocity offsets errors. This is attributable to eddy currents and Maxwell gradients, which can be corrected by gelatin- or water-based phantom acquisition as the current gold standard [7]. Maxwell gradient effects are predominantly corrected during analysis, whilst eddy currents tend to be adjusted for by active-shielded gradient coils and pre-emphasis. Although these potential errors are small in terms of the absolute number (~1–2 cm/s), they can theoretically cause up to 10 % error in shunt measurement due to the summation of velocities needed in calculating volume flow [5]. In clinical practice, correction of background offset areas with phantom acquisition is not routinely carried out.

Scanners produced by various manufacturers demonstrate variations in offset behaviour and across different slice orientations for small changes to a scanning protocol, towards which adjustments have been implemented by automatic correction of Maxwell gradients during post-processing. Rolf et al. [8] demonstrated that offsets due to eddy currents may never be completely abolished by acquisition optimisation, thereby necessitating post-processing techniques. Optimisation has to be performed on a per scanner per protocol basis, in view of variations of velocity offset errors across different manufacturers. It is pivotal that the vessel of interest is positioned at the magnet iso-centre to minimise velocity offset errors (i.e. with zero offset along the head–foot direction). Interpolation of the static tissue in the chest wall can also be employed to estimate the velocity offset, although this is not yet validated across different systems. Jet velocity in residual stenotic lesions (such as pulmonary stenosis) should be measured through a plane located carefully to transect the core of the jet, immediately downstream of the orifice. It is worth noting that CMR-measured jet velocities are accurate and reliable only in the presence of a coherent jet core with central, high velocity and low shear region of sufficient size to contain entire voxels [9].

Contrast-Enhanced MR Angiography

Contrast-enhanced MR angiography (CE-MRA) may help illustrate the anatomy of the RV outflow tract and PA and is particularly valuable in the assessment of major aortopulmonary collateral arteries and patency of previous surgical shunts. It is typically acquired with a single breath hold without cardiac gating.

Three-Dimensional Balanced SSFP

3D bSSFP imaging is useful for visualisation of anomalous coronary artery anatomy, the nature of which may alter planned surgery in ~4 % of TOF cases [10]. Also the proximal relationships of the coronary arteries to the RVOT are important in determining suitability for percutaneous PVR procedures and preprocedure planning.

Late Gadolinium Enhancement Imaging

Late gadolinium enhancement (LGE) imaging exploits the propensity of chelated gadolinium to persist in myocardial scar and fibrotic tissue after its concentration begins to diminish in the bloodstream. This manifests as areas of bright myocardial enhancement, in contrast to dark healthy myocardium. LGE imaging is usually performed as a 2D stack of breath-hold inversion-prepared segmented gradient-echo acquisitions with inversion time (TI) adjustment to compensate for gadolinium wash-out throughout the study. Alternate R-wave gating allows for almost complete recovery of the longitudinal magnetisation between sequence repeats and improves contrast between normal and abnormal tissue and reduces the effects of cardiac arrhythmia. In patients with faster or irregular heart rates, gating on every 3rd R wave may improve image quality. In-plane resolution of standard sequences is typically 1.2–1.8 × 1.2–1.8 mm, with a slice thickness of 6–8 mm in a breath hold of ~12 s. The TI varies from patient to patient and depends on the dose of gadolinium and the time after administration. For experienced operators this individualised approach with meticulous inversion time adjustment remains the best [11]. The presence, extent and location of gadolinium enhancement should be reported with respect to the clinical context.

Gadolinium imaging is well established for clinical application in the detection of ventricular thrombus, in the delineation of infarcted myocardium in coronary artery disease and in establishing the aetiology of cardiomyopathies and systemic conditions such as sarcoidosis and amyloidosis and has prognostic value in ischaemic heart disease, hypertrophic cardiomyopathy and dilated cardiomyopathy. Myocardial fibrosis demonstrated with LGE CMR has an emerging role in TOF assessment. Specific pitfalls of LGE CMR in TOF [12] include sternal wires obscuring regions of interest in the RV, the thin RV wall in the outflow tract and related partial volume effects and impaired CMR quality in patients with previous transcatheter coil embolisation of major aortopulmonary collateral arteries, which can render the images non-diagnostic in some instances. Artefact may also arise from 'ghosting' caused by cerebrospinal fluid, which can be overcome by the placement of pre-saturation bands over the spinal cord. In ACHD LGE CMR [12], positive findings should be demonstrated in 'phase-swapped' images so that myocardial enhancement, and potentially in both diastole and systole and or in more than one plane (i.e. in cross-cut views), avoids false positives. Imaging planes unnecessary for ischaemic heart disease imaging, such as oblique RV views, may have a high diagnostic yield in TOF and care must be taken not to abandon the study promptly not having waited long enough for LGE to be well demonstrated. Inversion times should also be strategically chosen to minimise false positives and negatives in interpreting LGE, and sequences need to be optimised to individual patient heart rate and breath-holding ability [12].

Suggested Approach to CMR Acquisition in Repaired TOF

Different CMR operators may have varying approaches to CMR in TOF, all of which are informative. In our experience the following approach is helpful as a starting point after which other data may need to be acquired depending on findings. Figures 9.1, 9.2, 9.3, 9.4, 9.5 and 9.6 are from one specific patient assessed with this approach.

Image acquisition in TOF should include:

1. *Multislice stacks* in transaxial, coronal and sagittal planes (with HASTE or single-shot bSSFP).
2. *Cines* of two-chamber, four-chamber and short-axis stacks; two views each of left and right (Fig. 9.1) ventricular outflow tracts, aortic valve views should be acquired for further evaluation of aortic root. Dedicated right pulmonary artery (RPA) and left pulmonary artery (LPA) views (cines and velocity mapping) should be obtained if there is suspicion of branch pulmonary artery obstruction. In our experience, long-axis oblique RV views showing the aorta in short axis, pulmonary valve and tricuspid valve which shows the RV outflow tract ('RV in and out'), a similar image plane with the aorta in long axis orientated more towards the body and apex of the RV ('RV oblique') and two-chamber right atrial right ventricular views perpendicular in orientation to the four-chamber view are useful for qualitative, regional RV assessment (Fig. 9.2). Additional 'cross-cut' cines may be required in the presence of tricuspid regurgitation or VSD to better delineate these lesions.
3. *Phase-shift velocity mapping* to derive *pulmonary regurgitation fraction*. Flow mapping for pulmonary regurgitation should be aligned perpendicular to the pulmonary trunk in at least two cine RVOT views. *In-plane RVOT velocity mapping* is not only useful to locate a subsequent throughplane velocity map appropriately for determination of *peak pulmonary velocity* but also useful to align the throughplane mapping for pulmonary regurgitation. A *subpulmonary valve level throughplane velocity map* is useful to demonstrate the size of the regurgitant jet. To determine cardiac output as well as identify any residual intracardiac shunt by calculation of *Qp*:*Qs*, an aortic throughplane velocity map should be acquired at the aortic sinotubular junction. Where appearances suggest potential branch PA stenosis, right and left PA throughplane velocity mapping should be performed to assess

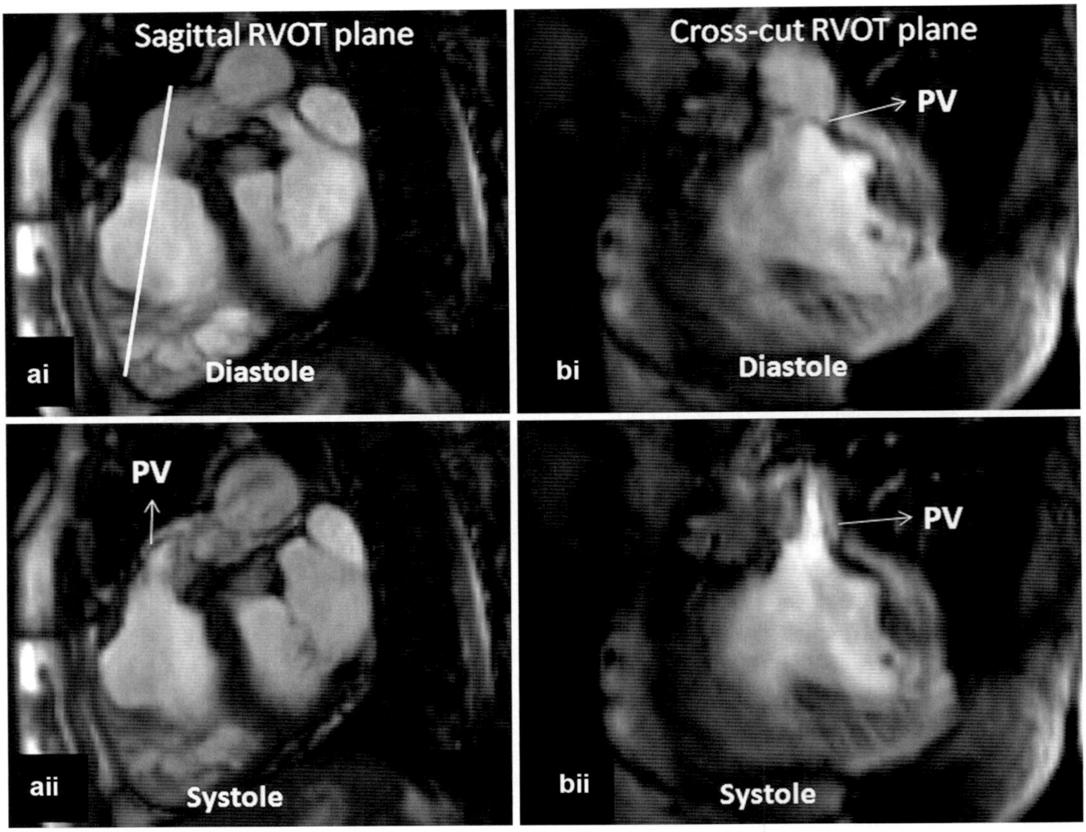

Fig. 9.1 RV–PA cine views. Still frame from sagittal right ventricle outflow tract (*RVOT*) cine in diastole (**ai**) and systole (**aii**) is shown. There is mild residual subpulmonary valve RVOT obstruction with maximum velocity 2.1 m/s. The cross-cut RVOT cine view (**b**) is from a plane perpendicular to the pulmonary valve (*PV*) and RVOT on the sagittal RVOT cine (*white bar*) and is shown in diastole (**bi**) and systole (**bii**). Note also there is mild kinking of the distal conduit used in the most recent surgery associated with a peak velocity 1.8 m/s

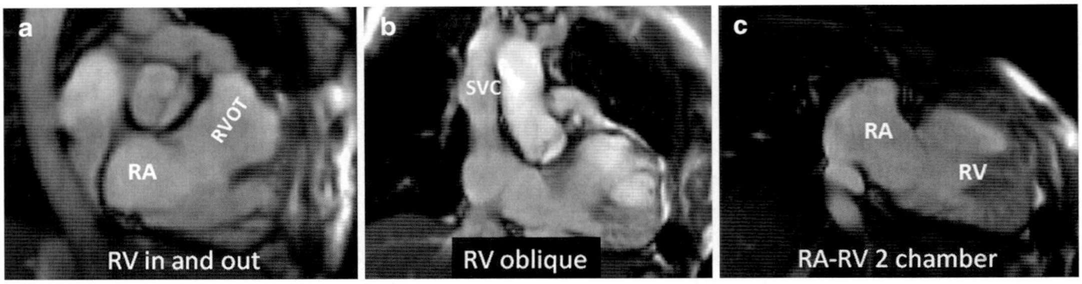

Fig. 9.2 Additional long-axis views. Examples of right ventricle (*RV*) in and out (**a**), RV oblique (**b**) and right atrial–right ventricular (*RA–RV*) long-axis (**c**) cine orientations are shown. (**a**) and (**b**) are useful for detecting ventricular septal defect patch leaks, right ventricle outflow tract (*RVOT*) regional wall motion abnormality and a dilated RV less apparent in four-chamber orientation and for subsequent piloting of late enhancement CMR. These views may show the akinetic area of the RVOT and may be useful views in addition to a four-chamber and basal short axis for assessment of tricuspid regurgitation. *SVC* superior vena cava

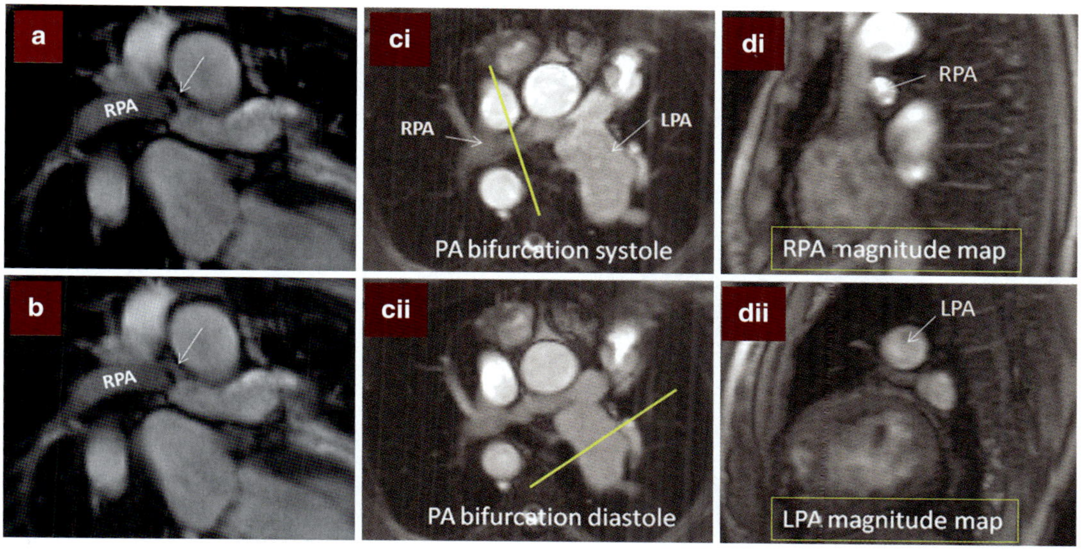

Fig. 9.3 Branch pulmonary artery (*PA*) assessment. (**a**) Shows discrete mid right pulmonary artery (*RPA*) stenosis in a TOF patient with previous history of Waterston shunt. The shear edges of the mid RPA jet (*arrow*) can be seen. The RPA measured 9 × 5 mm at the level of stenosis where peak velocity was 2 m/s. (**b**) is a corresponding in-plane phase velocity map with right–left orientation useful to help determine the area of peak velocity and for subsequent peak velocity throughplane mapping location. (**c**) Images are of the PA bifurcation in systole (**ci**) and diastole (**cii**) showing relative lack of pulsatility of the RPA versus the left pulmonary artery (*LPA*) which is also dilated. The *yellow bar* in (ci) and (cii) shows the planes used to locate the throughplane RPA velocity map (magnitude image **di**) and LPA velocity map (magnitude image **dii**), respectively. Regions of interest drawn throughout the cardiac cycle on the corresponding phase encoded velocity maps can be used to determine the blood flow through the RPA and LPA and to subsequently calculate differential lung perfusion. In this case percentage RPA:LPA flow was reversed at 40:60. The features are of moderate RPA stenosis

preferential branch PA blood flow (Fig. 9.3). In unilateral pulmonary stenosis, this helps assess severity. Normal differential pulmonary blood flow is RPA:LPA 60 %:40 %.

(a) Further clinically directed imaging should encompass *3D data* from CE-MRA and or 3D bSSFP (Fig. 9.4).
(b) *Late gadolinium imaging* for myocardial fibrosis (Fig. 9.5).

Specific Considerations for CMR Reporting in TOF

Pulmonary Regurgitation and Other Valvar Assessments

CMR plays an important role in the assessment of pulmonary regurgitation, which is common two to three decades after repair of TOF (Fig. 9.6). Pulmonary regurgitation is implicated in progressive RV dysfunction, arrhythmia and sudden cardiac death. Free pulmonary regurgitation is whereby there is no effective valvar function apparent both with anatomical features on cine imaging and when forward and reverse flow jets on in-plane velocity mapping are equal in diameter. Free pulmonary regurgitation may be tolerated without symptoms for decades and is typically associated with a regurgitant fraction of approximately 30–40 % (in the absence of additional distal branch or peripheral PA stenosis). This discrepancy with aortic regurgitation assessment is for two reasons. Firstly, as in the Fontan circulation, forward pulmonary flow can occur in the absence of an RV due to the effects of inspiration and also because the left ventricle ejects blood out of the thoracic cavity creating a negative pressure that sucks blood into the PA. Secondly, the pulmonary microvascular resis-

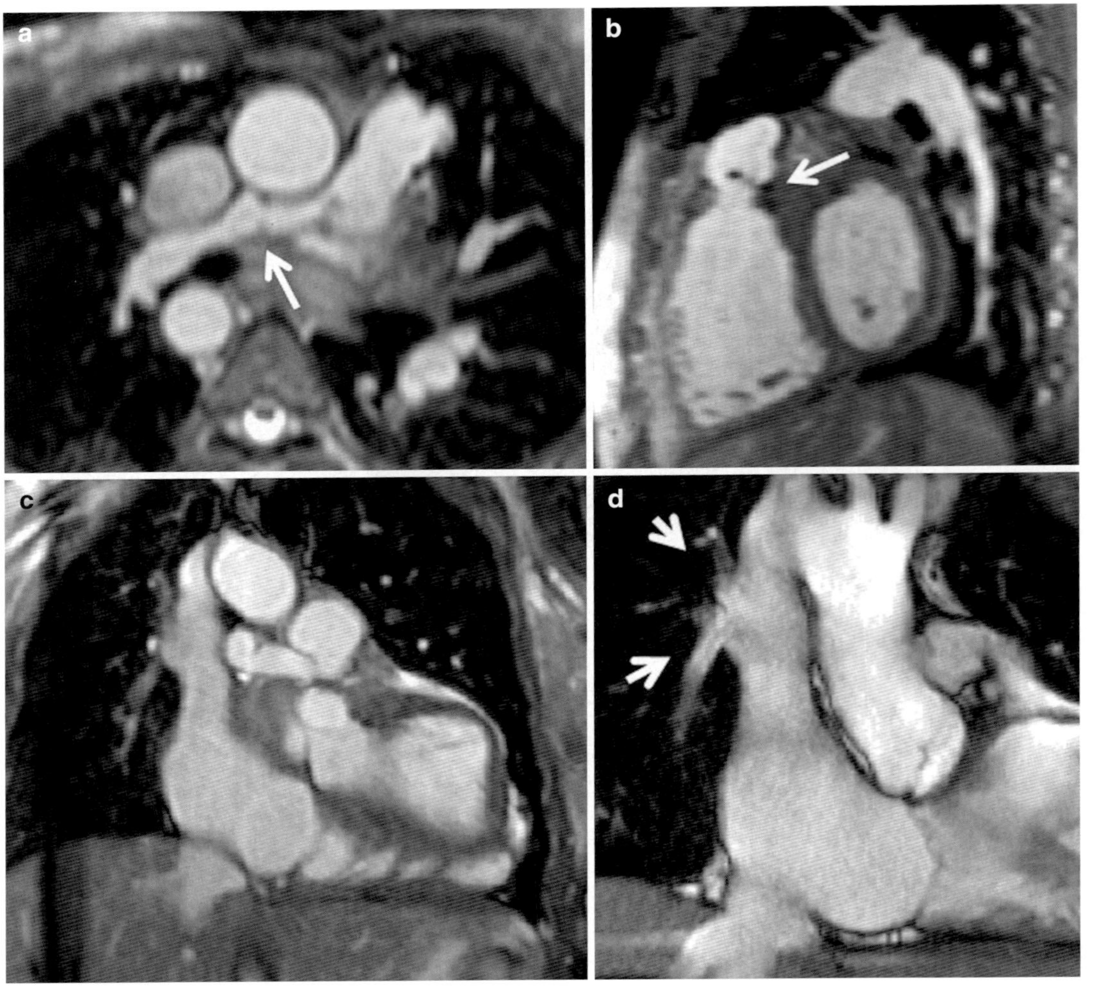

Fig. 9.4 Utility of 3D assessment. Still images from 3D balanced steady-state free precession (bSSFP) acquisition in diastole in transaxial (**a**), sagittal (**b**) and coronal (**c**) orientations. (**a**) Shows the distorted small right pulmonary artery (RPA) (*arrow*). (**b**) Shows a fixed pulmonary valve leaflet (*arrow*). (**c**) Shows anomalous right pulmonary venous drainage to the superior vena cava and a small field of view cine (**d**) was subsequently piloted to show the right upper lobe pulmonary vein and right middle lobe pulmonary vein returning to the superior vena cava (*arrows* in d). This was associated with a Qp:Qs of 1.3:1. The 3D data set was very useful to delineate the two small anomalous right-sided pulmonary venous vessels

tance is low and situated relatively near to the heart. As a result RV systole moves blood through the pulmonary microcirculation including capillaries into the low pressure pulmonary veins. Flow that passes through alveolar capillaries does not pass back again in diastole as there is no significant reversal of gradient. Thus, the magnitude of the regurgitant fraction is limited unless there are additional factors such as branch PA stenosis which may increase regurgitation leading to progressive RV dysfunction [13]. The calculated pulmonary regurgitant fraction may be lower despite ineffective valve function if there is valvar or subvalvar RVOT obstruction or an incompliant RV but higher if there is distal pulmonary stenosis and pulmonary hypertension (rare in this condition but could be present related to, e.g. a previous Waterston shunt) or with increased pulmonary arterial compliance [14]. Arguably, pulmonary regurgitant volume may be more relevant

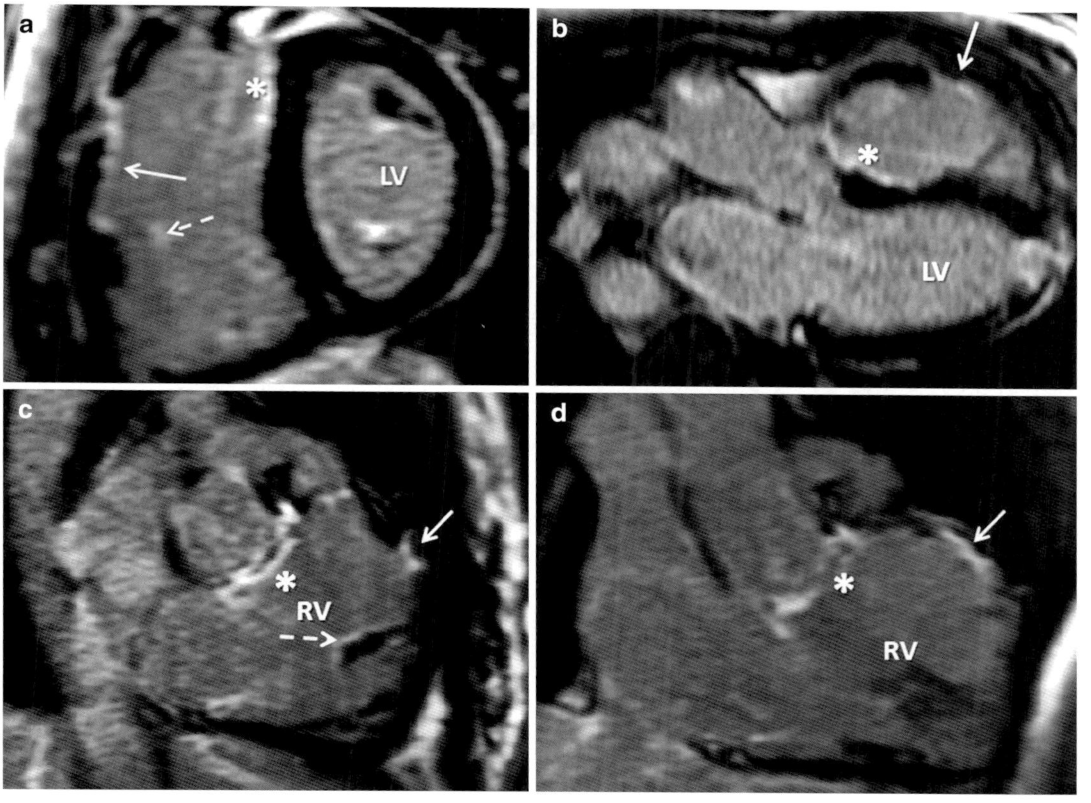

Fig. 9.5 Need for long-axis right ventricle (*RV*) views for late contrast enhancement (*LGE*) in TOF. A mid short-axis view is shown late after administration of intravenous gadolinium (**a**) demonstrating right ventricle outflow tract (*RVOT*) LGE with endocardial extension in the anterior RV free wall. There is also ventricular septal defect (*VSD*) site scar (*asterisk*) and both LV papillary muscles have LGE. In one view, it is not possible to clearly ascertain whether other faint enhancement is all due to the tricuspid valve. (**b**) Shows the VSD patch site scar (*asterisk*) and RVOT scar (*solid arrow*) as well as LGE in the left ventricle (*LV*) apex consistent with apical vent. (**c** and **d**) Show VSD patch scar (*asterisk*), small-degree RVOT scarring (*solid arrow*) and scarring in RV trabeculation (*dotted arrow*) confirmed in another RV in and out images in systole and after phase swap. This small LGE focus is also seen in image (a) (*dotted arrow*)

[15]. Pulmonary regurgitation also varies with respiration [16]. Serial scans allow monitoring of the severity of pulmonary regurgitation in tandem with the effects of chronic volume overload on biventricular haemodynamics and function. Once pulmonary regurgitation is moderate or severe, clinical decision-making with regard to timing of pulmonary valve implantation is influenced by RV volumes. PVR improves biventricular mechanics and patient symptoms (Fig. 9.7).

Tricuspid regurgitation may be found in association with dilatation of the RV related to pulmonary regurgitation and less commonly in isolation due to damage at surgery or congenitally dysplastic tricuspid valve. Dedicated cross-cuts of jets on cines will be needed, and the degree of regurgitation can be assessed from a throughplane flow image of the regurgitant jet and from tricuspid regurgitant fraction (difference between RV stroke volume and forward flow in the PA at pulmonary trunk velocity mapping divided by total RV stroke volume and expressed as a percentage). Aortic regurgitation may be associated with aortic root dilatation and can be quantified by aortic regurgitant fraction calculated from velocity mapping located at the sinotubular junction. Mitral regurgitation is rare.

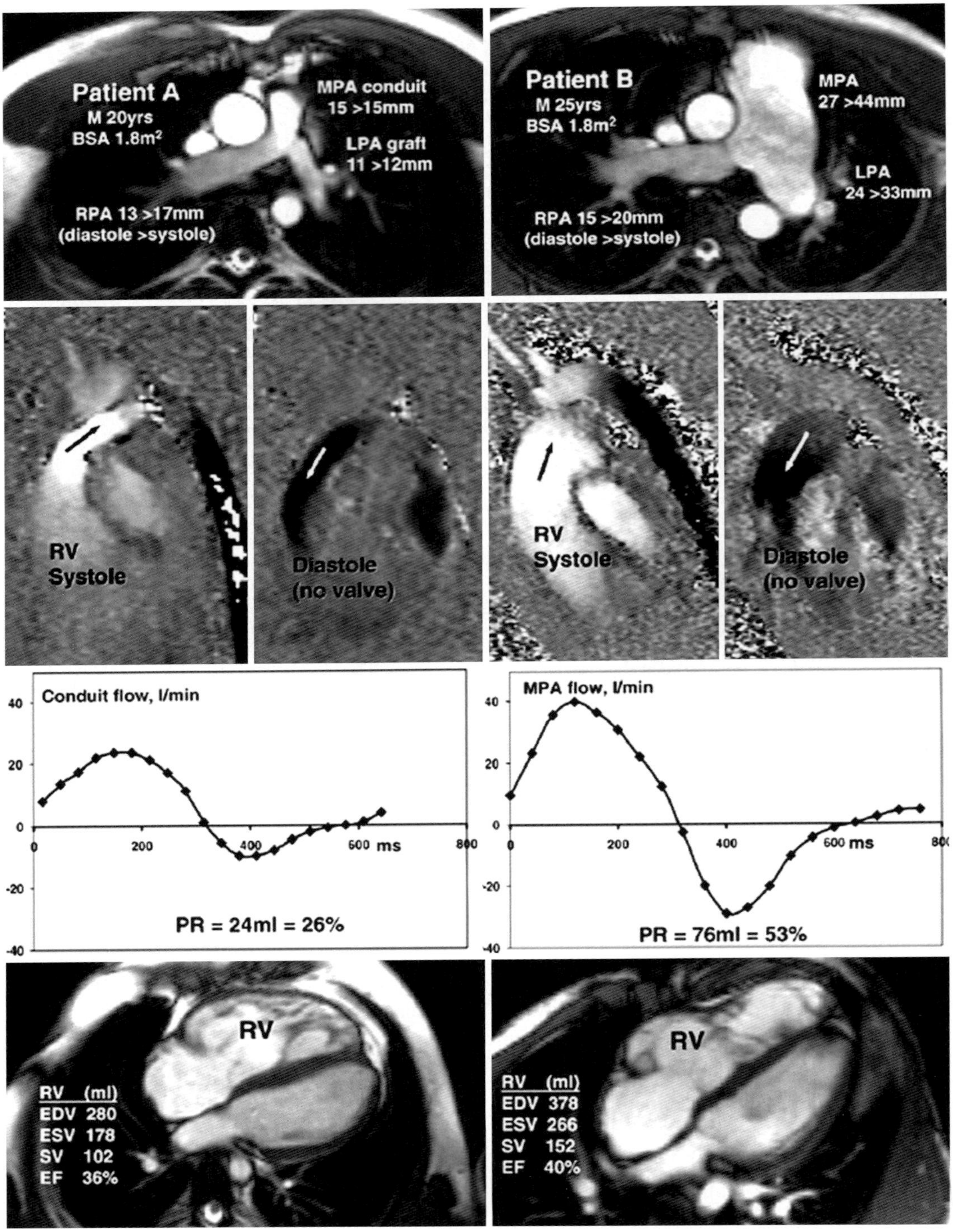
Patient A
M 20yrs
BSA 1.8m²
MPA conduit
15 >15mm
LPA graft
11 >12mm
RPA 13 >17mm
(diastole >systole)
Patient B
M 25yrs
BSA 1.8m²
MPA
27 >44mm
LPA
24 >33mm
RPA 15 >20mm
(diastole >systole)
RV
Systole
Diastole
(no valve)
RV
Systole
Diastole
(no valve)
Conduit flow, l/min
PR = 24ml = 26%
MPA flow, l/min
PR = 76ml = 53%
ms
RV
RV (ml)
EDV 280
ESV 178
SV 102
EF 36%
RV
RV (ml)
EDV 378
ESV 266
SV 152
EF 40%

Global and Regional Ventricular Function Assessment and Ventricular–Ventricular Interaction

CMR makes a very valuable assessment of both right and left ventricular function. Geometrical assumptions that are relied upon using echocardiography are totally unsuitable to the tripartite RV that unlike the left does not approximate an ellipsoid shape. Furthermore, in TOF the RV is yet more complex due to alterations from surgical intervention. Volumes, mass and ejection fraction for the RV are not encumbered by geometrical assumptions when using CMR for analysis.

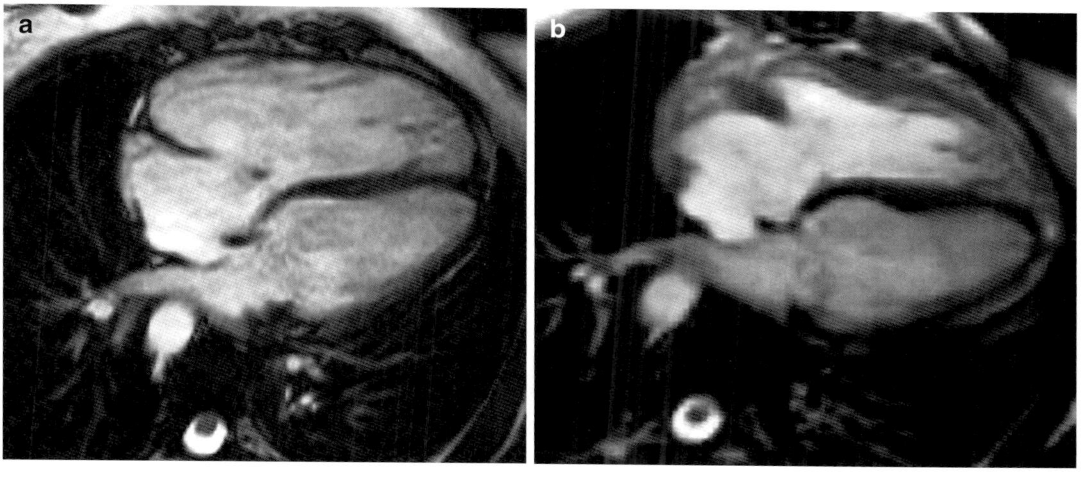

Fig. 9.7 Effect of pulmonary valve regurgitation on biventricular mechanics. Diastolic frame from four-chamber cine preceding pulmonary valve replacement for pulmonary regurgitation in the setting of TOF (**a**) compared with diastolic four-chamber cine after pulmonary valve replacement (**b**). In image **b** versus **a**, the right ventricle can be seen to have reduced in size, there is no longer a small jet of tricuspid regurgitation, and left ventricular diastolic filling appears to have increased

Fig. 9.6 Differing pulmonary regurgitation fraction with ineffective pulmonary valve in TOF. CMR studies in two patients, neither with an effective pulmonary valve but with different amounts of pulmonary regurgitation. Patient A (*left panels*) with TOF was repaired using a right ventricle (*RV*) to pulmonary artery (*PA*) homograft conduit with graft augmentation of the proximal LPA. Patient B (*right panels*) with similar body surface area, born with pulmonary and subpulmonary stenosis and a ventricular septal defect, had patch reconstruction of the RVOT aged 2 years. Cine imaging (*upper row*) showed marked differences of size and expansion of the proximal pulmonary arteries, replaced by a conduit and graft in patient A but dilated and expansile in patient B, as indicated by the end-diastolic peak systolic diameter measurements shown. In-plane, vertically encoded velocity maps aligned with the RV outflow tract (*second row*) show no effective valve action in diastole. Flow curves (*third row*) were plotted from retrospectively gated acquisitions of velocities through planes transecting the proximal main PA or conduit, giving the regurgitant volumes and fractions. The peak systolic velocity was 3 m/s in the conduit of patient A and 1 m/s in the main PA of patient B. Patient A had a higher heart rate and a less dilated RV as shown by the four-chamber cines and right ventricular volume measurements (*bottom row*). *M* male, *BSA* body surface area, *MPA* main pulmonary artery, *RPA* right pulmonary artery, *LPA* left pulmonary artery, *RV* right ventricle, *PR* pulmonary regurgitation, *EDV* end-diastolic volume, *ESV* end-systolic volume, *SV* stroke volume, *EF* ejection fraction (From Kilner et al. [14] with permission)

Therefore, for volumetric function quantification, CMR is a gold standard for the RV. As discussed below, it is also highly suitable to assessment for regional RV abnormality most commonly affecting the outflow tract in TOF. There is interest in so-called ventricular interaction in TOF. Certainly RV volumes and function relate to LV volumes and function in this condition [17, 18], which may be explained by a number of factors, some of which are perhaps unsurprising. These include shared pericardium, a parallel circulation, a shared septum and interdigitation of the RV and LV myocardial fibres. It seems that in the late follow-up of repaired TOF, LV dysfunction may be a consequence of RV dysfunction.

Global Assessment of Ventricular Volumes, Mass and Function

There is no doubt that CMR is the gold standard technique for right as well as left ventricular volume assessment and no other technique has as excellent a reproducibility. This quality of CMR is the reason fewer patients are needed to power clinical trials [19]. However, there are important differences in approaches and measurements made by different operators across various institutions. Awareness of these is important to determine the applicability of published literature to the individual patient in an individual institution. Defining the valve planes may be ambiguous. The pulmonary valve may be absent or just a small remnant. The basal short-axis slice may include right atrial tissue even in systole when the RV is dilated. In the context of a heavily trabeculated ventricle, the volumes may be operator dependent. Whether the approach chosen is a transaxial ventricular volume stack or short axis and whether the trabeculations are excluded from the blood pool or ignored, each operator and centre requires a robust and reproducible protocol. A transaxial stack approach has been argued for because some operators have found it more reproducible and certainly it may be easier to determine the tricuspid valve plane. An argument in favour of a short-axis approach is that TOF is a biventricular disease. LV dysfunction is an important predictor of mortality, though it is likely to develop late and partly as a consequence of RV dysfunction. Given right as well as left ventricular volumes are valuable, having an approach that may be easier for the RV but requiring the LV to be measured at a different time with a different data set adds time and biological variability to the CMR study. In TOF, RV assessment is as pertinent as the left but poses challenges in accurately assessing the thin myocardium and coarse trabeculations, which increase towards the apex. These complex trabeculations increase in the presence of RV hypertrophy and can be difficult to visualise and outline individually. Ignoring RV trabeculations may be a more rapid and reproducible way [20] to approach ventricular volume assessment. However, not only may this be inaccurate for RV mass measurement but as others have also stated, this leads to incorrectly large volume estimates for the RV and prohibits the internal validation of stroke volumes through comparison with aortic and pulmonary flow volumes [21]. Our own practice is to exclude trabeculations from the blood pool (Fig. 9.8). Careful demarcation of the borders of the RV can give highly reproducible results even in the context of complex operated RVs in TOF. [22] Whilst reproducible with a single experienced operator, this method is labour intensive and requires at least 30 min per patient. However, for research, this degree of reproducibility enabled adequate powering of a randomised controlled trial in repaired TOF with chronic pulmonary regurgitation to assess the effects of ramipril (the APPROPRIATE study) [23].

Consistency between serial measurements should be optimised through standardisation of scanning approaches and protocols and regular quality assurance. Practically, because intraobserver variability is lower [22], it may be important for a single operator to remeasure a previous CMR scan at the time of a current report to be certain if there is true change in RV ventricular volumes. Awareness of technical issues regarding acquisition and analysis is important as RV volume measurements are pivotal to clinical decision-making regarding the indications for pulmonary valve implantation in asymptomatic patients and assessment of the haemodynamic benefits of surgery.

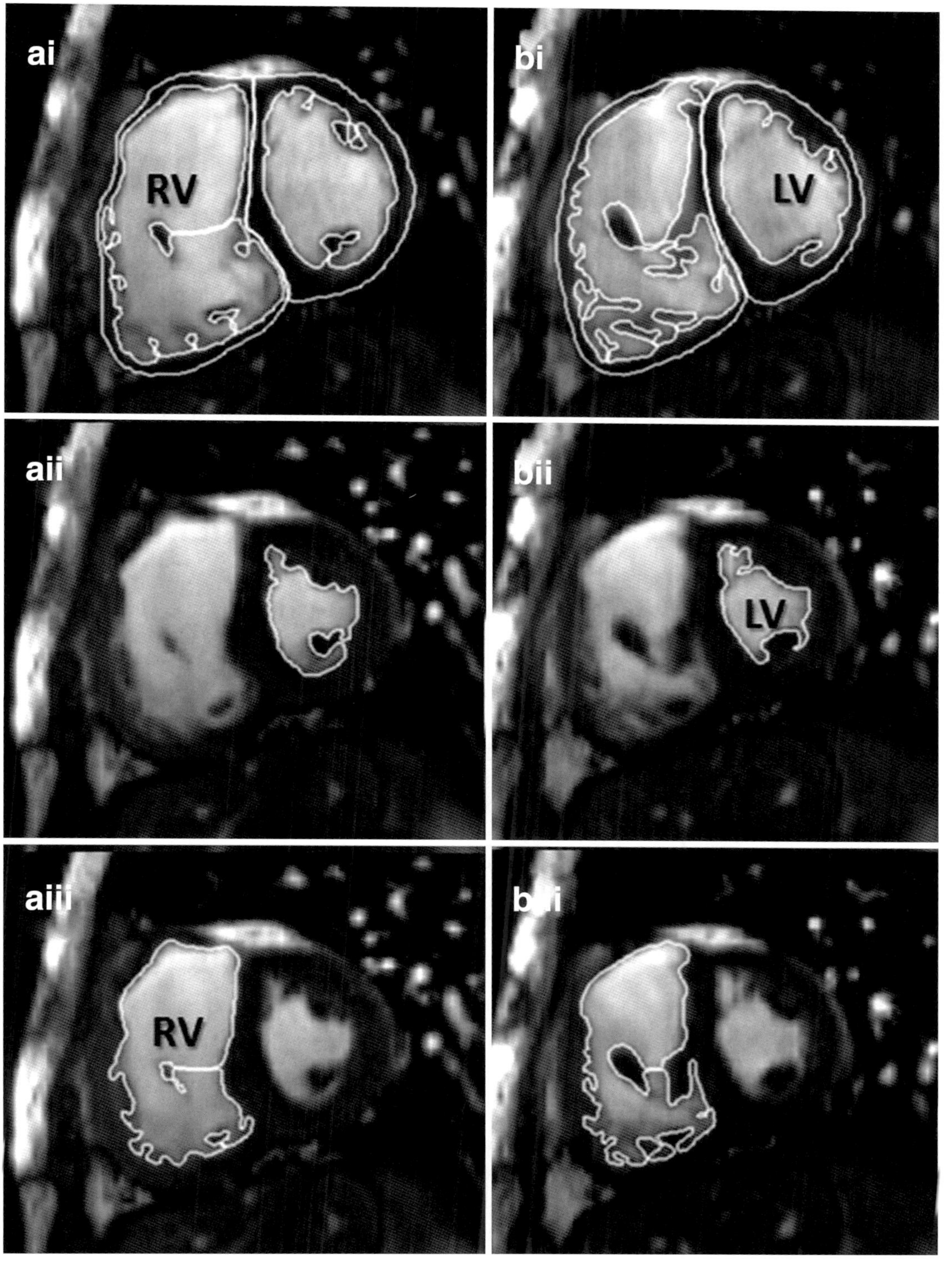

Fig. 9.8 Example of contouring right ventricle (*RV*) volumes in TOF. Manual planimetry of short-axis contiguous slices from base to apex of the heart has proven highly reproducible for research in our centre. Trabeculations will be excluded from the blood pool and included in the ventricular mass. In this example at levels a and b, RV end systole (**aiii** and **biii**) was in a different frame from left ventricular end systole (**aii** and **bii**) consistent with the patient having wide right bundle branch block. End diastole (**ai** and **bi**) for both ventricles are synchronous. *LV* left ventricle

Numerous contributions have been made to the literature in the last 10 years describing the value of CMR RV volume assessment for determining indications for pulmonary valve replacement [24–32] though still more data are needed to determine optimal timing in asymptomatic TOF patients. Oosterhof et al. have implied surgical PVR should be carried out before RV end-diastolic volume exceeds 160 mL/m^2 or RV end-systolic volume >82 mL/m^2 as these thresholds predict return of RV volumes to normal size following PVR [30]. Another group found RV end-systolic volume <90 mL/m^2 to be a predictor of normal RV size and function postoperatively [33]. The implication is that beyond this degree of RV dilatation, there is limited reversibility of RV dilatation and dysfunction. Other authors suggest PVR might be indicated even earlier before RV end-diastolic volume exceeds 150 mL/m^2 [28, 31]. In a number of centres, an RV:LV diastolic volume ratio of ≥2:1 is also considered significant. Consensus has been established amongst ACHD clinicians that the previous clinical management of operating on repaired TOF patients later when symptoms are established is too late.

European Society of Cardiology (ESC) Guidelines for ACHD [34] advocate pulmonary valve replacement in symptomatic TOF patients with severe pulmonary regurgitation and/or stenosis with RV systolic pressure >60 mmHg/TR velocity >3.5 m/s with a Class 1 indication. In asymptomatic patients, Class IIa indications for pulmonary valve intervention in the presence of severe pulmonary regurgitation and/or stenosis are:

- An objective decrease in exercise capacity has been demonstrated.
- Progressive RV dilatation on CMR.
- Progressive RV systolic dysfunction.
- Progressive (at least moderate) tricuspid regurgitation.
- RVOT obstruction with RV systolic pressure >80 mmHg/TR velocity >4.3 m/s.
- Sustained atrial and/or ventricular arrhythmias.

These guidelines are not prescriptive with regard to nonserial CMR measures. In our centre RV:LV ratio ≥2:1 with RVEDVi >150 mL/m^2 usually prompts multidisciplinary discussion of elective pulmonary valve implantation which is an individualised decision based also on non-CMR-based data such as objectively measured exercise capacity.

Regional Assessment of the RV Including Akinetic Outflow Tract Regions

In older patients, reflecting the earlier era of TOF repair, akinetic and or aneurismal areas in the RVOT are common and present even in the absence of patch reconstruction of the RVOT [17] (Fig. 9.9). Given the limits of the RV are the tricuspid and pulmonary valves, any akinetic or aneurismal region in the RVOT is included in the ventricular volumes. Such akinetic and or aneurismal regions are adverse not only as they relate to RV systolic dysfunction [17] but also because they cause conduction delay within the RV contributing to prolonged QRS duration [35] and are associated with scar [36, 37]. These dilated or dyskinetic RVOT regions therefore lower the calculated ejection fraction as they are included in the ventricular volume. The disadvantage of including them is that small progressive reductions in function of the contractile RV beneath the akinetic area may be masked. A reproducible method to characterise the function of these regions separately is, however, not widely available. We report a simple linear measurement based on the sagittal RVOT view. We use this feasible measure to help describe the relative contribution of outflow tract pathology to impaired RV ejection fraction and to describe size. Recently a prospective follow-up study for clinical outcomes demonstrated that larger akinetic area length predicted sustained ventricular arrhythmia [38]. Routine views such as four-chamber cine may be misleadingly normal, whereas long-axis views (RV outflow tract, LV outflow tract, oblique RV views) are more likely to show wall thinning and regional motion abnormality because the primary pathology is of the RV infundibulum.

Global and Regional LV Dysfunction

LV regional wall motion abnormality may be present in TOF. A small area (<1 cm) at the apex may be present and related to apical

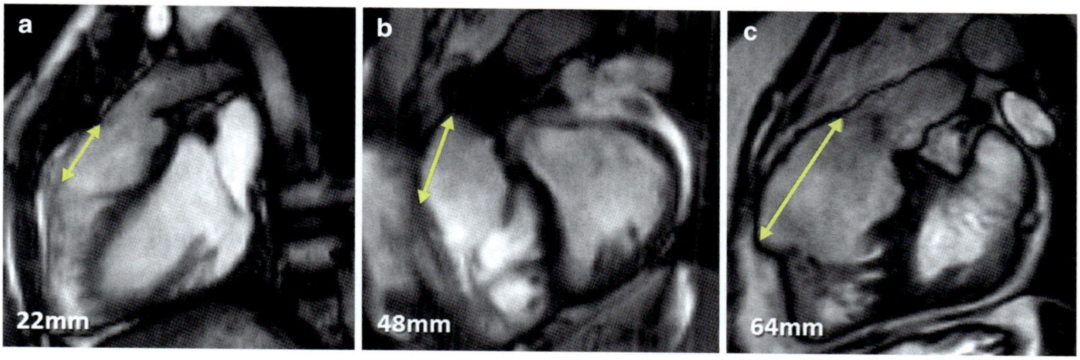

Fig. 9.9 Right ventricle outflow tract (RVOT) akinetic area in TOF. Examples of simple linear RVOT measurements in sagittal RVOT planes in TOF patients A, B and C are shown. These measurements should be taken after also reviewing the left ventricular outflow tract plane as well as the short-axis stack. Not all akinetic areas are necessarily associated with RVOT patching and muscle bundle resection alone can result in thinning and regional wall motion abnormality. Artefact in the pulmonary trunk of patient B is due to previous percutaneous pulmonary valve implantation

vent insertion at the time of surgery in order to deair the heart. However, more extensive abnormalities have been noted and associated with scarring either in small localised areas or in a larger anteroapical distribution [36]. Local injury at the time of vent insertion, damage to coronary arteries perioperatively and anomalous coronary artery disease or coronary embolism could explain this regional scarring. Global LV dysfunction may also be a late consequence of RV dysfunction due to ventricular–ventricular interaction as discussed above. Additionally, aortic valve regurgitation, late repair, residual ventricular septal defects, prolonged cardiopulmonary bypass and acquired heart disease including hypertension and coronary artery disease may have a role.

Right Atrial Area

Right atrial dilatation is associated with atrial arrhythmia, the most common arrhythmia burden in TOF and associated with morbidity [39]. Maximum right atrial area from four-chamber cine CMR indexed to body surface area appears to be a useful predictor of future atrial arrhthmogenesis [38] which may be corroborated in future studies. Dilated right atrium is associated with restrictive RV physiology [38] and tricuspid regurgitation.

Branch Pulmonary Artery Stenosis

Branch PA stenosis is a potential therapeutic target in repaired TOF, and meticulous cine plane selection should be undertaken to obtain left and right PA views, in addition to a PA bifurcation view. 3D CMR is useful for imaging discrete branch PA stenosis especially in complex bifurcation pathology and for imaging distal PA lesions. In-plane images of branch PA stenoses can be utilised to plan alignment of through-plane views for assessment of peak velocity in stenotic regions. A combination of anatomical findings, distal pulsatility on cine imaging and the results of differential lung perfusion calculated from velocity mapping in each branch PA is used to determine degree of pulmonary stenosis. Flow through branch pulmonary arteries is measured to determine differential lung perfusion. Throughplane velocity mapping is usually aligned in the mid branch PA perpendicular to the walls in two cine views. This method shows good agreement with radionuclide lung perfusion imaging [40] but avoids the ionising radiation inherent to nuclear imaging. There is usually preferential blood flow to the right lung such that in the normal circulation, 60 % of main PA blood flow goes to the right lung and 40 % to the left. In addition, reduced distal pulsatility suggests more functionally significant stenosis.

Aortic Assessment in the Repaired TOF Patient

Note should be made whether the aorta is right or left sided. Aortopathy is recognised in TOF, with aortic root dilatation greater in patients with unrepaired or late repair of TOF and pulmonary atresia. Progressive aortic root dilatation seems to occur in a subset of patients [41] and lead to aortic regurgitation, which may require surgical intervention. Rare case reports have been made of aortic dissection in very dilated aortas in TOF. This process is related to early left-sided volume overload prior to repair and intrinsic abnormalities of the aortic wall including cystic medial necrosis [41, 42]. Dilatation affects the ascending aorta, not just the aortic root in some patients, and CMR imaging should include at least 2 cine views for serial assessment of the aorta (Fig. 9.10). 3D CMR may be useful in the follow-up of patients with known aortopathy. Care must be taken to document where measures are taken and whether measurements are taken in systole or diastole.

Assessment of Major Aortopulmonary Collateral Arteries (MAPCAs)

3D CE-MRA with bSSFP and fat suppression will provide robust visualisation of MAPCAs with clear delineation of spatial relationship of MAPCAs in relation to surrounding structures in addition to their course, origin and pulmonary connections. Noninvasive CMR findings have been shown to correlate completely with transcatheter and surgical findings [43] and potentially to be more accurate than cardiac catheterisation [44].

Dual-source computer tomography (CT) angiography provides complementary information to CMR assessment of MAPCAs, with shorter examination times and high spatial resolution, although exposure to ionising radiation needs to be considered in CHD patients requiring lifelong follow-up and serial imaging. CT angiography is the imaging modality of choice in patients with pacemakers who require imaging surveillance for MAPCAs.

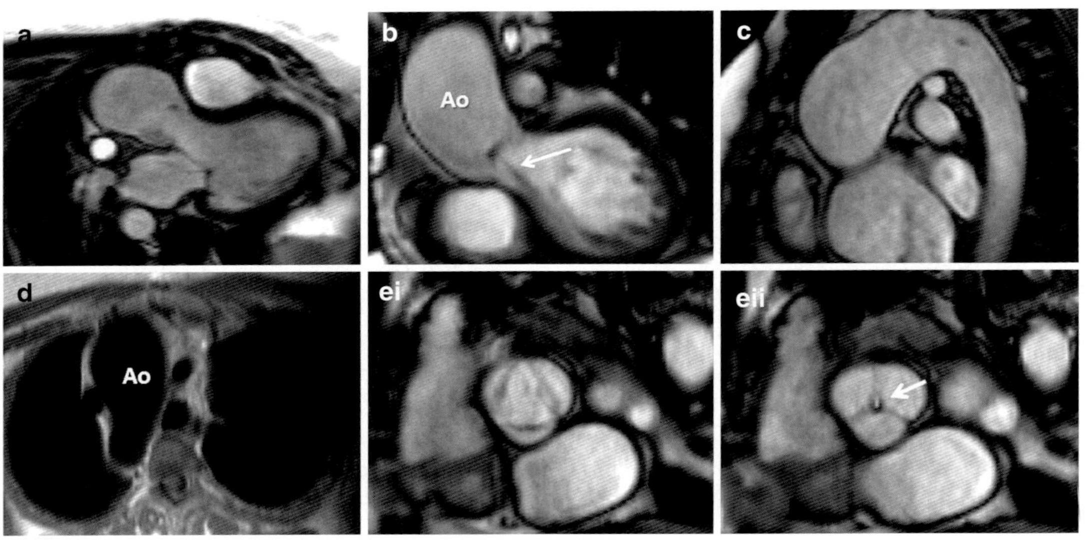

Fig. 9.10 Dilated aorta in TOF. A dilated aorta (*Ao*) in the setting of adult repaired TOF is shown in left ventricular outflow tract (**a**), coronal cross-cut left ventricular outflow tract (**b**) and ascending and arch (**c**) cine views. The maximum dimension at right pulmonary artery level could not have been documented without cross-sectional imaging and was 48 mm. The aortic arch was right sided (**d**). The aortic valve (**ei**) showed failure of central coaptation of the valve leaflets (**eii**) allowing aortic regurgitation (*arrow*). The diastolic still frame in b shows the jet of aortic regurgitation (*arrow*) in which, from multiple views, stroke volume difference and aortic regurgitation fraction were mild to moderate in severity

Anatomy of Coronary Arteries in TOF

CMR three-dimensional angiography delineates the origin and proximal course of the coronary arteries, whilst CT coronary angiography can provide detailed reconstructions of the coronary tree. These imaging modalities facilitate anatomical identification and provide spatial information to minimise the risk of damage or dissection during planned valve surgery or transcatheter pulmonary valve implantation.

Coronary anomalies are common in TOF, occurring in 5–12 % of patients in reported series [10]. A common important coronary anomaly (~4 % of patients) [10] is an anomalous left anterior descending arising from right coronary artery or right sinus of Valsalva and coursing anterior to the RVOT. This is important as if identified pre-repair, the surgical approach preferred may be the insertion of an RV–PA conduit to bypass the native RVOT–PA connection and avoid coronary arterial damage (Fig. 9.11). This anatomy may also make a percutaneous pulmonary valve approach unsuitable [45]. Other anomalies include a single coronary artery typically arising from the left coronary system and less commonly coronary to bronchial artery anastamoses and coronary fistulas.

ECG-gated CT is the imaging modality of choice for coronary anomalies with sensitivity

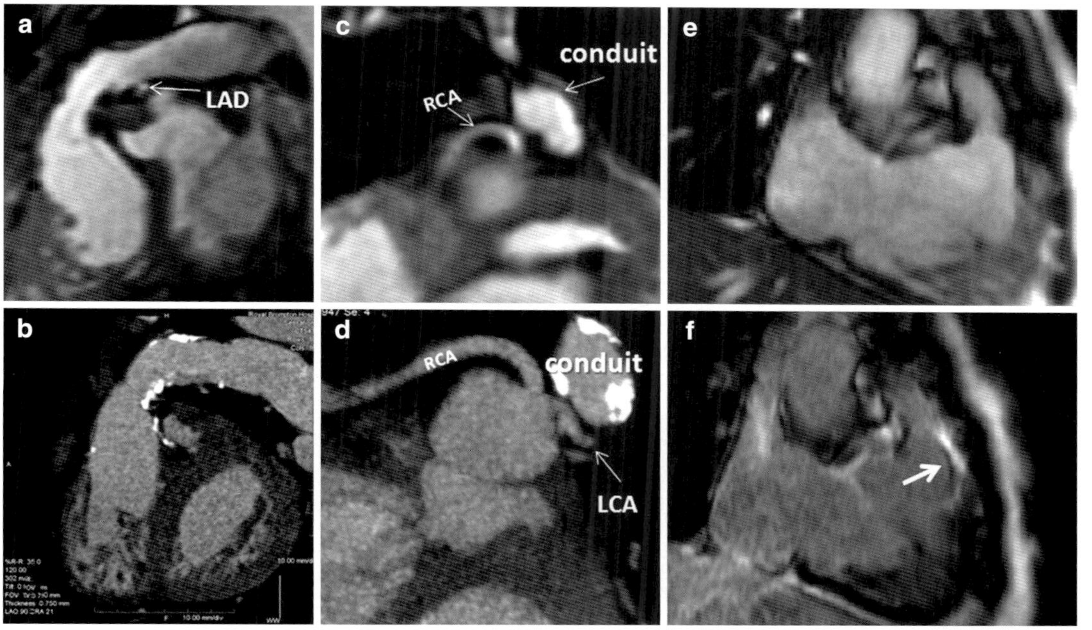

Fig. 9.11 Conduit assessment. Single image from 3D balanced steady-state free precession (**a** and **c**) and corresponding cardiac CT post-contrast images (**b** and **d**) in a TOF patient with pulmonary atresia variant and previous right ventricle to pulmonary artery (RV–PA) homograft repair being considered for percutaneous pulmonary valve implantation (PPVI) for severe pulmonary regurgitation and stenosis. The conduit was easily imaged by both techniques. From the interventionalist's viewpoint, knowledge of the relationships of proximal coronary arteries to the conduit and the preprocedure knowledge of the calcium distribution inform judgements in the catheter laboratory. In this case, the right coronary artery (*RCA*) passed close to a narrow part of the conduit, an area that warrants target intervention to relieve obstruction. The decision made was that it was reasonable to proceed with attempted PPVI knowing there was an increased chance the procedure might be abandoned after selective cannulation and imaging of the coronary arteries simultaneous with balloon dilatation. In fact, the patient underwent successful PPVI. However, transcatheter therapy for valve implantation does not address inherent undesirable qualities of the RV outflow tract, a substrate for future ventricular arrhythmia. Image (**e**), a still frame from an RV oblique cine and its corresponding late enhancement image (**f**) show enhancement in the RV outflow tract (*arrow*) (Non-CMR data with kind permission of Drs Michael Rubens and Anselm Uebing, Royal Brompton Hospital). *LCA* left coronary artery

80–90 % [46] as it is able to both delineate calcium and provide high spatial resolution information regarding the coronary arteries, both of which may be desirable for the invasive cardiologist planning a transcatheter intervention. CMR provides complementary information about the origin and proximal course of the coronary arteries and 3D bSSFP can usually also assess relationships of coronary arteries to the previous sternotomy or RVOT.

Residual Intracardiac Shunts and Right Ventricular Outflow Tract Obstruction

VSD patch leaks in repaired TOF patients may have haemodynamic consequences amenable to percutaneous or surgical intervention. LV outflow tract, RV in and out, RV oblique and short-axis cine views should be routinely scrutinised for jets suggestive of shunts. Cross-cutting relevant short-axis images where there is a suspected jet core can be performed to visualise the intracardiac shunt. Commonly a residual patch leak may be best seen in RV in and out or RV oblique cine views which show the surgical patch beneath the aortic valve. Other residual VSD locations can be demonstrated including from previously operated or unoperated additional VSDs (Fig. 9.12). Shunt calculation (Qp:Qs) should be undertaken to determine if haemodynamically significant shunt is present.

Residual RVOT obstruction (peak velocity 3 m/s or more) may be subvalvar, valvar or supravalvar. Phase velocity mapping in addition to cines plays a valuable role in identifying the level of stenosis and determining the most significant level of stenosis where there is multilevel RV outflow obstruction.

Other Associated Morphological Lesions

Certain additional associated lesions such as left superior vena cava to coronary sinus, atrial septal defect or additional inlet muscular VSD are not uncommon and should be actively sought. As discussed elsewhere in the chapter, right aortic arch is common and coronary artery anomalies may be clinically relevant. An atrioventricular septal defect – usually in the setting of Down syndrome – can coexist with tetralogy in which case the atrioventricular valves may need dedicated assessments.

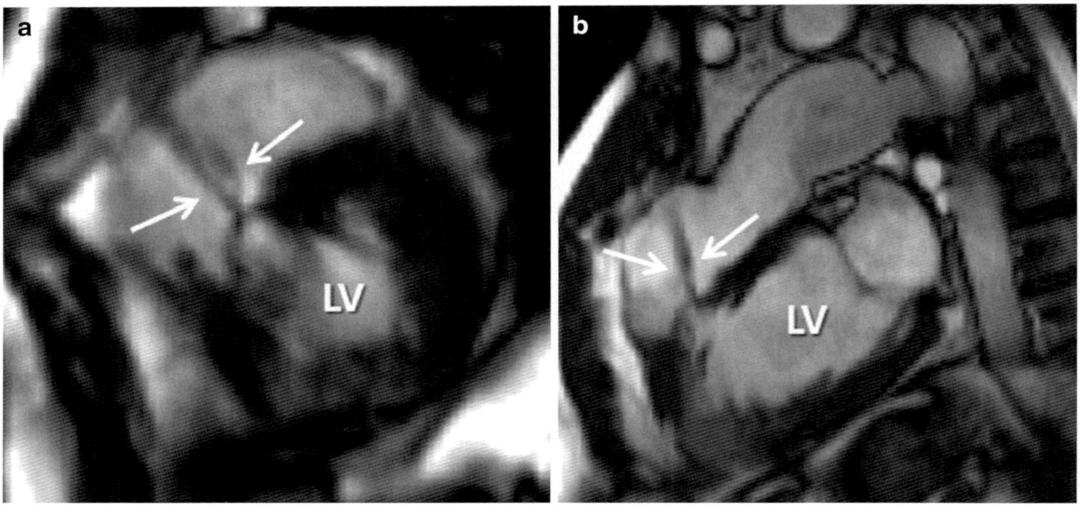

Fig. 9.12 Residual ventricular septal defect (VSD) in TOF patient. An unusual remaining VSD is seen in this patient located in the muscular septum which has possibly been previously patched. The VSD jet (*arrows*) is seen in short-axis (**a**) and right ventricle oblique (**b**) cine views. *LV* left ventricle

Current and Future Roles for LGE CMR in Arrhythmia Prediction in TOF

LGE CMR as a marker of focal myocardial fibrosis may prove to be an important risk factor for tachyarrhythmia and other adverse clinical features in TOF as cross-sectionally more extensive RV LGE was shown to correlate with clinical arrhythmia presentation [36]. In our study of 92 TOF patients, RV LGE was found routinely in patterns and locations consistent with previous surgery but with highly variable extent. These included RVOT free wall which may relate to previous ventriculotomy, RV muscle bundle resection or RVOT patching, the site of perioperative apical vent insertion in the LV and in the outlet septum at the site of previous VSD patching and suturing (Fig. 9.13). Additionally, 'remote' RV LGE was seen in a significant minority of patients in the body of the RV and in areas remote from direct surgical incision and related to higher prevalence of arrhythmia; thus expected site LGE may have differing importance for prediction of arrhythmia than expected site RV LGE. Faint LGE was commonly seen in the inferior and or superior right–left ventricular insertion point. In this context the appearance of LGE is likely to be secondary to RV hypertrophy exaggerating the normally occurring myocardial features of the insertion region as others have described [47]. These were therefore excluded from the semi-quantitative scoring of RV LGE extent used for analysis. The extent of RV LGE in the repaired TOF patient correlated to risk factors for adverse clinical outcomes [36]. Specifically, LGE in right and left ventricles in repaired TOF patients is related to increased age, later age at repair, ventricular dysfunction (RV and LV), restrictive RV physiology, exercise intolerance, neurohormonal activation and clinical presentation with tachyarrhythmia (Fig. 9.14). The latter is highly suggestive of a potential clinical role for LGE CMR in risk stratification for sudden cardiac death and malignant arrhythmias in TOF patients. Of note, LV LGE was also present to an unexpected extent in a subgroup of patients and unrelated to obstructive coronary disease (Fig. 9.15). Commonly, evidence of perioperative apical vent insertion was seen underlining the technique's sensitivity, but other unexpected non-apical vent LV LGE was also seen in a smaller number of patients [36]. The latter, when more extensive, seemed to be anteroapical, but LV LGE, confined to very small mid LV wall areas and papillary muscle, was also seen [36]. To support the view that LGE CMR may have a future role in risk assessment for arrhythmia in ACHD, a recent study in a heterogeneous group of CHD patients correlated lack of LGE with inability to induce ventricular tachycardia at invasive electrophysiology study [48]. Our preliminary work has shown correlation of CMR RV LGE with low-voltage areas at electrophysiology study (Fig. 9.16). Others have also shown that RV LGE is present in TOF patients and associated with regional wall motion abnormality, impaired systolic function and impaired exercise capacity [37]. However, our own previous study of the value of LGE CMR in TOF was cross-sectional and as yet there are no prospective studies of clinical outcomes in longitudinal follow-up to help ascertain the precise prognostic role of LGE CMR in TOF. Furthermore, we cannot know how much LGE is due to early insult from preoperative cyanosis and perioperative factors or whether there is ongoing progressive increase in LGE related to age and adverse haemodynamics.

Future Applications

Whether LGE CMR will prove to have incremental value, when applied to the clinical evaluation of TOF patients compared with ventricular volume and function assessment and other easier and more widely available markers of risk, remains to be proven in longitudinal prospective studies. If LGE CMR and other CMR features contribute in large prospective studies to better identification of patients at most risk of premature death, this will allow referral for surgical, transcatheter or electrophysiological intervention including implantation of an automated internal cardiac defibrillator to be expedited where appropriate and avoidance of the risks and significant morbidity [49–52]. CMR is not only being used in determining indications for

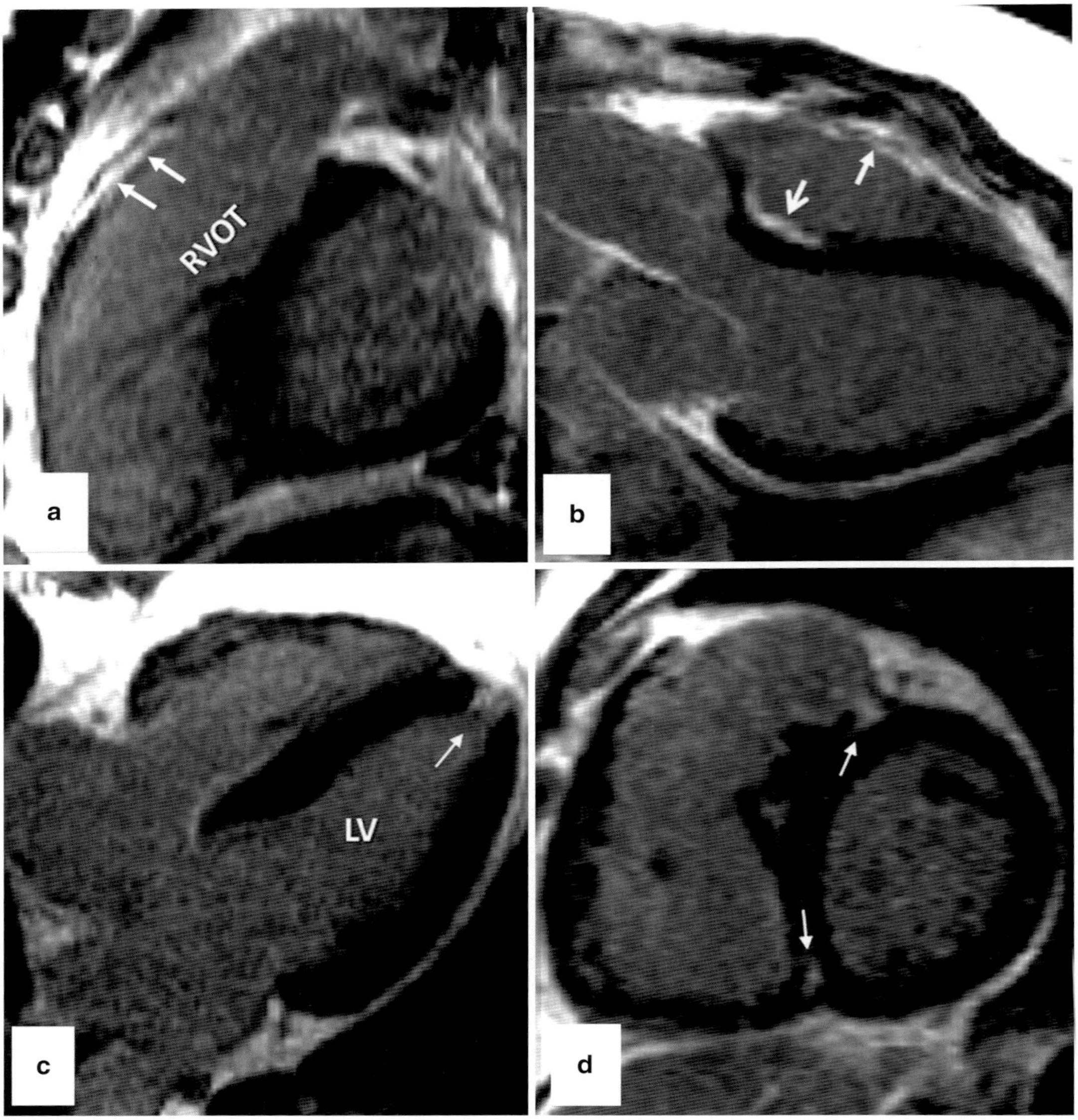

Fig. 9.13 Typical late gadolinium enhancement (*LGE*) locations in adults after TOF repair. Regions affected appear white with LGE in contrast to the black appearance of normal myocardium. Typical sites of LGE in adults after repaired TOF include the anterior wall of the right ventricle outflow tract (*RVOT*) (**a** and *upward pointing arrow* **b**), the region of surgical patching of the ventricular septal defect (b; *downward pointing arrow*), the site of apical vent insertion in the left ventricle (*LV*) where this was part of previous surgery (**c**) and the inferior (*lower arrow*) and superior (*upper arrow*) RV–LV insertion points (**d**), which is very common and not counted in the analysis of extent of LGE (From Babu-Narayan et al. [35] with permission)

procedures and in preprocedure planning but also to innovate newer devices such as implantable valves and predict their success [53–55]. Future roles for CMR in TOF with respect to real time advances for interventional CMR, CMR use in electrophysiological procedures, CMR 4D flow assessment and CMR myocardial assessment with tagging, speckle tracking, T1 mapping or tractography are likely to evolve but currently remain primarily for use in a research setting.

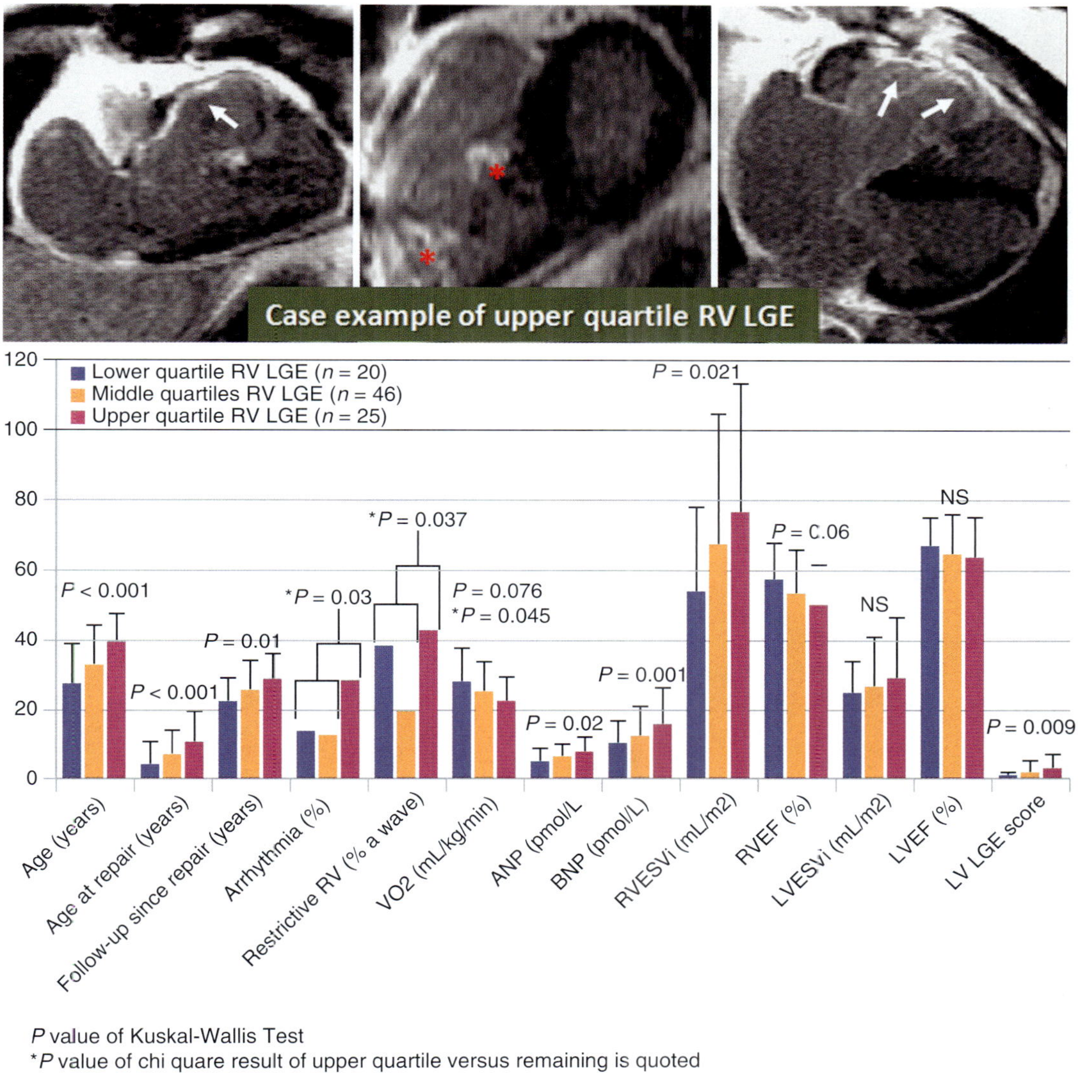

Fig. 9.14 More extensive right ventricle (*RV*) late gadolinium enhancement (*LGE*) relates to adverse clinical features. The *top row* shows a right atrial–right ventricular long-axis, short-axis and four-chamber views in a patient with extensive RV LGE. LGE corresponded to akinesia of the anterior wall on cine imaging, extending more inferiorly than is commonly seen, hence, also seen in the four-chamber view (*arrows*). LGE of the trabeculated RV myocardium was present (*asterisk*). Differences in clinical, neurohormonal and CMR variables between patients classified according to lower-quartile, middle-quartiles and upper-quartile RV LGE extent score are illustrated in the bar chart below. More extensive RV LGE was associated with increased age, later repair, longer follow-up, presentation with clinically documented arrhythmia, restrictive RV physiology defined by anterograde flow in the pulmonary artery with pulse wave echo Doppler present throughout the respiratory cycle, impaired peak oxygen consumption at cardiorespiratory exercise testing, increased atrial and brain natriuretic peptides, increased RV end-systolic volume, impaired RV ejection fraction, increased left ventricle (*LV*) end-systolic volume, impaired LV ejection fraction and increased LV LGE (Adapted from Babu-Narayan et al. [35] with permission)

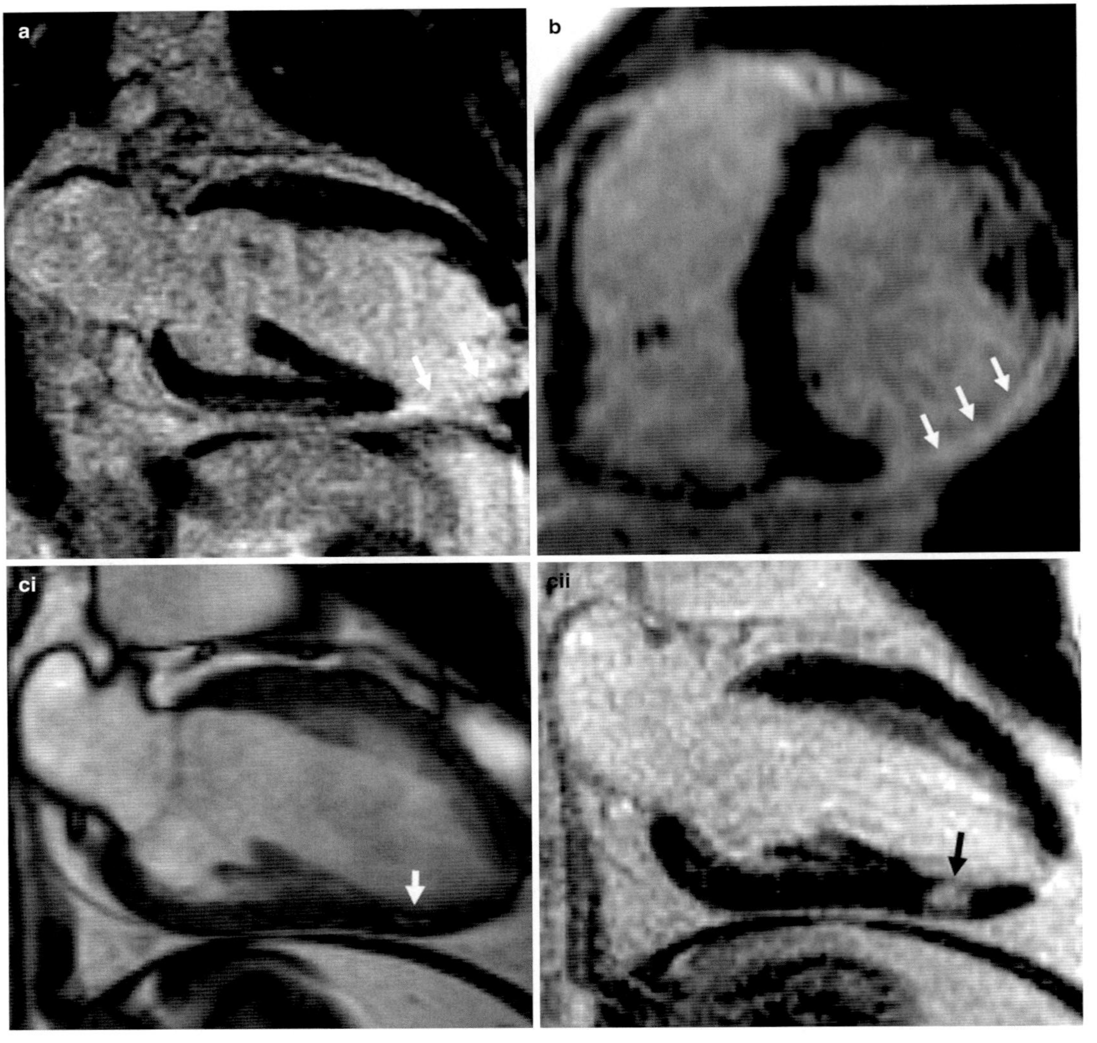

Fig. 9.15 LV late gadolinium enhancement patterns in TOF. Examples of LV LGE late after TOF repair. Images illustrating unexpected LV infarction (*arrows*) in 2 different patients (**a** and **b**). (**c**) Shows a further example of localised LV LGE (*arrows*) in ci and cii another patient. The cine frame in (**ci**) and corresponding LGE image in (**cii**) suggest fibrofatty change in this region (From Babu-Narayan et al. [35] with permission)

Fig. 9.16 Right ventricle (*RV*) late gadolinium enhancement (LGE) associated with RV regional wall motion abnormality and scar at subsequent electrophysiology study. RVOT cine still frames in diastole (**ai**) and systole (**aii**) demonstrate an akinetic area (*arrows*) in the RVOT which corresponds to RV LGE (*arrows*) on inversion recovery sequences late after administration of gadolinium (**aiii**, **aiv**). A contrast-enhanced MR angiography (CE-MRA) was segmented to provide a 3D volume reconstruction for image integration in the electrophysiological procedure (**bi**). From a 3D LGE data set (still frame from 3D (bi) *inset*), the RVOT scar was also segmented and registered to the CE-MRA image (*arrows*) in bi and bii. CMR imaging was integrated with fluoroscopy (**bii**). The magnetic catheter and RV apex catheter used in the procedure are seen (**bii**). Ventricular tachycardia was induced near to the anatomical scar defined by CMR with unstable haemodynamics. Ablation at this site rendered ventricular tachycardia non-inducible

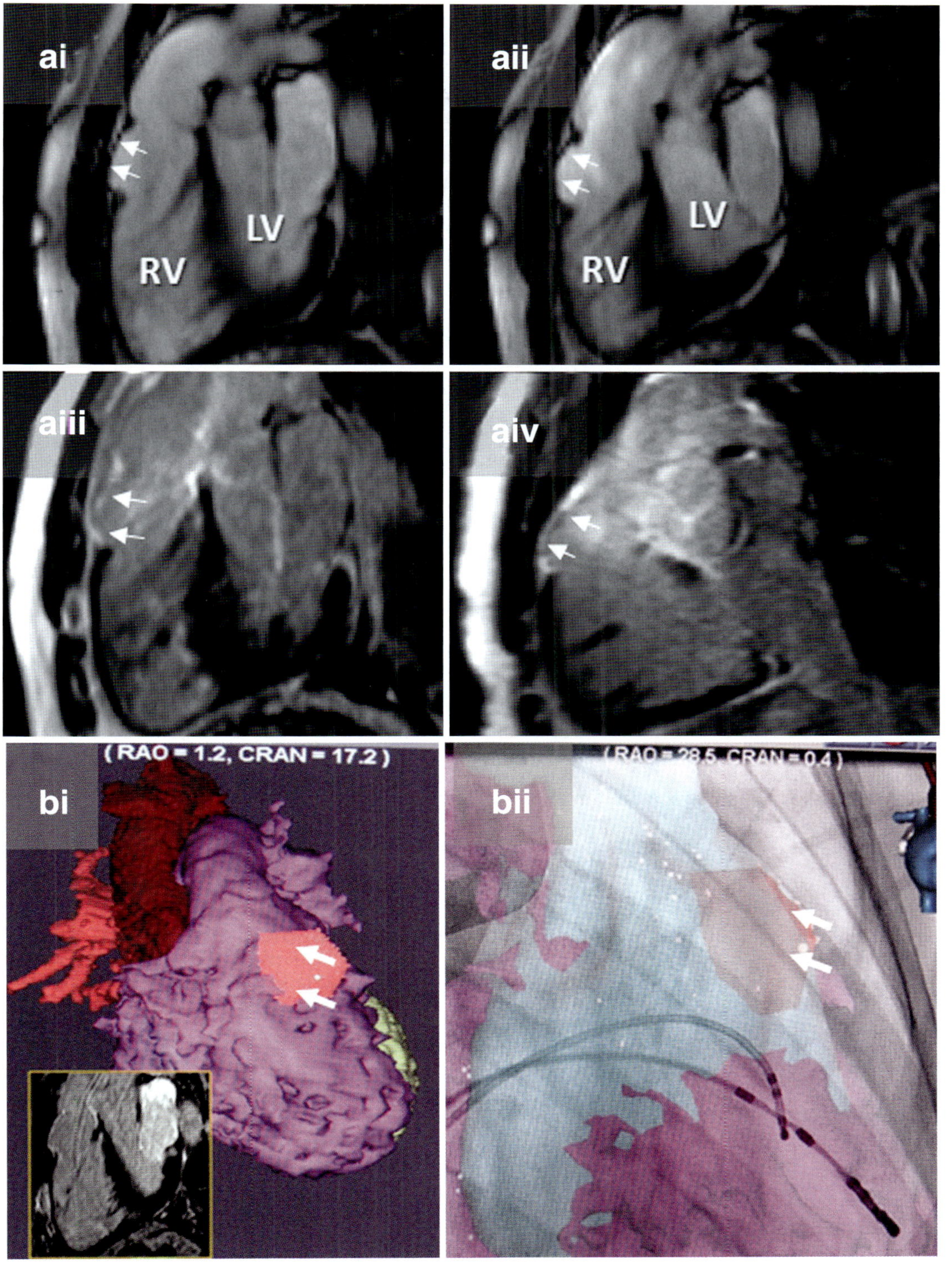
ai
RV
LV
aii
RV
LV
aiii
aiv
(RAO = 1.2, CRAN = 17.2)
bi
bii

Acknowledgments Sonya Babu-Narayan is supported by the British Heart Foundation. This work was supported by the NIHR Cardiovascular Biomedical Research Unit of Royal Brompton and Harefield NHS Foundation Trust and Imperial College London. This report is independent research by the National Institute for Health Research Biomedical Research Unit Funding Scheme. The views expressed in this publication are those of the authors and not necessarily those of the NHS, the National Institute for Health Research or the Department of Health.

References

1. Shinebourne EA, Babu-Narayan SV, Carvalho JS. Tetralogy of Fallot: from fetus to adult. Heart. 2006;92(9):1353–9.
2. Babu-Narayan SV GM. Tetralogy of Fallot. In: Gatzoulis MA, Webb GD, Daubeney PEF, editors. Diagnosis and management of adult congenital heart disease. 2nd ed. Philadelphia: Elsevier Press; 2011. p. 316–28.
3. Gatzoulis MA, Balaji S, Webber SA, Siu SC, Hokanson JS, Poile C, Rosenthal M, Nakazawa M, Moller JH, Gillette PC, Webb GD, Redington AN. Risk factors for arrhythmia and sudden cardiac death late after repair of tetralogy of Fallot: a multicentre study. Lancet. 2000;356(9234):975–81.
4. Hoffmann A, Engelfriet P, Mulder B. Radiation exposure during follow-up of adults with congenital heart disease. Int J Cardiol. 2007;118(2):151–3.
5. Ernst S, Babu-Narayan SV, Keegan J, Horduna I, Lyne J, Till J, Kilner PJ, Pennell D, Rigby ML, Gatzoulis MA. Remote-controlled magnetic navigation and ablation with 3D image integration as an alternative approach in patients with intra-atrial baffle anatomy. Circ Arrhythm Electrophysiol. 2012;5(1):131–9.
6. Kilner P, Babu-Narayan SV. Adult congenital heart disease. In: Higgins CB, de Roos A, editors. MRI and CT of the cardiovascular system. 2nd ed. Philadelphia: Lippincott Williams & Wilkins; 2005. p. 429–40.
7. Gatehouse PD, Rolf MP, Bloch KM, Graves MJ, Kilner PJ, Firmin DN, Hofman MB. A multi-center inter-manufacturer study of the temporal stability of phase-contrast velocity mapping background offset errors. J Cardiovasc Magn Reson. 2012;14:72.
8. Rolf MP, Hofman MB, Gatehouse PD, Markenroth-Bloch K, Heymans MW, Ebbers T, Graves MJ, Totman JJ, Werner B, van Rossum AC, Kilner PJ, Heethaar RM. Sequence optimization to reduce velocity offsets in cardiovascular magnetic resonance volume flow quantification – a multi-vendor study. J Cardiovasc Magn Reson. 2011;13:18.
9. Kilner PJ, Gatehouse PD, Firmin DN. Flow measurement by magnetic resonance: a unique asset worth optimising. J Cardiovasc Magn Reson. 2007;9(4):723–8.
10. Dabizzi RP, Caprioli G, Aiazzi L, Castelli C, Baldrighi G, Parenzan L, Baldrighi V. Distribution and anomalies of coronary arteries in tetralogy of Fallot. Circulation. 1980;61(1):95–102.
11. Kim RJ, Shah DJ, Judd RM. How we perform delayed enhancement imaging. J Cardiovasc Magn Reson. 2003;5(3):505–14.
12. Babu-Narayan SV. The role of late gadolinium enhancement cardiovascular magnetic resonance in the assessment of congenital and acquired heart disease. Prog Pediatr Cardiol. 2010;28:11–9.
13. Kilner PJ. Pulmonary resistance in cardiovascular context. Int J Cardiol. 2004;97 Suppl 1:3–6.
14. Kilner PJ, Balossino R, Dubini G, Babu-Narayan SV, Taylor AM, Pennati G, Migliavacca F. Pulmonary regurgitation: the effects of varying pulmonary artery compliance, and of increased resistance proximal or distal to the compliance. Int J Cardiol. 2009;133(2):157–66.
15. Wald RM, Redington AN, Pereira A, Provost YL, Paul NS, Oechslin EN, Silversides CK. Refining the assessment of pulmonary regurgitation in adults after tetralogy of Fallot repair: should we be measuring regurgitant fraction or regurgitant volume? Eur Heart J. 2009;30(3):356–61.
16. Johansson B, Babu-Narayan SV, Kilner PJ. The effects of breath-holding on pulmonary regurgitation measured by cardiovascular magnetic resonance velocity mapping. J Cardiovasc Magn Reson. 2009;11:1.
17. Davlouros PA, Kilner PJ, Hornung TS, Li W, Francis JM, Moon JC, Smith GC, Tat T, Pennell DJ, Gatzoulis MA. Right ventricular function in adults with repaired tetralogy of Fallot assessed with cardiovascular magnetic resonance imaging: detrimental role of right ventricular outflow aneurysms or akinesia and adverse right-to-left ventricular interaction. J Am Coll Cardiol. 2002;40(11):2044–52.
18. Geva T, Sandweiss BM, Gauvreau K, Lock JE, Powell AJ. Factors associated with impaired clinical status in long-term survivors of tetralogy of Fallot repair evaluated by magnetic resonance imaging. J Am Coll Cardiol. 2004;43(6):1068–74.
19. Bellenger NG, Davies LC, Francis JM, Coats AJ, Pennell DJ. Reduction in sample size for studies of remodeling in heart failure by the use of cardiovascular magnetic resonance. J Cardiovasc Magn Reson. 2000;2(4):271–8.
20. Winter MM, Bernink FJ, Groenink M, Bouma BJ, van Dijk AP, Helbing WA, Tijssen JG, Mulder BJ. Evaluating the systemic right ventricle by CMR: the importance of consistent and reproducible delineation of the cavity. J Cardiovasc Magn Reson. 2008;10:40.
21. Hughes ML, Muthurangu V, Taylor A. Cardiovascular MR imaging—indications, techniques and protocols. Prog Pediatr Cardiol. 2010;28:3–10.
22. Babu-Narayan SV, Bouzas B, Broberg CS, Kilner PJ. Interstudy reproducibility of right and left ventricular volume and mass measurements by cardiovascular magnetic resonance in repaired tetralogy of Fallot patients. J Cardiovasc Magn Reson. 2005;7(1):153.
23. Babu-Narayan SV, Uebing A, Davlouros PA, Kemp M, Davidson S, Dimopoulos K, Bayne S, Pennell DJ,

Gibson DG, Flather M, Kilner PJ, Li W, Gatzoulis MA. Randomised trial of ramipril in repaired tetralogy of Fallot and pulmonary regurgitation: the APPROPRIATE study (Ace inhibitors for Potential PRevention Of the deleterious effects of Pulmonary Regurgitation In Adults with repaired TEtralogy of Fallot). Int J Cardiol. 2012;154(3):299–305.
24. Therrien J, Siu SC, McLaughlin PR, Liu PP, Williams WG, Webb GD. Pulmonary valve replacement in adults late after repair of tetralogy of Fallot: are we operating too late? J Am Coll Cardiol. 2000;36(5):1670–5.
25. Therrien J, Provost Y, Merchant N, Williams W, Colman J, Webb G. Optimal timing for pulmonary valve replacement in adults after tetralogy of Fallot repair. Am J Cardiol. 2005;95(6):779–82.
26. van Straten A, Vliegen HW, Hazekamp MG, Bax JJ, Schoof PH, Ottenkamp J, van der Wall EE, de Roos A. Right ventricular function after pulmonary valve replacement in patients with tetralogy of Fallot. Radiology. 2004;233(3):824–9.
27. Vliegen HW, van Straten A, de Roos A, Roest AA, Schoof PH, Zwinderman AH, Ottenkamp J, van der Wall EE, Hazekamp MG. Magnetic resonance imaging to assess the hemodynamic effects of pulmonary valve replacement in adults late after repair of tetralogy of Fallot. Circulation. 2002;106(13):1703–7.
28. Buechel ER, Dave HH, Kellenberger CJ, Dodge-Khatami A, Pretre R, Berger F, Bauersfeld U. Remodelling of the right ventricle after early pulmonary valve replacement in children with repaired tetralogy of Fallot: assessment by cardiovascular magnetic resonance. Eur Heart J. 2005;26(24):2721–7.
29. Khambadkone S, Coats L, Taylor A, Boudjemline Y, Derrick G, Tsang V, Cooper J, Muthurangu V, Hegde SR, Razavi RS, Pellerin D, Deanfield J, Bonhoeffer P. Percutaneous pulmonary valve implantation in humans: results in 59 consecutive patients. Circulation. 2005;112(8):1189–97.
30. Oosterhof T, van Straten A, Vliegen HW, Meijboom FJ, van Dijk AP, Spijkerboer AM, Bouma BJ, Zwinderman AH, Hazekamp MG, de Roos A, Mulder BJ. Preoperative thresholds for pulmonary valve replacement in patients with corrected tetralogy of Fallot using cardiovascular magnetic resonance. Circulation. 2007;116(5):545–51.
31. Frigiola A, Tsang V, Bull C, Coats L, Khambadkone S, Derrick G, Mist B, Walker F, van Doorn C, Bonhoeffer P, Taylor AM. Biventricular response after pulmonary valve replacement for right ventricular outflow tract dysfunction: is age a predictor of outcome? Circulation. 2008;118(14 Suppl):S182–90.
32. Geva T, Gauvreau K, Powell AJ, Cecchin F, Rhodes J, Geva J, del Nido P. Randomized trial of pulmonary valve replacement with and without right ventricular remodeling surgery. Circulation. 2010;122(11 Suppl):S201–8.
33. Baumgartner H, Bonhoeffer P, De Groot NM, de Haan F, Deanfield JE, Galie N, Gatzoulis MA, Gohlke-Baerwolf C, Kaemmerer H, Kilner P, Meijboom F, Mulder BJ, Oechslin E, Oliver JM, Serraf A, Szatmari A, Thaulow E, Vouhe PR, Walma E. ESC guidelines for the management of grown-up congenital heart disease (new version 2010). Eur Heart J. 2010;31(23):2915–57.
34. Uebing A, Gibson DG, Babu-Narayan SV, Diller GP, Dimopoulos K, Goktekin O, Spence MS, Andersen K, Henein MY, Gatzoulis MA, Li W. Right ventricular mechanics and QRS duration in patients with repaired tetralogy of Fallot: implications of infundibular disease. Circulation. 2007;116(14):1532–9.
35. Babu-Narayan SV, Kilner PJ, Li W, Moon JC, Goktekin O, Davlouros PA, Khan M, Ho SY, Pennell DJ, Gatzoulis MA. Ventricular fibrosis suggested by cardiovascular magnetic resonance in adults with repaired tetralogy of Fallot and its relationship to adverse markers of clinical outcome. Circulation. 2006;113(3):405–13.
36. Wald RM, Haber I, Wald R, Valente AM, Powell AJ, Geva T. Effects of regional dysfunction and late gadolinium enhancement on global right ventricular function and exercise capacity in patients with repaired tetralogy of Fallot. Circulation. 2009;119(10):1370–7.
37. Bonello B, Kempny A, Uebing A, Li W, Kilner P, Diller G, Pennell D, Ernst S, Shore D, Babu-Narayan S. Right atrial area and right ventricular outflow tract akinetic region length predict sustained tachyarrhythmia in repaired tetralogy of Fallot. Eur Heart J Cardiovasc Imaging. 2012;13 Suppl 1:i40–1.
38. Khairy P, Aboulhosn J, Gurvitz MZ, Opotowsky AR, Mongeon FP, Kay J, Valente AM, Earing MG, Lui G, Gersony DR, Cook S, Ting JG, Nickolaus MJ, Webb G, Landzberg MJ, Broberg CS. Arrhythmia burden in adults with surgically repaired tetralogy of Fallot: a multi-institutional study. Circulation. 2010;122(9):868–75.
39. Sridharan S, Derrick G, Deanfield J, Taylor AM. Assessment of differential branch pulmonary blood flow: a comparative study of phase contrast magnetic resonance imaging and radionuclide lung perfusion imaging. Heart. 2006;92(7):963–8.
40. Niwa K, Siu SC, Webb GD, Gatzoulis MA. Progressive aortic root dilatation in adults late after repair of tetralogy of Fallot. Circulation. 2002;106(11):1374–8.
41. Tan JL, Davlouros PA, McCarthy KP, Gatzoulis MA, Ho SY. Intrinsic histological abnormalities of aortic root and ascending aorta in tetralogy of Fallot: evidence of causative mechanism for aortic dilatation and aortopathy. Circulation. 2005;112(7):961–8.
42. Prasad SK, Soukias N, Hornung T, Khan M, Pennell DJ, Gatzoulis MA, Mohiaddin RH. Role of magnetic resonance angiography in the diagnosis of major aortopulmonary collateral arteries and partial anomalous pulmonary venous drainage. Circulation. 2004;109(2):207–14.
43. Geva T, Greil GF, Marshall AC, Landzberg M, Powell AJ. Gadolinium-enhanced 3-dimensional magnetic resonance angiography of pulmonary blood supply in patients with complex pulmonary stenosis or atresia: comparison with x-ray angiography. Circulation. 2002;106(4):473–8.
44. Sridharan S, Coats L, Khambadkone S, Taylor AM, Bonhoeffer P. Images in cardiovascular medicine. Transcatheter right ventricular outflow tract

intervention: the risk to the coronary circulation. Circulation. 2006;113(25):e934–5.
45. Gartner RD, Sutton NJ, Weinstein S, Spindola-Franco H, Haramati LB. MRI and computed tomography of cardiac and pulmonary complications of tetralogy of Fallot in adults. J Thorac Imaging. 2010;25(2): 183–90.
46. Bradlow WM, Assomull R, Kilner PJ, Gibbs JS, Sheppard MN, Mohiaddin RH. Understanding late gadolinium enhancement in pulmonary hypertension. Circ Cardiovasc Imaging. 2010;3(4):501–3.
47. Tsai SF, Chan DP, Ro PS, Boettner B, Daniels CJ. Rate of inducible ventricular arrhythmia in adults with congenital heart disease. Am J Cardiol. 2010;106(5):730–6.
48. Witte KK, Pepper CB, Cowan JC, Thomson JD, English KM, Blackburn ME. Implantable cardioverter-defibrillator therapy in adult patients with tetralogy of Fallot. Europace. 2008;8:926–30.
49. Yap SC, Roos-Hesselink JW, Hoendermis ES, Budts W, Vliegen HW, Mulder BJ, van Dijk AP, Schalij MJ, Drenthen W. Outcome of implantable cardioverter defibrillators in adults with congenital heart disease: a multi-centre study. Eur Heart J. 2007;28(15):1854–61.
50. Berul CI, Van Hare GF, Kertesz NJ, Dubin AM, Cecchin F, Collins KK, Cannon BC, Alexander ME, Triedman JK, Walsh EP, Friedman RA. Results of a multicenter retrospective implantable cardioverter-defibrillator registry of pediatric and congenital heart disease patients. J Am Coll Cardiol. 2008;51(17):1685–91.
51. Khairy P, Harris L, Landzberg MJ, Viswanathan S, Barlow A, Gatzoulis MA, Fernandes SM, Beauchesne L, Therrien J, Chetaille P, Gordon E, Vonder Muhll I, Cecchin F. Implantable cardioverter-defibrillators in tetralogy of Fallot. Circulation. 2008;117(3): 363–70.
52. Schievano S, Petrini L, Migliavacca F, Coats L, Nordmeyer J, Lurz P, Khambadkone S, Taylor AM, Dubini G, Bonhoeffer P. Finite element analysis of stent deployment: understanding stent fracture in percutaneous pulmonary valve implantation. J Interv Cardiol. 2007;20(6):546–54.
53. Schievano S, Migliavacca F, Coats L, Khambadkone S, Carminati M, Wilson N, Deanfield JE, Bonhoeffer P, Taylor AM. Percutaneous pulmonary valve implantation based on rapid prototyping of right ventricular outflow tract and pulmonary trunk from MR data. Radiology. 2007;242(2):490–7.
54. Schievano S, Coats L, Migliavacca F, Norman W, Frigiola A, Deanfield J, Bonhoeffer P, Taylor AM. Variations in right ventricular outflow tract morphology following repair of congenital heart disease: implications for percutaneous pulmonary valve implantation. J Cardiovasc Magn Reson. 2007;9(4):687–95.
55. Gatzoulis MA, Clark AL, Cullen S, Newman CG, Redington AN. Right ventricular diastolic function 15 to 35 years after repair of tetralogy of Fallot. Restrictive physiology predicts superior exercise performance. Circulation. 1995;91(6):1775–81.

Transposition of the Great Arteries

10

Farhood Saremi

Many adults with congenital heart disease (CHD) have limited knowledge of their heart disease and heart history. It is not uncommon to encounter adult patients with transposition of the great arteries (TGA) that have not seen a physician in many years. Radiologist and cardiologist need to understand image findings and the anatomy of the repair and the potential late complications associated with it. In this chapter, these issues will be reviewed. Table 10.1 shows anatomic definitions relevant to the TGA, and Table 10.2 defines morphological characteristics of the ventricles for correct identification.

Transposition of the Great Arteries

TGA is a common cyanotic defect seen in newborns with an incidence of about 1 per 5,000 live births [1]. It is seen in 5 % of CHD [2]. It is due to embryologic defect of conotruncal septum rotation resulting in ventriculoarterial discordance. Almost all patients with this defect who reach adulthood have had prior reparative cardiac surgery, although some with a large ventricular septal defect (VSD) and subpulmonic stenosis can survive with Eisenmenger physiology [3]. Without treatment, 95 % of these patients die in the first year, mainly from hypoxemia. Patients who have undergone atrial-level repair for TGA comprise an important group of adults with CHD. It is estimated there to be approximately 9,000 patients in the United States currently alive with an atrial-level repair [4, 5].

F. Saremi, MD
Department of Radiology, Cardiothoracic Section, University of Southern California, USC Keck Hospital, 1500 San Pablo St., Los Angeles, CA 90033, USA
e-mail: fsaremi@usc.edu

Morphology

In typical TGA, the atria and ventricles are in the usual position (Fig. 10.1). It is also known as D-TGA; the "D-" refers to the dextroposition of the bulboventricular loop [i.e., the position of the right ventricle (RV), which is on the right side]. In this anomaly the aorta and associated coronary arteries arise anteriorly from the RV and the pulmonary artery arises posteriorly from the left ventricle (LV). The aorta also tends to be on the right and anterior, and the great arteries are parallel rather than crossing as they do in the normal heart (56 %) [6] (Figs. 10.2 and 10.3). The second most common arrangement is with the aorta just anterior to the pulmonary artery (26 %); the rarest fetal variant is side-by-side arrangement. In Massoudy et al.'s [7] study of 200 cadaveric hearts with TGA, five categories for the relationships of the great arterial trunks were found. The aorta could be anterior and to the right of the pulmonary trunk (75 %), directly anterior (10 %), anterior and to the left (3 %), side by side with the aorta to the right (10 %), or posterior and to the right (2 %). The latter arrangement is also called normal relations, albeit with discordant

F. Saremi (ed.), *Cardiac CT and MR for Adult Congenital Heart Disease*,
DOI 10.1007/978-1-4614-8875-0_10, © Springer Science+Business Media New York 2014

Table 10.1 Anatomic definitions relevant to the TGA

Transposition of the great arteries (TGA)	Aorta arising entirely above the right ventricle and pulmonary artery more than 50 % above the left ventricle. Complete TGA is usually D-TGA with the aorta on the right side of the pulmonary valve designated as {S, D, D} in Van Praagh classification. The S stands for atrial situs solitus (normal). The first D is for a D-looped right ventricle. The second D stands for the right-sided aortic valve. L-TGA (the aorta to the left side of the pulmonary valve) is seen in situs inversus
Transposition with pulmonary atresia	Right ventricular aorta with pulmonary atresia often termed double outlet right ventricle with pulmonary atresia
Congenitally corrected transposition of the great arteries (ccTGA)	Atrioventricular discordance and ventriculoarterial discordance (Double discordance) resulting in normal physiology circulation {S, L, L}. The first L stands for an L-looped right ventricle. The second L stands for the position of the aortic valve, which is anterior and to the left of the pulmonary valve. ccTGA is usually L-TGA in situs solitus and D-TGA in situs inversus
Anatomically corrected malposition (ACM) of the great arteries	The aortic origin lies to the left of the pulmonary trunk when there is situs solitus and concordant ventriculoarterial connection. Parallel arterial trunks, instead of the normal spiral relationship of the aorta and the pulmonary trunk
Crisscross heart or twisted atrioventricular connection	Rare anomaly as a result of rotation of ventricular mass along its long axis causing supero-inferior relationship of the ventricles with the morphological right ventricle located superiorly. The right atrioventricular axis appears orthogonal, rather than parallel, to the left atrioventricular axis. It may be seen with all kinds of atrioventricular and ventriculoarterial connections. Many have discordant ventriculoarterial connections
Subarterial infundibulum (conus)	Four possible types: subpulmonary infundibulum (normal), subaortic infundibulum (TGA or ccTGA), bilateral infundibulum (ACM of the great arteries, double outlet right ventricle), and bilaterally absent conus (double outlet left ventricle). Typically, in the absence of infundibulum, an arterial-atrioventricular valvular fibrous continuity exists. The presence of conus under a semilunar valve usually indicates that the vessel originates from the right ventricle
Ventricular loop	D-loop: refers to the normal rightward (D=dextro) loop or bend of the embryonic heart tube and indicates that the morphological RV inflow tract is on the right side of the morphological LV (right hand topology) L-loop: refers to a leftward (L=levo) loop or bend of the embryonic cardiac tube resulting in the inflow portion of the morphological right ventricle being to the left of the morphological left ventricle (left hand topology)
Loop rule	In complex cases, it may be difficult to characterize a right or left ventricle. In general, in the presence of a right-sided aortic valve, the right ventricle is located to the right of the left ventricle (D-loop), and in the presence of a left-sided aortic valve, the right ventricle is located to the left of the left ventricle (L-loop)
Atrioventricular connection	Five types exist: concordant (normal), discordant, ambiguous, double inlet, and absent right or left connection. Concordant, discordant, and ambiguous connections are used when two ventricles are present, whereas double inlet and absent right (or left) connections are used for a univentricular heart. Concordant cardiac loops are the D-loop with situs solitus and the L-loop with situs inversus. Discordant cardiac loops are L-loop with situs solitus and D-loop with situs inversus
Ventriculoarterial connection	Double arterial trunk may have concordant connection (normal), discordant connection (TGA), double outlet right ventricle (the great vessels arise from the right ventricle), and double outlet left ventricle (the great vessels arise from the left ventricle). Single outlet can exist as a common arterial trunk, a single pulmonary trunk with atresia of the aortic trunk, or a single aortic trunk with pulmonary atresia
Position of the atrioventricular valves	It is correlated with the orientation of the ventricular loop . In a D-loop, the tricuspid valve is located to the right of the mitral valve; in an L-loop, it is to the left of the mitral valve. In general, the mitral valve is associated with the morphological left ventricle, and the tricuspid valve is associated with the morphological right ventricle

ventriculoarterial connections [8] (Fig. 10.4). In regard to the orientation of the sinuses of the aorta relative to those of the pulmonary trunk, in most cases, the commissures between the valvular leaflets face each other at the sinotubular junctions. Commissural mismatch is uncommon

Table 10.2 Morphological characteristics of the ventricles

	Right ventricle	Left ventricle
Trabeculations	Coarse and thick at the apex	Thickened wall
Moderator band	Starts from the ventricular septum and extend towards the apex	None
Atrioventricular valve	Tricuspid	Mitral
Septal valve leaflet	Apical position of the septal tricuspid leaflet	Mitral-aortic valvular fibrous continuity
Papillary muscle	Medial papillary muscle attaching to the septum. Anterior papillary muscle continuous with the moderator band	Anterosuperior and posteroinferior papillary muscle. No septal papillary muscle
Infundibulum	Usually exists	Usually absent

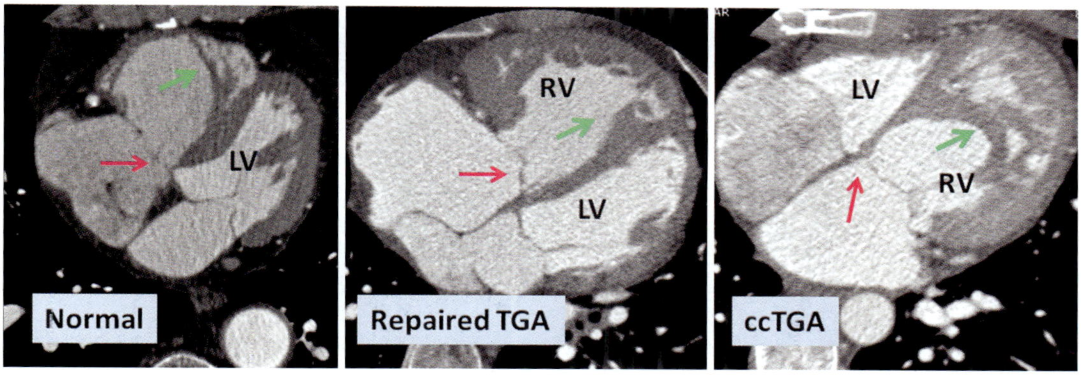

Fig. 10.1 Axial views of the heart demonstrate the orientation of heart in thorax, ventricular arrangement and the atrioventricular valves position in normal, repaired transposition of great arteries (*TGA*), and congenitally corrected TGA (*ccTGA*). The cardiac crux has a mirror image appearance in ccTGA. The moderator band of morphological right ventricle (*RV*) is shown by *green arrows*. In the RV the septal leaflet of tricuspid valve (*pink arrows*) is attached to the septum 1 cm closer to the apex compared to the mitral valve (*pink arrows*). Further apical migration of the tricuspid valve is common in ccTGA. *LV* morphological left ventricle

(13 %) and may have surgical implications during arterial switch [7] (Fig. 10.5).

About two-thirds of TGA patients have simple transposition and may only have a small patent ductus arteriosus (PDA) and/or a patent foramen ovale (PFO) (Fig. 10.6). The presence of other cardiac lesions constitutes complex transposition. These include large PDA, atrial septal defect (ASD), VSD (22 %) [9], or coarctation of the aorta (4 %) [5, 10]. Rightward (more common) or leftward displacement of the outlet septum frequently results in subaortic or subpulmonary stenosis, respectively, and is frequently associated with a perimembranous VSD [11, 12]. Subaortic stenosis due to either deviation of the outlet septum or prominence of the ventriculo-infundibular fold and septoparietal trabeculations can occur.

Postsurgical TGA

If there is no atrial defect or VSD, the cyanotic neonate with TGA will not survive the first few days of life without some early intervention. As the first intervention, TGA babies may be treated with percutaneous Rashkind atrial balloon septostomy procedure to create a more sizable atrial septal defect to allow mixing of systemic and pulmonary venous return [13]. This procedure can improve their oxygenation until definitive surgery is performed. Early attempts at surgical repair of TGA were aimed at physiologic correction, because techniques for anatomic repair were not available. The surgical techniques of an atrial switch for patients presenting with TGA were described by Senning in 1959 [14] and by

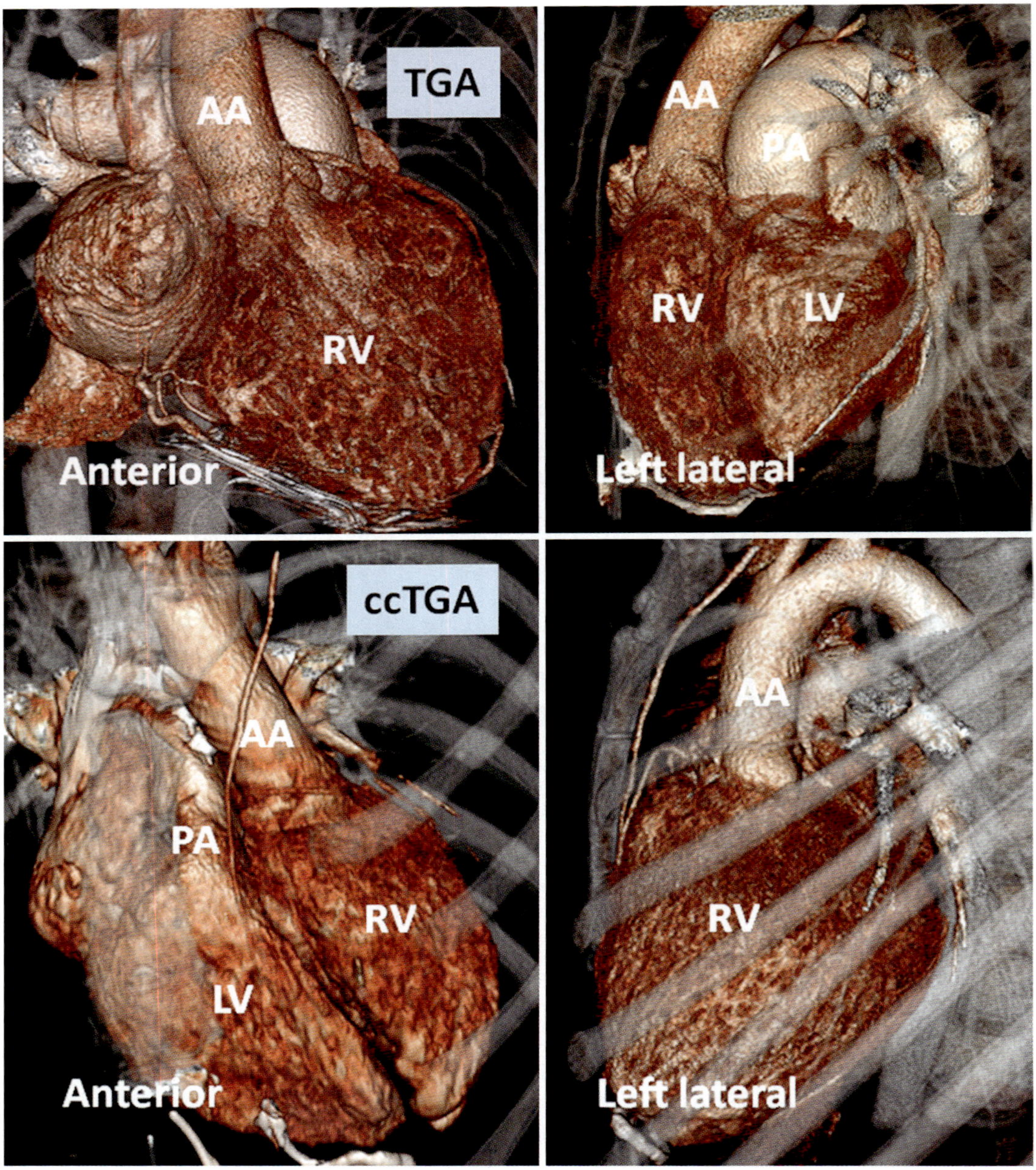

Fig. 10.2 Anterior and left lateral intrathoracic orientation of the heart in TGA and ccTGA. Note the anterior/posterior arrangement of the ventricles in TGA and their side-by-side position in ccTGA. In ccTGA, the morphological right ventricle (*RV*) forms the left lateral cardiac margin (levoposition). In TGA, the ascending aorta (*AA*) is located on the right anterior aspect of the main pulmonary artery (*PA*). *LV* morphological left ventricle

Mustard in 1964 [15]. By the 1980s, late complications of these repairs including sinus node dysfunction, atrial flutter, systemic ventricular dysfunction, baffle leak, and stenosis of the superior vena cava (SVC) baffle had become well recognized [16]. These complications, along with advances in cardiac surgery, led to the adoption of the neonatal arterial switch operation (ASO), which is now standard therapy for TGA [17–19].

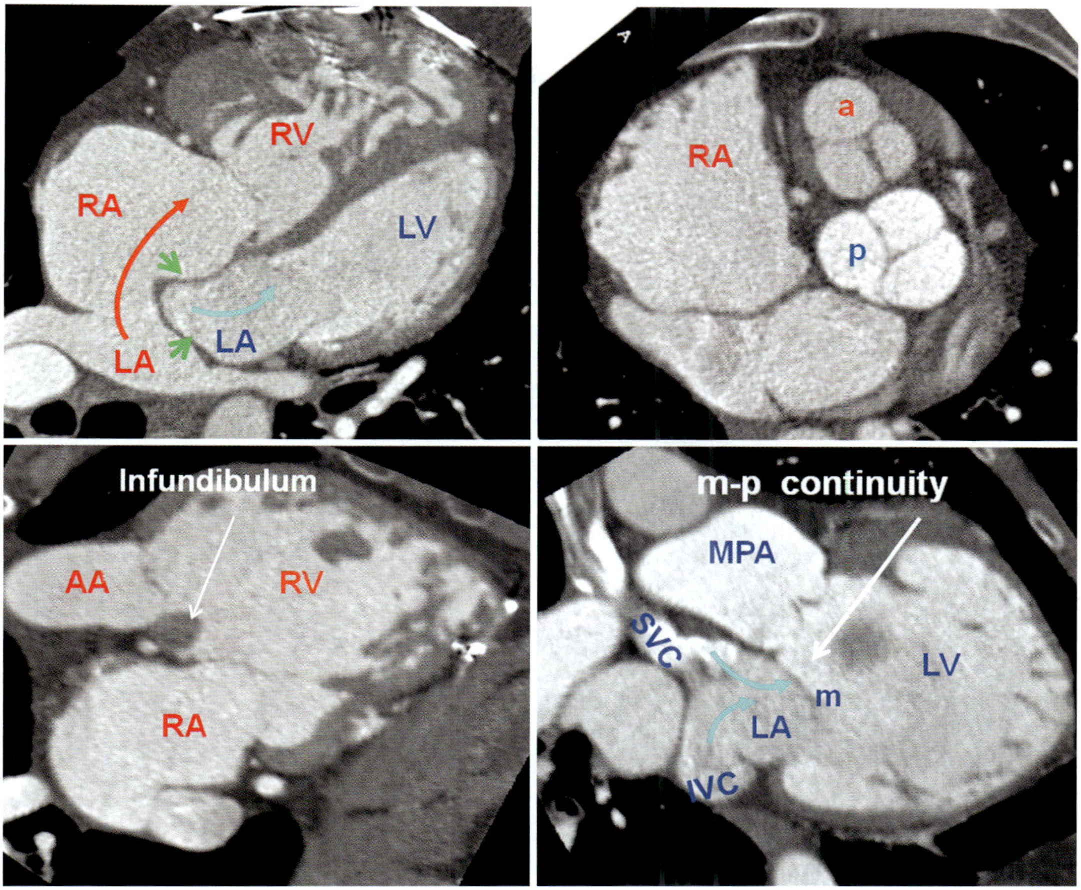

Fig. 10.3 Heart morphology in transposition of great arteries (*TGA*) status post atrial switch. Intra-atrial baffle (*green arrowhead*) diverts oxygenated blood of the left atrium (*LA*) into the right atrium (*RA*) (*red arrow*). Cardiac crux is normal. The morphological right ventricle (*RV*) works as systemic ventricle and appears hypertrophied. In TGA the aortic valve (*a*) is located anterior and to the left of the pulmonary valve (*p*) in most cases. The pulmonary valve is sitting between the two atria. The RV infundibulum is not well developed and there is fibrous continuity between the mitral (*m*) and the pulmonary (*p*) valves. *AA* ascending aorta, *IVC* inferior vena cava, *MPA* main pulmonary artery, *SVC* superior vena cava. *LV* left ventricle, *blue arrows* showing caval (non systemic) flow

Intra-atrial Baffle

In the Senning repair, two longitudinal incisions are made through lateral walls for the right and left atria. A flap made from the atrial septum is sewn to the free wall of the left atrium (LA) between the left atrial appendage and pulmonary veins, isolating the pulmonary veins behind it. If the flap is not large enough, it may obstruct left pulmonary veins at their orifices. The posterior and anterior edges of the incision through the lateral wall of the right atrium are then sutured to the free margin of the atrial septum and the left atrial incision, respectively, to reroute the deoxygenated caval blood to the mitral valve and the oxygenated pulmonary venous blood to the tricuspid valve. In Mustard technique which is less complicated, the baffle is created by intra-atrial sewing of a trouser-shaped patch of pericardium or synthetic material to the atrial walls (Fig. 10.7). In Mustard, the atrial septum must be excised as much as possible. At the end, the right atrium may be enlarged by a pericardial or a synthetic patch (Fig. 10.8). In both techniques the anatomic LV continues to act as the pulmonary pump and the anatomic RV acts as the systemic pump (Figs. 10.9 and 10.10). The Senning and Mustard repairs still have a small

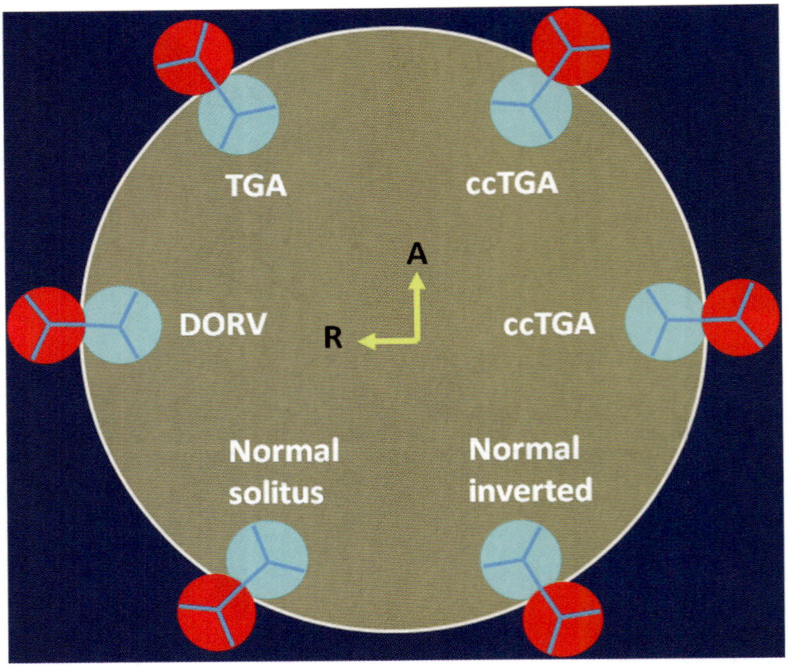

Fig. 10.4 Schematic representation of the aortic (*red*) and pulmonary (*blue*) valve relationships. Variability between the presented alignments is common

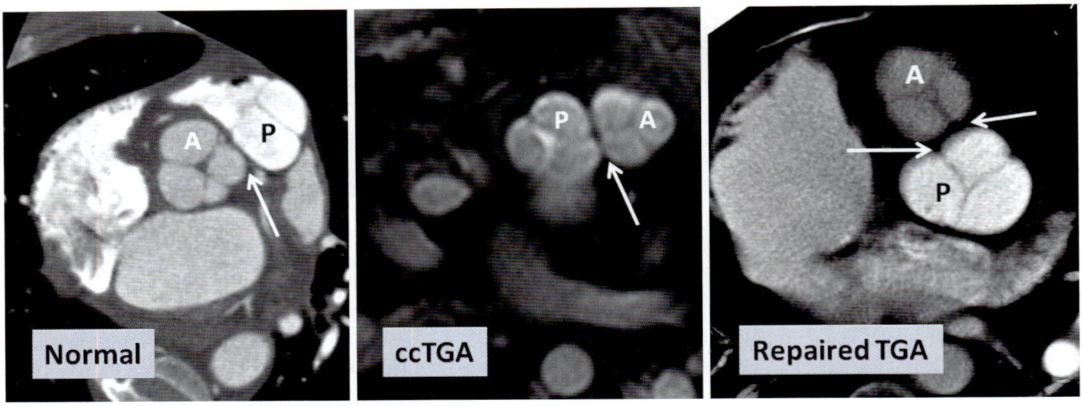

Fig. 10.5 Commissural malalignment of the aortic (*A*) and pulmonary (*P*) valves in TGA (shown by *arrows*). In normal heart and ccTGA, the intervalvular commissures are well aligned. Although uncommon, mismatch between aortic and pulmonary valves can occur in TGA patient which may have surgical implication for arterial switch operation

Fig. 10.7 Illustration of Mustard procedure. (**a**) The interatrial septum is removed through a right atrial incision. (**b**) A trouser-shaped patch of pericardium is created. (**c**) A baffle is formed by suturing the patch to the right atrial wall, the ostia of the inferior vena cava (*IVC*) and superior vena cava (*SVC*), and the anterior margin of atrial septal window to reroute the deoxygenated caval blood to the mitral valve and the oxygenated pulmonary venous blood (*red arrows*) to the tricuspid valve. Note in this example the coronary sinus ostium is not covered by the patch. Some surgeons may leave the coronary sinus to drain to the systemic venous atrium to lower possible suturing damage to the conduction system

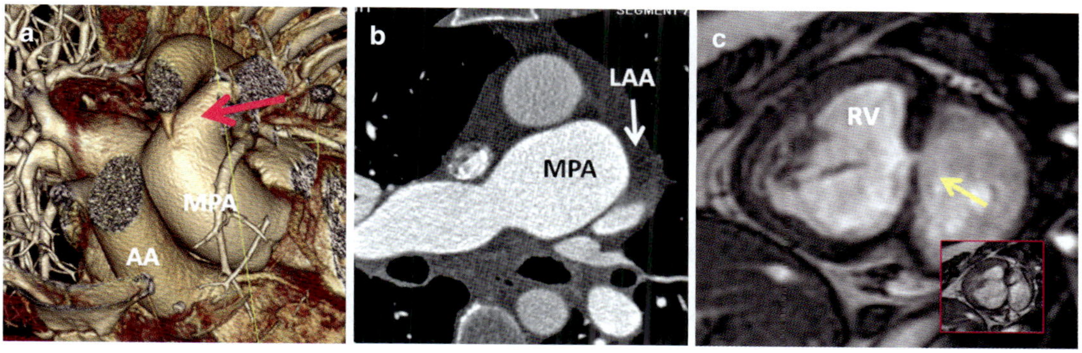

Fig. 10.6 Associated findings in repaired TGA. (**a**) Small patent ductus arteriosus (*pink arrow*). *AA* ascending aorta, *MPA* main pulmonary artery, *RV* right ventricle, inset box is systolic image showing the shunt as a dark line extending into the left ventricle. (**b**) Enlarged pulmonary arteries due to pulmonary hypertension. Note incomplete opacification of the left atrial appendage (*LAA*) suggestive of atrial fibrillation. (**c**) Recurrent small ventricular septal defect (*arrow*)

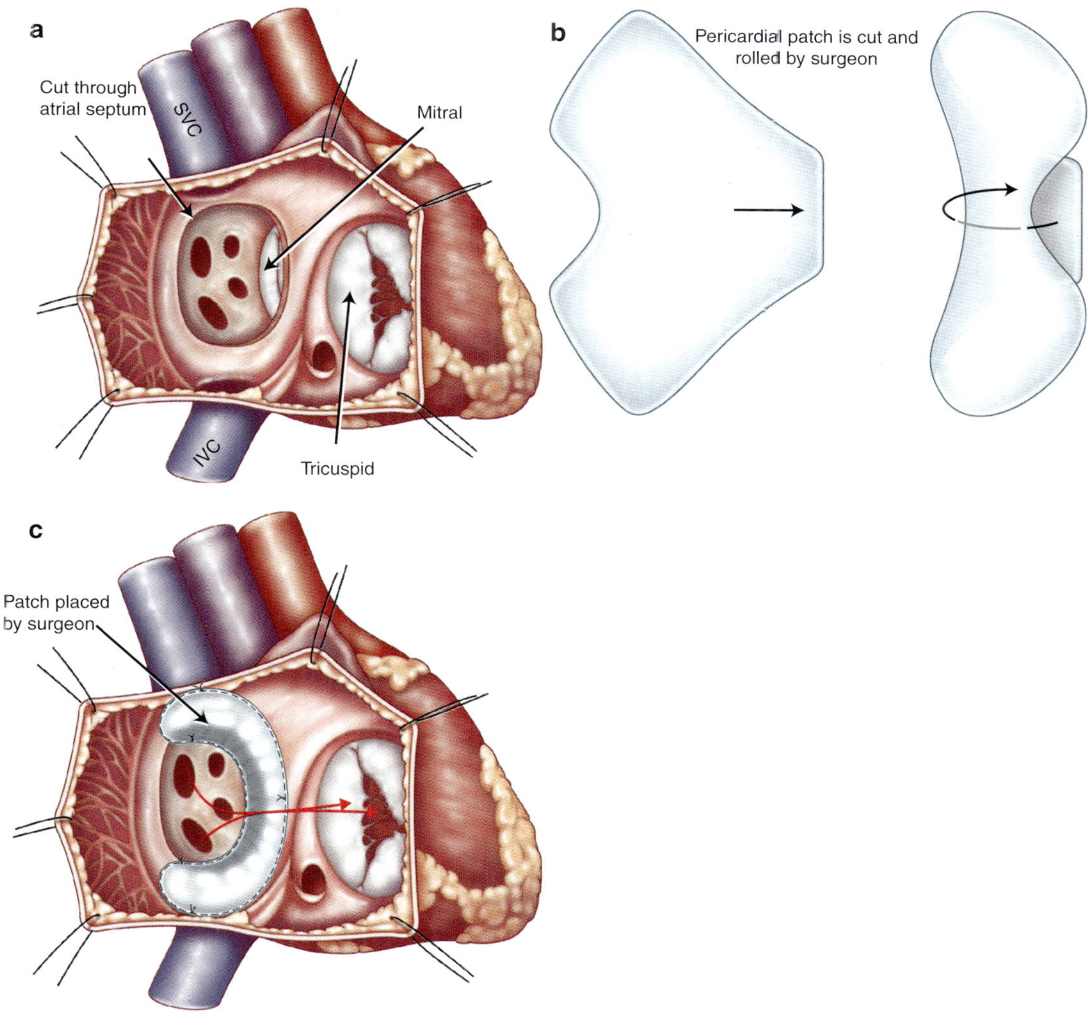

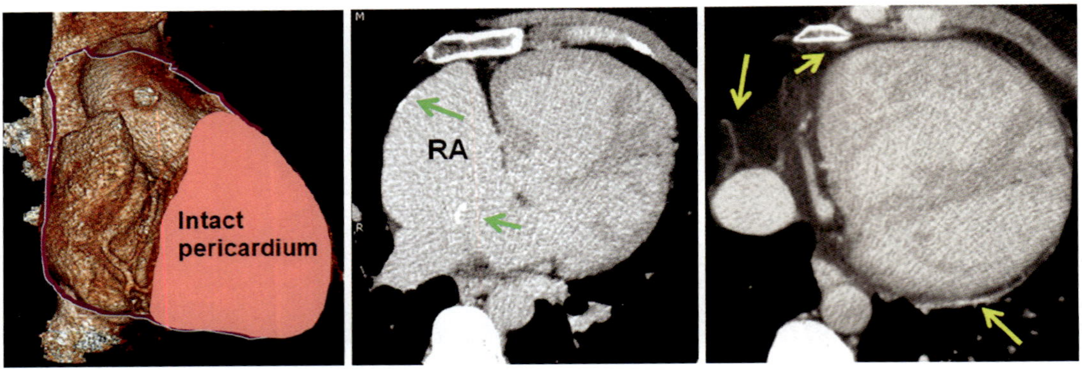

Fig. 10.8 Pericardiectomy to prepare a pericardial patch for Mustard surgery. A large part of the right pericardium is usually removed. It is mostly used for baffle construction. Part of it can be used to repair or enlarge the right atrial wall. The left anterior and posterior pericardium remain intact (*yellow arrows*). Note calcified foci at the surgical sites of the right atrial wall and interatrial baffle (*green arrows*)

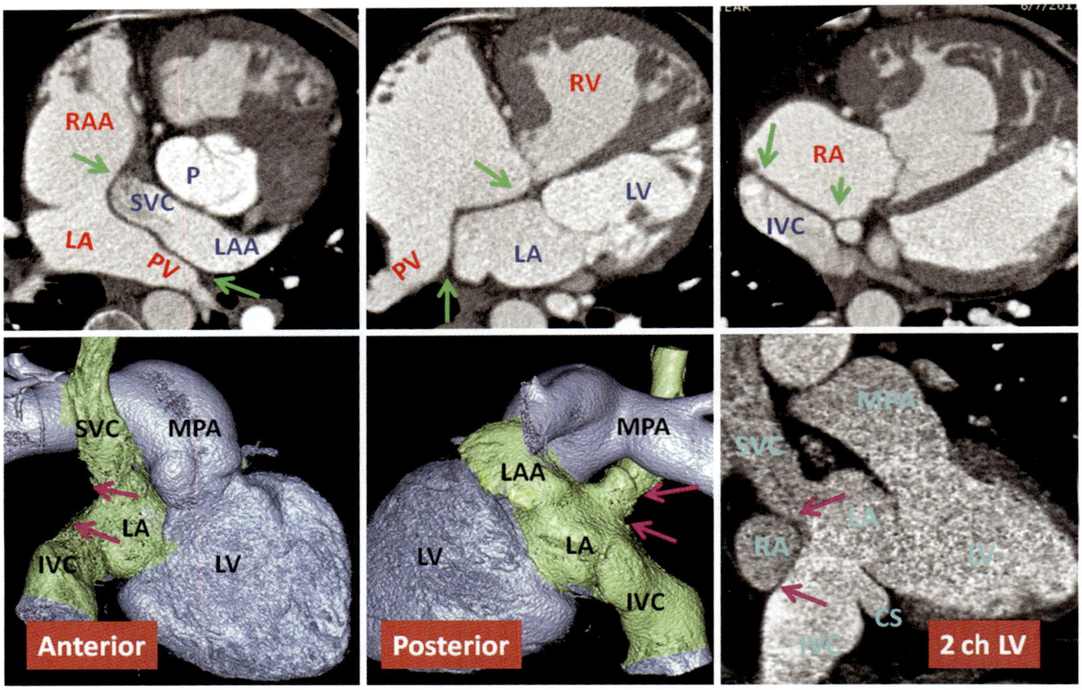

Fig. 10.9 *Upper row*: Intra-atrial baffle boundaries in transposition of great arteries (*TGA*) after atrial switch operation. The pericardial baffle covers the ostia of the SVC and IVC and from there extends into the left atrium (*LA*), dividing atrium into inner (venous) and outer (systemic) chambers. The baffle then attaches to the lateral wall of the LA between the pulmonary veins (*PV*) and left atrial appendage (*LAA*) ostia. Points of suturing of the patch, marked by *green arrows*, include superior (SVC ostium), inferior (*IVC*), midline (remainder of atrial septum at cardiac crux), and lateral (free wall of the left atrium). *Lower row*: nonsystemic circulation of TGA. The intra-atrial baffle location is shown by *pink arrows*. The structures participating in nonsystemic circulation include the SVC, IVC, LAA, anterior wall of LA, left atrial vestibule, mitral ring, morphological LV, and pulmonary arteries. Color-coded images show no connection to the coronary sinus. The coronary sinus (*CS*) may be covered by the baffle and becomes part of the nonsystemic circulation. This is shown in sagittal two-chamber (*2ch*) CT in a different patient. *IVC* inferior vena cava, *LV* left ventricle, *MPA* main pulmonary artery, *P* pulmonary artery, *RA* right atrium, *RAA* right atrial appendage, *RV* right ventricle, *SVC* superior vena cava

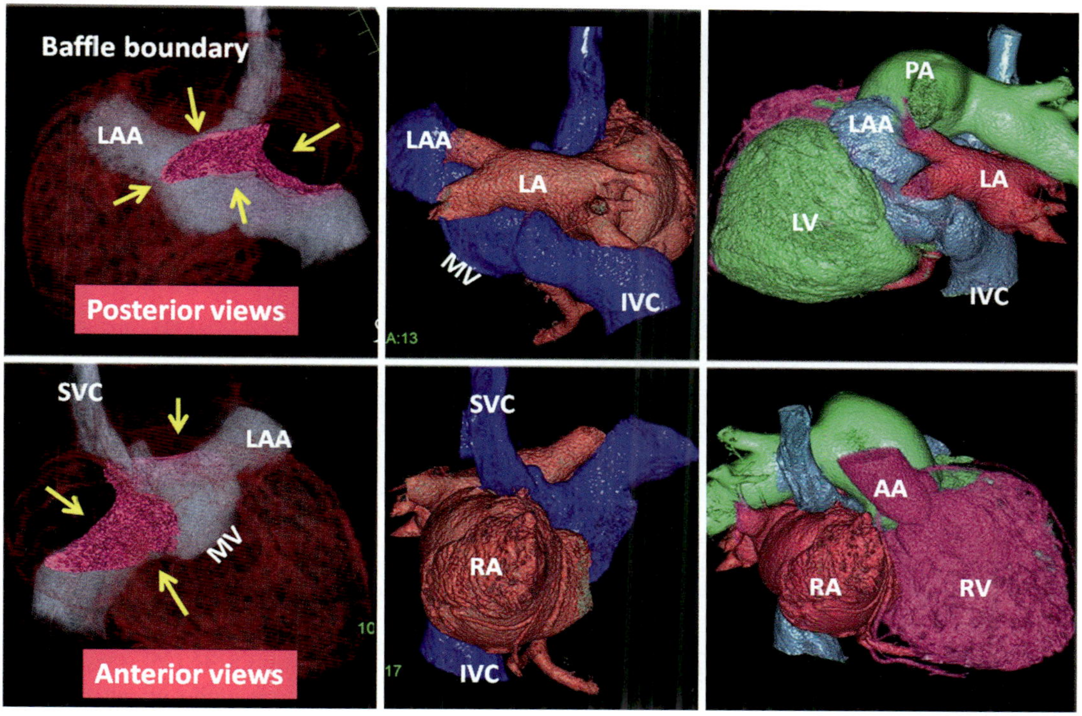

Fig. 10.10 The status of atrial baffle after atrial switch for transposition of great arteries. The boundaries of intra-atrial baffle are shown by *yellow arrows* on volume-rendered CT images. Homogenous enhancement of both atria was achieved using a double injection CT technique. As a result of modest attenuation values throughout the heart chambers, high-quality three-dimensional images can be reconstructed. After atrial switch non-oxygenated blood of the IVC and SVC is diverted into the vestibule of left atrium (*LA*), the left ventricle (*LV*), and finally the main pulmonary artery (*MPA*). The oxygenated blood of the venous part of LA enters the right atrium (*RA*), the right ventricle (*RV*), and the ascending aorta (*AA*). *IVC* inferior vena cava, *LAA* left atrial appendage, *MV* mitral valve location, *SVC* superior vena cava

role in the treatment of TGA in patients with fixed subpulmonary obstruction and as part of the "double-switch" type of repair used in the treatment of congenitally corrected transposition of great arteries (ccTGA).

Arterial Switch: Jatene Procedure

With improvements in critical care and technical skill, the Jatene arterial switch has become the optimal surgery of TGA and can be performed in early weeks of life [17, 18]. To restore the ventriculoarterial relationships, the coronary arteries are excised from the aorta, followed by transection and switch of the ascending aorta and the pulmonary artery. To reduce the risk of coronary artery kinking before their reimplantation, the pulmonary artery is relocated anterior to the aorta (the Lecompte maneuver) (Fig. 10.11). The pulmonary artery may be augmented by using pericardial patch to prevent the possibility of stenosis. Patients with anomalous coronary arteries are not good candidates for the Jatene procedure. In cases in which TGA is associated with a VSD and subpulmonary stenosis, the Rastelli procedure is the preferred method of repair. This procedure consists of a patch closure of the VSD to the aortic valve and placement of a conduit between the RV and the pulmonary arteries [20]. After the Rastelli operation, assessment of possible stenosis or incompetence of the RV-to-PA conduit, LV outflow tract flow, biventricular function, and possible residual shunt is needed. This is probably best achieved by cardiac MRI. After the Mustard or Senning procedure, adults

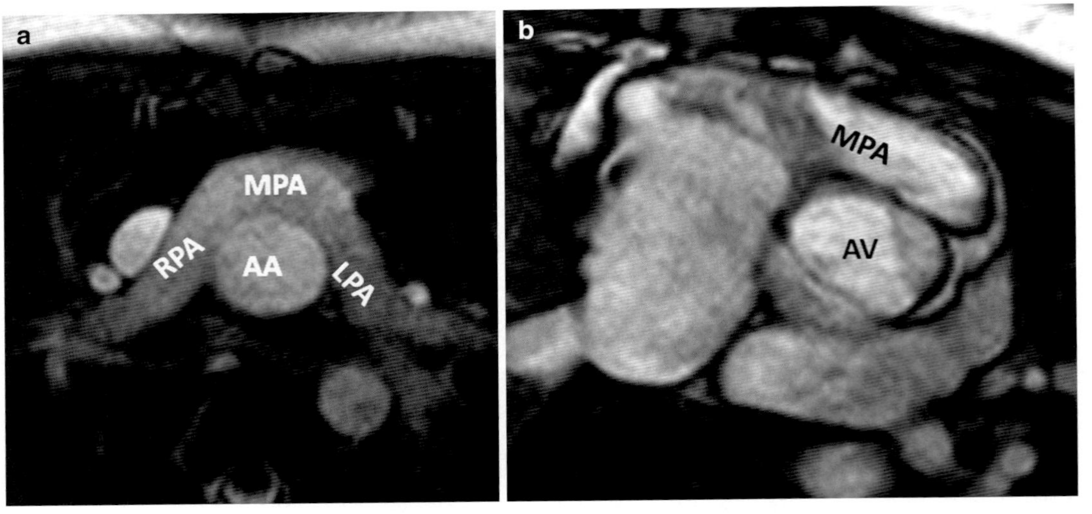

Fig. 10.11 Pulmonary artery appearance after Jatene arterial switch procedure. (**a**) Axial MRI and (**b**) Short-axis MRI show retrosternal course of main pulmonary artery (*MPA*). Dilated aortic annulus (neoaorta) is shown in (b). *AA* ascending aorta, *AV* aortic valve, *LPA* left pulmonary artery, *RPA* right pulmonary artery

with TGA may develop right ventricular failure and require consideration of new therapies. A 2-stage pulmonary artery banding and ASO may be performed as an alternative to heart transplantation (Fig. 10.12).

Postsurgical Complications

Complications After Atrial Switch

Baffle-related complications are a frequent cause of reoperation and account for 30 % of reoperations in patients with history of Mustard operation and 5 % of Senning operation [21–24]. The reason for a higher incidence of baffle-related complications in the Mustard group may be seen in the use of synthetic material or folding of excessive baffle material. Early complications include baffle obstruction or leak and vena cava obstruction [21, 24]. Late surgical complications include leak and pulmonary and/or systemic venous pathway stenosis [24].

Baffle Stenosis. The systemic venous pathway obstruction occurs more often after Mustard repair (15 %) than after the Senning procedure (1.4 %) [22], but there is a trend towards greater obstruction of the pulmonary venous pathway in those who have undergone the Senning procedure (7.6 % versus 3.8 %) [25]. Obstruction of the pulmonary venous pathway can manifest as pulmonary venous hypertension and pulmonary edema. The site of obstruction is typically between the inferior vena cava (IVC) baffle limb and the lateral atrial wall. Less commonly, the left pulmonary veins can become obstructed, causing left-sided edema. Both the superior and inferior caval baffle limbs can develop stenosis, but the SVC limb is more frequently affected (Fig. 10.13). With MR and CT the site of stenosis can be easily identified. The degree of stenosis can also be quantified using MR velocity encoding. Severe stenosis is defined as narrowing on cine images with a peak velocity of over 1.5 m/s and a damped and continuous flow curve. Mild stenosis is defined when the flow is pulsatile and peak velocity in early diastole not exceeding 1 m/s [26]. In chronic SVC stenosis, patients are often asymptomatic, as they may develop collateral flow into the chest wall and paravertebral veins with retrograde drainage into the IVC [27]. Patients may also develop persistent pleural effusions or chylothorax. Chronic stenosis of the IVC is not well tolerated owing to subsequent hepatic congestion and ascites. Venous stenosis can often be treated with transcatheter-delivered stents [28] (see Fig. 25.11). Pulmonary venous pathway obstruction after Mustard is often identified using phase-contrast imaging that demonstrates increased venous flow velocity or loss of normal phasic flow patterns. However, in the setting of severe obstructions, pulmonary arterial blood flow is redistributed towards the unaffected side resulting in very low venous flow on the affected side masking flow acceleration. In this situation, measuring pulmonary artery flow can be helpful. In case of left pulmonary vein obstruction, arterial flow will be redistributed with more flow shifting to the right side. Reversed diastolic flow in the ipsilateral artery (in the absence of pulmonary regurgitation) and continuous flow in the contralateral pulmonary artery may be seen in severe pulmonary vein obstruction [29].

Baffle Leaks. Leaks in the intra-atrial baffle are more common with Mustard than with Senning repairs. Small defects in the wall of baffle are common and usually hemodynamically insignificant

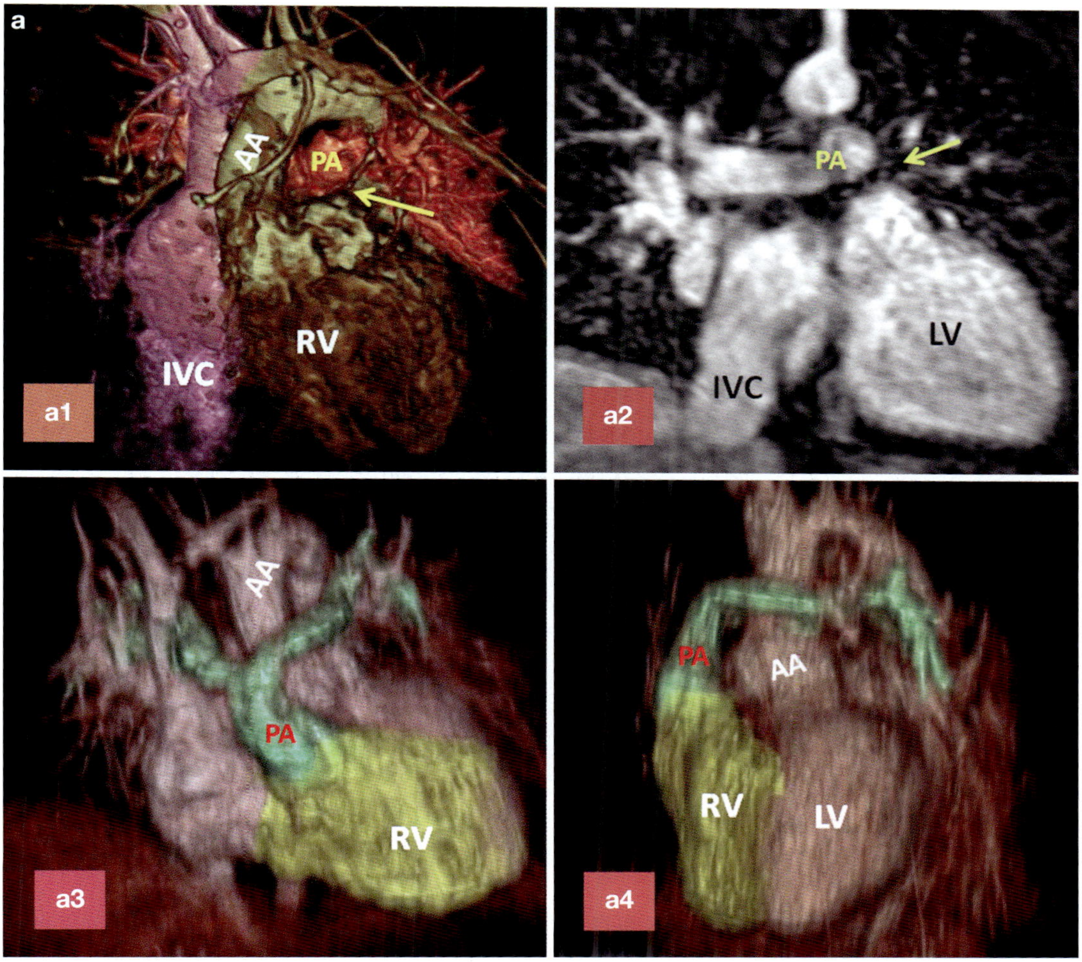

Fig. 10.12 (**a**) A 26-year-old patient with post Mustard TGA, complete correction was performed after 2-stage pulmonary artery banding and arterial switch operation. (**a1**) and (**a2**) are MR angiograms after pulmonary banding. The pulmonary band creates a dark signal on MR angiogram (*yellow arrow*). Note anterior position of the ascending aorta (*AA*). (**a3**) and (**a4**) are MR angiogram after arterial switch performed 1 year after pulmonary banding. Note anterior position of the pulmonary artery (*PA*). (**b**) A 25-year-old female status post Mustard TGA before (**b1** and **b3**) and 6 months after (**b2** and **b4**) pulmonary artery (*PA*) banding showing improved left ventricular (*LV*) function as shown by ventricular dilatation and decreased septal straightening. The right ventricle (*RV*) load is diminished. Stenosis of the main pulmonary artery at level of banding is shown (*arrows*). *IVC* inferior vena cava

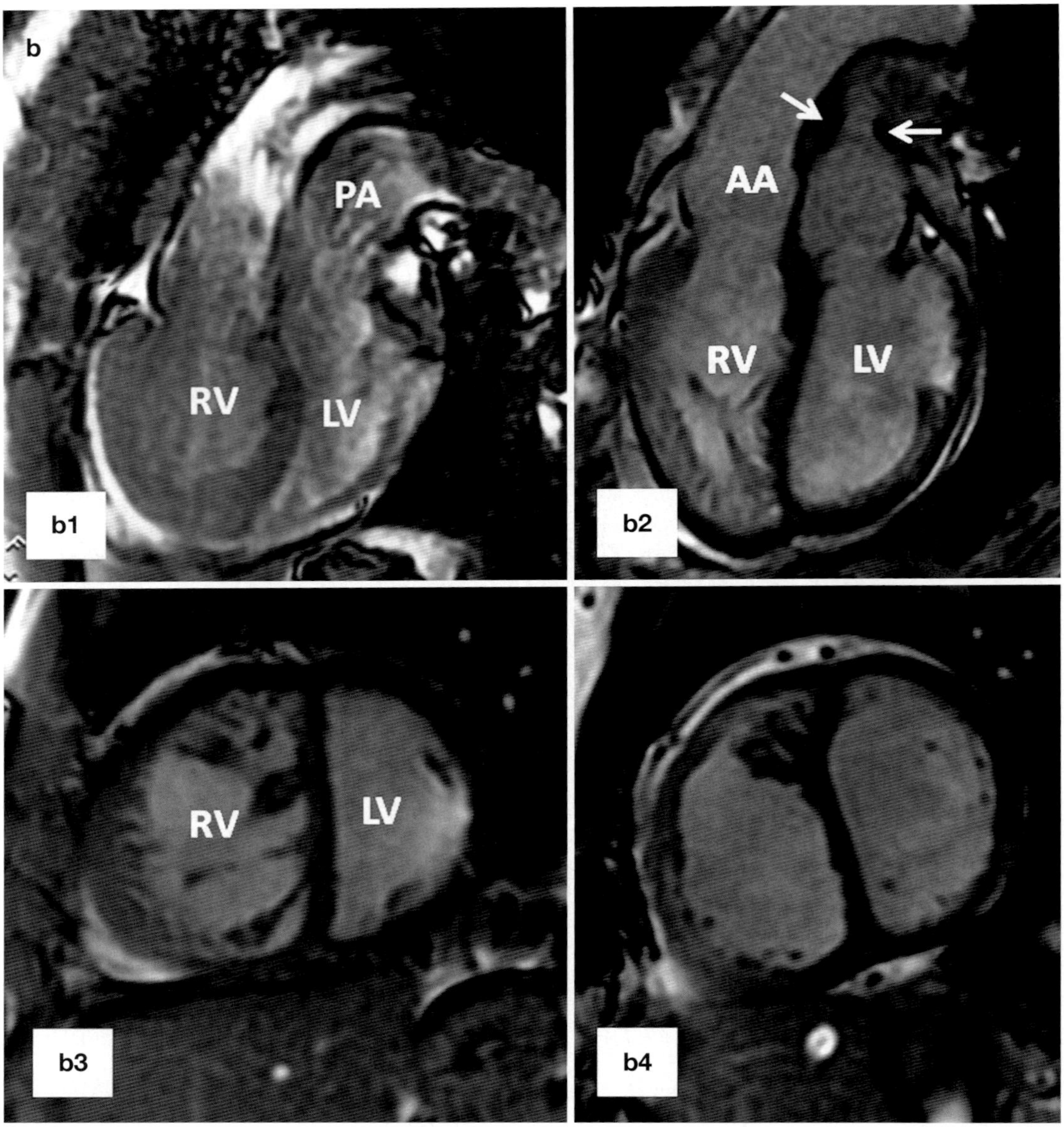

Fig. 10.12 (continued)

(Fig. 10.14). However, small defects can increase the risk of paradoxical embolus and cerebrovascular event, especially in patients with history of tachyarrhythmias or in the presence of an endocardial pacemaker (see Fig. 30.13, extracardiac complications). In order to decrease this risk, all TGA patients who require pacemaker implantation typically undergo a thorough pre-procedural imaging evaluation to assess for the presence of a baffle leak. Complex anatomy of the interatrial septum after atrial switch can make detailed analysis of the baffle difficult (Fig. 10.10). Although transesophageal echocardiography can provide most information required to evaluate these cases, in many cases it is not conclusive and additional diagnostic tests are necessary for final decision making. CT is known for its ability to show detailed anatomic structures. It is fast and

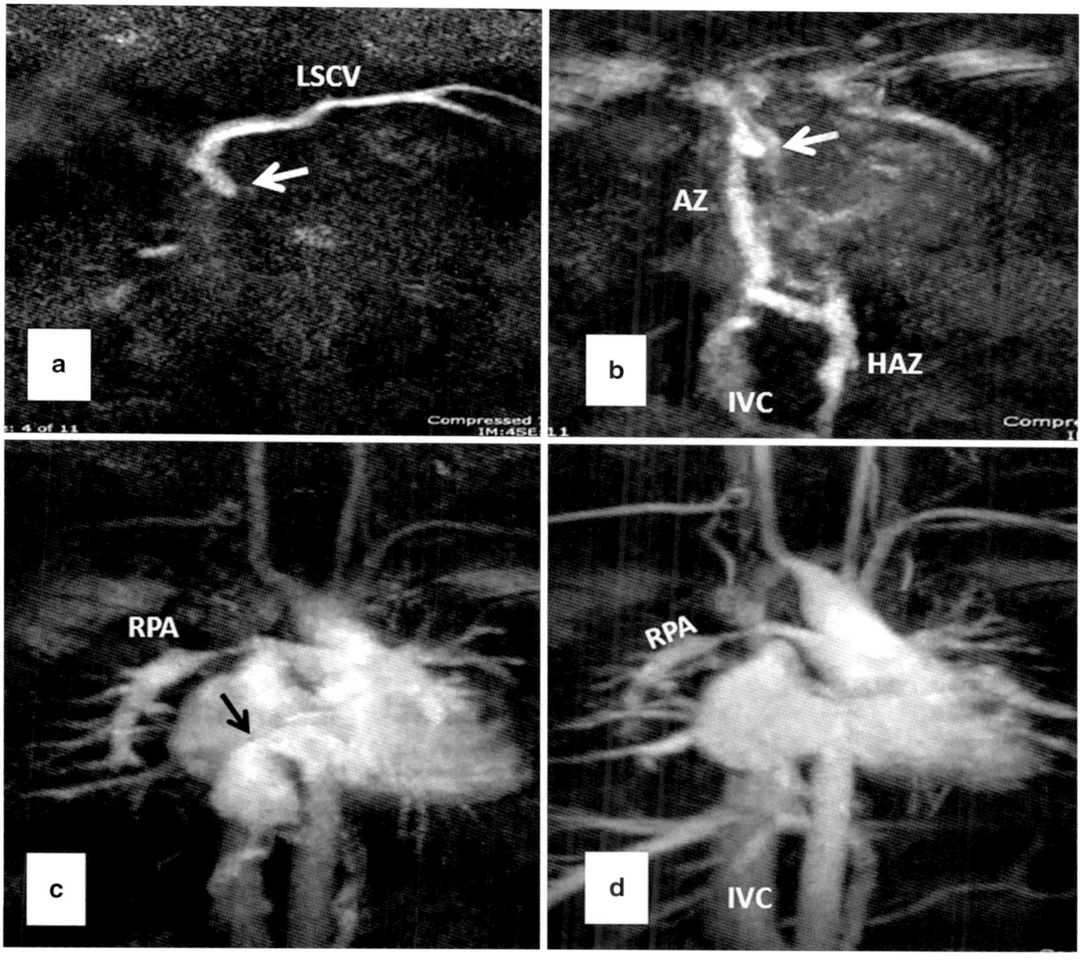

Fig. 10.13 Serial MR angiography images (**a**–**d**) show severe superior caval baffle stenosis (*white arrows*) causing shift of contrast injected from left subclavian vein (*LSCV*) into the azygos (*AZ*), hemiazygos (*HAZ*), and inferior vena cava (*IVC*) (**a** and **b**). Mild stenosis of the inferior caval baffle is also shown (*black arrow* in **c**). Note stenosis of the right pulmonary artery (*RPA* in **c** and **d**) and occlusion of the proximal right subclavian artery as sequelae of a Blalock-Taussig shunt (Courtesy of Tiffanie R. Johnson MD, Section of Pediatric Cardiology, Riley Hospital for Children, Indiana University)

easy to interpret (Figs. 10.9 and 10.10). However, special injection technique is required to show both sides of the baffle without much streak artifacts (Fig. 10.10). CT has also the advantage of showing additional anatomic problems including a patent ductus arteriosus or anomalous venous return (Fig. 10.6). When the LV is enlarged, it is important to rule out a significant pathway leak with predominant systemic-to-nonsystemic shunt (equivalent of RV enlargement in concordant heart chambers with an ASD). Baffle leaks can sometimes be treated with placement of occluder devices [30] (see Fig. 30.13, extracardiac complications). The combination of a baffle leak proximal to a baffle stenosis will exacerbate nonsystemic-to-systemic shunting and leads to desaturation, especially with exercise.

Other Complications. Direct operative trauma to the sinus node or damage to its blood supply and scar lines across the atrium have been suggested as the principal causes of sinus node dysfunction in both types of atrial switch operations [7, 31].

Atrial flutter is not uncommon after Mustard repair [22, 31]. Long-term neurologic complications include stroke and seizures, often related to thromboembolic events (see Fig. 30.14, extracardiac complications). Right (systemic) ventricular failure with secondary tricuspid valve insufficiency is common [23, 25]. These patients can develop progressive cardiomegaly and may ultimately require end-stage heart failure management, including cardiac transplant [25]. Less common complications include pulmonary arterial hypertension (6 %), residual VSD, and dynamic subpulmonary stenosis [32–34] (Fig. 10.6). A mild degree of subpulmonary stenosis is common in patients with TGA following atrial-level repair [32]. More-severe subpulmonary stenosis after baffle reconstruction is rare and can be treated with a left ventricle-to-pulmonary artery valved conduit [33].

Complications After Arterial Switch

Compared to atrial switch, the rate of dysrhythmias is less [35]. Complications that may be seen at imaging after an arterial switch procedure include main pulmonary artery and branch pulmonary artery obstruction, aortic root dilatation with aortic regurgitation, right ventricle outflow tract (RVOT) obstruction, and coronary artery stenosis [36, 37]. The most frequent types of stenosis are discrete pulmonary narrowing at the anastomosis and the right pulmonary artery segmental stenosis because they are draped across the aorta behind the sternum. Dilatation of the neoaortic root is also common, but hemodynamically significant neoaortic valve regurgitation is uncommon [38]. Increased dimensions of the aortic annulus lead to loss of coaptation of the aortic valve leaflets and varying degrees of central aortic regurgitation (Fig. 10.11a). Reduced elasticity of the proximal aorta, reduced LV systolic function, and increased LV dimensions as measured with MRI are frequently observed these patients [39]. It has been reported that there is a substantial risk of early and late coronary artery occlusion or stenosis in patients undergo-

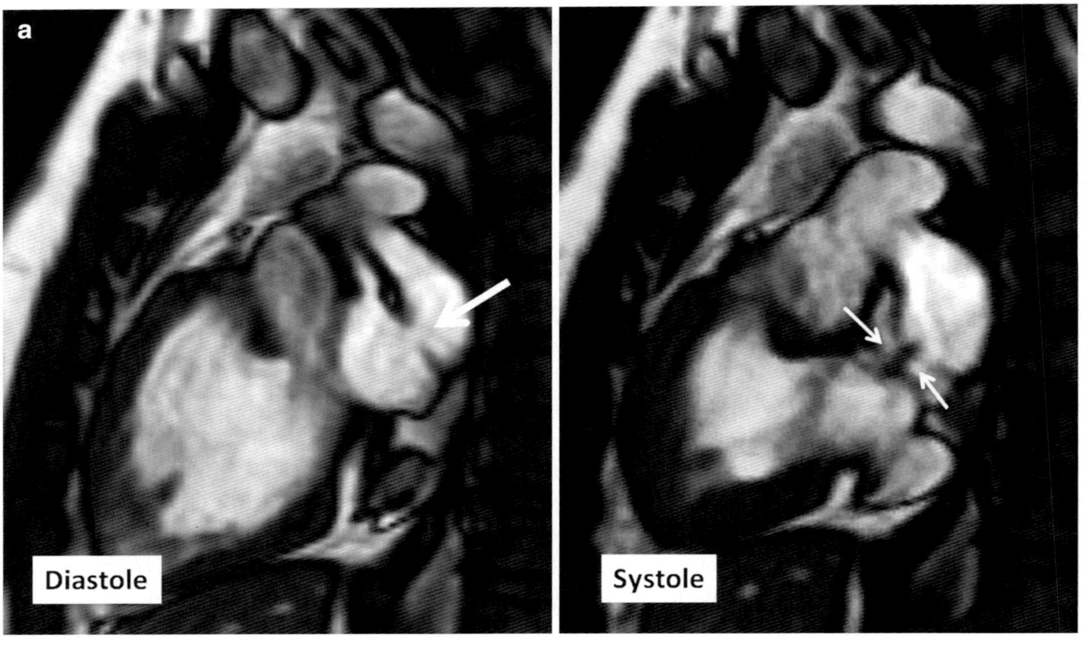

Fig. 10.14 (**a**) Two-chamber long-axis cine MR images show an atrial baffle small defect of atrial baffle show a small defect in diastole (*large arrow*) and a shunt (*small arrows*) though it during ventricular systole. (**b**) Baffle leak shown by CT angiography. (**b1**) is sagittal cut through the caval veins and (**b2–b4**) are axial images at three levels of baffle. Contrast arrival through the superior limb of baffle shows a defect (between *green arrows*) at superior caval limb between the superior vena cava (*SVC*) and right atrial appendage causing small right to left shunt. *IVC* inferior vena cava, *LA* left atrium, *RA* right atrium, *LV* left ventricle, *RV* right ventricle

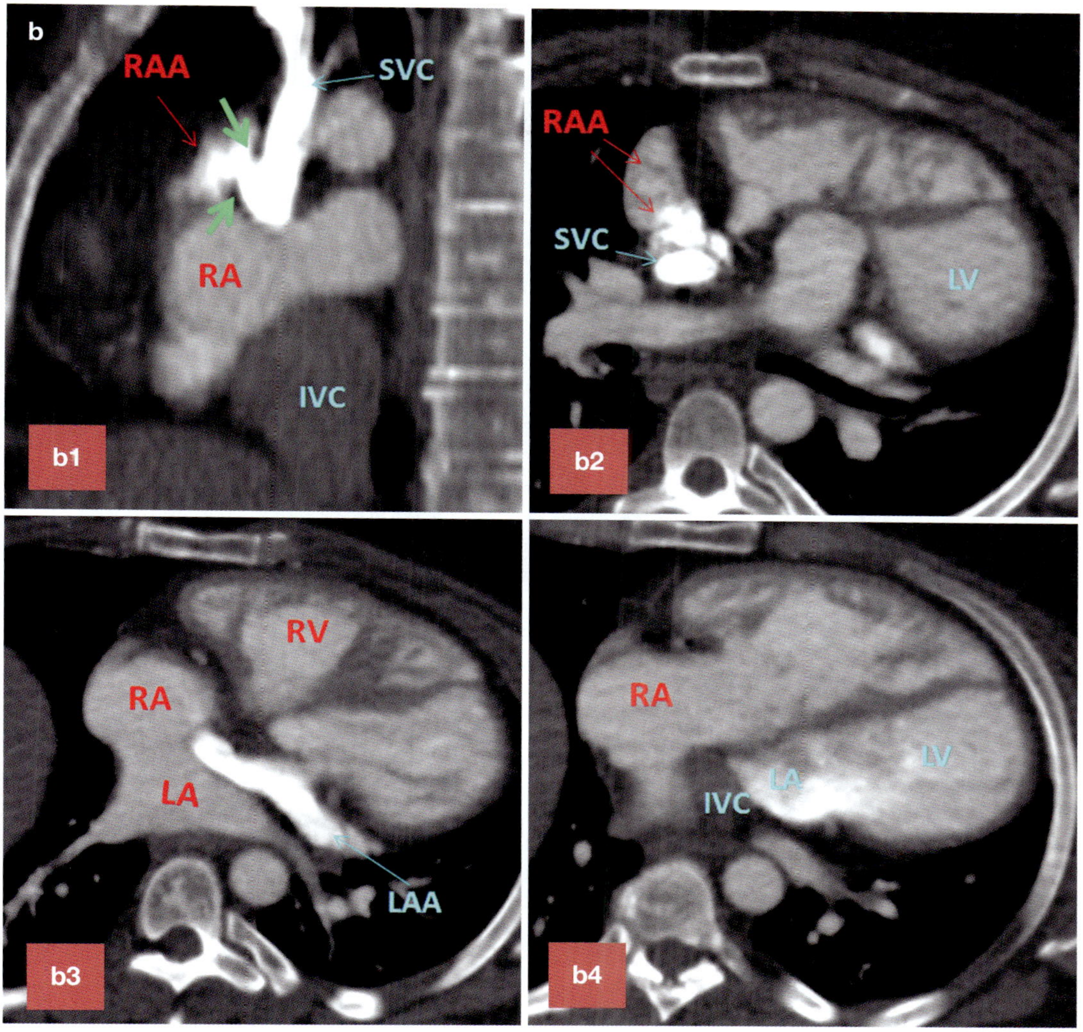

Fig. 10.14 (continued)

ing an arterial switch procedure. Most of these patients are asymptomatic, at least initially [40]. Because the RVOT and the pulmonary arteries are positioned immediately behind the sternum after the arterial switch procedure, transthoracic echocardiography is a poor method for evaluating obstructive lesions in these vessels. The anatomic and functional significance of such obstructions can be more accurately assessed with MR imaging by using a combination of techniques including cine imaging, gadolinium-enhanced MR angiography, and velocity-encoded MRI [41]. In patients in whom the presence of coronary ischemia is suspected, coronary CT angiography is the imaging modality of choice. However, coronary MR angiography is also useful for the noninvasive investigation of proximal segments of the coronary arteries [42].

Conversion to Arterial Switch

If the systemic RV is failing after an intra-atrial repair, morphologically left ventricular reconditioning and an arterial switch operation is an alternative to cardiac transplantation in selected patients [43]. The first step in such an approach is a surgically placed pulmonary artery band

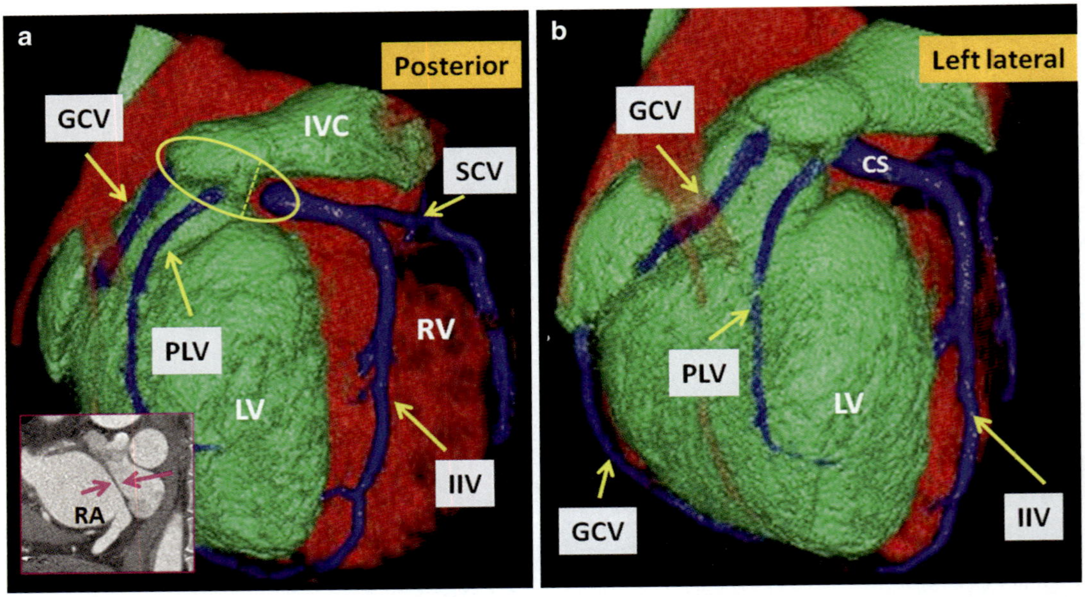

Fig. 10.15 TGA status post Mustard operation. Posterior (**a**) and left lateral (**b**) views of the heart show anatomic distribution of the coronary veins. The coronary sinus (within the *yellow circle*) appears divided into two parts by the intra-atrial baffle (*pink arrows*). For this reason, the great cardiac vein (*GCV*) and the posterolateral vein (*PLV*) are opened into the nonsystemic atrial conduit, and the inferior interventricular vein (*IIV*) and the small cardiac vein (*SCV*) follow the normal path and drain into the coronary sinus (*CS*) and systemic conduit. Note veins draining into the systemic circulation are larger due to increased intra-atrial pressure of the systemic side. The inferior vena cava (*IVC*) is shown connecting into the nonsystemic atrial conduit. *LV* left ventricle, *RA* right atrium, *RV* right ventricle (systemic)

(average 1 year). This is necessary because the LV rapidly becomes deconditioned when exposed to the low-resistance pulmonary circuit, losing its ability to generate systemic pressure. Pulmonary artery banding provides adequate LV training if done at an early age, but results in older patients may not be satisfactory [44]. After banding, MRI is used to evaluate ejection fraction, ventricular mass, and tricuspid valve function. With increasing morphological LV pressure after banding, a shift in the interventricular septum and reduction of the tricuspid regurgitation and right ventricle dysfunction are expected. Later the atrial baffle can be taken down, the pulmonary artery band removed, and the arterial switch procedure performed [44] (Fig. 10.12).

Anatomic Variability of Coronary Vessels

Anomalous origin of the coronary artery is not uncommon in TGA patients and may cause problem during arterial switch operation [7]. In adult patients with the history of atrial switch, these anomalies can be seen in diagnostic tests including MRI and CT and could be of surgical significance at the time of anatomic conversion surgeries (Fig. 10.15). In Massoudy et al.'s study [7], the frequency of the potentially relevant surgical features in a large series of autopsied hearts was reported. In 60 % of cases, the right coronary artery (RCA) arose from the right sinus and the left anterior descending (LAD) and left circumflex arteries from the left sinus. In 10 % the LAD originated from the right sinus, taking a retropulmonary course in 50 %, interarterial in 10 %, and preaortic in 40 %. High takeoff above or at the level of sinotubular junction was seen in 16 %. Juxtacommissural origin of coronary arteries, intramural or tangential takeoff, and commissural mismatch of arterial trunks are relatively rare but can lead to accidental injury when the aorta is transected during arterial switch [45]

(Fig. 10.5). Furthermore, other features, such as retropulmonary course of the left coronary artery or origin of both the RCA and the LAD from the right sinus, have been shown to be important [46]. These abnormal features can now be diagnosed with accuracy using cardiac CT angiography. With MRI diagnostic-quality images of the coronary ostium and proximal coronary artery, course can be obtained [42]. Anomalies of the coronary veins are rare. However, in patients with intra-atrial baffle after Senning of Mustard operations, part of the coronary sinus tributaries may be divided between the right and left atria (Fig. 10.15). In patients with systemic right ventricle, the coronary veins draining into the right atrium are enlarged.

CT and MR Techniques

CT Study of the Baffle and RV Function

Current standard practice for ECG-gated CT angiography of the heart involves injection from an upper extremity vein into the SVC. Noncontrast blood from the IVC mixing with high-density contrast injected through the SVC frequently produces artifacts that obscure anatomic detail of the right heart particularly the right atrium. This makes detailed assessment of anatomy of the right atrium and cavoatrial junctions difficult, especially in complicated situations such as surgically corrected congenital cardiac malformations. In our institution we adopted a modified injection protocol using dual extremity contrast injections which provides artifact free images of the right heart. We have used this technique in selected patients with repaired TGA to evaluate anatomy of the heart including the atrial baffle (Fig. 10.10). Dual injection technique has been used for Fontan shunt using peripheral veins of lower and upper extremities with some limitations related to contrast dilution [47]. Using our technique, a 20 gauge angiocatheter needle is inserted into the antecubital vein, and a second needle (similar size but longer in length) will be placed in a femoral vein under ultrasound guidance, local anesthesia, and sterile conditions. Contrast injection steps are as follows: 80 mL of nondiluted iodinated contrast is injected, followed by 30 mL of saline using a standard dual-barrel injector in the femoral vein at a rate of 4 mL/s. Ten seconds after injection of femoral contrast, 50–70 mL of 40 % contrast diluted with saline (20 mL of contrast mixed with 50 mL of saline) is injected manually or using a second power injector in the antecubital vein at 3 mL/s. Scan is triggered at 150 Hounsfield units in the descending aorta near the tracheal bifurcation.

MR Techniques

Currently, transthoracic echocardiography is the imaging modality of choice for the preoperative diagnosis and assessment of TGA. The main role of MRI is in the diagnosis of postoperative complications, particularly those that develop as the child grows older. Cardiac MRI is an excellent noninvasive imaging modality and may be repeated every 2–4 years for serial monitoring of ventricular function and baffle integrity in detail [48]. Unfortunately, many patients have pacemakers, which currently contraindicates MRI, although this circumstance might change in the future. In patients with a pacemaker, CT may be a better choice, especially for the assessment of anatomy and complication related to surgery. The goals of MRI after an atrial switch procedure include evaluations of the function and size of the ventricles, careful assessment of the intra-atrial baffle for leak and stenosis, atrioventricular valves for regurgitation, and outflow tracts for obstruction. In post arterial switch, additional objectives of MRI include careful evaluation of pulmonary arteries for stenosis and the neoaorta for dilatation and valve regurgitation. Assessment of the RV function is very important in patients with atrial switch, and MRI is the method of choice for functional evaluation of the RV and follow-up studies [49]. In one study comparing MRI and echocardiography, transthoracic echocardiography underestimated right ventricular ejection fraction compared to cardiac MRI [48]. Table 10.3 demonstrates cardiovascular MR imaging protocol for TGA patients. For cardiac function, following obtaining localizer images of the heart, a segmented balanced steady-state free precession sequence (b-SSFP) with retrospective

Table 10.3 Comprehensive cardiovascular MRI protocol for TGA and ccTGA patients

2-Dimensional axial, sagittal, and coronal stacks of single-shot fast spin-echo images (dark blood) and balanced steady-state free precession (b-SSFP) (bright blood) covering the chest
Axial cine b-SSFP imaging in multiple contiguous sections from the level of the diaphragm to the level of the aortic arch to allow dynamic evaluation of the pulmonary venous baffles, qualitative assessment of ventricular and atrioventricular valve function, and assessment of the aorta and pulmonary arteries
Oblique coronal and sagittal cine b-SSFP imaging in multiple contiguous sections parallel to the SVC and IVC in post atrial switch (to allow detection of a systemic venous baffle obstruction or leak) and parallel to the right ventricle outflow tract (RVOT) and left ventricle outflow tract (LVOT) in cases after arterial switch (ideally, two orthogonal views each for the RVOT and LVOT to assess stenosis)
Short-axis, two-chamber (left), and four-chamber cine b-SSFP imaging for quantitative analysis of right and left ventricular function
3-Dimensional gadolinium-enhanced MR angiography (time resolved), coronal orientation
Short-axis, two-chamber (left), and four-chamber delayed myocardial enhancement
Velocity-encoded MR imaging of the aortic root and main pulmonary artery for measurement of pulmonary flow relative to aortic flow (Qp:Qs) and if indicated over baffle defect (shunt quantification) and branch pulmonary arteries (stenosis assessment) or any suspected narrowed region

electrocardiographic gating is used for short- and long-axis views. Short-axis slices perpendicular to the ventricular septum are obtained encompassing the entire heart during end-expiratory breath holds. Typical parameters are flip angle, 50–70°; repetition time, 3–4 ms; echo time, 1–2 ms; 8 mm slice thickness; and 1–2 mm inter-slice gap. A temporal resolution of 40–50 ms can be achieved. In patients who have difficulty holding their breath, a single-shot version of this technique can be used as an alternative to the segmented form of data acquisition. Delayed gadolinium-enhanced MRI can be used to detect myocardial fibrosis in the systemic RV and should be carefully analyzed in the baseline and follow-up MR studies [50]. Time-resolved contrast-enhanced MR angiography is an easy, fast, and reliable technique for the assessment of anatomy and shunt and can be added to any MRI protocols for patients with CHD [51]. In post atrial switch it may be able to show moderate baffle limb stenosis and wall defects causing shunt [26]. The imaging sequence will be started simultaneously with the power injection of 10 mL of gadolinium-based contrast followed by 20 mL of saline solution into an antecubital vein at a rate of 4–5 mL/s. A three-dimensional fast gradient echo sequence is used. At 1.5 T, coronal or axial 3D data set (coronal for baffle stenosis and axial for baffle leak) can be acquired in 5–6 s and repeated (i.e., 4–5 times) during one breath hold. The following parameters are generally used: TR/TE, 1.9/0.7; flip angle, 20°; matrix, variable; slice thickness, 4 mm; number of slices, variable; and parallel imaging with acceleration factor of 2. Background signal will be suppressed by the subtraction of the first baseline data set from the subsequent data sets.

Systemic Right Ventricular Dysfunction

The RV is able to turn functionally, and maybe structurally, into a LV (Fig. 10.16). The RV functions as the systemic pumping chamber in hypoplastic left heart syndrome, ccTGA, and post atrial switch TGA. Medium-term survival in patients with a systemic RV is relatively good; however, long-term outcome is unknown and decisions on the timing of operation depend on RV function. Accurate analysis of RV anatomy, volumes, and function and the degree of systemic atrioventricular valve regurgitation is important and. all patients should have a periodic assessment of ventricular function by echocardiography and/or MRI. The importance of having an accurate and reproducible diagnostic tool for the evaluation and follow-up of systemic RV volumes and function is evident, and cardiac MRI is the gold standard and should be performed at least every 2–4 years. The MRI method of volumetric measurements is very important. Trabeculations in the systemic RV cavity are

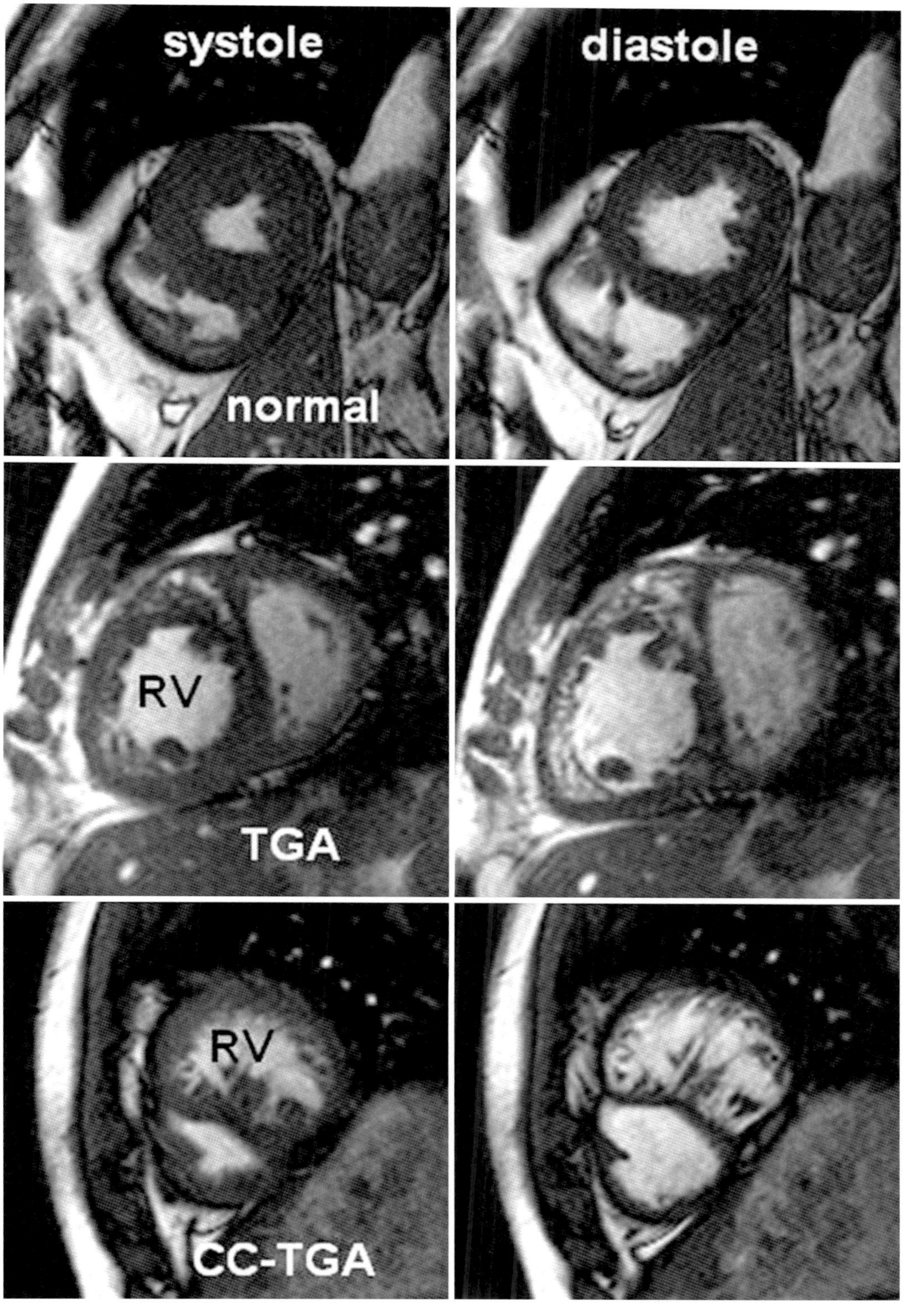

Fig. 10.16 Comparison of the right ventricle (*RV*) morphology during systole with diastole in normal condition, transposition of great arteries (*TGA*) (post atrial baffle), and congenitally corrected TGA (*ccTGA*). Overtime, the systemic RV function and morphology can change and become similar to a left ventricle. Note rounding and hypertrophy of the RV in TGA. In ccTGA the morphological RV (systemic RV) is thickened and the interventricular septum is straightened

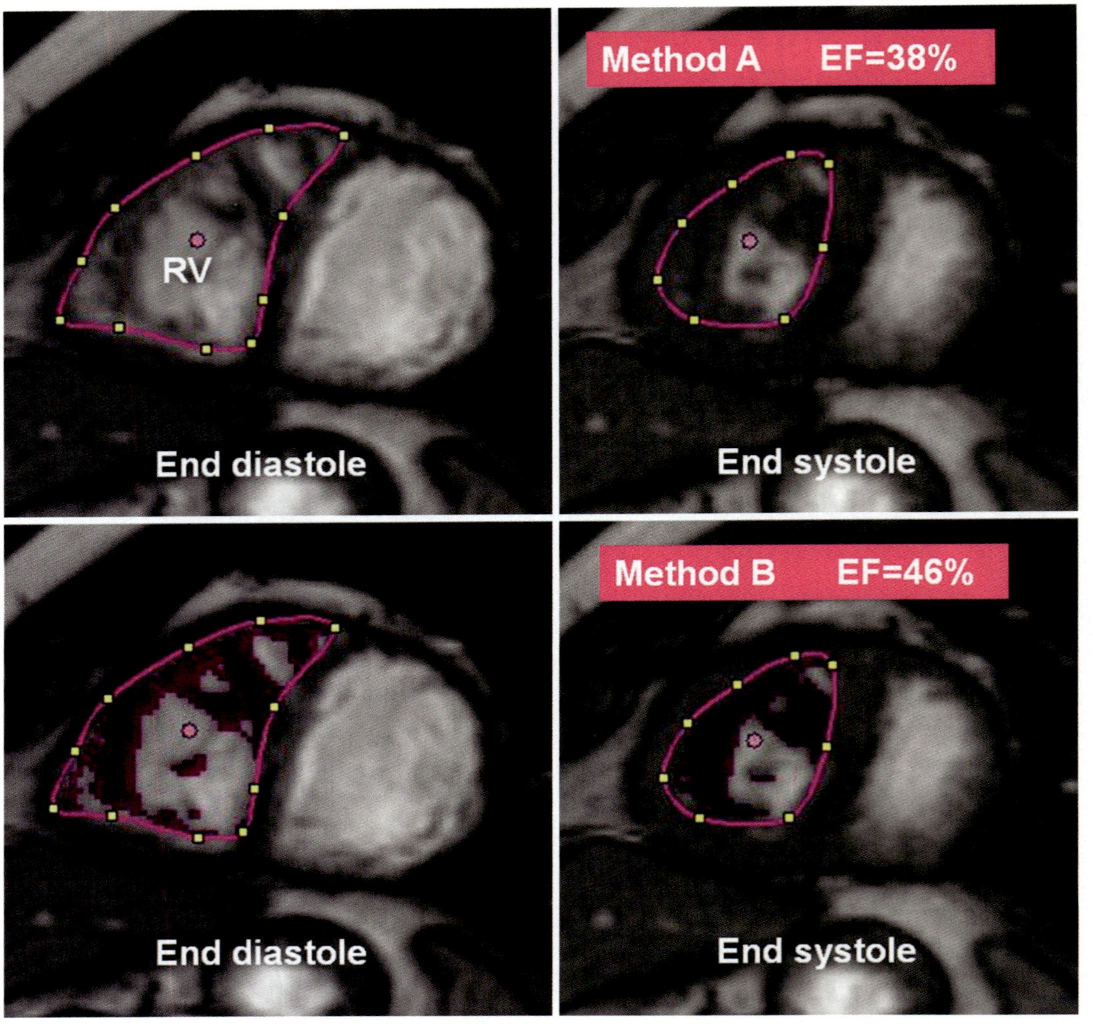

Fig. 10.17 MRI shows two different methods of the right ventricle (*RV*) volume analysis in a patient with systemic RV due to TGA status post Mustard surgery. Simpson method (short-axis images) is used in both methods. Method A (*upper row*) shows the inclusion of trabeculations and papillary muscles in the ventricular cavity. Method B (*lower row*) shows exclusion of those structures. Ejection fraction is underestimated in method A. Method B appears to be more accurate. Trabeculations are numerous towards the apex of the RV and partial volume averaging blurs boundaries and method A may be a more reproducible approach. It is important to use a single method for longitudinal follow-ups

large and very crowded near the apex and placing region of interest outside the trabeculations is probably the easier approach. Although the influence of papillary muscles and trabeculations on measured ventricular volumes of normal heart is not significant [52], including those structures in measurements of systemic RV may lead to a significantly higher end-diastolic and end-systolic volumes and lower calculated ejection fraction [53] (Fig. 10.17). Whatever method is selected needs to be consistent for the follow-up examinations [54]. Most current volumetric techniques use the Simpson's method. In this technique, the volume is calculated from a stack of parallel planes, usually in the short-axis orientation. This method can be accurate for the left ventricle, but it may underestimate the RV volumes (possibly due to incomplete coverage of the

RV outflow tract) when compared to advanced three-dimensional techniques using image data acquired from combinations of views (short and long axes) to reconstruct the RV [55]. The major advantage of using cross-references between long- and short-axis images, as compared with analysis based on short-axis-only images, is the ease of determining the planes of the tricuspid and pulmonary valves (Fig. 10.18). This advantage is likely responsible for the slightly higher reproducibility of measurements compared to older software. However, we should be careful when using new volumetric analysis methods because most reports on normal values and those obtained in repaired CHDs are based on volumetric analysis of short-axis images. The assessment of the extent of myocardial fibrosis with delayed post contrast MRI may be of prognostic value and can be associated with RV dysfunction, poor exercise tolerance, arrhythmia, and progressive clinical deterioration. In the study of Broberg et al. [56], the fibrosis index values were highest in systemic RV patients and correlated with end-diastolic volume index and ventricular ejection fraction.

TGA and RV Function

Despite good long-term survival of near 80 % after atrial switch procedures [21–24], deterioration of the systemic ventricle function is seen in up to 50 % of patients [57, 58]. The exact cause of RV dysfunction is unclear. A shift in the systemic RV free wall from longitudinal to circumferential shortening is seen when compared with the normal RV. This contraction pattern resembles that of the normal LV and may be explained by alterations in ventricular geometry and/or myocardial hypertrophy (Fig. 10.16). In contrast to the normal LV, ventricular torsion is essentially absent and strain rate is reduced. RV dyssynchrony and regional functional dysfunction at rest are common [59, 60]. Continuous exposure of the RV to a high-resistance systemic circulation results in a compensatory RV hypertrophy. This may lead to decreased myocardial perfusion and ischemia, scar, and failure due to mismatch between RV blood supply and systemic RV work [61]. Abnormal response to stress by dobutamine or exercise testing is common [62, 63]. Regions of delayed gadolinium enhancement due to focal fibrosis are described in the RV myocardium of 60 % of patients late after atrial switch [50]. In contrast, the results from Fratz et al. in a relatively younger group did not support this [64].

In Babu-Narayan et al.'s MR study, the presence and extent of scar regions in systemic RV correlate directly with the degree of RV hypertrophy and inversely with RV systolic function [50]. Enhancement patterns include localized full-thickness RV anterior wall enhancement, small patchy areas of enhancement, and VSD closure site (see Fig. 7.31). Enhancement at RV free wall insertion to the septum appears to be a common benign finding and due to continuous pressure overload. The systemic atrioventricular valve (anatomic tricuspid valve) insufficiency is common in systemic RV failure and appears to be related annular dilatation [60]. Pulmonary banding and arterial switch operation may improve coaptation of the systemic valve [65].

Systemic RV in Congenitally Corrected Transposition of the Great Arteries (ccTGA)

The RV also supports the systemic circulation in patients with ccTGA [66, 67]. Long-term outcome is not normal even in ccTGA patients without associated lesions due to a propensity to develop RV dysfunction and tricuspid valve regurgitation [68, 69]. More than one-third of patients with no significant associated heart defect may develop congestive heart failure by the fifth decade [70]. As explained earlier, the factors responsible for accelerated systemic RV dysfunction include ventricular geometry, perfusion abnormality, ischemia, and impaired contractility [71–73]. Although an uncommon finding, delayed post contrast MRI is helpful to show the extent of myocardial scar in ccTGA patients [62]. A subendocardial pattern of enhancement may suggest coronary artery disease. Comparing systemic RV of post atrial baffle TGA and ccTGA, it is shown that atrial baffles restrict a rise in stroke volume under dobutamine stress in TGA patients [74]. The subgroups of

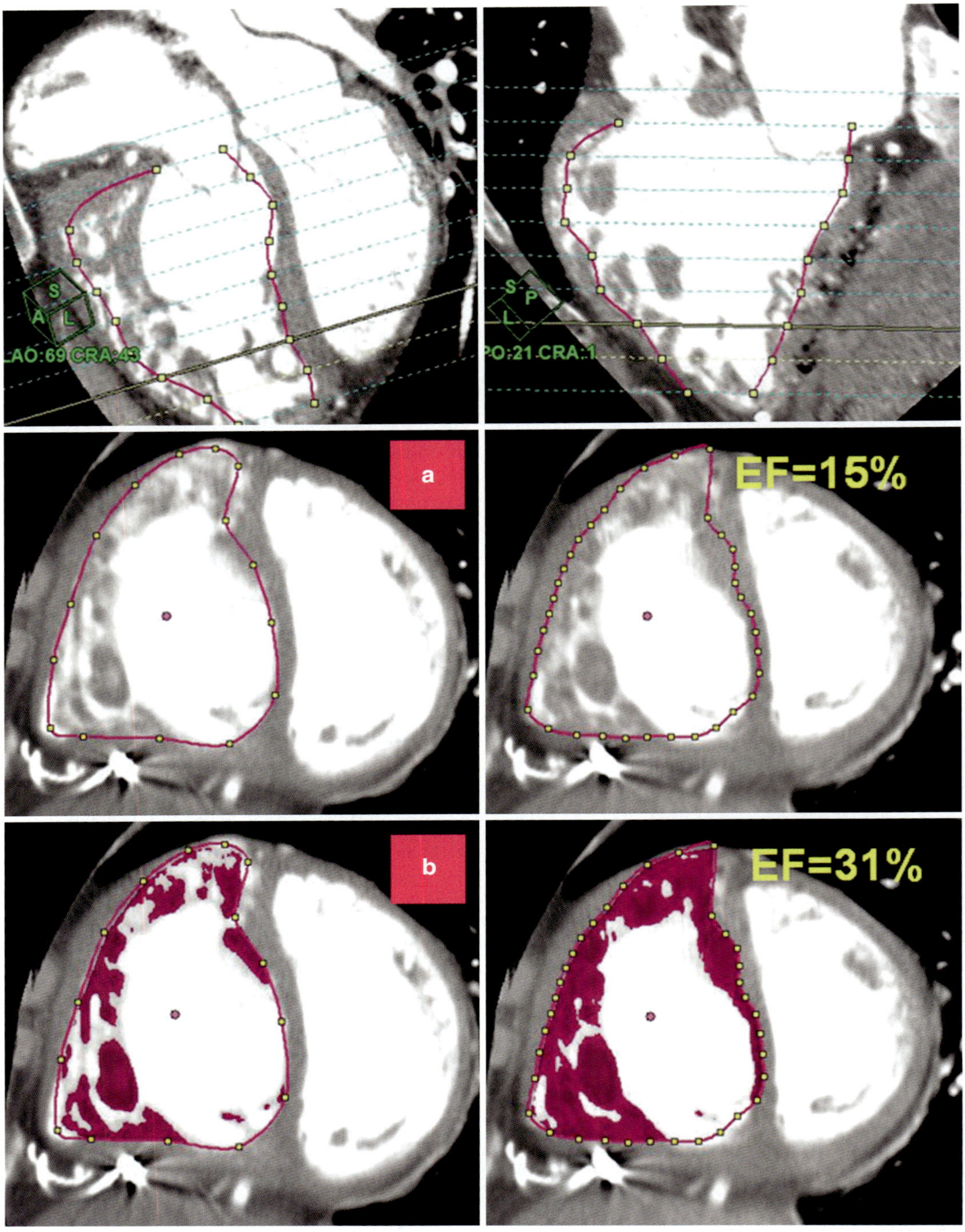

Fig. 10.18 CT images of two different methods of the systemic right ventricle (RV) volume analysis in a patient with markedly dilated systemic RV due to TGA status post Mustard surgery. In both methods three-dimensional data is used to accurately measure RV indices. In method A, trabeculations are included (EDV = 340, EF = 15 %), and in method B, trabeculations are excluded (EDV = 267, EF = 31 %). Tracing the short-axis views with access to the long-axis views may increase the accuracy of RV volume analysis by improving localization of the atrioventricular border

ccTGA patients with favorable anatomy and no history of surgery have better cardiac indices and good survival than repaired patients [75].

Congenitally Corrected Transposition of the Great Arteries

ccTGA was first described by Von Rokitansky in 1875 [76]. It is rare and comprises <1 % of all forms of CHD [2, 77–79]. The anomaly is characterized by discordant connections at atrioventricular and ventriculoarterial levels (double discordance) resulting in normal physiology circulation. It is also known as L-loop transposition of the great arteries, physiologically corrected transposition, or ventricular inversion. The L-loop signifies that the morphological RV is on the left side of the morphological LV (left-handed topology) [67] (Figs. 10.1 and 10.2). In this condition, the systemic venous return reaches the pulmonary circulation through the right-sided LV, and the pulmonary venous return reaches the aorta through the left-sided RV. ccTGA is not cyanotic and may be discovered incidentally in asymptomatic patients. However, it is not a benign condition, and late complications are common that warrant careful, long-term follow-ups [80].

Morphology

In ccTGA, the morphologically LV is sitting between the right atrium and the pulmonary trunk and the morphologically RV connects the left atrium to the aorta. Imaging characteristics that help locate the RV include coarse trabeculations, septomarginal trabeculations, septal origin of the moderator band, and the location of the medial papillary muscle complex on the interventricular septum. In contrast, the trabeculae of the LV are usually thin and the two papillary muscles are attached only to the free wall (Fig. 10.1). In the presence of LV noncompaction, its morphology can be confusing and difficult to differentiate from the RV.

The atrioventricular valve remains concordant with the associated ventricle. Therefore, the mitral valve remains on the nonsystemic side of circulation and the tricuspid valve serves on the systemic side. With this arrangement, when the interventricular septum is intact, there is reversed off setting of the septal attachments of the leaflets of the atrioventricular valves at the crux of the heart, with the tricuspid valve on the systemic side attached closer to the apex [78]. The crux anatomy facilitates recognition of atrioventricular morphology because the septal leaflet of the tricuspid valve is always closer to apex (Fig. 10.1). In presence of a VSD, however, this reversed offsetting can be lost. The morphologically LV outflow tract is demarcated by fibrous continuity between the leaflets of the pulmonary and mitral valves, and the presence of the subaortic infundibulum helps to identify the morphologically RV (Fig. 10.19). The ventricles are positioned side by side and the ventricular septum lies in a more anteroposterior position (Fig. 10.2). Excessive tilting produces a supero-inferior relation of the ventricles, the so-called crisscross heart [81]. The two arterial trunks are parallel rather than crossing as they do with concordant ventriculoarterial connections, and the aorta is usually located on the left of the pulmonary trunk. The pulmonary valve is wedged between the atrial septum and the mitral valve. In a small number of patients with usual atrial arrangement, the aorta can be found in directly anterior or right anterior to the pulmonary trunk.

Dextrocardia is present in 25 % of ccTGA patients (Fig. 10.20). In hearts with an intact ventricular septum, the membranous septum can be large [82] (Fig. 10.21). Associated abnormalities are common [67, 83]. The most common anatomic associations include VSD in almost 80 % of cases [67, 80] and pulmonary stenosis in approximately 75 % of cases [80] (Fig. 10.20). The majority of VSDs are perimembranous. Large VSD can cause a systemic-to-pulmonary shunt; however, this is usually balanced because of the protective effect of coexisting pulmonary outflow tract stenosis. Subvalvular pulmonary stenosis is more common than valvular and can be due to muscular hypertrophy, presence of a fibrous shelf on the septum, or aneurysm of the membranous septum (Fig. 10.21). Pulmonary

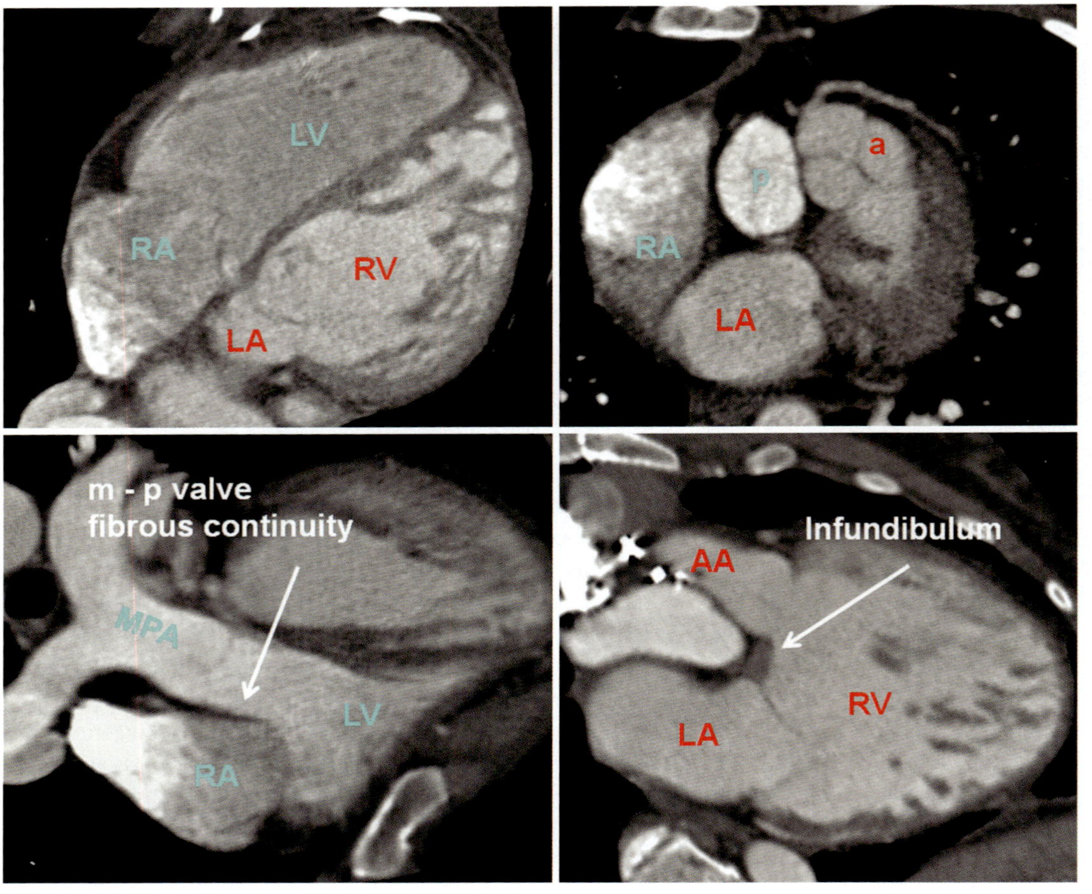

Fig. 10.19 Morphology of congenitally corrected transposition of great arteries (ccTGA). In ccTGA the ventricles are congenitally switched with the left ventricle (*LV*) is located behind the sternum. The pulmonary (*p*) and aortic (*a*) valves are side by side with the aorta on the left. This anatomic arrangement of great arteries is very uncommon in TGA (<10 %). The pulmonary artery in ccTGA arises directly from the LV with direct fibrous continuity between the mitral (*m*) and pulmonary (*p*) valves. The right ventricle (*RV*) infundibulum is not well formed or is very short (*white arrow*). *AA* ascending aorta, *LA* left atrium, *MPA* main pulmonary artery, *RA* right atrium

atresia is rarely seen and usually repaired by a right ventricle-pulmonary conduit (Fig. 10.20). Tricuspid valve anomalies, including dysplasia, straddling, or Ebstein-like malformation, also are common and are reported in up to 40 % of patients [80]. Smaller percentage of patients with ccTGA have no intracardiac defect and may remain asymptomatic until age 40–50. Even without an associated abnormality, most patients with ccTGA develop rhythm disturbances, systemic atrioventricular valve regurgitation, and moderately impaired systemic ventricular function causing congestive cardiac failure [84] (Fig. 10.22). The role of MRI or CT in these cases is mainly in the assessment of systemic RV function and associated tricuspid regurgitation. By the age of 45 years, half of the patients with associated lesions, and one-third of those without significant associated lesions, present with dysfunction of the systemic RV [70, 84]. Progressive atrioventricular block occurs in up to one-third of adult patients [85] and 45 % of patients may require pacemakers. The anatomic basis for this block is related to abnormal alignment of the atrial and ventricular septal structures with an abnormally placed AV node [82].

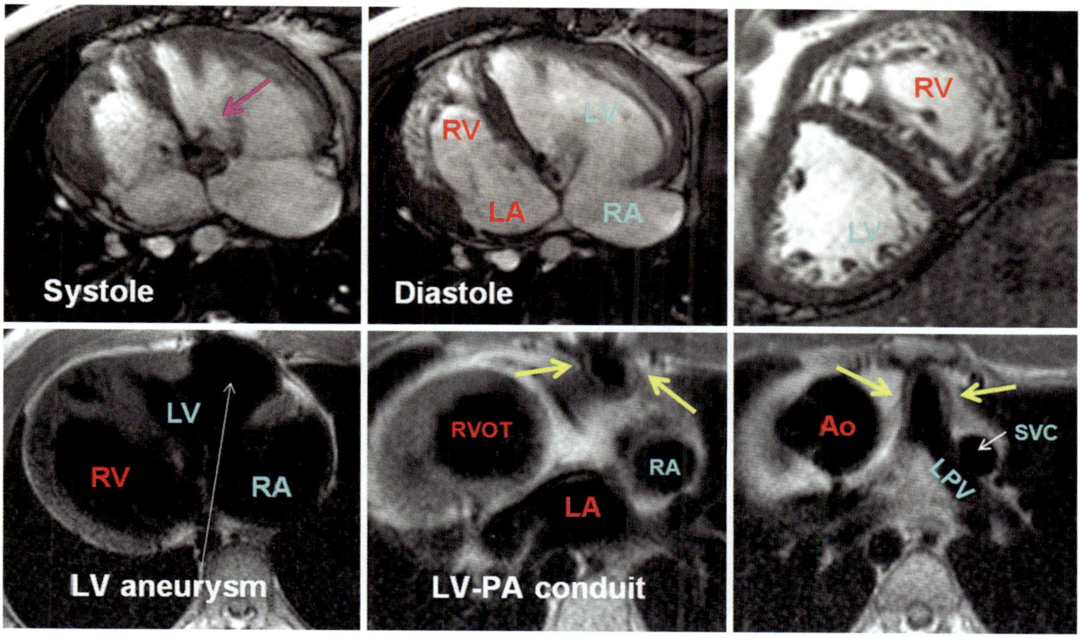

Fig. 10.20 Complex congenitally corrected transposition of great arteries (ccTGA), with dextrocardia, situs inversus, and status post left ventricle (*LV*) to pulmonary artery (*PA*) conduit for pulmonary atresia {I, D, D}. The jet of residual small perimembranous ventricular septal defect (*pink arrow*) is seen in the systolic image. The LV-to-PA conduit (*yellow arrows*) measured 1.5, cm and there was an LV aneurysm just proximal to the conduit measuring 5 cm. The right (systemic) ventricle (*RV*) is hypertrophied but the systolic function was good. The LV is hypertrophied and enlarged, and the aorta (*Ao*) is dilated. *LA* left atrium, *RA* right atrium, *SVC* superior vena cava, *RVOT* right ventricle outflow tract

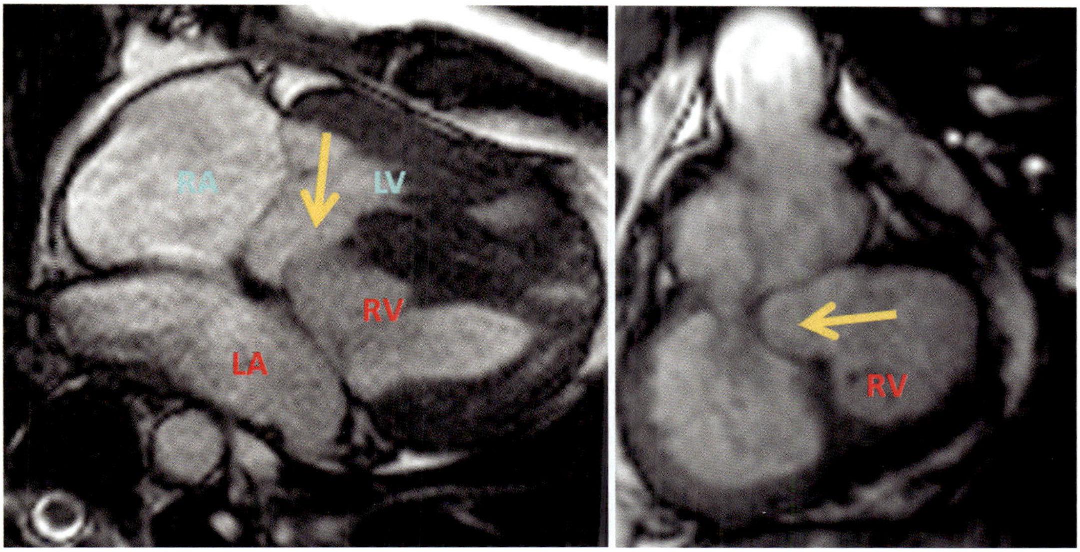

Fig. 10.21 Large aneurysmal membranous septum in congenitally corrected transposition of great arteries (ccTGA) causing mild narrowing of the LV outflow tract. In ccTGA the atrioventricular conduction system is abnormally positioned due to the malalignment of the atrial and ventricular septal structures; the gap is usually filled by an extensive membranous septum (*arrows*) when the septal structures are intact. *LA* left atrium, *LV* left ventricle, *RA* right atrium, *RV* right ventricle

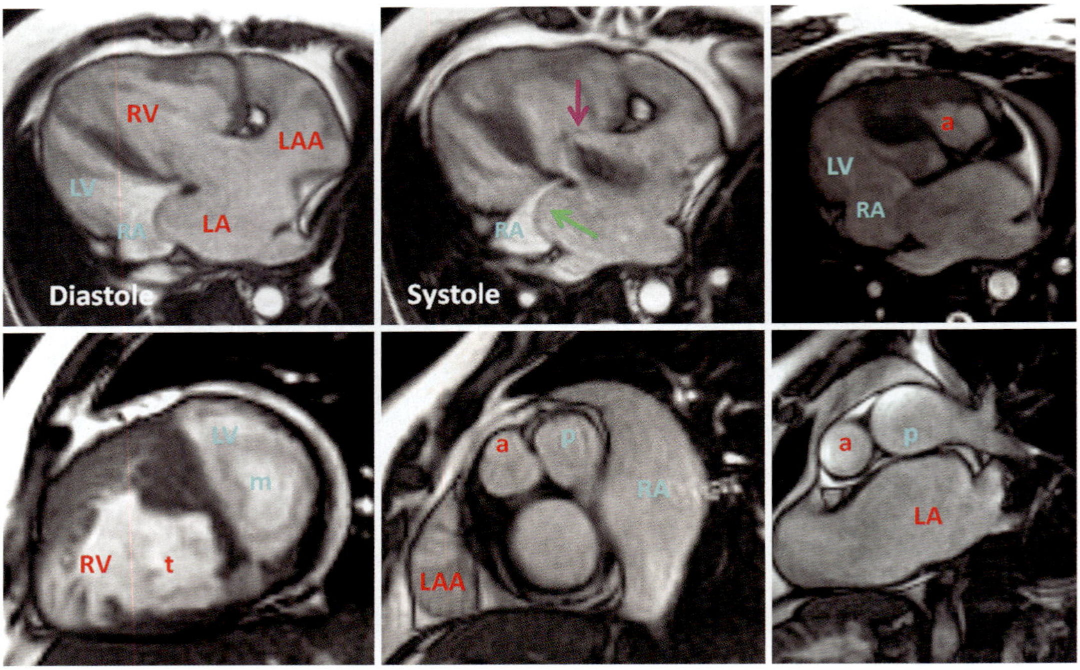

Fig. 10.22 A 38-year-old female with congenitally corrected transposition of great arteries (ccTGA) and dextrocardia (S, L, L). In *upper row* are long-axis four-chamber and in *lower row* are short-axis MR images. Major problem was moderate to severe tricuspid regurgitation (*pink arrow*). The right ventricle (*RV*) and left atrium are dilated and RV outflow tract is thickened. Interatrial septum (*green arrow*) is bulging to the right atrium (*RA*). Systemic RV is retrosternal and on the left side of the *LV* (levoposition). The aortic (*a*) valve is anterior and on the left side (levoposed) of the pulmonary (*p*) valve. *m* mitral valve, *t* tricuspid valve, *LAA* left atrial appendage

Imaging Techniques

Diagnosis of ccTGA can be made by conventional angiography, echocardiography, CT, and MRI. Conventional angiography is invasive and mostly used for cardiac catheterization, assessment of the coronary arteries, or interventional procedure. The indications for cardiac catheterization are limited nowadays, since echocardiography and MRI better delineate the anatomy, ventricular function, and the severity of the systemic valve regurgitation (Figs. 10.22 and 10.23). The need for evaluation of the coronary arteries or the aortic arch, complex pulmonary atresia, or pulmonary venous abnormalities are better indications for a cardiac CT angiography study. Evaluation of the coronary arteries should also be performed in older patients prior to any surgical repair to study their anatomy and distribution and to evaluate for coronary arterial disease and osteal stenosis.

Although echocardiography is frequently used in children, comprehensive anatomic and functional analysis cannot be easily obtained, especially in adults and those who had previous surgery. In these patients, CT or MRI are usually preferred methods to complete the examination. The number of adult patients with ccTGA who need CT or MRI for early detection of complications has been increasing, due to better imaging techniques as well as increasing life expectancy of these patients [86, 87].

The imaging protocols for ccTGA imaging are similar to TGA (Table 10.3). Major advantages of CT over MRI are the ease of technique, high spatial resolution, and that it can be used in patients with a pacemaker [88, 89]. CT is advantageous over MRI in delineation of the coronary anatomy [88]. MRI is the technique of choice for functional assessment of the systemic RV. MRI permits quantification of systemic and pulmonary

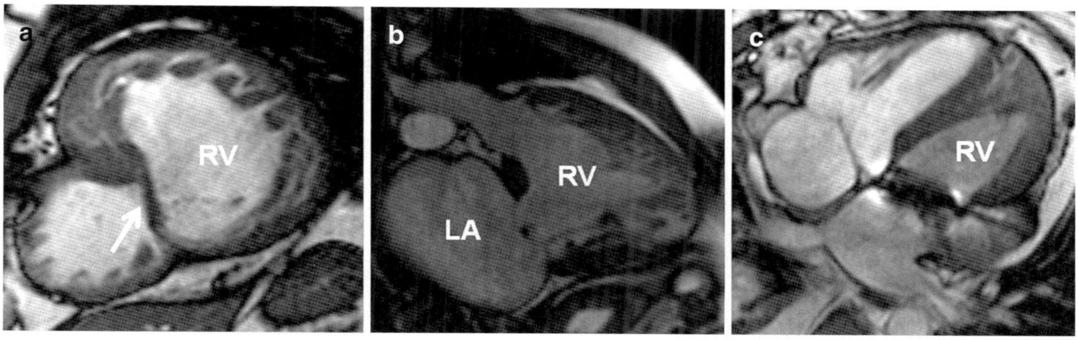

Fig. 10.23 (**a**) and (**b**) Congenitally corrected transposition of great arteries (ccTGA) status post ventricular septal defect repair (*arrow* in **a**) showing markedly dilated right ventricle (*RV*) and left atrium (*LA*). The tricuspid valve appears thickened and prolapsed. Moderate tricuspid regurgitation was shown. (**c**) Status post repair of tricuspid regurgitation with a St. Jude mechanical prosthesis

blood flows and shunt analysis by using velocity-encoded cine sequences. However, MRI study can be time-consuming and requires patient cooperation. Performing a comprehensive MR examination needs skilled technologists who are familiar with congenitally malformed hearts so that imaging planes are optimized during the procedure.

Postsurgical ccTGA

Indications for surgery include large VSD, pulmonary stenosis, systemic atrioventricular valve regurgitation, and complete heart block [68, 90]. The anatomic details encountered will ultimately determine the surgical repair. Replacement of the systemic atrioventricular valve is usually recommended should the valve regurgitation become severe (Fig. 10.23). Double-switch anatomic repair is achieved with Mustard procedure combined with an arterial switch operation. Pulmonary banding may be performed before anatomic repair to prepare the LV to function as a systemic ventricle. It is recommend that in adolescence an LV systolic pressure close to 100 % systemic pressure is required before restoring the LV to the systemic circulation [91]. Additional recommended criteria include an LV mass to LV volume ratio of greater than 1.5 or an LV wall thickness and mass that is normal for a systemic LV using established echocardiographic or MRI values [73]. Anomalous coronary arterial anatomy can be a relative contraindication to the double switch. For patients with a VSD and pulmonary stenosis, a Rastelli procedure with LV-to-aortic baffle and RV-to-pulmonary artery conduit can be performed [90]. Late failure of the systemic RV in the latter group has led to the increasing use of combined Rastelli and atrial switch procedures [68, 92]. Imaging evaluation of post double-switch patients may again involve assessment of problems with the atrial baffle, tricuspid valve regurgitation, those related to arterial switch including coronary arterial obstruction or stenosis, aortic regurgitation, and pulmonary artery stenosis.

Anatomic Variability of Coronary Arteries

The coronary arteries arise from the two aortic sinuses that are adjacent to the pulmonary trunk. In most cases, the epicardial distribution of the arteries follows their respective ventricles. Therefore, the morphological left main coronary artery arises from the right aortic sinus and bifurcates into the anterior descending and circumflex arteries, and the morphological right coronary artery originates from the left aortic sinus, giving rise to the marginal branches [93, 94]. The systemic RV is then perfused by a single right coronary artery which may not be large resulting in

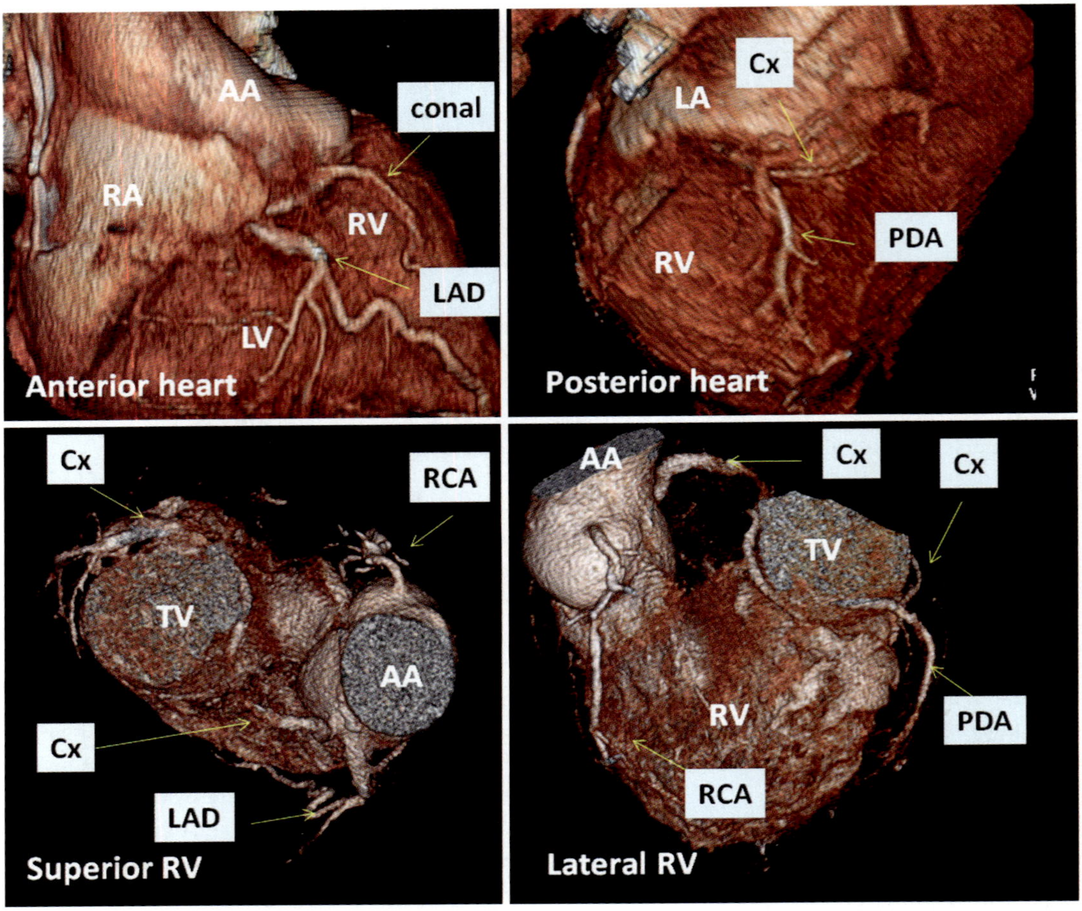

Fig. 10.24 Typical orientation of the coronary arteries in congenitally corrected transposition of great arteries (ccTGA). Three branches arise from a right anterior sinus including the left circumflex (*Cx*), the left anterior descending artery (*LAD*), and a large conal branch supplying the anterolateral wall of morphological right ventricle (*RV*). The Cx is dominant in this case and forms the posterior descending artery (*PDA*). The right coronary artery (*RCA*) originates from a posterior sinus and continues as acute marginal branch. *AA* ascending aorta, *LA* left atrium, *PA* pulmonary artery, *LV* left ventricle, *TV* tricuspid valve

perfusion abnormality and decreased coronary artery reserve [72] (Fig. 10.24). A relatively large conal branch supplying the RVOT is common (60 %). Conal branch may arise from the left main artery [94]. Anomalies in origin, course, and distribution of the coronary arteries are not uncommon, and knowledge of their presence can help determine the most appropriate surgical approach for anatomic correction surgery. Ismat et al. showed coronary artery abnormalities in 40 % of patients that could have complicated anatomic surgical repair including single coronary artery, eccentric ostia, and high-riding artery above the intercoronary commissure [94] (Fig. 10.25). In another coronary artery anatomy study of ccTGA patients [95], there was little deviation from a standard branching pattern, but early branching and RV muscle bridging, as well as malalignment of the aortic and pulmonary sinuses, occurred frequently. Typical coronary distribution is also reported in most ccTGA angiography studies by Dabizzi et al. [96]. Atherosclerotic coronary artery disease may be seen in adult CHD, and knowledge of the anatomic distribution may be important for coronary artery bypass surgery or transcatheter stenting [97].

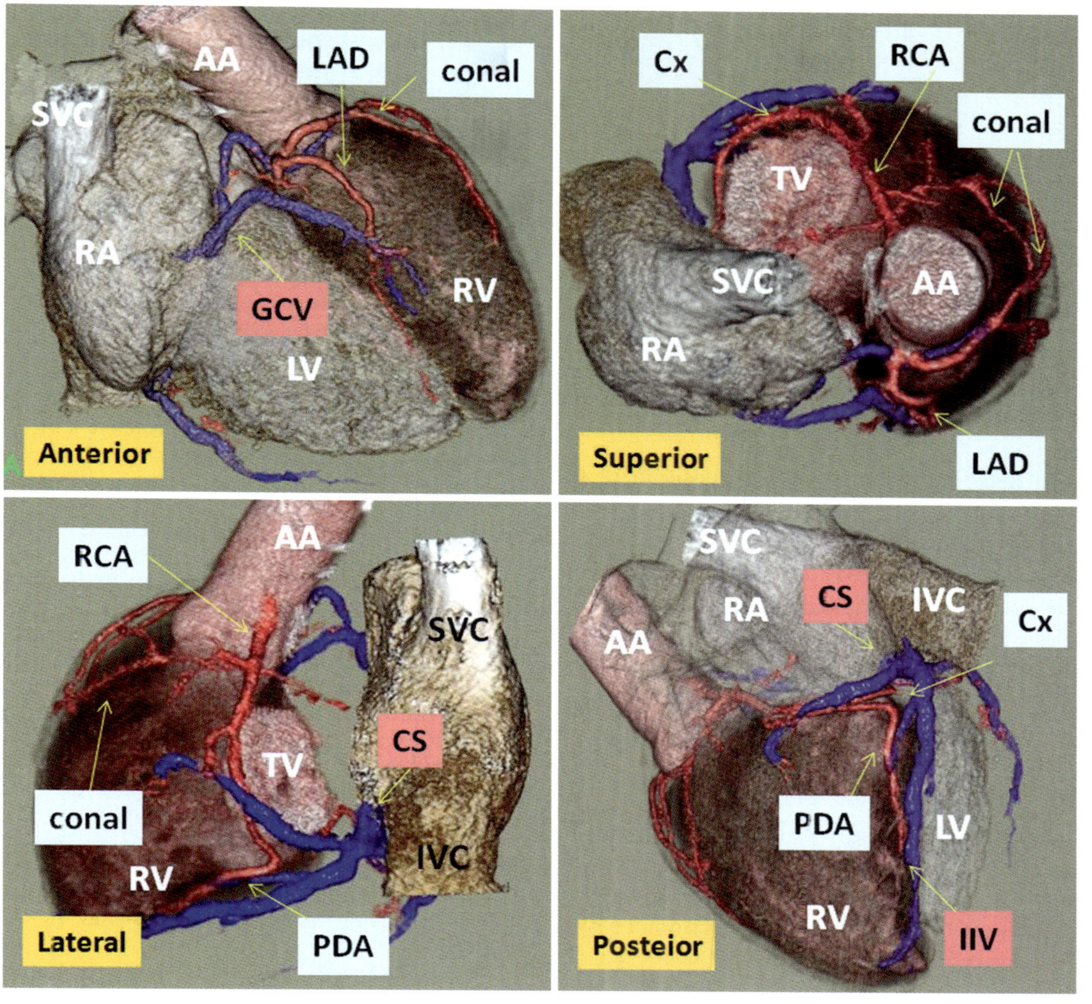

Fig. 10.25 Congenitally corrected transposition of great arteries (ccTGA); coronary artery and vein anatomy. The left anterior descending (*LAD*) artery arises from the right coronary cusp and runs in the anterior interventricular groove. Conal branches arise from the LAD and right coronary artery (*RCA*). The RCA is high riding and originates above a posteriorly located aortic sinus and runs around the tricuspid valve (*TV*) to form the circumflex artery (*Cx*) and gives rise to the posterior descending artery (*PDA*). The great cardiac vein (*GCV*) drains directly into the right atrium (*RA*). The coronary sinus (*CS*) is formed by confluence of the inferior interventricular vein (*IIV*) and two ventricular veins. Note short posterior left ventricular vein. *AA* ascending aorta, *IVC* inferior vena cava, *PA* pulmonary artery, *LV* left ventricle, *RV* systemic right ventricle, *SVC* superior vena cava

The Cardiac Veins

ccTGA patients are at increased risk for systemic ventricle dysfunction, arrhythmias, and valvular complications and may benefit from resynchronization pacing, pacemaker placement, or radiofrequency ablation [98, 99]. Furthermore, abnormal anatomic course of the coronary venous system is common in these patients (Fig. 10.25). Bottega et al. reported different coronary sinus variants in 14 % of ccTGA hearts including atresia, abnormal location below the level of the Eustachian valve, and multiple ostia [100]. The ventricular venous drainage was also abnormal and followed the morphological RV. Preprocedure knowledge of these anatomic variants may be important for effective transvenous cardiac interventions. For example, stimulation of the morphological RV may be difficult because of the relatively small and short lateral epicardial veins [100] (Fig. 10.25). However, large collateral vessels from the morphological RV draining into the interventricular vein may be used, or in certain circumstances, enlarged Thebesian veins can be directly cannulated. Cardiac CT venography is an effective method in demonstration of these variants [101].

Anatomically Corrected Malposition of the Great Arteries

The anatomically corrected malposition of the great arteries is a rare CHD with ventriculoarterial "concordance" but abnormal aortopulmonary relationship [102–104]. Bilateral subaortic and subpulmonary infundibula are seen in 50 % of cases [103]. Knowing this anomaly is important as it could be mistaken with TGA. The arterial trunks arise from their morphologically appropriate ventricles, and they exit from the base of the ventricles in a parallel rather than helical fashion. Imaging consideration should focus on the associated anomalies, ASD, VSD, and RVOT obstruction [105]. Anomalous origin of the coronary arteries is very common, especially a single or dual origin of the coronary arteries from the right coronary aortic sinus [103].

References

1. Fyler DC. Report of the New England regional infant cardiac program. Pediatrics. 1980;65(Suppl): 376–461.
2. Samanek M, Voriskova M. Congenital heart disease among 815,569 children born between 1980 and their 15-year survival: A prospective Bohemia survival study. Pediatr Cardiol. 1999;20:411–7.
3. Liebman J, Cullum L, Belloc NB. Natural history of transposition of the great arteries: anatomy and birth and death characteristics. Circulation. 1969;40:237–62.
4. Hoffman JI, Kaplan S, Liberthson RR. Prevalence of congenital heart disease. Am Heart J. 2004;147(3): 425–39.
5. Love BA, Mehta D, Fuster VF. Evaluation and management of the adult patient with transposition of the great arteries following atrial-level (Senning or Mustard) repair. Nat Clin Pract Cardiovasc Med. 2008;5(8):454–67.
6. Paladini D, Volpe P, Sglavo G, et al. Transposition of the great arteries in the fetus: assessment of the spatial relationships of the arterial trunks by four-dimensional echocardiography. Ultrasound Obstet Gynecol. 2008;31(3):271–6.
7. Massoudy P, Baltalarli A, de Leval MR, et al. Anatomic variability in coronary arterial distribution with regard to the arterial switch procedure. Circulation. 2002;106(15):1980–4.
8. Van Praagh R, Perez-Trevino C, Lopez-Cuellar M, et al. Transposition of the great arteries with posterior aorta, anterior pulmonary artery, subpulmonary conus and fibrous continuity between aortic and atrioventricular valves. Am J Cardiol. 1971;28: 621–31.
9. Lange R, Hörer J, Kostolny M, Cleuziou J, et al. Presence of a ventricular septal defect and the Mustard operation are risk factors for late mortality after the atrial switch operation: thirty years of follow-up in 417 patients at a single center. Circulation. 2006;114(18):1905–13.
10. Hornung TS, Derrick GP, Deanfield JE, Redington AN. Transposition complexes in the adult: a changing perspective. Cardiol Clin. 2002;20:405–20.
11. Hoyer MH, Zuberbuhler JR, Anderson RH, del Nido P. Morphology of ventricular septal defects in complete transposition. Surgical implications. J Thorac Cardiovasc Surg. 1992;104(5):1203–11.
12. Milanesi O, Ho SY, Thiene G, Frescura C, Anderson RH. The ventricular septal defect in complete transposition of the great arteries: pathologic anatomy in 57 cases with emphasis on subaortic, subpulmonary, and aortic arch obstruction. Hum Pathol. 1987;18(4): 392–6.
13. Rashkind WJ, Miller WW. Creation of an atrial septal defect without thoracotomy: a palliative approach to complete transposition of the great arteries. JAMA. 1966;196:991–2.
14. Senning A. Surgical correction of transposition of the great vessels. Surgery. 1959;45:966–80.
15. Mustard WT. Successful two-stage correction of the transposition of the great vessels. Surgery. 1964;55:469–72.
16. Dos L, Teruel L, Ferreira IJ, et al. Late outcome of Senning and Mustard procedures for correction of transposition of the great arteries. Heart. 2005;91: 652–6.
17. Jatene AD, Fontes VF, Paulista PP, et al. Anatomic correction of transposition of the great vessels. J Thorac Cardiovasc Surg. 1976;72:364–70.
18. Lecompte Y, Zannini L, Hazan E, et al. Anatomic correction of transposition of the great arteries. J Thorac Cardiovasc Surg. 1981;82:629–31.
19. Foran JP, Sullivan ID, Elliott MJ, de Leval MR. Primary arterial switch operation for transposition of the great arteries with intact ventricular septum in infants older than 21 days. J Am Coll Cardiol. 1998;31:883–9.
20. Bautista-Hernandez V, Marx GR, Bacha EA, del Nido PJ. Aortic root translocation plus arterial switch for transposition of the great arteries with left ventricular

outflow tract obstruction: intermediate-term results. J Am Coll Cardiol. 2007;49(4):485–90.
21. Wilson NJ, Clarkson PM, Barratt-Boyes BG, et al. Long-term outcome after the mustard repair for simple transposition of the great arteries. 28-year follow-up. J Am Coll Cardiol. 1998;32(3):758–65.
22. Moons P, Gewillig M, Sluysmans T, et al. Long term outcome up to 30 years after the Mustard or Senning operation: a nationwide multicenter study in Belgium. Heart. 2004;90:307–13.
23. Oechslin E, Jenni R. 40 Years after the first atrial switch procedure in patients with transposition of the great arteries: long-term results in Toronto and Zurich. Thorac Cardiovasc Surg. 2000;48:233–7.
24. Sarkar D, Bull C, Yates R, Wright D, Cullen S, Gewillig M, Clayton R, Tunstill A, Deanfield J. Comparison of long-term outcomes of atrial repair of simple transposition with implications for a late arterial switch strategy. Circulation. 1999;100:II-176–81.
25. Khairy P, Landzberg MJ, Lambert J, O'Donnell CP. Long-term outcomes after the atrial switch for surgical correction of transposition: a meta-analysis comparing the Mustard and Senning procedures. Cardiol Young. 2004;14(3):284–92.
26. Johansson B, Babu-Narayan SV, Kilner PJ, Cannell TM, Mohiaddin RH. 3-Dimensional time-resolved contrast-enhanced magnetic resonance angiography for evaluation late after the mustard operation for transposition. Cardiol Young. 2010;20(1):1–7.
27. Cohen MD, Johnson T, Ramrakhiani S. MRI of surgical repair of transposition of the great vessels. AJR Am J Roentgenol. 2010;194(1):250–60.
28. Brown SC, Eyskens B, Mertens L, Stockx L, Dumoulin M, Gewillig M. Self expandable stents for relief of venous baffle obstruction after the Mustard operation. Heart. 1998;79(3):230–3.
29. Matthews CE, Hussain T, Miles C, et al. Left-sided pulmonary venous pathway obstruction after mustard operation. Congenit Heart Dis. 2013;8(1):66–70.
30. Klein AJ, Kim MS, Salcedo E, Fagan T, Kay J. The missing leak: a case report of a baffle-leak closure using real-time 3D transoesophageal guidance. Eur J Echocardiogr. 2009;10(3):464–7.
31. Gatzoulis MA, Walters J, McLaughlin PR, Merchant N, Webb GD, Liu P. Late arrhythmia in adults with the mustard procedure for transposition of great arteries: a surrogate marker for right ventricular dysfunction? Heart. 2000;84(4):409–15. 19.
32. Theissen P, Kaemmerer H, Sechtem U, et al. Magnetic resonance imaging of cardiac function and morphology in patients with transposition of the great arteries following Mustard procedure. Thorac Cardiovasc Surg. 1991;39 Suppl 3:221–4.
33. Schmid FX, Morales M, Stark J. Left ventricular outflow tract obstruction in TGA: treatment with LV-to-PA valved conduit. Ann Thorac Surg. 1995;59(1):201–4.
34. Yehya A, Lyle T, Pernetz MA, McConnell ME, Kogon B, Book WM. Pulmonary arterial hypertension in patients with prior atrial switch procedure for d-transposition of great arteries (dTGA). Int J Cardiol. 2010;143(3):271–5.
35. Mussatto K, Wernovsky G. Challenges facing the child, adolescent, and young adult after the arterial switch operation. Cardiol Young. 2005;15 suppl 1:111–21.
36. Quaegebeur JM, Rohmer J, Ottenkamp J, et al. The arterial switch operation: an 8-year experience. J Thorac Cardiovasc Surg. 1986;92:361–84.
37. Losay J, Touchot A, Serraf A, et al. Late outcome after arterial switch operation for transposition of the great arteries. Circulation. 2001;104(12 suppl 1):I121–6.
38. Schwartz ML, Gauvreau K, del Nido P, Mayer JE, Colan SD. Long-term predictors of aortic root dilation and aortic regurgitation after arterial switch operation. Circulation. 2004;110(11 suppl 1):II128–32.
39. Grotenhuis HB, Ottenkamp J, Fontein D, et al. Aortic elasticity and left ventricular function after arterial switch operation: MR imaging – initial experience. Radiology. 2008;249(3):801–9.
40. Legendre A, Losay J, Touchot-Koné A, et al. Coronary events after arterial switch operation for transposition of the great arteries. Circulation. 2003;108 suppl 1:II186–90.
41. Gutberlet M, Boeckel T, Hosten N, et al. Arterial switch procedure for D-transposition of the great arteries: quantitative midterm evaluation of hemodynamic changes with cine MR imaging and phase-shift velocity mapping—initial experience. Radiology. 2000; 214(2):467–75.
42. Taylor AM, Dymarkowski S, Hamaekers P, et al. MR coronary angiography and late-enhancement myocardial MR in children who underwent arterial switch surgery for transposition of great arteries. Radiology. 2005;234(2):542–7.
43. Benzaquen BS, Webb GD, Colman JM, Therrien J. Arterial switch operation after Mustard procedures in adult patients with transposition of the great arteries: is it time to revise our strategy? Am Heart J. 2004; 147(3):E8.
44. Poirier NC, Yu JH, Brizard CP, Mee RB. Long-term results of left ventricular reconditioning and anatomic correction for systemic right ventricular dysfunction after atrial switch procedures. J Thorac Cardiovasc Surg. 2004;127(4):975–81.
45. Wernovsky G, Mayer Jr JE, Jonas RA, et al. Factors influencing early and late outcome of the arterial switch operation for transposition of the great arteries. J Thorac Cardiovasc Surg. 1995;109:289–301.
46. Sim EKW, van Son JAM, Edwards WD, et al. Coronary artery anatomy in transposition of the great arteries. Ann Thorac Surg. 1994;57:890–4.
47. Greenberg SB, Bhutta ST. A dual contrast injection technique for multidetector computed tomography angiography of Fontan procedures. Int J Cardiovasc Imaging. 2008;24:345–8.
48. Ho JG, Cohen MD, Ebenroth ES, et al. Comparison between transthoracic echocardiography and cardiac magnetic resonance imaging in patients status post

atrial switch procedure. Congenit Heart Dis. 2012;7(2):122–30.
49. Lorenz CH, Walker ES, Graham Jr TP, Powers TA. Right ventricular performance and mass by use of cine MRI late after atrial repair of transposition of the great arteries. Circulation. 1995;92(9 Suppl):II233–9.
50. Babu-Narayan SV, Goktekin O, Moon JC, et al. Late gadolinium enhancement cardiovascular magnetic resonance of the systemic right ventricle in adults with previous atrial redirection surgery for transposition of the great arteries. Circulation. 2005;111(16):2091–8.
51. Mohrs OK, Petersen SE, Voigtlaender T, et al. Time-resolved contrast-enhanced MR angiography of the thorax in adults with congenital heart disease. AJR Am J Roentgenol. 2006;187(4):1107–14.
52. Papavassiliu T, Kuhl HP, Schroder M, Suselbeck T, Bondarenko O, Bohm CK, Beek A, Hoffman MM, van Rossum AC. Effect of endocardial trabeculae on left ventricular measurements and measurement reproducibility at cardiovascular MR imaging. Radiology. 2005;236:57–64.
53. Winter MM, Bernink FJ, Groenink M, et al. Evaluating the systemic right ventricle by CMR: the importance of consistent and reproducible delineation of the cavity. J Cardiovasc Magn Reson. 2008;10:40.
54. Kilner PJ, Geva T, Kaemmerer H, Trindade PT, Schwitter J, Webb GD. Recommendations for cardiovascular magnetic resonance in adults with congenital heart disease from the respective working groups of the European Society of Cardiology. Eur Heart J. 2010;31(7):794–805.
55. Moroseos T, Mitsumori L, Kerwin WS, et al. Comparison of Simpson's method and three-dimensional reconstruction for measurement of right ventricular volume in patients with complete or corrected transposition of the great arteries. Am J Cardiol. 2010;105(11):1603–9.
56. Broberg CS, Chugh SS, Conklin C, Sahn DJ, Jerosch-Herold M. Quantification of diffuse myocardial fibrosis and its association with myocardial dysfunction in congenital heart disease. Circ Cardiovasc Imaging. 2010;3(6):727–34.
57. Hucin B, Voriskova M, Hruda J, Marek J, Janousek J, Reich O, Skovranek J. Late complications and quality of life after atrial correction of transposition of the great arteries in 12 to 18 year follow-up. J Cardiovasc Surg (Torino). 2000;41:233–9.
58. Kirjavainen M, Happonen JM, Louhimo I. Late results of senning operation. J Thorac Cardiovasc Surg. 1999;117:488–95.
59. Chow PC, Liang XC, Lam WW, Cheung EW, Wong KT, Cheung YF. Mechanical right ventricular dyssynchrony in patients after atrial switch operation for transposition of the great arteries. Am J Cardiol. 2008;101(6):874–81.
60. Roos-Hesselink JW, Meijboom FJ, Spitaels SE, et al. Decline in ventricular function and clinical condition after Mustard repair for transposition of the great arteries (a prospective study of 22–29 years). Eur Heart J. 2004;25(14):1264–70.
61. Millane T, Bernard EJ, Jaeggi E, et al. Role of ischemia and infarction in late right ventricular dysfunction after atrial repair of transposition of the great arteries. J Am Coll Cardiol. 2000;35:1661–8.
62. Tops LF, Roest AA, Lamb HJ, et al. Intraatrial repair of transposition of the great arteries: use of MR imaging after exercise to evaluate regional systemic right ventricular function. Radiology. 2005;237(3):861–7.
63. Tulevski II, Lee PL, Groenink M, et al. Dobutamine-induced increase of right ventricular contractility without increased stroke volume in adolescent patients with transposition of the great arteries: evaluation with magnetic resonance imaging. Int J Card Imaging. 2000;16(6):471–8.
64. Fratz S, Hauser M, Bengel FM, et al. Myocardial scars determined by delayed-enhancement magnetic resonance imaging and positron emission tomography are not common in right ventricles with systemic function in long-term follow up. Heart. 2006;92(11):1673–7.
65. van Son JA, Reddy VM, Silverman NH, Hanley FL. Regression of tricuspid regurgitation after two-stage arterial switch operation for failing systemic ventricle after atrial inversion operation. J Thorac Cardiovasc Surg. 1996;111(2):342–7.
66. Davlouros PA, Niwa K, Webb G, Gatzoulis MA. The right ventricle in congenital heart disease. Heart. 2006;92(Suppl):i27–38.
67. Allwork SP, Bentall HH, Becker AE, et al. Congenitally corrected transposition of the great arteries: morphologic study of 32 cases. Am J Cardiol. 1976;38:910–23.
68. Graham Jr TP, Bernard YD, Mellen BG, et al. Long-term outcome in congenitally corrected transposition of the great arteries: a multi-institutional study. J Am Coll Cardiol. 2000;36:255–61.
69. Blume E, Chung T, Hoffer FA, Geva T. Anatomically corrected malposition of the great arteries {S, D, L}. Circulation. 1998;97:1207.
70. Dimas AP, Moodie DS, Sterba R, Gill CC. Long-term function of the morphological right ventricle in adult patients with congenitally corrected transposition of the great arteries. Am Heart J. 1989;118:896.
71. Fogel MA, Weinberg PM, Fellows KE, Hoffman EA. A study in ventricular-ventricular interaction. Single right ventricles compared with systemic right ventricles in a dual-chamber circulation. Circulation. 1995;92:219–30.
72. Hauser M, Bengel FM, Hager A, et al. Impaired myocardial blood flow and coronary flow reserve of the anatomical right systemic ventricle in patients with congenitally corrected transposition of the great arteries. Heart. 2003;89:1231–5.
73. Hornung TS, Bernard EJ, Jaeggi ET, Howman-Giles RB, Celermajer DS, Hawker RE. Myocardial perfusion defects and associated systemic ventricular dysfunction in congenitally corrected transposition of the great arteries. Heart. 1998;80(4):322–6.
74. Fratz S, Hager A, Busch R, et al. Patients after atrial switch operation for transposition of the great

arteries can not increase stroke volume under dobutamine stress as opposed to patients with congenitally corrected transposition. Circ J. 2008;72(7):1130–5.
75. Dodge-Khatami A, Tulevski II, Bennink GB, et al. Comparable systemic ventricular function in healthy adults and patients with unoperated congenitally corrected transposition using MRI dobutamine stress testing. Ann Thorac Surg. 2002;73(6):1759–64.
76. Von Rokitansky K. Pathologisch-anatomische Abhandlung. Vienna: W. Braumuller; 1875. p. 83–6.
77. Li W, Hornung TS, Francis DP, et al. Relation of biventricular function quantified by stress echocardiography to cardiopulmonary exercise capacity in adults with Mustard (atrial switch) procedure for transposition of the great arteries. Circulation. 2004;110:1380–6.
78. Warnes CA. Transposition of the great arteries. Circulation. 2006;114:2699–709.
79. Ferencz C, Rubin JD, McCarter RJ, Brenner JI, Neill CA, Perry LW, Hepner SI, Downing JW. Congenital heart disease: prevalence at livebirth. Am J Epidemiol. 1985;121:31–6.
80. Connelly MS, Liu PP, Williams WG, Webb GD, Robertson P, McLaughlin PR. Congenitally corrected transposition of the great arteries in the adult: functional status and complications. J Am Coll Cardiol. 1996;27(5):1238–43.
81. Freedom RM, Culham G, Rowe RD. The criss-cross heart and superoinferior ventricular heart, an angiographic study. Am J Cardiol. 1978;42:620–8.
82. Wallis GA, Debich-Spicer D, Anderson RH. Congenitally corrected transposition. Orphanet J Rare Dis. 2011;6:22.
83. Friedberg DZ, Nadas AS. Clinical profile of patients with congenitally corrected transposition of the great arteries: a study of 60 cases. N Engl J Med. 1970;282:1053–9.
84. Presbitero P, Somerville J, Rabajoli F, Stone S, Conte MR. Corrected transposition of the great arteries without associated defects in adult patients: clinical profile and follow up. Br Heart J. 1995;74(1):57–9.
85. Huhta JC, Maloney JD, Ritter DG, Ilstrup DM, Feldt RH. Complete atrioventricular block in patients with atrioventricular discordance. Circulation. 1983;183:1374.
86. Nikolaou K, Alkadhi H, Bamberg F, Leschka S, Wintersperger BJ. MRI and CT in the diagnosis of coronary artery disease: indications and applications. Insights Imaging. 2011;2(1):9–24.
87. Lembcke A, Koch C, Dohmen PM, et al. Electrocardiographic-gated multislice computed tomography for visualization of cardiac morphology in congenitally corrected transposition of the great arteries. J Comput Assist Tomogr. 2005; 29:234–7.
88. Kantarci M, Koplay M, Bayraktutan U, Gundogdu F, Ceviz N. Congenitally corrected transposition of the great arteries: MDCT angiography findings and interpretation of complex coronary anatomy. Int J Cardiovasc Imaging. 2007;23(3):405–10.
89. Goo HW, Park IS, Ko JK, Kim YH, Seo DM, Park JJ. Computed tomography for the diagnosis of congenital heart disease in pediatric and adult patients. Int J Cardiovasc Imaging. 2005;21:347–65.
90. Reddy VM, McElhinney DB, Silverman NH, Hanley FL. The double switch procedure for anatomical repair of congenitally corrected transposition of the great arteries in infants and children. Eur Heart J. 1997;18(9):1470–7.
91. Duncan BW, Mee RB, Mesia CI, et al. Results of the double switch operation for congenitally corrected transposition of the great arteries. Eur J Cardiothorac Surg. 2003;24:11–9.
92. Langley SM, Winlaw DS, Stumper O, et al. Midterm results after restoration of the morphologically left ventricle to the systemic circulation in patients with congenitally corrected transposition of the great arteries. J Thorac Cardiovasc Surg. 2003;125(6):1229–41.
93. Uemura H, Ho SY, Anderson RH, et al. Surgical anatomy of the coronary circulation in hearts with discordant atrioventricular connections. Eur J Cardiothorac Surg. 1996;10:194–200.
94. Ismat FA, Baldwin HS, Karl TR, Weinberg PM. Coronary anatomy in congenitally corrected transposition of the great arteries. Int J Cardiol. 2002;86(2–3):207–16.
95. McKay R, Anderson RH, Smith A. The coronary arteries in hearts with discordant atrioventricular connections. J Thorac Cardiovasc Surg. 1996;111:988–97.
96. Dabizzi RP, Barletta GA, Caprioli G, Baldrighi G, Baldrighi V. Coronary artery anatomy in corrected transposition of the great arteries. J Am Coll Cardiol. 1988;12(2):486–91.
97. Stulak JM, Dearani JA, Burkhart HM, Ammash NM, Phillips SD, Schaff HV. Coronary artery disease in adult congenital heart disease: outcome after coronary artery bypass grafting. Ann Thorac Surg. 2012;93(1):116–22.
98. Anderson RH, Becker AE, Arnold R, et al. The conduction tissues in congenitally corrected transposition. Circulation. 1974;50:911–23.
99. Diller GP, Okonko D, Uebing A, et al. Cardiac resynchronization therapy for adult congenital heart disease patients with a systemic right ventricle: analysis of feasibility and review of early experience. Europace. 2006;8:267–72.
100. Bottega NA, Kapa S, Edwards WD, et al. The cardiac veins in congenitally corrected transposition of the great arteries: delivery options for cardiac devices. Heart Rhythm. 2009;6(10):1450–6.
101. Saremi F, Muresian H, Sánchez-Quintana D. Cardiac veins: comprehensive radio-anatomical classification, and review of variants and clinical implications using MDCT. Radiographics. 2012;32(1):E1–32.
102. Van Praagh R, Van Praagh S. Anatomically corrected malposition of the great arteries. Br Heart J. 1967;26:112.
103. Cavalle-Garrido T, Bernasconi A, Perrin D, Anderson RH. Hearts with concordant ventriculoarterial

connections but parallel arterial trunks. Heart. 2007;93:100–6.
104. Dalvi B, Sharma S. Anatomically corrected malposition: report of six cases. Am Heart J. 1993;126: 1229–32.
105. Huang SC, Chiu IS, Lee ML, Wu CS, Chiu HH, Chang CI, Wu MH, Wang JK. Coronary artery anatomy in anatomically corrected malposition of the great arteries and their surgical implications. Eur J Cardiothorac Surg. 2011;39(5):705–10.

Univentricular Heart

11

François-Pierre Mongeon, François Marcotte,
and Paul Khairy

The Univentricular Heart in Adults

A univentricular heart, or univentricular atrioventricular (AV) connection (UAVC), is not a single lesion but a broad term encompassing congenital malformations leading to single ventricular physiology, a very rare condition where one dominant ventricle supports both circulations. Tricuspid atresia is the classic example and the most common variety of UAVC. Other varieties include double-inlet right or left ventricle, mitral atresia, hypoplastic left heart syndrome, unbalanced common AV canal, pulmonary atresia, and heterotaxy syndromes. Heterotaxy syndromes refer to disorders of lateralization whereby the arrangement of abdominal and thoracic viscera differ from normal and mirror image of normal [1].

F.-P. Mongeon, MD, SM • F. Marcotte, MD, FRCPC
Non-Invasive Cardiology Service and Adult Congenital Heart Disease Center, Montreal Heart Institute, 5000 Bélanger Street, Montreal, QC H1T 1C8, Canada
e-mail: francois.pierre.mongeon@umontreal.ca; francois.marcotte@icm-mhi.org

P. Khairy, MD, PhD (✉)
Electrophysiology Service and Adult Congenital Heart Disease Center, Montreal Heart Institute, 5000 Bélanger Street, Montreal, QC H1T 1C8, Canada
e-mail: paul.khairy@cardio.chboston.org

Nomenclature and Classification

A univentricular heart is defined by the entire atrial input being committed to a single chamber in the ventricular mass [2]. The AV relationship may be double inlet or with absence of right or left AV connection [2]. The dominant ventricle may be of left, right, or undetermined morphology. A rudimentary ventricular chamber may or may not be present [2]. The ventriculo-arterial (VA) relationship may be concordant, discordant (transposition), double outlet, or single outlet (with atresia of one of the semilunar valves) [2]. The term single ventricle may cause some confusion since hearts that function as a single chamber may possess two anatomic chambers [3]. While it may indicate the absence of a rudimentary chamber, the term single ventricle is less useful for anatomic description. However, it may be used to explain that, physiologically, a unique pumping chamber is present. The above definitions would exclude hearts with two well-developed but nonseptable ventricles. However, the natural history or surgical management of patients with such lesion may lead to an Eisenmenger syndrome or completion of a Fontan operation. Principles outlined in this chapter may be of use to image these patients.

Prevalence

The prevalence of UAVC is estimated to be 0.03 per 1,000 adults and 0.13 per 1,000 children [4]. The higher prevalence in children likely reflects

F. Saremi (ed.), *Cardiac CT and MR for Adult Congenital Heart Disease*,
DOI 10.1007/978-1-4614-8875-0_11,

the success of the last decades in pediatric cardiac surgery; therefore, the number of adults with UAVC is expected to increase in the coming years.

Surgical Palliation

Survival to adulthood without repair is possible for patients with UAVC. It may result in Eisenmenger syndrome with the complications of chronic cyanosis and pulmonary hypertension. However, patients with double-inlet left ventricle (LV) and perfectly balanced circulations may survive to the sixth decade with good functional capacity and preserved ventricular function [5]. General objectives of surgical management are to provide unobstructed systemic outflow, unobstructed systemic and pulmonary venous return, and controlled pulmonary blood flow [1]. Imaging of these procedures will be discussed at length in the second part of this chapter. Pulmonary blood flow may initially be provided by a systemic-to-pulmonary shunt, such as a classic or modified Blalock-Taussig shunt (Fig. 11.1a) between the ipsilateral subclavian and pulmonary artery, or by a bidirectional cavopulmonary anastomosis (Glenn shunt, Fig. 11.1b). Aortopulmonary collaterals may require unifocalization in staged procedures [1]. Unrestricted pulmonary flow may require banding of the pulmonary artery to prevent pulmonary hypertension and allow later completion of a Fontan operation. The Fontan operation separates the pulmonary and from systemic circulation. Three main subtypes of Fontan circuit (Fig. 11.1a–c) have been proposed since its original description in 1971 for palliation of tricuspid atresia [6]. The Fontan has evolved from a valved conduit between the right atrium (RA) and PA to a total cavopulmonary connection, with an intracardiac or extracardiac tunnel. Most adults have either a direct RA to PA anastomosis or an intra-atrial tunnel from the inferior vena cava to the right PA with a Glenn shunt. In the presence of a left superior vena cava, bilateral Glenn shunts are used in a modification called the Kawashima operation. Criteria have been proposed to select patients for Fontan completion. They also serve as a reminder of conditions that should be maintained to keep the Fontan circuit functioning in the long term. Deciding on candidacy for Fontan completion in adults is beyond the scope of this chapter, but suffice it to say that Fontan circuits

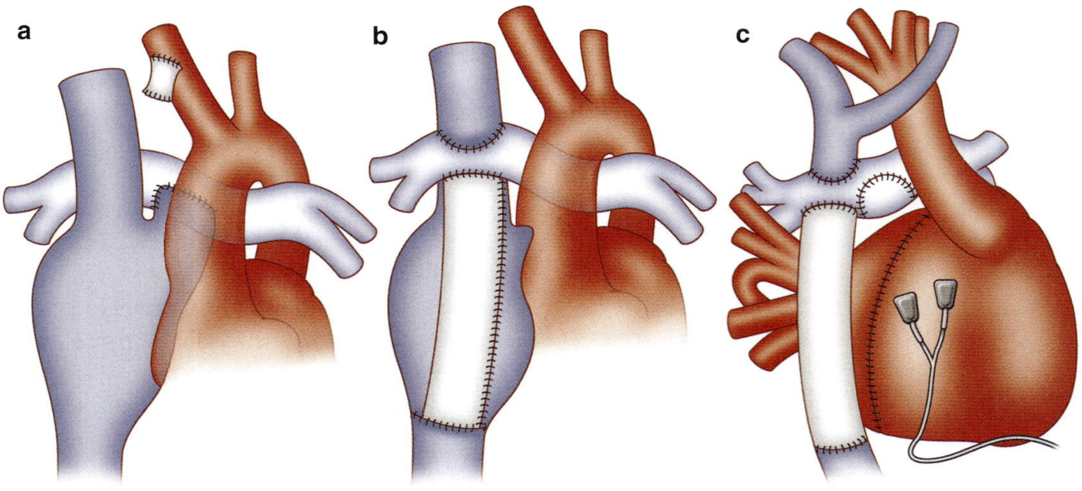

Fig. 11.1 Variations of Fontan surgery are illustrated. In a classic Fontan right atrium-to-pulmonary artery anastomosis (**a**) is performed. In (a), the modified Blalock-Taussig shunt, shown in white, was taken down and oversewn. (**b**, **c**) Demonstrate total cavopulmonary connections formed by a superior cavopulmonary anastomosis (bidirectional Glenn shunt) and completed by either an intracardiac lateral tunnel (**b**) or extracardiac conduit (**c**) Fontan operation. In (c), permanent atrial epicardial pacemaker leads are illustrated in *grey* (From Khairy et al. [1] with permission)

function more efficiently if the mean PA pressure is less than 15 mmHg, the systemic ventricular ejection fraction is normal, the systemic AV valve is competent, and the pulmonary arteries are not distorted.

A particular sequence of staged palliation was proposed in 1983 for hypoplastic left heart syndrome and is termed the Norwood operation [7]. The syndrome is a combination of aortic valve atresia, mitral atresia or stenosis, a diminutive or absent LV, and severe hypoplasia of the ascending aorta and aortic arch. The diminutive ascending aorta and aortic arch are reconstructed with anastomosis to the proximal main PA, establishing unobstructed flow from the right ventricle (RV) to the aorta. A systemic-to-pulmonary shunt ensures pulmonary blood flow until completion of the Fontan circuit within 2 years of life [7]. An increasing number of patients with a Norwood repair will reach adulthood.

Long-Term Outcomes of the Fontan Operation

One study found that, after a median of 12.2 years, 29.1 % of patients with Fontan palliation had died [8]. Fontan revisions and conversions were performed in 1.9 and 8 % of patients, respectively [8]. Major causes of attrition were thromboembolic, heart failure, and sudden deaths [8]. Another series reported outcomes in 499 consecutive Fontan patients [9]. Survival rates at 1, 5, and 10 years were 82, 74, and 71 % [9]. The most important risk factor for mortality was right ventricular dominance [9]. Other risk factors included AV valve regurgitation, not having transposition, and heterotaxy [9]. In a multicenter study, the combination of clinically relevant arrhythmias, atriopulmonary or AV connection, and signs of heart failure was associated with 25 % mortality by 3 years [10].

Imaging Findings and Protocols

In this section, we will review the comprehensive approach to cardiac magnetic resonance (CMR) and cardiac computed tomography (CCT) imaging for a patient with UAVC. The common feature to all forms is an intracardiac admixture of systemic and pulmonary venous blood leading to systemic desaturation with either reduced or excessive pulmonary blood flow. The clinical management strives to rectify pulmonary blood flow and separate the systemic and pulmonary venous returns, essentially rendering the heart an arterial blood pumping chamber to the aorta, while systemic venous blood is directed toward the pulmonary arteries for reoxygenation (the Fontan procedures). Most adult patients will have benefited from palliation with a Fontan operation. Therefore, the baseline anatomy should be described, but findings associated with the long-term evolution of the Fontan operation are equally, if not more, important.

Given their ability to depict cardiac anatomy in three dimensions, CMR and CCT are widely used in the diagnosis and management of patients with complex congenital cardiac diseases, including UAVC. Unlike echocardiography these techniques provide a wide field of view and are not limited by acoustic windows. Notwithstanding these advantages, the complexity and variety of UAVC still warrant a thorough understanding of complex congenital heart disease and the clinical questions relevant to each case. The imaging specialist should obtain the maximal available clinical documentation of the patients' anatomy and surgical and interventional history prior to planning a CMR or CCT study. In the pediatric population and in experienced hands, CMR and echocardiography may be sufficient to successfully plan Fontan surgery, avoiding the risks and the radiation exposure of cardiac catheterization and CCT [11, 12]. Their respective strengths and weaknesses are summarized in Table 11.1 [13]. The major weakness of CMR or CCT is its current inability to directly measure pulmonary pressures and resistances, information easily obtained by catheterization.

Preparation for CMR and CCT

For each patient, a chest X-ray should always be obtained prior to CMR or CCT to provide basic

Table 11.1 Comparison of cardiac MRI and CT for imaging of patients with univentricular atriopulmonary connection

	Cardiac MRI	Cardiac CT
Advantages	Radiation-free	Superior spatial resolution (<1 mm)
	Superior temporal resolution (20–30 frames/s)	Well tolerated (infrequent claustrophobia)
	Good spatial resolution (1–2 mm)	Short examination duration (a few minutes)
	May be performed without contrast	Compatible with ferromagnetic implants (pacemakers, valves)
Disadvantages	Incompatible with ferromagnetic implants (e.g., pacemakers)	Radiation exposure (3–15 mSv)
	Artifact from compatible implants (artificial valves and clips)	Requires contrast infusion
	Claustrophobia (10 %)	Artifact from metal implants (pacemakers, artificial valves, and clips) and calcium
	Long examination duration (45–90 min)	Low temporal resolution (10–15 frames/s)
Utility in UAVC	Great vessel (arterial and venous) and cardiac segment morphology	Great vessel (arterial and venous) and cardiac segment morphology
	Global and regional ventricular function	Coronary arteries
	Valvular function	Alternative for global ventricular function assessment
	Blood flow (volume and velocity) assessment	

Legend: *UAVC* univentricular atrioventricular connections, *mSv* millisievert

anatomic landmarks and evidence of prior surgical interventions, such as pacemaker and pacemaker leads, artificial valves, stents, and surgical clips. Some items may hinder image quality, particularly in gradient-recalled echo (GRE) imaging as opposed to black-blood fast spin echo (BB FSE) or as in the case of pacemakers represent a relative contraindication to CMR and prompt referral to CCT. Although CMR and CCT techniques are based on diametrically opposed imaging principles, important features are shared by the two modalities for UAVC imaging such that many of the principles discussed for CMR imaging will also apply to CCT imaging. Comments specific to CCT imaging will be covered in the last section with examples provided throughout. In addition to clinical and basic X-ray information, vital signs should be taken prior to examination, especially systemic oxygen (O_2) saturation measured by pulse oximetry, as cyanotic patients may have difficulties performing extended breath holds. Although standard CMR imaging planes and sequences generally capture the most clinically important findings, close collaboration between physician and technologist is essential to tailoring the examination to each patient's needs, as anatomies are markedly heterogeneous and unforeseen findings are frequent. All examinations must strive to obtain the maximum clinically useful information in the shortest time possible, since these individuals frequently have reduced functional (and breath hold) tolerance. Efforts should be directed toward ensuring that the experience remains positive, especially considering that follow-up studies are often required.

Native UAVC Anatomy and Evaluation of the Unoperated Patient

Determining AV and VA connections and function as well as characterizing ventricular morphology and function are fundamental issues to address by CMR or CCT. Often, such characterization has been performed by the pediatric cardiology and radiology imaging team and is clearly documented prior to referral. However, in the odd case of a patient unknown to your center, an organized and systematic approach can provide extremely important and sometimes lifesaving information to the care team. As described in the segmental or sequential approaches, anatomic structures must first be described by their intrinsic anatomic characteristics, second on their position, and third in their relationship to other parts of the heart and circulation [14].

Cardiac Chamber Anatomy

The RA almost always receives flow from the inferior vena cava (IVC) and superior vena cava (SVC), unless a cavopulmonary anastomosis has been created or a conduit implanted. Connection to the ostium of the coronary sinus is the hallmark of an anatomic RA. The left atrium (LA) usually receives the pulmonary veins that may vary in number and drainage type.

Ventricular morphology determines the nature of the AV valve such that the RV is associated with the tricuspid valve and the LV with the mitral valve. Semilunar valve identification is determined by the connecting great vessel. Determining ventricular morphology is sometimes challenging but certain features are fairly typical for each ventricle (Table 11.2). A dominant ventricle of LV morphology shows a rather posterior or inferiorly situated cavity with relatively smooth walls and AV valve to semilunar valve fibrous continuity or proximity, even if either valve is atretic. An accompanying hypoplastic ventricle of RV morphology typically lies anterosuperiorly to the dominant LV. A dominant ventricle of RV morphology appears more trabeculated (although a hypertrophied overloaded LV can have a similar appearance) with fibrous discontinuity between the AV valve and semilunar valve. Demonstrating AV valve and semilunar valve continuity may be challenging in the straight axial projection, as this relationship is supero-inferior and often requires coronal and sagittal or even double-oblique correlations. From a practical perspective, ventricular looping may be determined by the right-hand technique. If the right hand is placed in the RV with the thumb directed toward the inflow, palm facing the septum, and the fingers point to the outflow, it is considered D-looping.

Double-inlet ventricular morphology can be well appreciated in axial or four-chamber views, showing both AV valves connecting to a single dominant ventricle with a severely hypoplastic accessory ventricle seen either anterosuperiorly (RV) or inferoposteriorly (LV). The annulus of each valve appears oriented toward the apex of a single ventricle, regardless of the coexistence of a smaller ventricle and ventricular septal defect (VSD). Again, AV-to-semilunar valve continuity is an important feature as is position (i.e., RV more often anterosuperior and LV more often inferoposterior). A double-inlet ventricle can be easily differentiated from an AV septal defect (AVSD) where two distinct ventricles can be identified apically despite the presence of a large inlet VSD and that each component of the AV valve is oriented toward a different apex.

Segmental Approach

Evaluation of the adult with UAVC by CMR or CCT shares several features with protocols established for echocardiography [15]. We thus describe visceral arrangement and cardiac anatomy in the following segments: systemic and pulmonary venous return, atria (including septum), AV valves, ventricles (including septum), semilunar valves, and great vessels (including aortopulmonary or collateral flow). At each level, key issues specific to UAVC include (1) mode of AV connection, (2) position and type of the accessory chamber, (3) outlet foramen obstruction, (4) AV valve abnormality, (5) positions of the great arteries and connections, (6) pulmonary obstruction, and (7) ventricular morphology [15]. Tables 11.3 and 11.4 summarize our anatomic and functional imaging objectives and protocols.

Table 11.2 Features of ventricular morphology

Feature	Right ventricle	Left ventricle
Position	Usually anterosuperior	Usually inferoposterior
AV valve to semilunar valve relationship	Discontinuity	Fibrous continuity
Trabeculation pattern	Coarse with a moderator band	Fine and bullet-shaped
Subarterial muscular conus	Present	Absent

Legend: *AV* atrioventricular

Table 11.3 CMR imaging sequences

Item (duration)	Objective	Sequence	Remarks
1 (2 min)	Establish basic thoracic, cardiac, and great vessel landmarks	Low resolution axial, sagittal, and coronal localizers (GRE or SSFP)	
2 (5 min)	Establish basic thoracic, cardiac, and great vessel landmarks	Medium resolution axial, sagittal and coronal (single-shot BB FSE)	Slice thickness 6–8 mm, gap 0–3 mm
3 (5 min)	Establish cardiac and great vessel landmarks and ventricular function	Axial cinema (balanced SSFP)	20 slices: thickness 6–8 mm, gap 0–3 mm
4 (3 min)	Establish cardiac and great vessel landmarks, atrial or veno-pulmonary connection, aortic branches, systemic-to-pulmonary shunts	Coronal cinema (balanced SSFP)	14 slices: thickness 6–8 mm, gap 0–3 mm
5 (2 min)	Establish cardiac and great vessel landmarks, atrial or veno-pulmonary connection	Sagittal cinema (balanced SSFP)	Ten slices: thickness 6–8 mm, gap 0–3 mm
6 (10 min)	Assess valvular and ventricular function	Vertical and horizontal oblique long axis, short-axis stack ± 3 and 4-chamber views (balanced SSFP)	Two long-axis slices, 10 short-axis, 12 long-axis 4 chamber, 13 chamber: thickness 6–8 mm, gap 0–1 mm
7 (2 min)	Great vessel and shunt morphology	Gadolinium contrast-enhanced angiography in coronal projection (fast GRE)	Cover aortic and pulmonary roots and descending aorta
8 (5 min)	Blood flow and velocity measurement of aortic, pulmonary and systemic and pulmonary venous flows	Phase-contrast velocity mapping in double-oblique views (fast GRE)	Aliasing velocities can be guided by echo imaging results
9 (5 min)	Detection of myocardial fibrosis by late gadolinium enhancement	Ventricular imaging in short and long-axis views (IR GRE)	Identical locations and views as in #6

Legend: *GRE* gradient-recalled echo, *SSFP* steady-state free precession, *BB FSE* black-blood fast spin echo, *IR* inversion-recovery prepared, *gap* distance between slices

The AV connection may be classified as (1) double inlet via 2 AV valves, (2) single inlet via one AV valve (with atresia of the other right or left AV valve), or (3) common inlet via a common AV valve [15]. The accessory chamber is part of the ventricular mass, but it does not receive at least half of an AV valve orifice. The accessory chamber is called an "outlet chamber" if it gives rise to one or both great arteries [15]. The VA connection may be described as (1) PA arising from the main outlet chamber and aorta arising from the outlet chamber, (2) aorta arising from the main outlet chamber and PA arising from the outlet chamber, (3) one great artery arising from the main ventricular chamber with atresia of the other semilunar valve, or (4) both great arteries arise from one chamber [15]. Once the connections have been identified, attention should turn to other structures.

Imaging Planes

As patients with UAVC often have thoracic deformities (e.g., rotoscoliosis) and abnormalities of situs and looping, a Cartesian basic three-plane (i.e., axial, coronal, and sagittal as used in CCT) approach often rewards the imaging specialist with useful extracardiac anatomic landmarks to determine cardiac structure arrangement or situs. Cardiac centered double-oblique planes similar to those used in echocardiography can thereafter be used for ventricular and valvular function measurement and depiction of conduit and great vessel anatomy as needed.

Table 11.4 CMR imaging objectives in Fontan patients

	Morphology	Function and flow measurement
Liver	Dilatation, nodular aspect suggestive of cirrhosis	
Systemic veins	Dilatation, veno-venous collaterals	Quantification of venous return by velocity mapping of IVC and SVC
Right atrium and Fontan conduit	Dilatation, presence of thrombus, residual shunt, or fenestration	Velocity mapping at RA to PA junction in classic APA
Pulmonary arteries	Anatomy, size, thrombus, arteriovenous fistulas	Quantification of PA flow by SSFP and velocity mapping in TCPC and lateral tunnel
Pulmonary veins and left atrium	Number of veins, obstruction by dilated RA	Quantification of total pulmonary blood flow by velocity mapping for each vein
AV valves and systemic ventricle	Type of AV and VA connection and ventricular situs	Quantitative ventricular function and volumes
Aorta and aortopulmonary collaterals	Anatomy of thoracic aorta and aortopulmonary collaterals originating from the descending aorta	Quantitative aortic root flow and pre-diaphragmatic flow

Legend: *IVC* inferior vena cava, *SVC* superior vena cava, *RA* right atrium, *PA* pulmonary artery, *APA* atriopulmonary anastomosis (classic Fontan), *SSFP* cinema in steady-state free precession, *TCPC* total cavopulmonary connection, *AV* atrioventricular, *VA* ventriculo-arterial

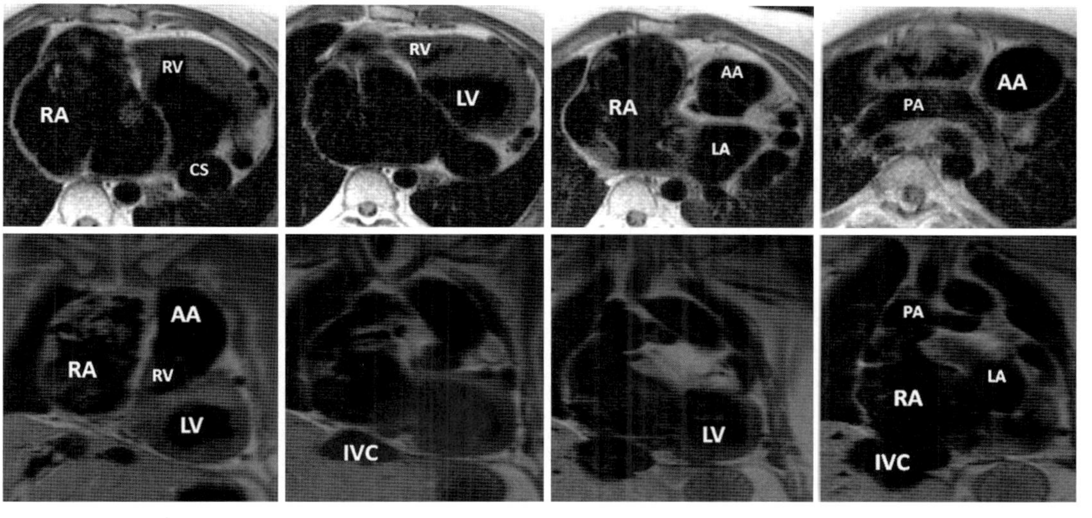

Fig. 11.2 Black-blood fast spin echo MR axial images from basal to apical levels (*upper row*) and coronal views from anterior to posterior (*lower row*) in a patient with tricuspid atresia, transposition of the great arteries, and bidirectional Glenn shunt. *AA* ascending aorta, *CS* coronary sinus, *IVC* inferior vena cava, *PA* pulmonary artery, *LA* left atrium, *RA* right atrium, *LV* left ventricle, *RV* right ventricle

Fast triplanar (axial, coronal, and sagittal) images in steady-state of free precession (SSFP) scout views are first obtained to establish cardiac and thoracic landmarks and the situs. This can be followed by either a basic (free-breathing or breath held) high-resolution BB FSE in the axial plane (Fig. 11.2), covering the upper abdomen to above the aortic arch (using 6–8 mm slices with 0–3 mm gaps), or a lower-resolution triplanar half-Fourier sequence (HASTE) FSE to confirm atrio-visceral arrangement, depicting liver, spleen, and stomach positions; bronchial and PA relationships; and important extracardiac findings such as lymphadenopathy, pulmonary nodules,

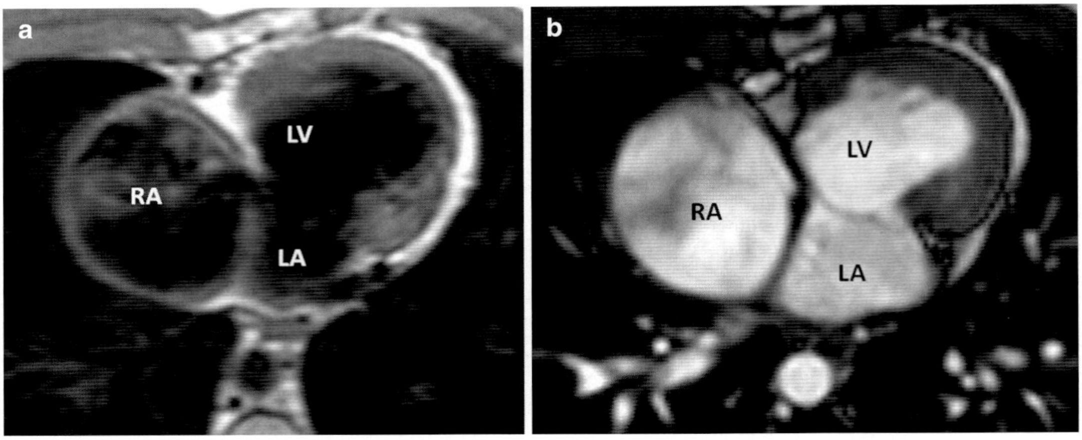

Fig. 11.3 (**a**) Insufficient blood pool nulling in black-blood fast spin echo in patient with tricuspid atresia with supero-inferior ventricles with intracavitary thrombus-like signal in the right atrium (*RA*), (**b**) same projection as (**a**) in bright-blood balanced steady-state free precession not showing thrombus within the RA. *LV* left ventricle, *LA* left atrium

and hepatosplenomegaly. Most often, usual arrangement (situs solitus) is seen, with the liver and IVC on the right side of the patient, a vertically oriented "right" main stem bronchus with anteriorly coursing right PA on the right, while the stomach and spleen and a horizontally oriented "left" main stem bronchus with a superiorly coursing left PA on the left-hand side. Mirror image (situs inversus) or ambiguous arrangements can occasionally be appreciated. In most cases, intracardiac anatomy can be depicted clearly without contrast in CMR based on the different relaxation properties of blood, muscle, and fat. Intravenous contrast is required for CCT.

Ventricular Volumes and Function

Since many UAVC patients present low cardiac output or flow rate, even the best black-blood FSE sequences may reveal abnormal intracavitary signals suggesting thrombus or mass, particularly in an enlarged RA (Fig. 11.3a). To prevent misinterpretation, we also use bright-blood single-shot SSFP sequences liberally using basic axial, sagittal, and coronal planes (6–8 mm slices with 0–2 mm gaps) to confirm basic anatomy, segmental relationships, and valvular and ventricular function and exclude intracardiac thrombus more specifically (Fig. 11.3b) [16]. Most patients are capable of breath holding to ensure proper image registration but occasionally we use respiration triggered gating if patients are fatigued or unable to hold their breath. With its 3D capabilities and excellent temporal and spatial resolution, CMR provides better noninvasive quantitative ventricular function assessment than echo or CCT.

Quantitative evaluation of ventricular function is a pivotal part of the assessment of adults with UAVC and is a crucial parameter in the outcome of patients converted to a Fontan circulation [17]. Ventricular systolic function can be addressed by obtaining short-axis slices planned from basic long-axis plane localizers. The dominant ventricle may have an unusual shape and the defined geometric assumptions may not hold. Therefore, evaluation of ventricular volume and function by CMR requires parallel tomographic images [17]. Commercially available calculation packages enable tracing end-diastolic and end-systolic endocardial and epicardial contours to determine ventricular volumes, mass, and ejection fraction. Although short-axis planes provide excellent blood to endocardial delineation of all myocardial segments, the major difficulty is in assessing the basal slices near the AV and semilunar valves as this plane moves back-and-forth toward the apex during the cardiac cycle (Fig. 11.4a). To include a slice in ventricular quantitation, the myocardium must be present for more than half (1/2) of the short-axis perimeter for a given slice to be used in volume calculations [18]. Accuracy and inter-study variability are dependent on

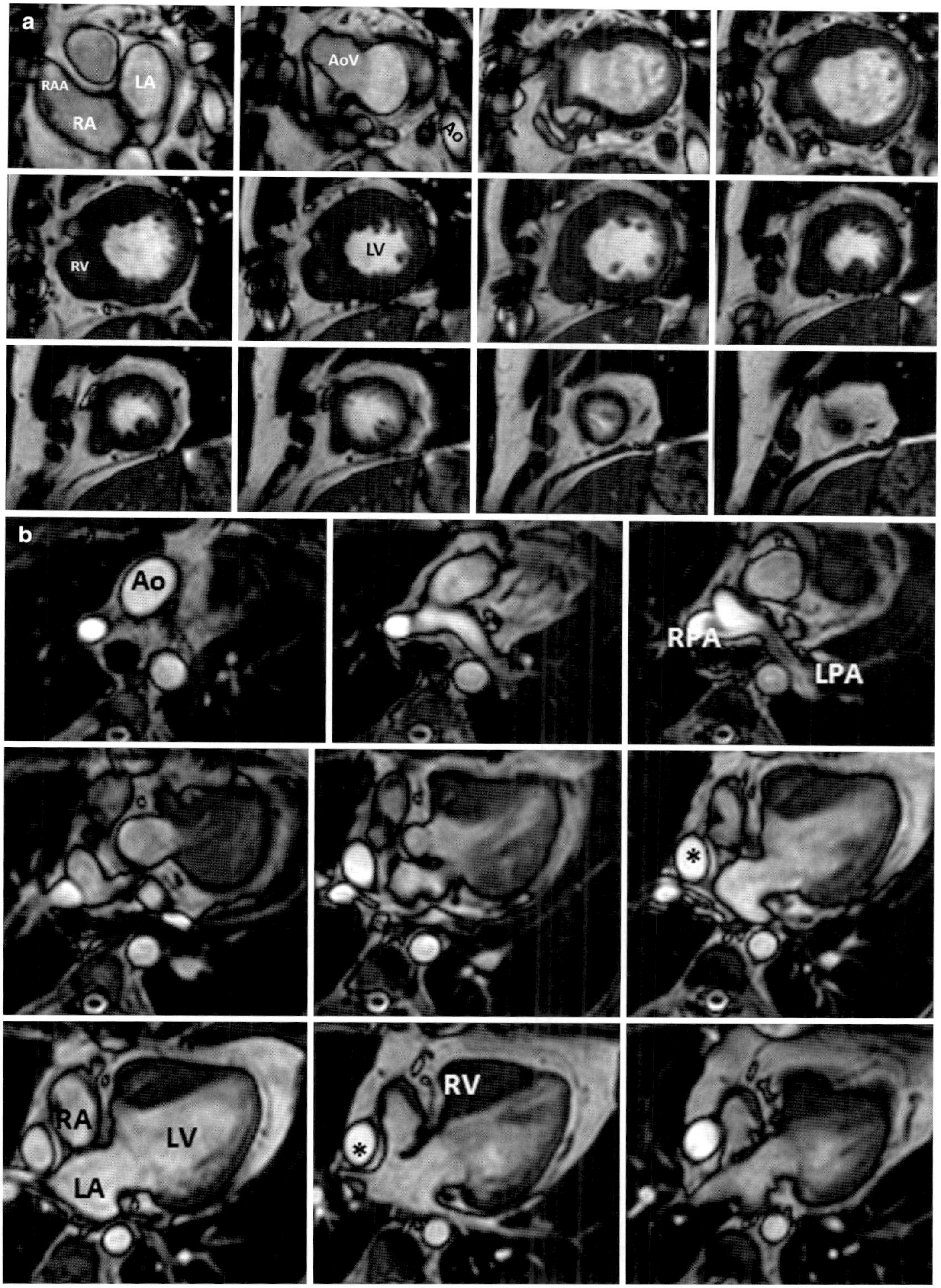

Fig. 11.4 Stack of short-axis (**a**) and four-chamber (**b**) sequential cine images using balanced steady-state free precession in a patient with tricuspid atresia. Hypoplastic right ventricle (*RV*) is best shown in short-axis views. Note absence of the tricuspid valve replaced by large fatty wedge in the right atrioventricular groove. Lateral Fontan tunnel (*asterisk*) is seen in (**b**). *AoV* aortic valve, *Ao* aorta, *RA* right atrium, *RAA* right atrial appendage, *LV* left ventricle, *LA* left atrium, *LPA* left pulmonary artery, *RPA* right pulmonary artery

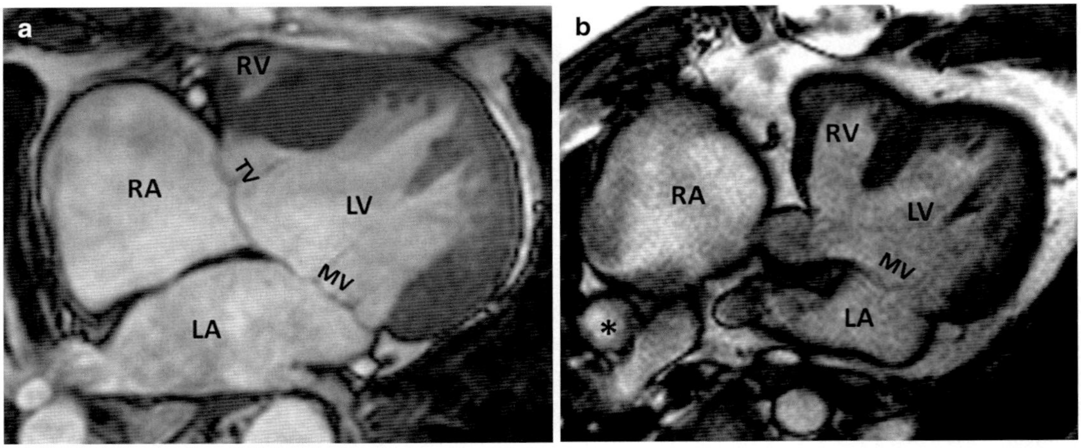

Fig. 11.5 (**a**) Double-inlet left ventricle in four-chamber view, showing clear delimitation of the plane of the atrioventricular valves. (**b**) Tricuspid atresia is shown for comparison. *RA* right atrium, *LV* left ventricle, *RV* right ventricle, *LA* left atrium, *TV* tricuspid valve, *MV* mitral valve, *asterisk* lateral Fontan tunnel

operator experience but can be within a 5 % margin of error in normals [19]. Long-axis views provide a better localization of AV the valve (Figs. 11.4b and 11.5) and semilunar valve function and planes and are particularly useful for the RV volume and function assessment but are limited in assessing the inferior wall function [20]. Inter-study variability is higher for the RV than for the LV and is also proportional to chamber dilatation and systolic dysfunction [21].

In UAVC, the dominant ventricle is most commonly of left morphology, followed by systemic right ventricles, and ventricles of undetermined morphology [22]. The majority of adult patients with UAVC have normal ventricular function, possibly reflecting a selection of patients with better late outcomes following childhood operations. Ammash et al. reported normal ventricular function in 11 of 13 adults with unrepaired UAVC [5]. In 62 adults with palliated or unrepaired UAVC, Angeli et al. found a mild decrease in the average systemic ventricular ejection fraction (52 %) with a range from 20 to 70 % [22]. There was no correlation between peak oxygen consumption and ejection fraction. The ventricle was also, on average, mildly dilated with a mean volume of 106 ± 448 mL/m^2 [22]. Patients undergoing heart transplant were all in functional class IV, had moderate to severe AV valve regurgitation, and an ejection fraction between 18 and 35 %. The anatomic type of the ventricle and specific lesion appear to influence survival. Best survival seems to occur in patients with double-inlet LV, transposition of the great arteries, and pulmonary stenosis, allowing streaming of blood flow from the LA to aorta [22].

Tricuspid Atresia

In patients with tricuspid atresia, severe RV hypoplasia is characteristic and quantitative dominant LV function should be measured as outlined above (Figs. 11.2 and 11.4). Many patients exhibit a mildly decreased LV ejection fraction following the Fontan operation with normal LV mass and volumes [23]. The addition of myocardial tagging has shed light on subtle abnormalities of reverse ventricular torsion in such patients [24]. If, despite the above views, questions persist on valvular function, intracardiac shunt, or ventricular quantitative function, we occasionally obtain a stack of long-axis oblique views in the four-chamber orientation determined from the available short-axis and long-axis localizers (Fig. 11.4b). Systemic venous and RA dilatation are generally present with the classic fatty wedge seen in the right AV groove on axial or long-axis four-chamber views (Fig. 11.4b). The RA receives the coronary sinus and has a broad- and triangular-shaped appendage. A large atrial septal defect (ASD) is the only outlet for the RA in the native form, and a VSD is the only possible intracardiac outlet to the PA with the dominant single and frequently dilated LV supporting both circulations. The LV characteristically appears as a smooth-walled ventricle with fibrous continuity between the AV (mitral) valve and the semilunar (aortic or pulmonary) valve. The small hypoplastic RV lies anteriorly and to the right. Mitral and aortic valve function is usually normal.

The three intracardiac morphological characteristics to demonstrate in tricuspid atresia are (1) VA connection, (2) VSD size, and (3) subpulmonary and pulmonary stenosis or atresia. In most cases (75 %), the VA connection is concordant, with the LV connected to the aorta and hypoplastic RV to the PA with a restrictive VSD and pulmonary and subpulmonary stenoses leading to profound cyanosis. In the remainder, VA discordance is seen (RV to aorta and LV to PA) (Fig. 11.2), usually with a nonrestrictive VSD between the LV and aorta and a normal pulmonary valve, leading to LV volume overload and, ultimately, pulmonary hypertension unless some form of early correction is provided.

Other Types of Univentricular AV Connections

A double-inlet ventricle is when both AV valves are connected to one dominant, usually left, ventricle with VA discordance and pulmonary stenosis protecting the pulmonary circulation and a VSD (bulboventricular foramen) leading to the subaortic (hypoplastic) ventricle (Figs. 11.5 and 11.6). Another form of UAVC is a supero-inferior twisting of the ventricles, so-called "crisscross" heart, where the LA empties into a right-sided LV with pulmonary atresia and a bulboventricular foramen leading into a small left-sided subaortic RV (Fig. 11.7). Finally, some patients with a very

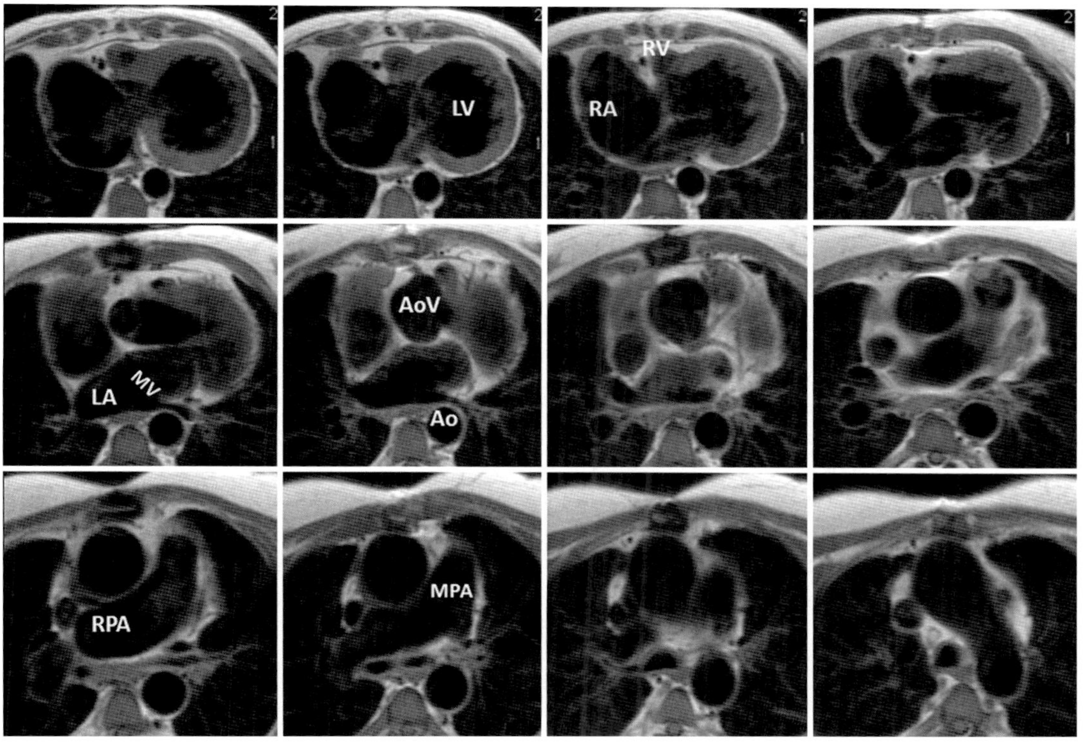

Fig. 11.6 CMR assessment of double-inlet ventricle using black-blood spin echo in the axial plane. *RA* right atrium, *LV* left ventricle, *RV* right ventricle, *LA* left atrium, *MV* mitral valve, *AoV* aortic valve, *Ao* aorta, *RPA* right pulmonary artery

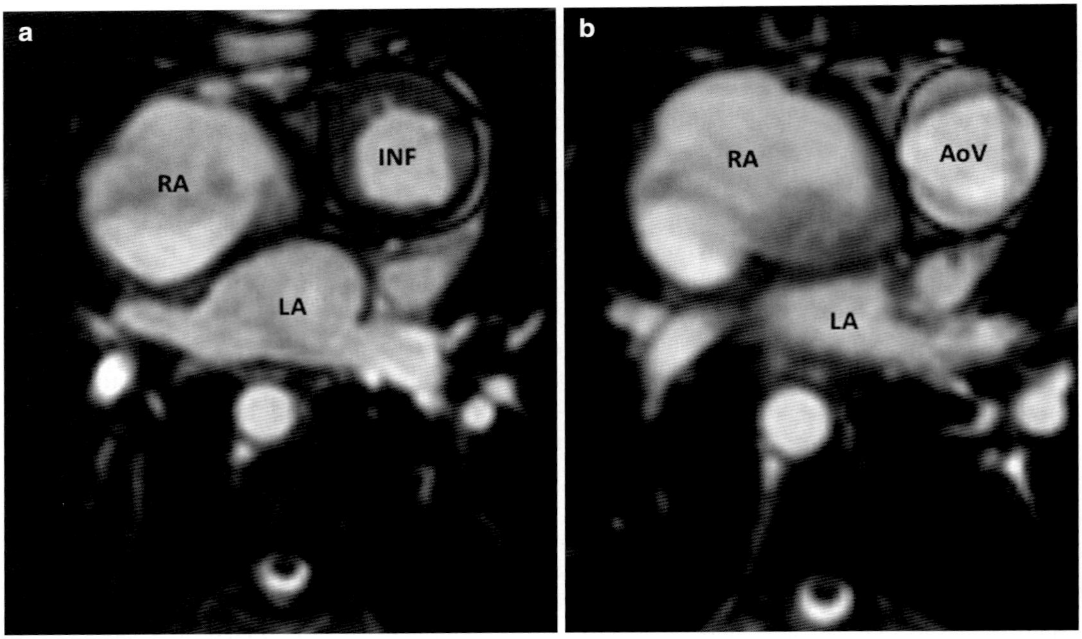

Fig. 11.7 CMR assessment of crisscross heart showing (**a**) the relationship of the left atrium (*LA*), right atrium (*RA*), and infundibulum (*INF*) and (**b**) the relationship of the LA, RA, and aortic valve (*AoV*)

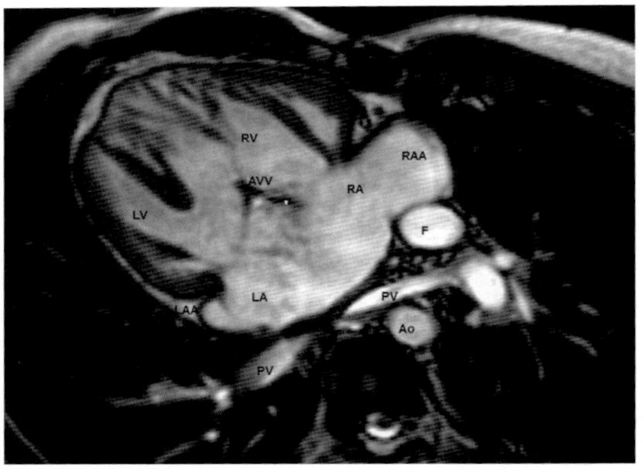

Fig. 11.8 Complete atrioventricular canal defect with dextrocardia in the four-chamber view showing a large atrial septal defect and a large ventricular septal defect, therefore functioning as a single ventricle physiology. *F* Fontan conduit, *RA* right atrium, *RAA* right atrial appendage, *RV* right ventricle, *LA* left atrium, *LAA* left atrial appendage, *AVV* atrioventricular valve, *asterisk* atrioventricular valve regurgitation, *LV* left ventricle, *Ao* aorta, *PV* pulmonary vein

large VSD or a complete AV canal defect with unbalanced ventricular morphology cannot undergo a biventricular repair and are managed a univentricular Fontan approach (Fig. 11.8). Long-axis axial and four-chamber views best depict double-inlet anatomy, valvular function, and extent of the VSD (Figs. 11.4 and 11.5). Ventricular outflow chamber obstruction was present in 14 % of patients with UAVC hearts in one series [15]. Subpulmonary obstruction was more common than subaortic obstruction.

Imaging UAVC from Native Anatomy to Palliative Surgical Procedures

In the native stage of UAVC, PA anatomy must be precisely depicted for patient management. The presence of reduced pulmonary blood flow will be palliated by systemic-to-pulmonary shunts, while nonrestrictive torrential pulmonary flow will require protection from pulmonary hypertension.

Systemic-to-Pulmonary Shunts

In a classic Blalock-Taussig shunt, the subclavian artery is anastomosed directly to the ipsilateral

PA. A modified Blalock-Taussig shunt is constructed by suturing a graft between the subclavian artery and PA. Absence of one subclavian artery is a common sequel of a classic Blalock-Taussig shunt, which usually has little clinical impact. There may be PA stenosis at the site of implantation of a classic or modified Blalock-Taussig shunt (see Fig. 10.13). Central shunts are placed between the ascending aorta and right PA (Waterston) or between the descending aorta and left PA (Potts). After closure, they may cause focal stenosis of the great arteries. Aortic arch imaging either in SSFP or by contrast-enhanced angiography in the coronal plane is the preferred view to demonstrate Blalock-Taussig or central shunt patency and the presence of native aortopulmonary collaterals (see section "Collaterals" below). A coronal view may also depict a Blalock-Taussig systemic-to-pulmonary shunt between the subclavian artery and ipsilateral PA. These shunts are usually closed at the time of the Fontan operation. However, they may remain patent and cause volume overload of the univentricular pumping chamber. If central shunts remain patent, they can cause unrestricted pulmonary flow and pulmonary hypertension. As PA size and pulmonary arterial resistance are crucial determinants of success in patients upgraded from a simple systemic-to-pulmonary shunt to the Fontan operation, CMR must provide precise characterization of pulmonary arteries and dimensions. In patients who do not undergo a Fontan operation, blood supply to the lungs may depend on the patency of a systemic-to-pulmonary shunt. It is, therefore, critical to ensure patency of these shunts in cyanotic UAVC patients.

Imaging of Fontan Procedures

In patients having undergone the Fontan operation, characterization of the type of surgery may be readily achieved by CMR. Historically, if the Fontan was constructed before the 1990s, it likely takes the form of a direct RA to PA or atriopulmonary anastomosis (APA), usually via the RA appendage. RA to PA Fontans are associated with giant pressure overloaded RAs (Fig. 11.9a). Modifications of the classic Fontan technique may be appreciated, such as the Björk operation, where the RA is anastomosed to a small hypoplastic RV outlet chamber in the hope of improving PA flow (Fig. 11.9b). In addition to causing systemic venous hypertension and, ultimately, cardiac cirrhosis, massive RA dilatation predisposes to supraventricular arrhythmias, increases the likelihood of stagnant flow and thrombus within the RA, and may compress right pulmonary veins that course posterior to the RA before entering the LA, thereby increasing pulmonary vascular resistance.

In the 1990s, a more streamlined type of conduit, called the lateral tunnel, was developed, partitioning the RA with a Dacron or Gore-Tex patch, to improve energy efficiency and reduce RA dilation (Fig. 11.10). Since the late 1990s, some centers have modified their approach be directing IVC flow to the PA by means of an entirely extracardiac conduit (Fig. 11.11) [25]. Unfortunately for CMR, many of these patients also had prophylactic epicardial pacing systems at the time of surgery such that CCT is favored over CMRs for subsequent investigation (see below). In all patients, Fontan conduit patency can first be determined from cine views and measured by velocity mapping. The remainder of this section will cover key topics in imaging UAVC patients who have undergone a Fontan-type palliation.

Phase-Contrast (PC) Velocity Mapping

In a fashion analogous to Doppler's fundamental role in echocardiography to measure blood velocity and flow in order to derive pressure gradients and cardiac output, background noise-corrected PC velocity mapping is an integral part of CMR examination in patients with UAVC. Such a technique has been shown superior to nuclear ventilation perfusion studies to determine pulmonary perfusion [26]. We use the available triplanar GRE and other double-oblique SSFP images to plan proper alignment of PC velocity mapping perpendicular to blood flow (Fig. 11.12). Comprehensive CMR assessment usually involves flow measurement at multiple levels. As pulmonary arterial flow can originate from multiple sources (e.g., subpulmonary

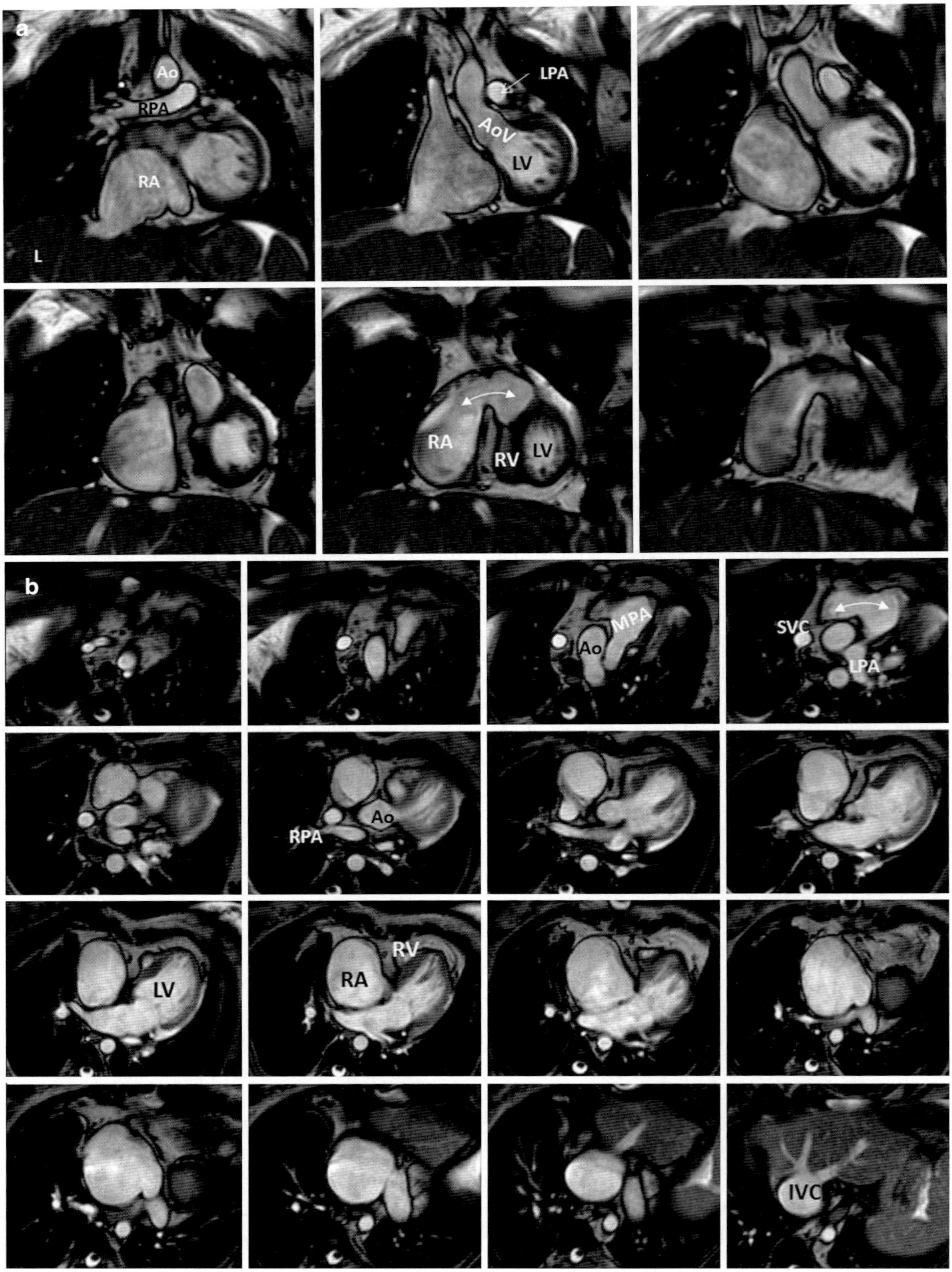

Fig. 11.9 (**a**) Classic atriopulmonary Fontan connection in coronal view. The right atrium is massively enlarged, but the right atrium-to-pulmonary artery anastomosis (*double-headed arrow*) is widely patent. (**b**) Björk modification of the Fontan operation with severely dilated right atrium in axial plane. The right atrium is anastomosed to a small hypoplastic right ventricular outlet chamber (*double-headed arrow*). *L* liver, *IVC* inferior vena cava, *RA* right atrium, *LA* left atrium, *AoV* aortic valve, *LV* left ventricle, *Ao* aorta; RPA, right pulmonary artery, *LPA* left pulmonary artery, *SVC* superior vena cava

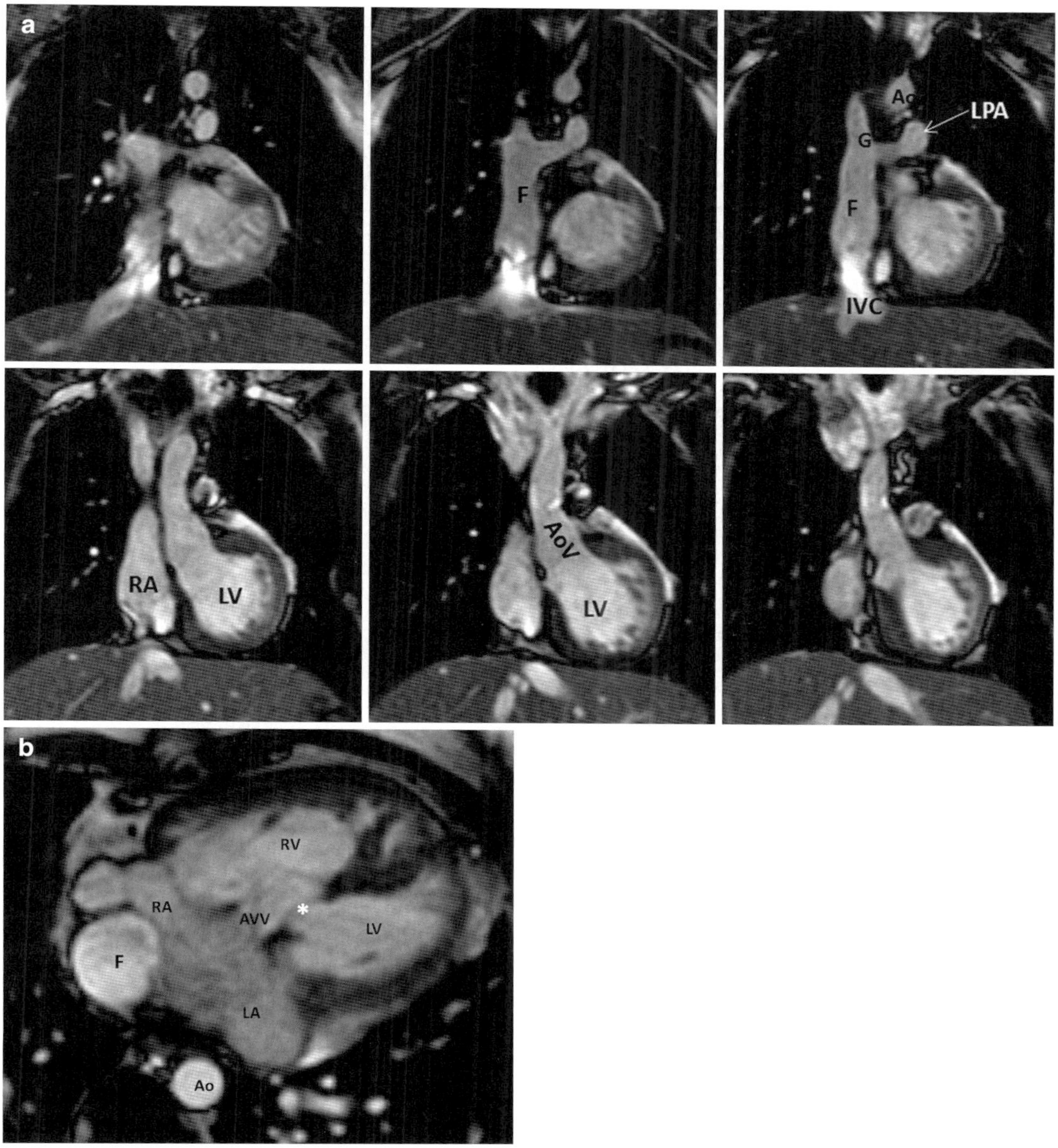

Fig. 11.10 CMR assessment of lateral tunnel (**a**) in coronal view in tricuspid atresia and (**b**) in long-axis four-chamber view in a patient with large AV canal defect, using steady-state free precession. The superior cavopulmonary anastomosis (bidirectional Glenn shunt) is seen in the *center and right top panel* images. *IVC* inferior vena cava, *F* Fontan conduit, *G* Glenn shunt, *RA* right atrium, *LA* left atrium, *AVV* atrioventricular valve, *AoV* aortic valve, *asterisk* ventricular septal defect, *LV* left ventricle, *Ao* aorta, *LPA* left pulmonary artery

ventricle, if present, native or surgically created shunts), quantification of total pulmonary blood flow may be challenging. Although we interrogate the main PA (and its proximal branches if discontinuous) in each patient, the most reliable way to quantify pulmonary blood flow may be to measure pulmonary venous flow returning to the LA, although pulmonary AV fistulas may drain directly to the LA. We also calculate flow at the level of the aortic root and compare it to the stroke volume obtained from the systemic ventricle in order to quantify AV valve regurgitation, in the absence of

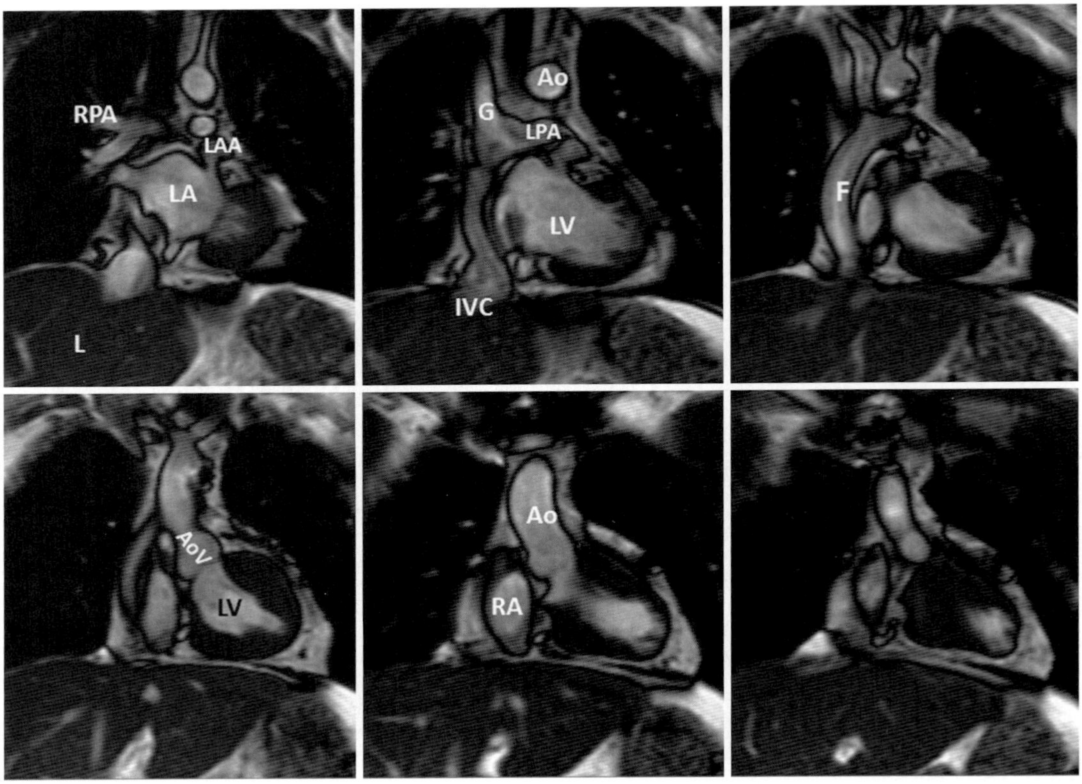

Fig. 11.11 CMR assessment of extracardiac Fontan conduit in coronal view using steady-state free precession. The total cavopulmonary connection combines a conduit between the inferior vena cava and right pulmonary artery (*top center and right panels*) and bidirectional Glenn shunt as superior cavopulmonary anastomosis (*top center panel*). *L* liver, *IVC* inferior vena cava, *F* Fontan conduit, *G* Glenn shunt, *RA* right atrium, *LA* left atrium, *LAA* left atrial appendage, *AoV* aortic valve, *LV* left ventricle, *Ao* aorta, *RPA* right pulmonary artery, *LPA* left pulmonary artery

significant interventricular shunting. Quantification of aortopulmonary collateral flow is also possible but more cumbersome (see below).

Pulmonary Arteries and Relative Lung Flows

PA banding may be required early in life to prevent pulmonary overcirculation until Fontan completion in patients with preserved antegrade pulmonary flow. Magee et al. found mild PA distortion to be present in 14 % of Fontan patients. In patients with severe PA distortion, one PA was implicated in 11 % and both in 4 % of patients [27]. Contrast-enhanced (CE) magnetic resonance angiography (MRA) allows tridimensional visualization of PA distortion or extrinsic compression [17]. CMR can also detect unrecognized pulmonary atresia [28]. Pulmonary arteries may also be small because their growth may fail to follow somatic growth after the Fontan operation [29]. PA flow and distensibility, but not PA area, are lower in Fontan patients than in controls [30]. Pulmonary arteries in Fontan patients also show evidence of endothelial dysfunction in the form of inadequate response to low-dose dobutamine and of variation in patterns of wall shear stress, as assessed by CMR [30]. Under low-dose dobutamine stress, total flow and peak flow rate increase, but stroke index does not [30]. In part, this may also be due to the absence of a subpulmonary pumping chamber. In controls, peak wall shear stress occurs during systole. In total cavopulmonary connection Fontans, there is no change in wall shear stress throughout the cardiac cycle, and in atriopulmonary connection Fontans, peak wall shear stress occurs in diastole [30].

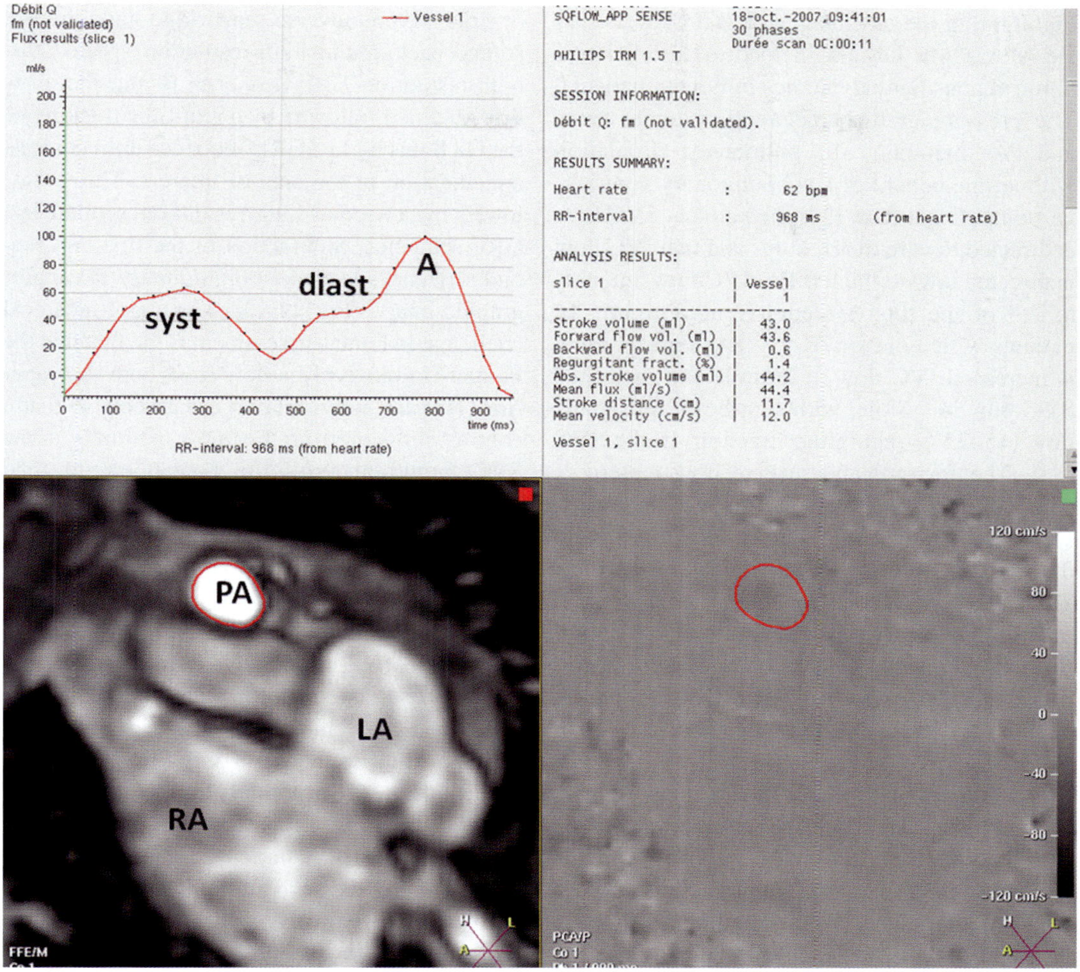

Fig. 11.12 CMR phase-contrast velocity mapping of Fontan conduit flow. *PA* pulmonary artery, *RA* right atrium, *LA* left atrium, *syst* systolic flow, *diast* diastolic flow, *A* flow from atrial contraction

Differences in wall shear stress may affect PA remodeling late after the Fontan operation.

VA connections and central PA anatomy are well shown by axial and coronal SSFP but small or peripheral PA vessels are best shown by contrast-enhanced MRA (see below) because of magnetic susceptibility between lung tissue and blood vessels. Various indices are used, generally indexing PA branch area or diameter to the body surface area (the Nakata index).

Systemic Venous Anatomy and Function

According to Magee et al. [27], 15 % of patients with univentricular hearts have a bilateral SVC connection. In that case, the Fontan circuit is constructed using bilateral SVC to PA connections (Glenn shunts). CMR or CCT studies should demonstrate patency of the systemic veins. If contrast enhancement is used, the injection and image acquisition should be appropriately timed to image the superior and inferior venae cavae. Systemic venous flow after Fontan is readily studied with phase-contrast CMR [17]. Multidimensional phase-velocity MRI and shear stress measurements by MRI have provided important insights into understanding of RA and Fontan physiology [31] and may help to assess advantages of different surgical approaches, highlighting the advantages of TCPC over classic APA. CMR has also helped to describe systemic venous hemodynamics in Fontan patients. The pressure gradient between systemic veins and PAs maintains the pulmonary circulation without the benefit of a subpulmonary ventricular pump. Fogel et al. [32] showed that SVC flow is directed toward the right PA and that IVC flow is directed toward the left PA. IVC flow amounts to 2/5 of the total systemic venous return. In patients with a classic (RA to PA) Fontan, there is increased IVC flow in diastole and increased SVC flow in systole, with significant retrograde flow (15–22 % regurgitant fraction) in the SVC [33]. The forward and reverse flow pattern in classic Fontans is energy inefficient in comparison to the continuous balanced flow throughout the cardiac cycle observed in patients with a TCPC [33]. Fontan patients with ascites or pleural effusions have a lower IVC return (1.5 L/min/m^2) and increased SVC to total caval flow ratio (0.56 vs. 0.35 in patients with better hemodynamics) [34]. Total caval flow decreases with age [34].

A coronal view usually best depicts a Glenn shunt [35, 36]. The Glenn shunt may be a classic unidirectional connection to the ipsilateral PA (elbow-shaped) or a bidirectional connection to both PAs (T-shaped), as depicted in Figs. 11.10, 11.11, and 11.13. Classic APC Fontan flow can be measured cranial to the RA to PA anastomosis and is generally phasic with predominantly diastolic flow and atrial kick augmentation (Fig. 11.12). As RA-propelled blood flow is sluggish, a signal void from spin dephasing is generally absent despite conduit stenosis. Conduit stenosis usually takes the form of a low velocity continuous flow. In classic APA Fontan conduits, PA flow measurement can be determined at the RA to PA junction in an oblique para-axial view. In the case of lateral tunnel or extracardiac Fontan with a bidirectional Glenn, each PA must be interrogated in a parasagittal plane to obtain total pulmonary flow.

To complete the UAVC and Fontan circuit assessment, 3D CE MRA using a gadolinium contrast agent is almost always performed, unless contraindicated (e.g., severe renal insufficiency or prior severe adverse reaction to gadolinium). A dry background high-resolution spoiled fast high-resolution GRE sequence of the thorax is first obtained followed by a real-time tracking of the Gd bolus by fast GRE sequence until contrast opacification of the area of interest. This is followed by a second high-resolution spoiled fast GRE sequence. Subtraction of the first and second sequences leads to a high-quality 3D angiographic image (Fig. 11.13). The major technical challenge in Fontan assessment is the fact that the Fontan circuit receives flow from both the superior (1/3) and inferior (2/3) caval veins so that a contrast infusion from the upper extremity to the SVC would underfill the Fontan circuit (and falsely suggest thrombus) on the first-pass acquisition, unless a second data set is obtained during the following systemic venous phase. An equilibrium study using an intravascular agent such as Gadofosveset may be of interest to delineate intricacies of the systemic venous return, including frequently encountered pulmonary arteriovenous and system-to-pulmonary veno-venous fistulas. The advantage of CE MRA over that produced by CCT is not only the lack of radiation but also the ability to record multiple imaging series at no extra radiation cost. Time-resolved MRA can provide such multiple images at different times of contrast opacification based on the relative stability of the thoracic great vessel structure. The technique works by overweighting acquisition of center of k-space data to follow contrast changes, while acquiring a framework of great vessel contours (k-space periphery) at baseline and throughout acquisition. This technique shortens total 3D imaging acquisition time, enabling multiple data sets to be acquired. The advantage of extracellular compared to intravascular agents is the possibility to perform late gadolinium enhancement (LGE) studies on the systemic ventricle (Fig. 11.14, see below). In patients with contraindications to CMR (e.g., pacemakers), a high-quality angiogram can be performed using iodinated-enhanced CCT, with proper timing of the contrast bolus, preferably in the late venous (with detection of contrast in the IVC) or portal phase. Overall, delayed images do not provide high-quality angiographic images.

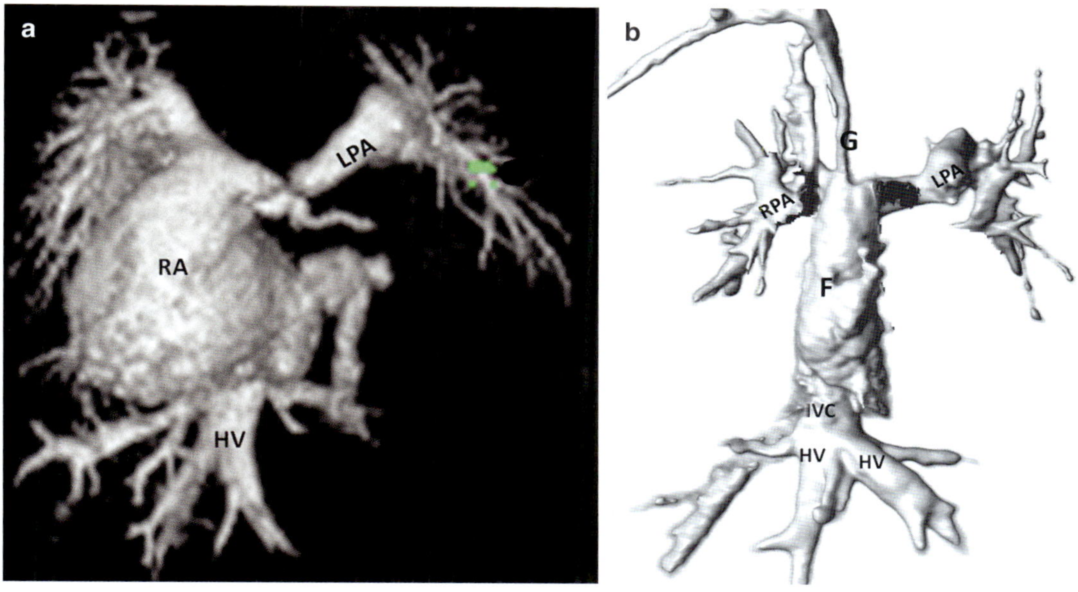

Fig. 11.13 Contrast-enhanced CMR angiography. (**a**) Anterior 3D projection of classic atriopulmonary Fontan. Right atrium (*RA*) is massively dilated. A prominent metal artifact in the area of prior stenting is present at the most proximal left pulmonary artery (*LPA*) causing pseudostenosis. (**b**) Anteroposterior or coronal projection of volume rendering of lateral tunnel and bidirectional T-shaped Glenn with hepatic veins and pulmonary arteries, respectively. *HV* hepatic vein, *IVC* inferior vena cava, *F* Fontan conduit, *G* Glenn shunt, *RPA* right pulmonary artery

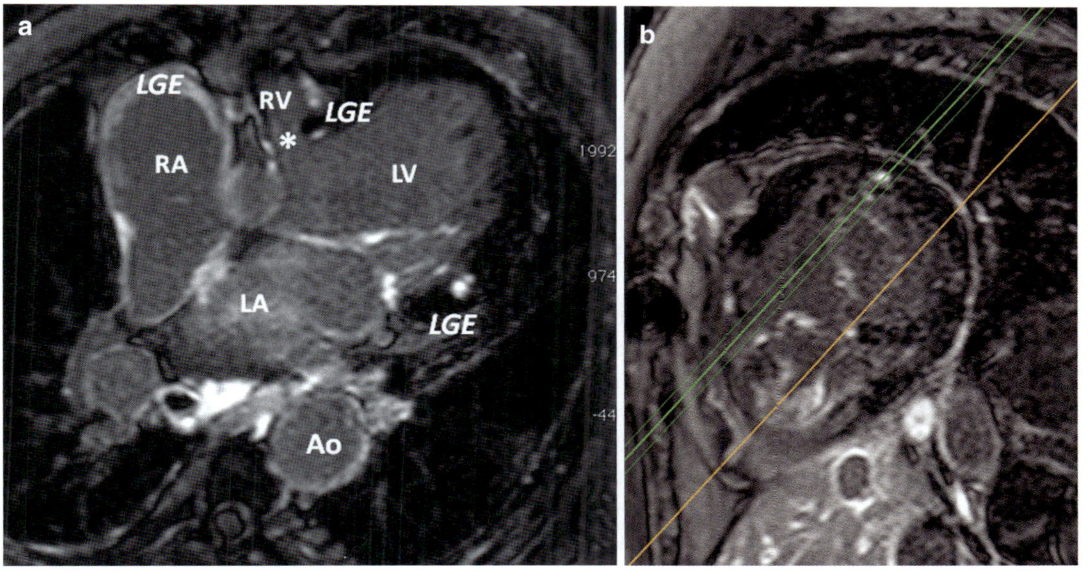

Fig. 11.14 CMR late gadolinium study of double-inlet left ventricle showing a scar within the myocardium of the anterolateral wall (**a**). The **b** shows an orthogonal view, with the reference line (*green line*) confirming the presence of late gadolinium enhancement as well as in septal crest and right atrial free wall. *RA* right atrium, *LV* left ventricle, *asterisk* ventricular septal defect, *RV* right ventricle, *LA* left atrium, *Ao* aorta, *LGE* late gadolinium enhancement

Thrombus

Thrombus formation may occur in the RA or at other sites such as a pulmonary root pouch from oversewing of the pulmonary valve in the course of a cavopulmonary connection. Thrombus formation is a risk factor for thromboembolic death [8]. In the RA, thrombus poses a risk of pulmonary emboli, while a PA stump predisposes to systemic emboli [37] (see Figs. 30.10 and 30.11). Atrial enlargement, arrhythmias, and sepsis are risk factors for thrombus formation [22]. Thrombus formation in a classic Fontan may justify conversion to a TCPC connection. The presence of thrombus can be readily seen by cine sequences, appearing as a wall-adherent hypointense round or sessile mass. The thrombotic nature of a mass may be demonstrated by rapid decline of signal intensity on T2*-weighted imaging. On contrast-enhanced CMR, a thrombus will not show enhancement on first-pass perfusion imaging and will appear as a low-signal mass using on LGE sequences using a long inversion time (600 ms) [38–40].

Pulmonary Venous Drainage and Obstruction

Close attention should be paid to pulmonary venous drainage, in particular, in patients with isomerism [17]. Compression of pulmonary veins by the giant RA may occur in patients with classic APC Fontans. Pulmonary venous obstruction can be demonstrated by long-axis axial or four-chamber views using cinema or black-blood imaging. To assess pulmonary veins, MRA or CTA may also be used. In an angiographic study, O'Donnell et al. characterized the following three patterns of pulmonary venous compression: (1) compression of the left lower pulmonary vein as it crosses anterior to the descending aorta and posterior to the atrium, (2) uninvolved upper lobe pulmonary veins, and (3) reduced flow in the PA to the affected lung [41]. Of note, lower pulmonary vein compression is usually ipsilateral to the aortic arch [41]. CMR was also sensitive to identify pulmonary vein stenosis but was only performed in seven patients [41]. Detailed reviews have previously described the CMR evaluation of pulmonary venous anatomy and flow [42].

Collaterals

After a TCPC, venous decompression channels may develop between the superior and inferior vena cava and RA, with progressive cyanosis. Magee et al. reported that 31 % of patients have systemic venous collaterals after bidirectional Glenn shunts [27]. Collaterals are associated with a significant gradient between the SVC and RA [27]. The most frequent decompressing venous channels are the azygos and hemiazygos veins, followed by pericardiophrenic, pericardial, paravertebral, and mediastinal veins [27]. Systemic venous decompression may also occur through internal mammary, chest wall, hepatic, superior intercostal, and cervical veins. In the study by Magee et al., 38 % of patients eventually underwent coil occlusion of collaterals.

Systemic-to-pulmonary collaterals may also develop after bidirectional cavopulmonary anastomosis in 59 % of patients, requiring intervention in 30 % of them [43]. Systemic-to-pulmonary collaterals cause volume overload of the systemic ventricle and flow at systemic pressure in the pulmonary system. Risk factors include a prior right-sided systemic-to-pulmonary shunt, lower ventricular end-diastolic volume and pulmonary vascular resistance prior to the Glenn shunt, and use of cardiopulmonary bypass during surgery [43]. Evaluation of collateral flow without CMR is impractical and relies on cross-sectional areas of collateral vessels or invasive measurements at the time of Fontan completion, on cardiopulmonary bypass. Cinema in SSFP can detect the presence of veno-venous or aorto-pulmonary collaterals [12, 44]. CMR allows noninvasive calculation of collateral flow either as ascending aorta flow minus total caval flow (superior + inferior caval flows) or as total pulmonary venous flow minus pulmonary artery flow (right + left pulmonary arteries flow) [44, 45]. However, these methods cannot distinguish between systemic-to-pulmonary collaterals flow and systemic-to-pulmonary venous collateral flow. Prakash et al. studied systemic-to-pulmonary collateral flow by CMR in patients with Fontans and at an earlier palliative stage [45]. Median systemic-to-pulmonary collateral flow indexed to body surface area was higher in the pre-Fontan group and decreased after the Fontan operation [45]. Systemic-to-pulmonary collateral flow also decreased with increasing age [45]. In Fontan patients, the highest quartile of systemic-to-pulmonary flow was associated with a higher ventricular end-diastolic volume [45]. Independent associations were found between systemic-to-pulmonary flow and pre-Fontan status, unilateral branch PA stenosis, hypoplastic left heart syndrome, and previous catheter occlusion of a systemic-to-pulmonary collateral vessel [45].

Schmitt et al. proposed a method to calculate pulmonary venous resistance in Fontan patients, taking collateral flow into account. Collateral flow is obtained by the difference between effective antegrade ascending aorta flow and the sum of antegrade right and left PA flows. Pulmonary venous resistance, therefore, is equal to the transpulmonary gradient divided by the sum of right and left pulmonary flows plus collateral flow [46]. Schmitt et al. also reported that collateral flow increases under dobutamine stress, with a decrease in pulmonary vascular resistance and no change in stroke volume [46]. The contribution of systemic-to-pulmonary flow to total pulmonary output was 13 % at rest and increased to >25 % under dobutamine stress [46].

Myocardial Fibrosis

LGE CMR allows detection of regional fibrosis in ischemic and nonischemic cardiomyopathy [47–50]. It signifies an increased partition coefficient of gadolinium in a given volume owing to the presence of scar from either necrosis (as in post myocardial infarction) or replacement fibrosis from ventricular strain or postoperative scar. The pattern of LGE allows distinction between various cardiomyopathies [51] and provides prognostic information [52]. In a retrospective review, Rathod et al. identified myocardial LGE, indicating regional fibrosis, in 28 % of Fontan patients [53]. It was independently associated with a lower ejection fraction, higher end-diastolic volume and ventricular mass, and non-sustained ventricular tachycardia [53]. LGE was transmural in 40 % of patients, subendocardial in 32 %, subepicardial in 20 %, and speckled in 12 % [53]. Transmural and subendocardial LGE is typical of myocardial infarction, while subepicardial enhancement is encountered in myocarditis. Circumferential subendocardial LGE is a pattern typical of endocardial fibroelastosis and was seen in 16 % of patients [53]. Fibrosis can be localized to areas of the myocardium, such as an infarction. It may also be generalized, leading to expansion of the myocardial extracellular space by diffuse collagen deposition [50]. Since it relies on a difference in signal intensity that may not exist if the fibrosis is diffuse, LGE imaging may only partially reflect the extent fibrosis. Gadolinium-based contrast agents enter the extracellular space and shorten the T1 of the whole myocardium. T1 mapping techniques that determine myocardial T1 have, therefore, allowed measurement of the fraction of myocardial volume occupied by extracellular space [54, 55]. Such techniques currently remain in the realm of research are close to clinical applications. They have been applied successfully to a variety of congenital heart defects. Patients with systemic right ventricles and cyanosis have the highest degree of diffuse fibrosis by this technique [56].

Liver Disease

Both CMR and CTC provide the opportunity to screen for signs of liver disease, even if the whole liver is not routinely included in CMR examination. Hepatopathy results from transmission of pulmonary pressure to the systemic veins. The most common findings by CCT or CMR in Fontan patients are abnormal parenchymal enhancement, hypervascular nodules, signs of cirrhosis and, rarely, hepatocellular carcinoma [57]. An example of liver congestion on a routine SSFP localizing sequence is shown in Fig. 11.15.

Cardiac CT (CCT) Imaging

With the expanded use of permanent pacing in patients with univentricular hearts, especially after palliative surgery, cardiac CT (CCT) is increasingly requested to help delineate cardiac structures and great vessel anatomy. Although

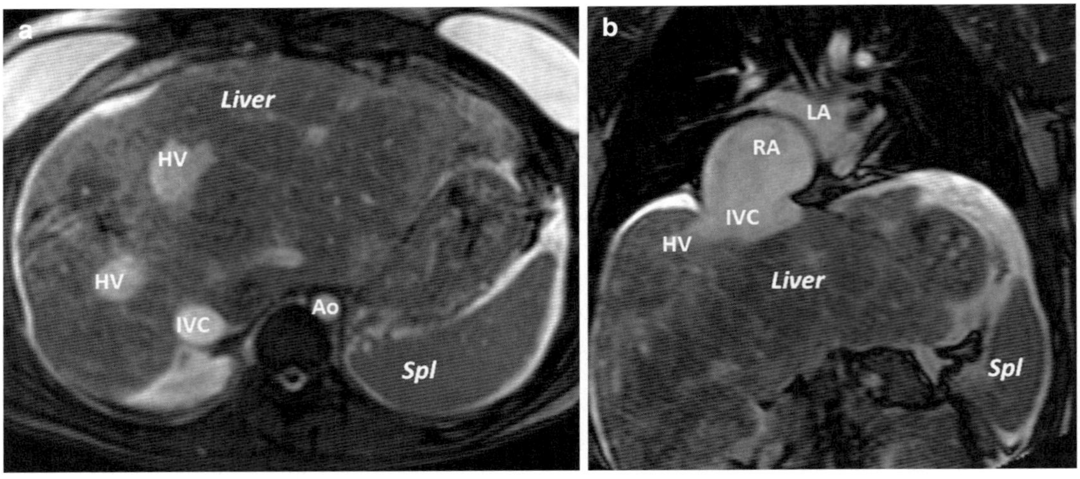

Fig. 11.15 CMR image of liver in a Fontan patient: (**a**) Axial plane and (**b**) coronal plane steady-state free precession. The liver is severely enlarged and appears nodular. Mild ascites is present. The inferior vena cava is markedly dilated. *IVC* inferior vena cava, *HV* hepatic vein, *RA* right atrium, *LA* left atrium, *Spl* spleen, *Ao* aorta

CMR and CCT employ drastically different techniques to generate images, the imaging philosophy remains similar. It begins with the segmental approach to describe the heart and great vessel from the standpoint of blood flowing from the veins and atria to the great vessel, with anatomy defined for each segment. Systemic and pulmonary venous return must be described precisely; AV connections and AV valve anatomy are next with ventricular morphology or situs and VA connections completing intracardiac anatomic assessments. Image acquisition is performed from the axial approach with computer-based reconstruction generating high-quality orthogonal and double-oblique planes similar to the ones obtained by echocardiography and CMR. The required time is much shorter but at the expense of exposure to radiation and iodinated contrast (with inherent risks of allergy and nephrotoxicity). Advantages of CCT also include a larger and shorter bore enabling claustrophobic patients to better tolerate this examination compared to CMR and better assessment of the coronary circulation. The main weakness of CCT compared to echo and CMR is in its lower temporal resolution limiting the ability of CCT to assess ventricular and valvular function (Table 11.1).

Contrast-enhanced gated CCT, although fraught with more radiation exposure, is the most comprehensive CT imaging mode, providing an estimation of ventricular function and vessel anatomy. Given the radiation exposure, the timing of a contrast-enhanced CCT examination rests on providing timely important answers to questions raised during echocardiographic follow-up, such as preoperative testing in the context of a failing Fontan circulation and contraindications or inability to undergo CMR examination.

As in contrast-enhanced CMR, in order to obtain complete Fontan circuit opacification, iodinated contrast must reach not only the SVC but also the IVC (Fig. 11.16). Timing is thus at a relatively late stage with triggering of image acquisition based on contrast detection in the IVC (also called portal phase). The CCT images thus obtained occur at equilibrium with contrast dilution in the arterial and venous beds, rendering interpretation of CCT an even greater challenge in the face of complex anatomy. Fontan conduit anatomy is particularly well depicted in the coronal plane, and the diagnosis of thrombus must be cautiously made in the presence of insufficient conduit opacification or low cardiac output with stasis (see Fig. 30.12).

In terms of field of view, image acquisition must cover the liver, extending cephalad to the base of neck vessels. Liver CT is among the best

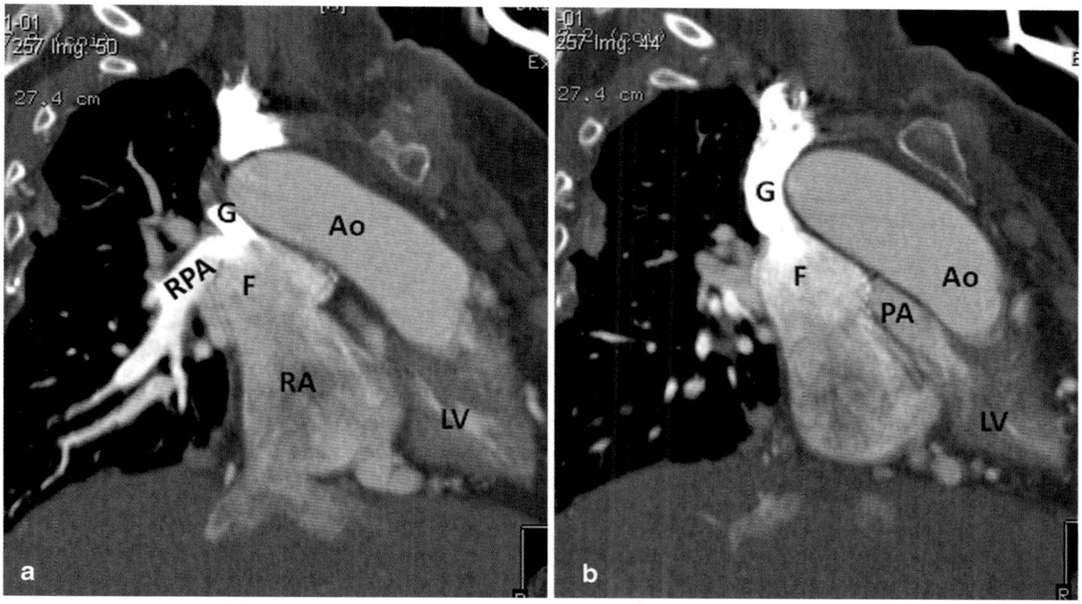

Fig. 11.16 Angio-CT depiction of a superior cavopulmonary anastomosis (Glenn shunt) in right anterior oblique projection. (**a**) Note that during this first-pass angiography, only the superior portion of the Fontan circuit is opacified. (**b**) Note the contrast visible in the superior vena cava, the hypoplastic left ventricle, and the transposition of the great arteries (anterior aorta). *F* Fontan, *G* Glenn shunt, *RA* right atrium, *Ao* aorta, *PA* pulmonary artery, *RPA* right pulmonary artery, *LV* left ventricle

techniques to diagnose and estimate the severity of cardiac cirrhosis [58]. Dilatation of systemic veins, including azygos and hemiazygos systems, is a frequent finding. Precise identification and description of veno-venous and arteriovenous collaterals is important as these may be responsible for significant systemic arterial desaturation (see Fig. 30.5). Atrial and ventricular dimensions and volumes can be determined by double-oblique plane reconstruction. Knowledge of CMR or echo prescription planes to generate long- and short-axis views is a definite advantage for cardiac radiologists, enabling multimodality comparisons to ultimately guide cardiovascular specialists to provide better patient care. Double-oblique reconstructions are cardiac rather than thorax centered. A stack of four-chamber views can be generated from a sagittal set. The central imaging plane should intercept the middle point of the mitral annulus and the LV apex. A stack of three-chamber views can be generated from a coronal set intercepting the center of the aortic and mitral annuli and the LV apex. A stack of short-axis views can be generated from a plane perpendicular to the four-chamber view. Despite the lower temporal resolution of CCT (10–15 vs. 20–30 phases per cardiac cycle in CMR), an estimate of ventricular function can be achieved if retrospective data acquisitions are obtained (at the cost of higher radiation doses), using commercially available software by tracing end-diastolic and end-systolic contours (as in CMR). Central PA anatomy is best demonstrated in the axial projection while peripheral segmental anatomy is best viewed in the coronal projection. Thoracic aortic anatomy and the presence of aortopulmonary collaterals from the descending aorta can be appreciated by combining axial, coronal, and sagittal views, provided the imaging planes extend cephalad enough. Objectives of the systematic diagnostic approach to UAVC by CCT are similar to CMR and provided in Table 11.4.

An important aspect of CCT imaging is the assessment of coronary arteries. The coronary anatomy can serve as an additional distinguishing

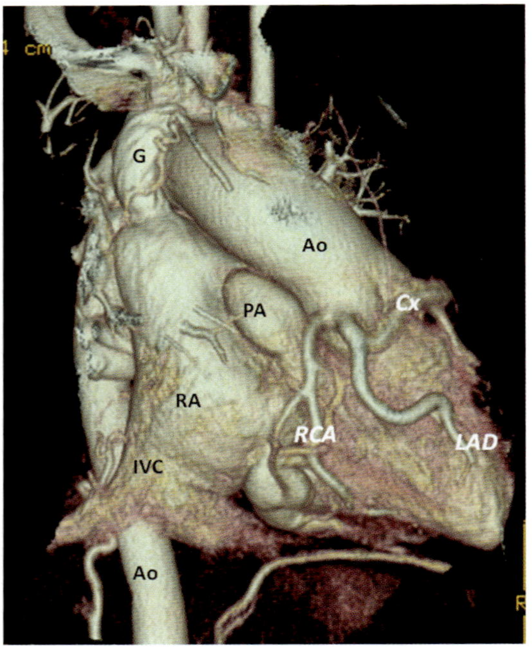

Fig. 11.17 CT tridimensional volume rendering depicting a univentricular heart with a dominant right ventricle, transposition of the great arteries, and a single coronary artery in right anterior oblique projection. *G* Glenn shunt, *RA* right atrium, *Ao* aorta, *PA* pulmonary artery, *RCA* right coronary artery, *LAD* left anterior descending artery, *Cx* circumflex artery, *IVC* inferior vena cava

feature in univentricular hearts, since coronaries usually follow ventricular situs. A morphological RV, even in the subaortic position, will generally be supplied by a single right coronary artery coursing in the AV groove. A morphological LV, even in the subpulmonary position, will be supplied by a left main artery rapidly branching into an anterior descending and circumflex artery coursing in interventricular and AV grooves, respectively (Fig. 11.17). Congenitally aberrant coronary arteries may, however, be encountered, especially in complex cases.

Conclusion

In summary, a systematic segmental approach provides the most comprehensive and clinically useful way to describe anatomy in complex congenital heart disease. CMR and CCT are second-line but critical techniques in the evaluation of patients with univentricular atrioventricular connections (UAVC), providing a relatively comprehensive noninvasive three-dimensional assessment of some of the most complex cardiac lesions known to man. A thorough knowledge of the anatomy, physiopathology, and natural history of these disorders is key to guiding imaging specialists in order to maximize the contribution of these techniques to the diagnosis and management of these complex conditions.

References

1. Khairy P, Poirier N, Mercier LA. Univentricular heart. Circulation. 2007;115:800–12.
2. Anderson RH, Tynan M, Freedom RM, Quero-Jimenez M, Macartney FJ, Shinebourne EA, Wilkinson JL, Becker AE. Ventricular morphology in the univentricular heart. Herz. 1979;4:184–97.
3. Vanpraagh R, Ongley PA, Swan HJ. Anatomic types of single or common ventricle in man. Morphologic and geometric aspects of 60 necropsied cases. Am J Cardiol. 1964;13:367–86.
4. Marelli AJ, Mackie AS, Ionescu-Ittu R, Rahme E, Pilote L. Congenital heart disease in the general population: changing prevalence and age distribution. Circulation. 2007;115:163–72.
5. Ammash NM, Warnes CA. Survival into adulthood of patients with unoperated single ventricle. Am J Cardiol. 1996;77:542–4.
6. Fontan F, Baudet E. Surgical repair of tricuspid atresia. Thorax. 1971;26:240–8.
7. Norwood WI, Lang P, Hansen DD. Physiologic repair of aortic atresia-hypoplastic left heart syndrome. N Engl J Med. 1983;308:23–6.
8. Khairy P, Fernandes SM, Mayer Jr JE, Triedman JK, Walsh EP, Lock JE, Landzberg MJ. Long-term survival, modes of death, and predictors of mortality in patients with Fontan surgery. Circulation. 2008;117:85–92.
9. d'Udekem Y, Xu MY, Galati JC, Lu S, Iyengar AJ, Konstantinov IE, Wheaton GR, Ramsay JM, Grigg LE, Millar J, Cheung MM, Brizard CP. Predictors of survival after single-ventricle palliation: the impact of right ventricular dominance. J Am Coll Cardiol. 2012;59:1178–85.
10. Diller GP, Giardini A, Dimopoulos K, Gargiulo G, Muller J, Derrick G, Giannakoulas G, Khambadkone S, Lammers AE, Picchio FM, Gatzoulis MA, Hager A. Predictors of morbidity and mortality in contemporary Fontan patients: results from a multicenter study including cardiopulmonary exercise testing in 321 patients. Eur Heart J. 2010;31:3073–83.

11. Fogel MA, Pawlowski TW, Whitehead KK, Harris MA, Keller MS, Glatz AC, Zhu W, Shore D, Diaz LK, Rome JJ. Cardiac magnetic resonance and the need for routine cardiac catheterization in single ventricle patients prior to Fontan: a comparison of 3 groups: pre-Fontan CMR versus cath evaluation. J Am Coll Cardiol. 2012;60:1094–102.
12. Ait-Ali L, De Marchi D, Lombardi M, Scebba L, Picano E, Murzi B, Festa P. The role of cardiovascular magnetic resonance in candidates for Fontan operation: proposal of a new algorithm. J Cardiovasc Magn Reson. 2011;13:69.
13. Marcotte F, Poirier N, Pressacco J, Paquet E, Mercier LA, Dore A, Ibrahim R, Khairy P. Evaluation of adult congenital heart disease by cardiac magnetic resonance imaging. Congenit Heart Dis. 2009;4:216–30.
14. Van Praagh R. The segmental approach clarified. Cardiovasc Intervent Radiol. 1984;7:320–5.
15. Huhta JC, Seward JB, Tajik AJ, Hagler DJ, Edwards WD. Two-dimensional echocardiographic spectrum of univentricular AV connection. J Am Coll Cardiol. 1985;5:149–57.
16. Casolo G, Rega L, Gensini GF. Detection of right atrial and pulmonary artery thrombosis after the Fontan procedure by magnetic resonance imaging. Heart. 2004;90:825.
17. Festa P, Ait Ali L, Bernabei M, De Marchi D. The role of magnetic resonance imaging in the evaluation of the functionally single ventricle before and after conversion to the Fontan circulation. Cardiol Young. 2005;15 Suppl 3:51–6.
18. Alfakih K, Plein S, Thiele H, Jones T, Ridgway JP, Sivananthan MU. Normal human left and right ventricular dimensions for MRI as assessed by turbo gradient echo and steady-state free precession imaging sequences. J Magn Reson Imaging. 2003;17:323–9.
19. Grothues F, Smith GC, Moon JC, Bellenger NG, Collins P, Klein HU, Pennell DJ. Comparison of interstudy reproducibility of cardiovascular magnetic resonance with two-dimensional echocardiography in normal subjects and in patients with heart failure or left ventricular hypertrophy. Am J Cardiol. 2002;90:29–34.
20. Alfakih K, Plein S, Bloomer T, Jones T, Ridgway J, Sivananthan M. Comparison of right ventricular volume measurements between axial and short axis orientation using steady-state free precession magnetic resonance imaging. J Magn Reson Imaging. 2003;18:25–32.
21. Mooij CF, de Wit CJ, Graham DA, Powell AJ, Geva T. Reproducibility of MRI measurements of right ventricular size and function in patients with normal and dilated ventricles. J Magn Reson Imaging. 2008;28:67–73.
22. Angeli E, Pace Napoleone C, Balducci A, Formigari R, Lovato L, Candini L, Oppido G, Gargiulo G. Natural and modified history of single-ventricle physiology in adult patients. Eur J Cardiothorac Surg. 2012;42(6):996–1002.
23. Eicken A, Fratz S, Gutfried C, Balling G, Schwaiger M, Lange R, Busch R, Hess J, Stern H. Hearts late after Fontan operation have normal mass, normal volume, and reduced systolic function: a magnetic resonance imaging study. J Am Coll Cardiol. 2003;42:1061–5.
24. Fogel MA, Weinberg PM, Gupta KB, Rychik J, Hubbard A, Hoffman EA, Haselgrove J. Mechanics of the single left ventricle: a study in ventricular-ventricular interaction II. Circulation. 1998;98:330–8.
25. Be'eri E, Maier SE, Landzberg MJ, Chung T, Geva T. In vivo evaluation of Fontan pathway flow dynamics by multidimensional phase-velocity magnetic resonance imaging. Circulation. 1998;98:2873–82.
26. Fratz S, Hess J, Schwaiger M, Martinoff S, Stern HC. More accurate quantification of pulmonary blood flow by magnetic resonance imaging than by lung perfusion scintigraphy in patients with Fontan circulation. Circulation. 2002;106:1510–3.
27. Magee AG, McCrindle BW, Mawson J, Benson LN, Williams WG, Freedom RM. Systemic venous collateral development after the bidirectional cavopulmonary anastomosis. Prevalence and predictors. J Am Coll Cardiol. 1998;32 502–8.
28. Brown DW, Gauvreau K, Powell AJ, Lang P, Colan SD, Del Nido PJ, Odegard KC, Geva T. Cardiac magnetic resonance versus routine cardiac catheterization before bidirectional Glenn anastomosis in infants with functional single ventricle: a prospective randomized trial. Circulation. 2007;116:2718–25.
29. Ovroutski S, Ewert P, Alexi-Meskishvili V, Holscher K, Miera O, Peters B. Hetzer R, Berger F. Absence of pulmonary artery growth after Fontan operation and its possible impact on late outcome. Ann Thorac Surg. 2009;87:826–31.
30. Robbers-Visser D, Helderman F, Strengers JL, van Osch-Gevers L, Kapusta L, Pattynama PM, Bogers AJ, Krams R, Helbing WA. Pulmonary artery size and function after Fontan operation at a young age. J Magn Reson Imaging. 2008;28:1101–7.
31. Morgan VL, Graham Jr TP, Roselli RJ, Lorenz CH. Alterations in pulmonary artery flow patterns and shear stress determined with three-dimensional phase-contrast magnetic resonance imaging in Fontan patients. J Thorac Cardiovasc Surg. 1998;116:294–304.
32. Fogel MA, Weinberg PM, Rychik J, Hubbard A, Jacobs M, Spray TL, Haselgrove J. Caval contribution to flow in the branch pulmonary arteries of Fontan patients with a novel application of magnetic resonance presaturation pulse. Circulation. 1999;99:1215–21.
33. Greenberg SB, Morrow WR, Imamura M, Drummond-Webb J. Magnetic resonance flow analysis of classic and extracardiac Fontan procedures: the seesaw sign. Int J Cardiovasc Imaging. 2004;20:397–405; discussion 407–8.
34. Ovroutski S, Nordmeyer S, Miera O, Ewert P, Klimes K, Kuhne T, Berger F. Caval flow reflects Fontan hemodynamics: quantification by magnetic resonance imaging. Clin Res Cardiol. 2012;101:133–8.
35. Fogel MA. Cardiac magnetic resonance of single ventricles. J Cardiovasc Magn Reson. 2006;8:661–70.

36. Fogel MA, Donofrio MT, Ramaciotti C, Hubbard AM, Weinberg PM. Magnetic resonance and echocardiographic imaging of pulmonary artery size throughout stages of Fontan reconstruction. Circulation. 1994;90:2927–36.
37. Lee SY, Baek JS, Kim GB, Kwon BS, Bae EJ, Noh CI, Choi JY, Lim HK, Kim WH, Lee JR, Kim YJ. Clinical significance of thrombosis in an intracardiac blind pouch after a Fontan operation. Pediatr Cardiol. 2012;33:42–8.
38. Barkhausen J, Hunold P, Eggebrecht H, Schuler WO, Sabin GV, Erbel R, Debatin JF. Detection and characterization of intracardiac thrombi on MR imaging. AJR Am J Roentgenol. 2002;179:1539–44.
39. Mollet NR, Dymarkowski S, Volders W, Wathiong J, Herbots L, Rademakers FE, Bogaert J. Visualization of ventricular thrombi with contrast-enhanced magnetic resonance imaging in patients with ischemic heart disease. Circulation. 2002;106:2873–6.
40. Weinsaft JW, Kim HW, Shah DJ, Klem I, Crowley AL, Brosnan R, James OG, Patel MR, Heitner J, Parker M, Velazquez EJ, Steenbergen C, Judd RM, Kim RJ. Detection of left ventricular thrombus by delayed-enhancement cardiovascular magnetic resonance prevalence and markers in patients with systolic dysfunction. J Am Coll Cardiol. 2008;52:148–57.
41. O'Donnell CP, Lock JE, Powell AJ, Perry SB. Compression of pulmonary veins between the left atrium and the descending aorta. Am J Cardiol. 2003;91:248–51.
42. Grosse-Wortmann L, Al-Otay A, Goo HW, Macgowan CK, Coles JG, Benson LN, Redington AN, Yoo SJ. Anatomical and functional evaluation of pulmonary veins in children by magnetic resonance imaging. J Am Coll Cardiol. 2007;49:993–1002.
43. McElhinney DB, Reddy VM, Tworetzky W, Petrossian E, Hanley FL, Moore P. Incidence and implications of systemic to pulmonary collaterals after bidirectional cavopulmonary anastomosis. Ann Thorac Surg. 2000;69:1222–8.
44. Grosse-Wortmann L, Al-Otay A, Yoo SJ. Aortopulmonary collaterals after bidirectional cavopulmonary connection or Fontan completion: quantification with MRI. Circ Cardiovasc Imaging. 2009;2:219–25.
45. Prakash A, Rathod RH, Powell AJ, McElhinney DB, Banka P, Geva T. Relation of systemic-to-pulmonary artery collateral flow in single ventricle physiology to palliative stage and clinical status. Am J Cardiol. 2012;109:1038–45.
46. Schmitt B, Steendijk P, Ovroutski S, Lunze K, Rahmanzadeh P, Maarouf N, Ewert P, Berger F, Kuehne T. Pulmonary vascular resistance, collateral flow, and ventricular function in patients with a Fontan circulation at rest and during dobutamine stress. Circ Cardiovasc Imaging. 2010;3:623–31.
47. Kim RJ, Shah DJ, Judd RM. How we perform delayed enhancement imaging. J Cardiovasc Magn Reson. 2003;5:505–14.
48. Kim RJ, Wu E, Rafael A, Chen EL, Parker MA, Simonetti O, Klocke FJ, Bonow RO, Judd RM. The use of contrast-enhanced magnetic resonance imaging to identify reversible myocardial dysfunction. N Engl J Med. 2000;343:1445–53.
49. McCrohon JA, Moon JC, Prasad SK, McKenna WJ, Lorenz CH, Coats AJ, Pennell DJ. Differentiation of heart failure related to dilated cardiomyopathy and coronary artery disease using gadolinium-enhanced cardiovascular magnetic resonance. Circulation. 2003;108:54–9.
50. Mewton N, Liu CY, Croisille P, Bluemke D, Lima JA. Assessment of myocardial fibrosis with cardiovascular magnetic resonance. J Am Coll Cardiol. 2011; 57:891–903.
51. Karamitsos TD, Francis JM, Myerson S, Selvanayagam JB, Neubauer S. The role of cardiovascular magnetic resonance imaging in heart failure. J Am Coll Cardiol. 2009;54:1407–24.
52. Cheong BY, Muthupillai R, Wilson JM, Sung A, Huber S, Amin S, Elayda MA, Lee VV, Flamm SD. Prognostic significance of delayed-enhancement magnetic resonance imaging: survival of 857 patients with and without left ventricular dysfunction. Circulation. 2009;120:2069–76.
53. Rathod RH, Prakash A, Powell AJ, Geva T. Myocardial fibrosis identified by cardiac magnetic resonance late gadolinium enhancement is associated with adverse ventricular mechanics and ventricular tachycardia late after Fontan operation. J Am Coll Cardiol. 2010;55:1721–8.
54. Flett AS, Hayward MP, Ashworth MT, Hansen MS, Taylor AM, Elliott PM, McGregor C, Moon JC. Equilibrium contrast cardiovascular magnetic resonance for the measurement of diffuse myocardial fibrosis: preliminary validation in humans. Circulation. 2010;122:138–44.
55. Jerosch-Herold M, Sheridan DC, Kushner JD, Nauman D, Burgess D, Dutton D, Alharethi R, Li D, Hershberger RE. Cardiac magnetic resonance imaging of myocardial contrast uptake and blood flow in patients affected with idiopathic or familial dilated cardiomyopathy. Am J Physiol Heart Circ Physiol. 2008;295:H1234–42.
56. Broberg CS, Chugh SS, Conklin C, Sahn DJ, Jerosch-Herold M. Quantification of diffuse myocardial fibrosis and its association with myocardial dysfunction in congenital heart disease. Circ Cardiovasc Imaging. 2010;3:727–34.
57. Wallihan DB, Podberesky DJ. Hepatic pathology after Fontan palliation: spectrum of imaging findings. Pediatr Radiol. 2013;43(3):330–8.
58. Kiesewetter CH, Sheron N, Vettukattill JJ, Hacking N, Stedman B, Millward-Sadler H, Haw M, Cope R, Salmon AP, Sivaprakasam MC, Kendall T, Keeton BR, Iredale JP, Veldtman GR. Hepatic changes in the failing Fontan circulation. Heart. 2007;93: 579–84.

12 Visceroatrial Situs in Congenital Heart Disease

Marinos Kontzialis, Hugo Spindola-Franco, and Linda B. Haramati

The visceroatrial situs describes the laterality and relative position of viscera, including the cardiac atria, the tracheobronchial tree, and the abdominal viscera [1]. Visceroatrial situs abnormalities are associated with congenital heart disease [2]. Mild forms of situs abnormalities may remain undiagnosed and can be incidentally discovered in adults on imaging, while other situs abnormalities are associated with severe congenital anomalies, which are fatal early in life unless treated. Determination of the visceroatrial situs and bulboventricular loop predicts the probability and type of congenital heart disease [3].

This chapter reviews the various configurations of visceroatrial situs and the segmental approach to cardiac anatomy described by van Praagh [4]. We present a methodical stepwise approach for determining the visceroatrial situs, the bulboventricular loop, and their associated anomalies [5]. With the advancement in the diagnosis and treatment of congenital heart disease, patients with situs abnormalities associated with severe congenital heart disease can survive into adulthood. Imaging is essential in diagnosing complications of their long-standing disease or its treatment. We will review the role of CT and MRI in imaging adult congenital heart disease and its relationship to anomalies of visceroatrial situs.

M. Kontzialis, MD
Department of Radiology and Radiological Science, The Johns Hopkins Hospital, Phipps B-112, 600 N. Wolfe Street, Baltimore, MD 21287, USA
e-mail: marinoskon@gmail.com

H. Spindola-Franco, MD
Department of Radiology, Albert Einstein College of Medicine, Montefiore Medical Center, 111 East 210 St., Bronx, NY 10467, USA
e-mail: hspindol@montefiore.org

L.B. Haramati, MD, MS (✉)
Cardiothoracic Imaging, Department of Radiology and Medicine, Albert Einstein College of Medicine, Montefiore Medical Center, 111 East 210 St., Bronx, NY 10467, USA
e-mail: lharamati@gmail.com

Thoracic and Abdominal Situs

In congenital heart disease, a segmental approach is used for the description of the cardiac anatomy, and an alphabetical nomenclature has been devised to describe each segment [4, 6]. The first step in the segmental approach described by van Praagh is the determination of the cardiac situs. Only the atria retain their laterality throughout cardiac embryogenesis, and therefore, the paired atria determine the cardiac situs [7]. Three distinct types of atrial situs exist: situs solitus {S,–,–}, situs inversus{I,–,–}, and situs ambiguus [8] or indeterminate situs{A,–,–} [9]. In situs solitus {S,–,–}, the morphologic right atrium is positioned to the right of the morphologic left atrium. Situs inversus {I,–,–} represents the mirror image of situs solitus with the morphologic right atrium to the left of the morphologic left atrium. In situs ambiguous {A,–,–}, the cardiac situs is neither situs solitus nor situs inversus, and

F. Saremi (ed.), *Cardiac CT and MR for Adult Congenital Heart Disease*,
DOI 10.1007/978-1-4614-8875-0_12, © Springer Science+Business Media New York 2014

Table 12.1 Types of visceroatrial situs

Situs solitus
Totalis (levocardia)
Mesocardia
Dextrocardia
Situs inversus
Totalis (dextrocardia)
Mesocardia
Levocardia
Heterotaxy
Polysplenia syndrome
Asplenia syndrome
Thoracoabdominal discordance

such situs is distinctively known as heterotaxy or isomerism (Table 12.1).

The next step in the segmental approach is the determination of the bulboventricular loop, which can be D-loop {–,D,–}, L-loop {–,L,–}, or X-loop {–,X,–}. With D-looping {–,D,–}, the bulboventricular tube bends and shifts to the right, placing the bulbus cordis, the precursor of the right ventricle, to the right of the primitive ventricle which is the precursor of the left ventricle. Therefore, in situs solitus with D-looping {S,D,–}, there is atrioventricular concordance with the right atrium connected to the right ventricle and the left atrium connected to the left ventricle (Fig. 12.1a). In early fetal development, the ventricular portion of the heart, the ventricular mass, is in the right hemithorax. Subsequently, the bulboventricular loop shifts to the left hemithorax, resulting in levoversion. In the case of partial shift of the bulboventricular loop to the midline or failure to shift to the left, the result is situs solitus with mesoversion and situs solitus with dextroversion, respectively.

In L-looping {–,L,–}, the heart tube folds and rotates to the left, which places the bulbus cordis to the left of the primitive ventricle. That means that the ventricular mass is in the left hemithorax, and the bulboventricular loop tends to rotate to the right hemithorax. Therefore, situs solitus with L-looping {S,L,–} results in atrioventricular discordance, with the right atrium connected to the left ventricle and the left atrium connected to the right ventricle (Fig. 12.1b) [10]. As above, the degree of shift of the cardiac mass determines the orientation (version) of the cardiac apex. Complete shift of the apex toward the right results in situs solitus with atrioventricular discordance and dextroversion; partial shift to the midline results in mesoversion and absence of shift results in levoversion. In a similar manner, formation of an L-loop (concordant loop) in cases of situs inversus results in atrioventricular concordance {I,L,–} (Fig. 12.1c), whereas a D-loop (discordant loop) results in atrioventricular discordance {I,D,–} (Fig. 12.1d). Therefore, a complete, partial, or a failure of shift of the cardiac apex to the right further classifies these forms into situs inversus with dextroversion, situs inversus with mesoversion, and situs inversus with levoversion [1, 7, 10].

In X-loop {–,X,–}, a single ventricle is present, and ventricular looping is undefined. Single ventricle or univentricular heart has three major presentations according to the trabecular pattern. If the pattern is similar to either the right or the left ventricle, then it is called single right or single left ventricle, respectively. If the trabecular pattern is indeterminate, then it is called single "undifferentiated" ventricle. The atrial connection is through a common atrioventricular valve (common inlet; AV canal) or through two atrioventricular valves (double inlet; right and left AV valves). Both atrioventricular valves may be patent (double inlet) or one may be often atretic (single inlet). Anatomically, the two valves are different from the tricuspid and mitral valves, and therefore, they should be referred to as right and left atrioventricular valve. The exit of flow of the main ventricular cavity into the great vessels may be direct or through a rudimentary outlet chamber. In single right ventricle, the exit is usually direct, whereas in single left ventricle, the exit is through a rudimentary chamber (outlet chamber). The outlet chamber can be anterior, superior and to the right (normally related), or anterior, superior, and to the left (inverted) of the base of the main cavity. It is uncommon for the outlet chamber to be in front of the main cavity. A bulboventricular foramen (ventricular septal defect; outlet foramen) connects the two chambers. The aorta and the pulmonary artery are almost always transposed (D- or L-malposition),

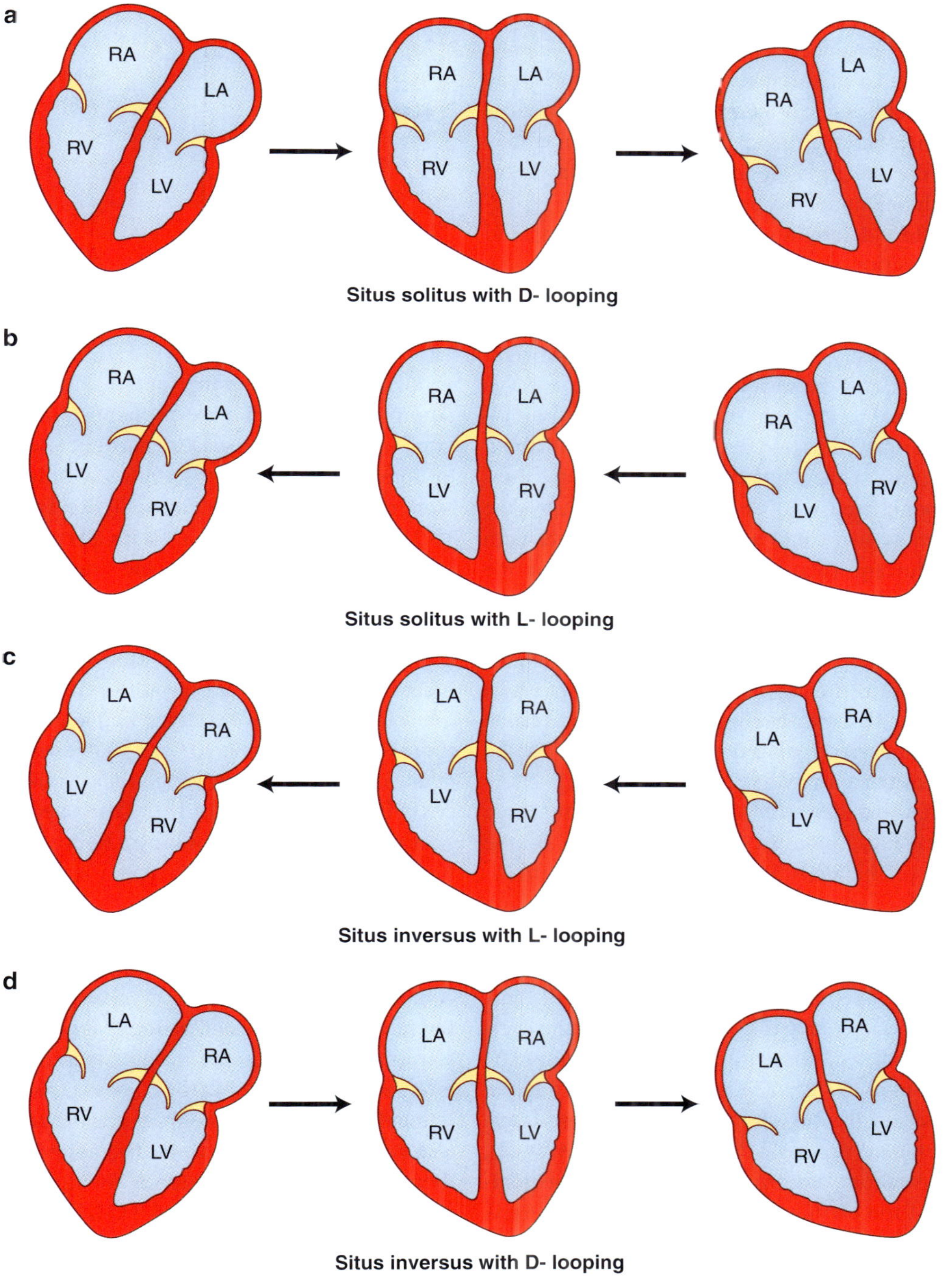

Fig. 12.1 Drawings demonstrate variations in looping and horizontal shift of the cardiac apex. (**a**) *Situs solitus with D-looping* resulting in atrioventricular concordance. The cardiac mass normally shifts from right to left, transitioning from dextroversion to mesoversion and finally to levoversion. (**b**) *Situs solitus with L-looping* resulting in atrioventricular discordance. The cardiac mass usually shifts from left to right resulting in dextroversion. (**c**) *Situs inversus with L-looping* results in atrioventricular concordance. The cardiac mass shifts from left to right, leading to dextroversion. (**d**) *Situs inversus with D-looping* results in atrioventricular discordance. The cardiac mass shifts from right to left, leading to levoversion. *RA* right atrium, *LA* left atrium, *RV* right ventricle, *LV* left ventricle

and both great vessels may arise from the rudimentary chamber or from the main cavity. Subvalvular or valvular pulmonary stenosis may be present, and restriction of the bulboventricular foramen may be found. The outlet foramen may straddle the right or left atrioventricular valve depending on its location.

After determining the cardiac situs and the position of the bulboventricular loop, the next step in the segmental approach is to identify the ventriculoarterial relationship [4, 6, 11]. Normally, the heart tube folds to the right {–,D,–}, and the developing ascending aorta is positioned to the right of the developing pulmonary artery in the truncus arteriosus with both structures at the same level. Growth in the subpulmonic free wall of the truncus elevates the pulmonic valve and advances it anteriorly with a rightward rotation; while resorption in the subaortic free wall results in the aortic-mitral fibrous continuity [12]. Therefore, normally the pulmonic valve is positioned anteriorly, superiorly, and to the left of the aortic valve (*solitus*) {–,–,S}. The mirror-image configuration results in an anteriorly placed pulmonic valve to the right of the aortic valve (*inversus*) {–,–,I}.

Defining the atrial situs (cardiac situs), the ventricular topology, and the position of the great vessels does not predict the atrioventricular and ventriculoarterial connections, which must be separately evaluated [4, 11]. Similarly, the orientation of the cardiac apex (ventricular mass) is independent of the position of the cardiac atria and depends on the degree of the horizontal shift of the cardiac mass. Defining the position of the cardiac apex after identification of the atrial situs and the cardiac loop determines the "version." The terms dextroversion, mesoversion, and levoversion indicate the position of the cardiac apex, when this structure is not in the usual location for the corresponding visceroatrial situs. The terms dextrocardia, mesocardia, and levocardia refer to the position of the heart within the thoracic cavity and, in common parlance, are used interchangeably with the version terminology. The cardiac situs is usually concordant with the thoracic situs (tracheobronchial tree) and the position of the ventricular mass (cardiac apex) and must be determined to predict the probability and type of congenital heart disease. There are two forms of determinate situs, situs solitus with levoversion or levocardia, the normal configuration {S,D,S}, and situs inversus with dextroversion or dextrocardia {I,L,I}, the mirror-image configuration.

Table 12.2 Congenital heart disease incidence for various configurations of visceroatrial situs

Situs configuration	Incidence (%)
Situs solitus totalis	0.8
Situs solitus mesocardia	0.8
Situs solitus dextrocardia	90
Situs inversus totalis	5
Situs inversus mesocardia	0.8
Situs inversus levocardia	95–100
Polysplenia	75
Asplenia	99–100

Interestingly, the degree of shift of the cardiac apex in the horizontal plane (the version) predicts the occurrence and complexity of congenital heart disease. Severe congenital heart disease is present in more than 90 % of people who have situs solitus with dextroversion and situs inversus with levoversion [1, 13]. The severity and occurrence rate is much lower in both situs solitus and situs inversus with mesoversion (Table 12.2).

The thoracic and abdominal organs are usually lateralized on either side of the midline. Situs solitus totalis {S,D,S} refers to the expected configuration of thoracic and abdominal organs with a trilobed right lung and a right-sided liver and inferior vena cava. The cardiac apex is toward the left and the spleen, the stomach and the aorta are also positioned on the left. In the case of normal thoracoabdominal concordance, the rate of congenital heart disease is 0.8 % [13]. The mirror-image configuration of thoracic and abdominal organs is referred to as situs inversus totalis {I,L,I} and has a 5 % incidence of congenital heart disease [13]. Approximately 20 % of the cases of situs inversus totalis are associated with Kartagener syndrome [14] comprised of the classic triad of situs inversus totalis, chronic sinusitis, and bronchiectasis [15]. Conversely, only half of the patients with primary ciliary dyskinesia have situs inversus [12, 13].

In the rare occasion of thoracoabdominal discordance (thoracic situs solitus with abdominal situs inversus or vice versa), there is high incidence of congenital heart disease [1, 16].

Heterotaxy Syndromes [1, 2, 17–19]

In situs ambiguus or heterotaxy, there is duplication of right- or left-sided structures and abnormal arrangement of organs and vessels, not in the expected configuration of situs solitus {S,D,S} or situs inversus{I,L,I}. Splenic abnormalities are a hallmark of heterotaxy, and there is a high association with complex anomalies of the cardiovascular system. Rather than a distinct set, there is a spectrum of anomalies. The two major forms of heterotaxy are polysplenia and asplenia or Ivemark syndrome [1].

Polysplenia is associated with multiple spleens and bilateral left-sided structures (left isomerism) (Fig. 12.2a) [1, 2, 20–22]. In contrast

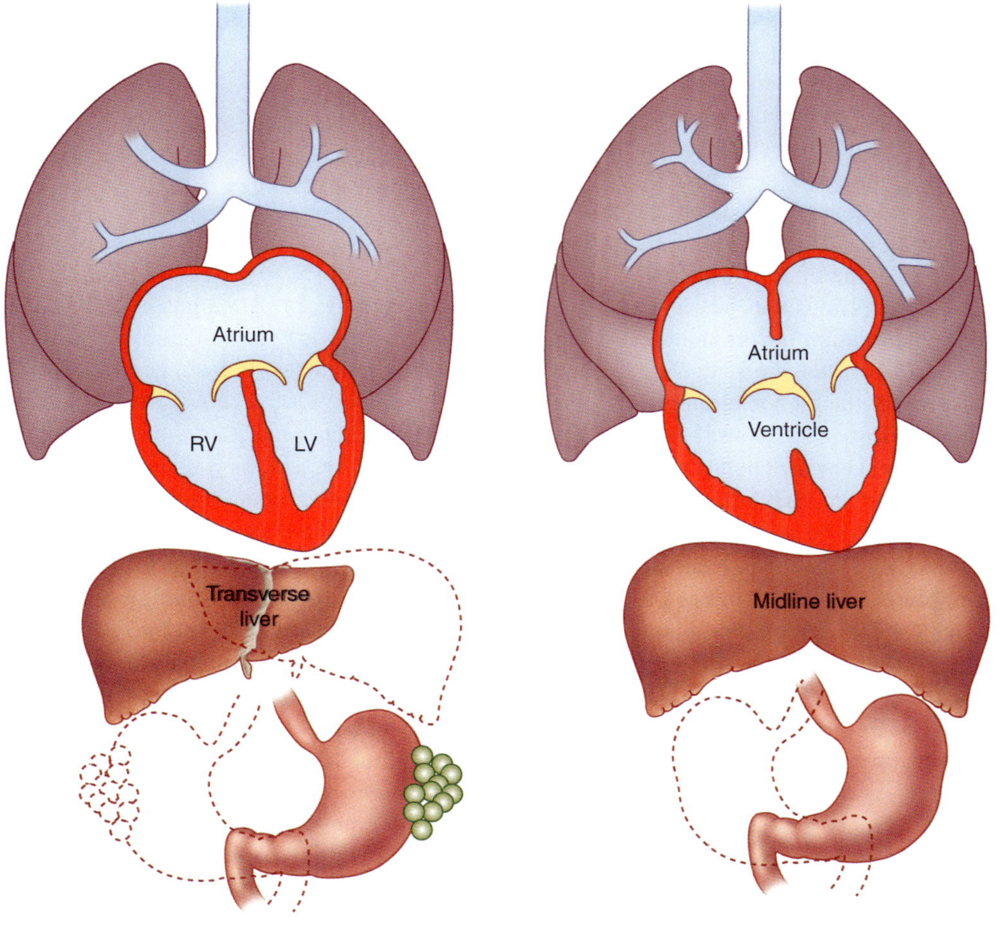

Fig. 12.2 Schematic diagrams of polysplenia and asplenia. (**a**) Polysplenia is characterized by bilateral bilobed lungs and bilateral hyparterial bronchi. Positions of multiple small rounded spleens and stomach are variable. Congenital heart disease occurs in 75 % of these patients and is usually mild. (**b**) Asplenia is characterized by bilateral trilobed lungs and bilateral eparterial bronchi. Liver is often midline, spleen is absent, and position of stomach is variable. Congenital heart disease is nearly universal. Associated cardiac defects are generally severe and include common atrium and single ventricle with pulmonary stenosis or atresia

to asplenia, polysplenia is more common in females and has a milder course, often presenting in childhood with a left to right shunt. However, some present in adulthood with an atrial septal defect and approximately 25 % of patients have no significant cardiac anomalies. Polysplenia is characterized by bilateral bilobed lungs and two hyparterial bronchi. A common atrium is usually present with morphologic characteristics of bilateral left atria. Congenital cardiac defects include endocardial cushion defects, double-outlet right ventricle, and left-sided obstructive lesions such as coarctation of the aorta, subaortic stenosis, or less commonly hypoplastic left heart syndrome. In contrast to asplenia, right ventricular obstruction and transposition of the great vessels are unusual, although minor forms of pulmonic stenosis have been described. Anomalous systemic and pulmonary venous drainage are seen, including partial anomalous pulmonary venous return, duplicated superior vena cava and azygos, or hemiazygos continuation of the inferior vena cava.

The gastric fundus can be right or left, and intestinal malrotation is common [23]. Multiple spleens are characteristic and can be seen on either side of the abdomen, resulting in the absence of Heinz and Howell-Jolly bodies on peripheral blood smear. The liver is usually midline or symmetric, and biliary and pancreatic abnormalities may be present (Table 12.3) [24].

Asplenia (Fig. 12.2b) is characterized by an absent spleen and duplication of right-sided structures (dextro isomerism, bilateral right sidedness) [1, 2, 25–28]. It is twice as common in males and has a high association with congenital heart defects (99–100 %) that present early in life and carry a grave prognosis. Unrecognized asplenia is only rarely encountered in adulthood. Congenital absence of the spleen is associated with immune deficiency, infections, and Heinz and Howell-Jolly bodies on peripheral blood smear.

Asplenia is associated with bilateral trilobed lungs and two eparterial bronchi. Anomalous systemic and pulmonary venous drainage are common, including bilateral superior venae cavae, total anomalous pulmonary venous return, and D- or L-malposition of the great arteries. There is usually a common atrium with anatomic characteristics suggestive of bilateral right atria or a large atrial septal defect. An atrioventricular canal (atrioventricular communis) is often present, as is a single ventricle or a large ventricular septal defect (bulboventricular foramen). If two atrioventricular valves are present, both may be patent or either one may be atretic. Right ventricular outflow tract obstruction is common, usually pulmonic stenosis or atresia, resulting in pulmonary undercirculation and cyanosis. Aortic stenosis or atresia is unusual in asplenia.

In the abdomen, the spleen is characteristically absent and the liver is usually midline. There is commonly ipsilateral course of the inferior vena cava and the aorta, resulting in their juxtaposition below the diaphragm [29]. The gastric bubble can be on either side of the midline, and there is a high occurrence of intestinal malrotation [23]. Other associations include agenesis of the gallbladder, annular pancreas, imperforate anus, horseshoe kidney, and urethral valves (Table 12.4).

Table 12.3 Polysplenia

Cardiovascular anomalies
Anomalous systemic venous connections (bilateral superior venae cavae) and interruption of the IVC with azygos continuation
Anomalous pulmonary venous return (partial or total of the cardiac variety)
Common atrium
Primum or secundum atrial septal defect
Ventricular septal defect often of the endocardial cushion type
Double-outlet right ventricle
Left-sided obstructive lesions (coarctation of the aorta, subaortic stenosis, hypoplastic left heart syndrome)
Cardiac malposition
Noncardiac anomalies
Bilateral hyparterial bronchi and bilobed lungs
Two or more spleens
Transverse or symmetric liver
Gallbladder anomalies including biliary atresia
Intestinal malrotation
Genitourinary abnormalities

From Spindola-Franco [1] with permission

Table 12.4 Asplenia

Cardiovascular anomalies
Bilateral superior venae cavae
Common atrium or a large atrial septal defect
Single ventricle or a large ventricular septal defect
AV communis (atrioventricular canal)
Transposition of the great arteries
Anomalous pulmonary venous return (either supracardiac or infracardiac)
Cardiac malposition
Midline crossing of the IVC just below the diaphragm to enter the systemic venous atrium
Common course of the IVC and the abdominal aorta
Severe pulmonary stenosis or atresia
Noncardiac anomalies
Bilateral eparterial bronchi and trilobed lungs
Absent spleen associated with Howell-Jolly bodies on peripheral blood smear and susceptibility to infections
Transverse or symmetric liver
Intestinal malrotation
Gallbladder agenesis
Annular pancreas
Imperforate anus
Horseshoe kidney
Ureteral and urethral valves

From Spindola-Franco [1] with permission

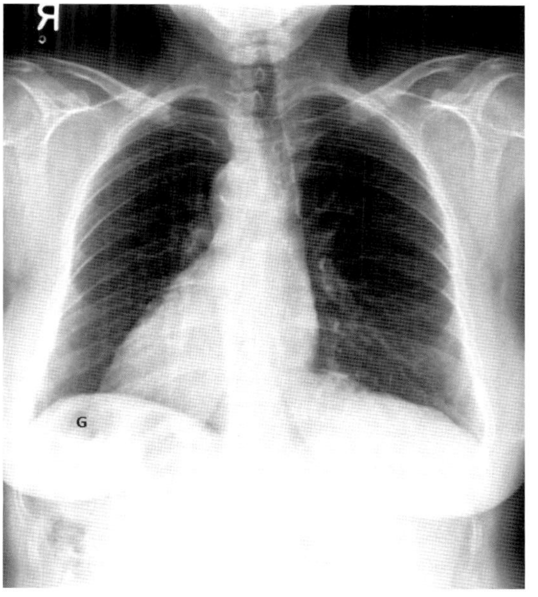

Fig. 12.3 A 60-year-old woman with situs inversus totalis and no associated congenital heart disease. There is tracheobronchial situs inversus with a right-sided hyparterial bronchus and a left-sided eparterial bronchus. Dextrocardia and right-sided aortic arch are present. The stomach (*G*) is in the right upper quadrant and the liver shadow is seen in the left upper quadrant

The Role of Imaging

The presentation of situs abnormalities in the adult depends largely on the underlying congenital heart disease and falls into two main groups. The first group includes patients who have situs abnormalities without congenital heart disease that can escape early diagnosis. This includes the majority of adults with situs solitus with mesocardia and situs inversus with mesocardia or dextrocardia (Fig. 12.3) and a minority of patients with polysplenia. Situs abnormalities associated with mild congenital heart disease, such as simple shunt lesions or complex congenital heart disease that is physiologically mild, such as corrected transposition of the great arteries, can also remain undiagnosed during childhood. They may present and become clinically apparent later in life, when long-standing disease and comorbidities unmask the underlying defect, or they may be incidentally detected on imaging [30]. Severe forms of congenital heart disease that are usually diagnosed prenatally or at birth and undergo treatment early in life comprise the second group. These patients present in adulthood for follow-up imaging or for imaging to help diagnose and treat symptoms related to their long-standing disease or its treatment.

In describing a patient's visceroatrial situs, the chest radiograph is useful to assess not only the location of the cardiac apex (ventricular mass) and gastric bubble but also the tracheobronchial situs, which is usually concordant with the atrial situs [1]. These structures are also well demonstrated on CT and MRI, which allow simultaneous evaluation of the abdominal viscera. Dextrocardia in adults can be associated with any form of situs and is present in up to half of patients with heterotaxy [9, 31]. When an anomaly of visceroatrial situs is identified, knowledge of the associated cardiac anomalies is key to making the appropriate findings and ultimately the correct diagnosis, which serves as a guide to patient management.

When CT or MRI is performed for a cardiac indication, it is typically to answer specific questions, since echocardiography remains the first-line cardiac imaging modality [32]. Tailoring the examination appropriately requires every effort to obtain relevant anatomic and surgical history and review of prior imaging. CT and MRI outperform echocardiography in demonstrating extracardiac vascular anatomy and systemic and pulmonary venous connections [33]. MRI is considered a reference standard for estimating ventricular volumes and function. Phase-contrast sequences for flow quantification are useful in documenting the presence or absence of shunts by calculating the pulmonary to systemic blood flow ratio (Qp:Qs) and regurgitant volumes and estimating the degree of stenosis [34]. There is increasing evidence that delayed enhancement and viability sequences have prognostic implications in these adults.

Situs solitus and situs inversus with mesocardia have the same rate of congenital heart disease as patients with normal situs or situs solitus totalis (0.8 %). However, when congenital heart disease is present, the diagnosis of corrected transposition of the great arteries should be considered [35]. Corrected transposition of the great arteries in patients with situs solitus totalis is L-transposition of the great arteries, while in situs inversus the same physiology occurs with D-transposition of the great arteries. In situs solitus with L-transposition {–,–,L}, asymmetric growth in the subaortic conus free wall and resorption in the subpulmonic conus free wall are usually associated with L-looping of the primitive heart tube, resulting in atrioventricular and ventriculoarterial discordance {S,L,L}. In situs inversus, the mirror image occurs {I,D,D}. In either scenario, the left atrium connects to the right ventricle, which in turn connects to an anteriorly located aorta with a subaortic conus. The right atrium connects to the left ventricle, which in turn connects to the posterior pulmonary artery, which is in fibrous continuity with the mitral valve. The aorta arises from the heart anterior and superior (to the left in situs solitus or to the right in situs inversus) of the pulmonary artery. Corrected transposition therefore represents a double discordance or "physiologically corrected" transposition.

These patients may present at any age with arrhythmias related to abnormal development of the conduction pathways. An intracardiac shunt is present in 60 %, most commonly a ventricular septal defect. When a shunt is absent, the initial diagnosis often comes to light in adulthood. Because their systemic ventricle is the right ventricle, patients with corrected transposition are at increased risk for developing heart failure and tricuspid insufficiency as they age. Surveillance MRI is recommended in these patients primarily to monitor the volumes and function of the systemic right ventricle on steady-state free precession (SSFP) cine images (Fig. 12.4). A dephasing jet of tricuspid insufficiency can be sought and the degree of tricuspid insufficiency can be estimated, if it is an isolated valvular abnormality, by calculating the differences in the left and right ventricular stroke volumes. Direct quantitation of atrioventricular valve regurgitation using phase-contrast MR is still an evolving technique. If the patient has a pacemaker or ICD, an ECG-gated cardiac CT can be performed to evaluate right ventricular volumes and function.

Typical findings of L-transposition of the great arteries should also be noted on cross-sectional imaging. The left-sided, systemic, morphologic right ventricle is heavily trabeculated and has a moderator band, while the right-sided, morphologic left ventricle is smooth walled. The aorta and pulmonary artery have a typical parallel course as they emerge from the heart with the aorta arising anterior and to the left of the pulmonary artery (Fig. 12.5).

The segmental anatomy in polysplenia is variable depending on the location of the heart and associated anomalies. With levocardia and normally related great arteries, it is {A,D,S}. Patients with polysplenia may initially present in adulthood with a left to right shunt, such as an atrial septal defect or partial anomalous pulmonary venous return, when the shunt becomes symptomatic or is detected incidentally on imaging. More typically, however, patients with polysplenia present in infancy or early childhood with an AV canal defect. Patients with polysplenia may

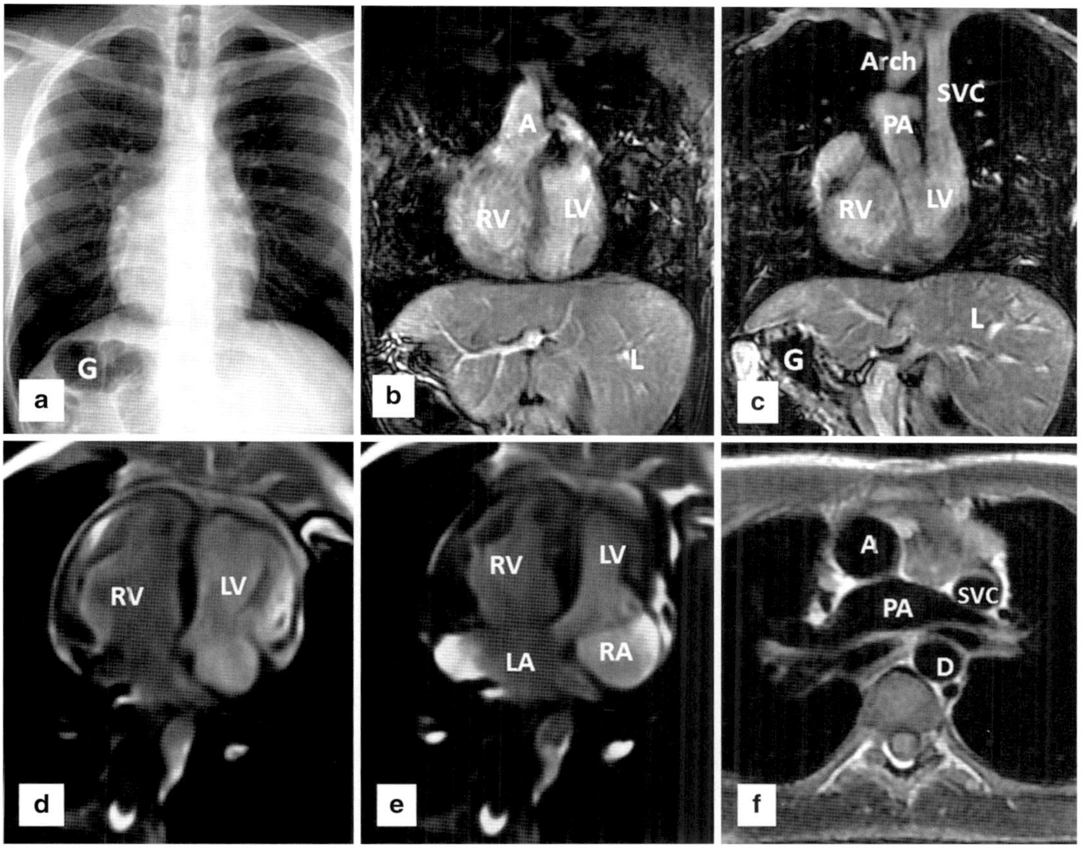

Fig. 12.4 A 20-year-old man with situs inversus and mesocardia who has congenitally corrected transposition of the great vessels (D-TGA). (**a**) PA radiograph demonstrates a right-sided hyparterial bronchus and a left-sided eparterial bronchus consistent with thoracic situs inversus. There is mesocardia. The stomach bubble is right sided and the aortic arch is left sided. (**b**, **c**) Coronal contrast-enhanced MRA images demonstrate a normal-sized heart with mesoversion. The ascending aorta (*A*) arises anteriorly from the trabeculated systemic right ventricle (*RV*). The pulmonary artery arises posteriorly from the smooth-walled left ventricle (*LV*). The liver (*L*) is left sided and the stomach (*G*) is right sided. (**d**, **e**) Axial steady-state free precession (SSFP) shows a right-sided morphologic left atrium (*LA*) connecting to a trabeculated right-sided RV. The right atrium (*RA*) is on the left connecting to the smooth-walled LV. (**f**) Axial black-blood image at the level of the pulmonary artery bifurcation shows the ascending aorta (*A*) to be anterior and to the right (*D-position*) of the pulmonary artery. A left-sided superior vena cava (*SVC*) drains into the right atrium. The descending aorta is on the left

also have physiologically neutral anomalies such as azygos continuation of the inferior vena cava or a duplicated inferior or superior venae cavae, which only become evident during catheter placement or as an incidental finding on imaging.

ECG-gated CT or MRI performs well in depicting the anatomy of an atrial septal defect. If it is a secundum type defect and repair with a closure device is contemplated, the adequacy of the rims must be described [30]. If the patient had repair of an atrial septal defect in childhood (Fig. 12.6), care should be taken to note the type of anomaly, the adequacy of the repair including integrity of the septum, the atrioventricular valve function, and the Qp:Qs, if MR is performed. As there may be multiple associated anomalies, other shunt lesions should be sought. The pulmonary and systemic venous anatomy should be scrutinized, as anomalies are common and superbly depicted on both CT and MR angiography (Fig. 12.7).

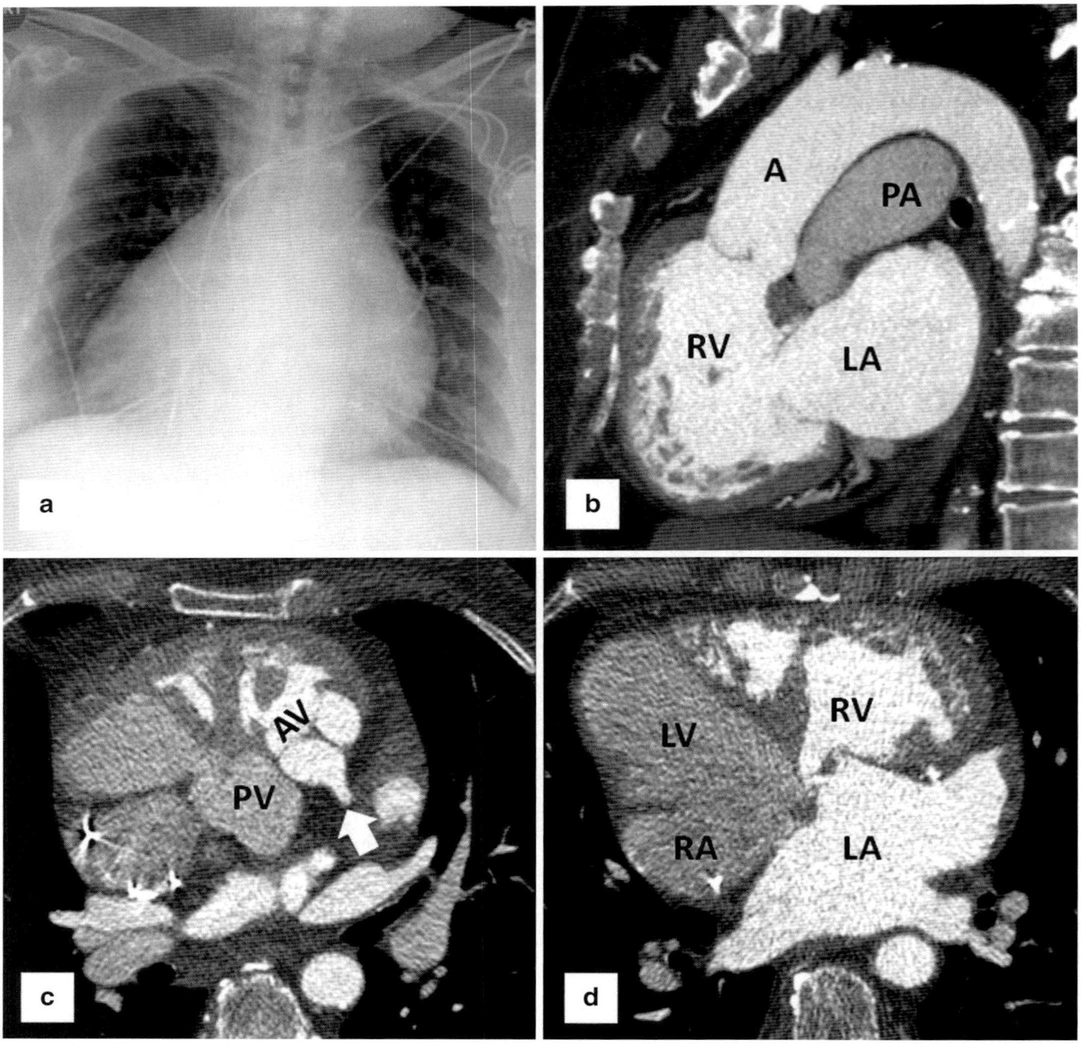

Fig. 12.5 A 60-year-old woman with situs solitus, mesocardia, and congenitally corrected transposition of the great arteries (L-TGA). (**a**) AP chest radiograph shows thoracic (tracheobronchial) situs solitus. There is mesocardia. (**b**) Oblique-sagittal multiplanar CT reconstruction shows the anterior trabeculated right ventricle (*RV*) giving rise to aorta (*A*), and there is characteristic parallel orientation of the great vessels. (**c**, **d**) Axial CT images demonstrate the aortic valve (*AV*) with a visible coronary artery (*white arrow*) anterior and to the left (L-position) of the pulmonary valve (*PV*). The left atrium (*LA*) connects to the trabeculated anterior RV and the right atrium (*RA*) to the smooth-walled posterior left ventricle (*LV*). *PA* pulmonary artery

Other findings of polysplenia should be sought and described on imaging. Bilateral hyparterial bronchi are evident on chest radiography and beautifully depicted on coronal CT and MR images (Figs. 12.6 and 12.8). The pulmonary arteries are similarly symmetric. Azygos continuation of the IVC is common (65 %) and associated with absence of the intrahepatic inferior vena cava [20]. Images of the upper abdomen will show multiple small round spleens. The liver is typically transverse. The stomach may be on either side.

Patients with situs anomalies who had more severe complex congenital heart disease diagnosed and treated during childhood are now surviving in larger numbers [36]. It is crucial to

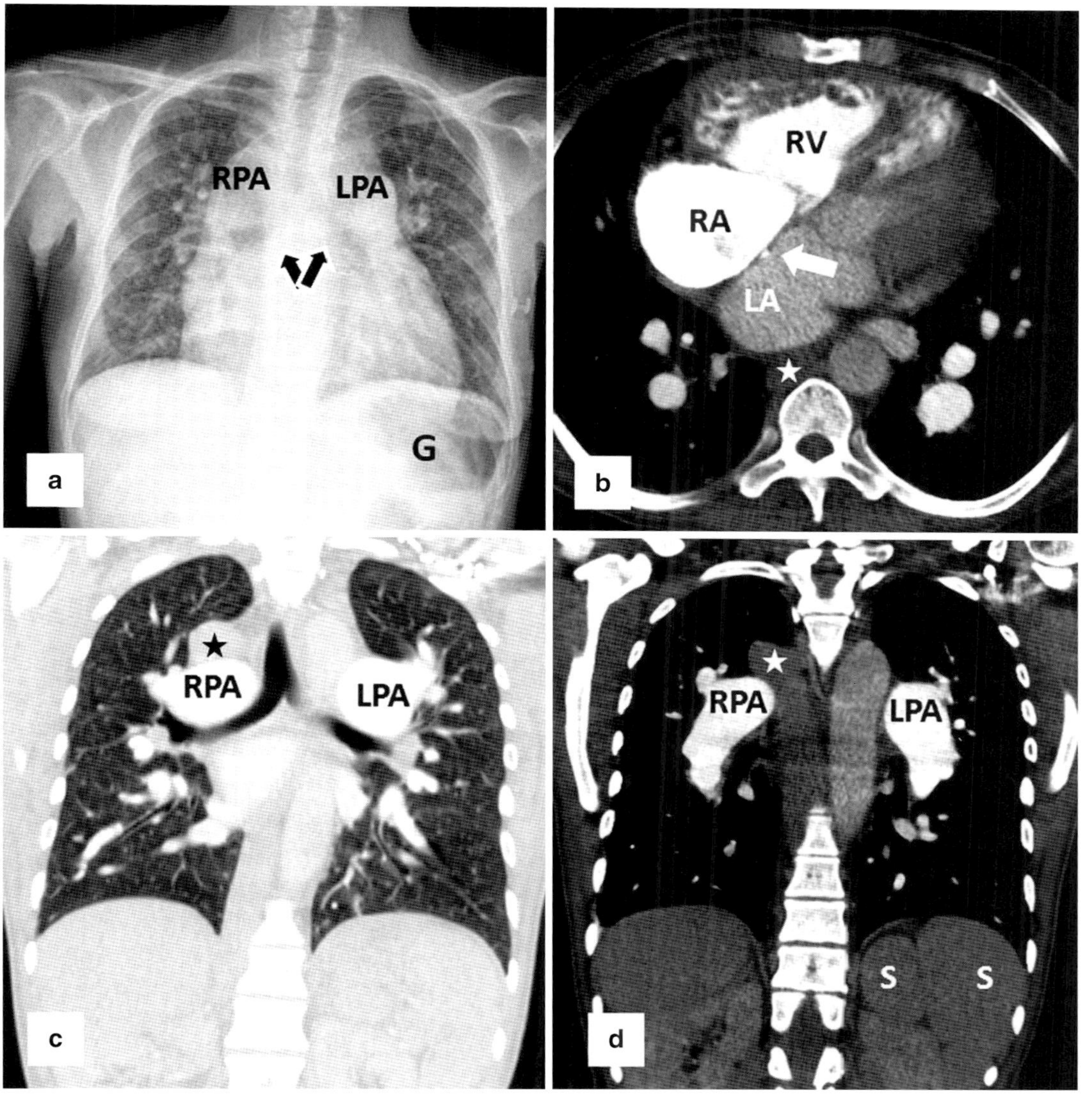

Fig. 12.6 A 39-year-old woman with polysplenia syndrome, who had repair of an atrial septal defect in childhood and presents with pulmonary hypertension. (**a**) Anteroposterior chest radiograph shows cardiomegaly with left-sided cardiac apex; the main bronchi are symmetric and hyparterial (*black arrows*), and the pulmonary arteries are dilated. The gastric bubble is on the left (*G*). (**b**) Axial CT demonstrates evidence of the atrial septal defect repair (*white arrow*) with dilatation and hypertrophy of the right ventricle consistent with pulmonary hypertension. The azygos vein is dilated (*star*). (**c**) Coronal CT in lung window depicts the symmetric hyparterial bronchi and pulmonary arteries. The azygos vein and arch (*star*) are dilated in this patient with azygos continuation of the inferior vena cava. (**d**) Coronal CT in soft tissue window shows multiple spleens in the left upper quadrant. Note the dilated pulmonary arteries. The unenhanced azygos vein and arch (*star*) are enlarged and similar in caliber to the contrast-enhanced aorta. *RA* right atrium, *RV* right ventricle, *LA* left atrium, *RPA* right pulmonary artery, *LPA* left pulmonary artery

know as much as possible about each patient's underlying diagnosis, surgical treatment, results of prior imaging, and the clinical question in order to properly tailor the MRI or less commonly CT examination. We will focus on a detailed discussion on several different situs configurations and the role of MRI and CT in evaluating adults with associated complex congenital heart

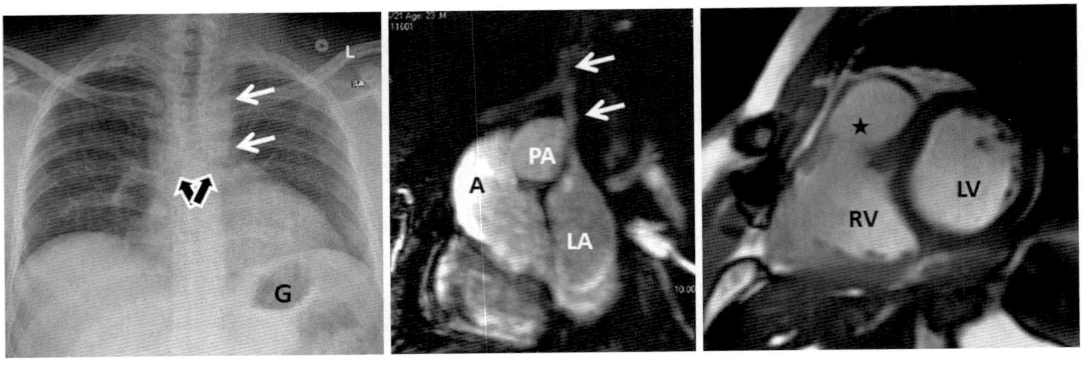

Fig. 12.7 A 23-year-old man with polysplenia and repaired tetralogy of Fallot. (**a**) PA radiograph shows levocardia and bilateral symmetric hyparterial bronchi (*black arrows*). There is an abnormal contour to the left upper mediastinum (*white arrows*). The stomach (*G*) is on the left. (**b**) Oblique-sagittal multiplanar reconstructed image from a contrast-enhanced MRA demonstrates a left-sided superior vena cava (*white arrows*) draining directly in the left atrium (*LA*) accounting for the left upper mediastinal border on radiograph and representing a small right to left shunt. The ascending aorta (*A*) and the pulmonary artery are also seen. (**c**) Still image from a short-axis cine MR in diastole shows a dilated right ventricle (*RV*) with deformity of the RV outflow tract (*star*), typical for repaired tetralogy of Fallot. *PA* pulmonary artery, *LV* left ventricle

disease: situs solitus with dextrocardia, situs inversus totalis, and asplenia.

Patients with situs solitus and dextrocardia or dextroversion have congenital heart disease in 90 % of cases, most commonly, complex anomalies associated with cyanosis such as tricuspid atresia or pulmonary stenosis or atresia [9]. Their segmental anatomy is typically {S,D,S}. Imaging evaluation of these patients depends on the underlying anomaly and surgical history. Some adults underwent only a palliative repair with a shunt, such as a Blalock-Taussig shunt (Fig. 12.9) [37]. This is particularly common in older patients, because of the limited surgical techniques available during their childhood or due to unfavorable anatomy, such as non-confluent central pulmonary arteries. In that scenario, MRI is usually performed to evaluate the shunt, quantify ventricular volumes and function, and assess the atrioventricular and ventriculoarterial valves.

Currently, patients with tricuspid atresia most often undergo a functional single ventricle repair, which results in a Fontan circulation (to be discussed in the asplenia section) [38]. Patients with tetralogy of Fallot or isolated pulmonary stenosis or atresia with confluent central pulmonary arteries generally undergo repair with valvotomy, transannular patch, or right ventricular to pulmonary artery conduit, depending on the underlying anatomy. These repairs generally result in distortion of the right ventricular outflow tract and pulmonary regurgitation (Fig. 12.7c); recurrent pulmonary stenosis may also develop [39, 40]. Currently, an adjusted right ventricular end-diastolic volume of 150 ml/m^2 may serve as a reference value for guiding pulmonary valve replacement [41]. MRI in these patients is performed to evaluate right ventricular volumes and function and left ventricular function, which can be impacted by right ventricular dysfunction (right ventricular-left ventricular interaction, as the ventricles share the septum and are encased by the pericardium). Other relevant information includes the pulmonary regurgitant volumes and fraction, which can be quantified on phase-contrast images. Delayed enhancement at the sites of surgical repair or elsewhere in the ventricles predicts a poorer prognosis [42].

Patients with situs inversus totalis usually do not have congenital heart disease, but when present (5 %), complete transposition of the great arteries must be considered (Fig. 12.10). These patients present in infancy with cyanosis, because they have atrioventricular concordance and ventriculoarterial discordance, i.e., two circuits in parallel. The physiology is the same as D-transposition, but, in situs inversus, complete transposition is L-transposition {I,L,L}. This

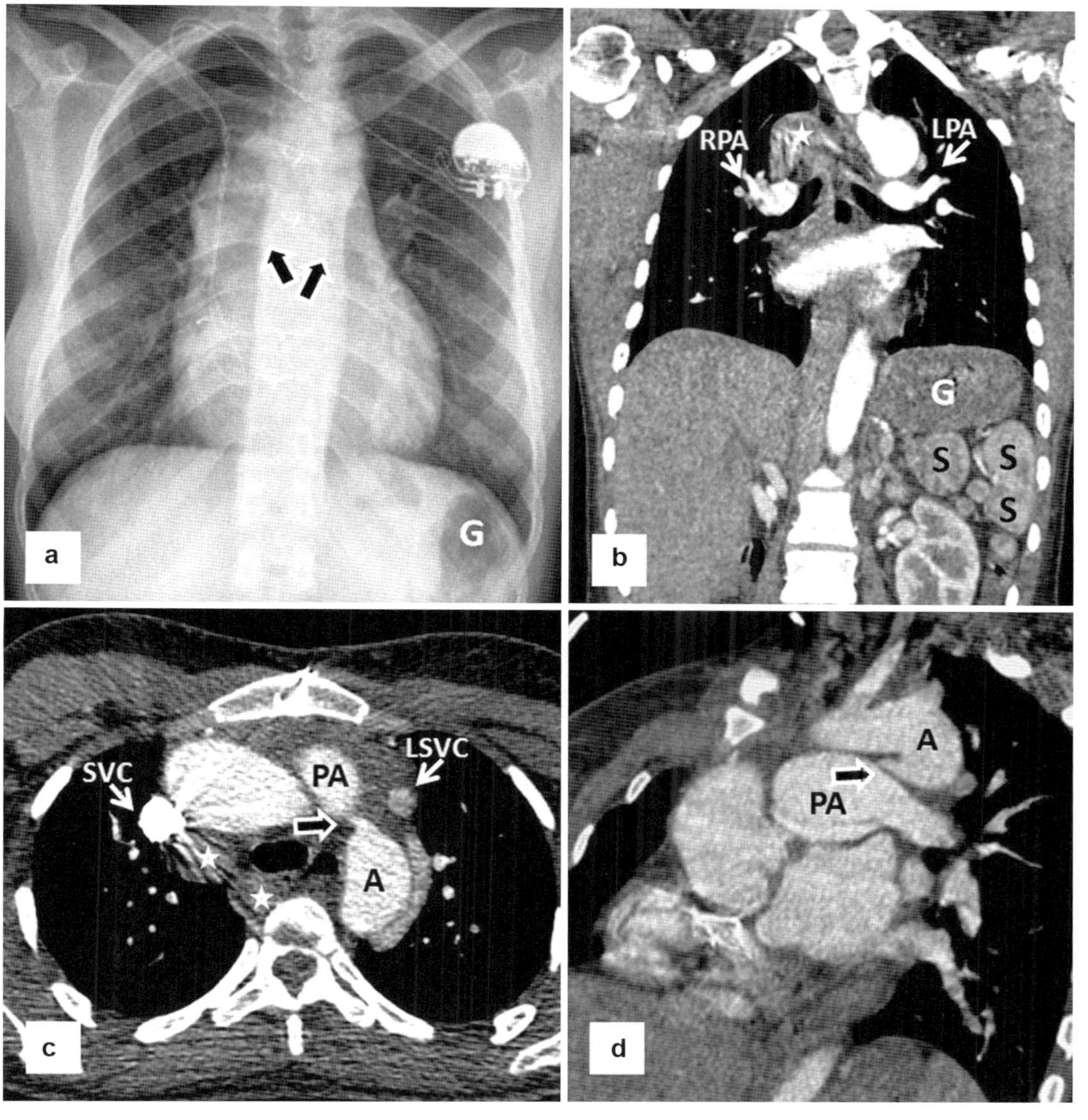

Fig. 12.8 A 24-year-old woman with polysplenia, who had an atrioventricular canal repaired in childhood. (**a**) PA radiograph shows bilateral hyparterial bronchial anatomy, typical of polysplenia (*arrows*). There is mild cardiomegaly with a left-sided cardiac apex. The stomach (*G*) is in the left upper quadrant. (**b**) Coronal CT reconstruction demonstrates the hyparterial bronchi inferior to the right and left pulmonary arteries (*RPA* and *LPA*, respectively). There is azygos continuation of the inferior vena cava and the azygos arch is enlarged (*). The stomach (*G*) is seen in the left upper quadrant, along with multiple small rounded spleens (*S*) with typical enhancement pattern. (**c**) Axial CT at the level of the carina demonstrates duplicated superior venae cavae with dilated azygos and hemiazygos veins draining into the larger right and smaller left cavae (*SVC* and *LSVC*), respectively. There is a small patent ductus arteriosus extending from the proximal descending aorta (*A*) to the proximal left pulmonary artery (*arrow*). (**d**) Oblique multiplanar CT reconstruction demonstrates the funnel-shaped patent ductus arteriosus with a larger aortic (*A*) and smaller pulmonary arterial communication (*arrow*). Star denotes azygos continuation of the inferior vena cava.

anomaly results from growth in the subaortic conus and resorption in the subpulmonic conus free wall [12]. The left-sided aorta with subaortic conus protrudes anteriorly and connects to the anatomic right ventricle. With resorption in the subpulmonic free wall, the right-sided pulmonary

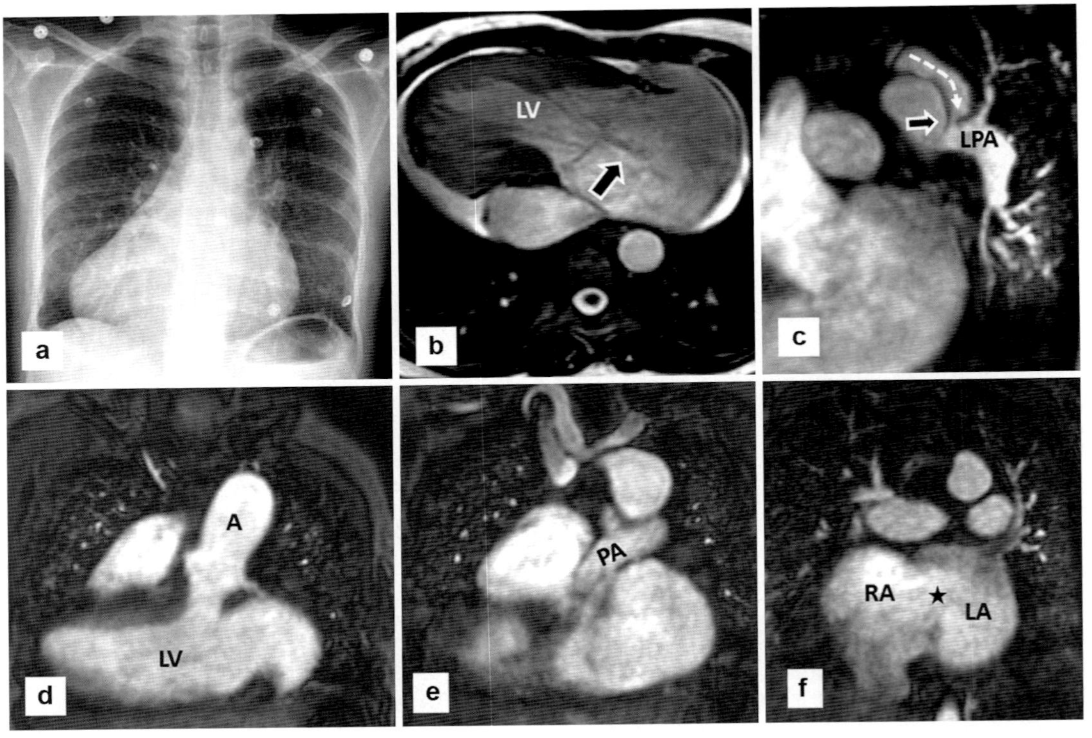

Fig. 12.9 A 51-year-old woman with situs solitus, dextrocardia, and tricuspid atresia status post classic left Blalock-Taussig shunt in childhood. (**a**) PA radiograph demonstrates situs solitus with a normal left-sided hyparterial bronchus and right-sided eparterial bronchus. The stomach bubble is on the left. There is dextrocardia and cardiomegaly. (**b**) Axial-balanced steady-state free precession (SSFP) image demonstrates a dilated and hypertrophied single left ventricle (*LV*) with a dephasing jet (*arrow*) into the dilated left atrium consistent with mitral regurgitation. There is a small high-signal intensity pericardial effusion. (**c**) Oblique reformat from the contrast-enhanced MRA demonstrates a patent left classic Blalock-Taussig (*white dashed arrow*) shunt with a severe stenosis (*arrow*) at its anastomosis with the left pulmonary artery (*LPA*). (**d–f**) Coronal contrast-enhanced MRA images show malposition of the great arteries with the ascending aorta (*A*) arising anterior and parallel to the stenotic main pulmonary artery. A large atrial septal defect (*star*) is also seen between the right and left atrium (*RA* and *LA*, respectively)

artery demonstrates pulmonary mitral fibrous continuity and connects to the morphologic left ventricle. The aorta is anterior, superior, and to the left of the pulmonary artery, and the great vessels are in parallel orientation as they emerge from the heart. The most common corrective surgery in adults with complete transposition is the atrial switch (Mustard or Senning) procedures, which were the dominant procedures during the 1970s and 1980s [43, 44]. A baffle at the atrial level directs blood from the systemic venous circulation (superior and inferior venae cavae) to the left ventricle and out through the pulmonary artery (Fig. 12.10). Complications of the atrial switch procedure include baffle leaks and stenosis [35]. Over the long term, failure of the systemic right ventricle is also a concern. MR or CT performs well in evaluating the patient after atrial switch [45]. It is crucial to image the superior and inferior systemic venous limbs of the baffle and the pulmonary venous return to rule out stenosis. This requires both early and later phase imaging in order to have adequate opacification of the inferior vena cava. Left and right ventricular wall motion and overall function is best assessed with SSFP cine MR imaging, although retrospectively ECG-gated CT can serve this function. The current favored surgery is the arterial switch, which came into clinical practice in the late 1980s [46]. The arterial switch is considered physiologically

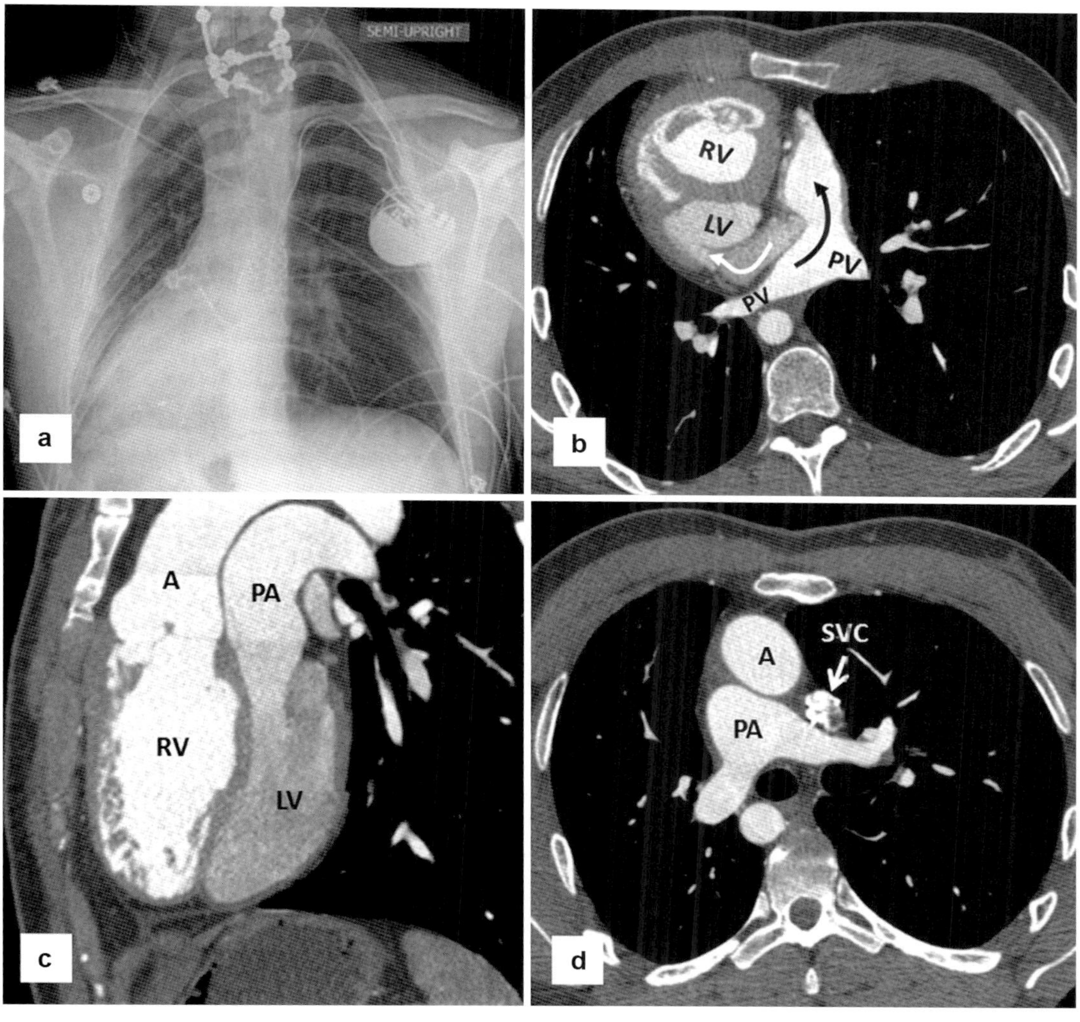

Fig. 12.10 A 28-year-old man with situs inversus totalis and complete transposition of the great arteries (L-TGA) status post atrial switch. (**a**) AP radiograph shows a right-sided hyparterial bronchus and a left-sided eparterial bronchus consistent with thoracic situs inversus. There is dextrocardia. The stomach bubble is right sided. (**b**) Axial CT image shows a normal-sized heart and dextrocardia. The interatrial baffle directs the systemic venous return into the left ventricle (*LV*) (*white arrow*). The pulmonary venous (*PV*) return (*black arrow*) is directed into the systemic right ventricle (*RV*). The hypertrophied, trabeculated systemic RV is anterior to the smooth-walled LV. (**c**) Sagital and (**d**) axial CT images demonstrate typical findings of complete transposition of the great arteries with the aorta (*A*) arising anteriorly from the trabeculated RV and the pulmonary artery arising posteriorly from the smooth-walled LV. The aorta (*A*) and the pulmonary artery (*PA*) are parallel and their normal spiraling orientation is absent. The aorta is anterior and to the left of the pulmonary artery. A left-sided superior vena cava (*SVC*) is present

favorable because the left ventricle becomes the systemic ventricle. This procedure is currently only seen in children and young adults [47]. Complications of arterial switch include coronary artery compression and myocardial infarction early on [48]. Later complications include pulmonary artery stenosis, particularly at the bifurcation. As the native pulmonary valve serves as the aortic valve, there is an increased risk of root dilatation and valve incompetence [45]. MR and ECG-gated CT angiography both perform well in demonstrating the aortic root, pulmonary artery, and coronary artery anatomy. MRI may be performed to evaluate valve and ventricular function and myocardial scars.

Many adults with asplenia have a single ventricle or severe anomalies that required a functional single ventricle repair, such as hypoplastic left heart, atrioventricular valve atresia, and double-outlet or double-inlet ventricle. The prognosis of most patients with a single functional ventricle used to be extremely poor until the introduction of staged surgical procedures [49]. The surgical goal for single ventricle patients is the complete separation of the systemic and pulmonary circulations with the single ventricle serving as the systemic pump and the pulmonary flow passively supplied by systemic venous return, thus establishment of Fontan circulation [38]. The first stage of the procedure is to establish adequate pulmonary circulation. Depending on the underlying anomaly, the pulmonary circulation may be inadequate, such as in pulmonary atresia, or may be excessive, such as in hypoplastic left heart. If the pulmonary circulation is inadequate, many patients will undergo a bidirectional Glenn shunt, which represents an end-to-side anastomosis of the superior vena cava to the right pulmonary artery [50]. If the pulmonary circulation is exuberant and the

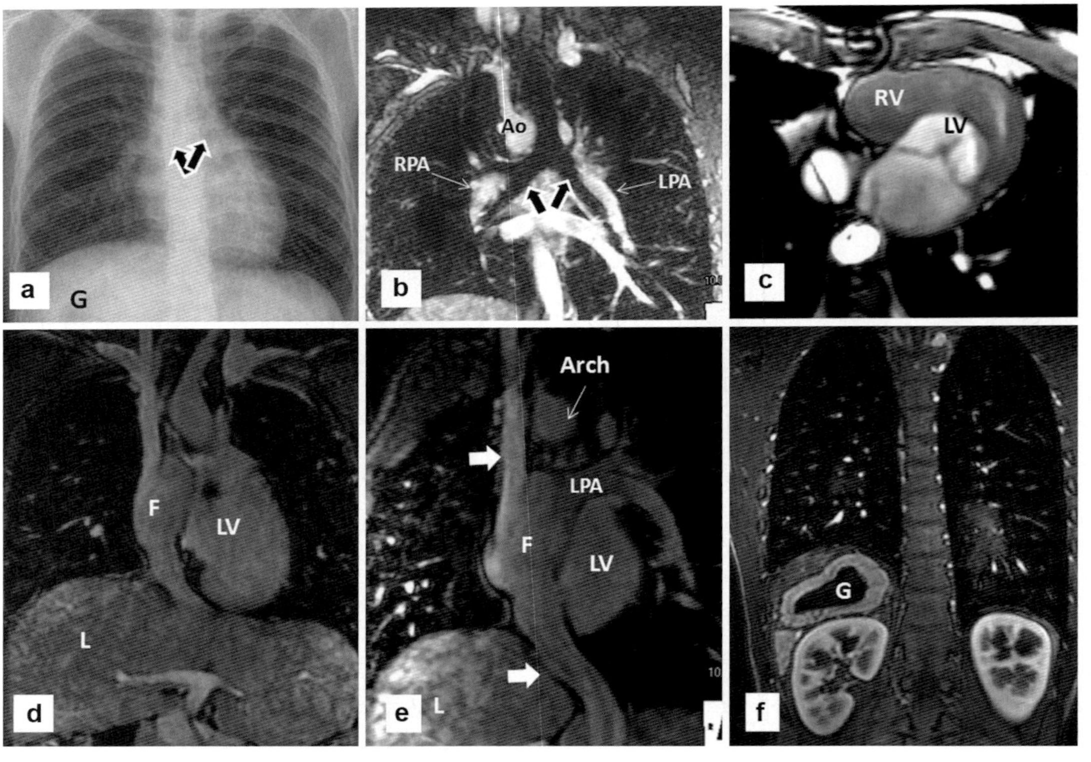

Fig. 12.11 A 26-year-old man with asplenia, tricuspid atresia, and single ventricle who underwent a variant of the classic Fontan repair with atriopulmonary anastomosis. PA radiograh (**a**) and coronal MR angiogram (**b**) demonstrate bilateral eparterial bronchi (*black arrows*) with right-sided aortic arch and right-sided gastric bubble. Axial systole and (**c**) axial balanced steady-state diastole balanced steady-state free precession (SSFP) images demonstrate levocardia and a single competent atrioventricular valve, which connects to the single left ventricle (*LV*). The right ventricle (*RV*) is a diminutive rudimentary chamber. (**d**, **e**) Coronal contrast-enhanced MRAs demonstrate patent atriopulmonary Fontan (*F*) directing the systemic venous return into the pulmonary arteries. There is adequate opacification of the superior and inferior limbs (*white arrows*) of the Fontan circuit, and the venous flow is unobstructed. Hepatic enhancement pattern is suggestive of cirrhosis. (**f**) There is characteristic absence of spleen from the left upper quadrant, and the stomach (*G*) is on the right. *Ao* aortic arch, *RPA* right pulmonary artery, *LPA* left pulmonary artery

systemic circulation is inadequate, the patient may initially undergo pulmonary artery banding plus surgery to establish adequate systemic arterial supply. In the second stage, a complete systemic venous to pulmonary artery circulation is established usually by placement of an intra- or extracardiac conduit connecting the inferior vena cava with the left or right pulmonary artery. Despite the improved outcomes with the staged surgical approach, the cavopulmonary Fontan circulation remains a palliative procedure. MRI using SSFP cine images can be performed to assess the size and function of the single ventricle and atrioventricular valve competence. Delayed gadolinium enhancement inversion recovery sequences are particularly useful for the evaluation of myocardial fibrosis. Single ventricle function can also be assessed on retrospectively ECG-gated CT. Unobstructed venous flow is crucial and stenosis usually develops along suture lines. When performing MR or CT angiography in patients with a Fontan circulation, adequate opacification of both the superior and inferior limbs of the Fontan circuit is tricky. Techniques include performance of both early and delayed phases of imaging or simultaneous contrast injection through upper and lower extremity veins. CT has higher spatial resolution than MR; MRI, however, allows flow quantification. The Fontan pathway should be assessed on MR using in-plane SSFP cine images (Fig. 12.11). Phase-contrast images should be performed to assess for Fontan pathway flow, systemic to pulmonary circulation shunting (Qp:Qs), and flow to the right and left lungs.

When performing CT or MRI in a patient with asplenia, besides evaluating the heart, other anomalies associated with asplenia should be sought and described. The tracheobronchial tree typically has bilateral right-sided lungs with three lobes and bilateral eparterial bronchi (Fig. 12.11). The patient will often have duplicated superior vena cava and a midline inferior vena cava. In the abdomen, the liver is typically transverse and the spleen is absent. The location of the stomach is variable and intestinal malrotation is usual. Pancreatic, biliary, and renal anomalies may also be present.

Conclusion

In conclusion, a systematic segmental approach is useful in defining the visceroatrial situs and cardiac anatomy. The clinical presentation of patients with situs abnormalities depends on the severity of the underlying congenital heart disease. Initial adult presentation of mild anomalies may be diagnosed on chest radiography or chest CT performed for other indications. Complex cardiac anomalies that were treated in childhood often merit imaging with cardiac MRI or CT tailored to assess for complications of long-standing disease or its treatment. Understanding abnormalities of visceroatrial situs and their associations is crucial to optimize imaging for proper diagnosis and as a guide to management.

References

1. Spindola-Franco H. Abnormalities of the visceroatrial situs. In: Spindola-Franco H, editor. Radiology of the heart: cardiac imaging in infants, children and adults. New York/Berlin/Heidelberg/Tokyo: Springer; 1985. p. 620–37.
2. Tonkin IL, Tonkin AK. Visceroatrial situs abnormalities: sonographic and computed tomographic appearance. AJR Am J Roentgenol. 1982;138(3):509–15.
3. Hernanz-Schulman M, Ambrosino MM, Genieser NB, et al. Pictorial essay. Current evaluation of the patient with abnormal visceroatrial situs. AJR Am J Roentgenol. 1990;154(4):797–802.
4. Van Praagh R. The importance of segmental situs in the diagnosis of congenital heart disease. Semin Roentgenol. 1985;20(3):254–71.
5. Ghosh S, Yarmish G, Godelman A, Haramati LB, Spindola-Franco H. Anomalies of visceroatrial situs. AJR Am J Roentgenol. 2009;193(4):1107–17.
6. Van Praagh R. Diagnosis of complex congenital heart disease: morphologic-anatomic method and terminology. Cardiovasc Intervent Radiol. 1984;7(3–4):115–20.
7. Angelini P. Embryology and congenital heart disease. Tex Heart Inst J. 1995;22(1):1–12.
8. Fulcher AS, Turner MA. Abdominal manifestations of situs anomalies in adults. Radiographics. 2002; 22(6):1439–56.
9. Maldjian PD, Saric M. Approach to dextrocardia in adults: review. AJR Am J Roentgenol. 2007;188(6 Suppl):S39–49; quiz S35–8.
10. Shaher RM, Duckworth JW, Khoury GH, Moes CA. The significance of the atrial situs in the diagnosis of positional anomalies of the heart. I. Anatomic and embryologic considerations. Am Heart J. 1967;73(1): 32–40.

11. Lapierre C, Dery J, Guerin R, Viremouneix L, Dubois J, Garel L. Segmental approach to imaging of congenital heart disease. Radiographics. 2010;30(2):397–411.
12. Van Praagh R. Normally and abnormally related great arteries: what have we learned? World J Pediatr Congenit Heart Surg. 2010;1(3):364–85.
13. Tonkin IL. The definition of cardiac malpositions with echocardiography and computed tomography. In: Friedman WF, Higgins CB, editors. Pediatric cardiac imaging. Philadelphia: Saunders; 1984. p. 157–87.
14. Imbrie JD. Kartagener's syndrome: a genetic defect affecting the function of cilia. Am J Otolaryngol. 1981;2(3):215–22.
15. Kartagener M, Stucki P. Bronchiectasis with situs inversus. Arch Pediatr. 1962;79:193–207.
16. Chacko KA, Krishnaswami S, Sukumar IP, Cherian G. Isolated levocardia: two cases with abdominal situs inversus, thoracic situs solitus, and normal circulation. Am Heart J. 1983;106(1 Pt 1):155–9.
17. Applegate KE, Goske MJ, Pierce G, Murphy D. Situs revisited: imaging of the heterotaxy syndrome. Radiographics. 1999;19(4):837–52; discussion 853–4.
18. Winer-Muram HT. Adult presentation of heterotaxic syndromes and related complexes. J Thorac Imaging. 1995;10(1):43–57.
19. Winer-Muram HT, Tonkin IL. The spectrum of heterotaxic syndromes. Radiol Clin North Am. 1989;27(6):1147–70.
20. Peoples WM, Moller JH, Edwards JE. Polysplenia: a review of 146 cases. Pediatr Cardiol. 1983;4(2):129–37.
21. Vossen PG, Van Hedent EF, Degryse HR, De Schepper AM. Computed tomography of the polysplenia syndrome in the adult. Gastrointest Radiol. 1987;12(3):209–11.
22. Winer-Muram HT, Tonkin IL, Gold RE. Polysplenia syndrome in the asymptomatic adult: computed tomography evaluation. J Thorac Imaging. 1991;6(2):69–71.
23. Ditchfield MR, Hutson JM. Intestinal rotational abnormalities in polysplenia and asplenia syndromes. Pediatr Radiol. 1998;28(5):303–6.
24. Gagner M, Munson JL, Scholz FJ. Hepatobiliary anomalies associated with polysplenia syndrome. Gastrointest Radiol. 1991;16(2):167–71.
25. Freedom RM. The asplenia syndrome: a review of significant extracardiac structural abnormalities in 29 necropsied patients. J Pediatr. 1972;81(6):1130–3.
26. Freedom RM, Fellows Jr KE. Radiographic visceral patterns in the asplenia syndrome. Radiology. 1973;107(2):387–91.
27. Ivemark BI. Implications of agenesis of the spleen on the pathogenesis of conotruncus anomalies in childhood; an analysis of the heart malformations in the splenic agenesis syndrome, with fourteen new cases. Acta Paediatr Suppl. 1955;44 Suppl 104:7–110.
28. Phoon CK, Neill CA. Asplenia syndrome: insight into embryology through an analysis of cardiac and extracardiac anomalies. Am J Cardiol. 1994;73(8):581–7.
29. Elliott LP, Cramer GG, Amplatz K. The anomalous relationship of the interior vena cava and abdominal aorta as a specific angiocardiographic sign in asplenia. Radiology. 1966;87(5):859–63.
30. Berko NS, Haramati LB. Simple cardiac shunts in adults. Semin Roentgenol. 2012;47(3):277–88.
31. Bartram U, Wirbelauer J, Speer CP. Heterotaxy syndrome – asplenia and polysplenia as indicators of visceral malposition and complex congenital heart disease. Biol Neonate. 2005;88(4):278–90.
32. Houston A, Hillis S, Lilley S, Richens T, Swan L. Echocardiography in adult congenital heart disease. Heart. 1998;80 Suppl 1:S12–26.
33. Haramati LB, Glickstein JS, Issenberg HJ, Haramati N, Crooke GA. MR imaging and CT of vascular anomalies and connections in patients with congenital heart disease: significance in surgical planning. Radiographics. 2002;22(2):337–47; discussion 348–9.
34. Rajiah P, Kanne JP. Cardiac MRI: part 1, cardiovascular shunts. AJR Am J Roentgenol. 2011;197(4):W603–20.
35. Warnes CA. Transposition of the great arteries. Circulation. 2006;114(24):2699–709.
36. Marelli AJ, Mackie AS, Ionescu-Ittu R, Rahme E, Pilote L. Congenital heart disease in the general population: changing prevalence and age distribution. Circulation. 2007;115(2):163–72.
37. Blalock A. Physiopathology and surgical treatment of congenital cardiovascular defects. Harvey Lect. 1945;41:90–116.
38. Jaquiss R, Imamura M. Single ventricle physiology: surgical options, indications and outcomes. Curr Opin Cardiol. 2009;24(2):113–8.
39. Gartner RD, Sutton NJ, Weinstein S, Spindola-Franco H, Haramati LB. MRI and computed tomography of cardiac and pulmonary complications of tetralogy of Fallot in adults. J Thorac Imaging. 2010;25(2):183–90.
40. Aggarwal S, Garekar S, Forbes TJ, Turner DR. Is stent placement effective for palliation of right ventricle to pulmonary artery conduit stenosis? J Am Coll Cardiol. 2007;49(4):480–4.
41. Therrien J, Provost Y, Merchant N, Williams W, Colman J, Webb G. Optimal timing for pulmonary valve replacement in adults after tetralogy of Fallot repair. Am J Cardiol. 2005;95(6):779–82.
42. Babu-Narayan SV, Kilner PJ, Li W, et al. Ventricular fibrosis suggested by cardiovascular magnetic resonance in adults with repaired tetralogy of Fallot and its relationship to adverse markers of clinical outcome. Circulation. 2006;113(3):405–13.
43. Senning A. Surgical correction of transposition of the great vessels. Surgery. 1959;45(6):966–80.
44. Mustard WT. Successful two-stage correction of transposition of the great vessels. Surgery. 1964;55:469–72.
45. Zwany SK, Lui GK, Scheinfeld MH, Levsky JM. Making complex adult congenital heart disease a little simpler. Semin Roentgenol. 2012;47(3):289–301.
46. Jatene AD, Fontes VF, Paulista PP, et al. Anatomic correction of transposition of the great vessels. J Thorac Cardiovasc Surg. 1976;72(3):364–70.
47. Lecompte Y, Zannini L, Hazan E, et al. Anatomic correction of transposition of the great arteries. J Thorac Cardiovasc Surg. 1981;82(4):629–31.

48. Legendre A, Losay J, Touchot-Kone A, et al. Coronary events after arterial switch operation for transposition of the great arteries. Circulation. 2003;108 Suppl 1: II186–90.
49. Khairy P, Fernandes SM, Mayer Jr JE, et al. Long-term survival, modes of death, and predictors of mortality in patients with Fontan surgery. Circulation. 2008;117(1):85–92.
50. Glenn WW. Circulatory bypass of the right side of the heart. IV. Shunt between superior vena cava and distal right pulmonary artery; report of clinical application. N Engl J Med. 1958;259(3):117–20.

13 Cardiac Shunts: ASD, VSD, PDA

Farhood Saremi

Atrial septum defects (ASDs), ventricular septum defects (VSDs), and patent ductus arteriosus (PDA) are common congenital heart defects in both children and adults [1–3]. Morphological classification of these anomalies is important for treatment decisions. Accurate morphological classification requires imaging technique that is able to identify the defect and define its site, size, and relationship to the structures forming its margins. Imaging technique should also be able to identify associated anomalies, the amount of shunt through the defect, and accurate analysis of the heart and valve functions. Echocardiography is a great method for diagnosis of intracardiac shunts with good resolution to image cardiac morphology in detail and can identify small intracardiac defects and measure the shunt volume. Cardiac MR provides a comprehensive assessment of intracardiac anatomy and accurately quantifies biventricular function and blood flow. Detections of small defects (i.e., apical VSD) may require high-resolution imaging and CT can be the preferred technique. Assessment of associated extracardiac anomalies such as anomalous venous return can be optimally done with CT. In this chapter, a complete review of the shunts and clinical applications of CT and MRI will be presented.

F. Saremi, MD
Department of Radiology, Cardiothoracic Section, University of Southern California, USC Keck Hospital, 1500 San Pablo St., Los Angeles, CA 90033, USA
e-mail: fsaremi@usc.edu

Interatrial Communications

Interatrial communications or ASDs present as an isolated abnormality or in association with other cardiovascular malformations. Generally, ASDs can be categorized into three major types including ostium secundum, ostium primum, and sinus venosus defects (Fig. 13.1). Unroofed coronary sinus (CS) can also be classified in this group although the abnormal defect is not directly related to the interatrial septum. Secundum ASD is the most common type and about two-thirds are seen in females. The exact cause is not clear and genetic factors may play a role. For example, ASD is the most common cardiac malformation of Holt-Oram syndrome and ostium primum defects are seen in 40 % of Down syndrome and may be associated with Ellis-Van Creveld and DiGeorge syndromes [1].

Developmental Considerations and Anatomy

In order to understand anatomy and different anomalies of the interatrial septum, it is necessary to be familiar with certain aspects of the atrial septation and the development of the sinus venosus and the pulmonary vein.

Embryology

Around the fourth week of development, the sinus venosus opens into the posteroinferior part of the common atrium in the midline and receives

F. Saremi (ed.), *Cardiac CT and MR for Adult Congenital Heart Disease*,
DOI 10.1007/978-1-4614-8875-0_13, © Springer Science+Business Media New York 2014

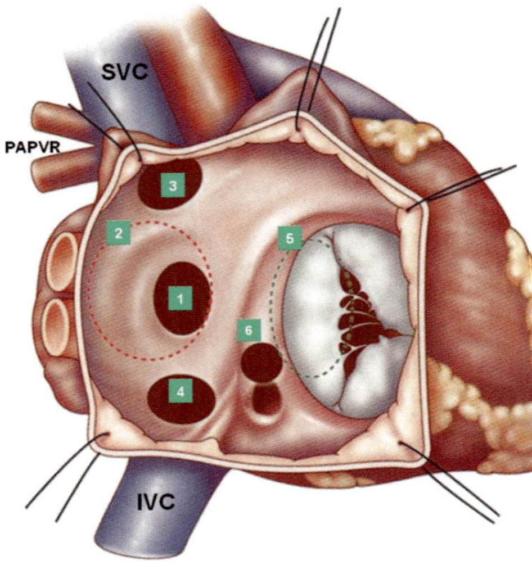

Fig. 13.1 Classifications of atrial septal defect (ASD): (*1*) secundum type 1, (*2*) secundum type 2 (*red circle*), (*3*) sinus venosus (superior), (*4*) sinus venosus (inferior), (*5*) atrioventricular septal (septum primum) defect (*green circle*), and (*6*) unroofed coronary sinus. *PAPVR* partial anomalous pulmonary venous return, *SVC* superior vena cava, *IVC* inferior vena cava

on each side the systemic (common cardinal veins), placental (umbilical), and vitelline (omphalomesenteric) blood by separate paired veins [4–6] (Fig. 13.2). At 5 weeks, the opening of the sinus venosus shifts into the right atrium (sinoatrial orifice) and is guarded by right and left venous valves which unite at the cephalic end of the orifice to form the septum spurium. The pulmonary vein enters the heart as a single structure (common pulmonary vein) with its orifice adjacent to the developing left atrioventricular (AV) junction.

The septum primum is also identifiable medial to the left venous valve and just to the right of the orifice of the common pulmonary vein. At 6 weeks, the liver has invaded the omphalomesenteric and umbilical veins, the umbilical veins have lost their connection with the sinus venosus, and the ductus venosus and intrahepatic portion of the inferior vena cava (IVC) are formed. With these changes, the sinus venosus now receives the two common cardinal veins and the IVC, formed by the termination of

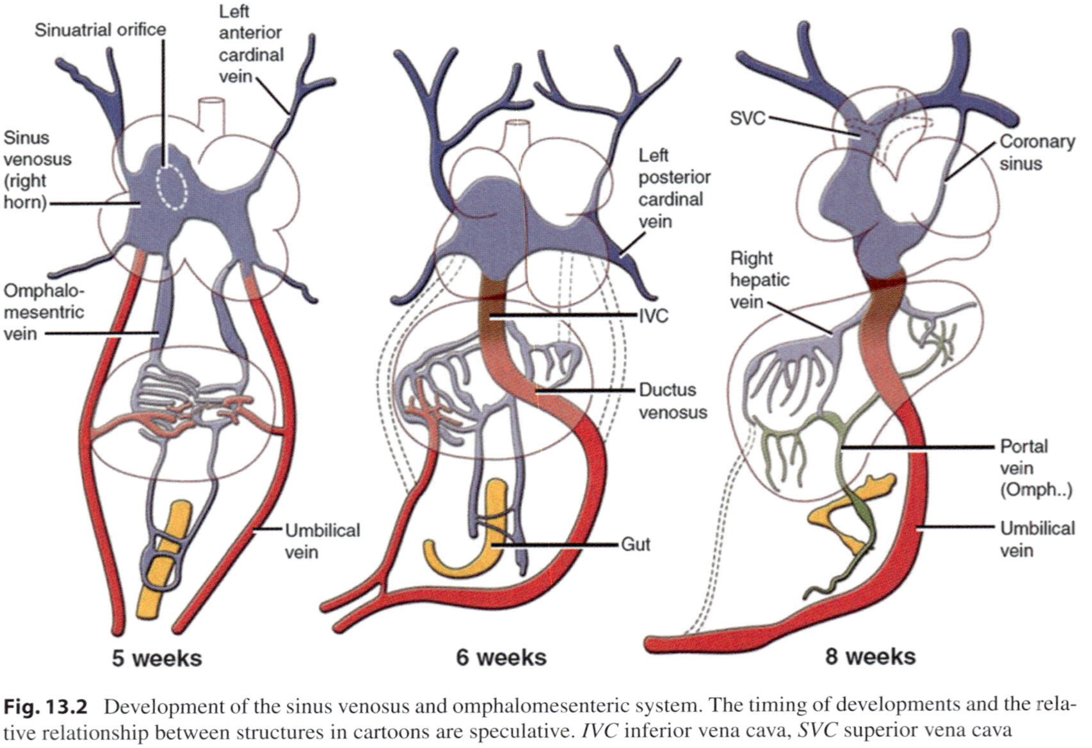

Fig. 13.2 Development of the sinus venosus and omphalomesenteric system. The timing of developments and the relative relationship between structures in cartoons are speculative. *IVC* inferior vena cava, *SVC* superior vena cava

the right omphalomesenteric vein (Fig. 13.2). These connections result in more enlargement of the right horn of sinus venosus. At this time, the septum primum has begun its growth from the roof of the atrial component, carrying on its leading edge a prominent mesenchymal cap. With time, the mesenchymal cap fuses with the atrioventricular cushions, dividing the AV canal into the prospective tricuspid and mitral valve orifices. The dorsal area of fusion grows into the heart tissue and vestibular spine develops which as it fuses with the primary atrial septum ensures that the pulmonary vein enters the cavity of the left atrium. Soon, the upper margin of the septum primum breaks to form a large secondary interatrial communication (ostium secundum or foramen ovale). In the seventh week, the septum secundum starts to form on the right side of the septum primum but the foramen ovale is still large. The septum secundum is nothing but infolding of the roof between the two atria (interatrial groove). The left common cardinal vein and the left horn of the sinus venosus regress, the latter forming the coronary sinus (CS). The superior vena cava (SVC), IVC, and CS now open into the posterior right atrium and find their final location, the so-called sinus venarum (Fig. 13.2). At 8 weeks, the "septum secundum" develops further. The interatrial groove deepens superiorly to separate the opening of the SVC to the right atrium and the attachments of the right pulmonary veins to the left atrium. The interatrial groove is filled by varying amount of extracardiac adipose tissue and is not a true septum. Its thickness determines the prominence of the fossa ovalis margin at its anterosuperior border. In general at 8 weeks, the incorporation of the sinus venosus into the right atrium and separation of the two atria are complete, and the common pulmonary vein has been taken into the left atrium.

By the ninth week, the left sinus valve disappeared. The residual of the septum spurium can be seen as a prominent trabeculation in right atrial appendage near the superior cavoatrial junction. Remnant of the left sinus valve may be seen on the right side of septum secundum on CT or echocardiography studies. The right venous valve will remain as the Eustachian and Thebesian valves guarding the ostia of the IVC and coronary sinus, respectively. By the 11th week, the right and left pulmonary veins have been taken into the left atrium which then contains four pulmonary orifices. As a reminder, the four pulmonary venous components, with separate orifices on both sides of the left atrial roof, do not achieve their definitive positions until after completion of atrial septation. In other words, the "septum secundum" is only seen at the stage when four pulmonary venous orifices are present.

Arial Septum

The normal atrial septum is made up of the floor and rims of the fossa ovalis, with the superior and posterior rims being infoldings of the atrial walls between the attachments of the caval veins to the right atrium and the ostia of the right pulmonary veins to the left atrium [7] (Fig. 13.3).

The floor of the fossa ovalis is formed by the septum primum. It is a relatively thin fibromuscular flap that, anterosuperiorly, overlaps an extensive muscular border, also known as "limbus" which is mainly formed by the septum secundum. In at least 70 %, the flap of fossa ovalis is adhered to the limbus. The inferoposterior border of the fossa ovalis continues directly into the wall of the IVC and its anteroinferior border is continuous with the epicardial fat squeezed between the atria and the ventricles at the AV junction (AV sandwich) (Fig. 13.3). The size of fossa ovalis and its margins may vary greatly. If the seal is incomplete, a patent foramen ovale (PFO) will remain at the anterosuperior quadrant of the rim orientated in a craniocaudal, dorsoventral, and right-to-left axis (Figs. 13.3 and 13.4). A PFO has been known to be a very common finding since 1930, when Thompson and Evans identified a "pencil-patent" defect (0.6–1.0 cm in diameter) within the atrial septum in 6 % of unselected autopsies and a "probe-patent" foramen (0.2–0.5 cm) in 29 % [8]. Hagen et al. found a PFO in 27 % of 965 autopsied hearts [9]. The incidence and size of PFO did not differ with gender but varied significantly with age; 34 % of PFOs occurred in the first three decades, 25 % in the fourth to eighth decades, and 20 % in the

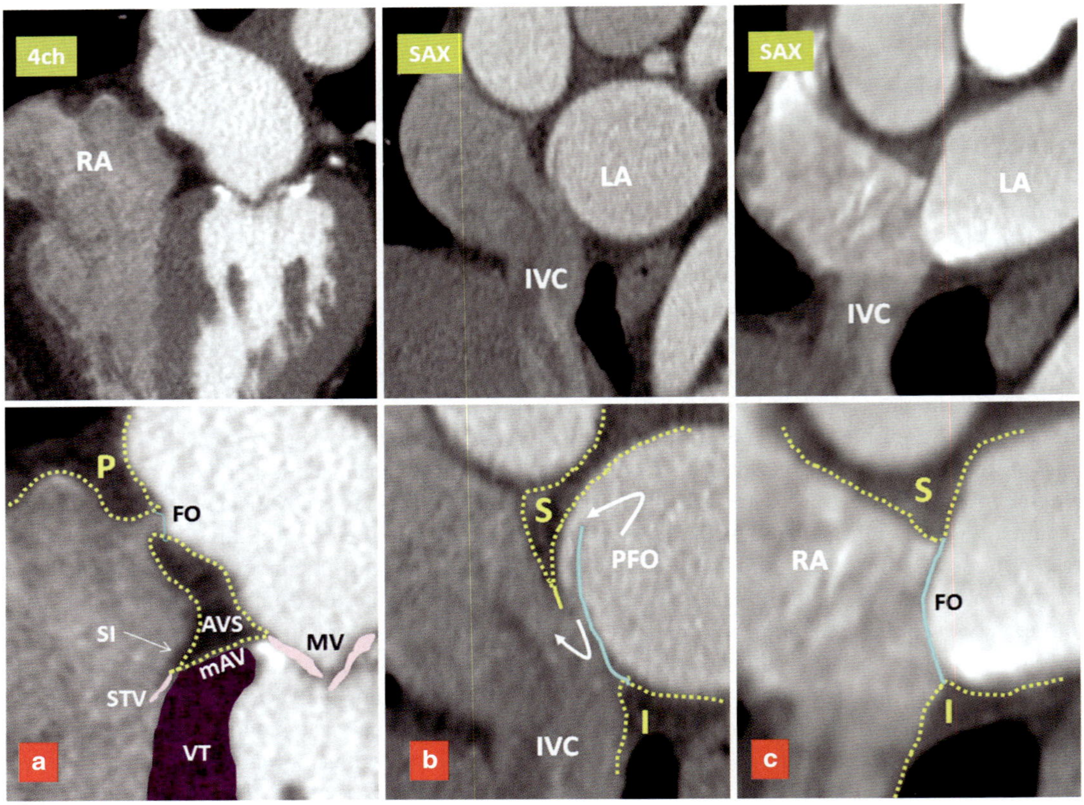

Fig. 13.3 Components of the interatrial septum. Upper row images are four-chamber (*4ch*) and short axis (*SAX*) images of three different patients. Lower row images include magnified views of the upper row images. The septum secundum forms the interatrial groove covering the superior (*S*), posterior (*P*), and inferior (*I*) margins of the fossa ovalis (*FO*). *Blue line* denotes the septum primum. (**a**) Small FO with fatty infiltration of the interatrial groove and atrioventricular sandwich (*AVS*). (**b**) Shows a patent foramen ovale (*PFO*). (**c**) Shows a large FO and a short interatrial groove. *IVC* inferior vena cava, *LA* left atrium, *mAV* muscular AV septum, *MV* mitral valve, *RA* right atrium, *SI* septal isthmus, *STV* septal leaflet of tricuspid valve, *VT* ventricular septum

ninth and tenth decades. The size of the PFO ranged from 1 to 19 mm (4.9 mm, mean) and increased progressively in size from a mean of 3.4 mm in the first decade to 5.8 mm in the tenth decade (perhaps because smaller defects seal with age).

Patent Foramen Ovale

PFO is probably the most common cause of right-to-left shunting in patients with paradoxical embolism [10, 11]. It is also an important mechanism by which an embolic stroke can develop in young patients and appears to be more common in larger PFOs [11]. The presence of shunting through the PFO not only depends upon the transatrial pressure gradient but also likely relates to anatomic features of the PFO; these include the size of opening into the right atrium, length of the PFO tunnel, and the extent of excursion of the flap membrane [11–14]. Moreover, the risk of stroke appears to be increased in the presence of structures that direct flow toward a PFO (i.e., prominent Eustachian valve) or hemodynamic changes that increase right-sided pressure (i.e., large pulmonary embolism). In a study performed by Natanzon and Goldman [14], the magnitude of right-to-left shunting was larger and the length of flap valve was shorter in patients with cryptogenic strokes as compared to those patients whose PFO was

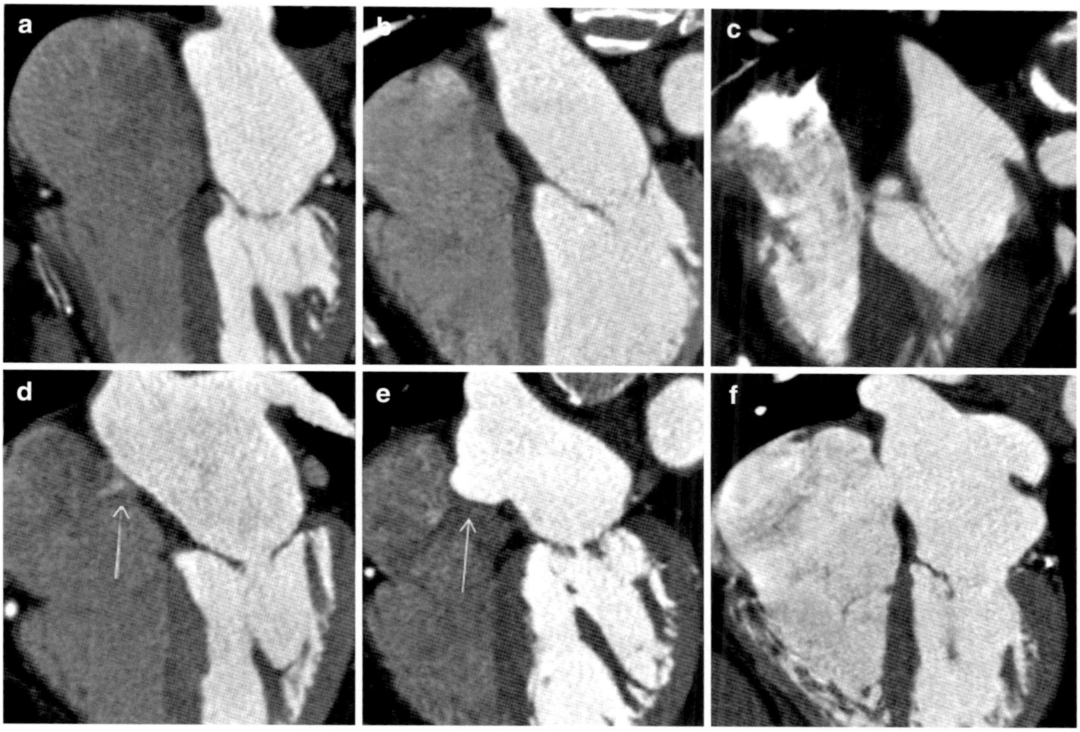

Fig. 13.4 Anatomic variations of the interatrial septum. (**a**) Straight thin line of septum is seen. No appreciable fat is seen in the interatrial groove. (**b**) Thickened interatrial groove due to fat accumulation. Fossa ovalis is well demarcated. (**c**) Severe fatty infiltration of the septum. Fossa ovalis is not seen. (**d**) Small PFO shunt is shown by *arrow*. (**e**) Aneurysm of the atrial septum (*arrow*). (**f**) Secundum ASD

incidentally found on transesophageal echocardiography (TEE). Similar findings have been reported with cardiac CT. In a recent multidetector CT (MDCT) study of asymptomatic individuals, 92 % of left-to-right shunts occurred with a PFO tunnel length of 6 mm or less in length [12]. When the flap length is very short, a bidirectional shunt is more probable. Patients with an atrial septal aneurysm (ASA) also have a very short PFO tunnel length. In a recent postmortem study by Ho et al. [13], two types of PFO were described: valve competent and valve incompetent. PFOs with a short, overlapping flap and with an ASA were classified as incompetent with high likelihood of bidirectional flow. Similar morphology has also been described using MDCT in patients with a short PFO tunnel length or those with an atrial septal aneurysm (ASA) [12] (Fig. 13.5).

Imaging Modalities in PFO Shunt

Imaging diagnosis of a shunt can be performed directly or indirectly. Direct assessment of an intracardiac shunt is mainly performed by echocardiography and MRI; for extracardiac shunts, CT or MR is commonly performed. Given its wide availability, noninvasive nature, and low cost, echocardiography is currently the most popular. With widespread use of cardiac CT for other indications, it has recently gained momentum for the analysis of intracardiac shunts and PFO. MRI enables direct flow quantification and provides valuable information about size, shape, location, and spatial relationship to other structures [15]. However, the present MRI technique may be inferior to contrast-enhanced TEE in detection of right-to-left PFO shunting (i.e., during Valsalva maneuver) and identification of ASA [15–17].

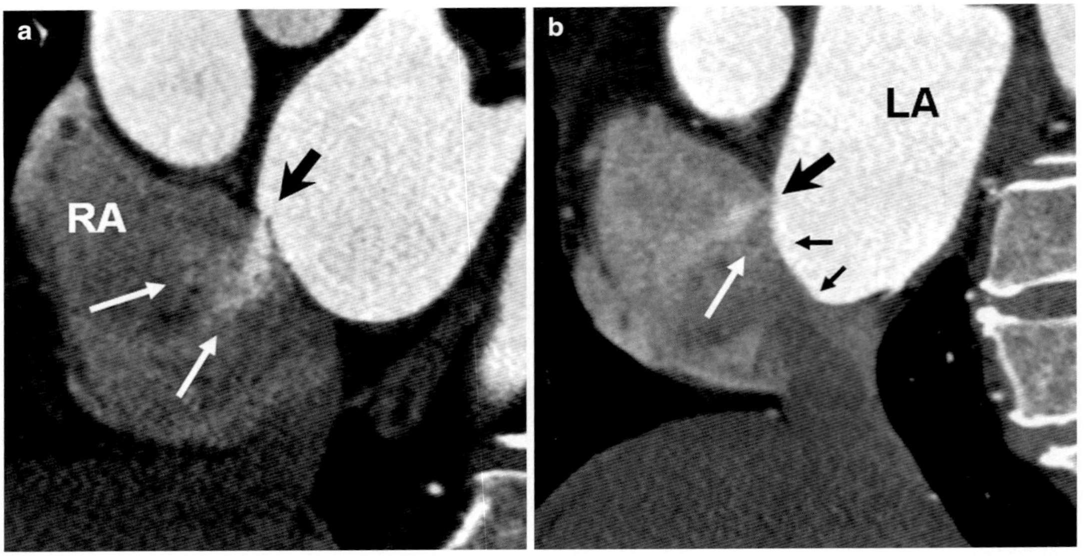

Fig. 13.5 Short axis images show incompetent valves in patent foramen ovale (PFO) with free flow of contrast through the opening (*white arrows*). (**a**) The free flap valve is too short to cover the superior rim of the septum secundum (*black arrow*). (**b**) Atrial septal aneurysm (*small arrows*) also demonstrates very short PFO tunnel (*large black arrow*) causing a left-to-right shunt (*white arrow*). *LA* left atrium, *RA* right atrium

Although TEE is a great modality to show a right-to-left shunt, most of shunts are positive only after the Valsalva maneuver [18]. Demonstration of a PFO tunnel by MDCT may predict the potential for a shunt. Only a limited number of studies have been performed comparing MDCT to TEE [12, 19]. Current CT techniques for coronary angiography are capable of showing a left-to-right shunt. This can be important as demonstration of a left-to-right shunt, particularly when a short flap valve length or ASA exists, indicates an incompetent valve mechanism with high likelihood of a bidirectional shunt (Fig. 13.5). Furthermore, no provocative test is necessary to demonstrate a left-to-right shunt with MDCT. Current techniques for placement of PFO closure devices rely on fluoroscopic landmarks combined with TEE or intracardiac echocardiography guidance [20]. CT has been used for localization of the fossa ovalis to aid for transseptal catheterization [21]. Given that a PFO is a 3-dimensional (3D) structure with dynamic opening and closing, describing the exact size with one simple dimension is not possible. With CT, scan-detailed 3D information can easily be obtained. CT can accurately demonstrate the relationship of important structures to the PFO including the distance to the aortic root, anomalous coronary artery course, and the location of the coronary sinus ostium. These information may be important before device closure placement [12].

Associated Findings with PFO

Chiari Network

The Chiari network represents coarse or fine fibers in the right atrium, arising from the Eustachian or Thebesian valve and strands within the right atrium connecting these valves with the crista terminalis, right atrial wall, or interatrial septum. It is a remnant of the embryonic right valve of the sinus venosus [22, 23] and should be differentiated from a large Eustachian valve by looking carefully for attachments to other parts of the right atrium. A Chiari network has been reported in 2–4 % of autopsy studies [23, 24] and is generally thought to not be of clinical significance. However, in rare instances, the network may be the site of thrombus

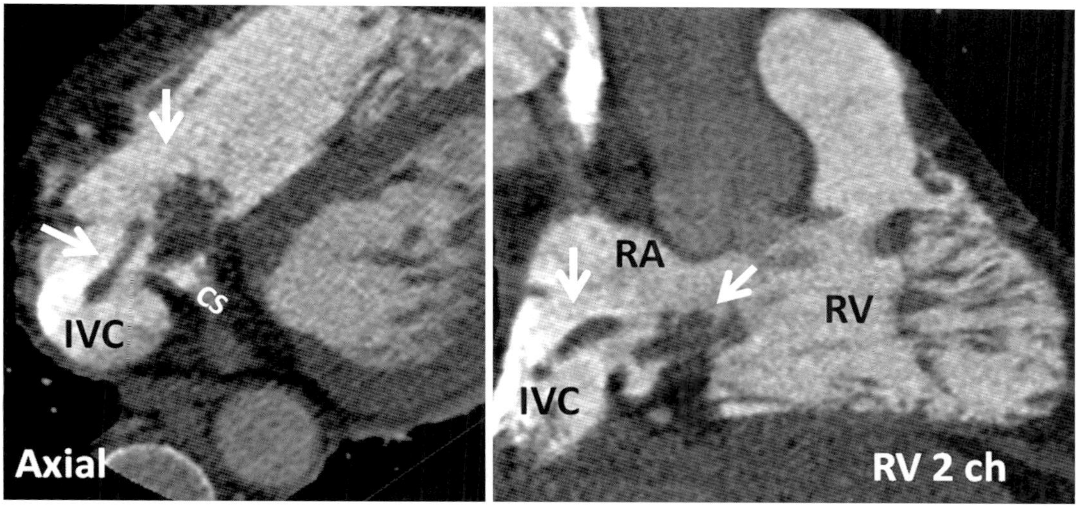

Fig. 13.6 Demonstration of Chiari network with dedicated CT of the right heart. Axial and right ventricle (*RV*) two-chamber (*2ch*) view show rounded and band-like structures (*arrows*) at the inferior cavoatrial junction attaching to the walls of inferior vena cava (*IVC*) and coronary sinus (*CS*) ostia. This was confirmed by echo which also showed possible thrombus covering the network. Patient had a history of right ventricle (*RV*) endocardial pacemaker. *RA* right atrium

formation [25] (Fig. 13.6). In a large study using TEE, a Chiari network was seen in 2 % [26]. Chiari network is frequently associated with a PFO (83 %), right-to-left shunting (55 %), and an ASA (24 %). Fine networks may be difficult to visualize with CT or MRI. With special right heart imaging techniques to clearly opacify the right atrium, a Chiari network may be seen in selected MDCT studies (Fig. 13.6).

Atrial Septal Aneurysm

An ASA is another important anatomic feature to consider in evaluating a PFO. The incidence of ASA is 4.6–10 % [27–29] by TEE. An ASA is associated with a PFO with a prevalence of 30–60 % [30–32] and is most likely associated with an increased rate of embolic events [33]. The prevalence of an ASA in patients with cerebral ischemia and normal carotid arteries is higher (28 %) than in patients without cerebral ischemia (10 %) [29]. An ASA can easily be assessed by CT and MRI. In one study with MDCT, an ASA was seen in 4 % of patients, and 63 % of patients with ASA were found to have a left-to-right shunt [12] (Fig. 13.5). An ASA is defined as a bulging of >15 mm beyond the plane of the atrial septum [34] and classified according to Hanley's diagnostic criteria by Pearson [33] into two types based on the direction and timing of protrusion. Generally, right atrial protrusion is the most common (76 %) and usually shows transient motion toward the left atrium during systole or with the Valsalva maneuver [33] (Fig. 13.7). Increased interatrial septum mobility is believed to enhance the probability of paradoxical embolism by mechanically directing blood flow from the IVC through the PFO into the left atrium.

Persistent Eustachian Valve in Adults

The Eustachian valve (EV), which guards the anterior-inferior aspect of the IVC, is a remnant of the embryonic right valve of the sinus venosus. Embryologically, the EV directs oxygenated blood from the IVC across the PFO into the systemic circulation [35] (Fig. 13.8). By directing the blood from the IVC to the interatrial septum, a persistent EV may prevent spontaneous closure of the PFO after birth and may, therefore, indirectly predispose to paradoxical embolism. A prominent EV is a common finding in CT or MRI studies of the heart and thorax and should not be mistaken with a thrombus.

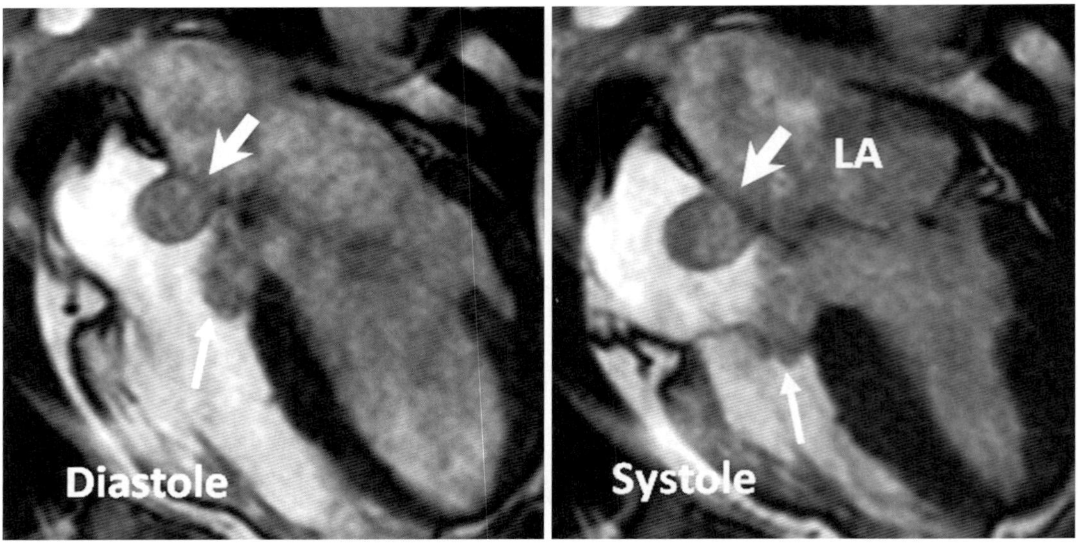

Fig. 13.7 Large atrial septal aneurysm (*thick arrows*) with persistent protrusion into the right atrium during cardiac cycle. A relatively large membranous septum aneurysm also exists (*thin arrows*)

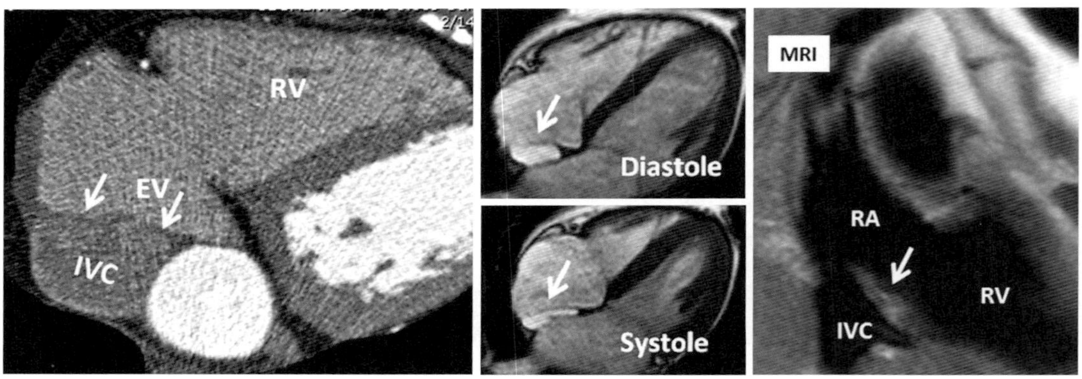

Fig. 13.8 Prominent Eustachian valve (*EV*) shown on axial CT and MR images (*arrows*). The EV guards the anterior-inferior aspect of the inferior vena cava (*IVC*). Note variation in morphology on systolic and diastolic images. *RA* right atrium, *RV* right ventricle

Cardiac MR Techniques

In general, MR protocols for intracardiac shunts contain most of the routine sequences. The choice of sequences and extent of coverage depend on the anatomy of interest. For example, in PDA analysis, MR angiography of the great vessels is necessary and the choice of cine and phase-contrast sequences can be individualized. As an another example, the entire chest is covered when looking for partial anomalous pulmonary venous return (PAPVR). An overview of MR protocol is listed below.

Protocol

Positioning

Scout images will be obtained in supine. Table repositioning will be made to place the anatomy of interest (i.e., interatrial septum) at the magnet isocenter.

Morphological Imaging

Two-dimensional axial, sagittal, and coronal images to define cardiovascular anatomy. Both dark- and bright-blood images are acquired with half-Fourier fast-spin-echo and balanced

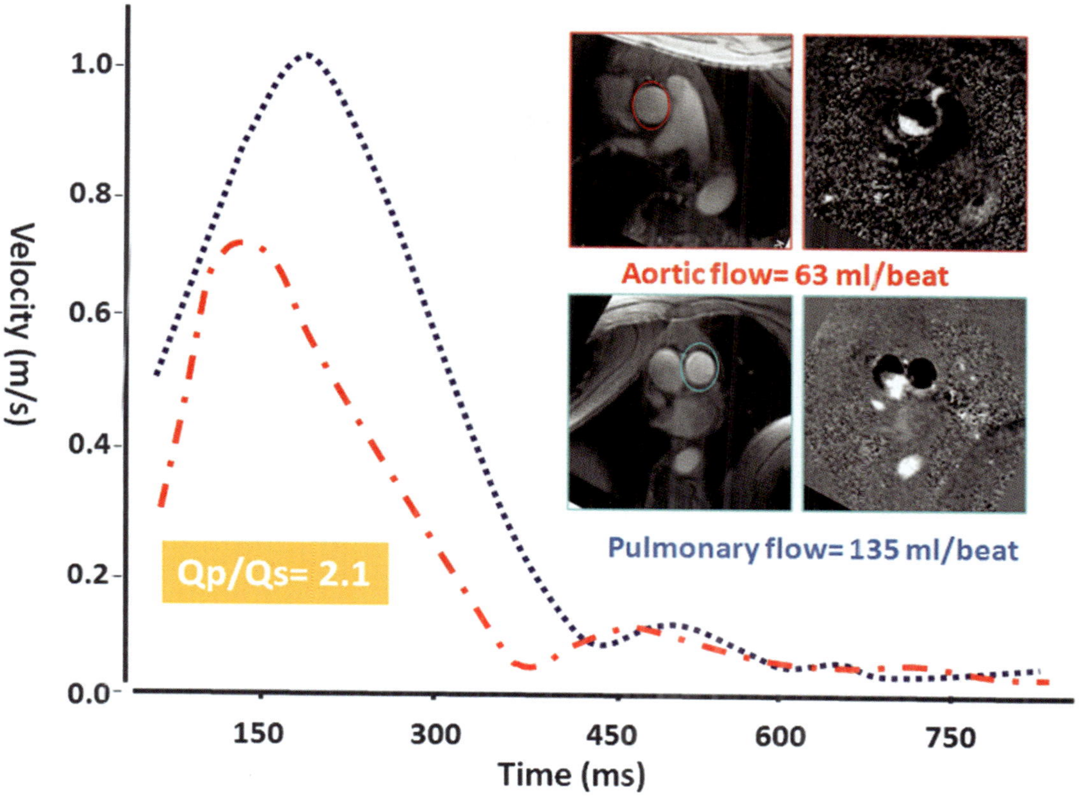

Fig. 13.9 Qp/Qs ratio assessment in a patient with ASD showing 2:1 shunt ratio. Slice position for phase-contrast MRI in the ascending aorta and pulmonary trunk is approximately 2.0 cm above the respected valve

steady-state free-precession (b-SSFP) sequences, respectively. Slice thickness of 6- and 2-mm interslice gap are enough.

Cine Imaging

It is for initial assessment of the intracardiac shunts and analysis of ventricular function. A segmented b-SSFP sequence is used with retrospective ECG gating during repeated 8-s breath holds (slice thickness, 8 mm; no gap). Standard long axis images will be obtained to cover the entire heart from the apex to the atrial base. In our institution, 4-chamber or axial views of the entire heart are obtained in all patients. With a matrix of 256, typical in-plane resolution is 1.7–1.4 mm. Temporal resolution will be 35 ms/phase.

Velocity-Encoded Imaging

Phase-contrast (PC) techniques include direct and indirect assessments of the shunt. Indirect assessment consists of comparing flow in the pulmonary artery (Qp) and aorta (Qs) (Fig. 13.9). Velocity-encoded images are generally acquired using a retrospective vector-ECG gating during repeated expiratory 12–18-s breath holds. Retrospective vector-ECG gating is used in almost all PC MR protocols to include end-diastolic flow. Breath hold technique is preferred to free breathing especially for direct assessment of shunt. For indirect shunt volume measurement, a free-breathing method with multiple measurements (number of excitations = 3–4) can be used to increase precision [36, 37].

Typical parameters are as follows: slice thickness, 5–6 mm; in-plane resolution, 1.5–2 mm; 18–20 reconstructed heart phases (temporal resolution, 25–30 ms/phase); flip angle 25°; and echo time, 2.8–3.0 ms. Velocity-encoding values differ depending on the anatomy and location and size of shunt. General values include 70–100 cm/s for

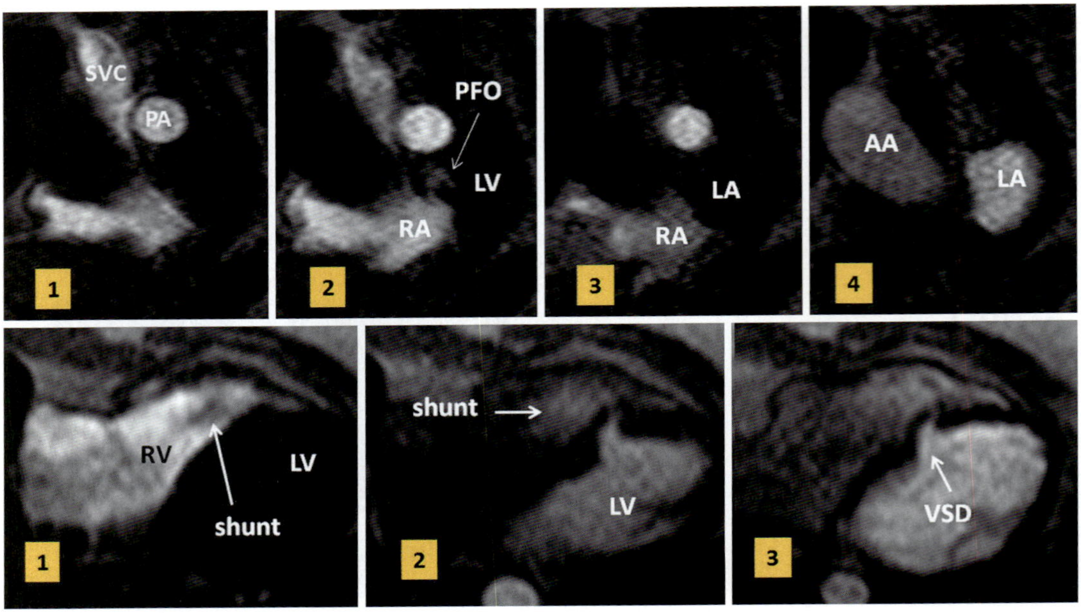

Fig. 13.10 *Upper row*: first-pass MR angiograms in a patient with patent foramen ovale (*PFO*). Short axis series during the Valsalva at atrial level show a small puff of contrast (*arrow*) from right to left at the level of PFO on the third image which disappeared on image 4. *Lower row*: small muscular ventricular septal defect (*VSD*) with left-to-right shunt is shown on first-pass MR angiogram. On the first image, non-enhanced blood is passed into the right ventricle (*RV*). On the second image, contrast-enhanced blood is shunted from the left ventricle (*LV*) into the right through a muscular VSD. *SVC* superior vena cava, *PA* pulmonary artery, *RA* right atrium, *LA* left atrium, *AA* ascending aorta

ASD, 100–200 for VSDs, 100–300 cm/s for PDA, and 150–250 cm/s for arteries.

MR Angiography (MRA)

Three-dimensional gadolinium-enhanced MRA using fast gradient-echo sequence provides further evaluation of any PAPVR. Coronal views are preferred to cover entire heart and major vessels. Alternatively, non-ECG-gated time-resolved MRA can be performed. In case of ASD, 10 mL of gadolinium-based contrast agent followed by a 20-mL saline flush at a flow rate of 5 mL/s will be injected and axial image is obtained. Shunts can be evaluated visually or by analysis of time-intensity curves extracted from measurements within the left atrium, right atrium, and pulmonary vein ostia. This technique has been described for diagnosis of patent foramen ovale during the Valsalva [15]. It can similarly be utilized in selected cases (without or with Valsalva) for diagnosis of other intracardiac shunts. Second alternative is a saturation-recovery gradient-echo sequence commonly used for myocardial perfusion imaging. It will be modified to a non-ECG-gated sequence to acquire continuous data at 6 frames per second during a proper Valsalva maneuver [17] (Fig. 13.10).

Shunt Quantification

MR velocity and flow quantification is mainly performed by PC velocity-encoding (VEC) sequences, which elicit contrast from the phase of a spin's transverse magnetization [38, 39] (Fig. 13.11).

TEE usually allows exact localization and sizing of the shunt defect. However, determination of shunt volumes by Doppler echocardiography has limitations [40]. TEE is semi-invasive and might have limitations in visualization of adjacent structures and anomalous venous return. Invasive oximetry using Fick's principle is the gold standard for the quantification of left-to-right shunting

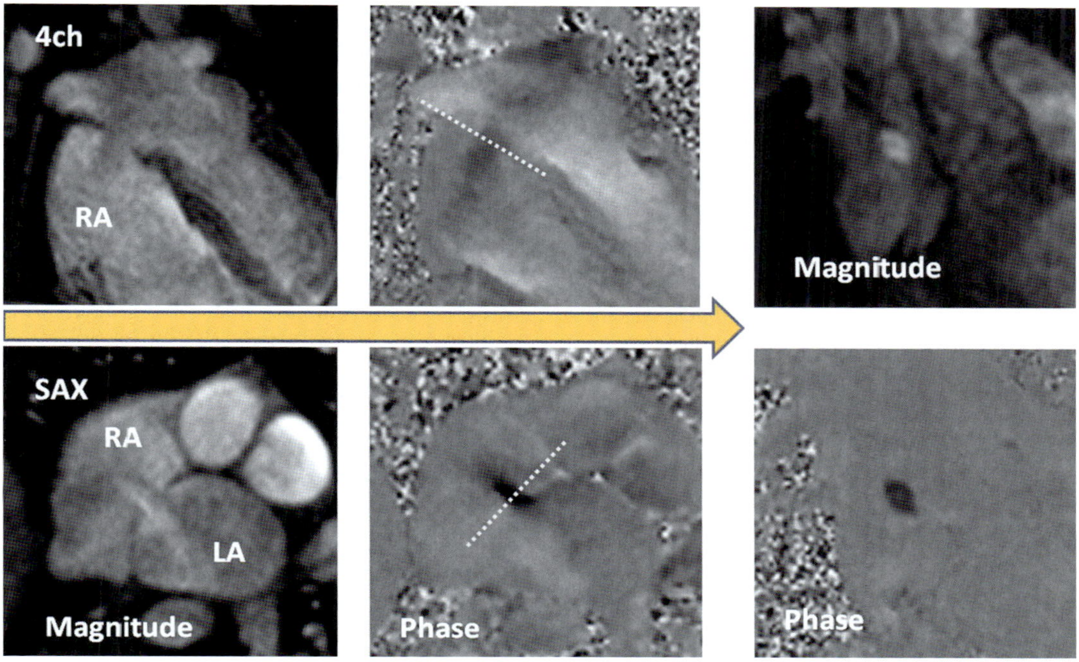

Fig. 13.11 Steps to obtain the optimal imaging plane for en face VEC MR of secundum ASD. It is important to know that the ASD flow direction is not often orthogonal to the plane of the interatrial septum and that the interatrial septum moves during cardiac cycle. To take into account these facts, two orthogonal phase-contrast images along the plane of shunt flow will be obtained. Using these reference planes, final phase-contrast image will be acquired perpendicular to the jet of flow close to the atrial septum and when the shunt flow is maximum. *LA* left atrium, *RA* right atrium

based on measurements of blood oxygenation but is not without limitations [41, 42].

In VEC MR, the phase of flowing protons relative to stationary protons along a magnetic gradient changes in proportion to flow velocity [38]. The change in phase angle is mapped on phase images, and flow velocity is computed with a standard formula. To determine flow volume across a shunt or vessel lumen, the spatial mean velocity of the area of interest is multiplied by the cross section of that area and repeated at each cine frame using automated or semiautomated methods available in most workstations. The region of interest around the blood vessel in each frame may require redrawing for motion and vessel compliance during the cycle. VEC MR imaging flow measurements taken at multiple (usually 16 or 32) evenly spaced points in the cardiac cycle can be plotted against time to construct a flow curve. The area under the curve can be integrated to derive flow volume for a given cardiac cycle.

Technical Considerations

Through-plane flow encoding of the septal defect or a vessel should be assessed in a plane perpendicular to main direction of flow. Underestimation of velocity and flow can result if the target structure is not imaged in a plane perpendicular to flow or if partial volume averaging occurs [43, 44]. Thick slices and volume averaging cause underestimation of flow. The estimation of flow can still be corrected up to 15° deviation from the orthogonal imaging plane. Up to this angle, the increase in vessel area is compensated for by the increase in partial volume effects [43]. Aliasing may occur if the selected velocity-encoding value is lower than the actual peak velocity at any time during the cardiac cycle. Care must be taken not to set the velocity-encoding values too high as this will increase the noise. Noise peaks may interfere with measurement of the peak velocity; however, the estimation of flow is less affected because the noise is averaged over cross-sectional area of the targeted structure [44, 45]. For small vessels, if the vessel diameter is less than 2–2.5 mm (four to eight pixels), accuracy of flow measurements may suffer [46]. Shimming of the magnet before scanning is necessary to compensate for local field inhomogeneity. Faster acquisition is the key to improve phase-offset errors that can occur between bipolar gradients in PC MR. Single breath hold probably causes less artifacts compared to long free-breathing acquisition that may take of 2–3 min. A recent study has shown higher value for pulmonary flow in breath hold technique compared with free-breathing method [47]. Low cardiac output value is expected in retrospective method compared with prospective technique. Therefore, same method should be used for follow-up examinations. In routine practice, the TE is kept short to minimize the time interval in which these phenomena can develop [48]. For technical reason, there is a limit to our ability to shorten the TE to a certain limit. Correct positioning of the patient is another important factor. It would cause less error when the anatomy of interest (i.e., interatrial septum) is placed as close as possible to the magnet isocenter [17]. Phase-offset errors such as those from nonlinear gradients increase with distance from the isocenter. With technological advances in MR imaging, faster data acquisition in single breath hold is possible. Parallel imaging techniques continue to improve and higher acceleration factor can be used in clinical practice. Unfortunately, parallel imaging accelerates acquisition at the expense of a lower signal-to-noise ratio. Therefore, combination with parallel imaging is only recommended when signal-to-noise ratio is not of critical importance for diagnostic image quality.

Aortic and Pulmonary Flow Quantification

VEC MR is an accurate method to measure the amount of shunt. Left-to-right shunting can be calculated indirectly by measuring flow Qp/Qs ration which is the ratio of right ventricle stroke volume to left ventricle stroke volume. For Qp/Qs ratio, VEC MR is shown to correlate well with echocardiography, invasive oximetry, and radionuclide angiography, although this approach does not provide information about the size, shape, or location of a defect [37, 46, 49–53]. Using VEC MR, a 5 % difference between flow in the ascending aorta and flow in the pulmonary artery in healthy individuals is calculated [49, 54]. Therefore, although Qp/Qs measurement by VEC MR may correlate with true shunt severity, this approach is limited when the shunt volume is small. In this case, direct shunt volume measurement is preferred.

Slice position in the ascending aorta is approximately 2.0–3.0 cm above the aortic valve and distal to the coronary arteries at the level of the right pulmonary artery (Fig. 13.9). Slice position in the pulmonary trunk is approximately 1.5–2.0 cm above the pulmonary valve but proximal to the bifurcation. Placing the imaging plane at level of valve should be avoided due to turbulent flow and valve motion. Some have suggested to place the aortic slice at level of coronary artery ostium to include coronary blood flow [55], although this level of slice selection does not seem to be a good choice as the cross-sectional area of the aorta at sinus of Valsalva especially at the level of left main coronary ostium is larger than the aorta above it and may interfere with correct flow calculations. Flow measurements in the ascending aorta distal to the coronary ostia would miss coronary blood flow. For this technical limitation, some have suggested to use Qp/Qs ratios of >1.75:1 as PC MRI threshold for surgery. In reality, diastolic flow into the coronary arteries is minimal (0.5 % of the cardiac output) [56] and even smaller than the errors expected from the PC technique of measurements to cause additional problem. Left-to-right shunts in ASD and VSD are calculated by the following formula: percentage of left-to-right shunt = (Qp–Qs)/Qp. In PDA, it would be (Qs–Qp)/Qs.

Direct Imaging of the Shunt

VEC MR analysis of the outflow tracts is simple, reliable, and straightforward in execution. In a recent study of 35 adult patients with ASD, VSD, and PDA, PC MRI was referenced to transthoracic echo and found to have 93 % specificity and 100 % sensitivity for description of

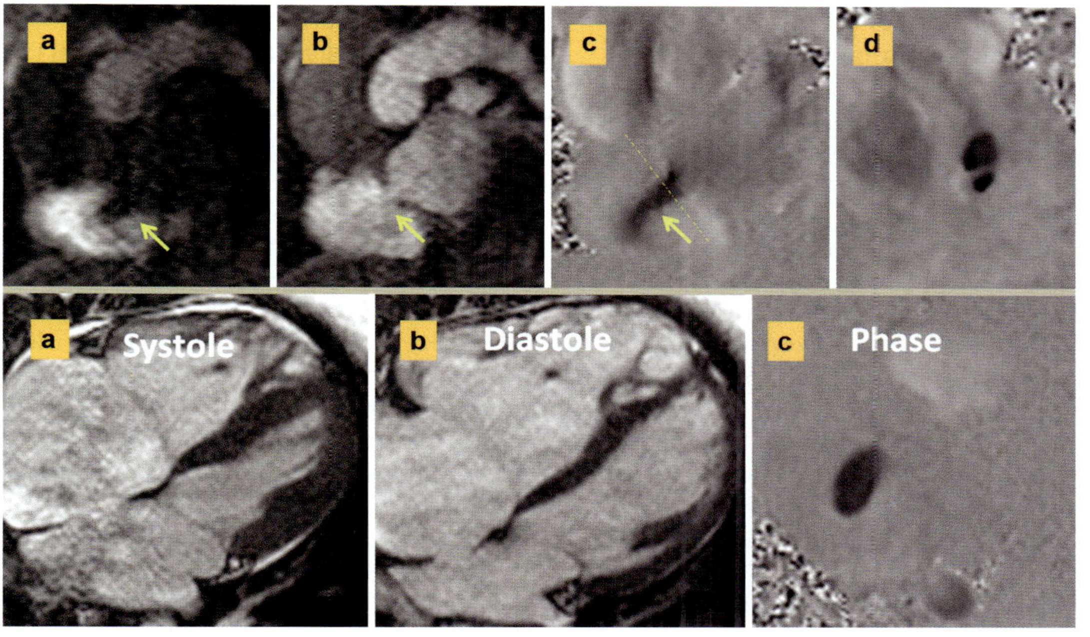

Fig. 13.12 Septum secundum ASD. *Upper row*: (**a** and **b**) are short axis first-pass MR angiographies at the level of ASD. Left-to-right shunt is shown as a negative band in the right atrium in (**a**). This is best confirmed on phase-contrast image (**c**). (**d**) Through-plane phase image shows a double-barrel ASD. *Lower row*: different case shows ASD diameters change with cardiac cycle. The maximum diameter is usually at ventricular systole (**a**) when the atria are largest. Smaller length is seen in diastole (**b**). Typical oval-shaped ASD at the time of maximal flow is shown in the phase image (**c**)

shunts with a Qp:Qs greater than 1.5 [57]. In contrast, direct measurement of shunt flow through the defect requires more experience and precision to get correct results. With direct shunt imaging, flow quantification, as well as size, and morphology analysis are possible which may have incremental clinical value especially for percutaneous closure candidates. The technique of direct en face shunt analysis is described in detail for ASD by Thompson et al. [17] and good correlations with echocardiography in adults were reported. In children, direct flow measurements may be difficult and inaccurate compared with Qp/Qs [37]. This is probably because in children higher heart and respiratory rates, along with higher peak velocities and smaller structures, can lead to increased error on VEC MR [51]. Newer sequences such as 4D phase-contrast sequence can improve visualization of cardiac shunts compared to conventional cardiac MR imaging.

The first step for direct shunt analysis is to review the cine images visually and determine whether flow can be detected (i.e., across the interatrial septum). If shunt is not visible on cine images, still PC images will be obtained at the level of septum to completely rule it out.

Velocity encoding is initially set low (60 cm/s) to ensure sensitivity for lower blood velocities.

Three contiguous through-plane PC slices will be acquired parallel to the septum with the middle cut in the septum. If the shunt is seen, through-plane VEC MR should be obtained perpendicular to the direction of shunt flow rather than simply perpendicular to the morphological plane of the septal defect [17]. To minimize errors, all phases of cine images will be reviewed and the imaging planes are prescribed at the time when the shunt flow is maximal (i.e., end-systole). Defect area is also measured by planimetry when shunt flow is maximal (Fig. 13.12).

Classification of Interatrial Communications

Secundum ASD

Secundum ASD is the most common ASD usually seen in middle-aged women [1]. It may be discovered in routine clinical examinations or imaging study of the heart as it is asymptomatic in 90 % of cases. Symptoms include palpitation, atypical chest pain, or those related to paradoxical embolism. Imaging demonstration of morphological variations in size, position, and shape of secundum ASD is important particularly since the widespread use of transcatheter closure techniques. Secundum ASD can be divided into two types depending on location [58]. Type one is the result of abnormal development of the septum primum [59] and is seen in 85 % of cases [58] (Fig. 13.13). In type one, the limbus is intact. The defect is usually oval shaped with a mean size of 1.8–2.8 cm on MR measurements [17]. The size of defect changes with cardiac cycle (Fig. 13.12). The defect area is usually reduced concentrically [60]. The most common location of defect is central with one or multiple holes (fenestrated) [58, 61]. Other variants include complete absence of the flap valve and an anterosuperior defect. Type two is less common (15 %). This type is characterized by abnormal development of the septum secundum or superior limbus of the fossa ovalis resulting in a superiorly located large ASD and an intact septum primum. The atrial roof without any substantial rim forms the superior border of the defect. This is in contrast to superior sinus venosus defects, in which the interatrial communication is located posterosuperior to the normally developed superior limbus. It seems that the two forms of secundum ASD have different pathogenesis.

Sinus Venosus Defects

Sinus venosus defects are relatively uncommon forms of interatrial communication (<15 %) [62, 63]. These abnormal venoatrial communications produce shunting between the two atria as a result of anomalous pulmonary venous connection to

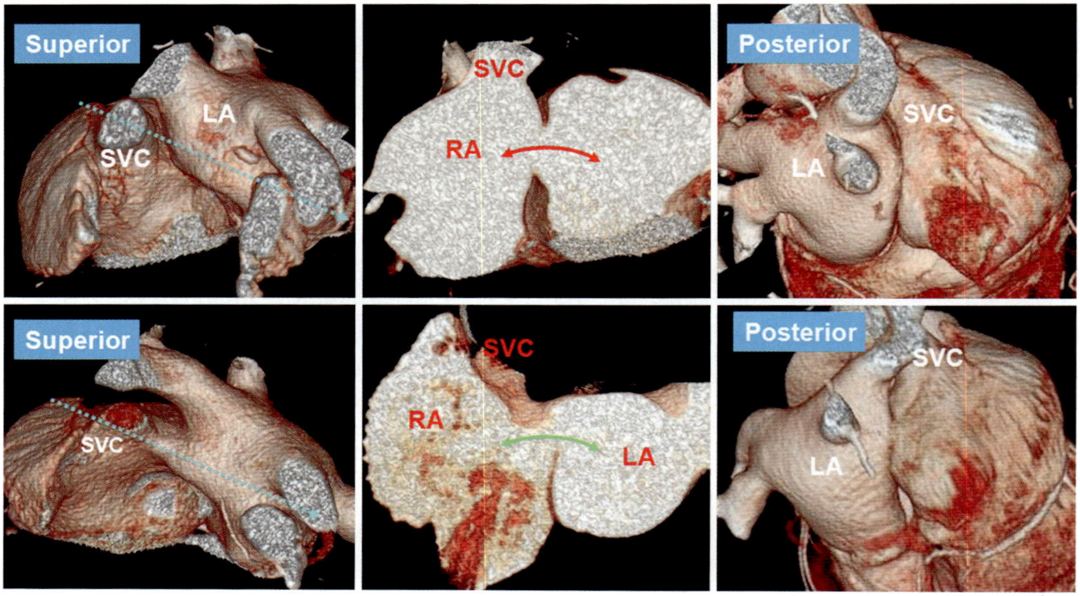

Fig. 13.13 Type 1 (*upper row*) and type 2 (*lower row*) of secundum ASD. Anterosuperior views show incomplete development of the interatrial groove in the superior aspect of the septum in type 2 secundum ASD causing a superiorly located defect (*curved green arrow*) and an intact septum primum compared with type 1 in which the defect is central in the septum primum (*curved red arrow*) but the superior groove is well formed. Note that posterior groove is relatively well developed in both conditions. *Dashed arrows* (*left images*) show the cross-sectional cuts through the ASD shown on the *middle images*

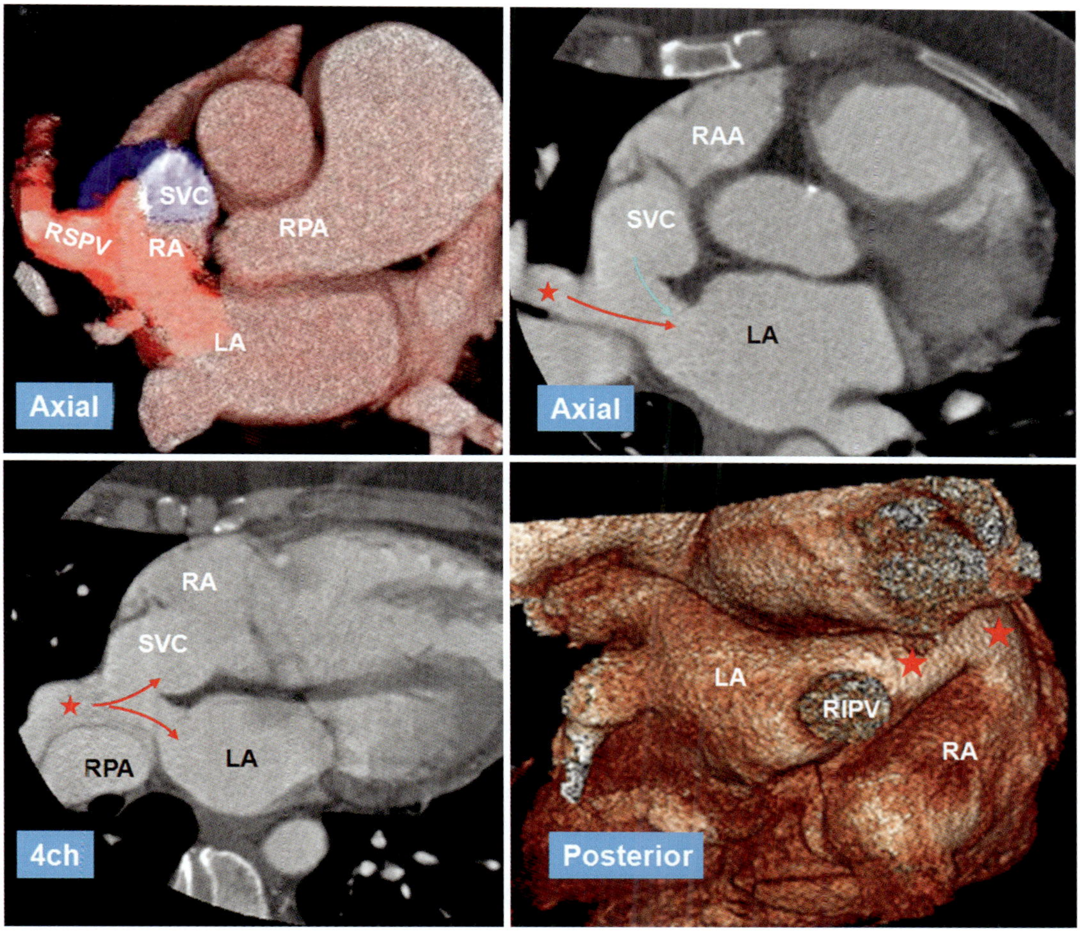

Fig. 13.14 CT images in 56-year-old female referred for evaluation of right heart enlargement and pulmonary hypertension showing sinus venosus defect as a result of anomalous connection of the right superior pulmonary vein (*RSPV*) (*red stars*) to the superior vena cava (*SVC*) while maintaining its connection to the left atrium (*LA*) (venous-venous malformation). Overriding of RSPV above the septal defect is shown on four-chamber view (*4ch*). Pulmonary flow (*red arrows*) and systemic SVC flow (*blue arrow*) can enter both atria. Posterior volume-rendered view shows RSPV bridging (*red stars*) between the two atria. *LA* left atrium, *RA* right atrium, *RIPV* right inferior pulmonary vein, *RPA* right pulmonary vein, *RAA* right atrial appendage

one of the caval veins (venous-venous malformation) while retaining its connection to the left atrium (Fig. 13.14) or an abnormal vena cava with a large hole at its ostium that overrides the intact rim of the fossa ovalis [64–67] (Fig. 13.15). The caval vein can therefore participate in the formation of a large interatrial communication outside the confines of the fossa ovalis. In other words, this anomaly would be correctly defined as an anomalous venoatrial communication rather than representing an interatrial communication.

Two variants are described, superior and inferior. The superior variant is related to the SVC and the inferior variant is in connection with the IVC. The inferior variant is rare and usually diagnosed in children [68]. The crucial anatomic and imaging diagnostic element is the establishment of the integrity of the rims of the oval fossa. Association with PAPVR exists in more than 90 % of cases [69], most commonly involving the right superior pulmonary vein. Involvement of the left pulmonary veins is rare. Abnormal pulmonary venous

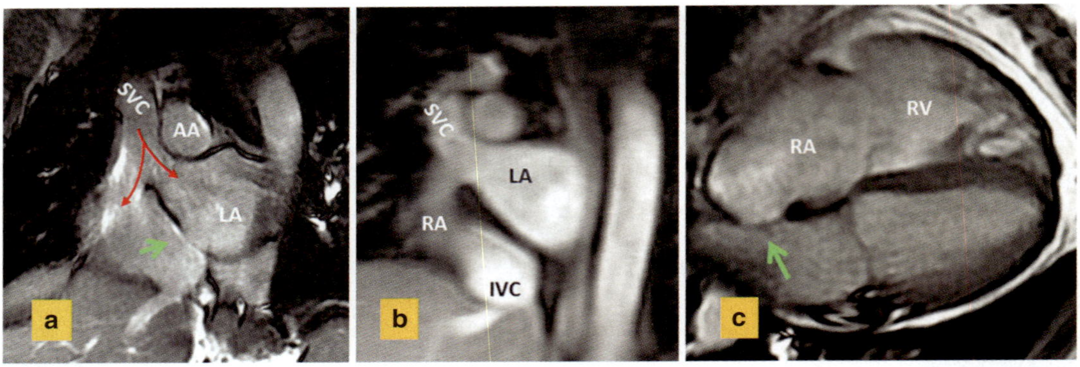

Fig. 13.15 Sinus venosus ASD in 55-year-old male with right heart enlargement. (**a**) Short axis cine view and (**b**) MR angiogram at basal level of the heart show the superior vena cava (*SVC*) riding over the superior septal defect with blood (*red arrows*) flowing into both the right atrium (*RA*) and the left atrium (*LA*). (**c**) Four-chamber view shows dilated RA and right ventricle (*RV*). Intact fossa ovalis is shown by *green arrows*. *AA* ascending aorta, *IVC* inferior vena cava

connections are not a prerequisite for diagnosis and can exist with other types of ASD. It is also possible for the SVC to remain connected to the right atrium only, without any overriding.

Sinus venosus defects may remain asymptomatic until the third or fourth decade of life despite substantial left-to-right shunting [1]. The hemodynamic abnormality is similar to other shuntings between the atria, and it is not possible based on clinical features to differentiate the sinus venosus defect from other forms of interatrial communications [70]. Increased blood flow through the right heart chambers may eventually lead to right ventricular failure. There is threefold greater risk of developing pulmonary arterial hypertension in patients with sinus venosus defects and developing it at younger age than patients with secundum ASD, which highlights the need for correct diagnosis [71].

Accurate demonstration of the abnormal anatomic pathway allows the surgeon either to patch or to baffle the pulmonary and caval pathways to the appropriate atrium without causing obstruction or permitting a residual shunt. Comprehensive imaging diagnosis of sinus venosus defect can be challenging. TEE is superior to the transthoracic approach in adults, with only one-quarter of the defects being correctly diagnosed in transthoracic echocardiography [72]. The majority of diagnostic difficulties arise from the poor acoustic windows. Even with TEE using conventional scan planes, the defect can be missed [73]. Demonstration of PAPVR with TEE is also challenging and in some cases can be frustrating especially for veins that connect to SVC more than 2 cm above the superior cavoatrial junction. Such information is crucial if surgical intervention is being considered. Adult patients with left-to-right shunting and enlarged right heart shown by transthoracic echocardiography should be further evaluated with MRI or CT (Fig. 13.14).

Both CT and MRI are great imaging methods to evaluate these abnormalities particularly for the diagnosis of anomalous pulmonary venous return [74, 75]. It is not uncommon to see a PAPVR with secundum ASD [66]. In an echocardiographic review by al Zaghal [66], 4 of 11 defects initially reported as superior type of sinus venous defect were found to be within the fossa ovalis with abnormal connection of the pulmonary veins to the right atrium in three cases. Therefore, distinction of the septal boundaries is crucial in providing solid criteria for diagnosis. Any problem in formation of superior part of interatrial septum will result in type 2 secundum ASD as described earlier (Fig. 13.13). Communications outside the confines of the true septum can take the form of sinus venosus defects, coronary sinus (CS) defects, and atrioventricular septal defect (AVSD) of "ostium primum" variety [66].

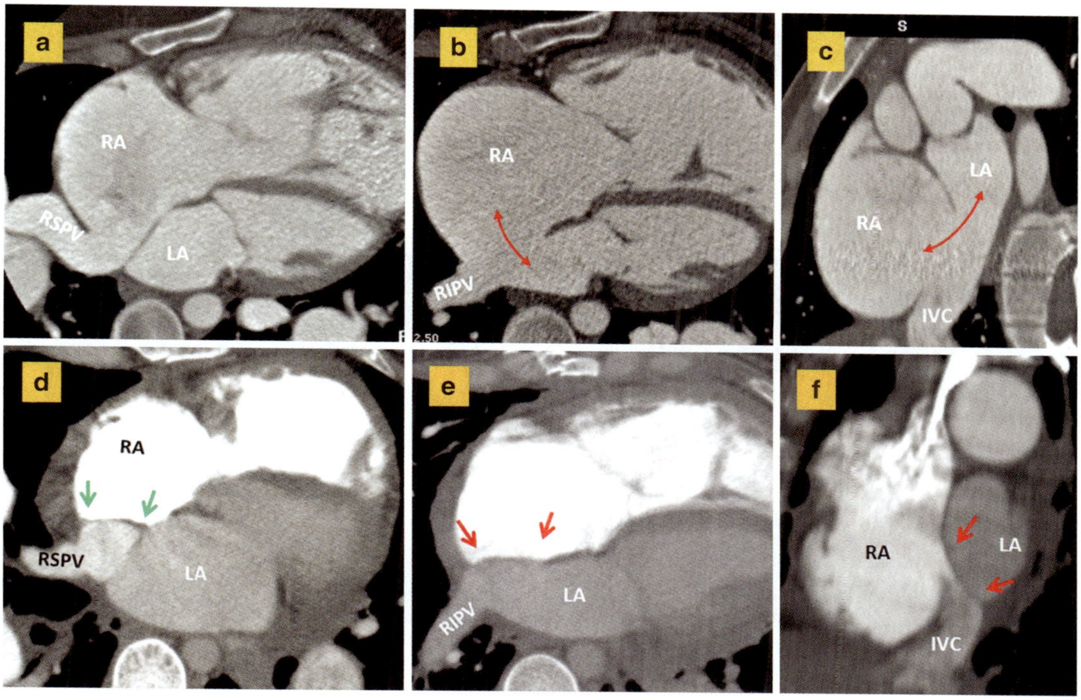

Fig. 13.16 (**a–c**) CT images before surgery show anomalous drainage of the right superior pulmonary vein (*RSPV*) into the right atrium (*RA*) in association with a large atrial septal defect (*double-headed arrows*) involving inferior aspect of the interatrial septum. Short axis image (**c**) shows large inferior septal defect and overriding of the inferior vena cava (*IVC*) over both atria making it difficult to differentiate a large secundum defect from an inferior sinus venosus defect. (**d–f**) Corresponding after surgery images show closure of the atrial septal defect (*between red arrows*) and baffling of the RSPV flow (*between green arrows*) into the left atrium. The right inferior pulmonary vein (*RIPV*) is normally draining into the left atrium (*LA*)

The diagnosis of inferior variant can be more difficult. Again, it is important to find the fossa ovalis rim intact. The Eustachian valve should not be mistaken with inferior border of the defect.

In contrast to superior variant, PAPVR is uncommon in the inferior sinus venosus defect [76], and overriding of the IVC appears to be the cause (Fig. 13.16). If the pulmonary vein participates in abnormal connection to the IVC, then it should continue its normal course to connect to the left atrium [67]. If the pulmonary vein did not maintain normal connection to the left atrium, the IVC would connect only to the right atrium, resulting in partial return to the IVC (scimitar) or the inferior right atrium.

Atrioventricular Septal Defect

Detailed AVSD is described in Chap. 17. In AVSD, the atria and the ventricles are separated by a common AV valve with one valve ring [77]. This common valve consists of five leaflets: a superior (anterior) bridging leaflet, an inferior (posterior) bridging leaflet, a left mural leaflet, a right mural leaflet, and a right anterolateral leaflet. A constant imaging feature is loss of normal offsetting of atrioventricular valves. Two morphologies are described, complete and partial [77]. Partial form is more common. In a complete AVSD, one single valve orifice exists. In the partial form, the free margins of the bridging leaflets are fused, creating two separate valve orifices sharing a common valve ring. Unlike a normal two leaflet mitral valve, in partial AVSD, the left AV valve (cleft mitral) has three leaflets. An intermediate or transitional AVSD is also described showing two valves with ASD and VSD. In complete AVSD, there is usually an ostium primum ASD and a large VSD between

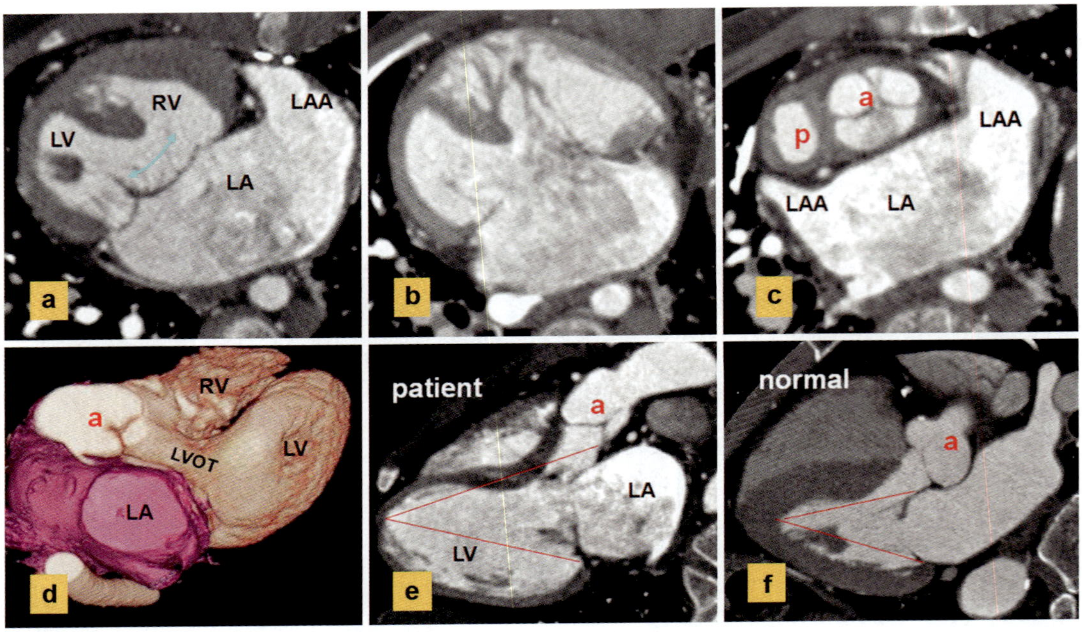

Fig. 13.17 CT images show a single atrium, left atrial isomerism, and dextrocardia. Status post-Fontan and main pulmonary artery exclusion. (**a**, **b**) Complete AVSD with a large inlet ventricular septal defect (*curved arrow*). (**c**) shows unwedging of the aortic root (*a*). (**d**, **e**) show elongation of the left ventricle (*LV*) outflow tract (*LVOT*) causing longer distance of the aortic valve to LV apex compared to the distance from apex to atrioventricular ring. Normally, the two distances are equal (**f**). (**f**) Normal example. *P* pulmonary, *LAA* left atrial appendage, *RV* right ventricle

the common valve and the crest of the interventricular septum. In a partial AVSD, the bridging leaflets fuse to the crest of the interventricular septum, leaving only an ostium primum ASD. They may also fuse with the atrial septum, leaving only a VSD. The potential for left-to-right shunting is related to the bridging leaflets being attached to the atrial septum, to the ventricular septum, or floating within the AVSD [77–80].

Another characteristic feature of AVSD is the anterior and rightward displacement of the aorta in relation to the common AV junction causing an "unwedged" aorta with a narrowed elongated left ventricle outflow tract (LVOT). LVOT elongation creates the characteristic "gooseneck deformity" on left ventriculography and unequal distances from the LV apex to the inlet and outlet valves. Normally, the two distances are equal (Fig. 13.17). Subaortic narrowing/stenosis is particularly notable in partial defects with an ostium primum ASD where the superior bridging leaflet is firmly fixed to the crest of the ventricular septum. Unwedging of aorta can lead to a displacement of the AV conduction tissue and its abnormality.

Most primum ASDs are relatively large and lead to right heart dilation. Because of the trileaflet nature of the left AV valve (the so-called cleft mitral valve), valvular regurgitation is common whereas valvular stenosis is rare [78]. A parachute-type or double-orifice "mitral" valve may be present [78]. Complex forms of AVSD are found in the majority of hearts with right atrial isomerism and in around half with left atrial isomerism. The former tends to have univentricular hearts, often with a common atrium, while the latter tends to have biventricular hearts [79] (Fig. 13.17). In atrial isomerism, the common AV valve usually has four leaflets: a large anterosuperior leaflet, two lateral leaflets, and a posteroinferior leaflet [80].

In most patients with AVSD, the ventricles are similarly sized (balanced AVSD). In a minority of cases, the common AV junction is committed to one ventricle leading to hypoplasia of the

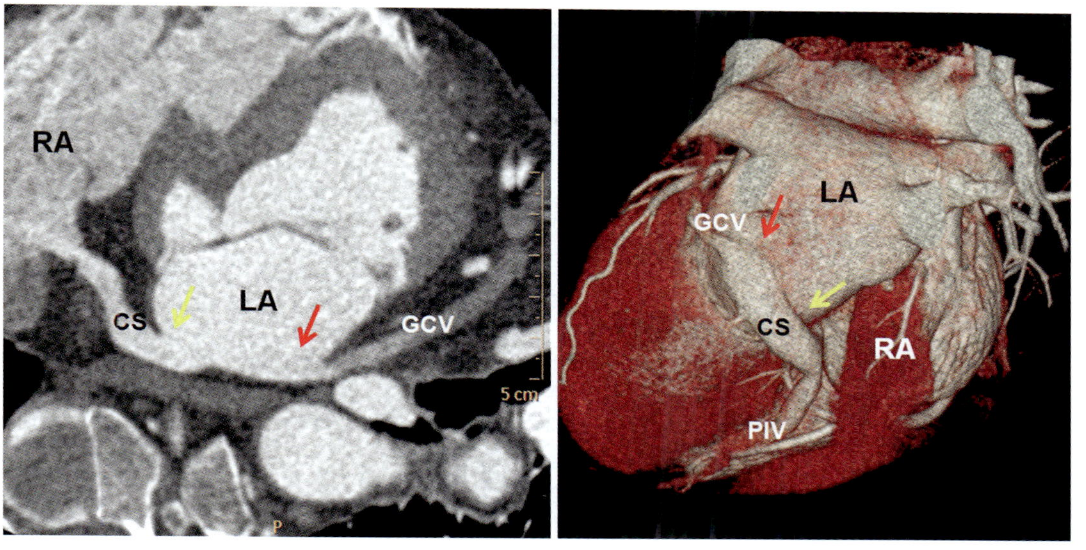

Fig. 13.18 Unroofed coronary sinus (*CS*) shown by CT. Large area of deficient CS roof (*between arrows*) is shown connecting its lumen with the left atrium (*LA*) cavity. No left superior vena cava was seen. The ostium of the CS connecting to the right atrium (*RA*) appears normal. *GCV* great cardiac vein, *PIV* posterior interventricular vein (Courtesy of Professor Se Hwan Kwon, College of Medicine, Kyung Hee University, Seoul, Republic of Korea)

opposing ventricle. Extreme commitment of the common AV junction to the left ventricle has been termed "double inlet LV with a common valve" [80]. Only a limited number of articles about MR and CT of AVSD exist. In one study of imaging analysis of AVSD, MRI was more accurate than echocardiography in predicting the size of the VSD and diagnosis of ventricular hypoplasia [81].

Fenestrated (Unroofed) Coronary Sinus

Anomalies of the coronary sinus may occur as isolated findings of little functional importance or as part of the spectrum of CHD findings. Fenestrated (unroofed) CS is rare and involves 1 % of all ASDs [82, 83]. Several anatomic variations have been described, ranging from complete absence of the walls between the CS and the left atrium to one or more partial fenestrations. In 2/3 of cases, partial communication is in the mid-portion and in 1/3 in the terminal portion of the CS (Fig. 13.18). In three-quarters of cases, there is either persistence of the left SVC or other findings of the CHD especially secundum ASD. It is relatively common in heterotaxy syndrome when there is isomerism of the left atrial appendages and in tricuspid atresia [84, 85] (see Chap. 31). In one series of partial CS fenestration, half of the cases were missed during previous cardiovascular surgery [84]. In adults, fenestrated CS is usually found incidentally as part of imaging workup of patients with history of surgery for CHD or as an isolated finding. Because of the small defect, the hemodynamic effect of the right-to-left shunting can be negligible. However, there is always the risk of stroke or brain abscess due to paradoxical embolism. Given the higher resolution and three-dimensional nature of reconstructed data, the diagnosis of CS fenestration may be easier in cardiac CT compared with MRI and echocardiography [86, 87].

ASD Closure

Indications for ASD closure are right atrial and right ventricular dilation, ASD size >1 cm, and Qp/Qs of 1.5 or greater. ASD closure is not recommended in severe pulmonary hypertension and very small defects. Small defects can be followed with imaging. Surgical closure is required for patients with ostium primum and sinus

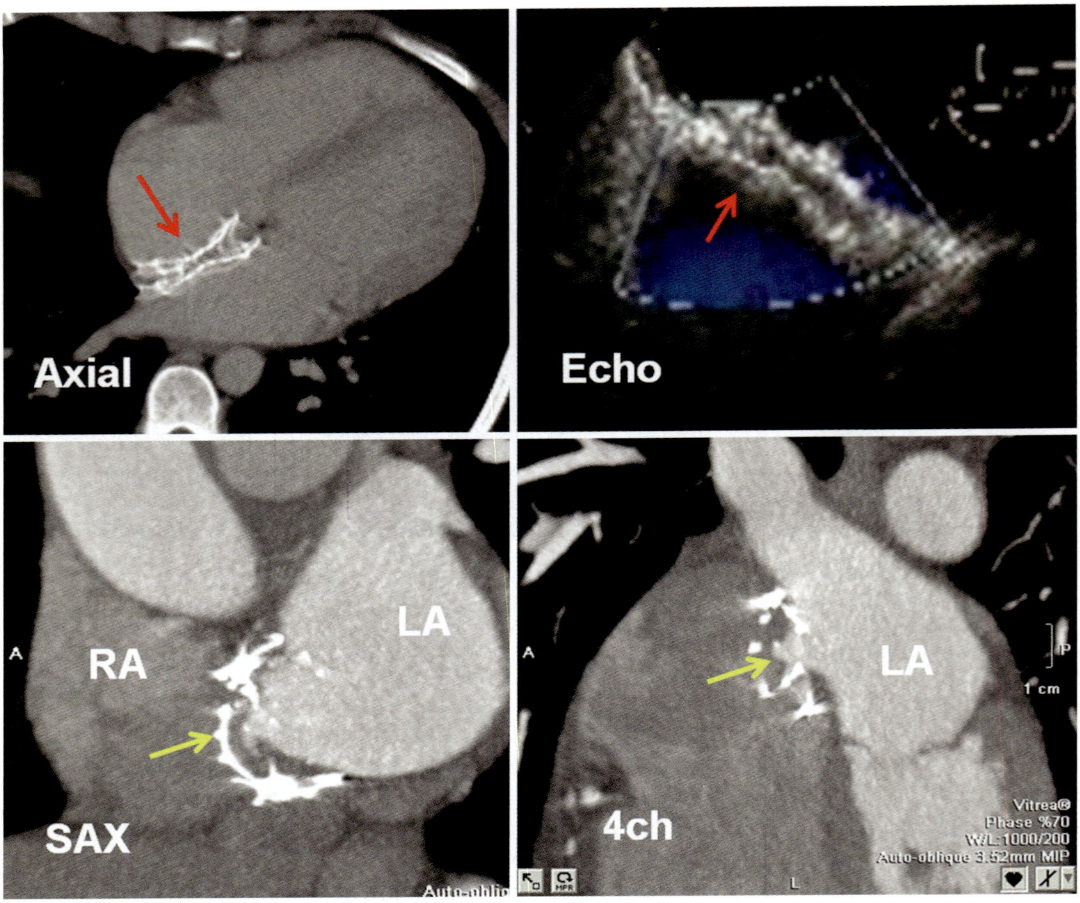

Fig. 13.19 Amplatzer septal occluders (*red arrows*) and Cardioseal device (*yellow arrows*) for ASD treatment are shown. *SAX* short axis, *4ch* four chamber, *LA* left atrium, *RA* right atrium

venosus ASDs as well as for patients with secundum ASDs with unsuitable morphology for device closure. A deficient rim of fossa ovalis and close proximity to the SVC, IVC, and CS may prevent successful closure [88, 89].

Different devices are available for ASD closure, although in the majority of centers the Amplatzer septal occluder and the Cardioseal device are used (Fig. 13.19). With the introduction of large Amplatzer devices (up to 40 m), the size of the defect no longer seems to be a limiting factor [89]. Device closure of secundum ASDs can produce rapid cardiac remodeling and decreased right atrial and ventricular volumes [90]. Residual small shunt after device closure is common and usually closes spontaneously in 1 year.

Both MR and CT have been used for pre- and post-transcatheter closure of ASDs and demonstrated some advantages over TEE [91, 92]. Demonstration of venous anomalous drainage is easier with these techniques. MDCT has been used as an alternative to TEE for evaluating Amplatzer septal occluders for ASD [92]. The metallic component of the occluder, which is a major problem for MRI and echocardiography, does not impair the diagnostic quality of MDCT scans (Fig. 13.19). MDCT is claimed to be helpful as it can reconstruct any plane owing to its volume image data nature and it is able to show residual defects, shunts, and device protrusions or migration that is not seen on TTE. MDCT is a good choice when TEE cannot provide convincing information. The most common operation for sinus venosus defects consists of patch closure of the defect with concomitant baffling of any associated PAPVR into the left atrium [93] (Fig. 13.16). Correction of the superior variety of defects is less problematic, although it can be difficult to separate the venous streams without producing venous obstruction [93]. Sinoatrial node injury is another complication.

Ventricular Septal Defect

The most common form of CHD in childhood is the VSD. It is found as a part of complex cardiac malformations in 50 % of patients and in 20 % as an isolated lesion [93–96]. Due to spontaneous and surgical closure, it is less common in adults. Still in adults, it is the second most common CHD after bicuspid aortic valve. Anatomic knowledge of the ventricles and the ventricular septum is the prerequisite for understanding different types of VSD. Detailed anatomy and pertinent terminologies of the RV and RVOT are described in Chap. 10. In this chapter, the ventricular septum anatomy will be reviewed.

Anatomy of Ventricular Septum

The interventricular (IV) septum can be divided into two morphological components, the membranous septum and the muscular septum [7]. The membranous septum is part of septal components of the AV junction. The septal components of the AV junction are important because they conduct the cardiac impulse from the atria to the ventricles [97]. At the crux of the heart, there is an area where tricuspid valve is attached to the septum closer to the ventricular apex than the mitral valve (Fig. 13.20). This relationship is inverted in congenitally corrected transposition of the great arteries (ccTGA) and the distance is longer in Ebstein anomaly. In this region, the cavity of the right atrium is separated from that of the LV by the AV muscular sandwich, also known as muscular AV septum. As stated by Anderson et al. [97], this area is not a true septum and similar to the interatrial groove is only filled with the epicardial fibrofatty tissue of inferior pyramidal space sandwiched between the atrial wall and the ventricular musculature. This can be clearly shown by CT [98] (Fig. 13.21). The membranous septum is small and is located at the base of the heart below the right and noncoronary cusps of the aortic valve. The membranous ventricular septum is divided by the attachment of the septal leaflet of the tricuspid valve into two components: the AV portion separating the left ventricle from the right atrium and the IV portion, attached to the muscular septum. The relative sizes of the two components are variable and determined by the site of attachment of the septal leaflet of the tricuspid valve to the membrane and the height of the posterior aortic sinus. The membranous septum can be large in ccTGA. The central fibrous body lies superior and anterior to the muscular AV septum. The central fibrous body is made up by the right fibrous trigone and the membranous septum and fuses the annuli of the tricuspid, mitral, and aortic valves [97]. Of surgical importance is the close proximity of the conduction system of the heart to the membranous septum. The AV node is located in apex of the triangle of Koch of the right atrium (formed by Eustachian ridge, the CS ostium, and the septal leaflet of the tricuspid valve). From another perspective, the AV node is below the nadir of the noncoronary sinus of the aortic valve on the right atrial side of the central fibrous body. The bundle of His exists the AV node and penetrates the right fibrous trigone and runs along the inferior margin of the IV component of the membranous septum underneath the septal attachment of the tricuspid valve before dividing into the left and right bundle branches. The bundle of His can be damaged by the sutures during repair of a perimembranous VSD. The left bundle branch fans out over the septum while the right bundle branch courses as a single trunk below the medial papillary muscle complex and then to the inferior borders of the septal and moderator bands until it reaches the anterior papillary muscle where it distributes to innervate the RV. The conduction system can also be at risk at the superior edge of a muscular inlet VSD, where the conduction system runs in the muscle between the VSD and the membranous septum.

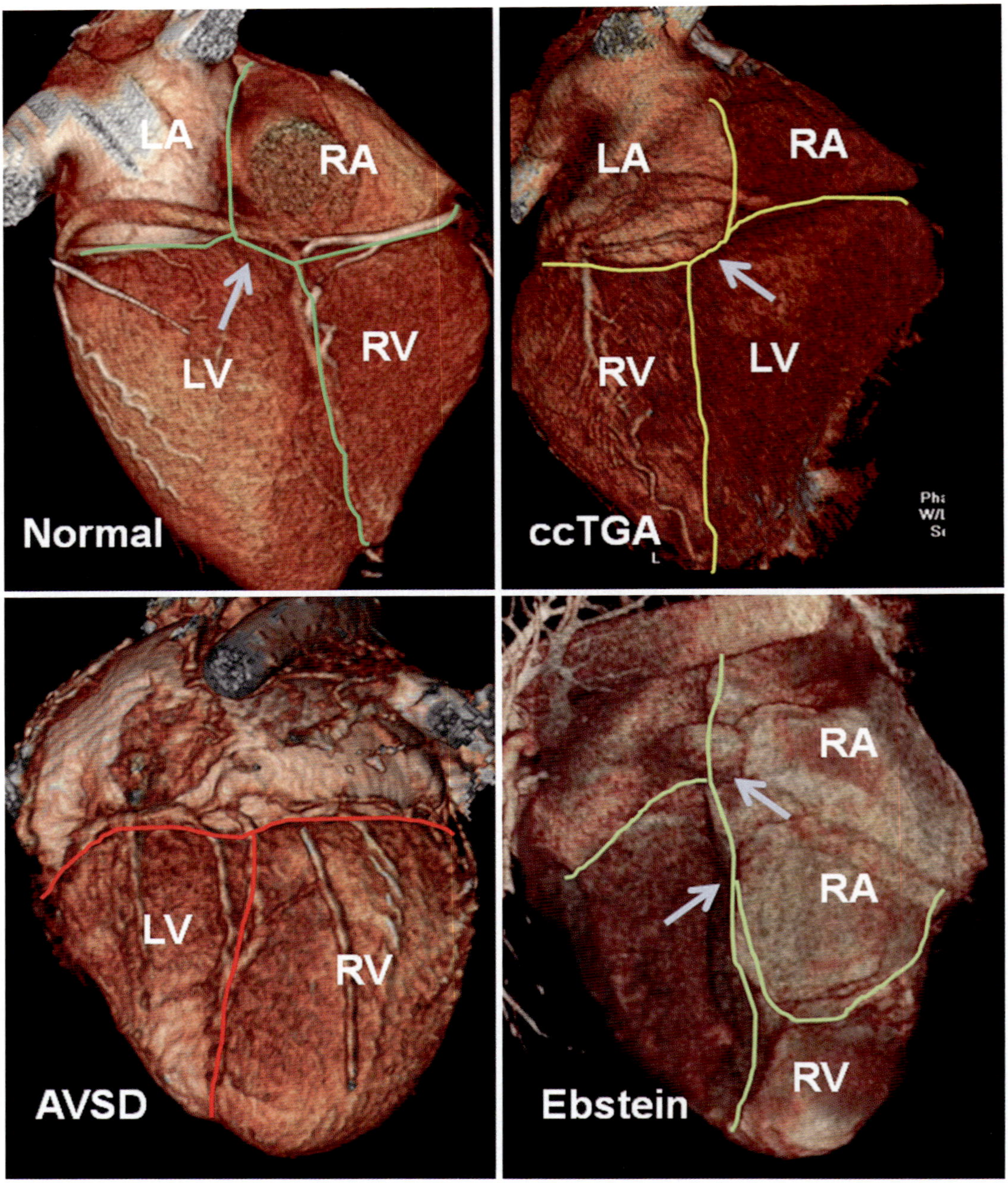

Fig. 13.20 External cardiac crux pattern in normal heart, congenitally corrected transposition of the great arteries (*ccTGA*), atrioventricular (AV) canal defect with single atrium, and Ebstein anomaly. External cardiac crux is an area in the posterior aspect of the heart where cardiac chambers show their maximum proximity (*arrow*). The vertical and horizontal lines in the cardiac crux are not perpendicular (*green lines*). In normal heart, the right AV groove is inferior to the left AV groove due to inferior position of the septal leaflet of tricuspid relative to the mitral valve. This relationship is reversed in ccTGA. There is no offset in the AV septal defect (*AVSD*) and the offset is huge in Ebstein due to apical migration of the tricuspid valve (*arrows*). *LA* left atrium, *LV* left ventricle, *RA* right atrium, *RV* right ventricle boundaries between heart chambers are shown by color line in each figure

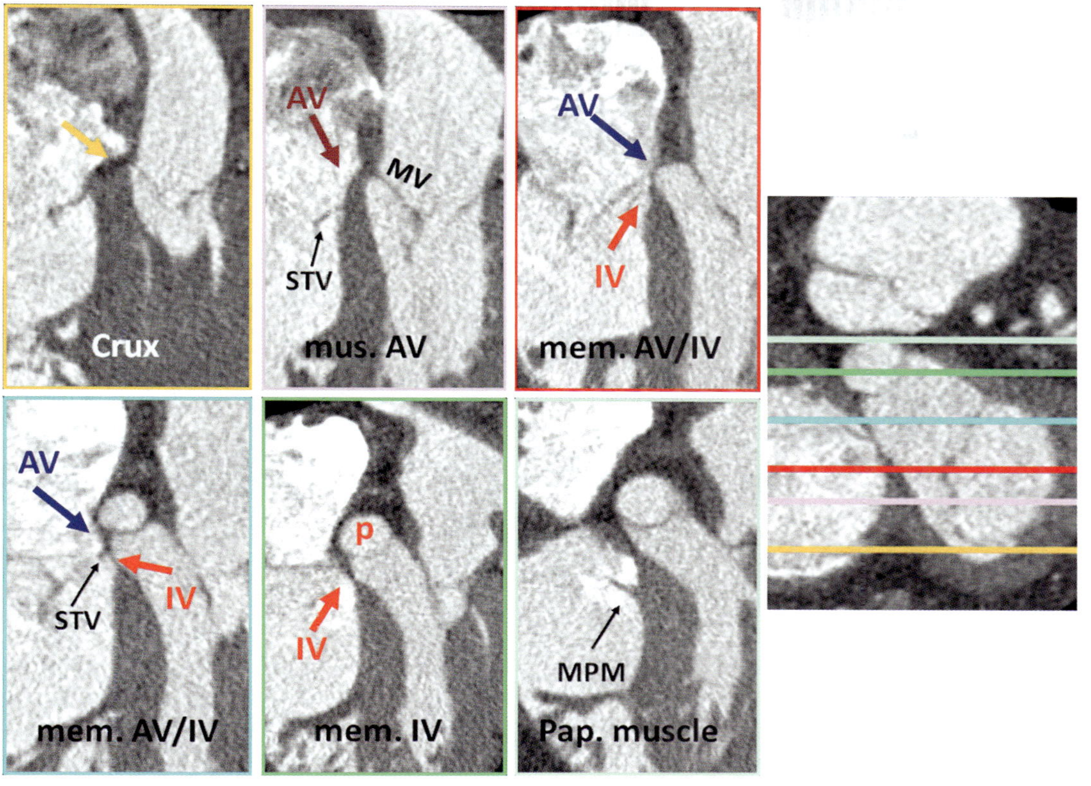

Fig. 13.21 The septal components of the atrioventricular (*AV*) junction. Four-chamber slices are reconstructed at the levels of internal cardiac crux, muscular (*mus.*) atrioventricular (*AV*) septum, membranous (*mem.*) AV septum, and membranous interventricular (*IV*) septum. Note the offset between the septal attachment of tricuspid valve (*STV*) and the mitral valve (*MV*) at muscular AV septum. The membranous septum itself is divided into two parts by the STV. Epicardial fibrofatty tissue is seen at the level of the cardiac crux sandwiched between the right atrial and left ventricular muscle walls (*mus. AV*). *MPM* medial papillary muscle, *p* posterior aortic sinus

The muscular septum can be divided into inlet, trabecular, and infundibular components. The inlet portion is inferoposterior to the membranous septum and extends from the AV junction to the chordal attachments of the AV valve. The trabecular component of septum is the largest part and extends to the apex. The infundibular septum separates the right and left ventricular outflow tracts.

Aneurysm of the Membranous Septum

The membranous septum can be thickened, perforated by one or many holes, or form an aneurysm. These are more likely to occur in the IV portion of the membranous septum in association with or as a result of a perimembranous defect. The etiology of this anomaly may be abnormal embryologic development or weakness of the affected tissues [99]. Aneurysms may limit intracardiac shunting and, in some cases, result in spontaneous defect closure. The characteristic outpouching or wind sock appearance on echocardiography or MRI results from aneurysmal distension to the right during ventricular systole (Fig. 13.7). Left-to-right shunt is usually shown only in systole (Fig. 13.22). Aneurysm of the IV membranous septum may be an uncommon occult cardiac source of systemic embolism [100]. Other associations include tricuspid regurgitation, obstruction to blood flow, endocarditis, and conduction disturbances [99].

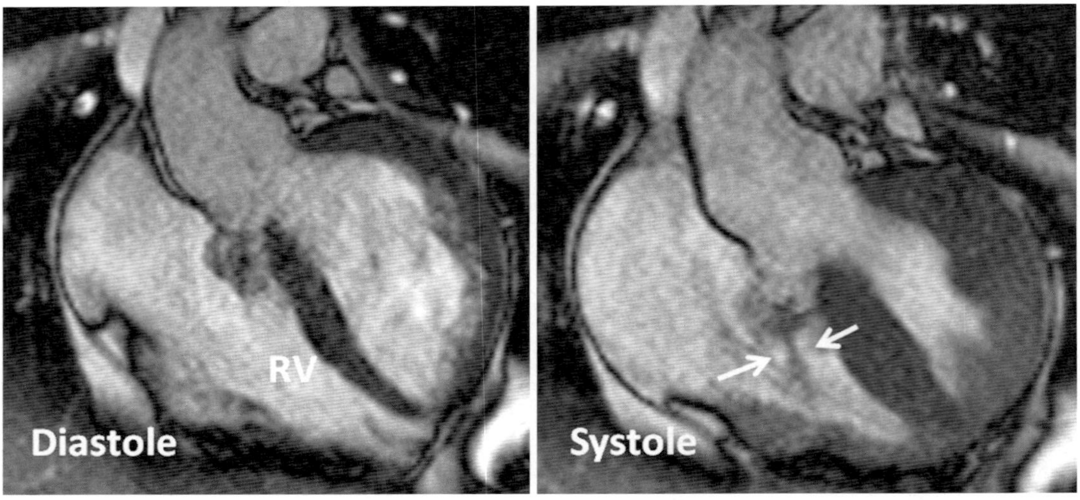

Fig. 13.22 Aneurysm of the interventricular membranous (*solid arrows*) with a small ventricular septal defect (*arrows*) best shown in systole. Aneurysms may limit intracardiac shunting and, in some cases, result in spontaneous defect closure. *RV* right ventricle

A defect in the AV membranous septum causing a shunt from the left ventricle to the right atrium is described as "Gerbode defect" [101, 102]. In congenital form, this usually represents a perimembranous VSD with a jet directed through a cleft in the tricuspid valve. An elongated sail-like anterior tricuspid leaflet in a perimembranous VSD may form an aneurysm and direct the shunt into right atrium. A consequence of this shunting can be right atrial enlargement. Acquired Gerbode defect has been described after bacterial endocarditis, trauma, and aortic root surgery (Fig. 13.23).

Classification of VSD

There are different classifications and nomenclature of VSDs, according to their location, that have been proposed and used [103, 104] (Fig. 13.24). Most classifications relate to the works done by Moulaert, Soto, and Anderson on cadaveric hearts [104, 105] and elegant echocardiography correlation on 280 cases of VSD later published by Sutherland et al. [106]. They divided VSDs into three groups: (1) perimembranous (70 %) including outlet (infundibular), muscular (trabecular), and inlet (AV canal defect) types, (2) subarterial (5 %), and (3) muscular including trabecular, outlet (infundibular), and inlet (25 %). A notable exception to this distribution is the high prevalence (30 %) of subarterial VSDs in the Asian population with VSDs [107].

Another popular classification was proposed by Capelli et al. based on two-dimensional (2D) echocardiography [108]. In their approach, the VSDs were simply grouped into subvalvular and muscular. The subvalvular group constitutes any VSDs partially bound by a valve and includes inlet, subtricuspid, subaortic, subarterial doubly committed, and subpulmonary. The muscular group was subclassified into outlet, central, and apical.

The most recent practical classification in use by the Society of Thoracic Surgeons (STS) is the one proposed by the American Heart Association Task Force on Practice Guidelines [96]: type 1 (conal, subpulmonary, infundibular, supracristal, and doubly committed juxta-arterial defects), type 2 (perimembranous, paramembranous, and conoventricular defects), type 3 (inlet and AV canal varieties), and type 4 (muscular VSDs).

Isolated defects of the membranous septum are surrounded by fibrous tissue without extension into adjacent muscular septum. These defects are uncommon in adults and probably are

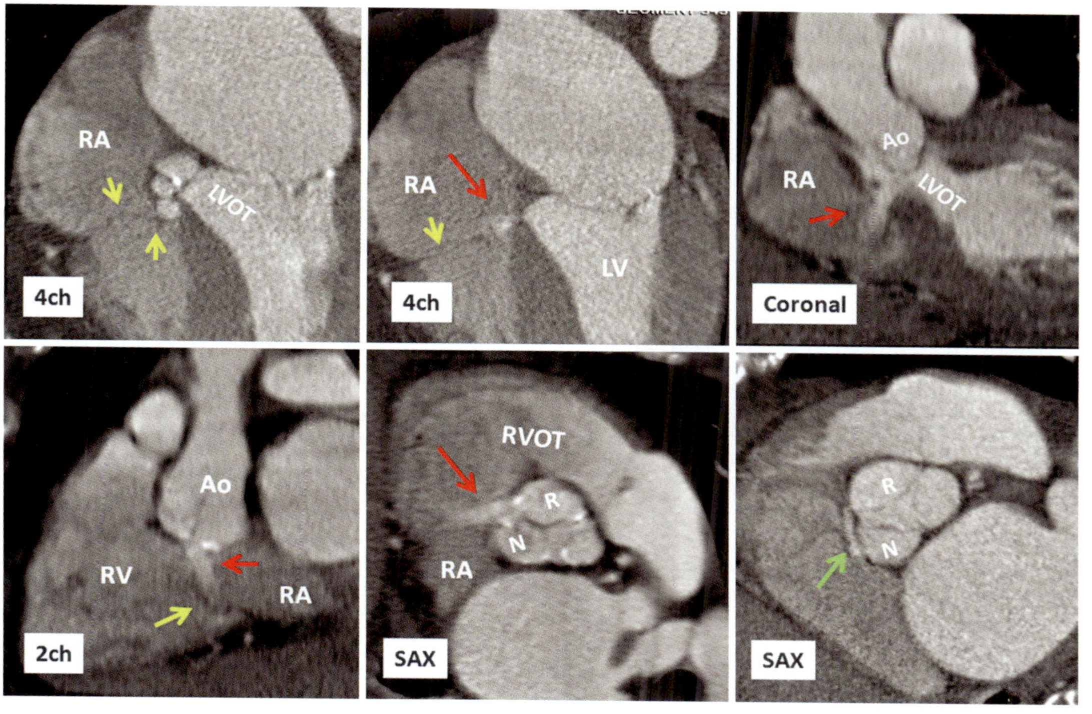

Fig. 13.23 Atrioventricular membranous defect (Gerbode) in a 73-year-old male with aortic valve disease. Calcified valve with vegetation and mild regurgitation was shown on echocardiography. Different projections of CT angiography show small membranous defect with shunt (*red arrows*) from the left ventricle (*LV*) into the right atrium (LA). The shunt was more obvious during diastole arising between the right coronary (*R*) and noncoronary (*N*) cusps. The level of tricuspid valve is shown by *yellow arrows*. Small collection of contrast (*green arrow*) between the aortic valve (*Ao*) and the RA is consistent with a small sinus tract. *LVOT* left ventricle outflow tract, *RVOT* right ventricle outflow tract, *RV* right ventricle, *4ch* four chamber, *2ch* two chamber, *SAX* short axis

sealed by tricuspid leaflet (Fig. 13.25). Defects that involve the membranous septum and surrounding muscles are called perimembranous, paramembranous, or infracristal. These are the most common VSDs and involve 70–80 % of cases [105]. Important criteria of diagnosis of perimembranous defects are subaortic location and fibrous continuity between the leaflets of the aorta and tricuspid valves (Fig. 13.26). Therefore, not every subaortic defect is perimembranous as it is common to see a fibrous tissue that separates the roof of defect from the aortic valve [109]. Subpulmonary extension occurs in large defects. Perimembranous defects are subpulmonary in hearts with discordant ventriculoarterial connection and there is fibrous continuity between the pulmonary and tricuspid valves. Perimembranous extensions of the defect are classified into the inlet, outlet, and muscular septa types. Large defects may involve all three components. The most common type is the outlet variant. Perimembranous outlet defects are located anterior to medial papillary muscle. Perimembranous inlet defects are also roofed by the AV valve and located posterior to the medial papillary muscle. Abnormalities of the tricuspid valve adjacent to a membranous or perimembranous VSDs can be in the form of an aneurysm partially or completely occluding the defect (Fig. 13.25). Although uncommon, prolapse of the right or noncoronary coronary sinus leaflets in perimembranous (subaortic) defects can cause aortic valve insufficiency (Fig. 13.27). This phenomenon is more common in subpulmonary infundibular VSDs.

Perimembranous trabecular defects are best seen at the most posterior aspect of a

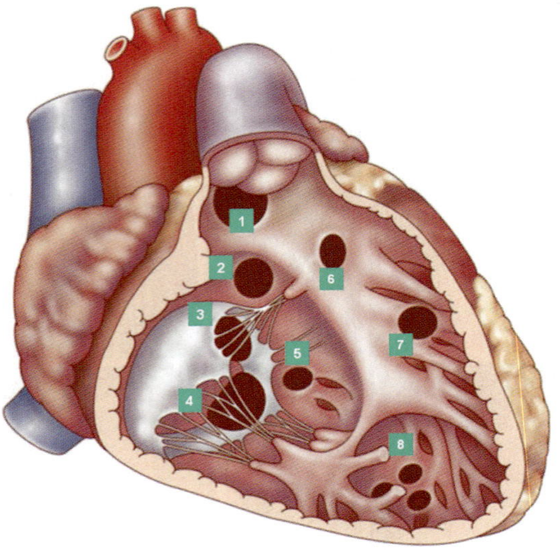

Fig. 13.24 VSD classification (right ventricular view). *1–4* are subvalvular defects. *1* Supracristal (doubly committed subarterial) defect. *2* Perimembranous outlet defect. *3* Perimembranous inlet defect. *4* Atrioventricular (septum primum) defect. *5–8* are muscular defects at inlet, outlet (infundibular) and anterior trabecular, and apical trabecular regions of the ventricular septum, respectively

four-chamber view of aortic root plane. In the normal heart, using two-dimensional echocardiography, it is difficult to locate the precise junction of membranous and trabecular septa but CT of the heart can easily localize it (Fig. 13.21). Blunting of the upper margin of the IV septum may indicate its involvement. Although perimembranous defect exists in isolation, it is most frequently associated with other defects (i.e., tetralogy of Fallot) (Fig. 13.26). From surgical point of view, the diagnosis of perimembranous VSD is important as it places the patient at risk of injury to conduction system at the time of surgery. The bundle of His passes along the inferior margin of perimembranous outlet VSD [109].

Perimembranous inlet defects (endocardial cushion defect) are roofed by the AV valve and characterized by absence of the AV muscular septum causing common level of insertion of the AV valve septal leaflets to central fibrous body (mitral-tricuspid continuity) (Fig. 13.28).

Muscular defects surrounded entirely by muscular rims may be subdivided into trabecular, outlet (infundibular), and inlet. Infundibular

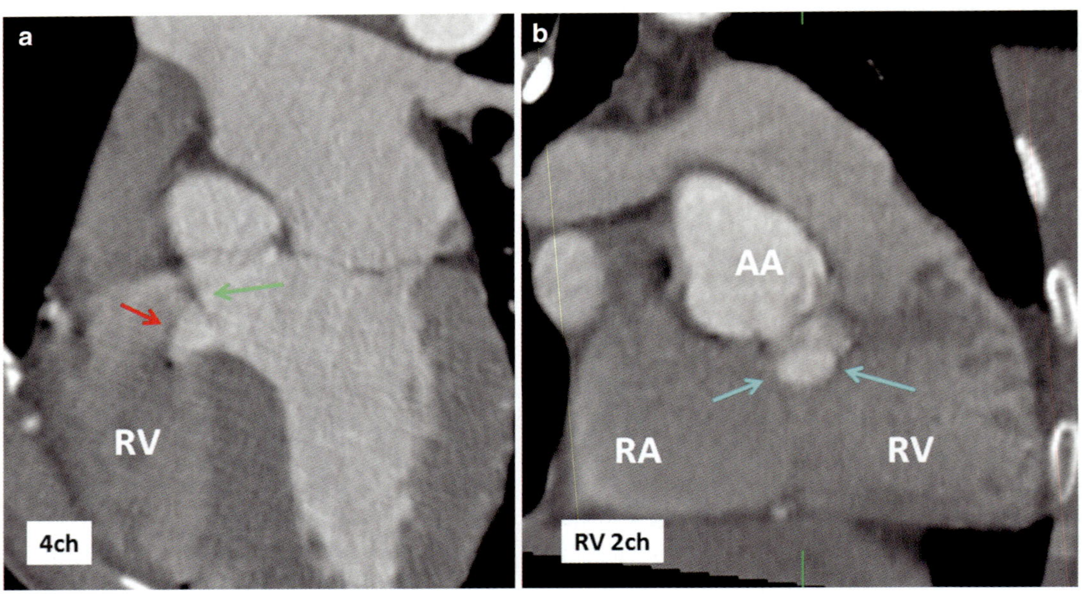

Fig. 13.25 (**a**) Four chamber and (**b**) 2 chamber of the right ventricle. Membranous VSD (*blue arrows*) protected and sealed by septal tricuspid leaflet (*red arrow*). Residual of the membrane is seen (*green arrow*). *AA* ascending aorta, *RA* right atrium, *RV* right ventricle, *4ch* four chamber, *2ch* two chamber

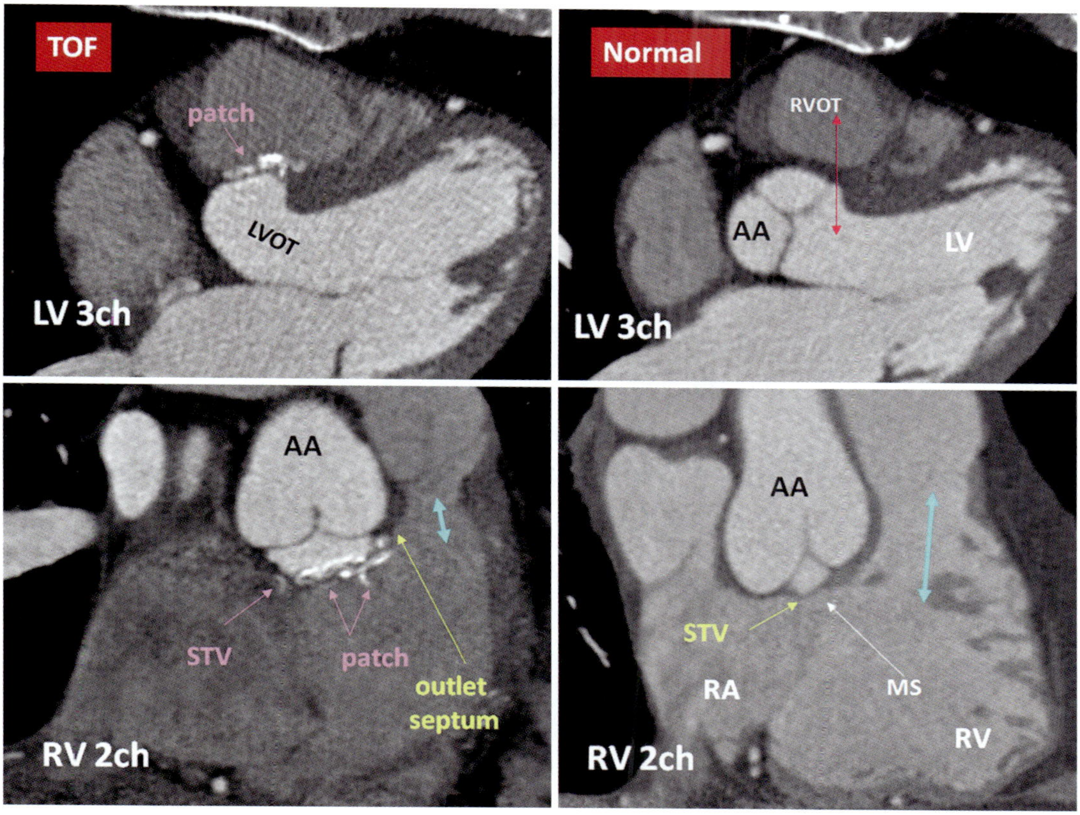

Fig. 13.26 Tetralogy of Fallot (*TOF*) versus normal heart. Left ventricle three-chamber (*LV 3ch*) and right ventricle two-chamber (*RV 2ch*) views of two subjects, one with repaired TOF and the second one with normal heart, are presented for comparison. In TOF, a subaortic perimembranous VSD is closed with a Dacron patch. The right ventricle outflow tract (*RVOT*) is short (*blue arrow*) and shows mildly thickened septoparietal trabeculations. No RVOT stenosis is seen (Eisenmenger defect). Malaligned outlet septum is seen displaced superiorly. The membranous septum (*MS*) is absent and the septal tricuspid (*STV*) leaflet is almost in fibrous continuity with the aortic leaflet. In 3ch view, the left ventricle outflow tract (*LVOT*) appears longer in TOF possibly due to dextroposition of the aortic root. Note the interventricular communication (closed by the patch) between the limbs of the septomarginal trabeculation. In normal heart, outlet septum is absent or involves a small portion of the crista supraventricularis crest (*double-headed red arrow*). *RA* right atrium, *RV* right ventricle, *LV* left ventricle, *AA* ascending aorta

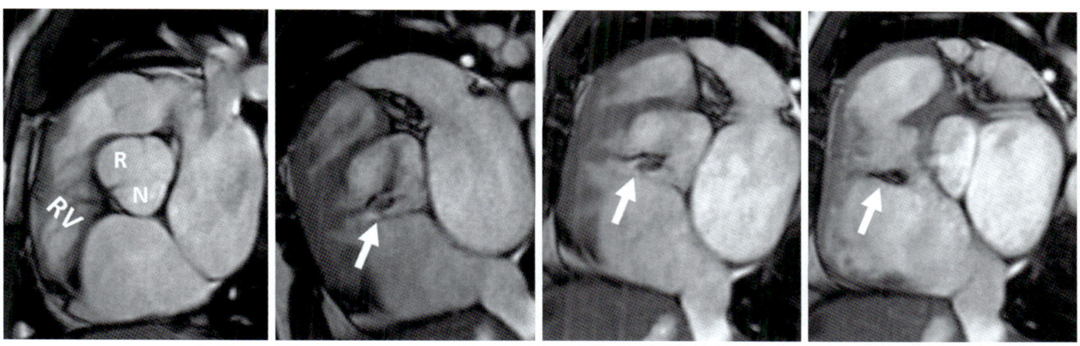

Fig. 13.27 A 35-year-old male with a small membranous VSD. Short axis MR images show aortic regurgitation between the right (*R*) and noncoronary (*N*) sinuses with the shunt (*arrows*) directed into the right ventricle (*RV*) through the membranous septum defect

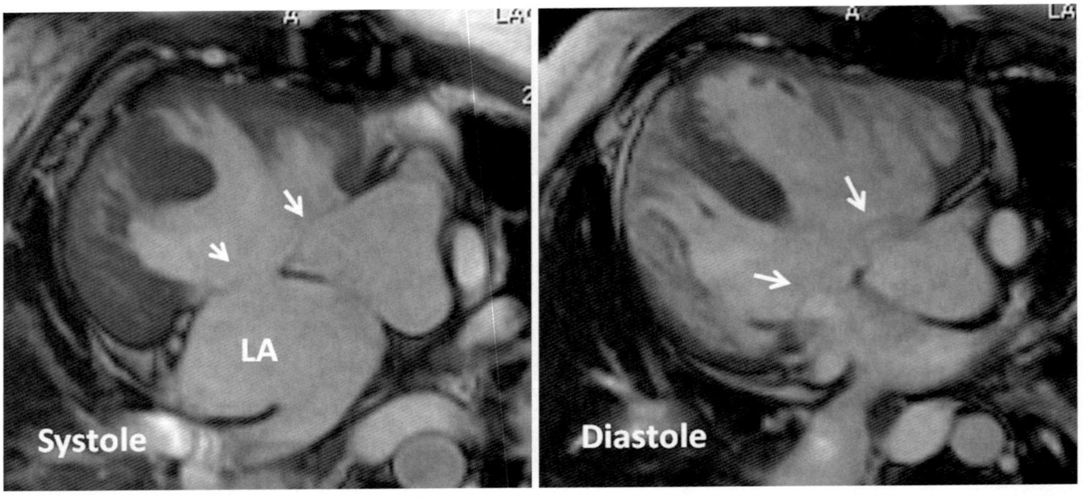

Fig. 13.28 Large perimembranous inlet (atrioventricular septal defect) with an intact atrial septum in a patient with dextrocardia, situs inversus, and azygos continuation of the inferior vena cava to the left superior vena cava. Note that the septal leaflets of the common atrioventricular valve (*arrows*) are attached at the same level to the central fibrous body

defects are the least common. Trabecular VSDs are the most common locations of muscular defects (Fig. 13.10). They are usually single but can be multiple and apical (Swiss cheese) [110]. Small VSDs in trabecular septum can be difficult to differentiate from myocardial clefts and large Thebesian sinuses (Fig. 13.29). The location of trabecular VSD can be subclassified as anterior, apical, and posterior [111]. The septomarginal trabeculation is the anatomic border between anterior muscular and posterior defects (Fig. 13.30). Apical defects are distal to the moderator band. Inlet muscular defects are posteriorly located beneath the medial papillary muscle but do not reach an arterial or AV valve, and there is normal pattern of septal AV valve insertions. Single trabecular defects and small multiple ("Swiss cheese") defects are difficult to find with echocardiography [106] and high-resolution cardiac CT may be the preferred method of diagnosis.

Defects in the infundibulum (conal, outlet, supracristal) can be muscular or subarterial. Outlet muscular VSD is found in the RVOT above or in a limb of septomarginal trabeculation. The superior border of this defect may extend up within the infundibular septum (Fig. 13.31). Infundibular muscular defect is best seen on short axis images at the level of RVOT. They can be small and easily be missed. Subarterial type of infundibular VSDs can be subpulmonary or doubly committed. Subpulmonary defects are often small and associated with prolapse of the right coronary cusp in older oriental patients, but is unusual in children <4 years of age. In subpulmonary defects, the infundibular septum exists but appears deficient. In doubly committed, subarterial defect is directly roofed by conjoined aortic and pulmonary valves at the same level (in 15 %, an offset exists) which are in fibrous continuity with no "outlet septum" between them [112] (Fig. 13.32). The inferior margin of defect is formed by the crest of the trabecular septum. Posteriorly, it may extend into the membranous septum (type 1) or may be covered by a muscle ridge (type 2). They are best seen on coronal or four-chamber planes of the heart passing through the aortic root. A fibrous raphe between the two arterial valves may be seen in doubly committed VSD that should not be mistaken with a hypoplastic outlet septum [112]. This defect may be isolated or as part of tetralogy of Fallot. In tetralogy of Fallot, the defect is mainly subaortic and pulmonary valve stenosis coexists. Subpulmonary VSD is an integral component of the Taussig-Bing anomaly (double outlet

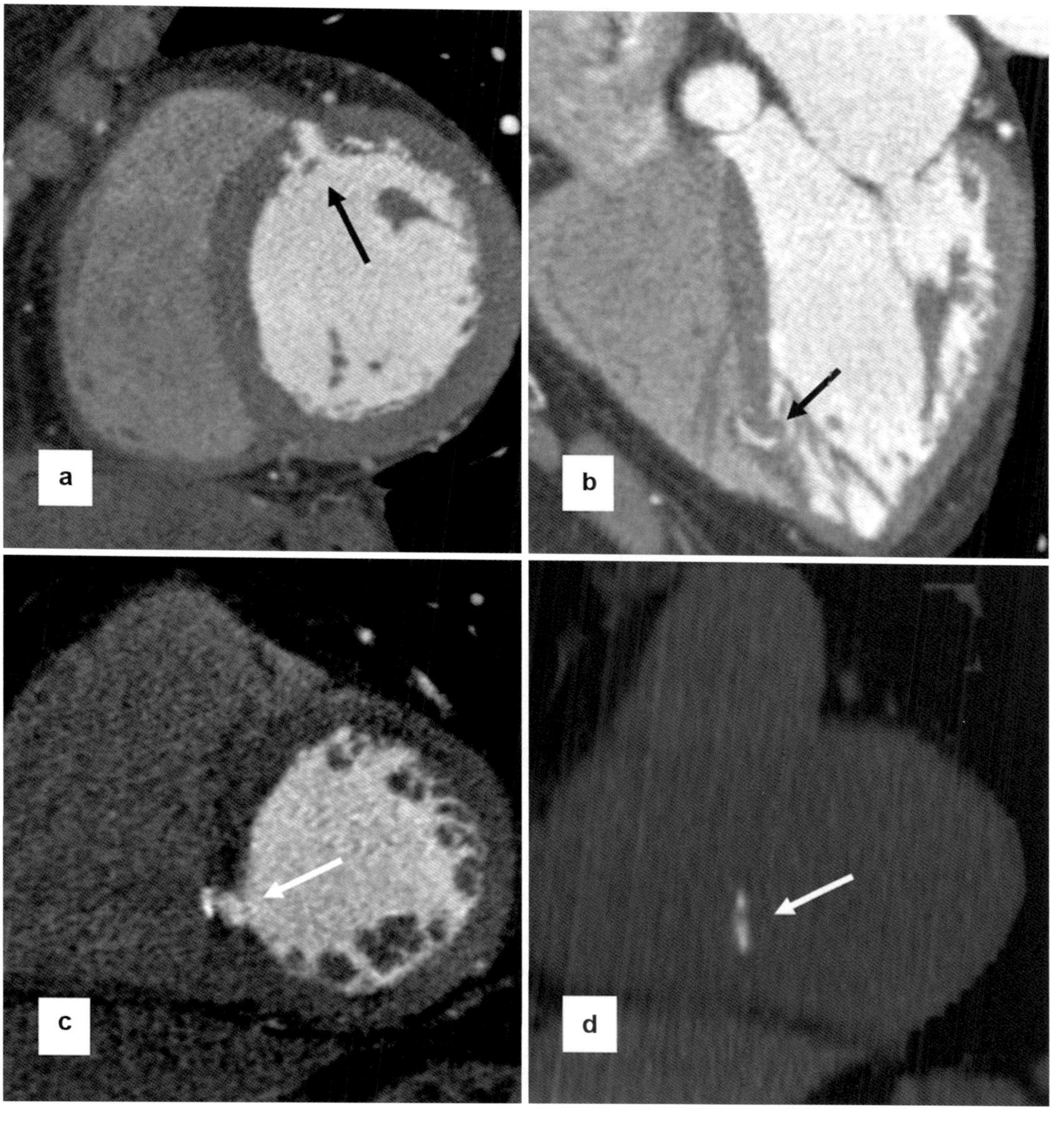

Fig. 13.29 Left ventricular septum filling defects. (**a**) Short axis CT shows diverticular appearance of a large Thebesian sinus (*arrow*). (**b**) Large venous sinus (*arrow*) in the apical septum. (**c**) Post- and (**d**) pre-contrast CT scans show residual cleft related to ventricular septal defect closing patch (*arrows*)

RV with subpulmonary VSD). It is important to remember that in normal heart, the outflow tracts are separated by ventriculoinfundibular fold and a true muscular septum cannot be identified or is very small [5] (Chap. 10). The subpulmonary infundibulum which supports the leaflets of the pulmonary valve produces the normal offsetting between the leaflets of the aortic and pulmonary valves. In the presence of a VSD between the two outlets, the septal morphology will be different and is characterized by the presence of a muscular bar named "outlet septum." This outlet septum forms the superior margin of the VSD and varies in length and thickness. In doubly committed defect, the ventriculoinfundibular fold is absent [112] (Fig. 13.32).

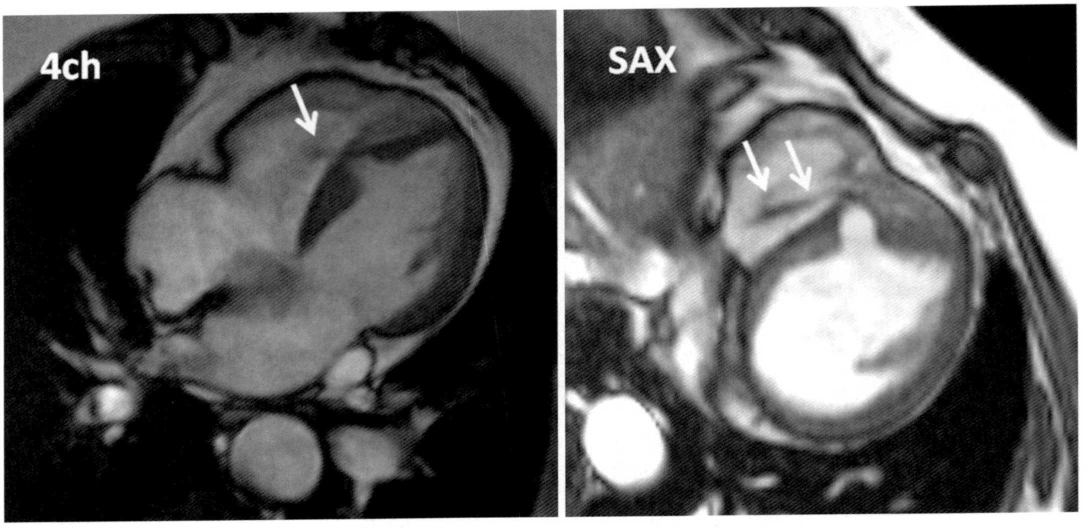

Fig. 13.30 Four-chamber (*4ch*) and short axis (*SAX*) cine images of cardiac MR show muscular ventricular septal defect in the anterior midportion of the trabecular septum causing a small left-to-right shunt (*arrows*)

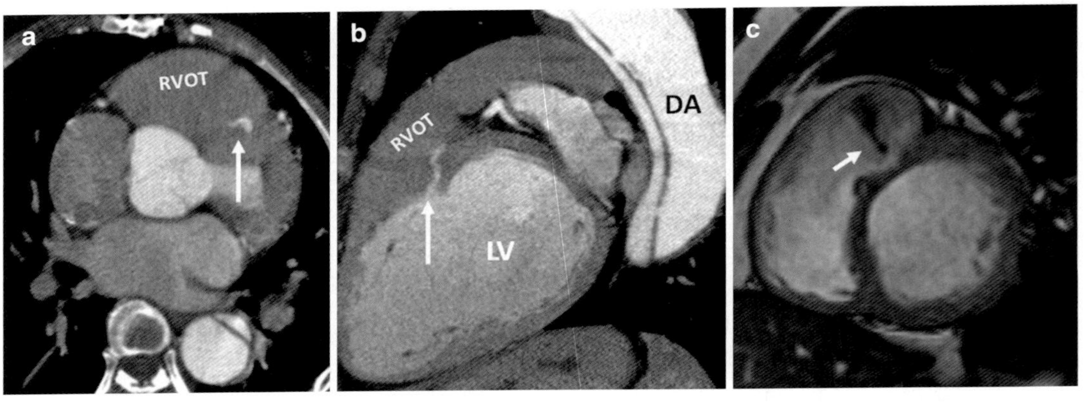

Fig. 13.31 (**a**, **b**) Axial and long axis CT images show that a small infundibular muscular ventricular septal defect (*arrows*) was incidentally found in this patient who admitted for treatment of descending thoracic aortic (*DA*) dissection. (**c**) Short axis MRI in a different patient shows the jet of left-to-right shunt into the right infundibulum (*small arrow*). *RVOT* right ventricle outflow tract, *LV* left ventricle

Infundibular and perimembranous outlet defects can be associated with various degrees of malalignment of the "outlet septum" and the remainder of the ventricular septum. Anterior or posterior deviation of the infundibular septum can cause right or left outflow tract obstruction, respectively. Fibroelastic bar or membranous tissue protruding from the left septal surface into the subaortic region can cause discrete short segment subaortic stenosis [113, 114]. In a VSD with subaortic stenosis, the rate of aortic arch interruption is higher. Subaortic stenosis may develop later after closure of VSD and repair of the aortic anomaly [115].

Imaging and Hemodynamic Assessment of VSDs

In addition to location, number, and sizes of defects, imaging data should include assessment of ventricular function and search for aortic valve

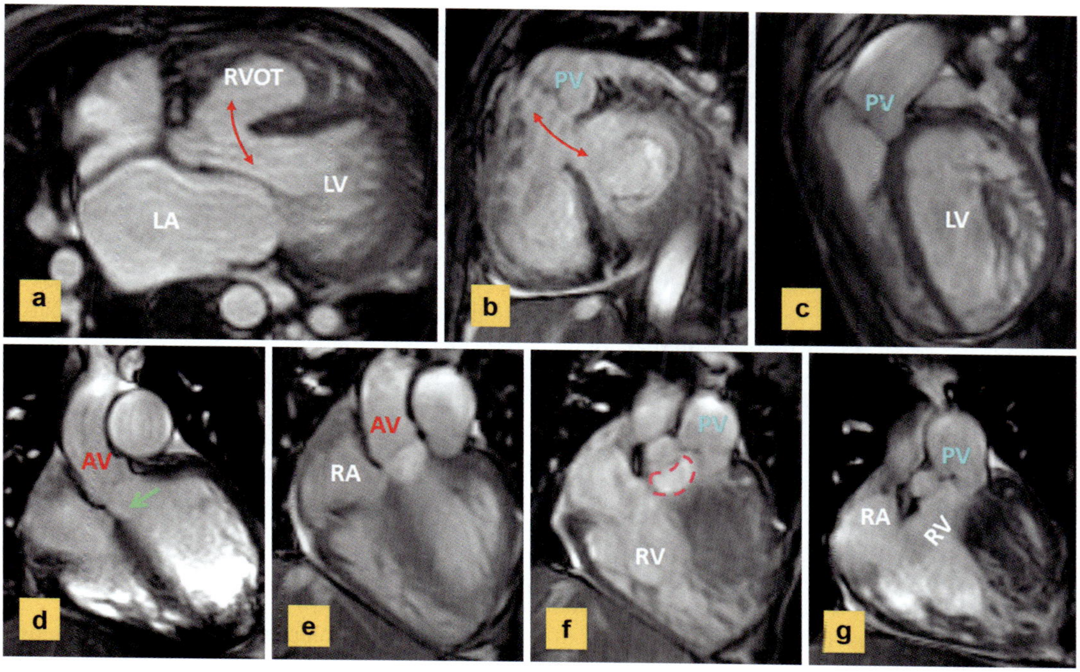

Fig. 13.32 Cine views of MRI in a 54-year-old male with left heart failure and pulmonary hypertension showing a subarterial ventricular septal defect (VSD). (**a**) Axial view shows the VSD and hypertrophied right ventricle outflow tract (*RVOT*). (**b**) Short axis at the level of mitral valve shows large VSD defect (*red arrow*). (**c**) Lateral view shows intact pulmonary valve (*PV*). There subpulmonary infundibulum is not developed. (**d–g**) are coronal images parallel to ventricular septum. The membranous septum is intact (*green arrow*). The VSD is mainly subaortic (**e**, **f**) with some subpulmonary component. The VSD area demarcated by *red circle* in (**f**), measured at 3.8 cm^2. The aortic valve (*AV*) and PV are at the same level. *RA* right atrium, *RV* right ventricle, *LA* left atrium, *LV* left ventricle

prolapse and/or regurgitation, outflow tract obstruction, and tricuspid regurgitation. Residual or recurrent VSDs in imaging studies of adults with repaired CHD are not uncommon. In adults with poor echocardiographic windows, TEE may be necessary. CT and MR are mainly recommended to confirm the anatomy of unusual VSDs such as inlet or apical defects not well seen by echocardiography as well as for the assessment of coexisting abnormalities in the pulmonary arteries, the pulmonary veins, and the aorta [109]. Diagnosis and correct localization of the perimembranous defects require detailed evaluation of the anatomic structures around them and multiplanar reconstructions to show their spatial location in the heart. For example, demonstration of fibrous continuity between the aorta and tricuspid valves is the key element for diagnosis of perimembranous defects. This can be best achieved with cardiac CT with special attention to technique of contrast administration to optimally show structures on both sides of the defect. A high-resolution imaging technique is required to show a small muscle bar between the valves and to distinct a muscular defect from a perimembranous defect.

Similar to ASD, noninvasive hemodynamic analysis of VSD can be obtained with echocardiography or MRI. CT can indirectly evaluate the amount of shunt by measuring the systemic and pulmonary flows using a retrospective ECG-gated technique. Direct measurement of shunt volume is not possible with CT; however, in selected cases, real-time visualization of the shunt can be achieved using a dynamic contrast-enhanced scan at the level of shunt. This will increase total radiation dose and is not routinely recommended.

The shunt volume in a VSD is determined largely by the size of the defect and the pulmonary vascular resistance. Without pulmonary hypertension or obstruction to the right ventricle, the direction of shunt is left to right and if large enough can cause left heart volume overload. In the setting of elevated pulmonary vascular resistance, RVOT obstruction due to hypertrophied muscles, or pulmonary stenosis, the shunt volume is limited and may be right to left, depending on the difference in pressure. Eisenmenger syndrome results from long-term left-to-right shunting, usually at higher shunt volumes [116] (Chap. 33).

VSD Closure

Muscular VSDs can undergo spontaneous closure as a result of muscular occlusion. Swiss cheese defects cannot close spontaneously and require surgery. The mechanism of closure of perimembranous defects is by apposition of tricuspid valve tissue, with or without formation of a septal aneurysm. Infundibular defects (doubly committed and subpulmonary) can close by prolapse of the right aortic cusp [117].

Spontaneous closure is otherwise rare. The pathophysiology of a VSD is determined by the size and location of defect. In restrictive VSD, the defect is smaller than the aortic annulus. In this type, the direction and volume of the shunt depends on the difference in systolic pressures of the ventricles [118]. Restrictive VSDs can be small or moderate in size. Small VSD is defined as <1 cm in size and left-to-right shunt of <50 % in the absence of pulmonary hypertension or pulmonary stenosis. The most common small defects in adults are perimembranous and subarterial [117]. Isolated small VSDs are considered benign and only need prophylaxis treatment for a low risk of endocarditis. Moderate-sized restrictive defects allow a large left-to-right shunt to cause left-sided volume overload, characterized by left atrium and left ventricle dilatation. Some pulmonary hypertension can exist [118]. In nonrestrictive VSD, the defect is large and ventricular pressures may equalize. The direction and volume of this shunt is determined by the difference in pulmonary and systemic vascular resistance. A nonrestrictive VSD is characterized by a large left-to-right shunt, left ventricle volume overload, and pulmonary hypertension resulting in Eisenmenger syndrome.

Generally, a Qp:Qs of 1.5:1 to 2:1, ventricular enlargement, pulmonary hypertension, or aortic regurgitation is an indication for surgery or transcatheter closure using Amplatzer VSD occluder [119–122]. Most common VSD surgeries in adults are perimembranous (70 %) and subarterial (25 %) [119].

Large apical muscular VSDs complicate management decisions, particularly when they occur in association with other congenital cardiac defects. Surgery for apical muscular VSDs is often suboptimal owing to difficulties in defect visualization, residual shunting, and ventricular dysfunction. Transcatheter closure is an alternative treatment [123].

Aortic cusp prolapse and aortic regurgitation can occur in more than 30 % of subarterial VSDs particularly in lesions larger than 5 mm. Aortic regurgitation is usually mild. It is more common in subpulmonary defect than subaortic perimembranous [107, 122]. In Lun et al. study, the coronary cusp prolapse in subpulmonic VSD was limited to the right cusp, and those in subaortic VSD were the right cusp, noncoronary cusp, or both [120]. Early surgical repair of the defect has been advocated. Subarterial defects <5 mm are usually asymptomatic and may incidentally be found during imaging workup [120] (Fig. 13.27).

Patent Ductus Arteriosus

Ductus arteriosus is a vascular connection between the aorta distal to the origin of the left subclavian artery and the superior margin of main pulmonary artery near the origin of the left pulmonary artery (Fig. 13.33). It originates from the distal left sixth embryonic arch and closes spontaneously within 48 h after birth. Persistence of the ductus after 3 months is called PDA [3, 124]. The incidence has been estimated to be as high as 1 in 500 and it is more common in females [125].

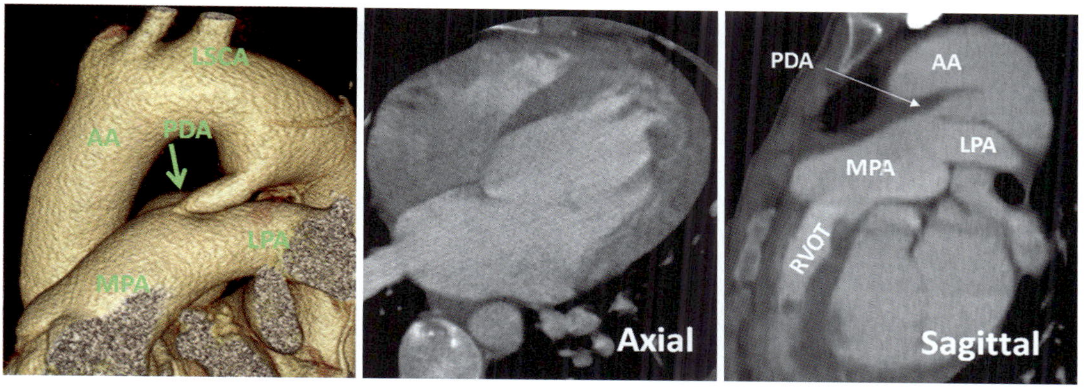

Fig. 13.33 Typical findings of patent ductus arteriosus (*PDA*). The PDA extends between the aorta distal to the origin of the left subclavian artery (*LSCA*) and the main pulmonary artery (*MPA*) near branching of the left pulmonary artery (*LPA*). It is usually less than 5 mm in diameter at the entrance into the MPA. Its origin from the aorta is larger and can be aneurysmal as shown in this case. There is volume overload of the left heart, hypertrophy of the right ventricle outflow tract (*RVOT*), and enlargement of the pulmonary arteries. *AA* ascending aorta

Clinical manifestations are usually determined by the size of PDA and the degree of left-to-right shunting. Regardless of the size, complications may arise, and imaging diagnosis is important. Long-standing left-to-right shunting results in pulmonary overcirculation, left heart volume overload, and progressive increase in pulmonary vascular resistance. In later stages, congestive heart failure or Eisenmenger syndrome can develop. It is not uncommon to find a small PDA in a patient with other congenital heart malformations (Fig. 13.34). A previously silent PDA may become symptomatic when combined with acquired conditions such as calcific aortic stenosis or ischemic heart disease [3]. Turbulent flow through the PDA can rarely lead to endothelial injury, complicated by infective or noninfective endocarditis and septic emboli [126].

Imaging diagnosis of a suspected PDA in adults can be difficult. Conversely, it is not uncommon to discover a silent PDA on routine CT or MR examinations. The information provided by imaging, such as the size, calcification, and morphology of the duct as well as the amount of left-to-right shunt, is crucial to the planning of optimal treatment. Different angiographic morphologies of PDA are classified by Krichenko et al. [127]. The most common morphology is "conical" with the aortic side larger than the pulmonary side (Fig. 13.33). Other variants include very short, long, tubular, and fusiform.

Traditionally, the initial noninvasive diagnostic investigation is performed with Doppler echocardiography [128]. In children, the size and morphology of the PDA can be predicted using Doppler echocardiography, but such assessment is not often possible in adults and MRI or CT may be required. TEE allows accurate diagnosis of shunt but it may not be the best technique for direct visualization of the PDA. Air in the left main bronchus can cause difficulty for TEE visualization of the PDA (Fig. 13.35). Intrabronchial balloon catheter filled with saline is used to overcome this limitation during intraoperative TEE [129]. Transcatheter occlusion has become the therapy of choice for treatment of PDA [130]; however, noninvasive imaging of PDA and judgment of indications for coil occlusion remain challenging. PDA closure is indicated for symptomatic adults with significant left-to-right shunting and for asymptomatic patients with significant shunting and evidence of left heart enlargement [3].

Both CT and MRI are accurate for morphological analysis of the PDA [131]. They both are useful for the assessment of associated abnormalities of the aortic arch such as vascular ring and right-sided aortic arch (Fig. 13.33). Demonstration of additional intracardiac lesions and anomalous venous return is easier with CT or MR. CT can

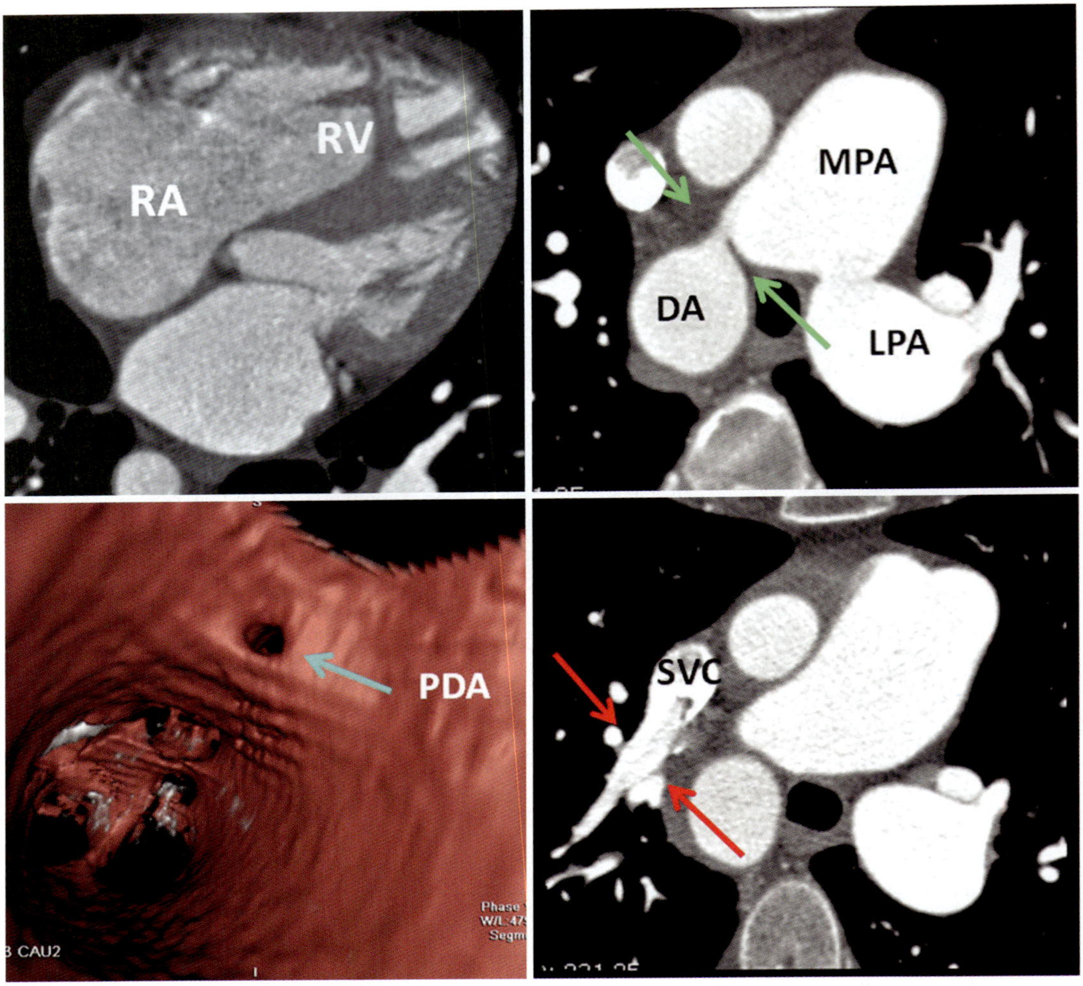

Fig. 13.34 A 37-year-old female scanned to further evaluate for right heart enlargement shown by echocardiography. Echo was reported negative for intracardiac shunt. CT angiography shows enlargement of the right atrium (*RA*), the right ventricle (*RV*), and the pulmonary arteries. Findings are consistent with pulmonary hypertension. A small short PDA was seen between a right-sided descending aorta (*DA*) and the main pulmonary artery (*MPA*) (*green arrows*). The origin of PDA is more toward the right pulmonary artery not the left pulmonary artery because of the right-sided position of the DA. The PDA orifice is clearly shown in CT endoscopy view of the aorta (*blue arrow*). Three anomalous pulmonary veins were found draining the right upper lung into the superior vena cava (*SVC*), one of those is shown in this case (*red arrow*). No intracardiac shunt was seen. It was concluded that pulmonary hypertension was the result of left-to-right shunting *arrows* at the level of anomalous pulmonary venous return rather caused by the small PDA. *LPA* left pulmonary artery

show calcification of the ductus better than MRI [131]. Patients with a heavily calcified duct or a duct exhibiting distortion or aneurysmal changes are not suitable candidates for surgery [132]. In large shunts, endovascular closure may also pose problems such as residual shunt or migration of the device [133]. In this situation, some reported endovascular stent graft as the preferred method of treatment [134]. Comprehensive imaging of aorta in these cases can be done with CT. Using

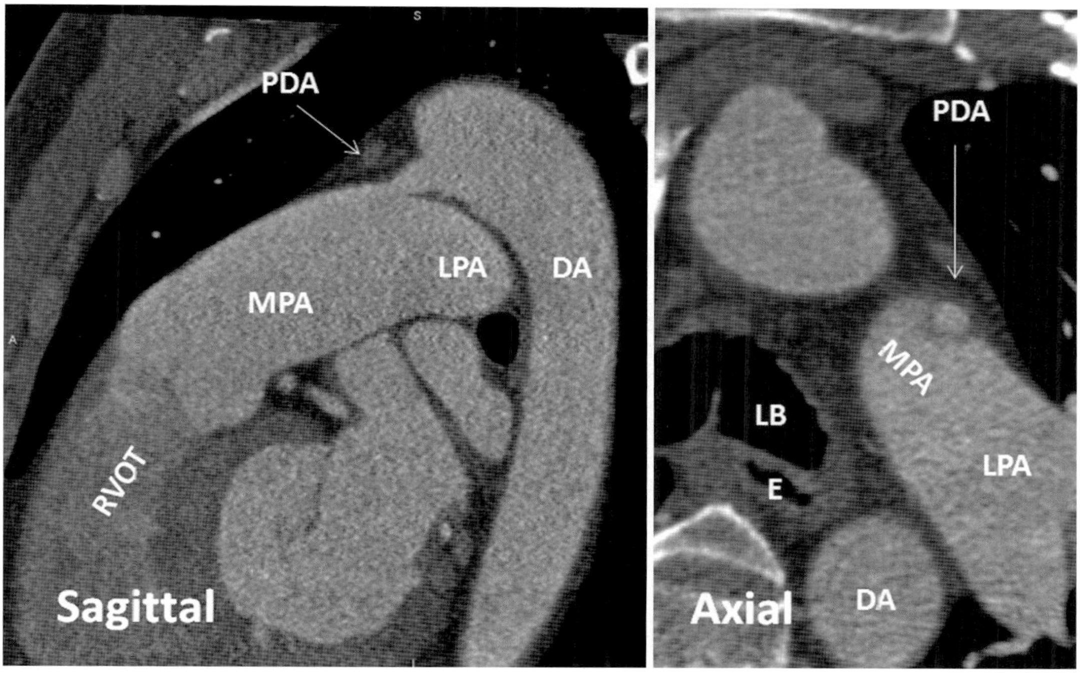

Fig. 13.35 The relation of the PDA with adjacent structures. The PDA is directed toward the main pulmonary artery (*MPA*). The left bronchus (*LB*) is interposed between the esophagus (*E*) and the left pulmonary vessels causing difficulty in visualization of the PDA orifice during transesophageal echocardiography. *DA* descending aorta, *LPA* left pulmonary artery, *RVOT* right ventricle outflow tract

CT anatomic relationship of the PDA and the left main bronchus can be reviewed before undertaking transcatheter closure, bearing in mind the assistance that the tracheal air shadow provides a fixed landmark during the transcatheter procedures (Fig. 13.34). Virtual endoscopy using CT data has been described as a useful technique in the assessment and treatment of PDA [135]. The anatomy of the orifice of the ductus and spatial relations of adjacent structures from both the aortic and pulmonary sides can be shown (Fig. 13.33). The mean angiographic diameter of the narrowest portion of a PDA can be as small as 3.2 (± 1.0) mm [127]. For this, high-resolution CT with at least 0.5-mm beam collimation is suggested to study these patients. To obtain high-quality images, an ECG-gated technique is preferred [131]. Dynamic assessment of the PDA shunt is possible with 64 or 320 slice scanners [136]. Overall, shunt analysis can be optimally performed with MRI or echocardiography. The jet of flow secondary to a PDA is directed preferentially toward the main pulmonary artery. For accurate results, collection of data with PC MRI should be perpendicular to direction of the PDA flow (Fig. 13.36). In PDA patients with high pulmonary vascular resistance and slow flow, the shunt may be very difficult to demonstrate. Additional image findings include ventricular septal flattening, right ventricular hypertrophy, high-velocity pulmonary regurgitation, tricuspid regurgitation, and left heart enlargement. Aneurysm of the ductus arteriosus is more common in children. In adult, it can be confused both clinically and radiologically with other masses in the aorticopulmonary window [137]. Large aneurysm can cause left vocal cord paralysis due to compression of the recurrent laryngeal nerve.

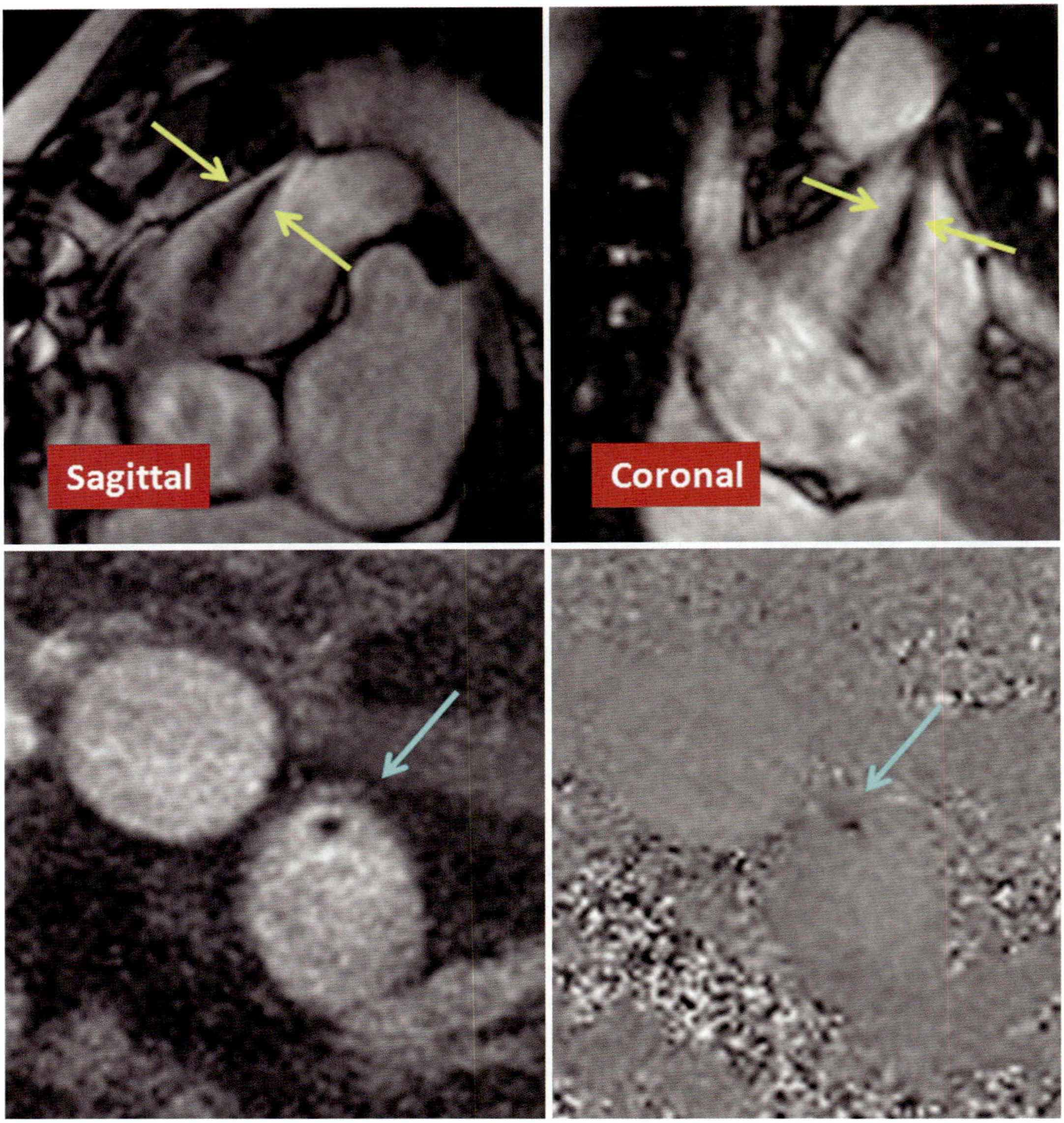

Fig. 13.36 MRI shows a small PDA (measured at 3 mm diameter) between the aorta and the main pulmonary artery. *Upper row* images are sagittal and coronal orthogonal cine images obtained for accurate localization of the shunt. *Lower row* demonstrates phase and magnitude MR images obtained through the shunt. There was a continuous left-to-right flow through the PDA with an easily identifiable jet into the main pulmonary artery (*yellow arrows*). Peak velocity through the PDA as measured with PC MR (*blue arrows*) was between 4.5 and 5.0 m/s. The main pulmonary artery is enlarged (4 cm). The heart was otherwise normal

References

1. Webb G, Gatzoulis M. Atrial septal defects in the adult: recent progress and overview. Circulation. 2006;114:1645–53.
2. Minette MS, Sahn DJ. Ventricular septal defects. Circulation. 2006;114:2190–7.
3. Schneider DJ, Moore JW. Patent ductus arteriosus. Circulation. 2006;114:1873–82.
4. Harley HR. The sinus venosus type of interatrial septal defect. Thorax. 1958;13(1):12–27.
5. Anderson RH, Webb S, Brown NA. Clinical anatomy of the atrial septum with reference to its developmental components. Clin Anat. 1999;12:362–74.

6. Anderson RH, Brown NA, Webb S. Development and structure of the atrial septum. Heart. 2002;88:104–10.
7. Anderson RH, Brown NA. The anatomy of the heart revisited. Anat Rec. 1996;246(1):1e7.
8. Thompson T, Evans W. Paradoxical embolism. Quart J Med. 1930;23:135–40.
9. Hagen PT, Scholz DG, Edwards WD. Incidence and size of patent foramen ovale during the first 10 decades of life: an autopsy study of 965 normal hearts. Mayo Clin Proc. 1984;59:17–20.
10. Webster MW, Chancellor AM, Smith HJ, et al. Patent foramen ovale in young stroke patients. Lancet. 1988;8601:11–2.
11. Homma S, Di Tullio MR, Sacco RL, Mihalatos D, Li Mandro G, Mohr JP. Characteristics of patent foramen ovale associated with cryptogenic stroke: a biplane transesophageal echocardiographic study. Stroke. 1994;25:582–6.
12. Saremi F, Channual S, Raney A, et al. Imaging of patent foramen ovale with 64-section multidetector CT. Radiology. 2008;249(2):483–92.
13. Ho SY, McCarthy KP, Rigby ML. Morphological features pertinent to interventional closure of patent oval foramen. J Interv Cardiol. 2003;16(1):33–8.
14. Natanzon A, Goldman ME. Patent foramen ovale: anatomy versus pathophysiology – which determines stroke risk? J Am Soc Echocardiogr. 2003;16(1):71–6.
15. Mohrs OK, Petersen SE, Erkapic D, Victor A, Schlosser T, Nowak B, Kauffmann G, Voigtlaender T, Kauczor HU. Dynamic contrast-enhanced MRI before and after transcatheter occlusion of patent foramen ovale. AJR Am J Roentgenol. 2007;188:844–9.
16. Nusser T, Hoher M, Merkle N, et al. Cardiac magnetic resonance imaging and transesophageal echocardiography in patients with transcatheter closure of patent foramen ovale. J Am Coll Cardiol. 2006;48:322–9.
17. Thomson LE, Crowley AL, Heitner JF, et al. Direct en face imaging of secundum atrial septal defects by velocity-encoded cardiovascular magnetic resonance in patients evaluated for possible transcatheter closure. Circ Cardiovasc Imaging. 2008; 1(1):31–40.
18. Sun JP, Stewart WJ, Hanna J, Thomas JD. Diagnosis of patent foramen ovale by contrast versus color Doppler by transesophageal echocardiography: relation to atrial size. Am Heart J. 1996;131(2): 239–44.
19. Kim YJ, Hur J, Shim CY, et al. Patent foramen ovale: diagnosis with multidetector CT – comparison with transesophageal echocardiography. Radiology. 2009; 250(1):61–7.
20. Koenig P, Cao QL, Heitschmidt M, Waight DJ, Hijazi ZM. Role of intracardiac echocardiographic guidance in transcatheter closure of atrial septal defects and patent foramen ovale using the Amplatzer device. J Interv Cardiol. 2003;16(1):51–62.
21. Graham LN, Melton IC, MacDonald S, Crozier IG. Value of CT localization of the fossa ovalis prior to transseptal left heart catheterization for left atrial ablation. Europace. 2007;9(6):417–23.
22. Chiari H. Uber Netzbildungen im rechten Vorhof des Herzens. Beitr Pathol Anat. 1897;22:1–10.
23. Gresham GA. Networks in the right side of the heart. Br Heart J. 1957;19:381–6.
24. Bhatnagar KP, Nettleton GS, Campbell FR, Wagner CE, Kuwabara N, Muresian H. Chiari anomalies in the human right atrium. Clin Anat. 2006;19(6):510–6.
25. Goedde TA, Conetta D, Rumisek JD. Chiari network entrapment of thromboemboli. congenital inferior vena cava filter. Ann Thorac Surg. 1990;49:317–8.
26. Schneider B, Hofmann T, Justen MH, Meinertz T. Chiari's network: normal anatomic variant or risk factor for arterial embolic events? J Am Coll Cardiol. 1995;26(1):203–10.
27. Schneider B, Hanrath P, Vogel P, Meinertz T. Improved morphologic characterization of atrial septal aneurysm by transesophageal echocardiography: relation to cerebrovascular events. J Am Coll Cardiol. 1990;16:1000–9.
28. Zabalgoitia-Reyes M, Herrerra C, Ghandi DK, Mehlman DJ, McPherson DD, Talano JV. A possible mechanism for neurologic ischemic events in patients with atrial septal aneurysm. Am J Cardiol. 1990; 66:761–4.
29. Mattioli AV, Aquilina M, Oldani A, Longhini C, Mattioli G. Atrial septal aneurysm as a cardioembolic source in adult patients with stroke and normal carotid arteries. A multicentre study. Eur Heart J. 2001; 22(3):261–8.
30. Mugge A, Daniel WG, Angermann C, et al. Atrial septal aneurysm in adult patients. A multicenter study using transthoracic and transesophageal echocardiography. Circulation. 1995;91(11):2785–92.
31. Schuchlenz HW, Weihs W, Horner S, Quehenberger F. The association between the diameter of a patent foramen ovale and the risk of embolic cerebrovascular events. Am J Med. 2000;109:456–62.
32. Olivares-Reyes A, Chan S, Lazar EJ, et al. Atrial septal aneurysm: a new classification in two hundred five adults. J Am Soc Echocardiogr. 1997; 10:644–56.
33. Pearson AC, Nagelhout D, Castello R, Gomez CR, Labovitz AJ. Atrial septal aneurysm and stroke: a transesophageal echocardiographic study. J Am Coll Cardiol. 1991;18:1223–9, 99.
34. Hanley PC, Tajik AJ, Hynes JK, et al. Diagnosis and classification of atrial septal aneurysm by two-dimensional echocardiography: report of 80 consecutive cases. J Am Coll Cardiol. 1985;6:1370–82.
35. Schuchlenz HW, Saurer G, Weihs W, Rehak P. Persisting eustachian valve in adults: relation to patent foramen ovale and cerebrovascular events. J Am Soc Echocardiogr. 2004;17(3):231–3.
36. Ley S, Ley-Zaporozhan J, Kreitner KF, et al. MR flow measurements for assessment of the pulmonary, systemic and bronchosystemic circulation: impact of different ECG gating methods and breathing schema. Eur J Radiol. 2007;61(1):124–9.
37. Beerbaum P, Korperich H, Barth P, Esdorn H, Gieseke J, Meyer H. Noninvasive quantification of left-to-right shunt in pediatric patients: phase-contrast cine mag-

netic resonance imaging compared with invasive oximetry. Circulation. 2001;103:2476–82.
38. O'Donnell M. NMR blood flow using multiecho, phase contrast sequences. Med Phys. 1985;12:59–64.
39. Chatzimavroudis GP, Zhang H, Halliburton SS, et al. Clinical blood flow quantification with segmented k-space magnetic resonance phase velocity mapping. J Magn Reson Imaging. 2003;17:65–71.
40. Boehrer JD, Lange RA, Willard JE, Grayburn PA, Hillis LD. Advantages and limitations of methods to detect, localize, and quantitate intracardiac left-to-right shunting. Am Heart J. 1992;124:448–55.
41. Daniel WC, Lange RA, Willard JE, Landau C, Hillis LD. Oximetric versus indicator dilution techniques for quantitating intracardiac left-to-right shunting in adults. Am J Cardiol. 1995;75:199–200.
42. Cigarroa RG, Lange RA, Hillis LD. Oximetric quantitation of intracardiac left-to-right shunting: limitations of the Qp/Qs ratio. Am J Cardiol. 1989;64:246–7.
43. Tang C, Blatter DD, Parker DL. Accuracy of phase-contrast flow measurements in the presence of partial volume effects. J Magn Reson Imaging. 1993;3:377–85.
44. Lotz J, Meier C, Leppert A, Galanski M. Cardiovascular flow measurement with phase-contrast MR imaging: basic facts and implementation. Radiographics. 2002;22(3):651–71.
45. Andersen AH, Kirsch JE. Analysis of noise in phase contrast MR imaging. Med Phys. 1996;23:857–69.
46. Hundley WG, Li HF, Lange RA, et al. Assessment of left-to-right intracardiac shunting by velocity-encoded, phase-difference magnetic resonance imaging: a comparison with oximetric and indicator dilution techniques. Circulation. 1995;91:2955–60.
47. Ley S, Fink C, Puderbach M, Zaporozhan J, et al. MRI Measurement of the hemodynamics of the pulmonary and systemic arterial circulation: influence of breathing maneuvers. AJR Am J Roentgenol. 2006;187(2):439–44.
48. Stahlberg F, Thomsen C, Sondergaard L, Henriksen O. Pulse sequence design for MR velocity mapping of complex flow: notes on the necessity of low echo times. Magn Reson Imaging. 1994;12:1255–62.
49. Kondo C, Caputo GR, Semelka R, Foster E, Shimakawa A, Higgins CB. Right and left ventricular stroke volume measurements with velocity en-coded cine MR imaging: in vitro and in vivo validation. AJR Am J Roentgenol. 1991;157:9–16.
50. Hoeper MM, Tongers J, Leppert A, Baus S, Maier R, Lotz J. Evaluation of right ventricular performance with a right ventricular ejection fraction thermodilution catheter and magnetic resonance imaging in patients with pulmonary hypertension. Chest. 2001;120:502–7.
51. Powell AJ, Tsai-Goodman B, Prakash A, Greil GF, Geva T. Comparison between phase-velocity cine magnetic resonance imaging and invasive oximetry for quantification of atrial shunts. Am J Cardiol. 2003;91:1523–5, A1529.
52. Mohiaddin RH, Underwood R, Romeira L, et al. Comparison between cine magnetic resonance velocity mapping and first-pass radionuclide angiocardiography for quantitating intracardiac shunts. Am J Cardiol. 1995;75:529–32.
53. Esmaeili A, Hohn R, Koch A, Vogl TJ, Hofstetter R, Abolmaali N. Assessment of shunt volumes in children with ventricular septal defects: comparative quantification of MR flow measurements and invasive oximetry. Clin Res Cardiol. 2006;95:523–30.
54. Evans AJ, Iwai F, Grist TA, et al. Magnetic resonance imaging of blood flow with a phase subtraction technique. Invest Radiol. 1993;28:109–15.
55. Goldberg A, Jha S. Phase-contrast MRI and applications in congenital heart disease. Clin Radiol. 2012;67(5):399–410.
56. Mymin D, Sharma GP. Total and effective coronary blood flow in coronary and noncoronary heart disease. J Clin Invest. 1974;53:363–73.
57. Debl K, Djavidani B, Buchner S, et al. Quantification of left-to-right shunting in adult congenital heart disease: phase-contrast cine MRI compared with invasive oximetry. Br J Radiol. 2009;82:386e91.
58. Blom NA, Ottenkamp J, Jongeneel TH, DeRuiter MC, Gittenberger-de Groot AC. Morphogenetic differences of secundum atrial septal defects. Pediatr Cardiol. 2005;26(4):338–43.
59. Biben C, Weber R, Kesteven S, et al. Cardiac septal and valvular dysmorphogenesis in mice heterozygous for mutations in the homeobox gene Nkx2-5. Circ Res. 2000;87:888–9.
60. Maeno YV, Benson LN, McLaughlin PR, Boutin C. Dynamic morphology of the secundum atrial septal defect evaluated by three dimensional transoesophageal echocardiography. Heart. 2000;83:673–7.
61. Ferreira SMAG, Ho SY, Anderson RH. Morphological study of defects of the atrial septum within the oval fossa: implications for transcatheter closure of left-to-right shunt. Br Heart J. 1992;67:316–20.
62. Ross DN. The sinus venosus type of atrial septal defect. Guy's Hosp Rep. 1956;105:376–81.
63. Davia JE, Cheitlin MD, Bedynek JL. Sinus venosus atrial septal defect. Am Heart J. 1973;85:177–85.
64. Brickner ME, Hillis LD, Lange RA. Congenital heart disease in adults- first of two parts. N Engl J Med. 2000;342:256–63.
65. Van Praagh S, Carrera ME, Sanders SP, Mayer JE, Van Praagh R. Sinus venosus defects: unroofing of the right pulmonary veins-anatomic and echocardiographic findings and surgical treatment. Am Heart J. 1994;128:365–79.
66. al Zaghal AM, Li J, Anderson RH, Lincoln C, Shore D, Rigby ML. Anatomical criteria for the diagnosis of sinus venosus defects. Heart. 1997;78(3):298–304.
67. Butts RJ, Crean AM, Hlavacek AM, et al. Venovenous bridges: the forerunners of the sinus venosus defect. Cardiol Young. 2011;21(6):623–30.
68. Crystal MA, Al Najashi K, Williams WG, Redington AN, Anderson RH. Inferior sinus venosus defect: echocardiographic diagnosis and surgical approach. Thorac Cardiovasc Surg. 2009;137(6):1349–55.
69. Kafka H, Mohiaddin RH. Cardiac MRI and pulmonary MR angiography of sinus venosus defect and

partial anomalous pulmonary venous connection in cause of right undiagnosed ventricular enlargement. AJR Am J Roentgenol. 2009;192:259–66.
70. Swan HJC, Kirklin JW, Becu LM, Wood EH. Anomalous connection of right pulmonary veins to superior vena cava with interatrial communications. Hemodynamic data in eight cases. Circulation. 1957;16:54–66.
71. Vogel M, Berger F, Kramer A, Alexi-Meshkishvili V, Lange PE. Incidence of secondary pulmonary hypertension in adults with atrial septal or sinus venosus defects. Heart. 1999;82:30–3.
72. Kronzon I, Tunick PA, Freedberg RS, Trehan N, Rosenzweig BP, Schwinger ME. Transesophageal echocardiography is superior to transthoracic echocardiography in the diagnosis of sinus venosus atrial septal defect. J Am Coll Cardiol. 1991; 17:537–42.
73. Pascoe RD, Oh JK, Warnes CA, Danielson GK, Tajik AJ, Seward JB. Diagnosis of sinus venosus atrial septal defect with transesophageal echocardiography. Circulation. 1996;94:1049–55.
74. Ferrari VA, Scott CH, Holland GA, Axel L, Sutton MS. Ultrafast three-dimensional contrast enhanced magnetic resonance angiography and imaging in the diagnosis of partial anomalous pulmonary venous drainage. J Am Coll Cardiol. 2001;37:1120–8.
75. Valente AM, Sena L, Powell AJ, Del Nido PJ, Geva T. Cardiac magnetic resonance imaging evaluation of sinus venosus defects: comparison to surgical findings. Pediatr Cardiol. 2007;28:51–6.
76. Plymale J, Kolinski K, Frommelt P, Bartz P, Tweddell J, Earing MG. Inferior sinus venosus defects: anatomic features and echocardiographic correlates. Pediatr Cardiol. 2013;34:322–6.
77. Anderson RH, Ho SY, Falcao S, et al. The diagnostic features of atrioventricular septal defect with common atrioventricular junction. Cardiol Young. 1998;8(1):33–49.
78. Smallhorn JF. Cross-sectional echocardiographic assessment of atrioventricular septal defect: basic morphology and preoperative risk factors. Echocardiography. 2001;18:415–32.
79. Arisawa J, Morimoto S, Ikezoe J, et al. Cross sectional echocardiographic anatomy of common atrioventricular valve in atrial isomerism. Br Heart J. 1989;62(4):291–7.
80. De Tommasi S, Daliento L, Ho SY, Macartney FJ, Anderson RH. Analysis of atrioventricular junction, ventricular mass, and ventriculoarterial junction in 43 specimens with atrial isomerism. Br Heart J. 1981;45(3):236–47.
81. Parsons JM, Baker EJ, Anderson RH, et al. Morphological evaluation of atrioventricular septal defects by magnetic resonance imaging. Br Heart J. 1990;64(2):138–45.
82. Quaegebeur J, Kirklin JW, Pacifico AD, Bargeron Jr LM. Surgical experience with unroofed coronary sinus. Ann Thorac Surg. 1979;27(5):418–25.
83. Ootaki Y, Yamaguchi M, Yoshimura N, Oka S, Yoshida M, Hasegawa T. Unroofed coronary sinus syndrome: diagnosis, classification, and surgical treatment. J Thorac Cardiovasc Surg. 2003;126(5):1655–6.
84. Attenhofer Jost CH, Connolly HM, Danielson GK, Dearani JA, Warnes CA, Jamil Tajik A. Clinical features and surgical outcome in 25 patients with fenestrations of the coronary sinus. Cardiol Young. 2007;17(6):592–600.
85. Matsuwaka R, Tomokuni T, Ishikawa S, Watanabe F, Matsushita T, Matsuda H. Partially unroofed coronary sinus associated with tricuspid atresia: an important associated lesion in the Fontan operation. Eur J Cardiothorac Surg. 1987;1:180–2.
86. Brancaccio G, Miraldi F, Ventriglia F, Michielon G, Di Donato RM, De Santis M. Multidetector-row helical computed tomography imaging of unroofed coronary sinus. Int J Cardiol. 2003;91:251–3.
87. Chaturvedi A, Dubinsky TJ, Maki JH. MR findings of a rare defect, coronary sinus ASD. Int J Cardiovasc Imaging. 2012;28(2):429–30.
88. Du ZD, Koenig P, Cao QL, et al. Comparison of transcatheter closure of secundum atrial septal defect using the Amplatzer septal occluder associated with deficient versus sufficient rims. Am J Cardiol. 2002;90:865–9.
89. Fischer G, Stieh J, Uebing A, et al. Experience with transcatheter closure of secundum atrial septal defects using the Amplatzer septal occluder: a single centre study in 236 consecutive patients. Heart. 2003;89: 199–204.
90. Veldtman GR, Razack V, Siu S, El-Hajj H, Walker F, Webb GD, Benson LN, McLaughlin PR. Right ventricular form and function after percutaneous atrial septal defect device closure. J Am Coll Cardiol. 2001;37:2108–13.
91. Rickers C, Jerosch-Herold M, Hu X, et al. Magnetic resonance image-guided transcatheter closure of atrial septal defects. Circulation. 2003;107(1):132–8.
92. Lee T, Tsai IC, Fu YC, Jan SL, Wang CC, Chang Y, Chen MC. MDCT evaluation after closure of atrial septal defect with an Amplatzer septal occluder. AJR Am J Roentgenol. 2007;188(5):W431–9.
93. Murphy JG, Gersh BJ, McGoon MD, et al. Long-term outcome after surgical repair of isolated atrial septal defect: follow-up at 27 to 32 years. N Engl J Med. 1990;323:1645–50.
94. Somerville J, Williams RG, Webb GD. Task force 1: the changing profile of congenital heart disease in adult life. J Am Coll Cardiol. 2001;37:1170–5.
95. Hoffman JI, Kaplan S, Liberthson RR. Prevalence of congenital heart disease. Am Heart J. 2004;147:425–39.
96. Warnes CA, Williams RG, Bashore TM. ACC/AHA 2008 guidelines for the management of adults with congenital heart disease: a report of the American College of Cardiology/American Heart Association Task Force on Practice Guidelines (writing committee to develop guidelines on the management of adults with congenital heart disease). Developed in collaboration with the American Society of Echocardiography, Heart Rhythm Society, International Society for Adult Congenital Heart Disease, Society for Cardiovascular Angiography and Interventions, and Society of Thoracic Surgeons. J Am Coll Cardiol. 2008;52(23): e143–263.

97. Anderson RH, Ho HY, Becker AE. Anatomy of the human atrioventricular junctions revisited. Anat Rec. 2000;260:81–91.
98. Saremi F, Krishnan S. Cardiac conduction system: anatomic landmarks relevant to interventional electrophysiologic techniques demonstrated with 64-detector CT. Radiographics. 2007;27(6):1539–65.
99. Tandon R, Edwards JE. Aneurysm like formations in relation to membranous ventricular septum. Circulation. 1973;47:1089–97.
100. Langer C, Horstkotte D, Piper C. Aneurysm of the membranous septum causes pre-syncopes and transient bilateral blindness. Eur Heart J. 2007;28(7):784.
101. Cheema OM, Patel AA, Chang SM, Shah DJ. Gerbode ventricular septal defect diagnosed at cardiac MR imaging: case report. Radiology. 2009;252(1):50–2.
102. Panduranga P, Mukhaini M. A rare type of Gerbode defect. Echocardiography. 2011;28(6):E118–20.
103. Becu LM, Fontana RS, DuShane JW, Kirklin JW, Burchell HB, Edwards JE. Anatomic and pathologic studies in ventricular septal defects. Circulation. 1956;14:349–64.
104. Moulaert AJ. Anatomy of ventricular septal defect. In: Anderson RH, Shineboume EA, editors. Paediatric cardiology 1977. Edinburgh/London: Churchill Livingstone; 1978. p. 113–24.
105. Soto B, Becker AE, Moulaert AJ, Lie JT, Anderson RH. Classification of ventricular septal defects. Br Heart J. 1980;43:332–43.
106. Sutherland GR, Godman MJ, Smallhorn JF, Guiterras P, Anderson RH, Hunter S. Ventricular septal defects: two dimensional echocardiographic and morphological correlations. Br Heart J. 1982;47:316–28.
107. Lue HC, Sung TC, Hou SH, et al. Ventricular septal defect in Chinese with aortic valve prolapse and aortic regurgitation. Heart Vessels. 1986;2(2):111–6.
108. Capelli H, Andrade JL, Somerville J. Classification of the site of ventricular septal defect by 2-dimensional echocardiography. Am J Cardiol. 1983;51(9):1474–80.
109. Baker EJ, Leung MP, Anderson RH, Fischer DR, Zuberbuhler JR. The cross sectional anatomy of ventricular septal defects: a reappraisal. Br Heart J. 1988;59(3):339–51.
110. Macé L, Dervanian P, Le Bret E, et al. "Swiss cheese" septal defects: surgical closure using a single patch with intermediate fixings. Ann Thorac Surg. 1999;67(6):1754–8.
111. Kirklin JK, Castaneda AR, Keane JF, Fellows KE, Norwood WI. Surgical management of multiple ventricular septal defects. J Thorac Cardiovasc Surg. 1980;80:485–93.
112. Griffin ML, Sullivan ID, Anderson RH, Macartney FJ. Doubly committed subarterial ventricular septal defect: new morphological criteria with echocardiographic and angiocardiographic correlation. Br Heart J. 1988;59(4):474–9.
113. Ozkutlu S, Saraçlar M, Alehan D, Yurdakul Y, Firat P, Tokel K. Subpulmonary and subaortic ridges in doubly committed subarterial ventricular septal defect: an echocardiographic study. Eur Heart J. 1996;17(6):935–9.
114. Newfeld EA, Muster AJ, Paul MH, Idriss FS, Riker WL. Discrete subvalvular aortic stenosis in childhood: study of 51 patients. Am J Cardiol. 1976;38:53–61.
115. al-Marsafawy HM, Ho SY, Redington AN, Anderson RH. The relationship of the outlet septum to the aortic outflow tract in hearts with interruption of the aortic arch. J Thorac Cardiovasc Surg. 1995;109(6):1225–36.
116. Niwa K, Perloff JK, Kaplan S, Child JS, Miner PD. Eisenmenger syndrome in adults: ventricular septal defect, truncus arteriosus, univentricular heart. J Am Coll Cardiol. 1999;34:223–32.
117. Neumayer U, Stone S, Somerville J. Small ventricular septal defects in adults. Eur Heart J. 1998;19(10):1573–82.
118. Backer CL, Winters RC, Zales VR, et al. Restrictive ventricular septal defect: how small is too small to close? Ann Thorac Surg. 1993;56:1014–8.
119. Mongeon FP, Burkhart HM, Ammash NM, et al. Indications and outcomes of surgical closure of ventricular septal defect in adults. JACC Cardiovasc Interv. 2010;3(3):290–7.
120. Lun K, Li H, Leung MP, Chau AK, Yung T, Chiu CS, Cheung Y. Analysis of indications for surgical closure of subarterial ventricular septal defect without associated aortic cusp prolapse and aortic regurgitation. Am J Cardiol. 2001;87:1266–70.
121. Fu Y-C, Bass J, Amin Z, et al. Transcatheter closure of perimembranous ventricular septal defects using the new Amplatzer membranous VSD occluder: result of the U.S. phase I trial. J Am Coll Cardiol. 2006;47:319–25.
122. Tomita H, Arakaki Y, Ono Y, Yamada O, Yagihara T, Echigo S. Impact of noncoronary cusp prolapse in addition to right coronary cusp prolapse in patients with a perimembranous ventricular septal defect. Int J Cardiol. 2005;101(2):279–83.
123. Kumar K, Lock JE, Geva T. Apical muscular ventricular septal defects between the left ventricle and the right ventricular infundibulum. Diagnostic and interventional considerations. Circulation. 1997;95(5):1207–13.
124. Cassels DE. The ductus arteriosus. Springfield: Charles C. Thomas; 1973.
125. Lloyd TR, Beekman III RH. Clinically silent patent ductus arteriosus. Am Heart J. 1994;127:1664–5.
126. Cerruto G, Mancuso L. Systemic and pulmonary embolization in a patient with patent ductus arteriosus. Eur J Echocardiogr. 2005;6(5):376–8.
127. Krichenko A, Benson LN, Burrows P, Moes CA, McLaughlin P, Freedon RM. Angiographic classification of the isolated, persistently patent ductus arteriosus and implications for percutaneous catheter occlusion. Am J Cardiol. 1989;63:877–9.
128. Andrade A, Vargas-Barron J, Rijlaarsdam M, Romero-Cardenas A, Keirns C, Espinola N. Utility of transesophageal echocardiography in the examination of adult patients with patent ductus arteriosus. Am Heart J. 1995;130(3 Pt 1):543–6.

129. Li YL, Wong DT, Wei W, Liu J. A new method for detecting the proximal aortic arch and innominate artery by transesophageal echocardiography. Anesthesiology. 2006;105:226–7.
130. Moore JW, George L, Kirkpatrick SE, et al. Percutaneous closure of the small patent ductus arteriosus using occluding spring coils. J Am Coll Cardiol. 1994;23:759–65.
131. Morgan-Jughes GJ, Marshall AJ, Roobottome C. Morphologic assessment of patent ductus arteriosus in adults using retrospectively ECG-gated multidetector CT. Am J Roentgenol. 2003;181:749–54.
132. Celermajer DS, Sholler GF, Hughes CF, Baird DK. Persistent ductus arteriosus in adults: a review of surgical experience with 25 patients. Med J Aust. 1991;155:233–6.
133. Wang JK, Liau CS, Huang JJ, Hsu KL, Lo PH, Hung JS, et al. Transcatheter closure of patent ductus arteriosus using Gianturco coils in adolescents and adults. Catheter Cardiovasc Interv. 2002;55:513–8.
134. Roques F, Hennequin JL, Sanchez B, Ridarch A, Rousseau H. Aortic stent-graft for patent ductus arteriosus in adults: the aortic exclusion technique. Ann Thorac Surg. 2001;71:1708–9.
135. Hayabuchi Y, Mori K, Kagami S. Virtual endoscopy using multidetector-row CT for coil occlusion of patent ductus arteriosus. Catheter Cardiovasc Interv. 2007;70(3):434–9.
136. Thai WE, Harper RW, Seneviratne S. Dynamic volume 320-slice CT in the assessment of patent ductus arteriosus for percutaneous closure. Heart. 2010;96(4):321.
137. Taneja K, Gulati M, Jain M, Saxena A, Das B, Rajani M. Ductal arteriosus aneurysm in the adult: role of computed tomography in diagnosis. Clin Radiol. 1997;52:231–4.

Atrioventricular Septal Defects

14

Nilda Espinola-Zavaleta, Luis Muñoz-Castellanos, and Aloha Meave-Gonzalez

In normal heart, the real atrioventricular septum separates the morphological right atrium from the anatomic left ventricle. It has two portions; the anterosuperior is membranous and the posteroinferior is muscular. The latter is located between the mitral annulus and the tricuspid annulus. The peripheral atrioventricular junction is constituted by an extension of epicardial fat between the walls of atria and ventricles [1]. In atrioventricular septal defect (AVSD) which is due to deficiency of myocardial tissue at AV junction, the membranous septum is absent and there is also a deficiency in the perimembranous muscular tissue.

AVSD has received numerous designations in the past including endocardial cushion defect, persistent embryonic atrioventricular canal, atrioventricular canal defect, and ostium primum atrial septal defect. Defect of the endocardial atrioventricular cushions [2, 3] is a nonspecific designation since it can include the absence of right atrioventricular connection and double inlet left ventricle. Persistent embryonic atrioventricular canal [4, 5] is also not a correct terminology since the defect is due to deficiency of septal structure at the level of the atrioventricular junction rather than the persistence of embryonic atrioventricular canal. Atrioventricular canal defect [6, 7] is also a generalized term since it can include hearts with absence of atrioventricular connection and Gerbode atrioventricular communication. This diverse nomenclature has been criticized and resulted in adoption of "atrioventricular septal defect" as the most suitable term [8]. In this chapter, anatomic features of AVSD will be discussed and its morphopathologic characteristics will be correlated with noninvasive imaging methods including echocardiography, magnetic resonance imaging (MR), and computed tomography (CT).

N. Espinola-Zavaleta, MD, PhD (✉)
Department of Echocardiography, ABC Medical Center, National Institute of Cardiology Ignacio Chavez, Juan Badiano N° 1, Colonia Sección XVI, Tlalpan, Mexico City CP:14080, Mexico
e-mail: niesza2001@hotmail.com

L. Muñoz-Castellanos, MD
Department of Embryology, National Institute of Cardiology Ignacio Chavez, Mexico City, Mexico

A. Meave-Gonzalez, MD
Department of Magnetic Resonance Imaging, National Institute of Cardiology Ignacio Chavez, Mexico City, Mexico

Cardiovascular Magnetic Resonance Unit, National Institute of Cardiology Ignacio Chavez, Mexico City, Mexico

Morphology and Classification

The pathognomonic feature of AVSD is that the septal absence of atrioventricular junction which results in the existence of a single common fibrous annulus within it can form a common atrioventricular valve or two separate valves which constitute the basis of the morphological classification [9, 10] (Fig. 14.1). In other words,

F. Saremi (ed.), *Cardiac CT and MR for Adult Congenital Heart Disease*,
DOI 10.1007/978-1-4614-8875-0_14, © Springer Science+Business Media New York 2014

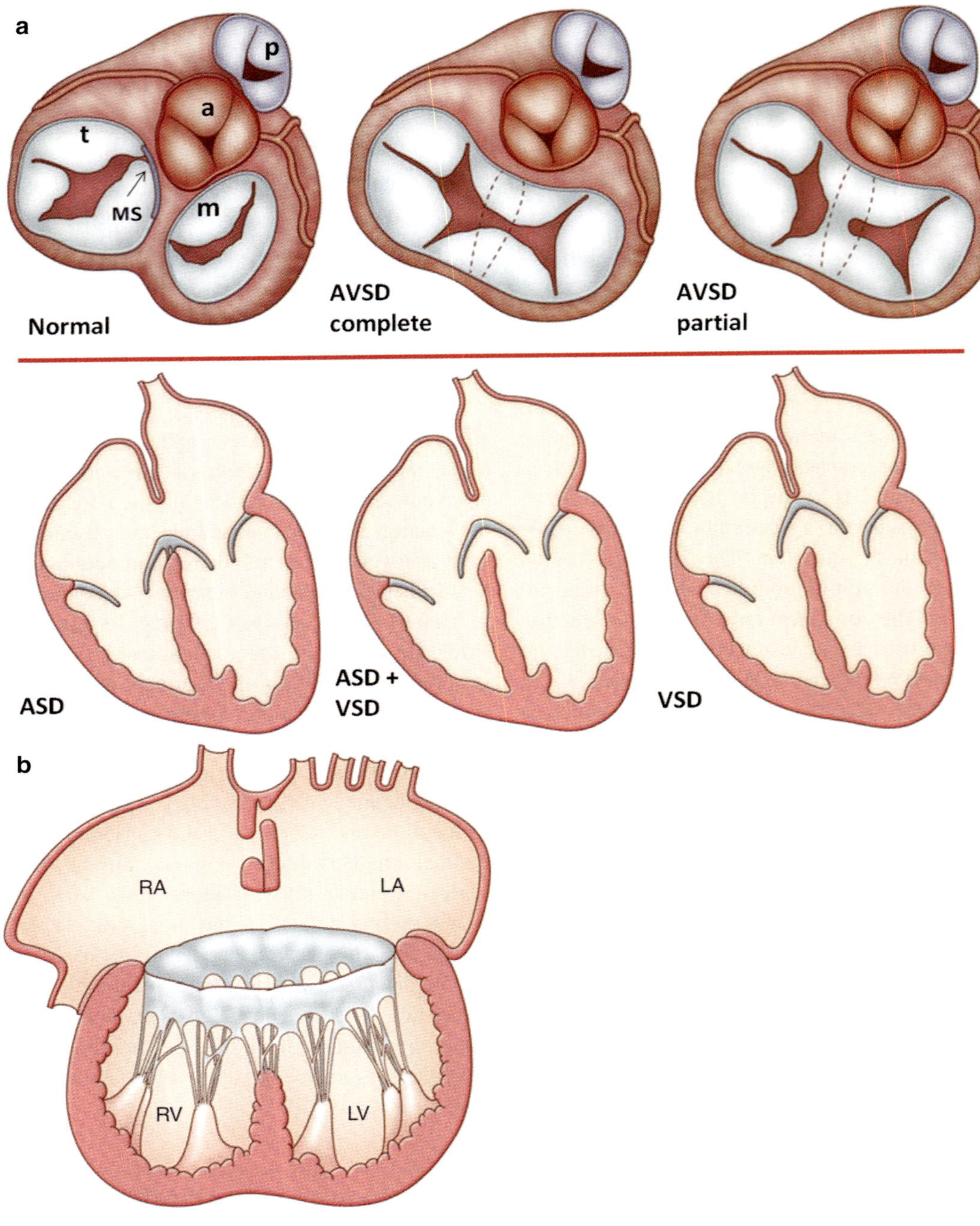

Fig. 14.1 (**a**) *Upper row*: comparison between mitral (*m*) and tricuspid (*t*) valves in normal heart versus atrioventricular septal defect (*AVSD*). Two types of AVSDs including common and partial (separate valves) are shown. Note the membranous septum (MS) position in normal heart and its absence in AVSD. Also note unwedged position of the aorta in AVSD. *Lower row*: different forms of shunting in AVSD are shown. In partial AVSD, only a septum primum atrial septal defect (*ASD*) exists. In complete form, both ASD and ventricular septal defect (*VSD*) usually exist. (**b**) Complete form of AVSD, Rastelli type A. *p* pulmonary valve, *LA* left atrium, *RA* right atrium, *MS* Membranous septum, *LV* left ventricle, *RV* right ventricle

both forms only differ by some modifications in valve leaflets morphology. In "common valve" variant (also known as complete form), the anterosuperior and posteroinferior bridging leaflets are separate causing a permeable interventricular communication, whereas in "two valve" morphology (also known as partial form), the bridging leaflets approach each other and conjoin by a tongue of tissue which is firmly fused to the crest of the ventricular septum sealing the interventricular septal communication [11, 12].

Both morphological types have the following pathological features:

1. Alteration of the fibrous skeleton of the heart characterized by the replacement of mitral and tricuspid fibrous rings by a common fibrous atrioventricular annulus. Trifoliate appearance of the left atrioventricular valve (cleft).
2. Absence of membranous septum and midline fibrous continuity between the left and right leaflets of the common valve. Fibrous continuity with aortic annulus may remain.
3. Unwedging of the aortic root.
4. A ventricular septal defect comprising perimembranous and inlet areas.
5. A relatively short ventricular inlet with an elongated outlet causing increased apex-aortic sigmoid distance (gooseneck). Inlet-outlet disproportion is more pronounced in complete form.
6. Excavated (scooped out) appearance of the ventricular septum which is more obvious in complete form.
7. Superior-inferior arrangement of left ventricle papillary muscles.
8. Posteroinferior displacement of the AV node.
9. Increased rate of the left ventricular outflow tract narrowing due to elongation of the outflow tract and adherence of the anterosuperior bridging leaflet to the scooped ventricular septum.

The interatrial septum is the least affected anatomy. In a large number of hearts, the interatrial septum has normal dimensions with no septal defect [13–15]. There are cases with AVSDs, in which the septal structures are intact and exhibit pathological stigmata of this malformation [16, 17].

An important feature in the diagnosis of AVSD is the type of insertion and the degree of extension of the anterosuperior bridging leaflet, which constitutes the basis for Rastelli type A, B, and C classification. Intermediate forms of insertion between A and B and between B and C and mixed forms have been described. In AVSD, when atrioventricular valves are removed, it is almost impossible to distinguish between the two basic types [8].

In the morphological diagnosis of AVSD, it is important to pay attention to associated anomalies in the hearts including the presence of a common atrium caused by absence of interatrial septation, the parachute insertions of part of the tensor apparatus of the common AV valve, tetralogy of Fallot with double outlet right ventricle [18], and the presence of double valve orifices both in half right and in half left of the common AV valve.

In the embryonic heart, the AV septum arises from growth, development, and fusion of the dorsal and ventral mesenchymal endocardial cushions of the AV canal, which divides it into two AV canals: left and right. On the cephalic part of the left AV canal, the annulus of the mitral valve is differentiated, and at the bottom of the right AV canal, the annulus of the tricuspid valve will be formed. The AV septum so formed has two ends; the cephalic end is associated with the transient foramen primum and the caudal end is related to interventricular septal defect. These two septal defects will be obliterated by fusion of the cephalic and caudal ends of the AV septum to the interatrial septal complex and the ventricular septum, respectively. The cephalic end of AV septum also bends to the left and differentiates into the central portion of the medial valve or anterior leaflet of the mitral valve. Many authors agree that AVSD originates by the lack of growth, development, and fusion of the dorsal and ventral endocardial cushions of the embryonic atrioventricular canal [12, 19]. There is also lack of growth of the ventricular septum and membranous septum causing inlet and perimembranous interventricular septal defect. These two facts explain all pathological stigmata which present the AVSD.

Imaging Techniques

Echocardiography has become the modality of choice for the complete assessment of AVSDs [20]. This technique includes all of the standard views to optimize imaging of specific structures. The subcostal views allow to determine abdominal and atrial situs. The long-axis view will determine the cardiac position within the thorax. Long- and short-axis views show the systemic venous and some of the pulmonary venous return and the size and location of any atrial septal defects. Both the right and left ventricular outflow tracts can be evaluated from these projections. A slow sweep in the short-axis view toward the apex will reveal the size and location of ventricular level shunts, the cross-sectional anatomy of the AV valves, and the location and number of left ventricular papillary muscles. This view is also good for the evaluation of ventricular function. From the short-axis plane, the transducer is rotated counterclockwise approximately 45° to assess AV valve morphology and attachments to the ventricular septum and papillary muscle anatomy. It is the best view to evaluate if the valve tissue is balanced over the two ventricles. The atrial and ventricular septal defects are best seen from the apical four-chamber view. A slow sweep from the apical window offers good visualization of the leaflet anatomy, AV valve attachments, defect size and location, and some information on the mechanism of AV valve regurgitation. This view is also used to measure ventricular length. The left ventricular outflow tract is imaged from the apical two-chamber view. Careful imaging of mitral valve attachments to the ventricular septum, in addition to color and spectral Doppler interrogation, is used to evaluate the presence of, and potential for, left ventricular outflow tract obstruction. Parasternal long-axis imaging gives another excellent view of the anatomy of the left ventricular outflow tract.

High parasternal imaging will complete the assessment of the branch pulmonary arteries and pulmonary venous return and the presence of patent ductus arteriosus and a left superior vena cava. The aortic arch should be imaged either from a high parasternal window or from the suprasternal notch. Long-axis imaging is used to evaluate for aortic arch obstruction. Short-axis views are used to determine aortic arch sidedness and the branching pattern of the brachiocephalic arteries and to exclude a vascular ring [15, 20].

The echocardiography provides precise images of the anatomic findings of this congenital malformation with details of the AVSD, the common AV valve or two separated AV valves, the relationships between the leaflets of the valves in both forms, septal structures and their defects, disproportion between the left ventricular inflow and outflow tracts, unwedged aorta, and the shunts that determine the clinical presentation. This anatomic information is of enormous value for the clinician in planning surgical treatment.

Recent studies demonstrate the incremental value of three-dimensional transthoracic echocardiography (3DTTE) over two-dimensional transthoracic echocardiography (2DTTE) in the evaluation of the AVSDs. Because the various morphological features of AVSDs could be viewed in three dimensions, a more comprehensive and accurate assessment of the size and extent of the septal defects; size, number, and abnormalities of AV valve leaflets (Fig. 14.2) and their attachment sites; as well as the relation of the valvular structures to the great vessels is provided by 3DTTE. In some cases, 3DTTE served to verify the findings seen on 2DTTE and, therefore, increased the confidence level with which various morphological features or abnormalities were detected. In others, 3DTTE substantially changes the morphological diagnosis by providing additional details not apparent on 2DTTE. The three-dimensional datasets also provide en face views of defects in the AV valves such as commissures, resulting in more accurate assessment of their size and extent. Such views are especially helpful when planning for surgical repair.

Color Doppler is useful not only in evaluating the three-dimensional extent of valvular regurgitant jets in the atrial chambers but also in providing en face views of the valve orifices, facilitating assessment of its exact size. This has the potential

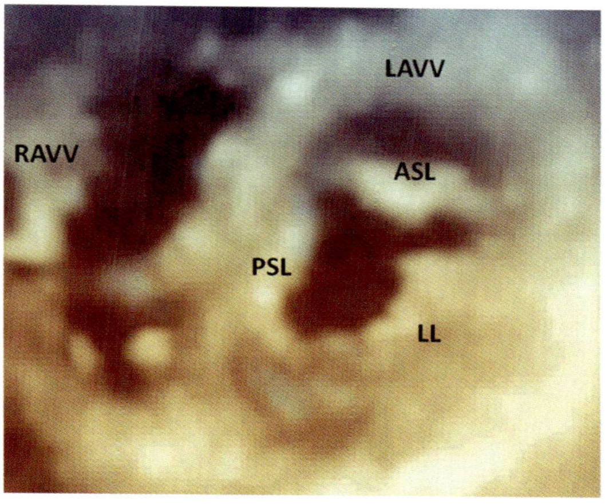

Fig. 14.2 Three-dimensional transthoracic echocardiography of an AVSD with two valves, showing a trifoliated atrioventricular structure in diastole. *RAVV* right atrioventricular valve, *LAVV* left atrioventricular valve, *PSL* posterior septal leaflet, *ASL* anterior septal leaflet, *LL* lateral leaflet

of providing a more accurate quantitative assessment of regurgitant volumes as compared to 2DTTE methods [15, 21, 22].

Echocardiography is limited, however, in the evaluation of certain portions of the aorta (particularly the ascending aorta and the transverse arch), the distal pulmonary arteries, the right ventricle, and the pulmonary veins. These are relative "blind spots" for the echocardiographer. MRI, unhindered by "blind spots," is excellent for the depiction of cardiac anatomy. In all cases of AVSD, the tricuspid and mitral valves originate at the same level. These findings are best seen on axial or four-chamber MR images. Cine MRI can demonstrate the presence of atrial and ventricular septal defects and valve regurgitation.

Cine MR sequences are used to obtain multiple images over the cardiac cycle at each anatomic location. Spin echo pulse sequences are usually used to produce images in which blood signal intensity is low and appears dark ("black blood" imaging). An ECG-gated velocity-encoded cine MRI (VEC MRI) sequence, a type of gradient echo sequence, can be used to measure blood flow velocity and quantify blood flow rate [23].

Multislice CT has important strengths in comparison with each of these imaging modalities, because it provides excellent anatomic information [24]. The primary disadvantage of CT is that it requires the use of ionizing radiation. Echocardiography, MRI, and CT are complementary in diagnosis of AVSD. Intracardiac anatomy is well depicted by all three modalities. Function and flow quantification are well assessed with Echocardiography and MRI. CT provides exquisite images of the great vessels and associated extracardiac anomalies [25].

Anatomo-Imaging Correlation

Anatomo-imaging correlation between heart specimens with AVSD and echocardiogram, MRI, and CT studies of patients with equivalent findings has demonstrated a high degree of precision that can be achieved with noninvasive imaging diagnosis [1].

The AVSDs can be found in any situs of the heart, situs solitus and situs inversus (Fig. 14.3), or in the isomeric positions of dextroisomerism or levoisomerism (Fig. 14.4). In all four situs positions, AVSD can occur in its two forms of common valve (Fig. 14.4) or two separate valves (Fig. 14.5). It is the relationships among the leaflets within the common AV junction that determine the number of AV orifices, while the relationships between the leaflets and the septal structures dictate the possible shunts that can be established between the two sides of the heart [14–17, 26]. Other anatomic characteristics that can be determined by noninvasive imaging include the interatrial or interventricular septal defects. Failure of closure of the ostium primum results in a large atrial septal defect, although in some cases the ostium primum is absent and the interatrial septum is complete [27]. The integrity of the atrial septum can be examined with a 4-chamber image at the level of the AV junction and the inferior portion of the atrial septum (Fig. 14.6). If the septum is complete, its inferior portion reaches the AV junction and there is no ostium primum defect (Fig. 14.6b, c). When the atrial septum is deficient, its inferior portion is far

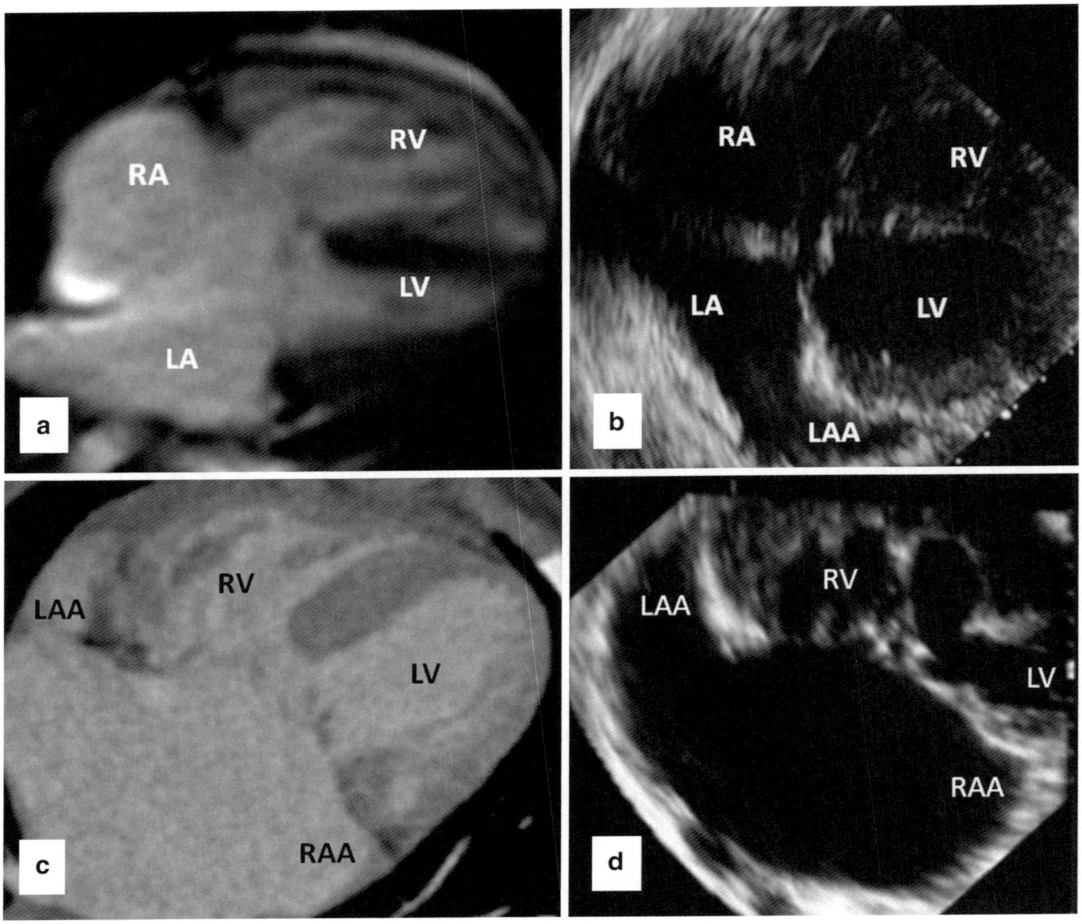

Fig. 14.3 *Upper row* images are four-chamber cine MRI (**a**) and transthoracic echocardiography (**b**) in AVSD with a common valve in atrial situs solitus. *Lower row* images are four-chamber cardiac CT (**c**) and transthoracic echocardiography (**d**) of an AVSD with a common valve and atrial situs inversus. *LA* left atrium, *RA* right atrium, *LV* left ventricle, *RV* right ventricle, *LAA* left atrial appendage, *RAA* right atrial appendage

above the plane of the AV junction and an ostium primum defect is present. Cases have been reported in the literature in which there are more than one atrial septal defect [14–16]. In those cases in which the atrial septum is fused with the leaflets of the common AV valve, a shunt would only be possible through a ventricular septal defect. Two cases are reported in the literature in which the septal defects were obliterated by fusion of the AV valve leaflets to the cardiac septa, and the patients had no septal defects [16, 17].

In cases of AVSD with a common AV valve and a ventricular septal defect, the mode of insertion of the right and left anterior leaflets determines the Rastelli types, a classification with significance for surgical correction. Rastelli types A, B, and C are shown in Fig. 14.7. Intermediate insertions between types A and B and mixed A and B insertions are shown in Fig. 14.8.

An important point is to determine the pattern of connection of common AV valve to the ventricular mass. If the valve is connected

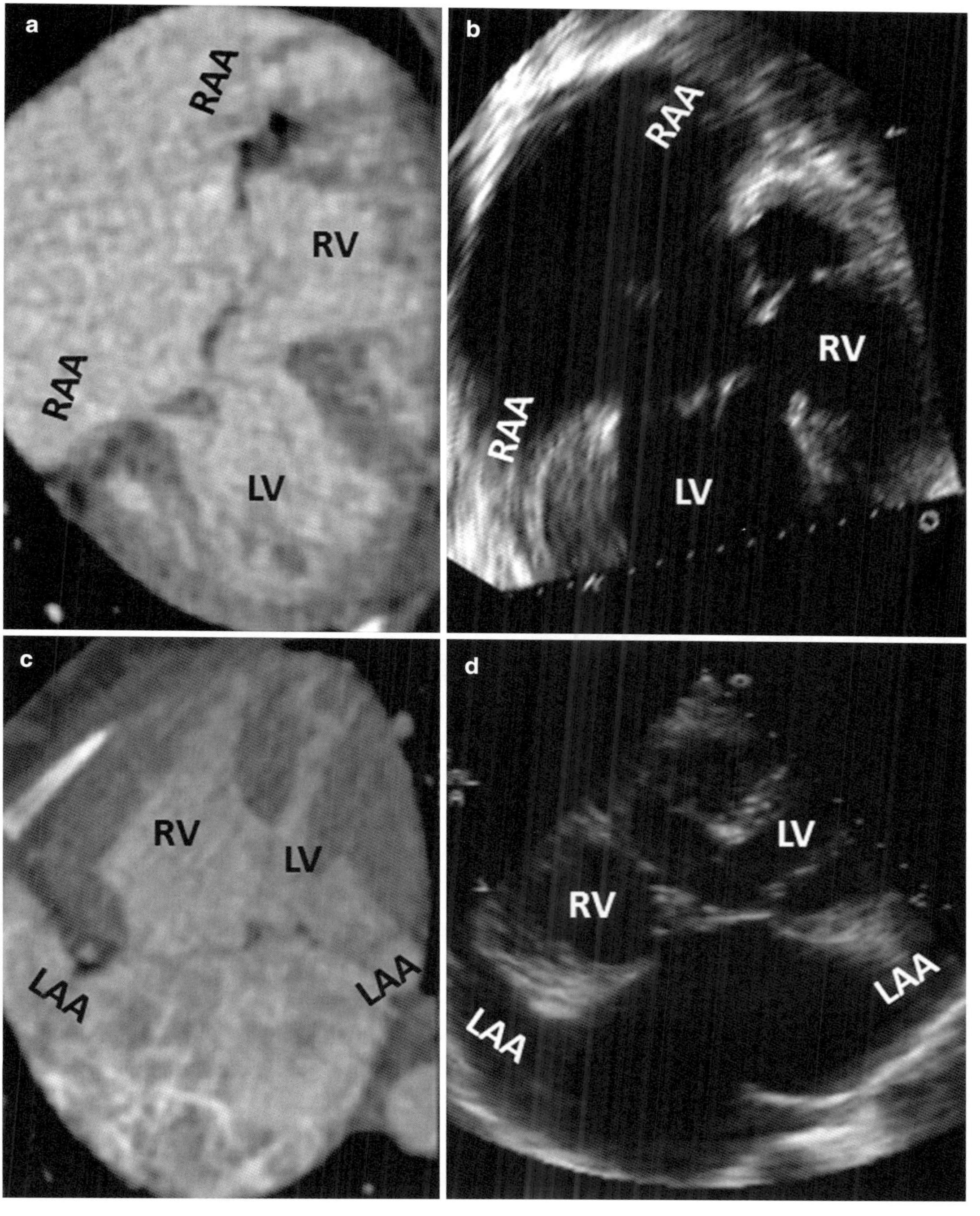

Fig. 14.4 *Upper row* images are four-chamber CT (**a**) and transthoracic echocardiography (**b**) of an AVSD with a common valve in dextroisomerism. *Lower row* images are four-chamber cardiac CT (**c**) and transthoracic echocardiography (**d**) of an AVSD with a common valve in levoisomerism. *LA* left atrium, *RA* right atrium, *LV* left ventricle, *RV* right ventricle, *LAA* left atrial appendage, *RAA* right atrial appendage

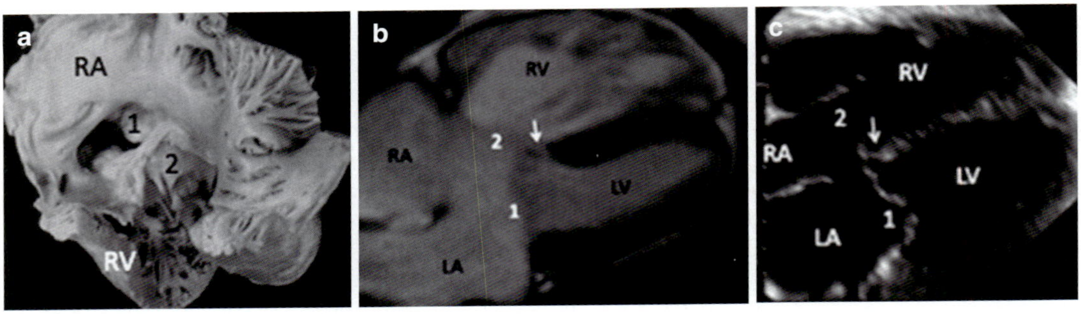

Fig. 14.5 Atrioventricular septal defect with two separate valves (*1* and *2*). (**a**) Anatomic specimen showing the right cardiac chamber and the two valves. (**b**) Four-chamber cine MR. (**c**) Four-chamber transesophageal echocardiography. The closure point of the ventricular septal defect is shown by *arrows*. Ostium primum atrial septal defect is shown between the two atria. *1*-left atrioventricular valve, *2*-right atrioventricular valve, *LA* left atrium, *RA* right atrium, *LV* left ventricle, *RV* right ventricle

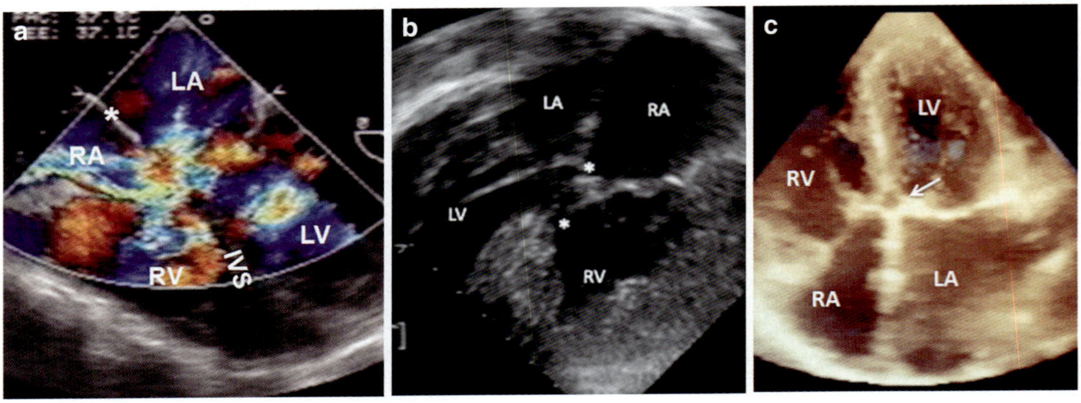

Fig. 14.6 (**a**) Color Doppler transesophageal echocardiogram shows shunt through the ostium primum defect and above the atrioventricular valve plane. The posterior part of interatrial septum is intact (*asterisk*). (**b**) Atrioventricular septal defect without ostium primum defect. Note that the interatrial septum reaches the atrioventricular plane; the superior *asterisk* shows the atrioventricular septal defect and the inferior one the ventricular septal defect. (**c**) Transthoracic 3D echocardiography showing AVSD with two valves and without ostium primum defect. The *arrow* points the closure of the ventricular septal defect. *IVS* interventricular septum, *LA* left atrium, *RA* right atrium, *LV* left ventricle, *RV* right ventricle

approximately with 50 % of its area on each ventricle, it is considered a balanced form (Fig. 14.9, upper row); if the valve is connected in more than 50 % to the left ventricle, it is considered left dominance (Fig. 14.9, middle row), and if the connection is made in more than 75 % to the left ventricle, it is considered double inlet left ventricle connection; when the common valve is connected in more than 50 % with the right ventricle, it is considered right dominance (Fig. 14.9, lower row), and if the valve is connected in more than 75 %, it is considered that this heart has double inlet right ventricle [18].

Another key characteristic of this cardiac anomaly that is present in both types with one and two valve orifices is an unwedged aorta with respect to the AV valves and elongation of the left ventricle outflow tract giving a "gooseneck" deformity appearance (Fig. 14.10). Gooseneck deformity will be best shown on 3-chamber CT or MRI views and on echocardiographic 5-chamber apical image. In this deformity, the length of inlet

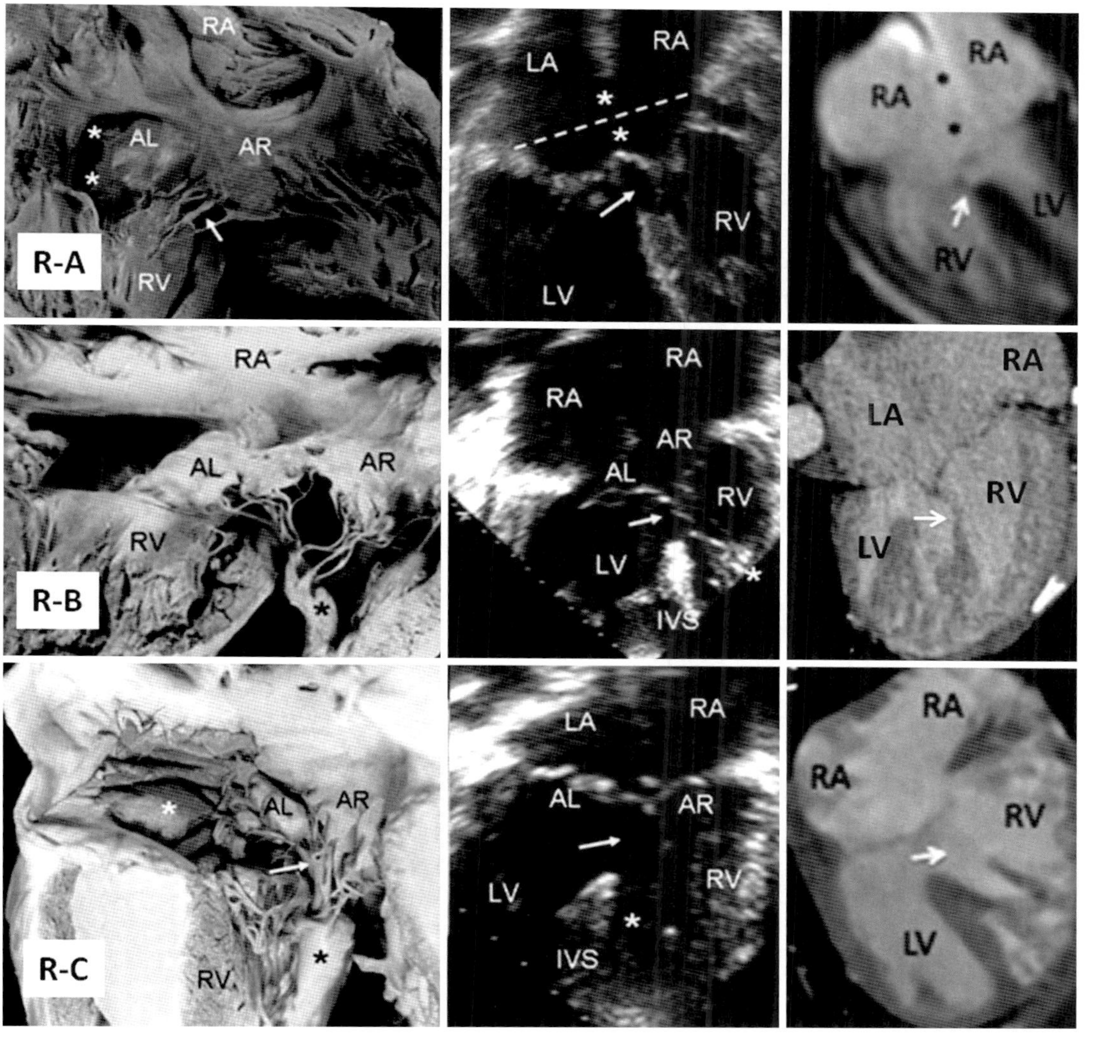

Fig. 14.7 Rastelli classification. Anatomic specimen (*left*), transthoracic echocardiography (*middle*), MRI (*upper right*), and CT (*right*) of different types are shown. *Upper row* shows Rastelli type A (*R-A*) in AVSD with a common valve. In R-A, the chordae tendineae of the anterior leaflets insert in the crest of the ventricular septum (*arrows*) causing the division of the common anterosuperior bridging leaflet into left and right components. As shown in this case, this chordal attachment pulls the plane of the AV valve down into the ventricular septal defect below the plane of the annulus. *Dotted line* indicates the common atrioventricular junction. *Superior asterisk* shows the foramen primum and the *inferior asterisk* shows the atrioventricular septal defect. *Middle row* shows Rastelli type B (*R-B*) in AVSD with a common valve. Rastelli type B is rare and involves anomalous papillary muscle chordal attachment from the right side of the ventricular septum (*arrows*) to the left side of the common anterosuperior bridging leaflet. Note the surgical patch in anatomic specimen (*asterisk*). *Lower row* shows Rastelli type C (*R-C*) insertion in AVSD with a common valve and dextroisomerism. Note the anterior bridging leaflet chordal insertion (*arrows*) into the RV free wall papillary muscle (*asterisk*). In Rastelli type C defects, the anterosuperior bridging leaflet is generally not divided and floats freely over the ventricular septum without chordal attachment to the crest of the ventricular septum. *AL* anterior left, *AR* anterior right, *IVS* interventricular septum, *LA* left atrium, *RA* right atrium, *LV* left ventricle, *RV* right ventricle

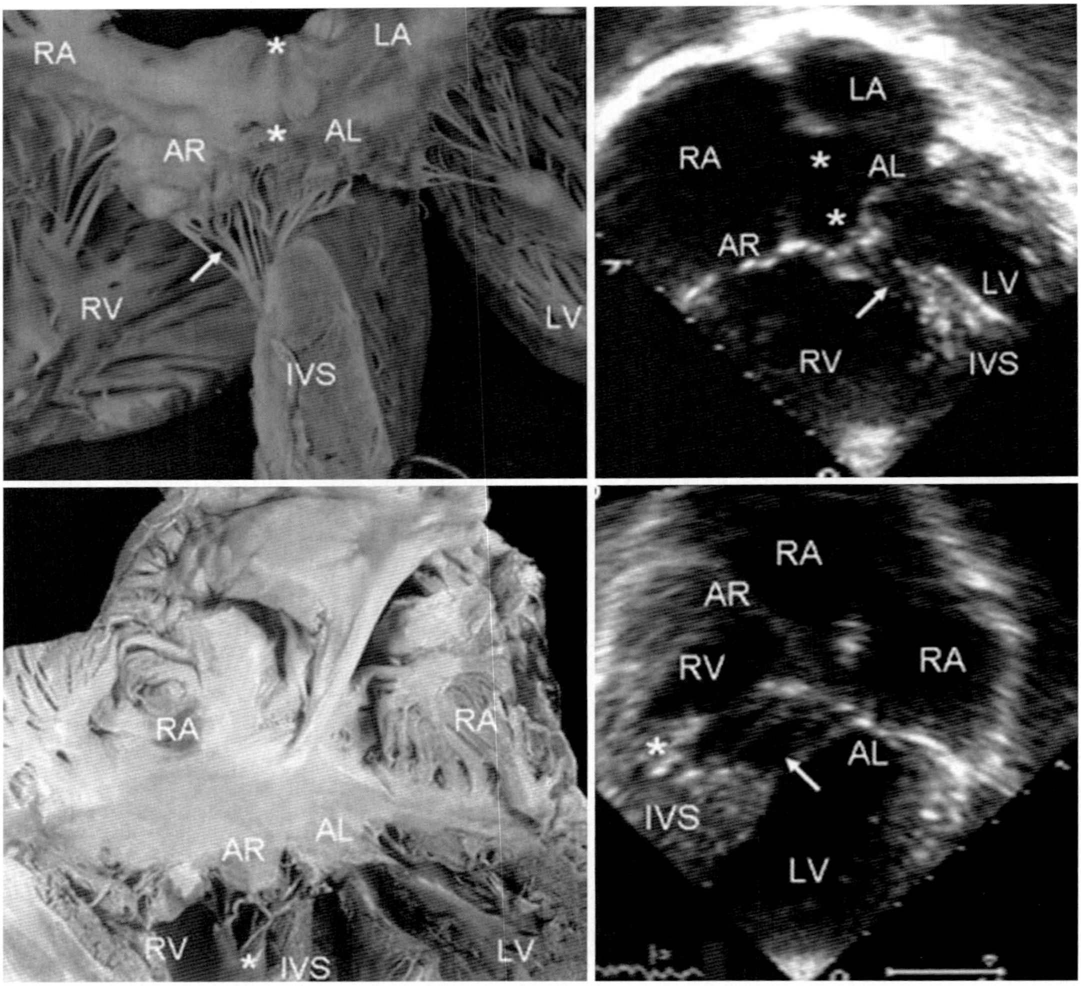

Fig. 14.8 Anatomic specimen (*left*) and transthoracic echocardiography (*right*) showing subtypes of Rastelli classification. *Upper row* shows AVSD with a common valve and intermediate chordal insertion between Rastelli types A and B. The ostium primum (*upper asterisk*) and the atrioventricular defect (*lower asterisk*) combine to form a large septal defect. The *arrow* points the interchordal spaces. *Lower row* images are AVSD with a common valve in dextroisomerism. There is mixed chordal insertions (*arrow*) of the anterior leaflets in the crest of the ventricular septum (Rastelli type A) and the papillary muscle (*asterisk*) adjacent to the ventricular septum (Rastelli type B). *AL* anterior left, *AR* anterior right, *IVS* interventricular septum, *LA* left atrium, *RA* right atrium, *LV* left ventricle, *RV* right ventricle

(AV ring) to apex is shorter than the length of outlet (aorta) to apex. This swan's neck shape constitutes a potential postoperative risk of obstruction [15, 28].

On occasion, the chordae tendineae of the anterior leaflet insert in the interior of the outflow tract causing partial obstruction (Fig. 14.11). The problems of clinical diagnosis can be solved by cross-sectional echocardiography and MRI that show the classic anatomic features of the AV defect [14, 15, 29]. Associated anomalies with AVSD include double outlet right ventricle with

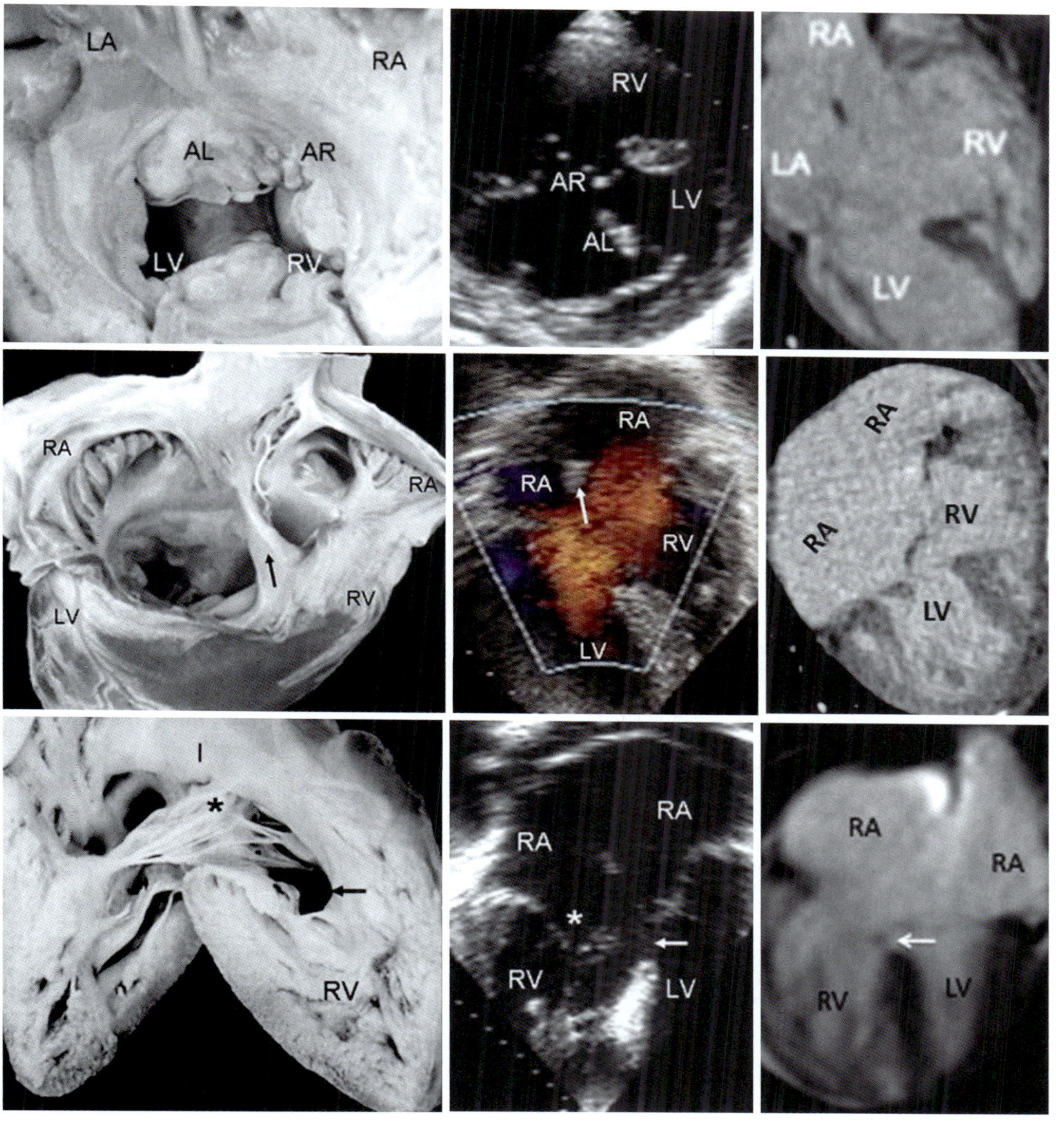

Fig. 14.9 Anatomic specimen (*left*), transthoracic echocardiography (*middle*), MRI (*upper* and *lower right*), and CT (*middle right*) of different types of ventricular sharing in AVSD. *Upper row* images show a balanced form of common valve. The common valve is equally shared by the two ventricles. *Middle row* images show common valve AVSD in dextroisomerism with left dominance. The valve ring is displaced toward the LV, and there is an interatrial band typical of this atrial situs (*arrows*). Color Doppler shows the shunt across the atrioventricular septal defect. *Lower row* images show common valve AVSD in dextroisomerism with right dominance. Note the preponderance of the connection of the common atrioventricular valve with the right ventricle with a double inlet. *AL* anterior left, *AR* anterior right, *IVS* interventricular septum, *LA* left atrium, *RA* right atrium, *LV* left ventricle, *RV* right ventricle

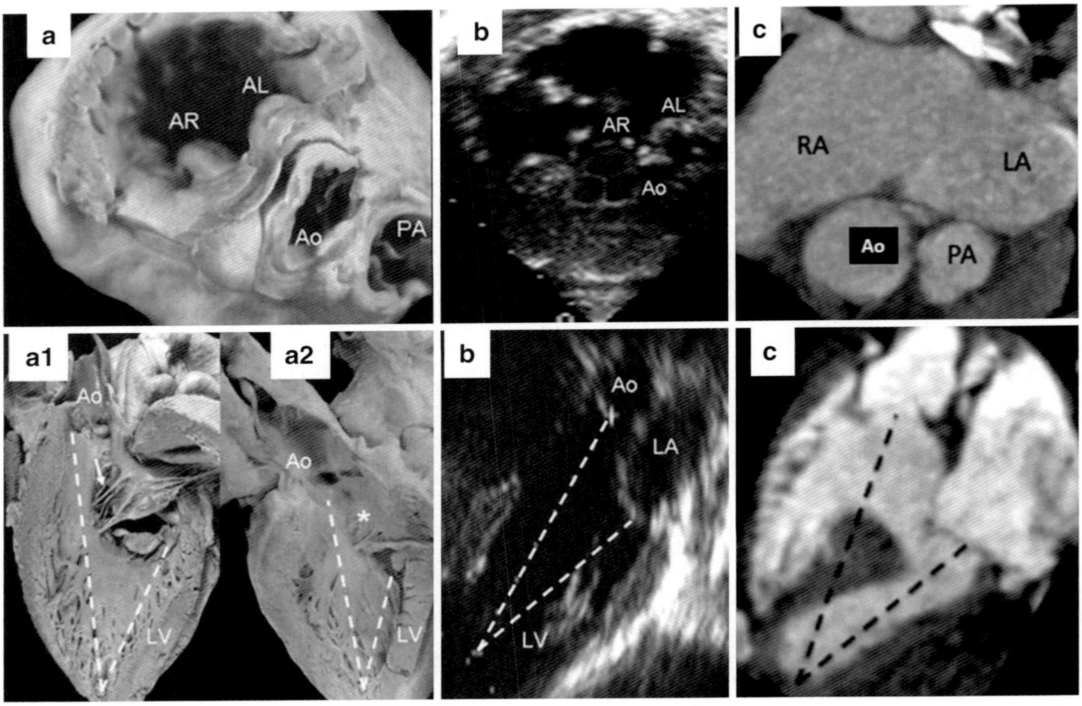

Fig. 14.10 Aortic unwedging and gooseneck deformity. Anatomic specimen (**a**), transthoracic echocardiography (**b**), and CT (**c**) images are shown. *Upper row* images show dilatation of the common atrioventricular ring with unwedging of the aortic valve (*Ao*). *Lower row* images show two anatomic specimens, one with a common atrioventricular valve (**a**1) and second with two atrioventricular valves (**a**2); in the latter, observe a continuous valve insertion on the crest of the ventricular septum, obliterating the ventricular septal defect (*asterisk*). Note shortened inflow tract and elongated outflow tract (*dotted line*) in both types. Disproportional inlet-outlet lengths are also shown on long-axis echocardiography and CT images. *AL* anterior left, *AR* anterior right, *LA* left atrium, *RA* right atrium, *LV* left ventricle, *PA* pulmonary artery

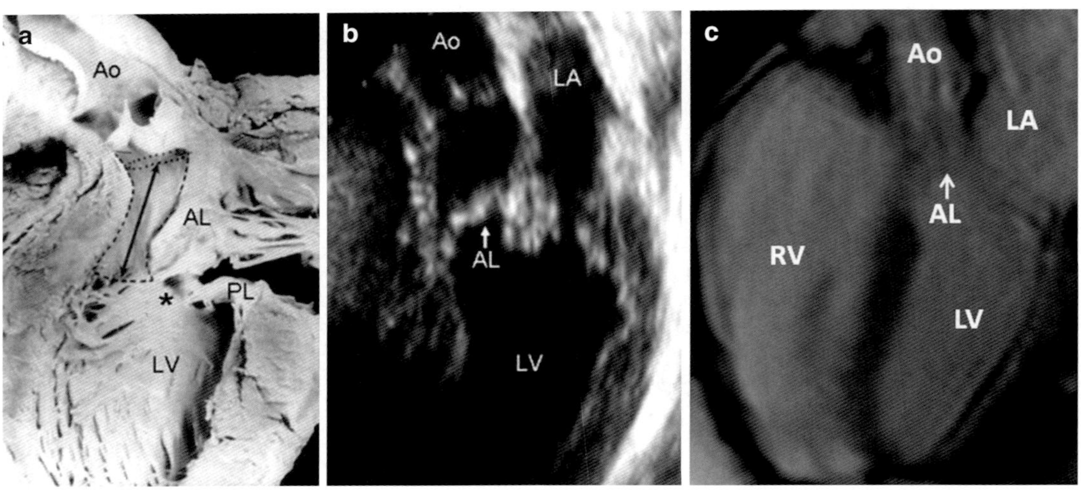

Fig. 14.11 Atrioventricular septal defect with two valve orifices. (**a**) Internal view of the left ventricle showing obstruction of the outflow tract by invasion of the left anterior leaflet of the left atrioventricular valve (*dotted lines* and *double-headed arrow*). The *asterisk* indicates the commissure between the septal anterior and posterior leaflets. (**b**) Parasternal long-axis echocardiographic image and (**c**) cine MR show similar features (*arrow*). *Ao* aorta, *AL* anterior left, *PL* posterior leaflet, *LA* left atrium, *LV* left ventricle, *RV* right ventricle

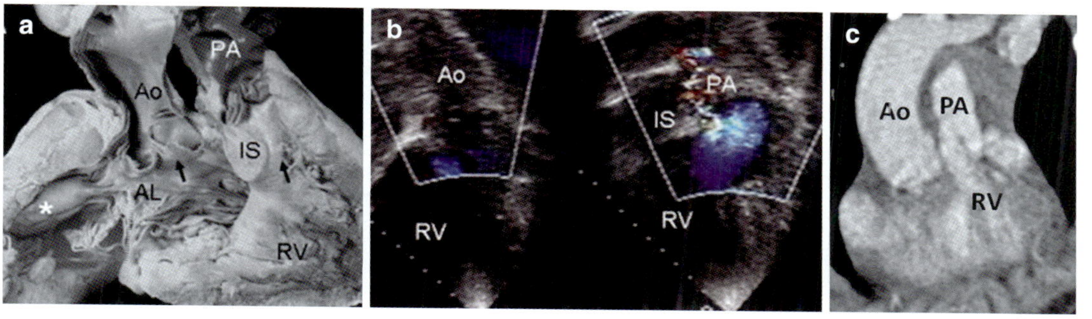

Fig. 14.12 Atrioventricular septal defect with common atrioventricular valve, double outlet right ventricle, and Fallot's tetralogy. (**a**) Anatomic specimen. (**b**) The echocardiographic image and (**c**) coronal CT show the findings. *Ao* aorta, *AL* anterior left, *IS* infundibular septum, *PA* pulmonary artery, *RV* right ventricle. * In (**a**) shows the anterior papillary muscle of the right ventricle. *Arrows* in (**a**) denote aortic and pulmonary outlets arising from the right ventricle.

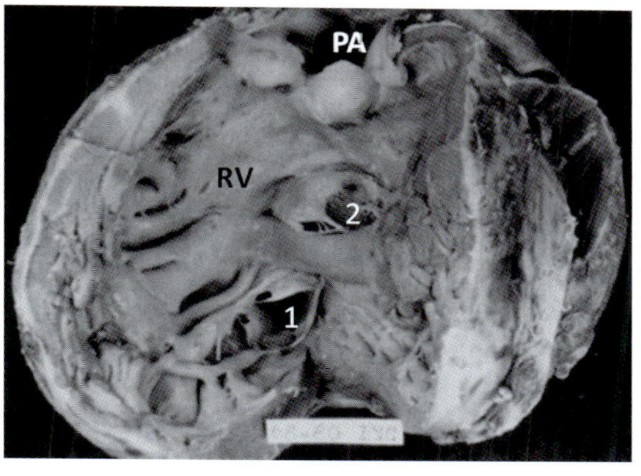

Fig. 14.13 Internal view of the right ventricle showing double tricuspid orifices (*1* and *2*) in an AVSD with a common valve. *PA* pulmonary artery, *RV* right ventricle

tetralogy of Fallot (Fig. 14.12) and double orifices in any half of the AV valve (Fig. 14.13) and common atrium (Fig. 14.14).

In conclusion, the spectrum of findings in AVSD is unified by the anatomic hallmarks of a common AV junction and deficient AV septation. An understanding of the anatomy of this congenital malformation is mandatory for clinical diagnosis by imaging. The anatomo-noninvasive imaging correlation between heart specimens and echocardiograms, CT, and MRI of patients with equivalent findings demonstrates the high degree of precision that can be achieved with noninvasive imaging diagnosis.

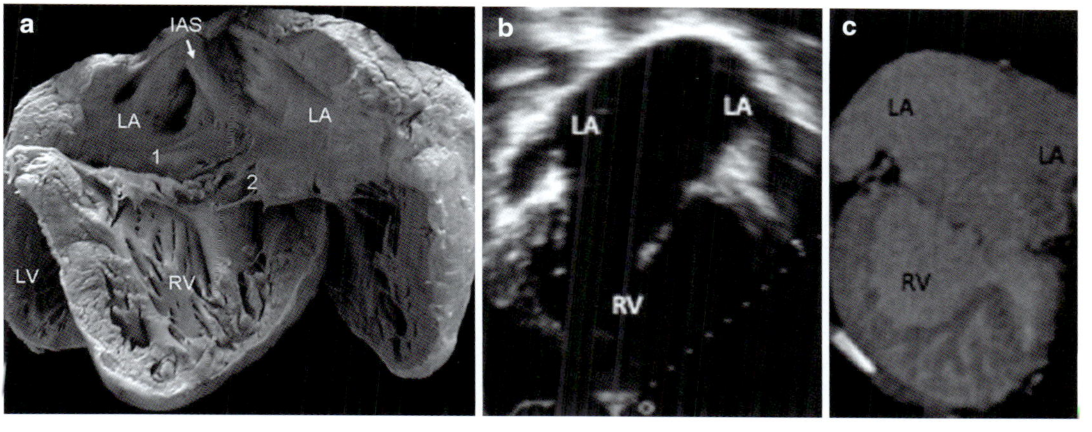

Fig. 14.14 Common atrium and levoisomerism with left (*1*) and right (*2*) atrioventricular valves in the anatomic specimen (**a**) and with a common atrioventricular valve in the echocardiographic study (**b**) and CT (**c**). *IAS* interatrial septum, *LA* left atrium, *RV* right ventricle, *LV* left ventricle

References

1. Espinola-Zavaleta N, Muñoz-Castellanos L, Kuri Nivon M, et al. Understanding atrioventricular septal defect: anatomoechocardiographic correlation. Cardiovasc Ultrasound. 2008;6:33–44.
2. Baron MG, Wolf BS, Van Mierop LHS. Endocardial cushion defects. Specific diagnosis by angiography. Am J Cardiol. 1964;13:162–75.
3. Blieden LC, Randall PA, Castaneda AR, et al. The "goose neck" of the endocardial cushion defect. Anatomical basis. Chest. 1974;65:13–7.
4. Edwards JE. The problem of mitral insufficiency caused by accessory chordae tendineae in persistent common atrioventricular canal. Mayo Clin Proc. 1960;35:299–306.
5. Girod D, Raghib G, Wang Y, et al. Angiocardiographic characteristics of persistent common atrioventricular canal. Radiology. 1965;85:442–7.
6. Somerville J. Clinical assessment of the function of the mitral valve in atrioventricular defects related to the anatomy. Am Heart J. 1966;71:701–11.
7. Emanuel RN, Anders JM, Moores EC, et al. Atrioventricular defects. A study of 92 families. Br Heart J. 1968;30:645–51.
8. Becker AE, Anderson RH. Atrioventricular septal defect: what's in a name? Thorac Cardiovasc Surg. 1982;83:462–9.
9. Piero GP, Leon MG, Wilkinson JG, et al. Morphology and classification of atrioventricular defects. Am Heart J. 1979;42:621–32.
10. Piccoli GP, Gerlis LM, Wilkinson H, et al. Morphology and classification of complete atrioventricular defects. Br Heart J. 1979;42:621–32.
11. Penkoske AA, Neches WH, Anderson RH, et al. Further observations on the morphology of atrioventricular septal defects. J Thorac Cardiovasc Surg. 1985;90:611–22.
12. Van Mierop LSH, Alley RD, Kausel HW, et al. The anatomy and embryology of endocardial cushion defects. J Thorac Cardiovasc Surg. 1962;43:71–83.
13. Gutgesell HP, Huhta JC. Cardiac septation in atrioventricular canal defect. J Am Coll Cardiol. 1986;8:1421–4.
14. Falcao S, Daliento L, Sy HO, et al. Cross sectional echocardiographic assessment of the extent of the atrial septum relative to the atrioventricular function in atrioventricular septal defect. Heart. 1999;81:199–205.
15. Mahle WT, Shivali GS, Anderson RH. Echo-morphological correlates in patients whit atrioventricular septal defects and common atrioventricular junction. Cardiol Young. 2006;3:43–51.
16. Silverman NH, Ho SY, Anderson RH, Smith A, et al. Atrioventricular septal defect with intact atrial and ventricular septal structures. Int J Cardiol. 1984;5:567–72.
17. Ho SY, Russell G, Gerlis LM. Atrioventricular septal defect with intact septal structures in a 74-year old. Int J Cardiol. 1990;26:371–3.
18. Tynan M, Becker AE, MaCartney FJ, et al. Nomenclature and classification in congenital heart disease. Br Heart J. 1979;41:544–54.
19. Van Mierop LHS. Pathology and pathogenesis of endocardial cushion defects. Surgical implication. In: Davis JC, editor. Second Henry Ford hospital international symposium on cardiac surgery. New York: Application Century Crofts; 1977. p. 201–7.
20. Levine JC, Geva T. Echocardiographic assessment of common atrioventricular canal. Prog Pediatr Cardiol. 1999;10:137–51.
21. Singh A, Romp RL, Nanda NC, et al. Usefulness of live/real time three-dimensional transthoracic echocardiography in the assessment of atrioventricular septal defects. Echocardiography. 2006;23:598–608.
22. Hlavacek AM, Crawford FA, Chessa KS, et al. Real-time three-dimensional echocardiography is useful in the evaluation of patients with atrioventricular septal defects. Echocardiography. 2006;23:225–31.
23. Geva T, Sahn DJ, Powell AJ. Magnetic resonance imaging of congenital heart disease in adults. Progr Pediatr Cardiol. 2003;17:21–39.
24. Cook SC, Raman SV. Multidetector computed tomography in the adolescent and young adult with congenital heart disease. J Cardiovasc Comput Tomogr. 2008;2:36–49.
25. Prakash A, Powel AJ, Geva T. Multimodality noninvasive imaging for assessment of congenital heart disease. Circ Cardiovasc Imaging. 2010;3:112–25.
26. Pahl E, Park SC, Anderson RH. Spontaneous closure of ventricular component of an atrioventricular septal defect. Am J Cardiol. 1987;60:1203–5.
27. Becker AE, Anderson RH. Pathology of congenital heart disease. London: Butterworth; 1981. p. 87–9.
28. Ebels T, Ho SY, Anderson RH, et al. The surgical anatomy of the left ventricular outflow tract in atrioventricular septal defect. Ann Thorac Surg. 1986;41:483–8.
29. Anderson RH, Ho SY, Falcao L, et al. The diagnostic features of atrioventricular septal defect with common atrioventricular junction. Cardiol Young. 1998;8:33–49.

15 Ebstein Anomaly

Daniel Tobler, Laura Jimenez Juan,
Andrew M. Crean, and Rachel M. Wald

Ebstein anomaly is a relatively rare lesion, which represents less than 1 % of all cases of congenital heart disease and has a prevalence of about 3–5 per 100,000 live births [1, 2]. Although Ebstein anomaly primarily relates to a malformation of the tricuspid valve with consequent effects on right ventricular development, there is, in fact, a wide variation of abnormalities and associated lesions which may have significant impact on disease prognosis. Ebstein anomaly is unique in that there is a broad spectrum of disease, varying from the severe neonatal form which continues to carry a dismal prognosis, even in contemporary series, to the milder form which may only become manifest in adult life, if at all.

Typically, the tricuspid valve septal leaflet is displaced in Ebstein anomaly, resulting in an 'atrialised right ventricle' and a 'functional right ventricle'. Significant tricuspid valve incompetence is often seen. Extent of tricuspid valve disease has been related to abnormalities in functional right ventricular size. Cardiovascular magnetic resonance imaging (CMR) is the cross-sectional imaging modality of choice for evaluation of cardiac anatomy and ventricular function in the adult with Ebstein anomaly. Cardiac computed tomography (CT) is an alternative imaging modality which is well suited for delineation of valve morphology, particularly in patients unable to undergo CMR.

Embryology and Morphology

Displacement of the Right Atrioventricular Junction

The sine qua non of Ebstein anomaly is apical displacement of the functional tricuspid annulus into the right ventricle in a spiral fashion such that the valve is displaced anteriorly and rightward. Embryologically, there is failure of delamination of the valve tissue from the underlying myocardium resulting in apical attachments of the mural (posterior) and septal leaflets. This apical displacement of the atrioventricular junction results in an inlet portion of the right ventricle which is attenuated resulting in two components: an

D. Tobler, MD
Congenital Heart Disease Program, Department of Cardiology, University Hospital Basel, Petersgraben 4, Basel CH-4031, Switzerland

L.J. Juan, MD
Department of Radiology, Sunnybrook Health Sciences Centre, University of Toronto, Toronto, ON, Canada

A.M. Crean, BSc, BM, MRCP, MSc, FRCR
Department of Medicine and Medical Imaging, Toronto Congenital Cardiac Centre for Adults, Peter Munk Cardiac Centre, University Health Network, University of Toronto, Toronto, ON, Canada

R.M. Wald, MD, FRCPC (✉)
Departments of Pediatrics, Medicine, Obstetrics/Gynecology and Medical Imaging, Toronto Congenital Cardiac Centre for Adults, Peter Munk Cardiac Centre, University Health Network, University of Toronto, Toronto, ON, Canada
e-mail: rachel.wald@uhn.ca

F. Saremi (ed.), *Cardiac CT and MR for Adult Congenital Heart Disease*,
DOI 10.1007/978-1-4614-8875-0_15, © Springer Science+Business Media New York 2014

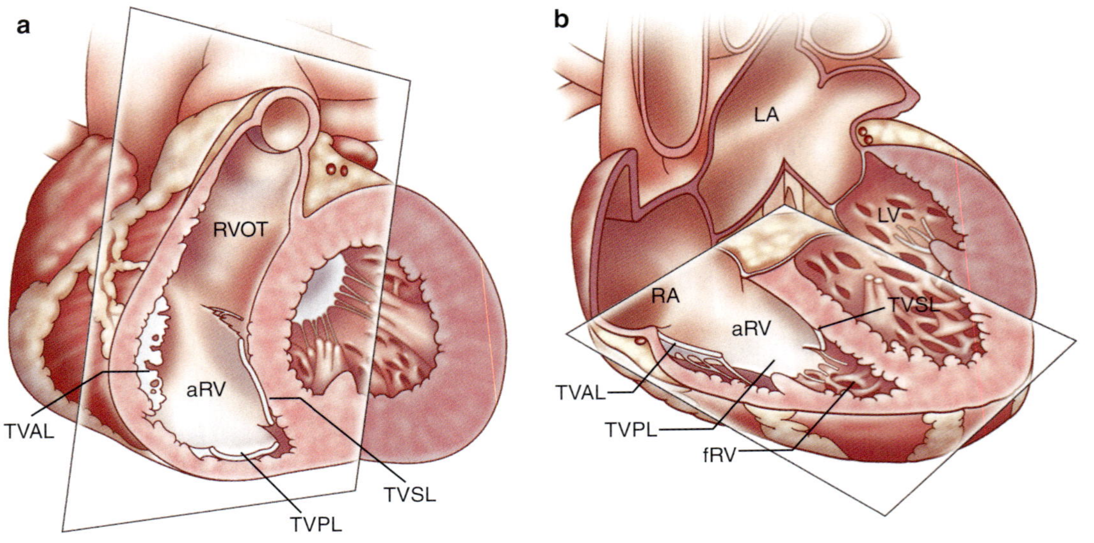

Fig. 15.1 Three-dimensional reproduction of the heart with Ebstein anomaly demonstrating views of the tricuspid valve from short-axis (panel **a**) and axial imaging (panel **b**). *aRV* atrialised right ventricle, *fRV* functional right ventricle, *RVOT* right ventricle outflow tract, *LA* left atrium, *LV* left ventricle, *RA* right atrium, *TVAL* tricuspid valve anterior leaflet, *TVPL* tricuspid valve posterior leaflet, *TVSL* tricuspid valve septal leaflet

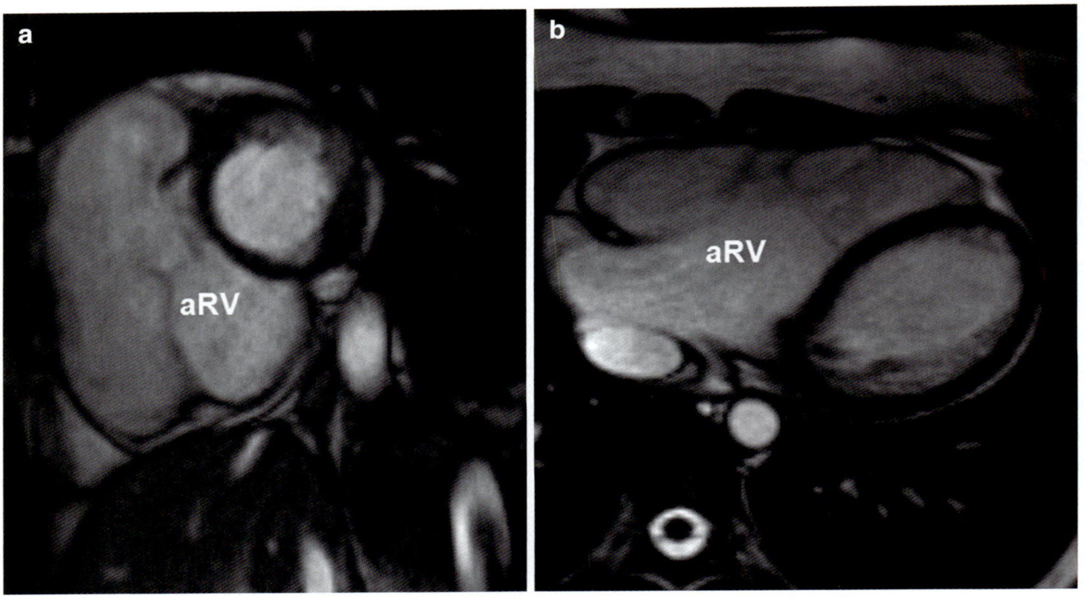

Fig. 15.2 Steady-state free-precession cine images of the atrialised right ventricle (*aRV*) in the short-axis view (**a**) and the axial view (**b**)

atrialised right ventricle and a *functional* right ventricle (Figs. 15.1, 15.2, and 15.3). The degree of adherence of the mural and septal leaflets determines the spectrum of disease severity, ranging from mild forms with minimal displacement of the septal leaflet to complete failure of delamination of the leaflets resulting in an imperforate membrane (tricuspid sac). In contrast, the anterior leaflet of the tricuspid valve is rarely displaced but is often redundant or 'sail-like' [3]. Of note, the

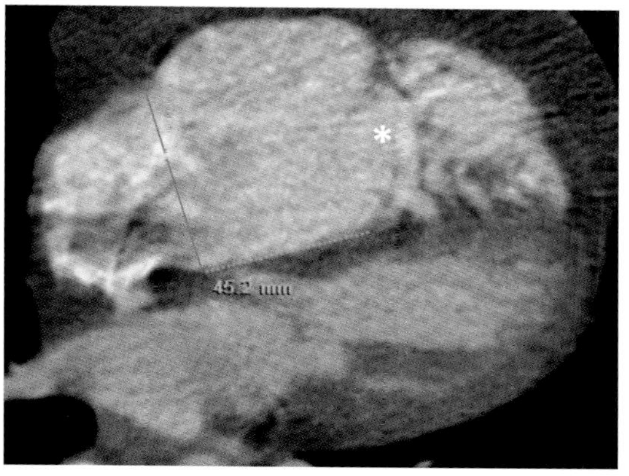

Fig. 15.3 Cardiac CT demonstrates severe dilatation of the right ventricle and apical displacement of the tricuspid valve by 45 mm compared to the mitral septal leaflet insertion. Note the distance between the tricuspid valve annular plane (*solid line*) and the tricuspid valve coaptation point (*asterisk*)

anatomically normal tricuspid valve demonstrates some apical displacement relative to the hinge-point of the mitral valve; however, this offset does not typically exceed 8 mm/m^2 [4, 5].

Morphology of the Tricuspid Valve Leaflets

At autopsy in 1866, Wilhelm Ebstein described an enlarged and fenestrated anterior leaflet of the tricuspid valve. The posterior and septal leaflets were hypoplastic, thickened and adherent to the right ventricle [6]. Indeed, the leaflets of the tricuspid valve are often thickened and dysplastic in the setting of Ebstein anomaly [7]. Fenestrations, particularly of the anterior leaflet, are often present. In addition, tethering of the anterior leaflet is often seen and is caused by chordal attachments to the ventricular free wall and/or displaced papillary muscles. The anterior leaflet is generally elongated and, if redundant, may obstruct the right ventricular outflow tract [5]. The malformed tricuspid valve leaflets often result in stenosis or regurgitation; however, the latter is far more common. The functional integrity of the tricuspid valve in Ebstein anomaly generally depends on several factors: (a) the degree of displacement of the right atrioventricular junction, (b) the extent of dysplasia and the presence/size of fenestrations, (c) the size and restriction of the anterior leaflet and/or (d) the dimension of the 'functional' tricuspid valve annulus. Of note, the degree of displacement of the right atrioventricular junction has important relevance for disease severity and ultimate prognosis in adult patients [8].

Development of the Right Heart Chambers

In addition to tricuspid valve disease, Ebstein anomaly is characterised by a wide spectrum of right ventricular development. In severe forms, the atrialised portion of the right ventricle can become disproportionally large, a finding which has been shown to be associated with poor prognosis in both children [9] and adults [8, 10]. The apex of the functional right ventricle is often heavily trabeculated although the myocardium itself may be thinned or even aneurysmal. In the extreme form, replacement of the myocardium with fibrous tissue has been observed [11]. Although hypoplasia of the functional right ventricle is often seen in neonates and young children with moderate to severe forms of Ebstein anomaly (as a result of downward displacement of the right atrioventricular junction), in adults, conversely, the indexed volume of the functional portion of the right ventricle is typically normal or may even be dilated [12–14]. In two recent studies, dilatation of the functional right ventricle was associated with the severity of tricuspid regurgitation suggesting a mechanistic link between valve insufficiency and enlargement of the functional right ventricle [14, 15] (Fig. 15.4). Unlike neonates, in these studies of adults, there was a linear relationship between the magnitude of apical displacement and the size of the functional right ventricle, likely reflecting an adaptive response to long-standing volume overload from tricuspid regurgitation.

Associated Cardiac Malformations

Numerous lesions can be seen in conjunction with Ebstein anomaly. Interatrial communications,

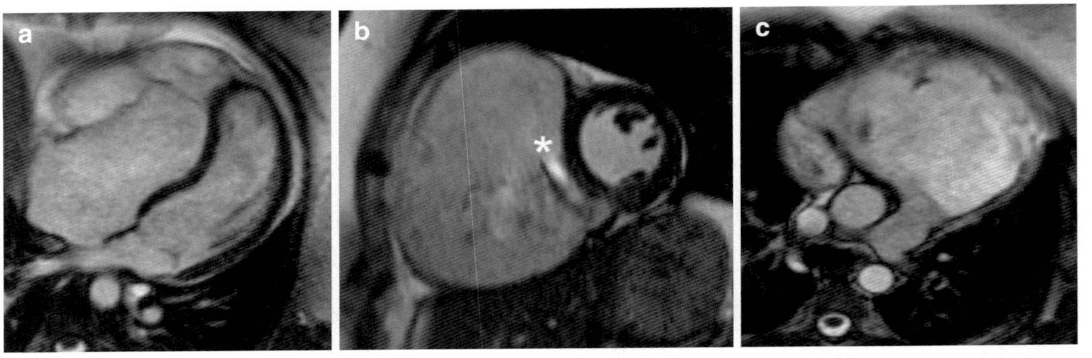

Fig. 15.4 Severe Ebstein anomaly in a 25-year-old woman. These steady-state free-precession cine MRI images demonstrate significant apical displacement of the septal leaflet in the 4-chamber view (**a**); severe tricuspid regurgitation (* indicates dephasing from a significant regurgitant jet) and severe right ventricular enlargement in the short-axis view (**b**); and marked dilation of the right ventricular outflow tract in the 4-chamber view (**c**). The end-diastolic volumes of the 'functional right ventricle' was 508 cc (244 cc/m^2) in the axial view consistent with severe enlargement (upper limit of normal, 103 cc/m^2 for a female)

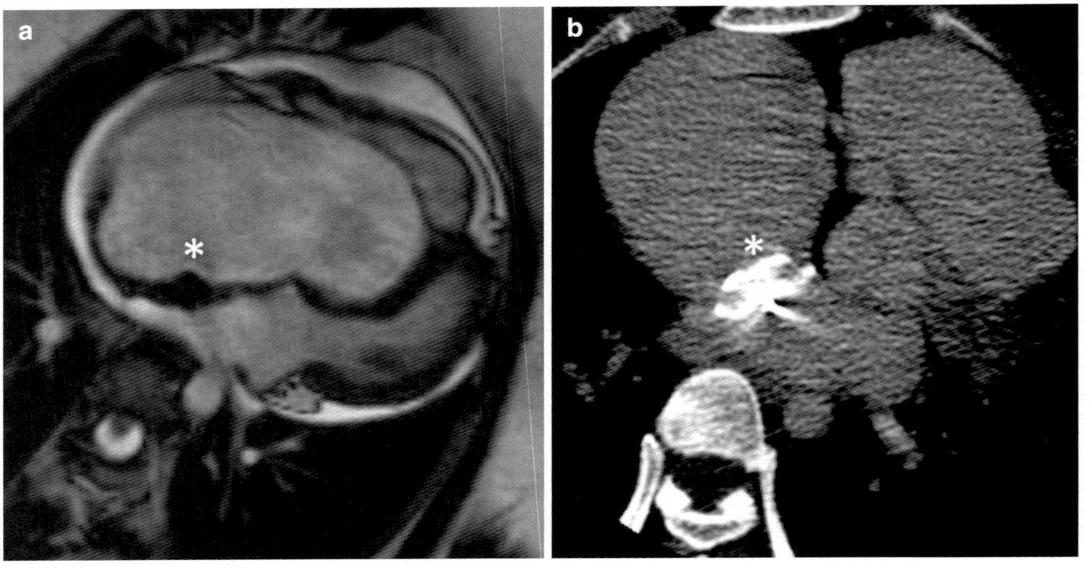

Fig. 15.5 A 32-year-old woman with severe Ebstein anomaly who developed significant cyanosis during pregnancy due to the presence of a patent foramen ovale (PFO). When cyanosis persisted postpartum, she underwent percutaneous device closure of her PFO with an Amplatzer septal occluder, shown here (*) in the 4-chamber view on steady-state free-precession cine MRI imaging (**a**) and in the axial view on non-contrast CT (**b**). Note the localised susceptibility artefact related to the device on MRI. After successful deployment of the device, there was full recovery of oxygen saturations

such as a secundum atrial septal defects or a patent foramen ovale, are the most common and are reported in more than 80 % of cases [16] (Fig. 15.5). Other associated findings include patency of the arterial duct, ventricular septal defects, pulmonary stenosis/atresia, bicuspid aortic valve, aortic stenosis/atresia, coarctation of the aorta and/or mitral valve defects (Fig. 15.6).

Congenitally corrected transposition of the great arteries (cc-TGA) is often associated with an Ebstein-like malformation of the tricuspid valve. In this condition, there are discordant

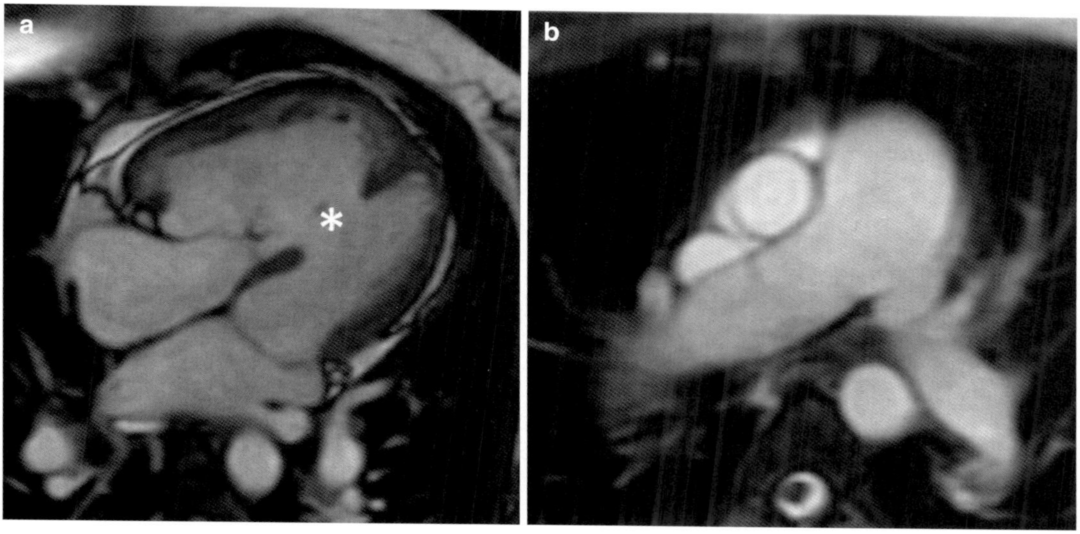

Fig. 15.6 A 22-year-old woman with mild Ebstein anomaly and severe pulmonary hypertension (Eisenmenger physiology) related to a large, unrepaired muscular ventricular septal defect (*). Based on her systemic pulmonary pressures, her right ventricle is hypertrophied (**a**) and the pulmonary arteries are enlarged (**b**). Her prognosis is determined by her pulmonary hypertension rather than her Ebstein anomaly

atrioventricular and ventriculo-arterial connections. The tricuspid valve is associated with the subaortic ventricle and, therefore, is exposed to higher pressure as compared with typical Ebstein anomaly with concordant atrioventricular connections where the tricuspid valve is associated with the subpulmonic ventricle. The dysplastic tricuspid valve in cc-TGA can occur without or with apical displacement of the septal and posterior leaflets. Unlike classic Ebstein anomaly, in cc-TGA, other typical features tend to be absent (i.e. there is no rotational displacement of the septal and posterior tricuspid leaflets, the anterior leaflet may not be elongated, adherence of the septal and posterior leaflets is limited, the atrialised portion of the right ventricular inflow is generally small, and the inlet portion of the right ventricular myocardium tends not to be dilated or thinned) [17–21].

Of note, left ventricular myocardial abnormalities and left heart lesions are commonly seen in Ebstein disease. In about 20 % of patients with Ebstein anomaly, noncompaction of the left ventricular myocardium has been described [22]. It is important to note that, despite potential links at the time of embryologic development, the extent of noncompaction does not mirror severity of Ebstein anomaly suggesting additional phenotypic modifiers (Fig. 15.7) [22, 23].

The apical displacement of the septal tricuspid valve leaflet may result in discontinuity of the central fibrous body and septal atrioventricular ring, creating a potential substrate for accessory pathway formation. Specifically, Wolff-Parkinson-White syndrome is seen and has been documented in up to 36 % of patients with Ebstein anomaly [24, 25]. In the adult population with further atrial enlargement, patients with Ebstein anomaly are predisposed to other supraventricular arrhythmias such as ectopic atrial tachycardia, atrial flutter or atrial fibrillation [25]. Ventricular arrhythmias (in the setting of myocardial fibrosis or in the context of left ventricular noncompaction) have been described, although are far less common than atrial arrhythmias. [22, 25]

Differential Diagnoses

The most common entities to consider in the differential diagnosis for Ebstein anomaly include tricuspid valve dysplasia and Uhl's anomaly.

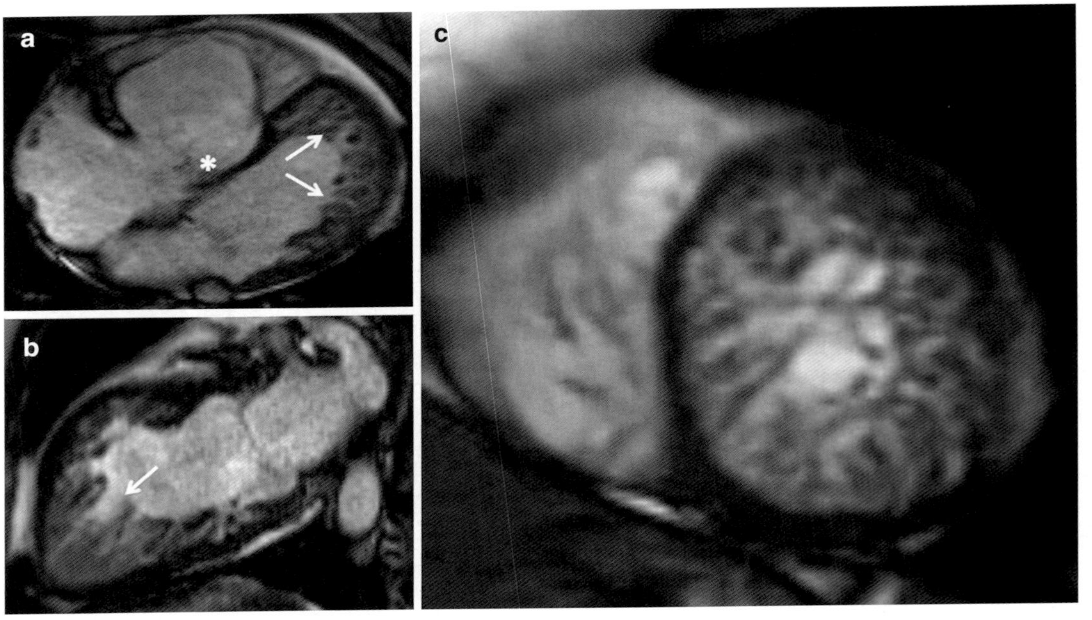

Fig. 15.7 A 40-year-old female with Ebstein anomaly of the tricuspid valve (*) associated with noncompaction of the left ventricle (noncompacted segments predominate at the left ventricular apex and free wall, *arrows*), on steady-state free-precession cine MR imaging in the 4-chamber view (**a**), 2-chamber view (**b**) and short-axis view (**c**)

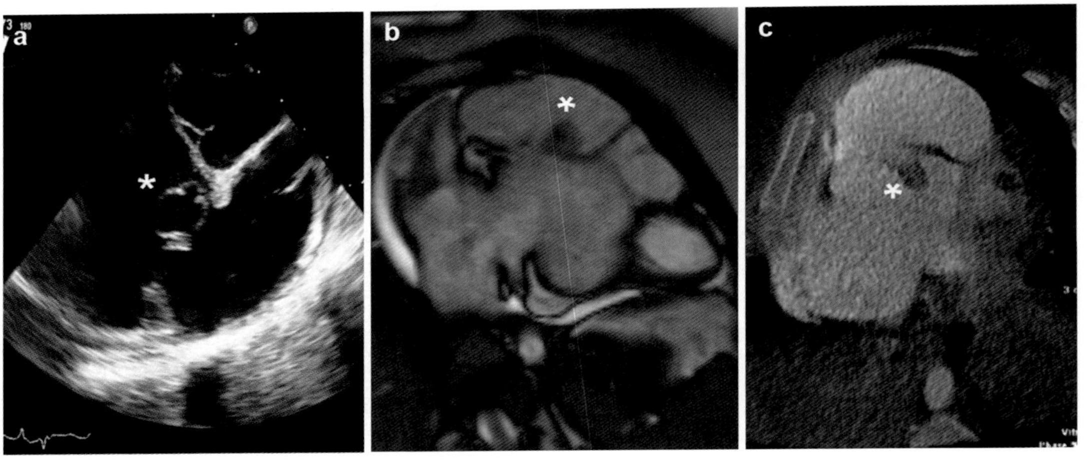

Fig. 15.8 Incidental finding of a cystic structure (*) (1.9 × 1.6 cm) related to the septal leaflet of the tricuspid valve, imaged on transthoracic echocardiography (**a**), cardiac MRI (**b**) and cardiac CT (**c**). Redundant tissue and other abnormalities of the valve leaflets are often seen in the setting of Ebstein anomaly

Tricuspid valve dysplasia is a condition defined as a spectrum of congenital anomalies of the tricuspid valve leaflets, chordae and papillary muscles often resulting in tricuspid regurgitation. Although the tricuspid valve may be dysplastic or redundant in the setting of Ebstein anomaly (Fig. 15.8), in the case of isolated tricuspid valve dysplasia, there is no apical displacement of the septal leaflet, and ventricular dysplasia is absent (in contrast to Ebstein anomaly). Uhl's anomaly is characterised by complete or partial absence of the myocardial layer of the right

ventricle. Unlike Ebstein anomaly, the tricuspid valve is not involved in the disease process. Uhl's anomaly is rarely associated with other cardiac malformations.

Clinical Presentation and Treatment Options

In the most extreme form of Ebstein anomaly, cyanosis and heart failure become apparent within the first days of life. Despite recent advances in surgical and medical treatment in congenital heart disease, symptomatic newborns with Ebstein anomaly continue to have dismal outcomes, even in contemporary series [26–28]. Perhaps as a consequence of high mortality in neonatal life, selection bias dictates that adult survivors of Ebstein anomaly will represent the milder form of the disease spectrum.

In milder forms of Ebstein anomaly, patients may be asymptomatic throughout adult life. Although adults may come to medical attention with signs of heart failure or symptomatic arrhythmia [10], fatigue and exercise intolerance are common presentations (Fig. 15.9). Indeed, peak oxygen uptake is reduced in most patients with Ebstein anomaly; the mean aerobic capacity (peak VO_2) in a meta-analysis of 230 patients (mean age 22.9 years, 51.5 % male) was about 21 ± 7 ml/min/

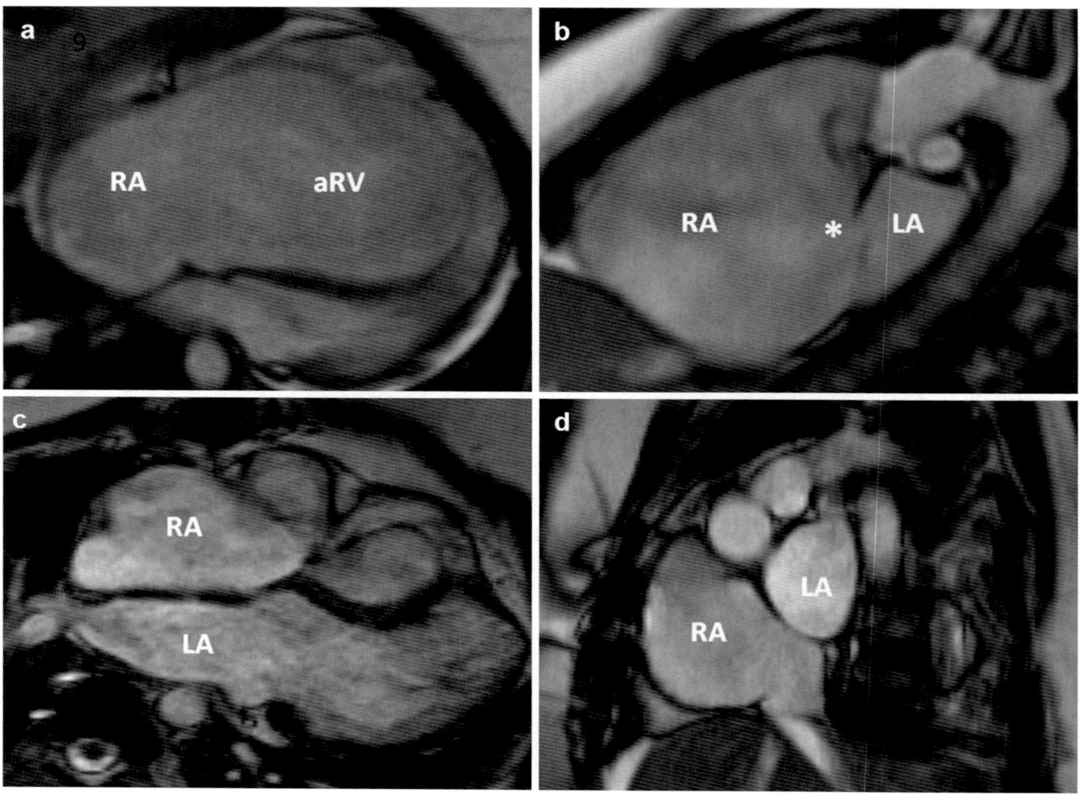

Fig. 15.9 A 26-year-old female with Ebstein anomaly of the tricuspid valve and secundum atrial defect was referred for surgical repair due to exercise intolerance, recurrent atrial arrhythmias and significant tricuspid insufficiency. Steady-state free-precession (SSFP) cine MRI images demonstrate anatomy before surgery (*top panels*) and after surgery (*lower panels*). Panels (**a**): 4-chamber SSFP view demonstrating apical displacement of the tricuspid valve and significant atrialisation of the right ventricle (*aRV*); (**b**) short-axis SSFP view through the atria demonstrating an enlarged right atrium (*RA*) and a secundum atrial septal defect (*); left atrium (*LA*) is diminutive. (**c**) 4-chamber SSFP view after surgical repair (including RA plication, RA Maze, secundum ASD closure and tricuspid valve repair); and (**d**) short-axis SSFP view demonstrating an intact atrial septum post suture closure of ASD

kg, and half of those studied had an aerobic capacity <60 % of predicted for normal [29]. Decreased aerobic activity has been associated with low resting oxygen saturation [30], a finding which is most often explained by a persistent right-to-left shunt at atrial level. Therefore, device closure may be indicated when cyanosis is present, despite the absence of severe tricuspid valve disease (Fig. 15.5) [31]. From an imaging perspective, aerobic capacity has been shown to have an inverse relationship with increased atrialised right ventricular volumes as measured using cardiac MRI [15].

Adults with Ebstein anomaly may first present with significant atrial and/or ventricular arrhythmias. In fact, arrhythmia was found to be a major contributor to late haemodynamic deterioration in the adult with Ebstein anomaly. In one study, arrhythmias were the most common reason for clinical presentation in unoperated adults with Ebstein anomaly (51 %) [8]. Patients who experience a significant arrhythmia should proceed to electrophysiologic testing and ablation therapy or surgical treatment of the arrhythmia if cardiac surgery is already indicated for haemodynamic reasons [31].

Contemporary practice guidelines suggest that surgical repair of the tricuspid valve be considered in the context of symptoms and at least moderate tricuspid valve dysfunction [31]. Additionally, PFO/ASD closure should be performed surgically at the time of valve surgery. [31] Currently, tricuspid valve repair is preferred over tricuspid valve replacement. Several surgical techniques have been described, and early and long-term results are reassuring with low in-hospital mortality [32, 33]. When valve repair is not feasible, prosthetic tricuspid valve replacement has shown to be a viable alternative (particularly in patients older than 50 years) with relatively low perioperative mortality [34]. Surgical outcome in tricuspid valve surgery in patients with Ebstein anomaly has been associated with various factors, including male sex, increased haemoglobin/hematocrit values, right and/or left ventricular dysfunction and/or presence of right heart obstructive disease (right ventricular outflow tract obstruction or hypoplastic pulmonary arteries) [35]. After surgical repair, aerobic capacity typically improves [30], and therefore guidelines suggest that symptomatic patients with Ebstein anomaly and at least moderate tricuspid regurgitation should proceed to operation [31]. In select circumstances, such as severe right heart disease including poor right ventricular contractility or extended atrialised right ventricle, a bidirectional cavopulmonary shunt may be inserted to off-load the right heart, considered a 'one and a half ventricle' repair. [36, 37] In rare cases, the right heart disease is severe enough to warrant a Fontan procedure, whereby the right heart is bypassed altogether and caval flow (both superior and inferior) is passively directed to the lungs (Fig. 15.10).

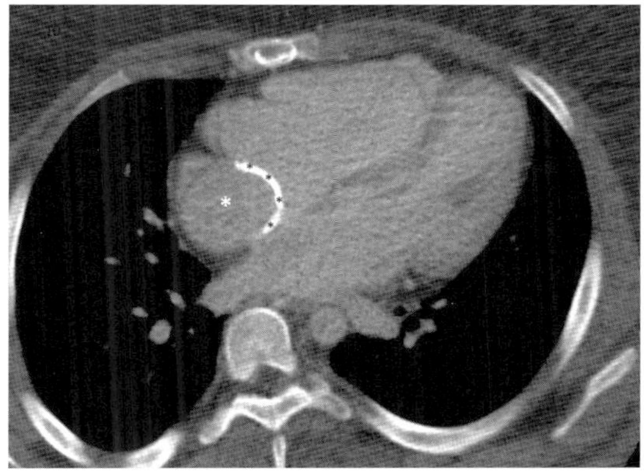

Fig. 15.10 A rare example of an adult patient having undergone Fontan palliation because of severe atrialisation of the right ventricle in Ebstein anomaly – there is severe displacement of the septal tricuspid leaflet towards the apex resulting in a large atrialised right ventricle component (aRV). The gated CT image has been acquired several minutes after contrast administration in order to allow full mixing of contrast and blood with the aim of ruling out thrombus within the lateral tunnel type of Fontan (*asterisk*). Unlike Fig. 15.3, which was acquired at an earlier time point after contrast injection, the tricuspid valve apparatus is harder to appreciate. The anterior component of the lateral tunnel is composed of synthetic material which routinely calcifies (*black asterisks*) with time

Imaging Techniques

Cardiac Magnetic Resonance Imaging

Virtually all aspects of Ebstein anatomy, with the exception of detailed valve morphology, can be well characterised using cardiovascular magnetic

resonance imaging (CMR). Steady-state free-precession (SSFP) cine imaging allows for precise delineation of degree of apical displacement of the tricuspid valve as well as volumetric and functional assessment of the ventricles [12]. Associated lesions, such as atrial level shunts, left heart valve abnormalities and presence of myocardial noncompaction are well seen on cine SSFP imaging; abnormalities in pulmonary arterial development, coarctation of the aorta or a residual ductus arteriosus are best characterised using magnetic resonance angiography. Quantification of an intracardiac shunt can be accurately determined through comparison of phase-contrast flow volumes through the main pulmonary artery and aorta. Severity of tricuspid regurgitation can be estimated when flow through the main pulmonary artery is indexed to the right ventricular stroke volume [14]. It should be noted that precise evaluation of tricuspid valve leaflets, chordal attachments and stenosis (if present) is best achieved using echocardiography due to superior spatial and temporal resolution as compared with conventional CMR.

Despite the widespread acceptance that CMR is considered the reference standard for assessment of right heart size and function [38, 39], relatively little was published on the CMR assessment of Ebstein anomaly until recently. It is only in the last few years that studies have explored assessment of the functional right ventricle using axial or short-axis views on cine SSFP imaging (Figs. 15.1 and 15.2) [12, 14]. Axial imaging seems to provide more consistent inter- and intraobserver measurements as compared with short-axis views which may be explained by the fact that the axial plane affords a better depiction of tricuspid valve displacement and point of leaflet coaptation [12]. That the functional right ventricle in the adult is not diminutive but is either normal in size or, more commonly, is enlarged when indexed for body surface area is a relatively new observation [12–14] and is likely explained by the presence of chronic tricuspid regurgitation (Fig. 15.4) [14, 15]. It should be noted that the precise role of CMR for risk stratification and preoperative assessment of the patient with Ebstein is incompletely defined and should serve as the focus of future research efforts.

At the University Health Network in Toronto, the first-time study of a patient with Ebstein anomaly includes the following sequences: 3 plane localisers, SSFP cine imaging in multiple planes (4-chamber stack, axial stack, short-axis stack and right ventricular 2-chamber view), gadolinium-enhanced magnetic resonance angiogram (time-resolved and conventional) and phase-contrast flow analysis (non-breath held) across the main pulmonary artery and ascending aorta. Follow-up CMR studies will not include magnetic resonance angiography or phase contrast flow sequences if additional cardiac abnormalities were not previously delineated using these sequences.

Although CMR is the cross-sectional imaging modality of choice to evaluate cardiac anatomy and ventricular function in patients with Ebstein anomaly, there are certain situations in which CMR cannot be performed. CMR is still considered a restricted modality due to its relatively limited availability and substantial cost. It is a long study which is often not tolerated by claustrophobic patients. CMR is contraindicated in patients with a permanent pacemaker, defibrillator or retained permanent epicardial pacing wires. Although not absolutely contraindicated in patients with severe arrhythmias, image quality is usually significantly impaired and may result in a nondiagnostic examination.

Cardiac CT

Cardiac CT is regarded as a partial alternative to CMR, since its ability to acquire data at an isotropic spatial resolution permits subsequent off-line reformatting into any anatomical plane desired. This allows precise visualisation of the position of the tricuspid valve, including chordae tendineae and papillary muscles as well as the trabeculated myocardium (Fig. 15.3) [40]. Newer generation multidetector scanners (≥64 MDCT) allow wider z-axis coverage, and with 320 MDCT, a volume of data covering the entire heart may be acquired in a single cardiac cycle – particularly useful in patients with atrial

fibrillation. Radiation dose is an appropriate concern when considering cardiac CT in a young population. However, modern scanning techniques have dramatically reduced the imparted radiation dose through a combination of size- and weight-based dose modulation, as well as with iterative reconstruction techniques that allow a relatively noisy data set (acquired at low dose) to be smoothed at the time of image reconstruction with acceptable final image quality. A complete single-phase image stack of the heart and great vessels can now usually be achieved with prospective triggering (X-ray tube turned on for only the diastolic portion of the cardiac cycle) at a dose of 1–2 mSv (average dose for a technetium SPECT study for comparison is 10–15 mSv). Ventricular function can be also obtained when data is acquired retrospectively – since this involves having the tube current on throughout one or more cardiac cycles, the dose increases in proportion. In most cases, therefore, function remains more appropriately assessed by CMR or echocardiography in all but the most challenging cases.

Intravenous injection of contrast is targeted to obtain good opacification of the right heart during image acquisition. The exact flow rate, total iodine volume and timing of the scan acquisition after the start of contrast injection are individually adjusted according to the precise clinical question. Intracardiac shunts (such as an atrial septal defect or a patent foramen ovale) may be appreciated particularly if a 'concentration gradient' is established between the right and left sides of the heart. This is most readily achieved with a dual-phase injection such that one atrium/ventricle is opacified with dense contrast, whilst the other is opacified with a mixture of iodine and normal saline. The difference in Hounsfield attenuation values between the two sides then allows shunted blood to be identified in the 'wrong' chamber – the effectiveness of this technique is particularly enhanced when a full cardiac cycle is acquired since the flow of blood through the hole in question becomes more apparent.

Although very uncommonly encountered, some patients with Ebstein anomaly require either Glenn shunt creation or even formal Fontan conversion in order to off-load a severely enlarged or impaired right ventricle (Fig. 15.10). In these circumstances cardiac CT may be useful both for preoperative planning and in the longer-term follow-up where adequate echocardiographic visualisation of the Fontan circuit (to exclude anatomical distortion or thrombus formation) is often challenging in adult patients.

In summary, cardiac CT – although not the modality of first choice for imaging Ebstein anomaly – is a reasonable method of assessing the valvular and atrioventricular components of this complex lesion where other methods have failed or are contraindicated. This can be done at low dose (1–2 mSv) with modern dose reduction strategies.

References

1. Samanek M, Voriskova M. Congenital heart disease among 815,569 children born between 1980 and 1990 and their 15-year survival: a prospective bohemia survival study. Pediatr Cardiol. 1999;20:411–7.
2. Correa-Villasenor A, Ferencz C, Neill CA, Wilson PD, Boughman JA. Ebstein's Malformation of the tricuspid valve: genetic and environmental factors. The baltimore-washington infant study group. Teratology. 1994;50:137–47.
3. Zuberbuhler JR, Allwork SF, Anderson RH. The spectrum of Ebstein's anomaly of the tricuspid valve. J Thorac Cardiovasc Surg. 1979;77:202–11.
4. Seward JB. Ebstein's anomaly: ultrasound imaging and hemodynamic evaluation. Echocardiography. 1993;10:641–64.
5. Edwards WD. Embryology and pathologic features of Ebstein's anomaly. Prog Pediatr Cardiol. 1993;2:5–15.
6. Ueber einen sehr seltenen Fall von Insuffizienz der Valvula tricuspidalis, bedingt durch eine angeborene hochgradige Missbildung derselben. Arch. Anat. Physiol. 1866;33:238–55.
7. Freedom RM, Mawson JB, Yoo SJ, Benson LN. Ebstein's malformation of the tricuspid valve, in Congenital Heart Disease: Textbook of Angiography, Armonk, NY: Futura Publishing Co, 1997;349–66.
8. Attie F, Rosas M, Rijlaarsdam M, Buendia A, Zabal C, Kuri J, Granados N. The adult patient with Ebstein anomaly. Outcome in 72 unoperated patients. Medicine. 2000;79:27–36.
9. Celermajer DS, Cullen S, Sullivan ID, Spiegelhalter DJ, Wyse RK, Deanfield JE. Outcome in neonates with Ebstein's anomaly. J Am Coll Cardiol. 1992;19:1041–6.
10. Celermajer DS, Bull C, Till JA, Cullen S, Vassillikos VP, Sullivan ID, Allan L, Nihoyannopoulos P,

Somerville J, Deanfield JE. Ebstein's anomaly: presentation and outcome from fetus to adult. J Am Coll Cardiol. 1994;23:170–6.
11. Celermajer DS, Dodd SM, Greenwald SE, Wyse RK, Deanfield JE. Morbid anatomy in neonates with Ebstein's anomaly of the tricuspid valve: pathophysiologic and clinical implications. J Am Coll Cardiol. 1992;19:1049–53.
12. Yalonetsky S, Tobler D, Greutmann M, Crean AM, Wintersperger BJ, Nguyen ET, Oechslin EN, Silversides CK, Wald RM. Cardiac magnetic resonance imaging and the assessment of Ebstein anomaly in adults. Am J Cardiol. 2011;107:767–73.
13. Lee CM, Sheehan FH, Bouzas B, Chen SS, Gatzoulis MA, Kilner PJ. The shape and function of the right ventricle in Ebstein's anomaly. Int J Cardiol. 2013; 167(3):704–10. doi:10.1016/j.ijcard.2012.03.062.
14. Fratz S, Janello C, Muller D, Seligmann M, Meierhofer C, Schuster T, Schreiber C, Martinoff S, Hess J, Kuhn A, Vogt M, Stern H. The functional right ventricle and tricuspid regurgitation in Ebstein's anomaly. Int J Cardiol. 2013;167(1):258–61. doi:10.1016/j.ijcard.2011.12.081.
15. Tobler D, Yalonetsky S, Crean AM, Granton JT, Burchill L, Silversides CK, Wald RM. Right heart characteristics and exercise parameters in adults with Ebstein anomaly: new perspectives from cardiac magnetic resonance imaging studies. Int J Cardiol. 2013; 165(1):146–50. doi:10.1016/j.ijcard.2011.08.004.
16. Danielson GK, Driscoll DJ, Mair DD, Warnes CA, Oliver Jr WC. Operative treatment of Ebstein's anomaly. J Thorac Cardiovasc Surg. 1992;104:1195–202.
17. Allwork SP, Bentall HH, Becker AE, Cameron H, Gerlis LM, Wilkinson JL, Anderson RH. Congenitally corrected transposition of the great arteries: morphologic study of 32 cases. Am J Cardiol. 1976; 38:910–23.
18. Silverman NH, Gerlis LM, Horowitz ES, Ho SY, Neches WH, Anderson RH. Pathologic elucidation of the echocardiographic features of Ebstein's malformation of the morphologically tricuspid valve in discordant atrioventricular connections. Am J Cardiol. 1995;76:1277–83.
19. Anderson KR, Danielson GK, McGoon DC, Lie JT. Ebstein's anomaly of the left-sided tricuspid valve: pathological anatomy of the valvular malformation. Circulation. 1978;58:I87–91.
20. Horvath P, Szufladowicz M, de Leval MR, Elliott MJ, Stark J. Tricuspid valve abnormalities in patients with atrioventricular discordance: surgical implications. Ann Thorac Surg. 1994;57:941–5.
21. Oechslin E. Physiologically 'Corrected' Transposition of the Great Arteries, in Echocardiography in Pediatric and Congenital Heart Disease: from Fetus to Adult (eds Lai WW, Mertens LL, Cohen MS, Geva T) Wiley-Blackwell, 2009;439–55.
22. Attenhofer Jost CH, Connolly HM, O'Leary PW, Warnes CA, Tajik AJ, Seward JB. Left heart lesions in patients with Ebstein anomaly. Mayo Clin Proc. 2005;80:361–8.
23. Sedmera D, Pexieder T, Vuillemin M, Thompson RP, Anderson RH. Developmental patterning of the myocardium. Anat Rec. 2000;258:319–37.
24. Khositseth A, Danielson GK, Dearani JA, Munger TM, Porter CJ. Supraventricular tachyarrhythmias in Ebstein anomaly: management and outcome. J Thorac Cardiovasc Surg. 2004;128:826–33.
25. Hebe J. Ebstein's anomaly in adults. Arrhythmias: diagnosis and therapeutic approach. Thorac Cardiovasc Surg. 2000;48:214–9.
26. Yetman AT, Freedom RM, McCrindle BW. Outcome in cyanotic neonates with Ebstein's anomaly. Am J Cardiol. 1998;81:749–54.
27. Wald RM, Adatia I, Van Arsdell GS, Hornberger LK. Relation of limiting ductal patency to survival in neonatal Ebstein's anomaly. Am J Cardiol. 2005;96:851–6.
28. Bove EL, Hirsch JC, Ohye RG, Devaney EJ. How I manage neonatal Ebstein's anomaly. Semin Thorac Cardiovasc Surg Pediatr Card Surg Annu. 2009:63–5.
29. Kempny A, Dimopoulos K, Uebing A, Moceri P, Swan L, Gatzoulis MA, Diller GP. Reference values for exercise limitations among adults with congenital heart disease. Relation to activities of daily life–single centre experience and review of published data. Eur Heart J. 2012;33:1386–96.
30. MacLellan-Tobert SG, Driscoll DJ, Mottram CD, Mahoney DW, Wollan PC, Danielson GK. Exercise tolerance in patients with Ebstein's anomaly. J Am Coll Cardiol. 1997;29:1615–22.
31. Baumgartner H, Bonhoeffer P, De Groot NM, de Haan F, Deanfield JE, Galie N, Gatzoulis MA, Gohlke-Baerwolf C, Kaemmerer H, Kilner P, Meijboom F, Mulder BJ, Oechslin E, Oliver JM, Serraf A, Szatmari A, Thaulow E, Vouhe PR, Walma E, Task Force on the Management of Grown-up Congenital Heart Disease of the European Society of Cardiology, Association for European Paediatric Cardiology, ESC Committee for Practice Guidelines. Esc guidelines for the management of grown-up congenital heart disease (new version 2010). Eur Heart J. 2010;31:2915–57.
32. Boston US, Dearani JA, O'Leary PW, Driscoll DJ, Danielson GK. Tricuspid valve repair for Ebstein's anomaly in young children: a 30-year experience. Ann Thorac Surg. 2006;81:690–5; discussion 695–6.
33. da Silva JP, da Silva Lda F. Ebstein's anomaly of the tricuspid valve: the cone repair. Semin Thorac Cardiovasc Surg Pediatr Card Surg Annu. 2012;15:38–45.
34. Attenhofer Jost CH, Connolly HM, Scott CG, Burkhart HM, Warnes CA, Dearani JA. Outcome of cardiac surgery in patients 50 years of age or older with Ebstein anomaly: survival and functional improvement. J Am Coll Cardiol. 2012;59:2101–6.
35. Brown ML, Dearani JA, Danielson GK, Cetta F, Connolly HM, Warnes CA, Li Z, Hodge DO, Driscoll DJ, Mayo Clinic Congenital Heart Center. The outcomes of operations for 539 patients with Ebstein anomaly. J Thorac Cardiovasc Surg. 2008;135: 1120–36. 1136.e1121–7.

36. Chauvaud S, Fuzellier JF, Berrebi A, Lajos P, Marino JP, Mihaileanu S, Carpentier A. Bi-directional cavopulmonary shunt associated with ventriculo and valvuloplasty in Ebstein's anomaly: benefits in high risk patients. Eur J Cardiothorac Surg. 1998;13:514–9.
37. Al-Najashi KS, Balint OH, Oechslin E, Williams WG, Silversides CK. Mid-term outcomes in adults with Ebstein anomaly and cavopulmonary shunts. Ann Thorac Surg. 2009;88:131–6.
38. Babar JL, Jones RG, Hudsmith L, Steeds R, Guest P. Application of mr imaging in assessment and follow-up of congenital heart disease in adults. Radiographics. 2010;30(4):1145.
39. Kilner PJ, Geva T, Kaemmerer H, Trindade PT, Schwitter J, Webb GD. Recommendations for cardiovascular magnetic resonance in adults with congenital heart disease from the respective working groups of the european society of cardiology. Eur Heart J. 2010;31:794–805.
40. Chandrashekhar G, Sodhi KS, Saxena AK, Rohit MK, Khandelwal N. Correlation of 64 row mdct, echocardiography and cardiac catheterization angiography in assessment of pulmonary arterial anatomy in children with cyanotic congenital heart disease. Eur J Radiol. 2012;81: 4211–7.

Hypertrophic Cardiomyopathy 16

Raymond H.M. Chan and Martin S. Maron

Hypertrophic cardiomyopathy (HCM) is a common genetic cardiomyopathy caused by mutations in genes which encode for the myofilament protein components of the sarcomere or the z-disc [1–4]. It has a prevalence of 1 in 500 in the general population and is a global disease affecting patients in all continents [5] and of both genders [6]. It is the leading cause of sudden death in young people, with an annual mortality rate of 1 % [7]. Since its first description over 50 years ago, the pathophysiology of the disease is still incompletely understood [8]. The disease is associated with tremendous heterogeneity with regard to its presentation, phenotype, and prognosis. The diagnosis for HCM is usually made clinically after symptom onset or cardiac events, but may also be found after routine 12-lead electrocardiogram (ECG), heart murmur on cardiac exam, or in family screening of probands.

R.H.M. Chan, MD, MPH, FRCP(C), BScPhm (✉)
Division of Cardiology,
Beth Israel Deaconess Medical Center,
PERFUSE Study Group, 330 Brookline Avenue,
East Campus SH 462, Boston, MA 02215, USA
e-mail: rhchan@bidmc.harvard.edu

M.S. Maron, MD
Cardiac CT and MRI, Division of Cardiology,
Hypertrophic Cardiomyopathy Center,
Tufts University School of Medicine,
Tufts Medical Center, 800 Washington St, #70,
Boston, MA 02111, USA
e-mail: mmaron@tuftsmedicalcenter.org

Imaging

Clinical diagnosis is confirmed through imaging using 2D echocardiography and/or cardiac MRI (CMR) or CT by identifying an increase in left ventricular (LV) wall thickness ≥15 mm (mean ~22 mm [normal ≤12 mm]) without a dilated LV chamber in absence of other cardiac or systemic disease processes (e.g., aortic stenosis, chronic hypertension) capable of producing the magnitude of hypertrophy [9]. In certain instances, such as patients with a family history of HCM, a maximal wall thickness ≥13 mm may be compatible with the diagnosis of HCM LV hypertrophy is most commonly asymmetric, with the most common location of increased wall thickness occurring in the contiguous area of the basal anterior septum and anterior wall [10] (Fig. 16.1), although there is tremendous heterogeneity in phenotypic expression, even in those with a common genotype. In addition, in close to 25 % of HCM patients, segments of LV hypertrophy can be separated by myocardial regions of normal thickness, i.e., noncontiguous pattern of LV hypertrophy. Concentric pattern of LV hypertrophy occurs very rarely in HCM (~1 %) [11, 12] (Fig. 16.2).

Characterization of Anatomy

LV Hypertrophy

CMR has the unique ability to acquire truly tomographic high-resolution images in any anatomic

F. Saremi (ed.), *Cardiac CT and MR for Adult Congenital Heart Disease*,
DOI 10.1007/978-1-4614-8875-0_16, © Springer Science+Business Media New York 2014

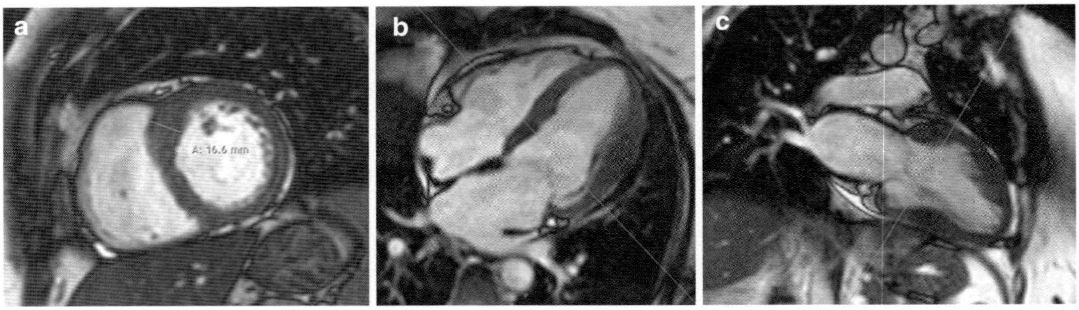

Fig. 16.1 Focal myocardial hypertrophy. Images in different planes (with corresponding scanlines) serve as a reference "road map" to pinpoint the location of focal hypertrophy and to precisely measure the true maximal wall thickness, a metric which has been associated with increased risk of cardiac events. (**a**) In this HCM patient, a basal short-axis slice shows a focal area of increased septal wall thickness confined to the anterior septum with normal wall thickness in other segments. Maximal wall thickness was 16.6 mm. Corresponding 4-chamber (**b**) and 2-chamber (**c**) views demonstrate the difficulty in appreciating the true geometry of the left ventricle walls without the short-axis slice

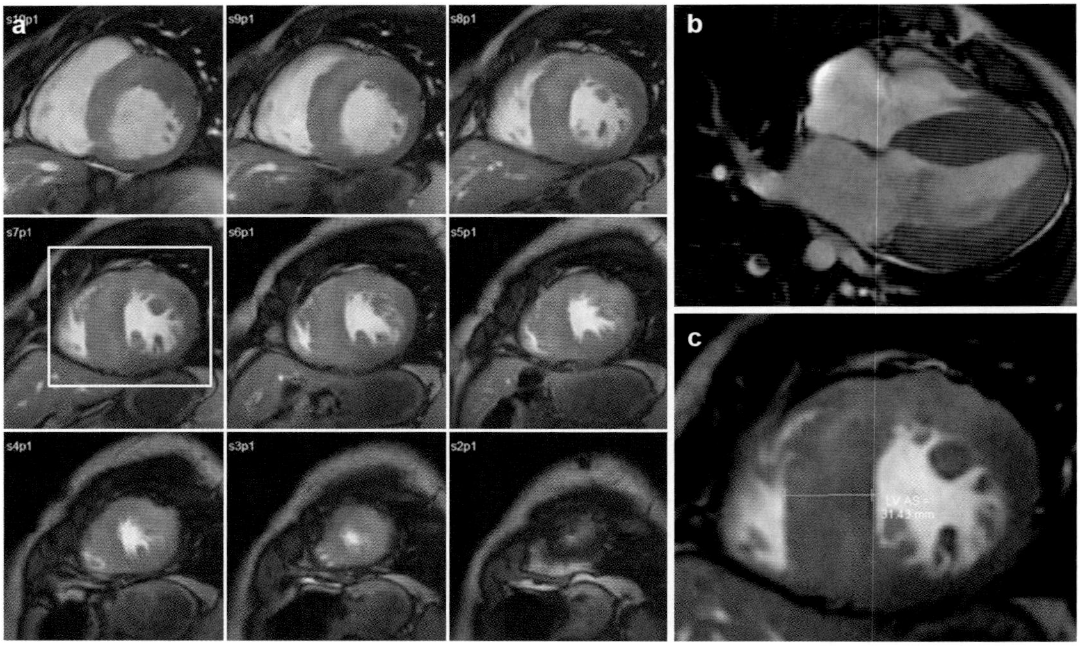

Fig. 16.2 Concentric hypertrophy on the left ventricle (LV). (**a**) Short-axis stack shows extreme hypertrophy in most segments. Note the relative sparing of the right ventricular walls. (**b**) 4-chamber slice showing the degree of hypertrophy in all of the LV walls. (**c**) Enlarged view of slice 7, showing maximal wall thickness of 31 mm. Overall LV mass was 311 g, with an LV mass index of 185 g/m^2. Based on this finding and after a balanced discussion with the patient, a prophylactic ICD was placed due to the high risk of sudden death associated with extreme hypertrophy

plane without ionizing radiation, thus making it a particularly useful tool for precisely characterizing the HCM phenotype. Balanced steady state free precession (SSFP) cine imaging sequences result in a sharp delineation of myocardial borders due to the high contrast between a relatively dark myocardium and bright blood pool. This allows for accurate measurements of wall thickness in any region of the LV chamber. By using contiguous short-axis slices, a clear and comprehensive presentation of the entire myocardial geometry from the base to apex can be achieved, resulting in precise and reproducible quantification of chamber volumes, LV mass, and systolic function (Figs. 16.1 and 16.2).

Focal areas of LV hypertrophy in the anterolateral free wall, apex, and posterior septum may not be well seen (or the extent underestimated) by echocardiography due to the inability to discriminate the epicardial borders of the heart from noncardiac structures, or due to anatomic interference from thoracic or pulmonary parenchyma (Fig. 16.3). Furthermore, there is evidence to suggest that in some HCM patients, echocardiography can substantially underestimate the magnitude of hypertrophy compared with CMR [13], particularly in patients with focal areas of increased LV wall thickness confined to the anterolateral wall [14] (Fig. 16.3c).

Apical HCM is characterized by hypertrophy of the myocardium, predominantly in the left ventricular apical area. This variant of HCM is rare in Western countries (1–2 %) but is common in Japanese and other Asian populations (up to 25 %). Typical features of apical HCM include giant negative T waves on ECG, mild symptoms, and a generally more benign course. Other morphological findings of this disease include cavity obliteration and apical sequestration (Fig. 16.3). Echocardiography has limitations for demonstration of the apex and may miss apical HCM. This limitation is not encountered with cardiac MRI.

CMR can also easily facilitate the identification of patients with massive hypertrophy (maximal wall thickness ≥30 mm) which is considered a high-risk feature and warrants consideration of primary prevention implantable cardioverter-defibrillator (ICD), even in the absence of any other risk markers (Fig. 16.2) [15]. CMR can identify myocardial crypts, which are more common in genotype-positive but phenotype-negative patients (i.e., without LV hypertrophy), and may help identify HCM family members to be considered for diagnostic genetic testing (Fig. 16.4) [16, 17].

LV mass calculated from planimetry of short-axis slices provides an excellent assessment of the overall extent of LV hypertrophy, as there is tremendous variability in the patterns of hypertrophy in regions remote from maximal LV wall thickness. LV mass is therefore a more robust measure of the overall extent of LV hypertrophy. There is recent evidence that marked increase in LV mass index may be more sensitive in predicting adverse outcome (including sudden death), while maximal wall thickness >30 mm was more specific [18]. However, its relevance as an independent marker for predicting adverse outcomes such as sudden death (SD) is still not well defined.

RV Hypertrophy

Precise delineation of right ventricular morphology has been challenging with echocardiography due to its complex three-dimensional geometry and its orientation within the thorax. The unique ability of CMR or CT to obtain or reconstruct images in any orientation provides tools for robust assessment of the RV. Recent studies have demonstrated increased RV wall thickness (≥8 mm) in over 1/3 of HCM patients, with an important proportion of patients who have an increased RV wall mass [19, 20].

In addition, approximately half of HCM patients will demonstrate hypertrophy of the septal band and the crista supraventricularis (Fig. 16.5) which is an RV muscle structure that is often positioned adjacent to the basal anterior septum [21–23]. As a result, it can sometimes be erroneously included in the measurement of the ventricular septum, which can lead to overestimations in LV maximal wall thickness. It is important to clarify the anatomy by carefully examining cine loops and seeing the crista move off the septum at various stages of the cardiac cycle. The morphological phenomena of hypertrophied crista supraventricularis and increased RV wall thickness support the principle that HCM is a disease process that can involve the right ventricle, rather than exclusively the LV.

LV Outflow Tract Obstruction

Subaortic obstruction in HCM is caused by anterior leaflet of the mitral valve (rarely the posterior leaflet) making contact with basal septum in mid-systole (SAM-septal contact) (Figs. 16.6 and 16.7). The Venturi effect was originally hypothesized to be the mechanism by which systolic anterior motion (SAM) of the mitral valve leaflet and chordal structures occurs. However, recent evidence has pointed to flow drag, which is the

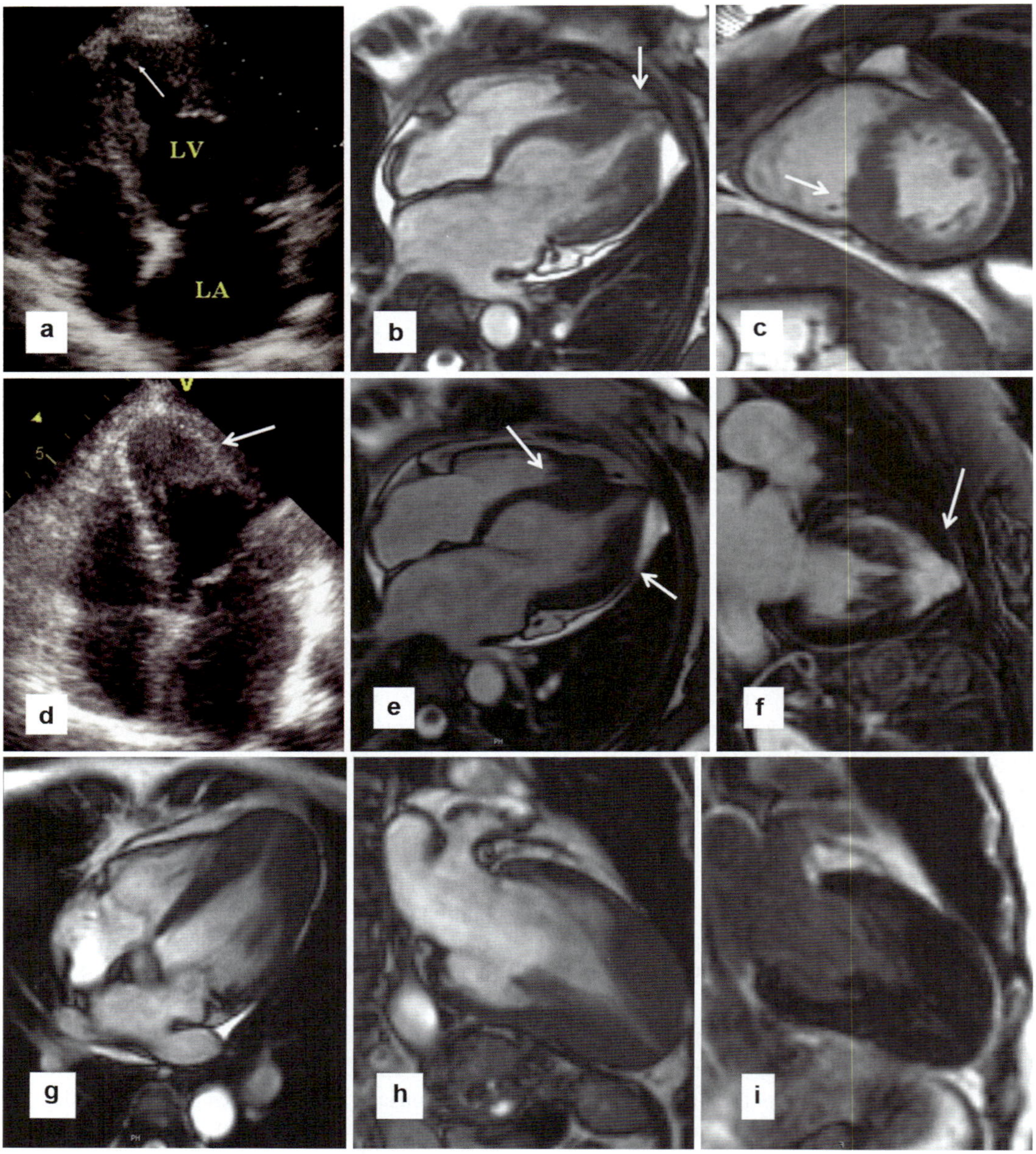

Fig. 16.3 Echocardiography weaknesses. (**a**, **b**) Patient with flipped T waves on lateral leads during a screening ECG leads to echocardiography, but was nondiagnostic due to incomplete visualization of the apex and apical lateral walls (**a**). In this case, steady state free precession (SSFP) MR (**b**) showed substantial hypertrophy at the apex as well as a small apical aneurysm (*arrow*). (**c**) Focal hypertrophy of the mid-inferior septum (*arrow*), which was underappreciated in echocardiography. (**e**, **f**) In a different patient, echocardiography suggested thickening of the apex (*arrow* in **d**); however, the endocardial borders were not clearly visualized. Corresponding 4-chamber cine slice (**e**) precisely delineating the degree and location of apical hypertrophy (*arrows*). Late gadolinium enhancement (LGE) imaging shows extensive enhancement in the apex and the anterior wall (*arrow*). (**g**–**i**) Patient with apical variant HCM without evidence of LGE. 4-chamber (**g**) and 2-chamber SSFP images clearly show the hypertrophy localized to the apex. 2-chamber late gadolinium enhancement (**i**) shows no abnormal enhancement

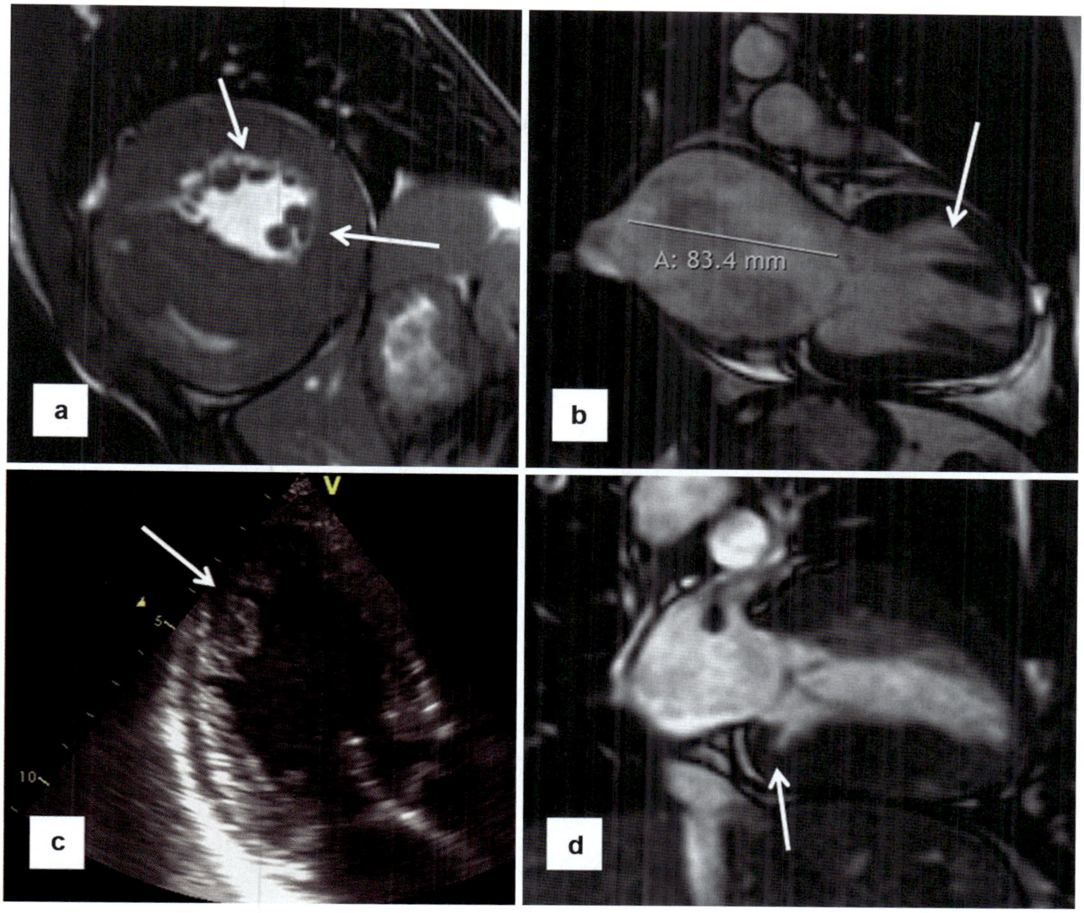

Fig. 16.4 Different phenotypic expressions of HCM. (**a**) Multiple accessory papillary muscles (*arrows*) seen on short-axis CMR. (**b**) End-stage HCM with left ventricle ejection fraction =30 %. Note the markedly enlarged left atrium and the presence of apicobasal bundle (*arrow*). (**c**) Myocardial crypts (*arrow*) seen in mid-inferolateral wall on echocardiogram in 3-chamber view. (**d**) Different patient with a myocardial crypt (*arrow*) seen in basal inferior wall

force of flow from a hyperdynamic ventricle, to be the primary hemodynamic force for pushing the mitral valve toward the septum. Hence, complete characterization of the mitral valve apparatus (including the chordal structures and papillary muscles), and their influence on the pathophysiology of LV outflow tract (LVOT) obstruction, has important therapeutic implications. There is also emerging evidence that the angle between LVOT and aortic root may be related with outflow tract gradient [24]. The elevated LV systolic pressures resulting from outflow tract obstruction lead to increased wall stress, venous congestion, myocardial ischemia, and mitral regurgitation. Fibrosis may lead to diastolic dysfunction and may also be a substrate for unstable arrhythmias (see discussion below on LGE).

Cine CMR can accurately locate in 3 dimensions the origin of high-velocity blood flow, frequently in the region of SAM-septal contact, which is visualized as a signal void from dephased blood (Fig. 16.6). Although SSFP sequences are less sensitive to dephasing from turbulent blood flow compared with gradient recalled echo (GRE) sequences, hemodynamically significant outflow tract gradients usually result in visually apparent signal voids to easily locate the origin of the obstruction. Phase contrast (PC) MR can

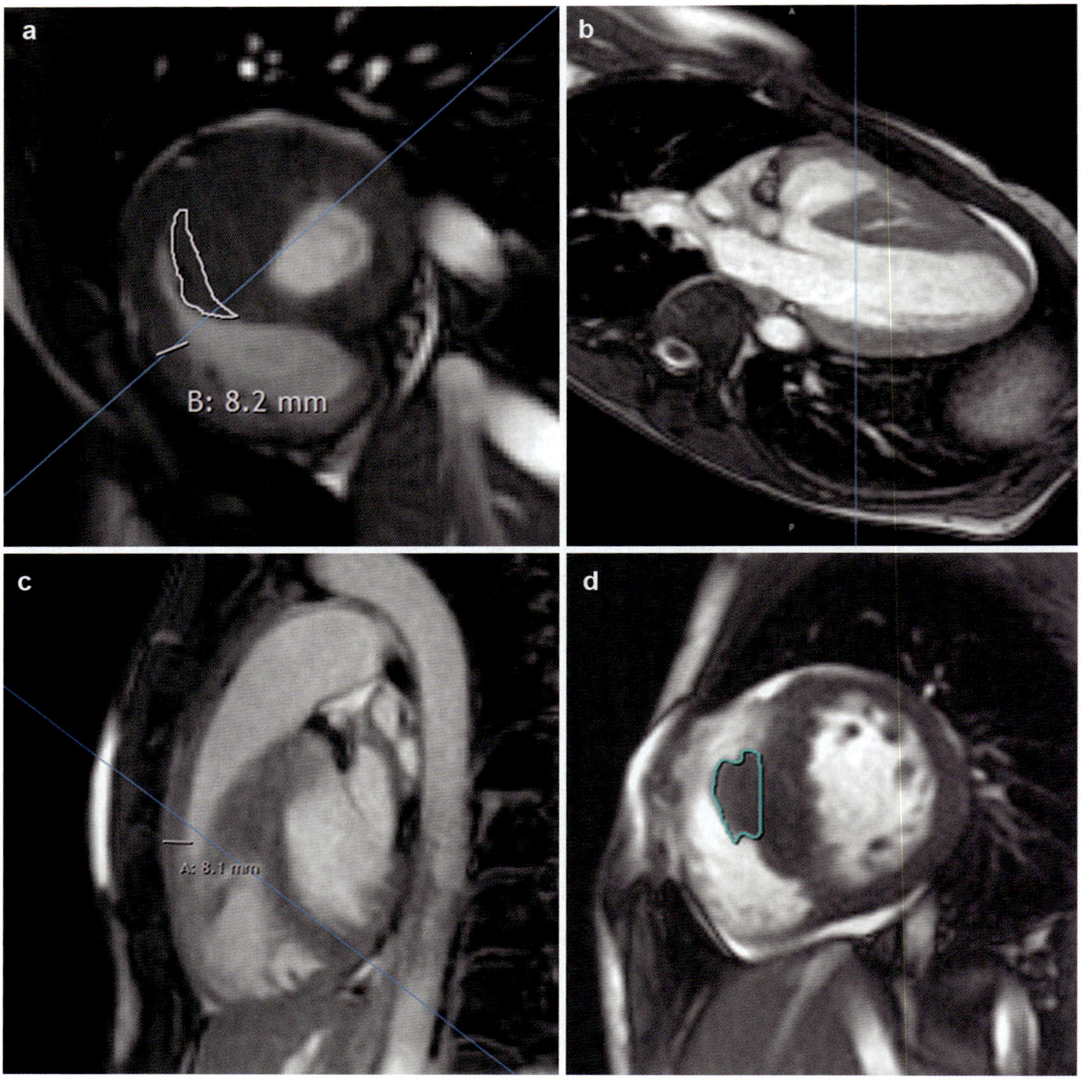

Fig. 16.5 Right ventricular (RV) septomarginal trabeculation and crista supraventricularis can be mistakenly incorporated in the intraventricular septum measurements. (**a**) HCM patient with very prominent septal band muscle (*outlined in white*), as well as increased thickness of right ventricular anterior free wall of 8.2 mm. Due to the location of this muscle adjacent to the septum, incorrect inclusion of its dimensions when measuring the left ventricle (LV) septal thickness may lead to overestimation of the maximum LV wall thickness. Close inspection of the cine short-axis stack confirms that this structure indeed moves away from the septum toward the RV cavity. Furthermore, views from other orientations with scanlines in (**b**) (modified 5-chamber view) and (**c**) (RV outflow tract view) confirm the location of the circumscribed area of thickness is in the right ventricular cavity rather than part of the septum. (**d**) Another patient with hypertrophied septomarginal trabeculation, with its structure outlined

be obtained if subaortic hypertrophic obstructive cardiomyopathy (HOCM) is suspected. For accurate measurements, it is important that the plane of PC image is adjusted perpendicular to jet of blood flow in subaortic region and the velocity encoding (VENC) value is set high enough to prevent aliasing. However, due to the superior temporal resolution of Doppler echocardiography,

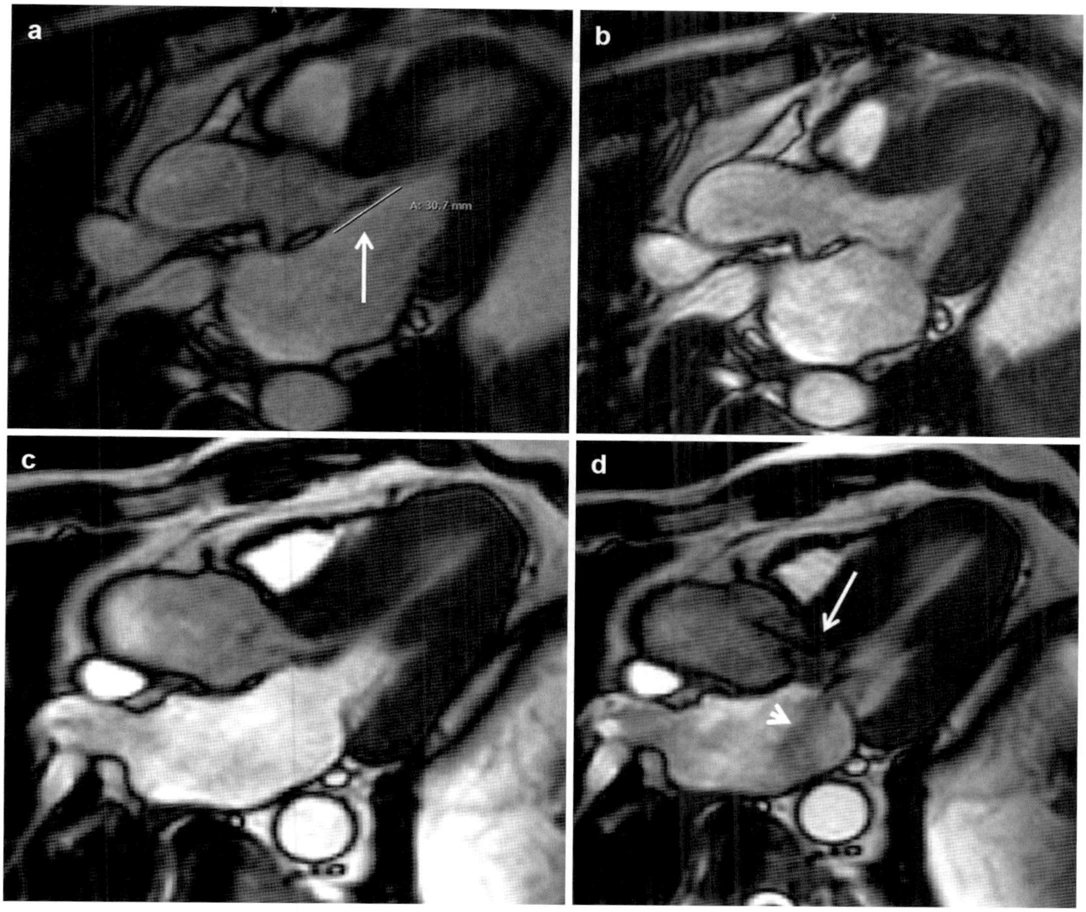

Fig. 16.6 Elongation of mitral valve leaflet length has been identified as a primary phenotypic abnormality in patients with HCM phenotype or genotype. (**a**) Patient with anterior mitral leaflet length of 31 mm (*arrow*), (**b**) Without systolic anterior motion or mitral regurgitation. (**c**) Patient with anterior mitral leaflet length of 31 mm and posterior mitral leaflet length of 23. (**d**) There was marked leaflet and chordal systolic anterior motion leading to an LVOT gradient of >80 mmHg. Note the dephasing jet indicative of turbulence through the LVOT (*arrow*) as well as dephased blood in left atrium (*arrowhead*) indicative of mitral regurgitation

it is preferable to use gradient measurements obtained from echocardiography when making treatment decisions.

Furthermore, fixed LVOT obstruction by a subvalvular membrane and aortic valve stenosis must be ruled out, usually through the use of echocardiography. The presence of an outflow tract gradient in the absence of SAM-septal contact is highly suggestive of a subaortic membrane.

Basal LVOT gradients ≥30 mmHg due to SAM-septal contact are a strong independent determinant of heart failure (HF) symptom progression, HF death, stroke death, and all-cause mortality [25]. The identification of obstruction at rest or following exercise opens up treatment options not available to nonobstructed patients, including surgery and alcohol septal ablation. Therefore, identifying obstruction is a critical issue in the diagnostic workup for HCM patients.

The limiting factor is the dynamic nature of LVOT obstruction [26, 27], where CMR can only assess a patient reliably under basal conditions. One-third of HCM patients will only have outflow obstruction transient during activity or provocation. Thus, clinical management decisions regarding

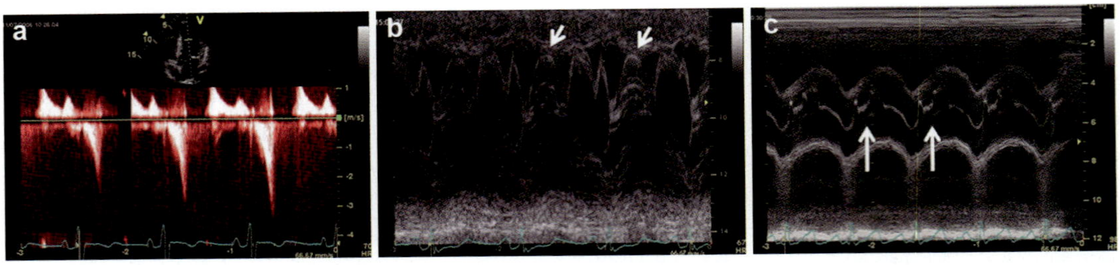

Fig. 16.7 Some classical echocardiographic findings found in HCM patients with left ventricle (LV) outflow tract obstruction, illustrating the anatomy and hemodynamic effects as a result of the obstruction. (**a**) Continuous wave Doppler through the LV outflow tract in 5-chamber view showing typical dagger-shaped flow indicative of dynamic obstruction. (**b**) M-mode through mitral valve leaflets in parasternal long axis showing valvular systolic anterior motion (*arrows*). (**c**) M-mode through aortic valve leaflets in parasternal long axis showing premature closure in mid-systole (*arrows*)

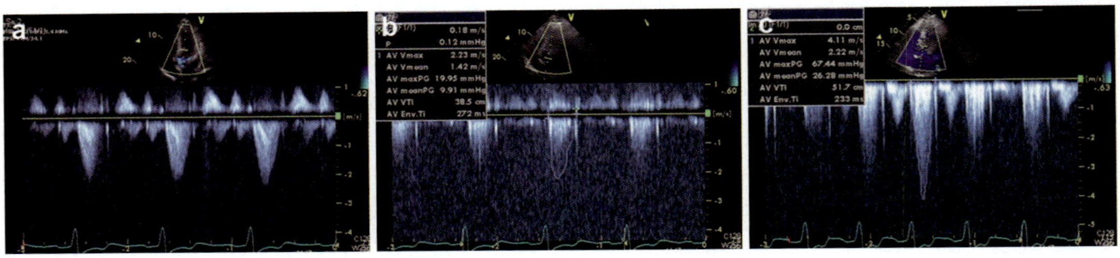

Fig. 16.8 Left ventricle (LV) outflow tract obstruction is a dynamic process. This is an echocardiogram of an HCM patient with marked dyspnea during exertion showing continuous wave Doppler gradients across LV outflow tract. (**a**) At rest – no significant gradient seen. (**b**) With Valsalva maneuver – no significant change in gradients. (**c**) During exercise – significant LV outflow tract obstruction with peak gradient >60 mmHg. Patient's symptoms were well controlled with titrating doses of beta-blockers

outflow obstruction should be predicated on measurements from echocardiography (with or without stress/provocative maneuvers) (Fig. 16.8) [28].

Papillary Muscles

Abnormalities in papillary muscle morphology are common, including papillary muscle hypertrophy, anteroapical displacement, double bifid, direct insertion into mitral leaflets, fusion to ventricular septum or free wall [11, 29–32], and accessory papillary muscles (including apicobasal muscle bundles [33]) (Fig. 16.9). Cardiac MR can be used to reliably characterize papillary muscle anatomy by accurately identifying their number, location, and position in the LV chamber (Fig. 16.10). When compared with controls, there appears to be an increased number of papillary muscles, in addition to an increased papillary muscle mass. Papillary muscle mass is related to overall LV mass index. However, subgroups of patients have normal LV mass but increased papillary muscle mass [30]. These observations broaden our understanding of HCM phenotype to include structures beyond the left ventricular wall and suggest that the same disease pathophysiology responsible for LV hypertrophy may also be involved in papillary muscle hypertrophy.

Certain abnormalities in papillary muscle anatomy have been shown to be related to LVOT obstruction. Papillary muscles appear to be positioned more anteriorly and closer to the ventricular septum in those with LVOT obstruction at rest and had more marked hypertrophy compared to those without obstruction [30]. Anteroapical displacement of anterolateral papillary muscles and double bifid papillary muscles have been found to be independently associated with significant outflow gradients, even after controlling for septal thickness [29]. Patients with significant outflow tract obstruction also have papillary muscles

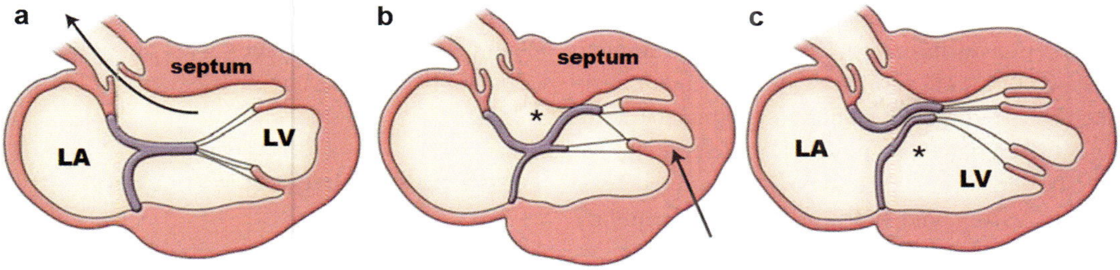

Fig. 16.9 Schematic of septum, papillary muscle, and mitral valve anatomy and their contribution to LV outflow tract obstruction and mitral regurgitation. (**a**) Normal papillary muscle and mitral valve location and length. Note the unimpeded flow through the LV outflow tract. (**b**) Anteroapical displacement of thickened papillary muscle (*arrow*), with lengthened anterior mitral valve leaflet (*) and thickened septum leading to significant outflow tract obstruction. (**c**) Double bifid papillary muscles with lengthened posterior mitral valve leaflet (*), leading to chordal and valvular systolic anterior motion, outflow tract obstruction, malcoaptation, and mitral regurgitation (Figures copyright Raymond H Chan)

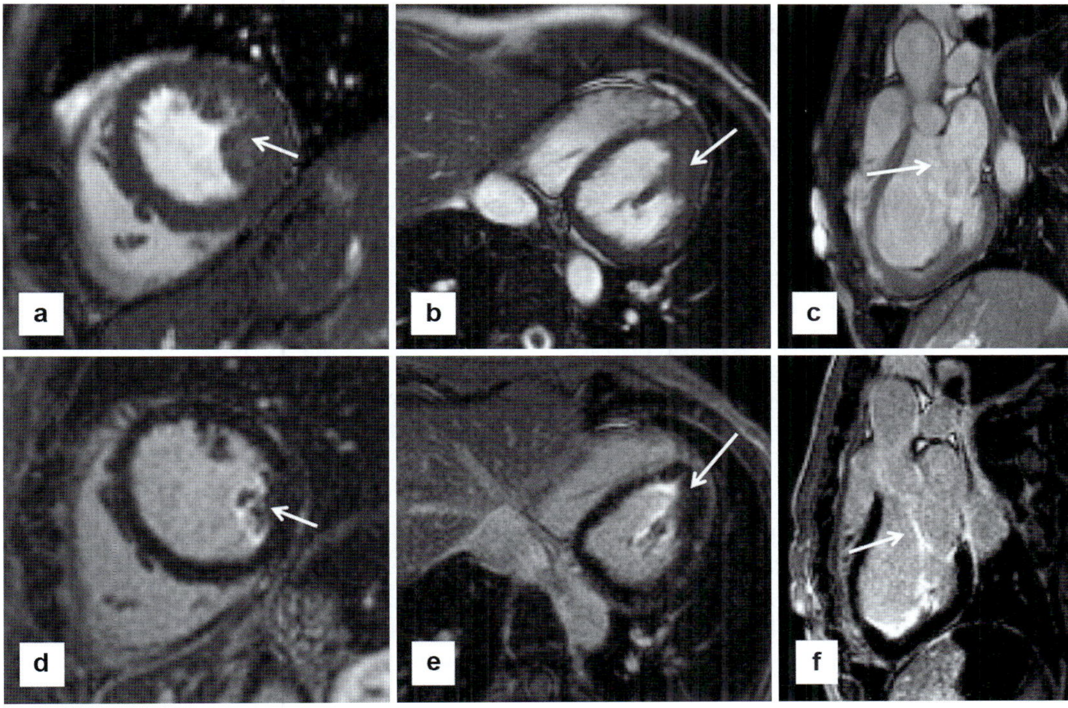

Fig. 16.10 Papillary muscle hypertrophy and mitral valve abnormalities are primary anatomic features of HCM, which affect more than the left ventricle (LV) walls. (**a**) Short-axis steady state free precession (SSFP) shows prominent size of posterior papillary muscle (*arrow*), despite relatively normal wall thicknesses. (**b**) Modified 4-chamber SSFP confirms marked enlargement of posterior papillary muscle (*arrow*). (**c**) LV outflow tract (LVOT) view shows elongated anterior mitral valve leaflet. (**d–f**) Show late gadolinium enhancement (LGE) imaging in corresponding views. Note enhancement seen in papillary muscle (**d**, **e**) and mitral valve leaflets (**f**) (*arrows*). The clinical significance of LGE in these structures is unknown

closer to the ventricular septum (Fig. 16.9) [30]. Prior to more widespread use of CMR, such abnormalities are often not well appreciated by echocardiography and thus missed and were only seen during surgery by direct inspection [22]. Papillary muscle mobility may also play an important role in dynamic LV outflow tract obstruction during exercise (Fig. 16.8). Complete visualization of papillary muscle anatomy is therefore a clinically important step in the management of patients with LVOT obstruction.

The above evidence supports the hypothesis that accessory and apically displaced papillary muscles contribute significantly to LVOT obstruction, by pulling the plane of the mitral valve toward the septum. As a result, they are often removed during surgery, and therefore, their identification by imaging can aid in preoperative surgical planning. Furthermore, CMR can identify anomalous papillary muscle insertion into the mitral valve, which can redirect patients toward surgery rather than alcohol septal ablation, since this abnormality causes mid-ventricular obstruction not amenable to percutaneous approach.

Mitral Valve Leaflet Anatomy

Mitral valve leaflets appear to be elongated independently of other morphological characteristics such as LV thickness or mass and may represent a primary phenotypic characteristic of HCM [34]. Such elongated leaflets play an important role in generating LV outflow tract gradients, particularly in those whose relative anterior mitral leaflet length exceeds twice that of the transverse LV outflow tract diameter (Fig. 16.6) [34]. The anterior mitral leaflet (AML) has more redundancy and mobility [35]. There is also a significant relationship between the ratio of AML length and LVOT diameter with length and the magnitude of outflow tract gradient. Extreme lengths of the AML may potentially produce mitral-septal obstruction even after extensive septal muscle resection. Increased mitral valve leaflet length may also serve as a marker of gene-positive status in HCM in family members without LV hypertrophy.

As a result of mitral leaflet malcoaptation due to systolic anterior motion (SAM), mitral regurgitation jets can also be seen as a signal void in the left atrium. These jets are often posteriorly directed due to relatively greater SAM of the AML compared to the posterior leaflet (Fig. 16.6). The regurgitant jet volume can be quantitated by comparing the left ventricular stroke volume by planimetry of SSFP images with the aorta flow obtained from phase contrast sequences.

Planning for Surgical Myectomy

Surgical myectomy is the gold standard for symptomatic relief in patients with significant LV outflow obstruction on maximal medical therapy [9]. As outlined above, CMR can be helpful by clear delineation of the relative three-dimensional anatomy of the LV outflow tract, mitral valve, and the subvalvular apparatus [28]. Accessory papillary muscles which may contribute to obstruction can be identified for planned removal. Important measurements for operative planning include maximal septal thickness, distance of maximum thickness from aortic annulus, and the apical extent of septal bulge. Careful CMR planning using multiple thin slabs with no gaps in the LV outflow tract orientation can be extremely helpful by providing precise and reproducible measurements. This anatomic information should supplement rather than supplant those obtained from transesophageal echocardiogram (TEE).

Evaluation After Alcohol Septal Ablation

Using late gadolinium enhancement imaging, CMR can objectively quantify the amount of necrosed tissue, as well as its location in relationship to the LVOT (Fig. 16.11). This may help in the assessment of patients who achieve suboptimal results after ablation or when gradients recur late after the procedure.

LV Apical Aneurysms

HCM patients with LV apical aneurysms are a previously under-recognized subgroup prior to more widespread use of CMR in these patients. Its prevalence is low at 2 % [36]. It is characterized by thin-walled, akinetic, or dyskinetic segments in the LV apex (Fig. 16.12). Often, these segments are

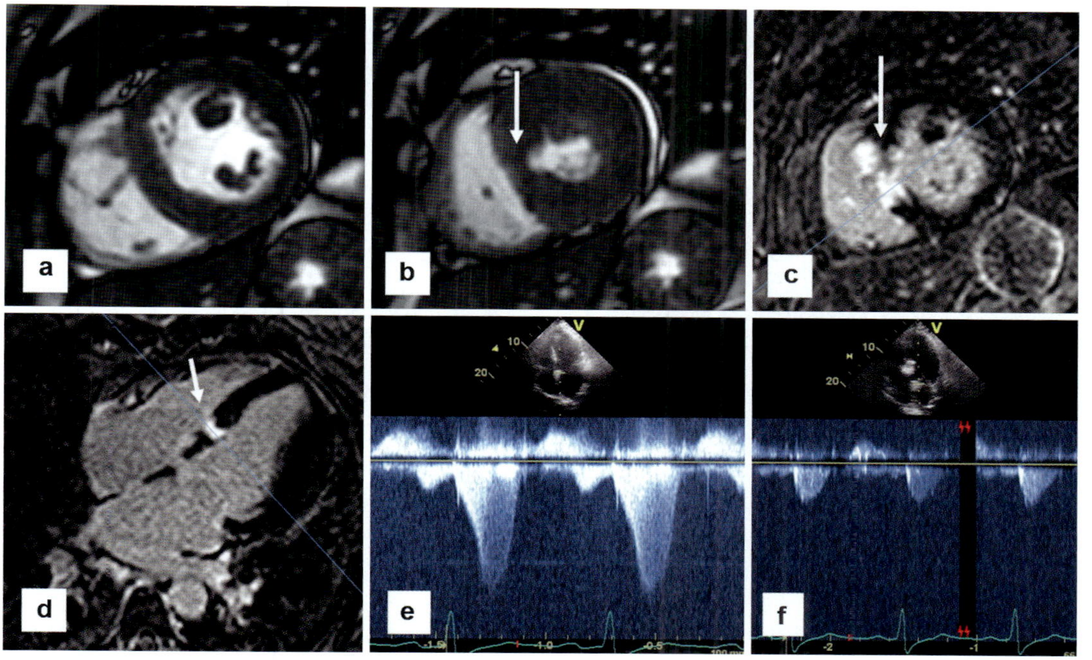

Fig. 16.11 Cardiac MR can be helpful in the evaluation of patients after alcohol septal ablation. These series of images are from a patient who had a successful alcohol septal 2 months prior to MR. (**a**) Short-axis steady state free precession (SSFP) slice showing small area of infarcted myocardium that fails to thicken during systole in (**b**) (*arrow*). Corresponding LGE imaging in short-axis (**c**) and 4-chamber view (**d**) showing focal area in the basal septum with bright transmural enhancement secondary to induced infarction from the alcohol septal ablation (*arrow*). (**e**) Prior to the alcohol septal ablation, continuous wave Doppler echocardiography shows a significant LVOT gradient well over 50 mmHg. (**f**) 2-month post-alcohol septal ablation, there is no clinically significant LVOT gradient

composed of fibrotic tissue which can be seen as a transmural pattern of late gadolinium enhancement (Fig. 16.13). Like apical hypertrophy, echocardiography may not reliably detect these aneurysms because of its technical limitations, where in one study the sensitivity was only 57 % [37].

Several mechanisms have been proposed, including genetic disposition, presence of myocardial bridging of the left anterior descending artery, and mid-cavitary obstruction causing elevated pressures leading to myocardial fibrosis. The true mechanism of aneurysmal formation is likely multifactorial, as each of the above characteristics has been shown to occur in a small minority of patients [37]. Mid-ventricular hypertrophic obstructive cardiomyopathy (HOCM) is characterized by asymmetric left ventricular hypertrophy and by a pressure gradient between basal and apical sites in the left ventricle. These patients are often symptomatic and prone to ventricular arrhythmias arising from the distal left ventricular aneurysm (Fig. 16.13).

Recent evidence shows that adverse event rates in the subgroup with apical aneurysms are substantial at ~10 % per year, including sudden death, ICD discharges, nonfatal thromboembolic stroke, progressive heart failure, and death [37]; thus, patients with apical aneurysms are considered a high-risk subgroup. Often, fibrosis can extend from the aneurysm to the periapical regions in the septum and free wall and may thus serve as a substrate for malignant dysrhythmias [38]. Patients should be considered for ICD implantation for primary prevention of sudden death, particularly those with extensive LGE [10]. Dyskinetic and akinetic segments may harbor pools of stagnant blood flow, leading to the formation of intracavitary thrombi and subsequent thromboembolic

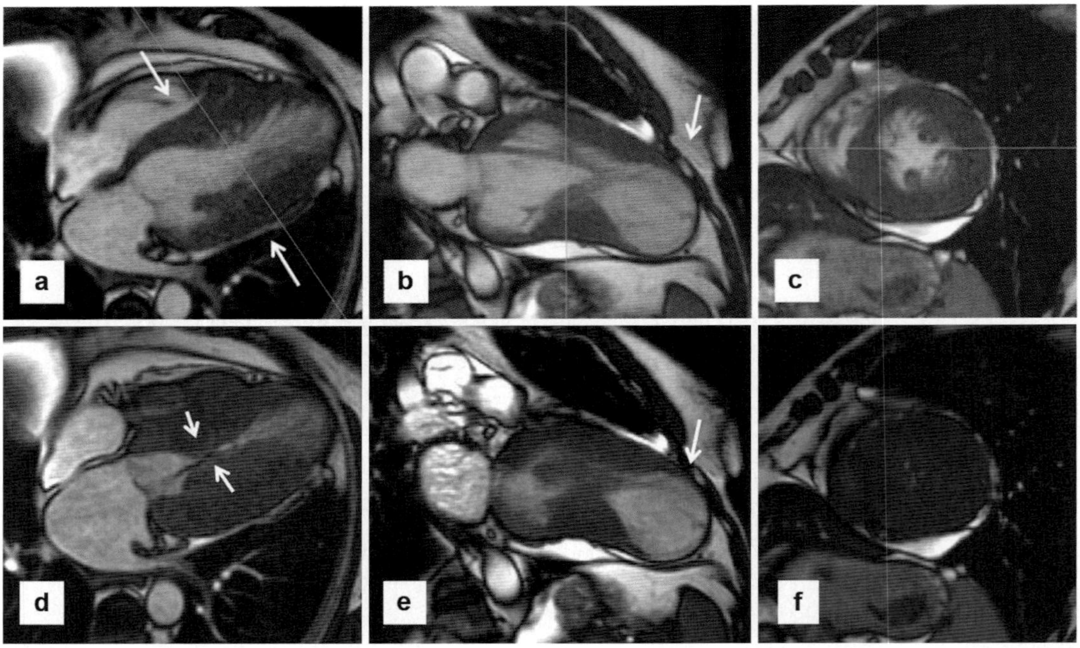

Fig. 16.12 Apical aneurysms. Patients with apical aneurysms represent a small subgroup of high-risk patients. Several mechanisms for aneurysm development have been proposed, including mid-cavitary obstruction. These series of steady state free precession (SSFP) images are from a patient with harsh systolic murmur and shortness of breath, diagnosed with hypertrophic cardiomyopathy with apical aneurysm and mid-cavitary obstruction, with intraventricular gradient >80 mmHg by echocardiogram. (**a**–**c**) Are diastolic and (**d**–**f**) are systolic views. 4-chamber slice (**a**) shows dramatic mid-ventricular hypertrophy (*arrows*) at end diastole and near obliteration of mid-cavity at systole with a jet of dephased blood (*arrows* in **d**) indicative of turbulent flow. 2-chamber views in systole (**b**) and diastole (**e**) showing noncontractile large apical aneurysm (*arrows*). Late gadolinium enhancement imaging did not show any evidence of enhancement, refuting the hypothesis that myocardial fibrosis and subsequent dilation is the mechanism of aneurysm formation

strokes. Among those with a sizable apical aneurysm, there may be a potential role for anticoagulation for stroke prophylaxis.

Fortunately, ventricular rupture is not common despite marked thinning of the myocardium at the apex; thus, prophylactic surgical resection is not warranted.

Tissue Characterization

Late Gadolinium Enhancement (LGE)

Current risk stratification algorithms for sudden cardiac death (SCD) in HCM are imprecise and not always definitive, as SCD occasionally occurs in patients without conventional risk factors (Fig. 16.14). Identification of additional markers to allow more precise selection of those patients who may benefit from primary prevention ICD therapy represents a major clinical aspiration in HCM. Recently, contrast-enhanced CMR with late gadolinium enhancement (LGE) has emerged as an imaging technique to noninvasively identify myocardial fibrosis in coronary artery disease and other cardiomyopathies, including HCM. The prognostic value of LGE in HCM patients has been the subject of immense interest since the first large study demonstrated a possible association between LGE and adverse events [39–44].

Pathophysiology of LGE

Myocardial fibrosis may be a manifestation of the repair process emanating from microvascular

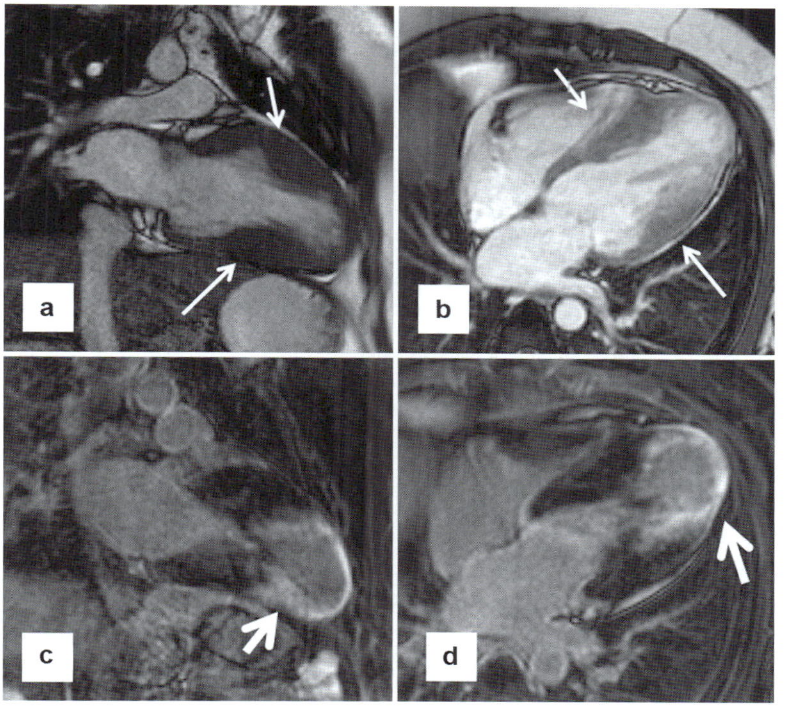

Fig. 16.13 Enhancing apical aneurysm. A young patient with hypertrophic cardiomyopathy and apical aneurysm presented with a recent stroke (presumed to be cardioembolic). (**a**, **b**) Focal hypertrophy in the mid-left ventricle (*arrows*), with a dyskinetic apical aneurysm. Corresponding late gadolinium enhancement (LGE) images on similar planes (**c**, **d**) show substantial enhancement of the left ventricle apex and the periapical regions (*arrows*)

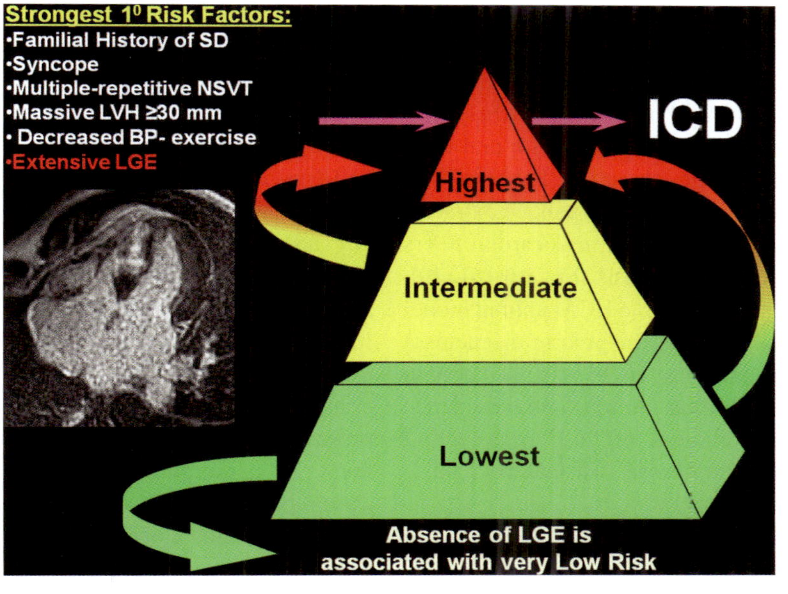

Fig. 16.14 Contrast-enhanced CMR with late gadolinium enhancement can be an arbitrator for implantable cardioverter-defibrillator (*ICD*) placement decisions in HCM patients whose risk remains ambiguous after assessment with conventional risk factors such as a familial history of sudden death, history of unexplained syncope, multiple episodes on non-sustained ventricular tachycardia, massive left ventricular hypertrophy (*LVH*), and abnormal blood pressure response to exercise. Furthermore, extensive late gadolinium enhancement (*LGE*) by itself can identify HCM patients at increased sudden death risk, in whom prophylactic ICD therapy would otherwise not be considered. Conversely, the absence of LGE is associated with low risk of sudden death (*SD*) and therefore a potential source of reassurance to patients. *NSVT* non-sustained ventricular tachycardia

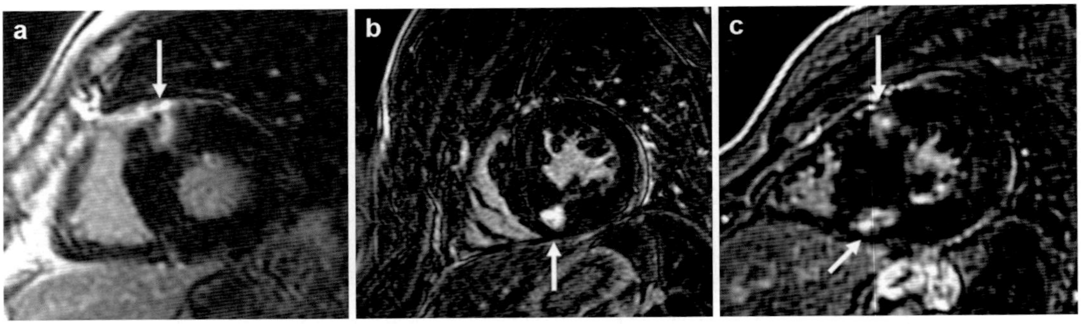

Fig. 16.15 Short-axis slices of late gadolinium enhancement (LGE) imaging, showing the classical "insertion point" enhancement described in various cardiomyopathies, including HCM. (**a**) Prominent LGE seen in isolation at the anterior RV insertion point (*arrow*), (**b**) at the inferior insertion point (*arrow*), and (**c**) at both the anterior and inferior insertion points (*arrows*)

dysfunction and silent ischemia in a large proportion of HCM patients. It has been postulated that LGE mostly represents such areas of myocardial fibrosis. However, much of the histopathological correlations with LGE imaging have been extrapolated from CMR-based animal models involving myocardial infarctions [45]. Only a small number of case reports with explanted end-stage HCM patients [44, 46] and small case series of patients who underwent myectomies [47, 48] have provided direct comparison of LGE to histopathology in HCM. Furthermore, it has been shown that the junction of the septum and right ventricular walls (the so-called RV insertion points) may in fact be areas of expanded extracellular space due to intersecting myocardial fibers rather than myocardial fibrosis (Fig. 16.15) [49]. There is currently no suitable HCM animal model available for study. Thus, the precise mechanism by which LGE occurs in HCM is still uncertain [50], but there is strong circumstantial evidence to support the paradigm of LGE representing areas of replacement fibrosis, particularly in end-stage HCM.

Pattern and Distribution of LGE

Prevalence of LGE is high, with a range between 40 and 80 % depending on patient population. Almost any pattern, distribution, and location of LGE can be observed in HCM (Fig. 16.16). Most commonly, it occurs in a patchy mid-wall distribution, usually involving segments with greatest degrees of hypertrophy [40, 44]. This is likely reflective of the severity of chronic microvascular ischemic damage leading to replacement fibrosis. Patients with greater maximal wall thickness and LV mass index tend to have greater extent of LGE [40, 44] (Fig. 16.17). LGE can be commonly localized to the RV insertion points, likely secondary to myocyte disarray and expansion of extracellular space rather than fibrosis (Fig. 16.15) [49]. As well, LGE can be found in the right ventricular wall and papillary muscles (Fig. 16.10). There is a strong inverse relationship between LVEF and the extent of LGE. Patients with end-stage HCM with depressed ejection fraction usually have extensive LGE seen in all segments (Fig. 16.18) [40, 44, 51]. LGE should not correspond to a coronary vascular distribution, unless there is concomitant coronary artery disease.

As the quantity of LGE may be small, contiguous stacks without gaps are needed to ensure proper sensitivity for small regions of enhancement. At a minimum, three orthogonal planes should be obtained: a short-axis stack with slice thickness of not more than 10 mm, 2-chamber view, and 4-chamber view. High-resolution (voxel size ≤1.4 mm) isotropic sequences can also be used if locally available and of sufficient image quality. Furthermore, it is crucial to cross-reference areas of enhancement simultaneously using scanlines in different imaging planes (Fig. 16.17) to exclude artifacts from blood pool and partial volume averaging, particularly in the

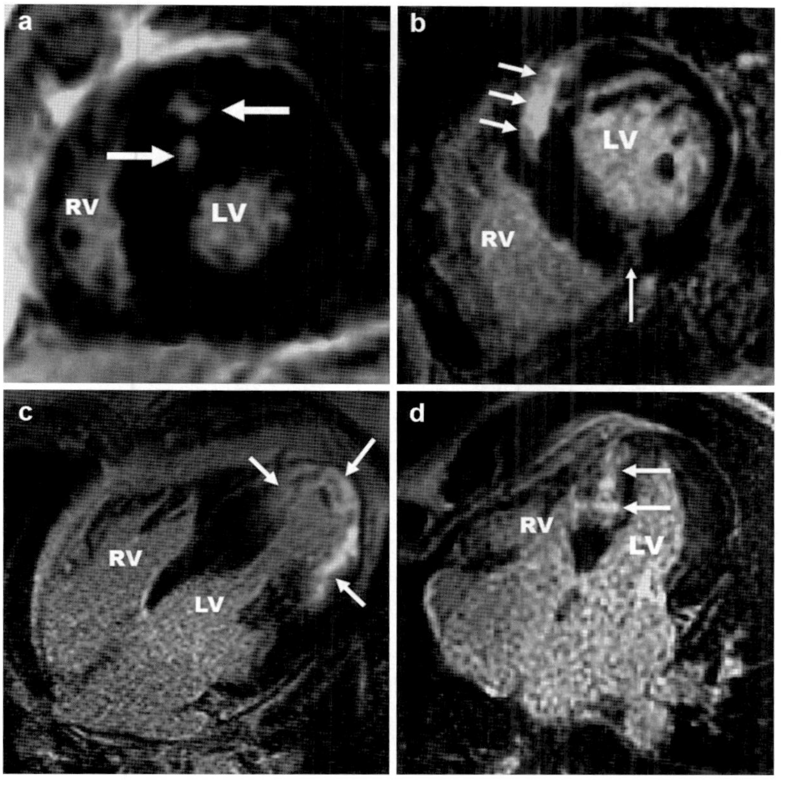

Fig. 16.16 Late gadolinium enhancement (LGE) patterns. Almost any pattern, distribution, and location of LGE can be observed in HCM. (**a**) Basal left ventricle (*LV*) short-axis image from an asymptomatic 29-year-old man with no conventional risk factors and focal areas of LGE confined to mid-myocardial anterior wall (*arrows*), encompassing 4 % of LV mass. (**b**) Mid-LV short-axis image from a 61-year-old woman, with substantial LGE (23 % of LV mass) involving basal anterior septum and contiguous anterolateral free wall (*thick arrows*) as well as a focal area at the intersection of the RV free wall and posterior septum (*thin arrow*). A short five beat run of NSVT on 24-h ambulatory Holter ECG was the only evidence for increased sudden death risk. Extensive LGE acted as an arbitrator for the decision to implant an ICD for primary prevention, which terminated an episode of rapid ventricular tachycardia 5 months later. (**c**) 4-chamber long-axis image from a mildly symptomatic 54-year-old man without conventional sudden risk factors, normal ejection fraction (60 %), and extensive, transmural LGE involving the distal posterior septum, apex, and lateral free wall (*arrows*) encompassing 36 % of LV mass. One year after implantable cardioverter-defibrillator (ICD) placement, this patient received an appropriate ICD shock for rapid monomorphic ventricular tachycardia. (**d**) 4-chamber long-axis image from a 29-year-old man with extensive LGE involving large portions of ventricular septum (*arrows*) encompassing 32 % of LV mass. Over the follow-up period, he developed the end-stage phase of HCM (EF <50 %) associated with progressive heart failure symptoms (NYHA class III), currently under consideration for heart transplantation

basal and apical areas. It is often helpful to use SSFP cine images as another source of reference, due to its high image contrast between dark myocardium and bright blood pool.

LGE and Risk of Adverse Events

Previous studies demonstrated that LGE is associated with ventricular arrhythmias [39–44]. LGE was shown to be an independent predictor of non-sustained ventricular tachycardia (NSVT), even after adjusting for age and maximal wall thickness [52]. These data suggest that LGE may be representative of the burden of arrhythmogenic substrate and perhaps contribute to the risk of lethal arrhythmias in HCM. This is supported by evidence that the presence of NSVT is associated with higher risks of sudden death, particularly in young patients [53].

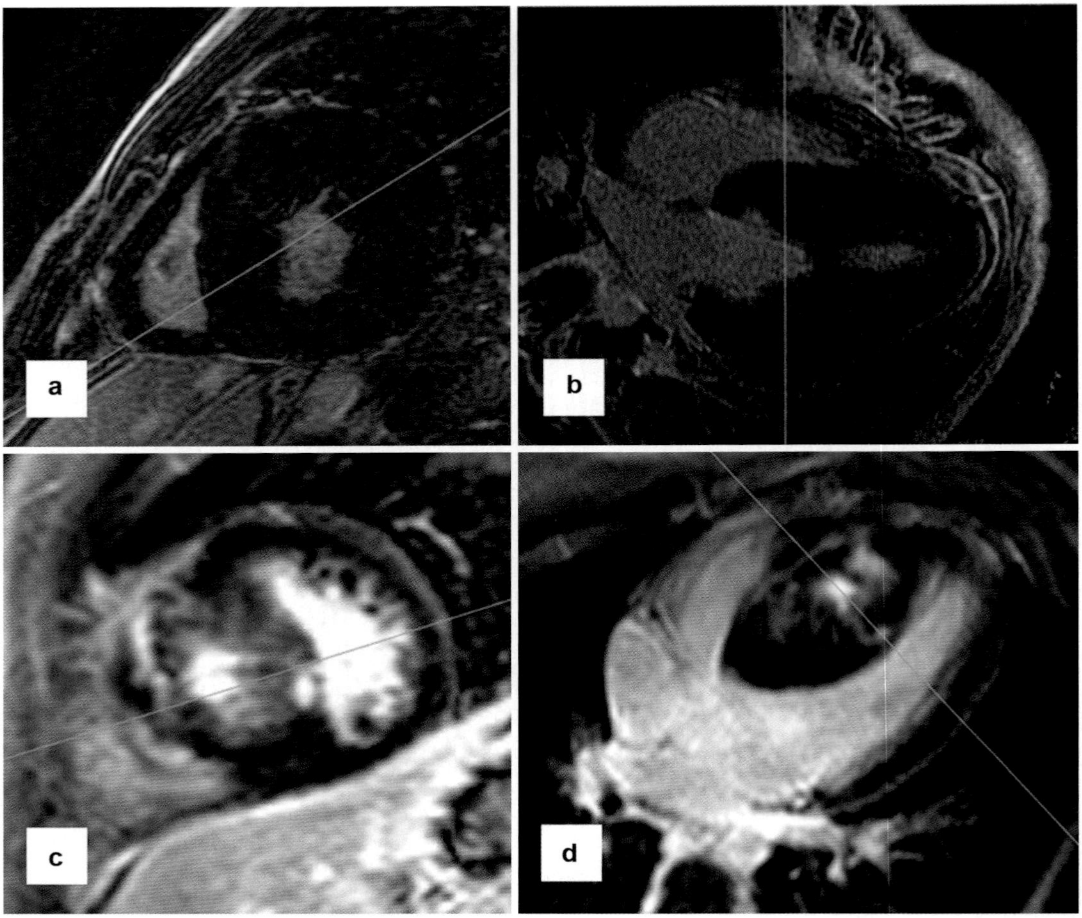

Fig. 16.17 Two patients with extreme hypertrophy, one with late gadolinium enhancement (LGE) and one without. (**a**, **b**) Late gadolinium enhancement imaging of patient with extreme hypertrophy with maximal wall thickness of 31 mm and LV mass of 481 g surprisingly shows complete lack of enhancement in short-axis slices (**a**), confirmed with 4-chamber (**b**) slice. (**c**, **d**) Second patient with extreme hypertrophy with maximal wall thickness of 44 mm and LV mass of 268 g showing extensive LGE in the short-axis slice (**a**) and 4-chamber slice (**b**). The LGE was seen in 33 g or 12 % of the LV mass

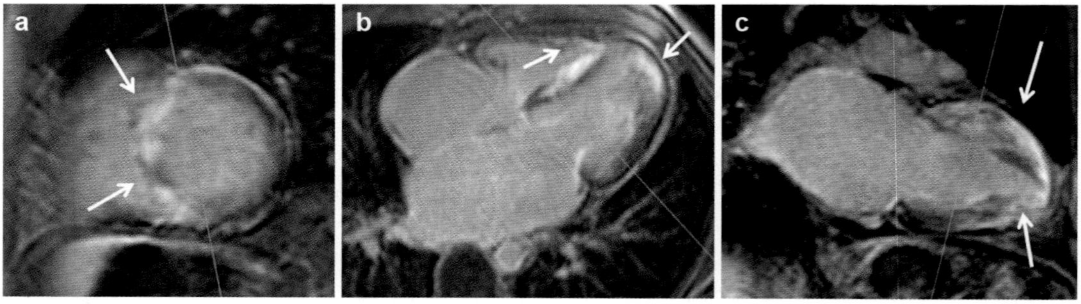

Fig. 16.18 Patients with end-stage HCM usually have extensive late gadolinium enhancement (LGE). In this end-stage HCM patient, late gadolinium enhancement imaging shows extensive enhancement encompassing well over 70 % of the entire LV myocardium. *Scanlines* indicate levels of corresponding slices. (**a**) Short-axis basal-mid-slice showing septum almost completely consisting of enhanced myocardium (*arrows*). (**b**) 4-chamber view shows enhancement in the RV and LV apices (*arrows*). (**c**) 2-chamber view shows enhancement of entire anterior wall and apex (*arrows*)

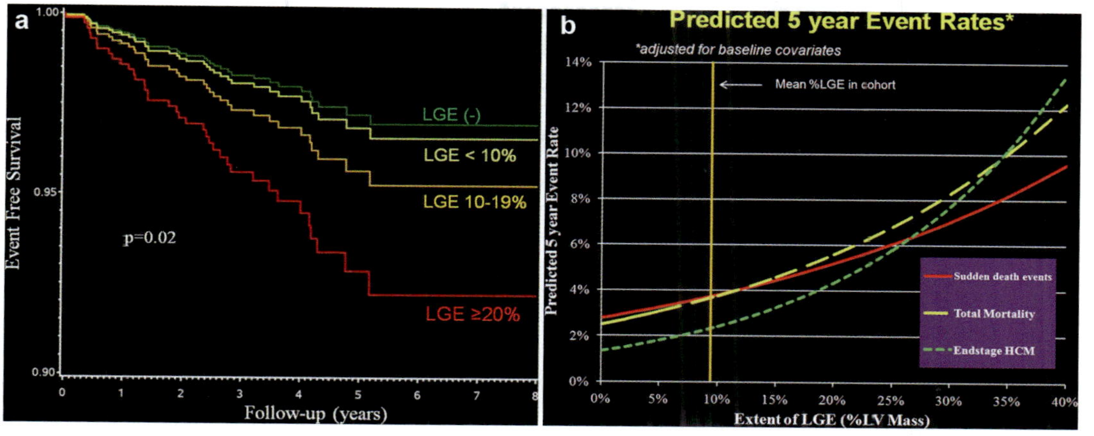

Fig. 16.19 (**a**) Predicted risk of sudden cardiac death events, stratified by the extent of late gadolinium enhancement (*LGE*). The extent of LGE is independently related to risk of sudden cardiac death events in HCM, even after adjusting for baseline risk factors and relevant covariates. (**b**) Risk of adverse events has a continuous independent relationship with the extent of LGE, including sudden death, development of end stage, and total mortality, even after adjusting for relevant baseline covariates

This has generated interest that LGE could serve as a novel risk marker for sudden death, thus improving current risk stratification strategies. Only four small short-term studies have examined the relationship between LGE and sudden death or appropriate therapy for ventricular tachycardia/fibrillation. However, all of the individual studies were underpowered to detect a significant relationship with sudden cardiac death, even when data were combined. It is important to note that these studies have focused entirely on the association between the *presence* of LGE and sudden death. However, the mere presence of any amount of LGE as a binary variable cannot practically be regarded as a risk marker, given that the reported prevalence of some LGE is up to 80 % of all HCM patients. Furthermore, this designation gives equal weight to LGE across a broad spectrum of amounts, from minimal to extensive.

More recently, results from a large prospective cohort study revealed a robust continuous relationship between the amount of LGE and sudden death risk in HCM patients with (as well as without) conventional risk factors (Fig. 16.19a) [51]. The absence of LGE itself was associated with low risk of SCD, representing a potential source of reassurance to patients with no other marker of increased risk. The data provides support for extensive LGE to be an independent prognostic marker for sudden death. The extent of LGE can also be used as an arbitrator in ICD decisions in patients in whom risk stratification remains ambiguous in the presence of possible conventional risk factors (Fig. 16.14). Furthermore, the extent of LGE also predicted development of end-stage HCM and all-cause mortality (Fig. 16.19b).

Intermediate signal-intensity LGE is thought to represent areas of tissue of heterogeneity, where there are islands of myocardium separated by fibrosis. This may potentially be important as these regions have been hypothesized to represent a more arrhythmogenic substrate, making one more likely to experience lethal arrhythmias [54]. While there is an association with ambulatory ventricular tachyarrhythmias in HCM [55], intermediate signal-intensity LGE does not appear to be a superior predictor for identifying high-risk patients for sudden death when compared with visually quantified or high-signal-intensity (i.e., >6 SD above normal mean SI of nulled myocardium) LGE (Fig. 16.20) [56]. The emergence of novel CMR techniques such as T1 mapping may provide an even more precise characterization of abnormal myocardial substrate in HCM [57].

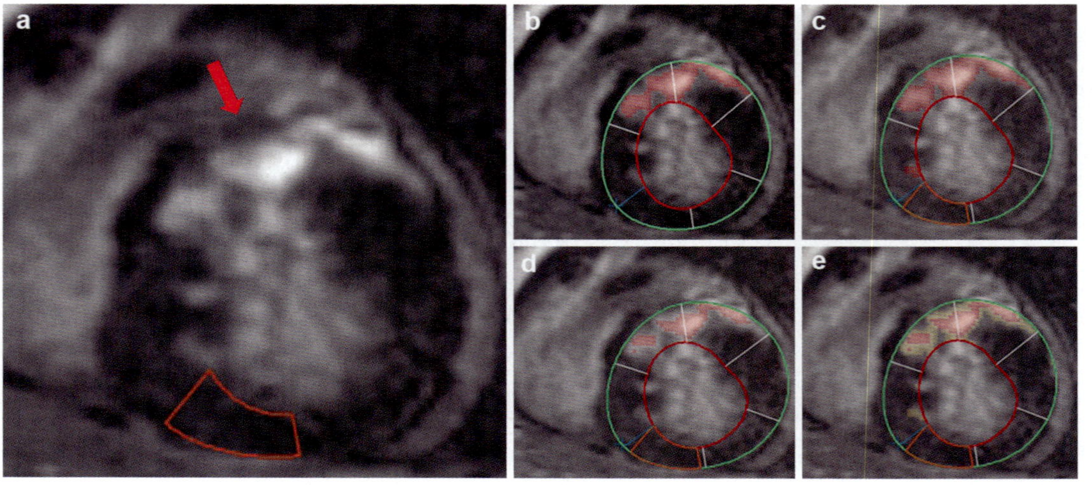

Fig. 16.20 These series of images illustrate the method to which intermediate signal-intensity (or "gray zone") enhancement is identified and quantified. (**a**) Mid-ventricular short-axis late gadolinium enhancement (LGE) image of 36-year-old man with considerable hyperenhancement (*red arrow*) in ventricular septum and anterior wall and a region of interest in normal myocardium (ROI; *orange box*) used to define thresholds for LGE. (**b**) Manual contouring of endocardial border (*red line*) and epicardial border (*green line*) of LV to define myocardium. *Red shading* denotes visually determined area of hyperenhancement. (**c**) Grayscale threshold ≥4SDs above signal intensity (SI) of the ROI (*red shading*), which includes both high- and intermediate-SI LGE. (**d**) High-SI LGE (*red shading*), defined by ≥6SD above SI of the ROI. (**e**) Intermediate-SI LGE (*yellow shading*), identified by subtracting LGE ≥4SD from ≥6SD (superimposed *red shading*)

Stress Perfusion CMR

CMR can be used to assess perfusion deficits and abnormalities of coronary blood flow [58]. Microvascular dysfunction has been well described in this disease and can be evaluated using multiparametric imaging with CMR [59]. It has been shown that ischemia identified by SPECT is associated with increased risk in HCM [60, 61]. Stress perfusion CMR may thus be considered as a further risk stratification tool; however, its role in the overall risk stratification strategy remains undetermined.

Differentiation of Athlete's Heart with HCM

A common clinical problem arises where physiological changes in the hearts of young competitive athletes may overlap phenotypically with a mild expression of HCM. This distinction is particularly important since HCM is the most common cause of sudden death in young competitive athletes [62]. Of these deaths, the vast majority occur during periods of severe exertion during training or competition. Accurate diagnosis has profound implications, as the misdiagnosis of disease may unnecessarily disqualify a patient from further participation and competition. On the other hand, proper identification of athletes with HCM can form the basis for disqualification from certain types of athletic activities in order to minimize risk.

Long-term athletic training (particularly in high-intensity endurance sports such as distance running, cycling, swimming, and rowing) can lead to increases in LV wall thickness, along with increases in LV end-diastolic volumes which leads to an increase in LV mass [63]. During such activities, cardiac output is greatly increased through physiological elevations in heart rate, stroke volume, and blood pressure, with a concomitant reduction in peripheral vascular resistance. Subsequently, the heart is subjected to predominantly a volume load, rather than a pressure load as experienced during

Table 16.1 Characteristics of athlete's heart versus hypertrophic cardiomyopathy (HCM)

Characteristic	Athlete's heart	HCM
LV end-diastolic dimension >55 mm	Present (>1/3 of highly trained elite male athletes), particularly in endurance athletes	Uncommon until the end stage with heart failure and systolic dysfunction
LV end-diastolic dimension <45 mm	Inconsistent with athlete's heart	If present, is supportive of diagnosis
Focal or "unusual" patterns of hypertrophy	Absent	Common
Degree of hypertrophy	Normal or mildly increased (≤12 mm), <2 % may be up to 16 mm	Average thickness ~20 mm, with small subgroup with substantial thickening >50 mm
Decreased thickness (~2–5 mm) within 3 months of deconditioning	Supportive of diagnosis	Absent
Left atrial enlargement	Absent	May be present
Peak oxygen consumption (VO_2) >110 %	Present	Absent
Late gadolinium enhancement	May be present, usually in small amounts in mid-myocardium and at RV insertion points, never extensive	Common (40–60 %), may be at RV insertion points but also elsewhere, occasionally (~10 %) extensive
Sarcomeric mutation on genetic testing	Absent	May be present (~40–50 %)
Family history of HCM	Absent	May be present
Abnormal ECG	May be present, thus not helpful	May be present
Right ventricular involvement	Absent	Occasionally present
Transmitral filling pattern on echocardiography	Normal	Decreased E wave, increased A wave, or may be normal

LV left ventricle, *RV* right ventricle, *ECG* electrocardiogram

isometric exercises such as weight lifting [64], thus leading to cavitary dilation. However, athletes engaging in either form of exercise tend to have increased LV cavity size compared with controls, a characteristic that is helpful in differentiating an athlete's heart from HCM, where cavity sizes tend to be small. Pathological changes such as severe left atrial enlargement and LV systolic and diastolic dysfunction should not occur in athlete's heart.

Cessation of systemic training in the athlete over a period of several months will cause regression of increased wall thickness but will not result in regression of hypertrophy in patients with HCM [65]. This method has been advocated as a method of differentiating between athlete's heart and HCM, since there should be no expected regression with detraining in true cardiac disease. Furthermore, the presence of greater than small amounts of LGE is highly suggestive of HCM and not athlete's heart.

Table 16.1 Lists of helpful findings which can help distinguish between athlete's heart and HCM

Differentiation of Hypertensive Heart Disease with HCM

A frequent diagnostic dilemma occurs when a patient with suspected HCM also has concomitant hypertension (Fig. 16.21). Typically, chronic hypertension produces concentric remodeling rather than asymmetric septal hypertrophy (ASH), although ASH is frequently encountered in elderly patients. Patients with a family history of HCM, ventricular hypertrophy in a nonhypertensive relative, or a positive genetic test may be supportive of a diagnosis of HCM. Treatment of hypertension may regress hypertrophy in those with hypertension. Hypertension rarely produces wall thickness >18 mm, while the average LV wall thickness in HCM is 21 mm. Strain metrics

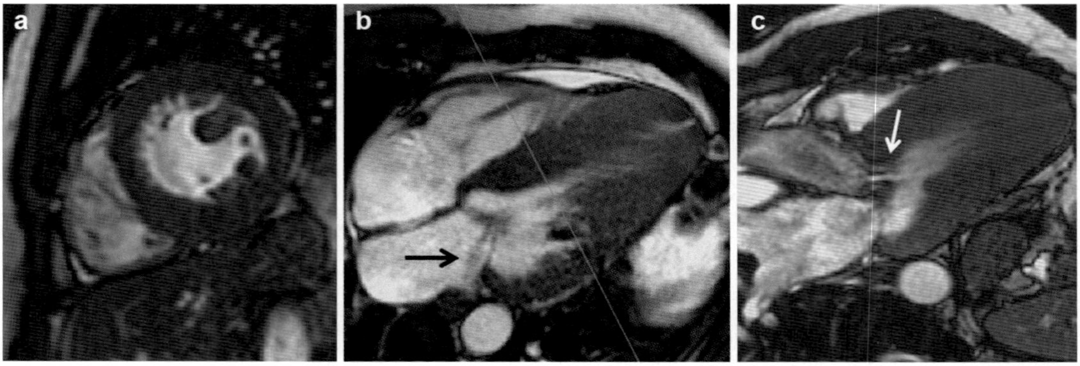

Fig. 16.21 Patient with genotype-positive HCM with concomitant hypertension. (**a**) Short-axis slice shows concentric thickening, with enlarged papillary muscle. (**b**) 4-chamber view shows a dephased jet of blood consistent with posteriorly directed mitral regurgitation (*arrow*). Note prominent hypertrophy in the apical region. *Scanline* represents level of the short-axis slice. (**c**) 3-chamber view in systole shows dephasing through left ventricle outflow tract (*arrow*), representing flow acceleration originating mitral leaflet tip secondary to chordal systolic anterior motion

from echocardiography and CMR are emerging as novel discriminatory tools [66–68].

Certain patterns of septal hypertrophy may be more prominent in HCM, such as reverse curvature and apical hypertrophy. Other patterns such as a sigmoid shape are more prominent in elderly hypertensive patients [69] and have been shown to be negative predictor of HCM genotype [70]. It also has to be noted that there may be significant overlap in phenotypes; therefore, diagnosis of hypertension does not necessarily preclude the diagnosis of HCM.

Differentiation of Metabolic and Infiltrative Cardiomyopathies and HCM

A variety of genetic diseases can produce phenotypes that may have myocardial geometry similar to HCM. The most common "non-sarcomeric" diseases include cardiac amyloidosis, Anderson-Fabry's disease, and Danon disease. Generally, most of these conditions produce symmetric rather than asymmetric hypertrophy, and LVOT obstruction is less common.

A systematic approach, including obtaining an accurate and complete family history, symptoms, physical examination, judicious use of imaging, and biochemical and genetic testing, is vital to the differential diagnosis between such diseases and hypertrophic cardiomyopathy. For example, CMR imaging can be used to identify patterns of LVH and LGE which can raise suspicion for diagnosis of HCM phenocopies. Molecular diagnosis can then be used as confirmatory tests for Danon and Fabry's disease, while biopsy should be considered for amyloid.

Anderson-Fabry's disease is an x-linked lysosomal storage disease where mutations in the α-galactosidase A gene lead to accumulation of glycosphingolipids in multiple organs, including the kidneys and heart. Cardiac manifestations are serious and progressive and may include left ventricular thickening, conduction abnormalities, dysrhythmias, and valve disease and are not usually detected until the third or fourth decade of life. Cardiac diseases are a major cause of death in patients with Fabry's [71]. Adults with this disease have LGE most commonly localized to the basal inferolateral wall, which would be an unusual distribution in HCM.

Danon disease is another x-linked lysosomal storage disease where mutations in the lysosome-associated membrane protein 2 (LAMP2) cause skeletal myopathy, developmental delay, and cardiomyopathy. Patients may present during adolescence with elevated creatine kinase, preexcitation pattern on ECG, left ventricular hypertrophy, and retinitis pigmentosa. Most patients die rapidly from

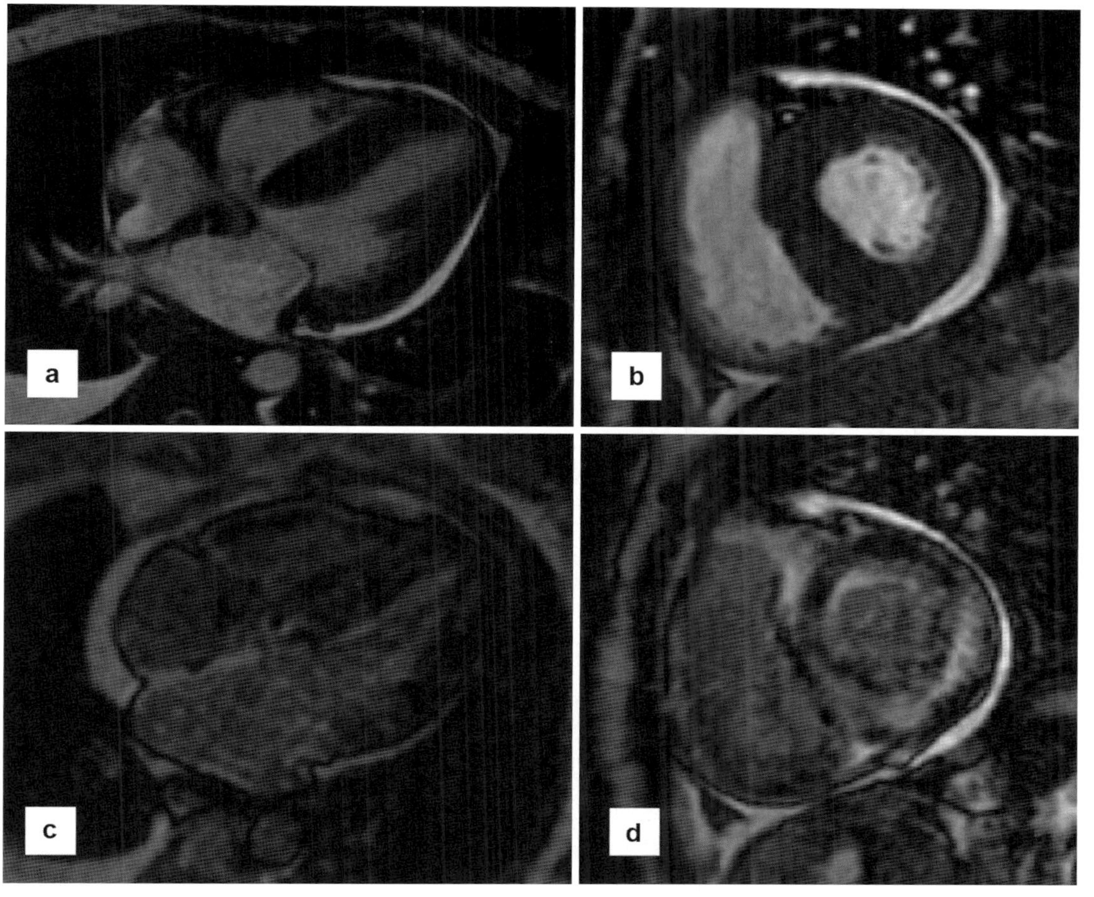

Fig. 16.22 Patient with biopsy-proven AL cardiac amyloidosis, showing several classical MR findings of amyloidosis. (**a**) 4-chamber steady state free precession (SSFP) showing diffuse thickening of LV myocardium and enlarged left atrium. Note small circumferential pericardial effusion and mild bilateral pleural effusions. (**b**) Short-axis SSFP slice showing symmetric thickening and small pericardial effusion. (**c**) Look-Locker T1 scout showing the typical "failure to null" appearance of myocardium despite varying inversion times from 100 to 500 ms. (**d**) Short-axis late gadolinium enhancement (LFE) imaging showing diffuse LGE as well as regions of subendocardial enhancement not in typical coronary distribution

heart failure (typically <25 years old), with a small proportion dying from sudden cardiac death [72].

Mutations in PRKAG2, the γ2 subunit of AMP-activated protein kinase (AMPK), can cause a syndrome of HCM, conduction abnormalities, and Wolff-Parkinson-White syndrome. However, this mutation does not seem to result in malignant consequences, such as sudden death and ventricular dilation [73].

Amyloidosis is caused by the abnormal deposition of insoluble amyloid proteins throughout the body, with cardiac involvement being more frequent in the AL and TTE subtypes. Amyloid deposition leads to diastolic dysfunction and restrictive cardiomyopathy, which ultimately progresses to heart failure. It is the leading cause of death for patients with AL amyloidosis. CMR shows a characteristic "failure to null" pattern in T1 scout during late gadolinium enhancement imaging, together with abnormal blood pool gadolinium kinetics. Patients may exhibit a pattern of global subendocardial LGE or patchy focal involvement in the LV myocardium. Supportive findings include enlarged atria (likely secondary to restrictive cardiomyopathy), pericardial effusion, and pleural effusions (Fig. 16.22).

Left Ventricular Noncompaction (LVNC)

Left ventricular noncompaction, or LVNC, was first reported in 1984 (Fig. 16.23) [74]. It was initially observed in echocardiography with the appearance of persistent myocardial sinusoids. Its prevalence is estimated to be between 0.05 and 0.24 %, with a wide range of ages at presentation with no predilection for any specific age [75]. Over half of all cases are male.

LVNC is hypothesized to be due to abnormal compaction of the myocardium during the fifth and eighth week of embryonic development. The trabecular layer of the ventricle has been observed to compact from the base to apex during development, from epicardium to endocardium, and from the septal to lateral wall. However, cases of acquired LVNC have been described, where infants whose echocardiograms did not show LVNC but were subsequently diagnosed with the disease later in life [76, 77].

Different genes found to be associated with LVNC include taffazin, β-dystrobrevin (DTNA), Cypher/ZASP (LDB3), lamin A/C (LMNA), SCN5A, MYH7, and MYBPC3 [78]. Much like HCM, there is considerable genetic heterogeneity associated with LVNC. As well, LVNC can exist concurrently with HCM or dilated cardiomyopathy [79]. Familial involvement ranges

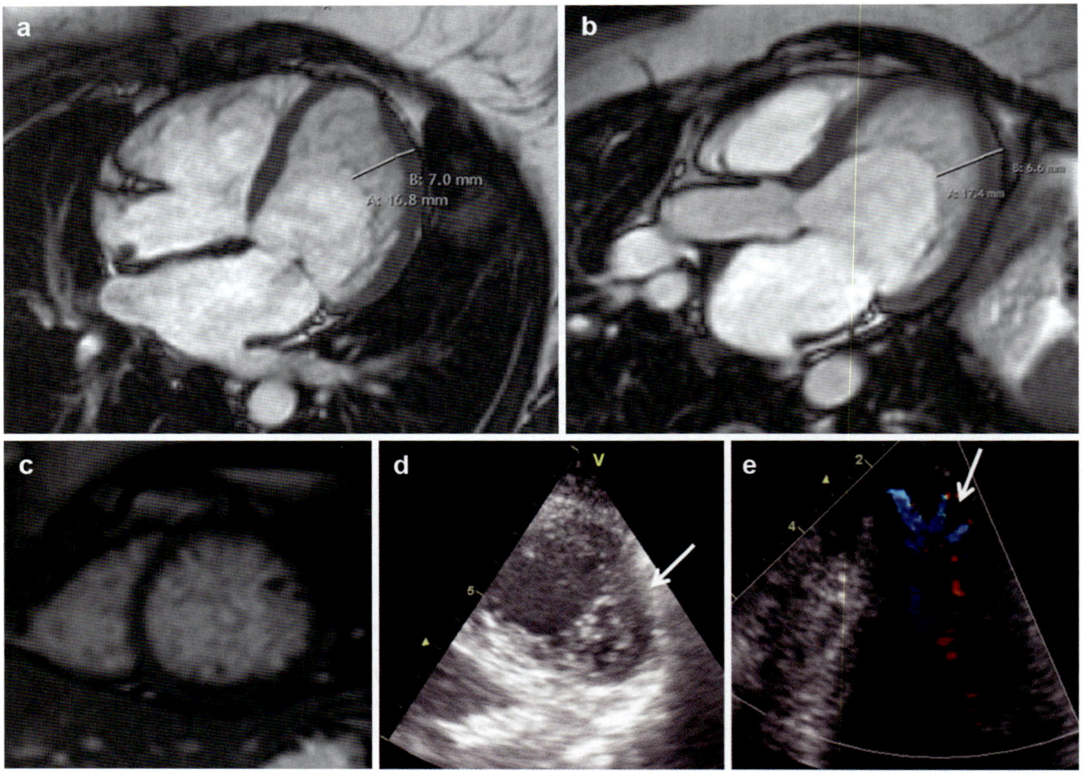

Fig. 16.23 Patient with suspected noncompaction on echocardiography. (**a**) 4-chamber slice shows large area of noncompacted myocardium, with a thickness ratio of 16.8/7 = 2.4 in relation to adjacent myocardium during diastole. (**b**) 3-chamber view of the same patient with a thickness ratio of 17.4/6.6 = 2.6. A maximum diastolic ratio of noncompacted versus compacted myocardium of >2.3–2.5 is required in three long-axis views. (**c**) Short-axis slice near the apex shows noncompacted myocardium filling the entire LV cavity. (**d**) Short-axis echocardiography near the apex shows echo-lucent matrix-like structure suggestive of noncompacted myocardium. (**e**) Color Doppler in 4-chamber orientation helps highlight blood flow in the recesses. There appear to be numerous prominent trabeculations with deep intertrabecular spaces. Alternatively, contrast echocardiography can be used

from 18 to 33 % [80–82]. Current guidelines recommend clinical screen of first-degree relatives of probands; however, genetic testing is not routinely recommended [83].

Echocardiography is the initial diagnostic test of choice, with contrast echo, transesophageal echo, and three-dimensional echo serving as useful adjuncts. There is no clear consensus on the echocardiographic diagnostic criteria for LVNC, as each threshold will have different sensitivities and specifies. The three most widely used criteria include:

1. Jenni criteria [84]: In parasternal short-axis view, end-*systolic* ratio >2 of noncompacted to compact layer; the absence of other coexisting structural abnormalities, plus numerous excessively prominent trabeculations and deep intertrabecular spaces; and recesses perfused by intraventricular blood seen by color Doppler
2. Chin criteria [85]: In parasternal short-axis view or apical views, end-*diastolic* ratio of compact layer to total thickness of LV <0.5
3. Stollberger criteria [75]: >3 trabeculations protruding from the LV free wall apically to the papillary muscles seen on one imaging plane; intertrabecular spaces perfused from the LV cavity shown by color Doppler

Different criteria have also been proposed, including combining the Jenni and Stollberger criteria or by quantifying along a continuum the noncompacted/compacted ratio and areas of noncompaction [86, 87].

Due to lower spatial resolution of echocardiography, and in its often suboptimal characterization of apical segments (where noncompacted areas are most commonly found), LVNC often goes undiagnosed or misdiagnosed as HCM or dilated cardiomyopathy. The superior image resolution and unlimited imaging planes make CMR a complementary (and often superior) tool in establishing the diagnosis. The Petersen criteria [88] in CMR require an end-*diastolic* ratio >2.3 of trabecular and compact layers (Fig. 16.23). These criteria have been shown to have high diagnostic accuracy to distinguish pathological LVNC from noncompaction seen in healthy, dilated, and hypertrophied hearts. Cardiac CT and contrast left ventriculography can also be useful if there is a need for concurrent delineation of coronary anatomy.

Asymptomatic patients do not need treatment but need to be followed, but all symptomatic patients should be followed closely. Incidence of NYHA class II/IV heart failure ranges from 35 to 44 % [80, 89]. Treatment of patients include medical therapy with beta-blockers, ACE inhibitors, and diuretics in those with systolic dysfunction [90]. Cardiac resynchronization therapy with or without an ICD is recommended for those on optimal medical therapy with LVEF <35 % and QRS >0.120 s [91]. Patients should also be monitored for ventricular arrhythmias, with ICD implantation in the appropriate patients. Prognosis depends on symptoms and LV ejection fraction.

References

1. Maron BJ, Maron MS, Semsarian C. Double or compound sarcomere mutations in hypertrophic cardiomyopathy: a potential link to sudden death in the absence of conventional risk factors. Heart Rhythm. 2012;9(1):57–63.
2. Konno T, Chang S, Seidman JG, Seidman CE. Genetics of hypertrophic cardiomyopathy. Curr Opin Cardiol. 2010;25(3):205–9.
3. Judge DP. Use of genetics in the clinical evaluation of cardiomyopathy. JAMA. 2009;302(22):2471–6.
4. Maron BJ, Maron MS. Hypertrophic cardiomyopathy. Lancet. 2013;381:242–55.
5. Maron BJ. Hypertrophic cardiomyopathy: an important global disease. Am J Med. 2004;116(1):63–5.
6. Olivotto I, Maron MS, Adabag S, et al. Gender-related differences in the clinical presentation and outcome of hypertrophic cardiomyopathy. J Am Coll Cardiol. 2005;46(3):480–7.
7. Maron BJ. Hypertrophic cardiomyopathy: a systematic review. JAMA. 2002;287(10):1308–20.
8. Teare D. Asymmetrical hypertrophy of the heart in young adults. Br Heart J. 1958;20(1):1–8.
9. Gersh BJ, Maron BJ, Bonow RO, et al. 2011 ACCF/AHA guideline for the diagnosis and treatment of hypertrophic cardiomyopathy: executive summary: a report of the American College of Cardiology Foundation/American Heart Association Task Force on Practice Guidelines. Circulation. 2011;124(24):2761–96.
10. Chan RH, Maron B, Olivotto I, et al. Prognostic utility of contrast-enhanced cardiovascular magnetic resonance in hypertrophic cardiomyopathy: an International Multicenter Study. J Am Coll Cardiol. 2012;59(13):E1570.

11. Klues HG, Schiffers A, Maron BJ. Phenotypic spectrum and patterns of left ventricular hypertrophy in hypertrophic cardiomyopathy: morphologic observations and significance as assessed by two-dimensional echocardiography in 600 patients. J Am Coll Cardiol. 1995;26(7):1699–708.
12. Maron MS, Maron BJ, Harrigan C, et al. Hypertrophic cardiomyopathy phenotype revisited after 50 years with cardiovascular magnetic resonance. J Am Coll Cardiol. 2009;54(3):220–8.
13. Maron MS, Lesser JR, Maron BJ. Management implications of massive left ventricular hypertrophy in hypertrophic cardiomyopathy significantly underestimated by echocardiography but identified by cardiovascular magnetic resonance. Am J Cardiol. 2010;105(12):1842–3.
14. Rickers C, Wilke NM, Jerosch-Herold M, et al. Utility of cardiac magnetic resonance imaging in the diagnosis of hypertrophic cardiomyopathy. Circulation. 2005;112(6):855–61.
15. Spirito P, Bellone P, Harris KM, Bernabo P, Bruzzi P, Maron BJ. Magnitude of left ventricular hypertrophy and risk of sudden death in hypertrophic cardiomyopathy. N Engl J Med. 2000;342(24):1778–85.
16. Maron MS, Rowin EJ, Lin D, et al. Prevalence and clinical profile of myocardial crypts in hypertrophic cardiomyopathy. Circ Cardiovasc Imaging. 2012;5(4):617–36.
17. Germans T, Wilde AAM, Dijkmans PA, et al. Structural abnormalities of the inferoseptal left ventricular wall detected by cardiac magnetic resonance imaging in carriers of hypertrophic cardiomyopathy mutations. J Am Coll Cardiol. 2006;48(12):2518–23.
18. Olivotto I, Maron MS, Autore C, et al. Assessment and significance of left ventricular mass by cardiovascular magnetic resonance in hypertrophic cardiomyopathy. J Am Coll Cardiol. 2008;52(7):559–66.
19. Maron MS, Hauser TH, Dubrow E, et al. Right ventricular involvement in hypertrophic cardiomyopathy. Am J Cardiol. 2007;100(8):1293–8.
20. Keeling AN, Carr JC, Choudhury L. Right ventricular hypertrophy and scarring in mutation positive hypertrophic cardiomyopathy. Eur Heart J. 2010;31(3):381.
21. Maron BJ, Dearani JA, Ommen SR, et al. The case for surgery in obstructive hypertrophic cardiomyopathy. J Am Coll Cardiol. 2004;44(10):2044–53.
22. Minakata K, Dearani JA, Schaff HV, O'Leary PW, Ommen SR, Danielson GK. Mechanisms for recurrent left ventricular outflow tract obstruction after septal myectomy for obstructive hypertrophic cardiomyopathy. Ann Thorac Surg. 2005;80(3):851–6.
23. Delahaye F, Jegaden O, De Gevigney G, et al. Postoperative and long-term prognosis of myotomy-myomectomy for obstructive hypertrophic cardiomyopathy: influence of associated mitral valve replacement. Eur Heart J. 1993;14(9):1229–37.
24. Kwon DH, Smedira NG, Popovic ZB, et al. Steep left ventricle to aortic root angle and hypertrophic obstructive cardiomyopathy: study of a novel association using three-dimensional multimodality imaging. Heart. 2009;95(21):1784–91.
25. Maron MS, Olivotto I, Betocchi S, et al. Effect of left ventricular outflow tract obstruction on clinical outcome in hypertrophic cardiomyopathy. N Engl J Med. 2003;348(4):295–303.
26. Geske JB, Sorajja P, Ommen SR, Nishimura RA. Left ventricular outflow tract gradient variability in hypertrophic cardiomyopathy. Clin Cardiol. 2009;32(7): 397–402.
27. Geske JB, Cullen MW, Sorajja P, Ommen SR, Nishimura RA. Assessment of left ventricular outflow gradient: hypertrophic cardiomyopathy versus aortic valvular stenosis. JACC Cardiovasc Interv. 2012;5(6): 675–81.
28. Nagueh SF, Bierig SM, Budoff MJ, et al. American Society of Echocardiography clinical recommendations for multimodality cardiovascular imaging of patients with hypertrophic cardiomyopathy: Endorsed by the American Society of Nuclear Cardiology, Society for Cardiovascular Magnetic Resonance, and Society of Cardiovascular Computed Tomography. J Am Soc Echocardiogr. 2011;24(5):473–98.
29. Kwon DH, Setser RM, Thamilarasan M, et al. Abnormal papillary muscle morphology is independently associated with increased left ventricular outflow tract obstruction in hypertrophic cardiomyopathy. Heart. 2008;94(10):1295–301.
30. Harrigan CJ, Appelbaum E, Maron BJ, et al. Significance of papillary muscle abnormalities identified by cardiovascular magnetic resonance in hypertrophic cardiomyopathy. Am J Cardiol. 2008;101(5):668–73.
31. Minakata K, Dearani JA, Nishimura RA, Maron BJ, Danielson GK. Extended septal myectomy for hypertrophic obstructive cardiomyopathy with anomalous mitral papillary muscles or chordae. J Thorac Cardiovasc Surg. 2004;127(2):481–9.
32. Shapiro LM, McKenna WJ. Distribution of left ventricular hypertrophy in hypertrophic cardiomyopathy: a two-dimensional echocardiographic study. J Am Coll Cardiol. 1983;2(3):43744.
33. Gruner C, Chan RH, Rowin EJ, et al. Left ventricular apico-basal muscle bundle identified by cardiovascular magnetic resonance imaging in patients with hypertrophic cardiomyopathy: implications for diagnosis and management. Circulation. 2012;126(21 Suppl), A14941.
34. Maron MS, Olivotto I, Harrigan C, et al. Mitral valve abnormalities identified by cardiovascular magnetic resonance represent a primary phenotypic expression of hypertrophic cardiomyopathy. Circulation. 2011;70:40–7.
35. Grigg LE, Wigle ED, Williams WG, Daniel LB, Rakowski H. Transesophageal Doppler echocardiography in obstructive hypertrophic cardiomyopathy: clarification of pathophysiology and importance in intraoperative decision making. J Am Coll Cardiol. 1992;20(1):42–52.
36. Fattori R, Biagini E, Lorenzini M, Buttazzi K, Lovato L, Rapezzi C. Significance of magnetic resonance imaging in apical hypertrophic cardiomyopathy. Am J Cardiol. 2010;105(11):1592–6.

37. Maron MS, Finley JJ, Bos JM, et al. Prevalence, clinical significance, and natural history of left ventricular apical aneurysms in hypertrophic cardiomyopathy. Circulation. 2008;118(15):1541–9.
38. Lim K-K, Maron BJ, Knight BP. Successful catheter ablation of hemodynamically unstable monomorphic ventricular tachycardia in a patient with hypertrophic cardiomyopathy and apical aneurysm. J Cardiovasc Electrophysiol. 2009;20(4):445–7.
39. Bruder O, Wagner A, Jensen CJ, et al. Myocardial scar visualized by cardiovascular magnetic resonance imaging predicts major adverse events in patients with hypertrophic cardiomyopathy. J Am Coll Cardiol. 2010;56(11):875–87.
40. Maron MS, Appelbaum E, Harrigan CJ, et al. Clinical profile and significance of delayed enhancement in hypertrophic cardiomyopathy. Circ Heart Fail. 2008;1(3):184–91.
41. Rubinshtein R, Glockner JF, Ommen SR, et al. Characteristics and clinical significance of late gadolinium enhancement by contrast-enhanced magnetic resonance imaging in patients with hypertrophic cardiomyopathy. Circ Heart Fail. 2010;3(1):51–8.
42. O'Hanlon R, Grasso A, Roughton M, et al. Prognostic significance of myocardial fibrosis in hypertrophic cardiomyopathy. J Am Coll Cardiol. 2010;56(11):867–74.
43. Kwon DH, Setser RM, Popovic ZB, et al. Association of myocardial fibrosis, electrocardiography and ventricular tachyarrhythmia in hypertrophic cardiomyopathy: a delayed contrast enhanced MRI study. Int J Cardiovasc Imaging. 2008;24(6):617–25.
44. Moon JCC, McKenna WJ, McCrohon JA, Elliott PM, Smith GC, Pennell DJ. Toward clinical risk assessment in hypertrophic cardiomyopathy with gadolinium cardiovascular magnetic resonance. J Am Coll Cardiol. 2003;41(9):1561–7.
45. Kim RJ, Fieno DS, Parrish TB, et al. Relationship of MRI delayed contrast enhancement to irreversible injury, infarct age, and contractile function. Circulation. 1999;100(19):1992–2002.
46. Papavassiliu T, Schnabel P, Schröder M, Borggrefe M. CMR scarring in a patient with hypertrophic cardiomyopathy correlates well with histological findings of fibrosis. Eur Heart J. 2005;26(22):2395.
47. Moravsky G, Ofek E, WIlliams L, Butany J, Rakowski H, Crean A. Cardiovascular magnetic resonance imaging with late gadolinium enhancement and histopathological correlation in hypertrophic cardiomyopathy. Circulation. 2011;124, A14546.
48. Kwon DH, Smedira NG, Rodriguez ER, et al. Cardiac magnetic resonance detection of myocardial scarring in hypertrophic cardiomyopathy: correlation with histopathology and prevalence of ventricular tachycardia. J Am Coll Cardiol. 2009;54(3):242–9.
49. Kuribayashi T, Roberts WC. Myocardial disarray at junction of ventricular septum and left and right ventricular free walls in hypertrophic cardiomyopathy. Am J Cardiol. 1992;70(15):1333–40.
50. Maron MS. Clinical utility of cardiovascular magnetic resonance in hypertrophic cardiomyopathy. J Cardiovasc Magn Reson. 2012;14(1):13.
51. Chan RH, Maron BJ, Olivotto I, et al. Prognostic utility of contrast-enhanced cardiovascular magnetic resonance imaging in hypertrophic cardiomyopathy: an International Multicenter Study. Circulation. 2012;126(21 Suppl), A13139.
52. Adabag S, Maron BJ, Appelbaum E, et al. Occurrence and frequency of arrhythmias in hypertrophic cardiomyopathy in relation to delayed enhancement on cardiovascular magnetic resonance. J Am Coll Cardiol. 2008;51(14):1369–74.
53. Monserrat L, Elliott PM, Gimeno JR, Sharma S, Penas-Lado M, McKenna WJ. Non-sustained ventricular tachycardia in hypertrophic cardiomyopathy: an independent marker of sudden death risk in young patients. J Am Coll Cardiol. 2003;42(5):873–9.
54. Yan AT, Shayne AJ, Brown KA, et al. Characterization of the peri-infarct zone by contrast-enhanced cardiac magnetic resonance imaging is a powerful predictor of post-myocardial infarction mortality. Circulation. 2006;114(1):32–9.
55. Appelbaum E, Maron BJ, Adabag S, et al. Intermediate-signal-intensity late gadolinium enhancement predicts ventricular tachyarrhythmias in patients with hypertrophic cardiomyopathy. Circ Cardiovasc Imaging. 2012;5(1):78–85.
56. Chan RH, Afilalo J, Maron BJ, et al. Prognostic utility of intermediate-signal-intensity late gadolinium enhancement in patients with hypertrophic cardiomyopathy. Circulation. 2012;126(21 Suppl), A17374.
57. Mewton N, Liu CY, Croisille P, Bluemke D, Lima JA. Assessment of myocardial fibrosis with cardiovascular magnetic resonance. J Am Coll Cardiol. 2011;57(8):891–903.
58. Kawada N, Sakuma H, Yamakado T, et al. Hypertrophic cardiomyopathy: MR measurement of coronary blood flow and vasodilator flow reserve in patients and healthy subjects. Radiology. 1999;211(1):129–35.
59. Petersen SE, Jerosch-Herold M, Hudsmith LE, et al. Evidence for microvascular dysfunction in hypertrophic cardiomyopathy: new insights from multiparametric magnetic resonance imaging. Circulation. 2007;115(18):2418–25.
60. Kaimoto S, Kawasaki T, Kuribayashi T, et al. Myocardial perfusion abnormality in the area of ventricular septum-free wall junction and cardiovascular events in nonobstructive hypertrophic cardiomyopathy. Int J Cardiovasc Imaging. 2012;28(7):1829–39.
61. Sorajja P, Chareonthaitawee P, Ommen SR, Miller TD, Hodge DO, Gibbons RJ. Prognostic utility of single-photon emission computed tomography in adult patients with hypertrophic cardiomyopathy. Am Heart J. 2006;151(2):426–35.
62. Maron BJ, Pelliccia A, Spirito P. Cardiac disease in young trained athletes. Insights into methods for distinguishing athlete's heart from structural heart disease, with particular emphasis on hypertrophic cardiomyopathy. Circulation. 1995;91(5):1596–601.
63. Maron BJ. Structural features of the athlete heart as defined by echocardiography. J Am Coll Cardiol. 1986;7(1):190–203.

64. Morganroth J, Maron BJ, Henry WL, Epstein SE. Comparative left ventricular dimensions in trained athletes. Ann Intern Med. 1975;82(4):521–4.
65. Fagard R. Athlete's heart. Heart. 2003;89(12): 1455–61.
66. Carasso S, Yang H, Woo A, Jamorski M, Wigle ED, Rakowski H. Diastolic myocardial mechanics in hypertrophic cardiomyopathy. J Am Soc Echocardiogr. 2010;23(2):164–71.
67. Kato TS, Noda A, Izawa H, et al. Discrimination of nonobstructive hypertrophic cardiomyopathy from hypertensive left ventricular hypertrophy on the basis of strain rate imaging by tissue Doppler ultrasonography. Circulation. 2004;110(25):3808–14.
68. Saito M, Okayama H, Yoshii T, et al. The differences in left ventricular torsional behavior between patients with hypertrophic cardiomyopathy and hypertensive heart disease. Int J Cardiol. 2011;150(3):301–6.
69. Lever HM, Karam RF, Currie PJ, Healy BP. Hypertrophic cardiomyopathy in the elderly. Distinctions from the young based on cardiac shape. Circulation. 1989;79(3):580–9.
70. Binder J, Ommen SR, Gersh BJ, et al. Echocardiography-guided genetic testing in hypertrophic cardiomyopathy: septal morphological features predict the presence of myofilament mutations. Mayo Clin Proc. 2006;81(4):459–67.
71. Mehta A, Beck M, Eyskens F, et al. Fabry disease: a review of current management strategies. QJM. 2010;103(9):641–59.
72. Arad M, Maron BJ, Gorham JM, et al. Glycogen storage diseases presenting as hypertrophic cardiomyopathy. N Engl J Med. 2005;352(4):362–72.
73. Bayrak F, Komurcu-Bayrak E, Mutlu B, Kahveci G, Basaran Y, Erginel-Unaltuna N. Ventricular preexcitation and cardiac hypertrophy mimicking hypertrophic cardiomyopathy in a Turkish family with a novel PRKAG2 mutation. Eur J Heart Fail. 2006;8(7):712–5.
74. Engberding R, Bender F. Echocardiographic detection of persistent myocardial sinusoids. Z Kardiol. 1984;73(12):786–8.
75. Stöllberger C, Finsterer J. Left ventricular hypertrabeculation/noncompaction. J Am Soc Echocardiogr. 2004;17(1):91–100.
76. Hofer M, Stöllberger C, Finsterer J. Acquired noncompaction associated with myopathy. Int J Cardiol. 2007;121(3):296–7.
77. Ichida F. Left ventricular noncompaction. Circ J. 2009;73(1):19–26.
78. Zaragoza MV, Arbustini E, Narula J. Noncompaction of the left ventricle: primary cardiomyopathy with an elusive genetic etiology. Curr Opin Pediatr. 2007;19(6):619–27.
79. Biagini E, Ragni L, Ferlito M, et al. Different types of cardiomyopathy associated with isolated ventricular noncompaction. Am J Cardiol. 2006;98(6):821–4.
80. Oechslin EN, Attenhofer Jost CH, Rojas JR, Kaufmann PA, Jenni R. Long-term follow-up of 34 adults with isolated left ventricular noncompaction: a distinct cardiomyopathy with poor prognosis. J Am Coll Cardiol. 2000;36(2):493–500.
81. Aras D, Tufekcioglu O, Ergun K, et al. Clinical features of isolated ventricular noncompaction in adults long-term clinical course, echocardiographic properties, and predictors of left ventricular failure. J Card Fail. 2006;12(9):726–33.
82. Xing Y, Ichida F, Matsuoka T, et al. Genetic analysis in patients with left ventricular noncompaction and evidence for genetic heterogeneity. Mol Genet Metab. 2006;88(1):71–7.
83. Hershberger RE, Lindenfeld J, Mestroni L, Seidman CE, Taylor MRG, Towbin JA. Genetic evaluation of cardiomyopathy–a Heart Failure Society of America practice guideline. J Card Fail. 2009;15(2):83–97.
84. Jenni R, Oechslin E, Schneider J, Attenhofer Jost C, Kaufmann PA. Echocardiographic and pathoanatomical characteristics of isolated left ventricular noncompaction: a step towards classification as a distinct cardiomyopathy. Heart. 2001;86(6):666–71.
85. Chin TK, Perloff JK, Williams RG, Jue K, Mohrmann R. Isolated noncompaction of left ventricular myocardium. A study of eight cases. Circulation. 1990;82(2): 507–13.
86. Belanger AR, Miller MA, Donthireddi UR, Najovits AJ, Goldman ME. New classification scheme of left ventricular noncompaction and correlation with ventricular performance. Am J Cardiol. 2008;102(1): 92–6.
87. Finsterer J, Stollberger C. Definite, probable, or possible left ventricular hypertrabeculation/noncompaction. Int J Cardiol. 2008;123(2):175–6.
88. Petersen SE, Selvanayagam JB, Wiesmann F, et al. Left ventricular non-compaction: insights from cardiovascular magnetic resonance imaging. J Am Coll Cardiol. 2005;46(1):101–5.
89. Lofiego C, Biagini E, Pasquale F, et al. Wide spectrum of presentation and variable outcomes of isolated left ventricular non-compaction. Heart. 2007;93(1):65–71.
90. Takano H, Komuro I. Beta-blockers have beneficial effects even on unclassified cardiomyopathy such as isolated ventricular noncompaction. Intern Med. 2002;41(8):601–2.
91. Epstein AE, Dimarco JP, Ellenbogen KA, et al. ACC/AHA/HRS 2008 Guidelines for device-based therapy of cardiac rhythm abnormalities. Heart Rhythm. 2008;5(6):e1–62.

17 The Right Myocardium

Fumiko Kimura and Nobuhisa Hagiwara

Congenital abnormalities of the right ventricular (RV) myocardium are rare and include arrhythmogenic right ventricular cardiomyopathy/dysplasia (ARVC/D) and Uhl's anomaly. Though rare, ARVC/D frequently appears in the differential diagnosis of patients with ventricular arrhythmia. We discuss magnetic resonance (MR) and computed tomography (CT) imaging techniques and various aspects of congenital abnormalities of the RV myocardium with special focus on ARVC/D.

Imaging Techniques

Although echocardiography is usually used for initial investigation of RV dysfunction, MR and CT imaging provide more detailed anatomic information. MR imaging allows for reproducible analysis of the RV function and measurement.

F. Kimura, MD (✉)
Department of Diagnostic Radiology, Saitama Medical University International Medical Center, 1397-1 Yamane, Hidaka-shi, Saitama 350-1298, Japan
e-mail: fkimura@saitama-med.ac.jp

N. Hagiwara, MD
Department of Cardiology, Tokyo Women's Medical University, 8-1 Kawada-cho, Shinjuku, Tokyo 162-0054, Japan
e-mail: mhagi@hij.twmu.ac.jp

MR Imaging Techniques

MR imaging protocol for ARVC/D contains cine imaging using balanced steady-state free precession (b-SSFP) technique, black blood double and triple (with fat suppression) inversion recovery (IR), and late gadolinium enhancement (LGE) using 2- (2D) or 3-dimensional (3D) segmented IR fast gradient-echo sequence.

Cine MR imaging is used to evaluate wall motion abnormalities (hypokinesis or dyskinesis) and measure volume and ejection fraction (EF) of both ventricles. Transaxial, standard long axis (2-, 3-, and 4- chamber), and short-axis views are commonly employed, and the addition of RV 2-chamber long-axis view is recommended to further evaluate the RV function [1]. Focal outpouching of the RV free wall (apical third of wall) is sometimes seen in normal subjects on transaxial views, but usually not on 4-chamber view [2]. Knowledge of variations in RV morphology and wall motion in normal subjects is important to avoid overdiagnosis of abnormalities [1].

Researchers disagree on the most suitable imaging plane for RV volumetric analysis using cine MR imaging. Volumetric measurement using transaxial rather than short-axis plane appears to be more accurate as most part of the RV outflow tract is incorporated in measurements using axial cuts [1, 3], but the use of short-axis plane allows measurement of both the RV and left ventricle (LV) volumes. The use of short-axis plane for the RV volume measurement requires

F. Saremi (ed.), *Cardiac CT and MR for Adult Congenital Heart Disease*,
DOI 10.1007/978-1-4614-8875-0_17, © Springer Science+Business Media New York 2014

correct placement of the basal short-axis slice immediately on the myocardial side of the tricuspid valve and careful exclusion of the right atrial cavity from the RV on the basal slice especially at end systole [1].

After acquisition of cine MR images, 5–7 mm transaxial or oblique transaxial black blood images (double IR fast spin echo) will be obtained and repeated using same-slice orientation after fat suppression (triple IR) to characterize myocardial fat. However, evidence of myocardial fat is sometimes unclear on MR imaging.

Diastolic LGE images are then obtained about 10–15 min after intravenous gadolinium contrast injection (0.1–0.2 mmol/kg). Using either transaxial or 4-chamber views in combination with short-axis series permits better evaluation of myocardial fibrosis of both ventricles. Thin slice thickness (5–6 mm) is recommended to improve detection of myocardial fibrosis of the RV wall.

CT Imaging Techniques

ECG-gated cardiac CT can be used to evaluate RV structural abnormality, providing superior spatial resolution to that of MR imaging to aid detection of myocardial fat and thinning of the RV free wall [4]. CT can also be used in patients with pacemaker or implantable cardioverter defibrillator. Radiation exposure, the greatest disadvantage of CT, can be reduced by lowering tube voltage and current as well as by taking advantage of newer dose reduction methods including, iterative reconstruction, prospective ECG-gating technique, and high-pitch helical scanning. However, prospective ECG triggering and high-pitch helical scanning methods are usually inadequate in patients with fast heart rate or arrhythmia. On the other hand, acquisition of all systolic and diastolic phases for analysis of volume and wall motion of the ventricles requires retrospective ECG gating which mandates higher radiation dose.

Patients whose heart rate exceeds 65 bpm require oral or intravenous beta-blocker administration before CT examination depending on the temporal resolution of the scanner. Oral nitroglycerin is not required when evaluation of the coronary artery is unnecessary. Noncontrast CT using prospective mid-diastolic ECG-gating is very useful for diagnosing ARVC/D by detecting small amounts of myocardial fat. Contrast-enhanced CT is crucial for evaluation of changes in cardiac structure and analyzing the LV and RV volumes. It can be performed using a prospective triggering scanning but may be replaced with retrospective ECG gating especially in patients with fast heart rate or arrhythmia or when volumetric analysis is desired. For post-contrast study, we administer an intravenous bolus of 350 or 370 mgI nonionic iodinated contrast material (0.8 mL × body weight) for 12 s followed by 30 mL of 50 % contrast material diluted with saline at 2–4 mL/s using a dual-syringe injector. Alternatively, we recommend slow infusion of 100 mL contrast material to evaluate RV structure only, but this may not be a great technique when assessment of the coronary arteries is also required.

Arrhythmogenic Right Ventricular Dysplasia/Cardiomyopathy

Pathogenesis and Definition

ARVC/D is a genetic disorder of the heart muscle with autosomal dominant inheritance in most cases and genetic variations in the desmosome-binding cells [5–7]. It is characterized by fibro-fatty replacement of the RV myocardium that leads to progressive alterations in RV ventricular size and function [5]. The disease generally involves the RV but has been known to involve the LV with some frequency early in the course of the disease, manifest parallel involvement of both ventricles, and occasionally demonstrates left dominance (early and prominent LV manifestation and relatively mild RV disease) [8, 9].

Clinical Features

Symptomatic ventricular arrhythmias and sudden death are the most common manifestations of ARVC/D. Less common presentations are right ventricular or biventricular heart failure. ARVC/D is an important cause of sudden cardiac death in young people, particularly athletes [10].

Disease progression can occur at any stage of life but is more likely after adolescence. The prevalence of disease increases greatly between 15 and 20 years of age [11]. ARVC/D occurs more commonly in males than in females [12]. The disease clinical manifestations vary. In early "concealed" phase, individuals are often asymptomatic but may be at risk of sudden cardiac death. In the overt "electrical phase," individuals manifest symptomatic arrhythmia, and conventional imaging clearly depicts abnormalities in the RV morphology. Later with progression of disease and diffuse involvement of the heart, biventricular heart failure from diffuse disease leads to a phenotype that may resemble dilated cardiomyopathy [5].

Diagnosis with 2010 International Task Force Criteria

Diagnosis of ARVC/D is currently based on criteria established by an International Task Force. The original 1994 criteria enabled confirmatory clinical diagnosis of ARVC/D that was highly specific but lacked sensitivity for early stage and familial diseases. In 2010, the original criteria were modified to include major and minor criteria that encompass global or regional dysfunction and structural alterations, characterization of wall tissue, repolarization abnormalities, depolarization/conduction abnormalities, arrhythmia, and family history (Table 17.1). The revised criteria added quantitative measures, particularly for imaging studies using 2D echo, MR imaging, and angiography. Diagnosis is fulfilled by the presence of 2 major criteria, 1 major criterion plus 2 minor criteria, or 4 minor criteria from these categories [5].

Table 17.1 International Task Force criteria for ARVC/D

I. Global or regional dysfunction and structural alterations
Major criteria by MRI:
Regional RV akinesia, dyskinesia, or dyssynchronous RV contraction and 1 of the following:
Ratio of RV end-diastolic volume to BSA ≥110 mL/m² (male) or ≥100 mL/m² (female)
Or RV ejection fraction ≤40 %
Minor criteria by MRI:
Regional RV akinesia, dyskinesia, or dyssynchronous RV contraction and 1 of the following:
Ratio of RV end-diastolic volume to BSA ≥100 to <110 mL/m² (male) or ≥90 to <100 mL/m² (female)
Or RV ejection fraction >40 to ≤45 %
II. Tissue characterization of wall
Fibrous replacement of the RV free wall myocardium in ≥1 sample, with or without fatty replacement of tissue on endomyocardial biopsy, plus one of the following major or minor criteria:
Major criteria: Residual myocytes <60 % by morphometric analysis (or <50 % if estimated)
Minor criteria: Residual myocytes 60–75 % by morphometric analysis (or 50–65 % if estimated)
III. Repolarization abnormalities
IV. Depolarization/conduction abnormalities
V. Arrhythmias
VI. Family history

From Marcus et al. [5] with permission
BSA body surface area

Histologic Features

The primary histologic feature of ARVC/D is segmental or diffuse transmural loss of the RV free wall myocardium and its replacement by fibrofatty tissue. Fibrofatty replacement occurs as a wave-front phenomenon that extends from the epicardium toward the endocardium (Fig. 17.1) [13]. One revised criterion involves fibrous replacement of the myocardium with or without fatty replacement of the tissue at endomyocardial biopsy and calls for quantification of residual monocytes to determine whether this is a major or minor diagnostic consideration (Table 17.1) [5].

The myocardium is commonly affected in the so-called triangle of dysplasia, which includes the outflow tract, inflow tract (inferior wall beneath the posterior leaflet of the tricuspid valve), and apex of the RV [5]. The RV free wall becomes thin and translucent in response to myocardial loss and fibrofatty replacement (Fig. 17.1). Nearly half of cases demonstrate saccular aneurysms at the apex and inferior wall of the RV [13,

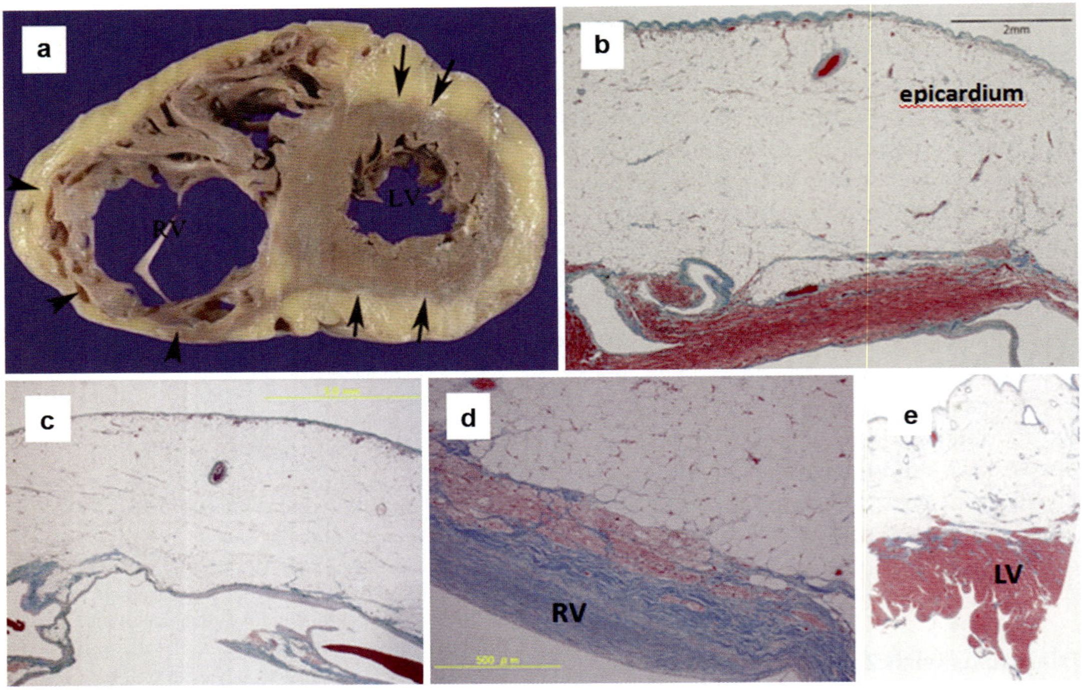

Fig. 17.1 Autopsy specimen of ARVC/D in a 67- year-old man who died of congestive heart failure. (**a**) Photograph of the cut surface of the heart shows marked thinning of the right ventricle (*RV*) free wall (*arrowheads*) with left ventricle (*LV*) involvement. (**b**, **c**) Low and (**d**) high power photomicrographs (Masson trichrome stain) of the RV lateral wall show fibrofatty myocardial replacement extending from the epicardium toward the endocardium. (**c**) Shows almost complete fibrofatty replacement of the RV myocardium. (**e**) Low power photomicrograph (Masson trichrome stain) also shows fibrofatty replacement from the epicardial side of the LV wall (From Kimura et al. [4] with permission)

14]. Histologic changes in the LV wall consist of transmural or predominantly subepicardial and mid-wall fibrofatty replacement that affects both the interventricular septum and the LV free wall either diffusely or, more often, regionally (Fig. 17.1). The wave front of the fibrofatty infiltration appears to extend from the outer to the inner layer of the LV wall, resembling the pattern of involvement of the RV free wall [15].

Imaging Findings

MR imaging findings are useful in diagnosing ARVC/D, and characteristic findings include dilatation of the RV, especially the RV outflow tract (RVOT) and part of the triangle of dysplasia in association with reduced RVEF and regional RV akinesia, dyskinesia, or aneurysm. Intramyocardial fat infiltration and thinning of the RV wall are common and usually coexist. Post-contrast images may show LGE of the RV free wall, ventricular septum, and/or LV free wall that suggests myocardial fibrosis [4–6, 8–10, 16] (Figs. 17.2, 17.3, and 17.4).

Cine MR imaging is widely used to measure RV size and EF and evaluate wall motion abnormality (Fig. 17.2). It enables diagnosis of early and subtle cases of ARVC/D by detecting regional wall motion abnormality, which is thought to precede global and systolic dysfunction during disease progression. Aneurysm of the RV free wall is also a characteristic finding on cine MR imaging, appearing as a focal outpouching of the wall. The revised criteria include qualitative and quantitative MR findings to diagnose global or regional dysfunction and structural alterations; ARVC/D diagnosis requires a combination of RV dilatation or reduced RVEF and regional wall motion abnormalities [5] (Table 17.1).

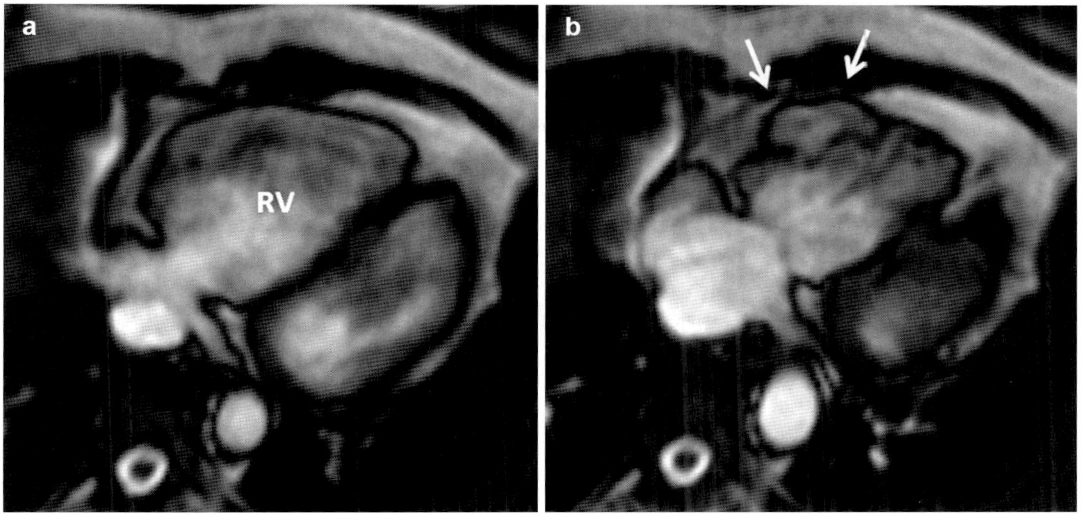

Fig. 17.2 ARVC/D according to the 2010 International Task Force criteria in a 50-year-old woman referred for evaluation of non-sustained ventricular tachycardia on Holter ECG. Cine MR imaging (**a** diastolic phase; **b** systolic phase) reveals systolic outpunching (dyskinesia) of the anterior wall of the RV (*arrows*)

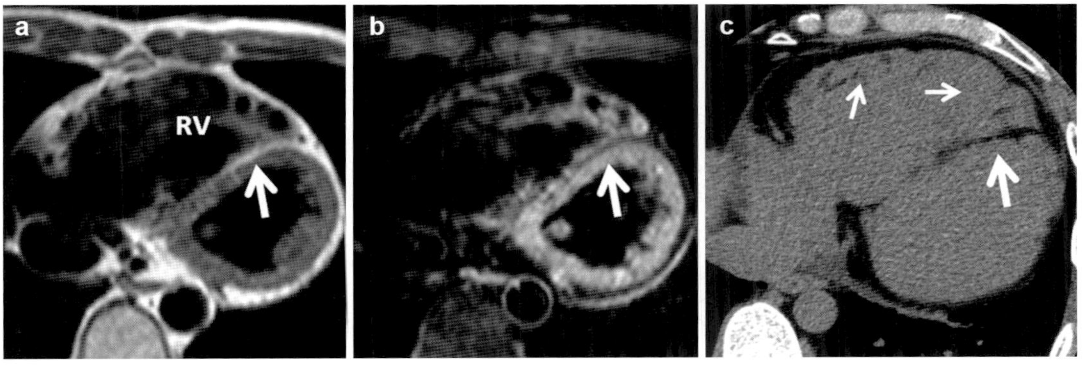

Fig. 17.3 ARVC/D according to the 2010 International Task Force criteria in a 41-year-old man referred for evaluation of congestive heart failure. Black blood MR images without (**a**) and with (**b**) fat suppression show dilatation of the right ventricle (*RV*) with a thin RV free wall and myocardial fat in the ventricular septum (*arrows*). Small amounts of fat in the RV trabeculae demonstrated on noncontrast CT (**c**) are difficult to discern on MR imaging (*small arrows*). CT also shows extensive fatty infiltration of the interventricular septum (*large arrow*) (From Kimura et al. [4] with permission)

It is important to know that the presence of RV myocardial fat is not specific to ARVC/D (Fig. 17.3) and appears to be but a common finding in elderly individuals and also in the scars of myocardium of patients with other cardiomyopathies [4]. Moreover, MR findings suggesting RV myocardial fat (high signal intensities on fast spin echo sequence) are least reproducible because of the thin RV myocardium and various artifacts related primarily to blood flow. Therefore, the Task Force does not include MR evidence of RV myocardial fat in its diagnostic criteria for ARVC/D.

MR imaging with LGE is a well-established mean of detecting myocardial fibrosis, but MR findings of myocardial fibrosis of the RV free wall (LGE) are not among the revised criteria, probably because of the limited spatial resolution of MR for detection of LGE in a thinned wall RV and scarce literature support on the utility of LGE for

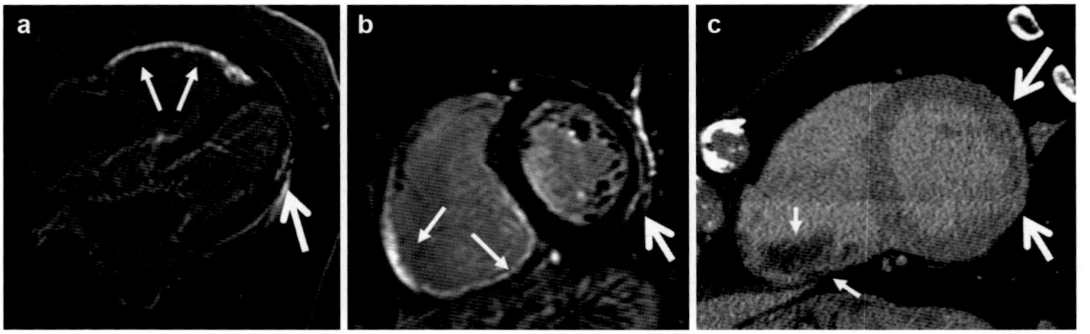

Fig. 17.4 ARVC/D according to the 2010 International Task Force criteria in a 78-year-old man referred for evaluation of syncope and non-sustained ventricular tachycardia on Holter ECG. MR images of 4-chamber (**a**) and short-axis (**b**) views show distinct LGE in the RV anterior and inferior walls (*thin arrows*) and the LV lateral wall (*thick arrow*). A delayed post-contrast short-axis CT image (**c**) also shows late enhancement of the LV lateral wall (*large arrows*), which is less distinct than the MR image. CT does not demonstrate the region of late enhancement of the RV wall. Thrombus is seen in the RV cavity (*small arrows*) (From Kimura and Nakajima [17] with permission)

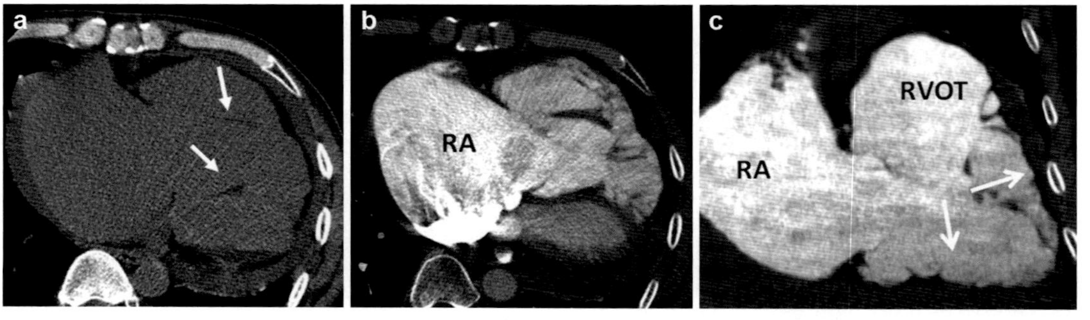

Fig. 17.5 Histologically proved ARVC/D in a 67-year-old man who died of congestive heart failure (same patient as in Fig. 17.1). Axial pre-contrast (**a**) and post-contrast (**b**) CT images and two-chamber RV image (**c**) of CT show a thin RV free wall with scalloped appearance (*arrows* in **c**) and scattered fat in the RV trabeculae and ventricular septum (*arrows* in **a**). Marked dilatation of the RV outflow tract (*RVOT*), inlet of the RV, and the right atrium (*RA*) is also shown (From Kimura et al. [4] with permission)

diagnosis of ARVC/D. We have found LGE with fat suppression and thin slice thickness (5 mm) useful in detecting myocardial fibrosis of the RV free wall (Fig. 17.4). Myocardial fibrosis (LV involvement) of the thicker LV wall is well demonstrated with LGE. LGE is most frequently seen in the subepicardial layer followed by the midwall of the LV myocardium. The anatomical locations of LGE in descending order are inferolateral wall, inferior wall-septal junction, inferior wall, septum, anterolateral wall, and anterior wall (Fig. 17.4) [8]. These anatomic distributions of LGEs correlate well with pathologic reports of ARVC/D [15].

CT images are useful in diagnosing ARVC/D, especially in patients with implantable cardioverter defibrillator. Although CT is not included in either the original or revised criteria, ACCF/SCCT/ACR/AHA/ASE/ASNC/NASCI/SCAI/SCMR 2010 appropriate use criteria for cardiac CT recognized the utility of CT in assessing RV morphology and patients with suspected ARVC/D [18]. Several characteristic CT findings of ARVC/D are reported including dilatation of the RV including outflow tract, thin RV free wall, myocardial fat in the RV trabeculae and moderator band, conspicuous trabeculae, and scalloped or bulging appearance of the RV free wall [4, 19] (Figs. 17.5 and 17.6). In our experience with CT scan in ARVC/D patients, the RV free wall is usually imperceptibly thin as

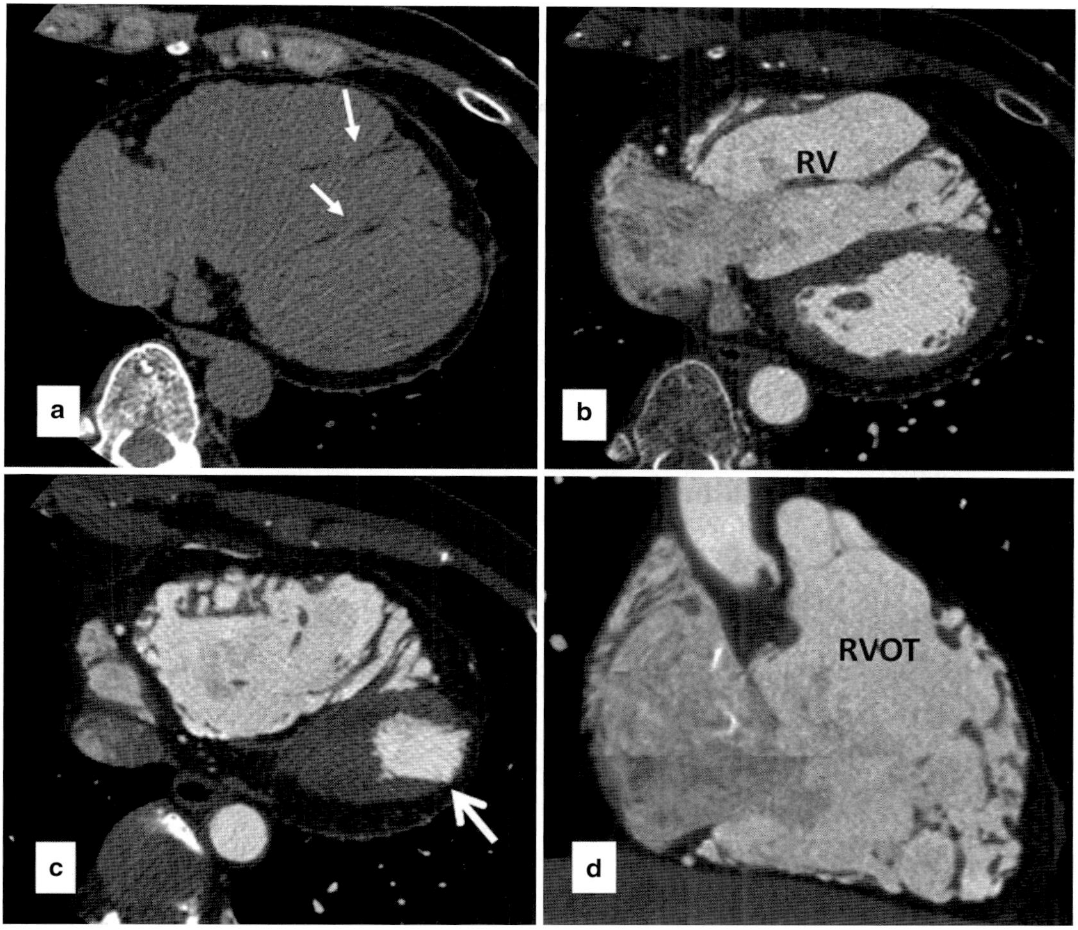

Fig. 17.6 ARVC/D according to the 2010 International Task Force criteria in a 62-year-old woman referred for evaluation of arrhythmia and RV enlargement. Pre-contrast CT (**a**) shows myocardial fat in the trabeculations and ventricular septum (*arrows*). Post-contrast axial (**b**, **c**) and RV two chamber (**d**) images show LV apical thinning (LV involvement) (*arrow*) and RV enlargement including the RV outflow tract (*RVOT*) as well as marked thinning and scalloping of the RV anterior and inferior walls (From Kimura and Nakajima [17] with permission)

a result of fibrofatty replacement extending from the epicardium toward the endocardium. On CT, fat is frequently seen in the ventricular septum, especially in the RV side of septum, and the LV involvement usually appears as areas of wedge-shaped or band-like fat deposition in the subepicardial LV free wall [4] (Figs. 17.5 and 17.6). Myocardial fat and wall thinning are more easily and precisely recognized with CT than MR imaging. The lower contrast resolution of CT compared with MR imaging limits its utility in detecting myocardial fibrosis using delayed enhancement (Fig. 17.4).

Differential Diagnosis

Several conditions that mimic ARVC/D demonstrate ventricular tachycardia of RV origin or imaging findings of RV structural abnormalities. From the clinical standpoint, RVOT tachycardia is one of the most important differential diagnoses, and cardiac sarcoidosis, idiopathic dilated cardiomyopathy, physiological myocardial fat, and Uhl's anomaly (discussed in the next section) show RV structural abnormality on CT or MR imaging and could be mistaken for ARVC/D.

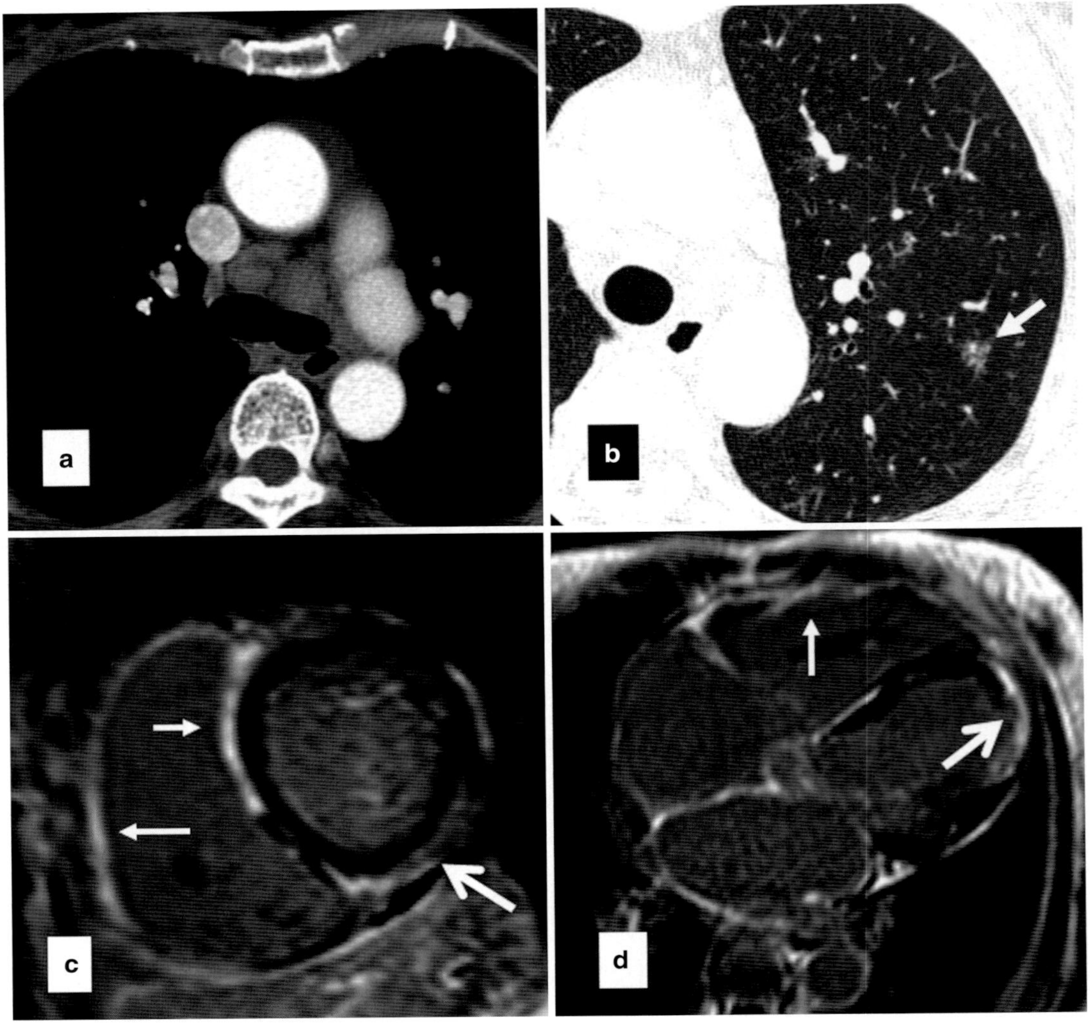

Fig. 17.7 Cardiac sarcoidosis in a 72-year-old woman referred for evaluation of palpitation and congestive heart failure. CT images of the chest (**a**, **b**) reveal mediastinal and hilar adenopathy and small nodules with perivascular distribution (*arrows* in **b**), suggesting thoracic involvement of sarcoidosis. Short-axis (**c**) and 4-chamber (**d**) MR views with fat suppression reveal intense LGE of the RV free wall contiguous from the RV side of the septum (*thin arrows* in **c** and **d**) and epicardial side of the LV (*thick arrows* in **c** and **d**)

Right Ventricular Outflow Tract Tachycardia

Differentiation of ARVD/C at its early stages from RVOT tachycardia, a usually benign and nonfamilial cardiac arrhythmia, remains clinically challenging. Reported MR findings of RVOT tachycardia vary. Tandri et al. reported that RVOT tachycardia usually shows no abnormalities in RV structure and function [20], whereas O'Donnell et al. reported minor MR imaging abnormalities in 54 % of these patients, including minute fatty infiltration and focal RV thinning without RV wall motion abnormality and RV dilatation [21].

Cardiac Sarcoidosis

RV-dominant cardiac sarcoidosis may mimic ARVC/D [22], with LGE of both the RV free wall and the RV side of basal ventricular septum, the latter a favorite site of sarcoidosis (Fig. 17.7).

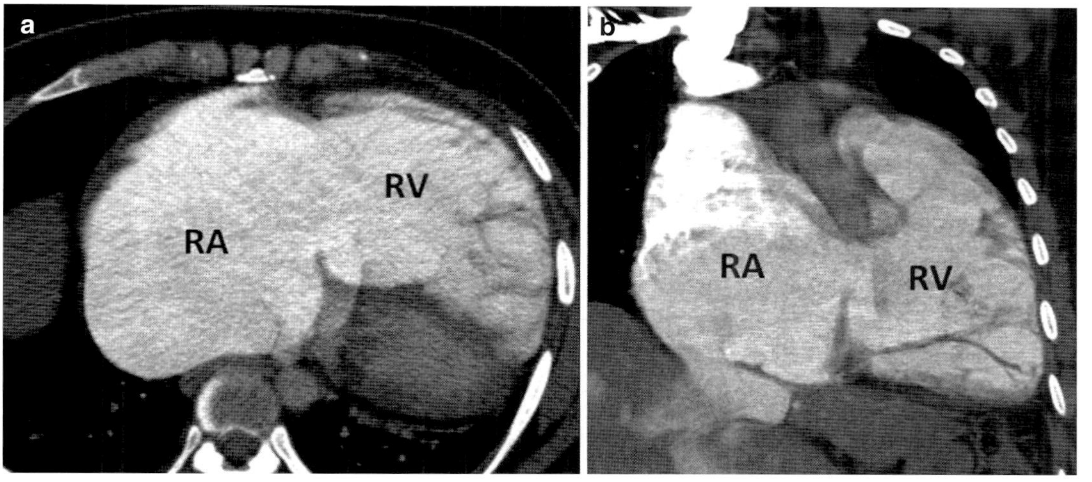

Fig. 17.8 A 38-year-old woman with right heart failure due to severe tricuspid insufficiency. Axial (**a**) and coronal (**b**) post-contrast CT images show markedly dilated thin-walled right ventricle (*RV*). The right atrium is also massively enlarged. The tricuspid valve was replaced with surgery, *RA* right atrium

Cine MR imaging shows abnormality of RV wall motion, such as regional akinesis or dyskinesis similar to that with ARVC/D. On CT, the presence of hilar and mediastinal lymphadenopathy and/or lung abnormality should alert the physician to consider sarcoidosis (Fig. 17.7). Though the presence of myocardial fat is a characteristic finding of ARVC/D, patients with sarcoidosis may also reveal myocardial fat associated with aging. Differentiation between RV-dominant sarcoidosis and ARVC/D may not be possible based on the revised ARVC/D criteria [22], and confirmation of cardiac sarcoidosis may require myocardial biopsy.

Dilated Cardiomyopathy and Valvular Causes of Right Heart Failure

Dilated cardiomyopathy (DCM) may be mistaken for ARVC/D, particularly when ARVC/D is associated with structurally advanced disease involving the LV. However, the LGE patterns of the LV wall in ARVC/D and DCM are quite different. LGE has a distinct pattern in ARVC/D involving the subepicardial myocardium of the LV inferolateral wall. In contrast, LGE pattern in DCM with myocardial scar is mostly mild in the LV midwall. Moreover, scalloping or regional dyskinesia of the RV free wall on cine MR favors diagnosis of ARVC/D. Right heart failure due to severe chronic tricuspid insufficiency may look similar to ARVD or Uhl's anomaly (Fig. 17.8).

Physiological Myocardial Fat and Adipositas Cordis (Cor Adiposum)

Physiological myocardial fat is a common and considered part of the aging process. Prevalence of 85 % is reported based on histologic analysis of patients who died of noncardiac causes [23]. It is frequently seen in the RVOT and RV free wall but sometimes involves the RV trabeculae, ventricular septum, and LV apex (Fig. 17.9) [4]. Adipositas cordis (cor adiposum) is a rare cardiomyopathy characterized by myocardial fatty infiltration of both ventricles in obese patients [24]. Pathologically, both conditions are similar and show fatty infiltration with dissociation of otherwise preserved myocardial fibers without myocardial loss and fibrosis. Adipositas cordis and physiological myocardial fat are generally considered benign, though patients with associated arrhythmias and restrictive cardiomyopathy are reported in patients with adipositas cordis [13, 24].

Differentiation between physiological fat or adipositas cordis and ARVC/D is not difficult. In ARVC/D, the RV free wall is usually

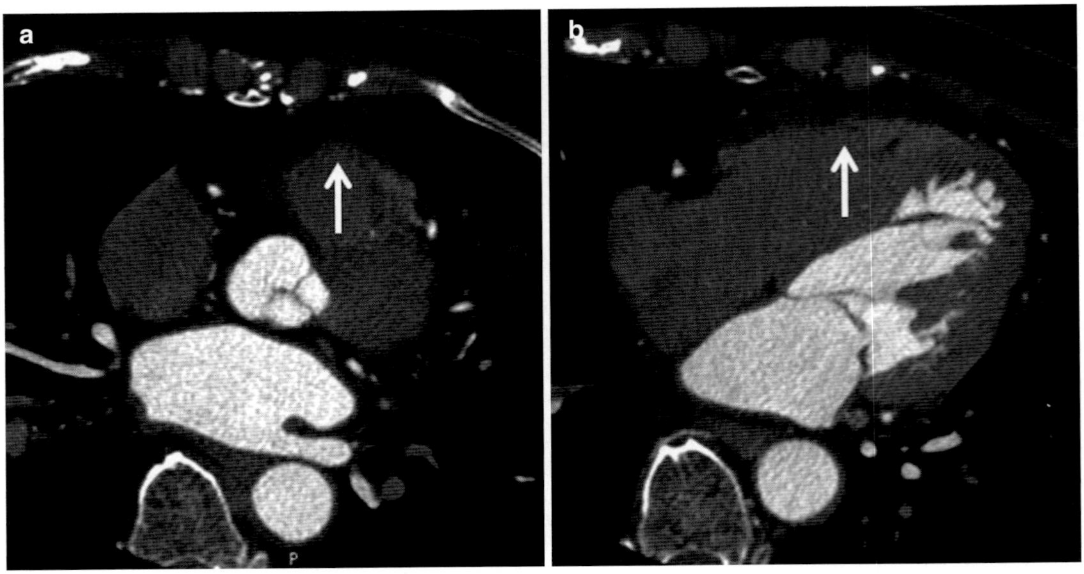

Fig. 17.9 Physiological myocardial fat in a 67-year-old woman referred for coronary artery evaluation because of chest pain. She was under medical treatment for hyperlipidemia. Axial images of contrast CT (**a**, **b**) show fatty infiltration of the RVOT (*arrow* in **a**), RV anterior wall, and trabeculation (*arrow* in **b**). Note thickening of the RVOT and RV free wall with fatty infiltration. CT also revealed no significant stenosis of the coronary arteries

almost imperceptibly thin as a result of fibrofatty replacement extending from the epicardium toward the endocardium (Figs. 17.5 and 17.6), whereas the wall maintains normal thickness or is sometimes thickened with physiological fat or adipositas cordis [4] (Fig. 17.9). The characteristic imaging findings of ARVC/D, such as RV enlargement with scalloped appearance of the RV free wall and RV wall motion abnormalities, also help differentiate patients from those with physiological fat deposition (Figs. 17.2, 17.5, and 17.6).

Uhl's Anomaly

Uhl's anomaly, another congenital abnormality of the RV, is extremely rare. It is characterized by the absence of myocardium in the RV free wall with no interposed adipose tissue or evidence of inflammatory cells or necrosis, normal tricuspid valve, and preserved septal and left ventricular myocardium [25]. The disease has been attributed to selective but unrestrained apoptosis of the right ventricular myocytes after complete cardiac development [26]. It often manifests initially with congestive heart failure, typically during infancy or childhood. Arrhythmia and conduction disturbance are not predominant features probably due to the absence of residual foci to initiate or transmit anomalous electrical activity [25]. Cardiac transplantation may be proposed when patients become refractory to medical treatment [27].

MR findings of Uhl's anomaly include an extremely dilated thin-walled RV and the absence of trabeculation (Fig. 17.10). The RV wall shows no fat infiltration. The septa, papillary muscles of the tricuspid valve, and left ventricular myocardium are intact. Cine MR images demonstrate no movement of the right ventricular wall [27].

Differentiation from ARVC/D

Uhl's anomaly is much less frequent than ARVC/D, and the median age of patients is lower [25]. ARVC/D is characterized by segmental or diffuse transmural loss of the myocardium caused by fibrofatty replacement, and trabeculation is sometimes hypertrophied,

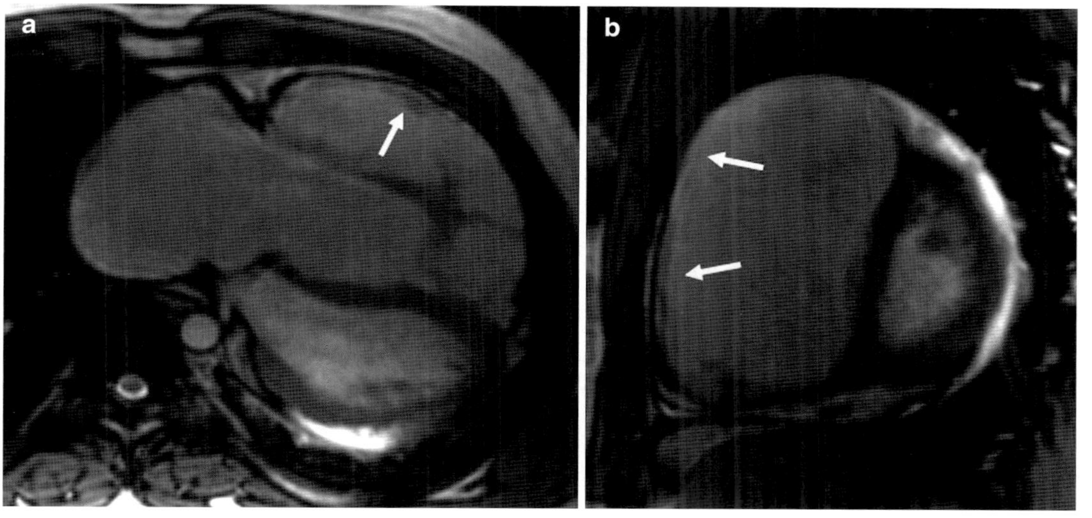

Fig. 17.10 Suspected Uhl's anomaly in a 31-year-old man admitted of RV enlargement at age 13. Cine MR images of the 4-chamber (**a**) and short-axis (**b**) views show marked dilation of the RV with thin free wall and regional absence of trabeculation (*arrows*). The ventricular septum, papillary muscles of the tricuspid valve, and left ventricle free wall appear intact. The left ventricle is normal in size (Courtesy of Dr. Masahiro Higashi, National Cerebral and Cardiovascular Center Hospital in Osaka, Japan)

whereas Uhl's anomaly shows no fibrofatty replacement and absence of trabeculation in the RV free wall. Moreover, clinical features differ between the two entities. The usual presentation of ARVC/D includes palpitation, syncope, ventricular tachycardia, heart block, or sudden death [25], while Uhl's anomaly presents with symptoms related to congestive heart failure.

Conclusion

Congenital abnormalities of the right ventricular (RV) myocardium are rare and include arrhythmogenic right ventricular cardiomyopathy/dysplasia (ARVC/D) and Uhl's anomaly. ARVC/D is a genetic heart muscle disorder characterized by enlarged thin-walled aneurysmal RV myocardium with fatty degeneration and wall motion abnormality. Uhl's anomaly is also characterized by enlarged thin-walled RV and paucity of myocardial trabeculation. Magnetic resonance (MR) imaging is commonly used to diagnose these diseases, but CT is useful in patients with implantable cardioverter defibrillator and for the assessment of myocardial fat or identifying RV free wall myocardial thinning.

References

1. Kramer CM, Barkhausen J, Flamm SD, Kim RJ, Nagel E. Standardized cardiovascular magnetic resonance imaging (CMR) protocols. Society for Cardiovascular Magnetic Resonance: Board of Trustees Task Force on Standardized Protocols. J Cardiovasc Magn Reson. 2008;10:35.
2. Fritz J, Solaiyappan M, Tandri H, et al. Right ventricle shape and contraction patterns and relation to magnetic resonance imaging findings. J Comput Assist Tomogr. 2005;29:725–33.
3. Clarke CJ, Gurka MJ, Norton PT, Kramer CM, Hoyer AW. Assessment of the accuracy and reproducibility of RV volume measurements by CMR in congenital heart disease. JACC Cardiovasc Imaging. 2012;5:28–37.
4. Kimura F, Matsuo Y, Nakajima T, et al. Myocardial fat at cardiac imaging: how can we differentiate pathologic from physiologic fatty infiltration? Radiographics. 2010;30:1587–602.
5. Marcus FI, McKenna WJ, Sherrill D, et al. Diagnosis of arrhythmogenic right ventricular cardiomyopathy/dysplasia: proposed modification of the task force criteria. Circulation. 2010;121:1533–41.
6. Sen-Chowdhry S, Prasad SK, Syrris P, et al. Cardiovascular magnetic resonance in arrhythmogenic right ventricular cardiomyopathy revisited: comparison with task force criteria and genotype. J Am Coll Cardiol. 2006;48:2132–40.
7. Sen-Chowdhry S, Syrris P, McKenna WJ. Role of genetic analysis in the management of patients

with arrhythmogenic right ventricular dysplasia/cardiomyopathy. J Am Coll Cardiol. 2007;50:1813–21.
8. Sen-Chowdhry S, Syrris P, Ward D, et al. Clinical and genetic characterization of families with arrhythmogenic right ventricular dysplasia/cardiomyopathy provides novel insights into patterns of disease expression. Circulation. 2007;115:1710–20.
9. Sen-Chowdhry S, Syrris P, Prasad SK, et al. Left-dominant arrhythmogenic cardiomyopathy: an under-recognized clinical entity. J Am Coll Cardiol. 2008;52:2175–87.
10. Tandri H, Bomma C, Calkins H, Bluemke DA. Magnetic resonance and computed tomography imaging of arrhythmogenic right ventricular dysplasia. J Magn Reson Imaging. 2004;19:848–58.
11. Nava A, Bauce B, Faliento L. Incidence and natural history. In: Nava A, Rossi L, Thiene G, editors. Arrhythmogenic right ventricular cardiomyopathy/dysplasia. Amsterdam: Elsevier; 1997. p. 17–23.
12. Marcus FI, Fontaine GH, Guiraudon G, et al. Right ventricular dysplasia: a report of 24 adult cases. Circulation. 1982;65:384–98.
13. Basso C, Thiene G. Adipositas cordis, fatty infiltration of the right ventricle, and arrhythmogenic right ventricular cardiomyopathy. Just a matter of fat? Cardiovasc Pathol. 2005;14:37–41.
14. Basso C, Corrado D, Rossi L, Thiene G. Morbid anatomy. In: Nava A, Rossi L, Thiene G, editors. Arrhythmogenic right ventricular cardiomyopathy/dysplasia. Amsterdam: Elsevier; 1997. p. 71–86.
15. Corrado D, Basso C, Thiene G, et al. Spectrum of clinicopathologic manifestations of arrhythmogenic right ventricular cardiomyopathy/dysplasia: a multicenter study. J Am Coll Cardiol. 1997;30:1512–20.
16. Tandri H, Saranathan M, Rodriguez ER, et al. Noninvasive detection of myocardial fibrosis in arrhythmogenic right ventricular cardiomyopathy using delayed-enhancement magnetic resonance imaging. J Am Coll Cardiol. 2005;45:98–103.
17. Kimura F, Nakajima T. Arrhythmogenic right ventricular cardiomyopathy/dysplasia. In: Kimura F, editor. Clinical cardiac computed tomography 12: cardiomyopathy evaluated by MDCT. Tokyo: Bunkodo Co., Ltd.; 2012. p. 47–52.
18. Taylor AJ, Cerqueira M, Hodgson JM, et al. ACCF/SCCT/ACR/AHA/ASE/ASNC/NASCI/SCAI/SCMR 2010 appropriate use criteria for cardiac computed tomography. A report of the American College of Cardiology Foundation Appropriate Use Criteria Task Force, the Society of Cardiovascular Computed Tomography, the American College of Radiology, the American Heart Association, the American Society of Echocardiography, the American Society of Nuclear Cardiology, the North American Society for Cardiovascular Imaging, the Society for Cardiovascular Angiography and Interventions, and the Society for Cardiovascular Magnetic Resonance. J Am Coll Cardiol. 2010;56:1864–94.
19. Hamada S, Takamiya M, Ohe T, Ueda H. Arrhythmogenic right ventricular dysplasia: evaluation with electron-beam CT. Radiology. 1993;187:723–7.
20. Tandri H, Bluemke DA, Ferrari VA, et al. Findings on magnetic resonance imaging of idiopathic right ventricular outflow tachycardia. Am J Cardiol. 2004;94:1441–5.
21. O'Donnell D, Cox D, Bourke J, Mitchell L, Furniss S. Clinical and electrophysiological differences between patients with arrhythmogenic right ventricular dysplasia and right ventricular outflow tract tachycardia. Eur Heart J. 2003;24:801–10.
22. Mohsen A, Panday M, Wetherold S, Jimenez A. Cardiac sarcoidosis mimicking arrhythmogenic right ventricular dysplasia with high defibrillation threshold requiring subcutaneous shocking coil implantation. Heart Lung Circ. 2012;21:46–9.
23. Lorin de la Grandmaison G, Le Bihan C, Durigon M. Assessment of right ventricular lipomatosis by histomorphometry in control adult autopsy cases. Int J Legal Med. 2001;115:105–8.
24. Rowin EJ, Yucel KE, Salomon R, Maron MS. Adipositas cordis: an uncommon cardiomyopathy identified by cardiovascular magnetic resonance. Circulation. 2010;122:2212–4.
25. Gerlis L. Uhl's anomaly. Orphanet encyclopedia. 2003. http://www.orpha.net/data/patho/GB/uk-uhl.pdf.
26. Greer ML, MacDonald C, Adatia I. MRI of Uhl's anomaly. Circulation. 2000;101:e230–2.
27. Otmani A, Leborgne L, Renard C, et al. Electrocardiogram, echocardiography, and magnetic resonance imaging characteristics in Uhl's disease. Circulation. 2007;115:e11–2.

CT in Pediatric Congenital Heart Disease

18

Hyun Woo Goo

Congenital heart disease includes an extremely diverse spectrum of congenitally malformed hearts leading to a variety of different hemodynamic consequences. The disease is often associated with anomalies of great vessels and airways and infrequently with those of other systems. Although the evaluation of simple defects, such as atrial septal defect (ASD) and ventricular septal defect (VSD), can be usually completed with echocardiography, supplementary imaging studies, such as computed tomography (CT), magnetic resonance imaging (MRI), and cardiac catheterization, are often required for the accurate diagnosis and optimal treatment of more complex defects. Among those supplementary imaging studies, the role of CT has greatly increased, thanks to recent technical evolutions [1–8].

In this chapter, scan techniques, radiation dose reduction techniques, and clinical applications of pediatric cardiac CT for congenital heart disease are comprehensively reviewed. Up-to-date knowledge and information on these topics, such as intracardiac, four-dimensional airway, and dual-energy evaluations, are included to provide radiologists, technologists, cardiologists, and cardiac surgeons with the contemporary status of pediatric cardiac CT.

H.W. Goo, MD
Department of Radiology and Research Institute of Radiology, Asan Medical Center, University of Ulsan College of Medicine, 88, Olympic-ro 43-gil, Songpa-gu, Seoul 138-736, South Korea
e-mail: hwgoo@amc.seoul.kr

Scan Techniques

Recent technical evolutions in cardiac CT can be summarized into longer z-axis coverage, faster gantry rotation speed, higher pitch, ECG-synchronized scanning, and various dose reduction techniques. Dose reduction techniques are described in a separate section. Because most corrective surgeries for congenital heart disease are undertaken early in their life, CT scan techniques should be adapted to free-breathing young children with high heart rates [5, 6]. Optimal scan techniques also may differ according to whether controlled ventilation with or without general anesthesia is available for cardiac CT. In addition, in setting up CT protocols, imagers should carefully consider which structures have to be included in the evaluation (Table 18.1).

Conventional non-ECG-synchronized spiral scanning has been used to evaluate extracardiac vascular and airway abnormalities of pediatric congenital heart disease [1–8]. Recently introduced high-pitch (up to 3.0–3.4; table feed, 41.1–46.6 cm/s) dual-source spiral scanning allows considerable reduction of cardiac and respiratory motion artifacts on non-ECG-synchronized cardiac CT [9, 10]. Nonetheless, ECG-synchronized scanning with either retrospective ECG gating or prospective ECG triggering should be performed for the evaluation of intracardiac structures and coronary arteries (Fig. 18.1). This has been proven by improved coronary artery visibility on ECG-synchronized cardiac CT in children with congenital heart disease [11–15]. ECG-synchronized

F. Saremi (ed.), *Cardiac CT and MR for Adult Congenital Heart Disease*,
DOI 10.1007/978-1-4614-8875-0_18, © Springer Science+Business Media New York 2014

Table 18.1 CT scan techniques for pediatric congenital heart disease according to target structures and a child's respiration status

Target structures	Scan mode	Respiration status
Extracardiac structures only	Non-ECG-synchronized spiral	Free breathing or breath holding
Intracardiac structures and coronary arteries	Prospectively ECG-triggered sequential	Free breathing (with or without respiratory triggering)
	Retrospectively ECG-gated spiral	Breath holding, controlled ventilation with or without general anesthesia, or free breathing (young children)
Dynamic evaluation of airways	Four-dimensional sequential (supplementary)	Free breathing
Regional lung perfusion (iodine) and ventilation (xenon)	Dual-energy spiral	Free breathing or breath holding

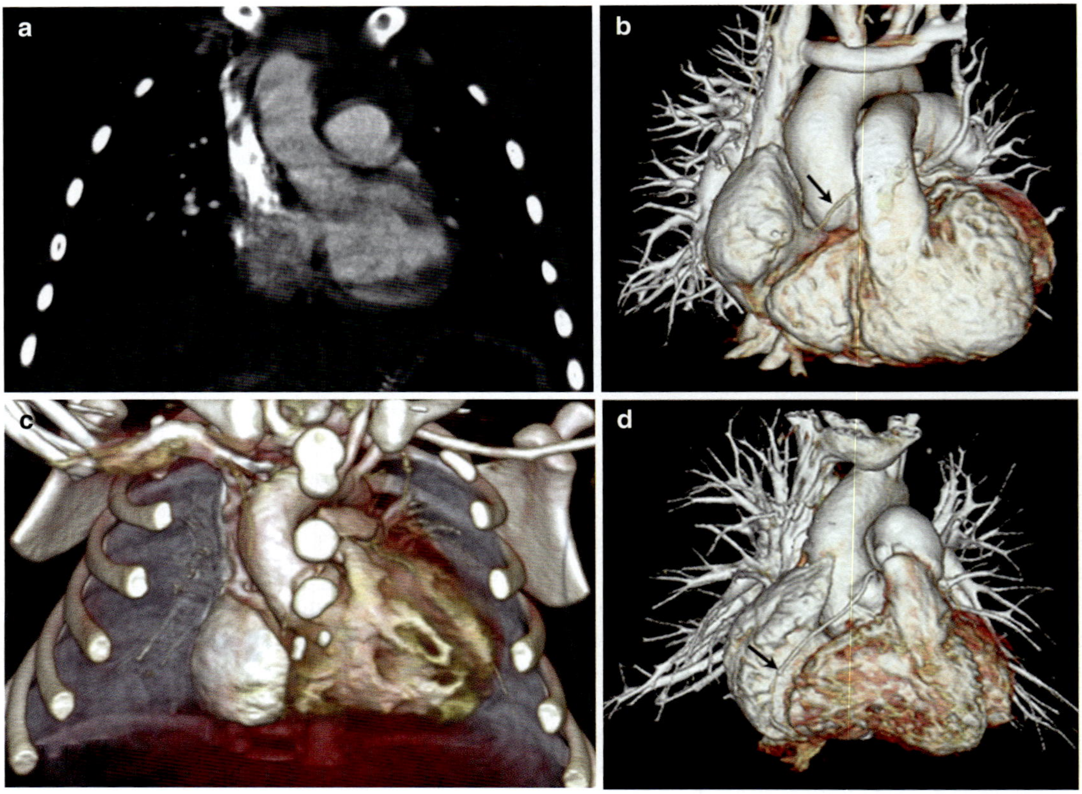

Fig. 18.1 CT scan techniques for pediatric congenital heart disease. (**a**) Coronal CT image acquired with breath-hold single-source non-ECG-synchronized spiral scanning in a 5-year-old girl shows cardiac pulsation artifacts. (**b**) Volume-rendered CT image acquired with free-breathing dual-source high-pitch non-ECG-synchronized spiral scanning in a 6-year-old girl reveals no discernible cardiac and respiratory motion artifacts. The right coronary artery (*arrow*) is faintly seen. (**c**) Volume-rendered CT image acquired with free-breathing dual-source prospectively ECG-triggered sequential scanning in a 2-day-old male newborn shows excellent image quality without cardiac and respiratory motion artifacts. (**d**) Volume-rendered CT image acquired with breath-hold dual-source retrospectively ECG-gated spiral scanning shows excellent image quality without cardiac and respiratory motion artifacts. The right coronary artery is clearly shown (*arrow*)

cardiac CT also allows more accurate identification and more detailed characterization of intracardiac abnormalities, e.g., potentially life-threatening coronary sinus ostial atresia with a persistent left superior vena cava (SVC) that has not been detected on cardiac CT [16].

The best cardiac phase with minimal cardiac motion should be selected for ECG-synchronized CT scanning [5, 6]. The mid-diastolic phase, the so-called diastasis, is chosen at low heart rates, while the end-systolic phase generally offers the best image quality at high heart rates (i.e., >75 beats/min). This heart rate-dependent best cardiac phase is attributed to the fact that the diastasis is decreased and eventually disappeared with increasing heart rate, and the end-systolic cardiac rest period tends to remain constant irrespective of heart rate. Single cardiac phase is usually sufficient for the morphologic evaluation, while multiphase scanning may be necessary for the accurate assessment of ventricular function, ventricular volumes, and coronary arteries at the expense of higher radiation dose.

High temporal resolution is beneficial for ECG-synchronized pediatric cardiac CT because most children have high heart rates. Currently, there are technical limitations to improve temporal resolution by increasing gantry rotation speed (0.27–0.35 s for single-source CT, 0.28–0.33 s for dual-source CT) and pitch. High gravitational (g) forces associated with fast gantry rotation speed (e.g., 17 g for 0.42 s rotation time, 33 g for 0.33 s rotation time) are close to a current mechanical upper limit. It is attributed to the fact that the g force is inversely proportional to the square of gantry rotation time. Theoretically, there are certain limits in increasing pitch in order to obtain gapless image data. In this respect, heart rate-dependent pitch, if available, is more beneficial than fixed low pitch. The highest temporal resolution, 75–83 ms, of ECG-synchronized scan is currently achieved with dual-source CT because only a quarter of gantry rotation is required for image reconstruction [9]. In contrast, at least a half of gantry rotation is needed for image reconstruction of ECG-synchronized scan using a single-source CT system.

Cine CT has been used to evaluate tracheobronchomalacia [17], air trapping [18], and subtle lung parenchymal abnormalities simply by reducing motion artifacts [19] in free-breathing children. With a longer longitudinal coverage of modern multi-detector row CT (MDCT) (4–16 cm for 64–320 detector rows), four-dimensional (4D) airway CT is increasingly used in clinical practice [5, 6, 20]. This 4D airway CT can overcome diagnostic pitfalls of conventional cine CT resulting from longitudinal motion of the airways and oblique course of the bronchi. In general, expiratory airway collapse greater than 50 % has been regarded as a diagnostic criterion of tracheobronchomalacia in children. A new diagnostic criterion, e.g., expiratory tracheal collapse of approximately 31–32 % in a study [17], and a quantitative analysis method should be developed for free-breathing children (Fig. 18.2).

Dual-energy CT is a recently highlighted scan mode acquired at two different tube voltages for material differentiation, e.g., iodine for perfusion and xenon for ventilation that is not readily seen on conventional single-energy CT [21]. Regional lung perfusion and ventilation can be assessed with dual-energy CT [22–27]. In children with congenital heart disease, dual-energy CT may be used for initial identification and follow-up of pulmonary embolism [22, 28] (Fig. 18.3) and for evaluation of airway anomalies or diseases. Radiation dose of dual-energy CT using a dual-source system is comparable to that of single-energy CT [21], whereas dual-energy CT using a single-source system with rapid tube voltage switching delivers substantially higher radiation dose [29]. The difference in radiation dose between the two dual-energy CT techniques should be cautiously considered in children.

Radiation Dose Reduction Strategies

To pursue the principle of as low as reasonably achievable in children, radiation dose of cardiac CT should be optimally minimized without compromising diagnostic image quality. In fact, submillisievert cardiac CT examination can be achieved by using available dose reduction strategies collectively, including body size-adapted dose settings, attenuation-based tube current modulation, optimally low tube voltage, ECG-controlled tube current modulation, minimal longitudinal coverage, and an iterative reconstruction algorithm [5, 6, 13, 15, 30].

First of all, radiation dose settings should be adjusted to individual body size. Body weight,

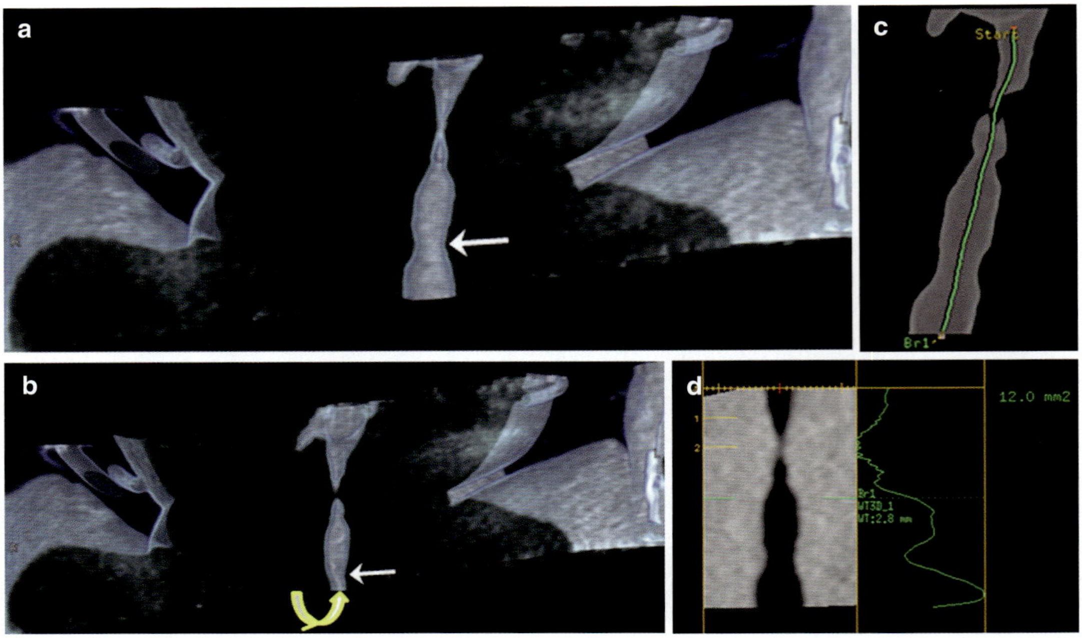

Fig. 18.2 Four-dimensional airway CT. Inspiratory (**a**) and expiratory (**b**) coronal volume-rendered CT images demonstrate a mild subglottic stenosis (*arrow*) and tracheomalacia (*curved arrow*). (**c**) The airway central axis (*green line*) is semiautomatically traced for quantitative analysis. (**d**) The cross-sectional areas of the airways were automatically measured along the airway central axis, which is mandatory for quantitative assessment of airway abnormalities, such as tracheobronchomalacia

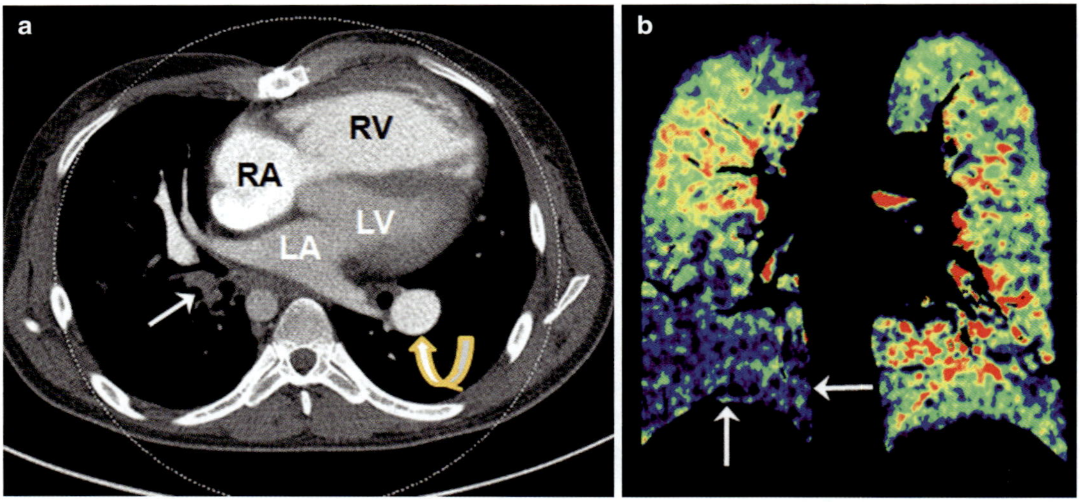

Fig. 18.3 Dual-energy CT for evaluating pulmonary embolism and lung perfusion. (**a**) Axial weighted average CT image in a 22-year-old man with repaired tetralogy of Fallot and recurrent pulmonary valve endocarditis shows obstructing pulmonary embolism (*arrow*) in the right lower lobe. The right ventricle (*RV*) appears enlarged and hypertrophic. A patent and dilated left pulmonary artery branch (*curved arrow*) is noted. (**b**) Coronal color-coded iodine map reveals a large perfusion defect in the right lower lobe (*arrows*). *RA* right atrium, *LA* left atrium, *LV* left ventricle

body mass index, cross-sectional dimensions, and mean body density can be used to develop a body size-adapted cardiac CT protocol [31–33]. In general, cross-sectional dimensions, such as body diameter and area, show better dose adaptation to body habitus than traditionally used body weight and body mass index do.

Tube current modulation should be used to reduce radiation dose of cardiac CT without degrading image quality [5, 6, 30–34]. It may be classified into angular, z-axis, and combined types according to modulation direction. For its proper use, we first need to understand that basic principles differ between vendors [35]. In a study [34], radiation dose of pediatric cardiac CT could be reduced by 9 ~ 26 % by using combined tube current modulation. The degree of dose reduction is influenced by tube voltage and scan direction [36]. More importantly, we must ensure patient positioning in the gantry isocenter to avoid adverse effects of improper positioning. We also should clearly recognize that tube current modulation is not truly automatic and it needs user-defined target image quality.

Low tube voltage provides not only potential for radiation dose reduction but also higher contrast-to-noise ratio of cardiac CT [30, 37]. Depending on body size and scan technique, 80 or 100 kV has been used for pediatric cardiac CT to have the benefits of low tube voltage. Additionally, 70 kV recently became available for pediatric cardiac CT. However, it should be noted that tube current saturation is more frequently reached during tube current modulation at low tube voltage, which limits the dose-reducing effect of tube current modulation [6, 30]. The use of lower pitch is a practical solution to this problem. In this respect, we have to ensure that low tube voltage for cardiac CT is truly dose efficient and optimal.

ECG-controlled tube current modulation or ECG pulsing is a useful dose-saving technique for retrospectively ECG-gated spiral CT scanning, in which the full dose is applied to the target cardiac phase and 4 or 20 % of the full dose is applied to the rest of the cardiac cycle [5, 6, 38]. Heart rate-adapted pitch may further reduce radiation dose with increasing heart rate [39]. In contrast, prospectively ECG-triggered sequential scanning is an intrinsically low-dose imaging technique [5, 6, 15].

Although required scan range of cardiac CT is quite variable according to clinical requests, it should be kept to the minimum. Overranging, i.e., unnecessary radiation exposure outside a scan range of multi-slice spiral CT, is directly proportional to beam collimation, reconstructed slice thickness, and pitch [40]. Because this overranging has a great impact on total radiation dose in pediatric cardiac CT, it should be reduced by using the adaptive collimation technology [41]. However, this adaptive collimation technology is not available for high-pitch dual-source spiral CT scanning, resulting in a greater radiation exposure. Therefore, this high-pitch scanning should be used only when the favorable risk-benefit ratio is expected.

Recently introduced iterative reconstruction algorithms have potential to reduce radiation dose of pediatric cardiac CT compared with conventional filtered back projection algorithms [42, 43]. Typical dose estimates of dose-optimized pediatric cardiac CT are below 1 mSv for single-source non-ECG-synchronized spiral scanning and prospectively ECG-triggered sequential scanning, 1–3 mSv for high-pitch dual-source spiral scanning, and 2–6 mSv for retrospectively ECG-gated spiral scanning in our institution. However, comprehensive single- or multicenter studies on radiation dose of pediatric cardiac CT are necessary to determine the current risk level of dose-optimized pediatric cardiac CT.

Clinical Applications

Recent technical innovations of cardiac CT expand clinical applications in patients with congenital heart disease. In addition to traditional applications including the evaluation of extracardiac great vessels, airways, and lungs, newer applications include the assessment of coronary arteries, conotruncal structures, intracardiac structures, cardiac function, ventricle volumetry, dynamic airway obstruction, and regional lung perfusion [44].

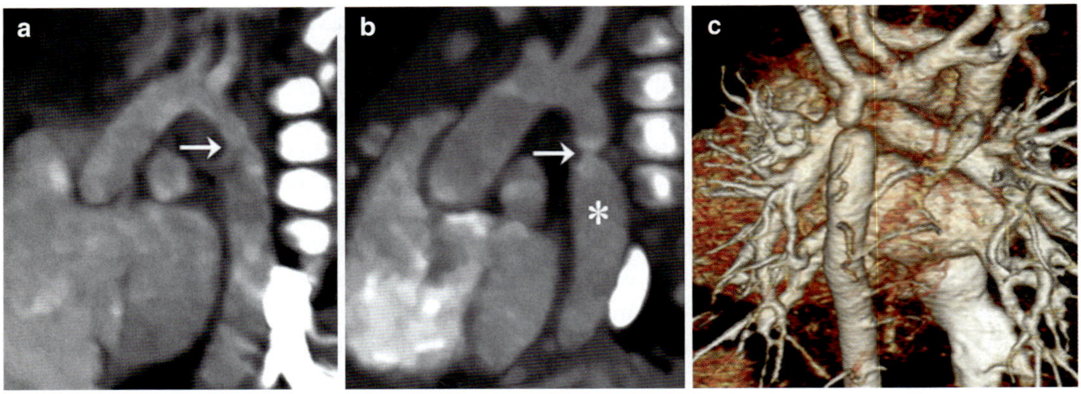

Fig. 18.4 Coarctation of the aorta. (**a**) CT image with an aortic arch view shows hypoplasia of distal arch and a minimal periductal stenosis (*arrow*). (**b**) Follow-up CT image demonstrates the development of a significant discrete narrowing (*arrow*) at the periductal area. The post-stenotic dilatation of the proximal descending thoracic aorta (*asterisk*) is noted. (**c**) Volume-rendered CT image with a posterior view reveals multiple collateral arteries connecting to the descending aorta, indicating significant aortic flow obstruction due to the coarctation of the aorta

Aorta

Anomalies of the aorta commonly include obstructive lesions in the aortic arch, such as coarctation of the aorta (CoA), interrupted aortic arch (IAA), and aortic arch atresia [45, 46]. In CoA, CT can avoid diagnostic pitfalls of echocardiography resulting from geometric distortion caused by a large patent ductus arteriosus (PDA). Because a periductal aortic stenosis in CoA is a dynamic process, monitoring of blood pressure difference between upper and lower extremities and echocardiographic follow-up are necessary although a patient is initially asymptomatic without a definite evidence of CoA. If there are equivocal findings on echocardiography, cardiac CT can provide the accurate diagnosis of CoA (Fig. 18.4). The presence of collateral arteries indicates long-standing, severe CoA, and these collateral arteries can be seen on cardiac CT as early as 3 months of age (Fig. 18.4). In CoA, the affected aortic arch may show various degrees of hypoplasia and elongation that may lead to modified surgical techniques to develop optimal geometry of the aortic arch and avoid postoperative left main bronchus narrowing.

Pseudocoarctation is characterized by tortuous elongation of a higher aortic arch without hemodynamically significant obstruction. In some cases showing pseudocoarctation on cardiac CT, cardiac catheterization may be necessary to exclude hemodynamically significant obstruction. Various degrees of progressive aneurysmal dilation of the aorta are shown in children with congenital connective tissue disorders, such as Marfan syndrome, Loeys-Dietz syndrome, and arterial tortuosity syndrome [47–49]. Cardiac CT can be used to detect and monitor cardiovascular complications in these connective tissue disorders (Fig. 18.5).

Among various types of aortic arch anomalies, common symptomatic vascular rings include double aortic arch and right aortic arch with an aberrant left subclavian artery (with or without Kommerell diverticulum) [50]. The arch anatomy and tracheal and esophageal compression can be accurately depicted on cardiac CT [51, 52]. The presence of the posterior ligamentum arteriosum contralateral to the aortic arch is closely related to the formation of vascular rings. However, the ligamentum arteriosum is not discernible on imaging. In this respect, the ligamentum arteriosum calcification, if detected, may be helpful to determine its location on cardiac CT [53]. Tracheomalacia may be complicated with these vascular rings before and more frequently after surgery [54–56]. Circumflex retroesophageal aorta makes surgical correction of aortic arch anomalies more difficult [57, 58] (Fig. 18.6).

In addition to the aortic arch, aortic stenosis may occur at supravalvular and valvular levels.

Supravalvular aortic stenosis, defined as a focal or diffuse narrowing of the aorta starting at the sinotubular junction, is commonly associated with Williams syndrome or may occur in nonsyndromic forms [59, 60]. Bicuspid aortic valve is seen in 3–8 % of patients with congenital heart disease and often associated with aortic stenosis and arteriopathy showing progressive dilation of the proximal aorta even in the absence of significant aortic stenosis [61]. In patients with aortic stenosis, cardiac CT may show anatomic features of valvular stenosis by planimetry, left ventricular hypertrophy, and dilation of the proximal aorta.

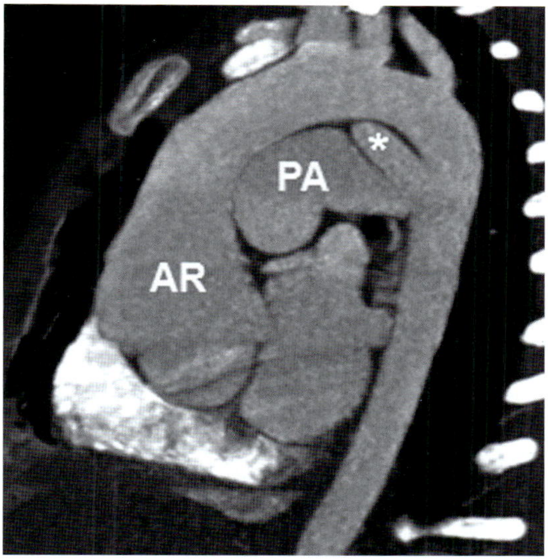

Fig. 18.5 A 2-year-old girl with Loeys-Dietz syndrome. CT image with an aortic arch view shows aortic root dilatation and annuloectasia. Other arteries, including the pulmonary arteries and aortic arch vessels, also show diffuse dilation. A patent ductus arteriosus (*asterisk*) is noted. *AR* aortic root, *PA* pulmonary artery

Pulmonary Artery

Obstructive pulmonary artery abnormalities, such as hypoplasia, stenosis, and atresia, can be shown on cardiac CT. These abnormalities are universally seen in patients with tetralogy of Fallot (TOF)/pulmonary atresia spectrum [62–64]. Juxtaductal left pulmonary artery stenosis often results in asymmetrically reduced left pulmonary vascularity on cardiac CT. Peripheral pulmonary artery stenosis is frequently seen in patients with Williams and Alagille syndromes [65, 66] (Fig. 18.7). In order to restrict pulmonary blood overflow resulting in pulmonary vascular disease, pulmonary artery banding is placed most commonly at the main pulmonary artery or at the branch pulmonary artery bilaterally as a hybrid procedure for

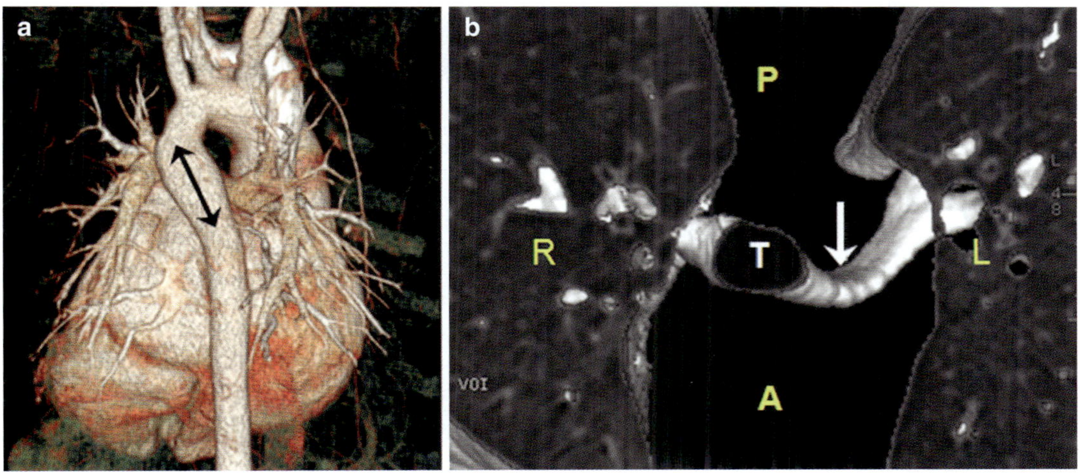

Fig. 18.6 Circumflex retroesophageal aorta. (**a**) Volume-rendered CT image with a posterior view shows the left aortic arch, a retroesophageal aortic segment (*arrow*), and the right-descending aorta. (**b**) Three-dimensional lung and airway CT image with a superior view reveals a left main bronchus narrowing (*arrow*) compressed by the aortic anomaly. *T* trachea, *A* anterior, *P* posterior, *R* right, *L* left

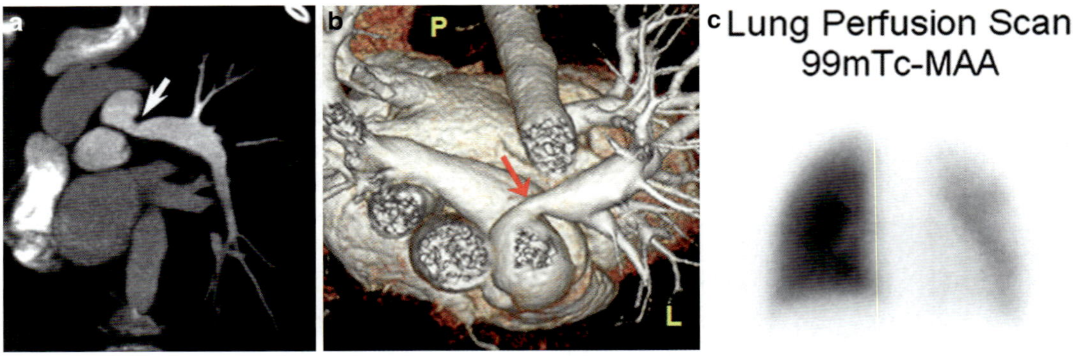

Fig. 18.7 A 7-year-old body with Alagille syndrome. Oblique coronal (**a**) and superior volume-rendered (**b**) CT views show a proximal left pulmonary artery stenosis (*arrow*). (**c**) Lung perfusion scintigraphy confirms diffusely decreased left-lung perfusion (25 % of total lung perfusion). *P* posterior, *L* left

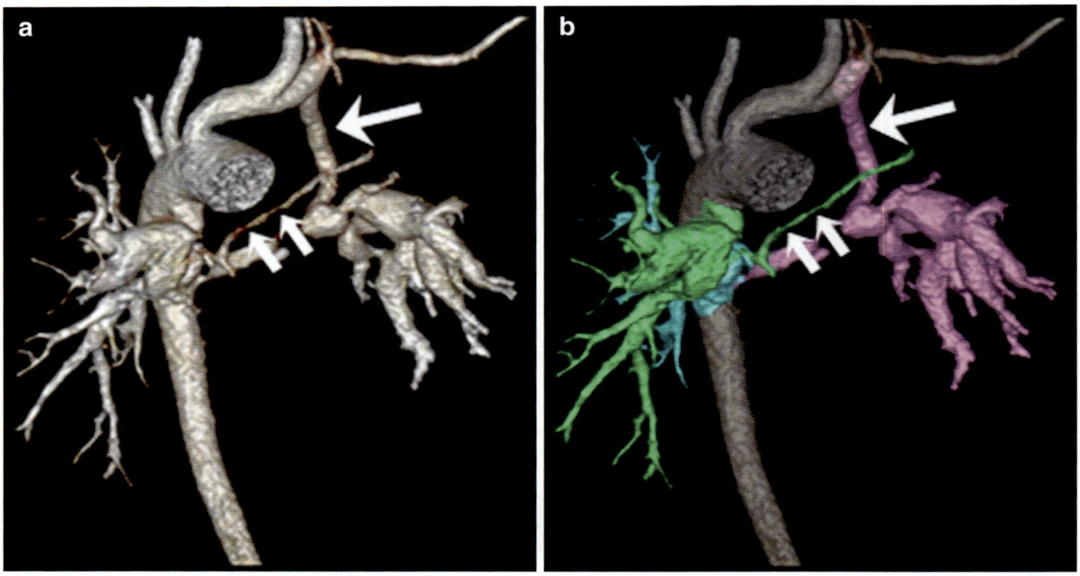

Fig. 18.8 Pulmonary atresia with major aortopulmonary collateral arteries (MAPCAs). (**a**) Volume-rendered CT image with an anterior view shows anatomic details of the tiny central pulmonary arteries (*short arrows*) and MAPCAs. A left modified Blalock-Taussig (LMBT) shunt (*long arrow*) is noted. (**b**) Color-coded volume-rendered image demonstrates three MAPCAs with different colors (*green*, *light blue*, and *purple*). The tiny central pulmonary arteries (*short arrows*) are connected to a green-colored MAPCA and a LMBT shunt (*long arrow*) is connected to a *purple-colored* MAPCA

hypoplastic left heart syndrome. Complications of this procedure, such as pulmonary artery stenosis resulting from impingement, distal migration, or scarring of the banding site and pulmonary artery pseudoaneurysm, can be identified on cardiac CT.

In pulmonary atresia, the systemic arterial source of pulmonary circulation may be single or multifocal, including a PDA or major aortopulmonary collateral arteries (MAPCAs). Anatomic details of the central pulmonary arteries and various systemic arterial sources, crucial for surgical planning of unifocalization, can be delineated on cardiac CT [67] (Fig. 18.8). Thanks to such CT road map of MAPCAs, procedure time of catheter angiography and possibility of overlooked MAPCAs can be substantially reduced. Nonetheless, conventional catheter angiography is necessary for identifying communications between pulmonary arterial feeders.

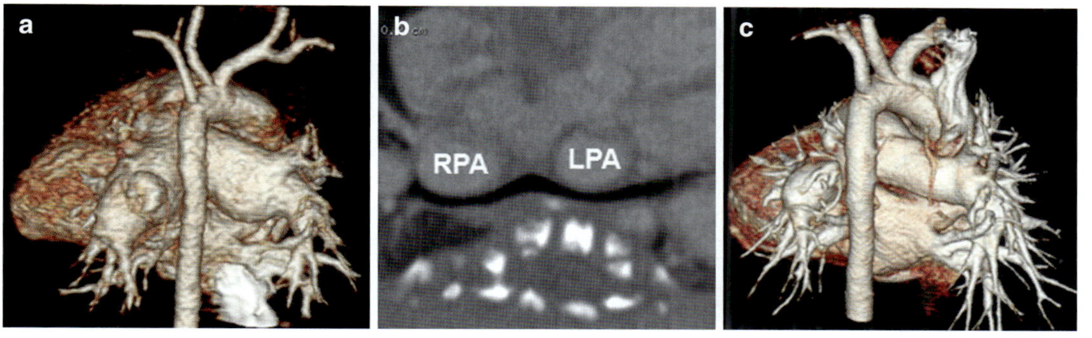

Fig. 18.9 Absent pulmonary valve syndrome. (**a**) Volume-rendered CT image with a posterior view shows aneurysmal dilatation of central pulmonary arteries. (**b**) Curved planar reformatted CT image along the bronchi demonstrates bilateral bronchial compressions by dilated central pulmonary arteries. (**c**) Volume-rendered CT image with a posterior view shows substantial decrease in size of dilated central pulmonary arteries after reduction pulmonary arterioplasty. *RPA* right pulmonary artery, *LPA* left pulmonary artery

Dilatation of the pulmonary arteries is commonly seen in patients with repaired TOF and absent pulmonary valve syndrome as a result of long-standing pulmonary regurgitation, or in patients with pulmonary arterial hypertension. In absent pulmonary valve syndrome, bronchial compression by severely enlarged central pulmonary arteries usually results in respiratory difficulties necessitating surgical treatments, such as reduction pulmonary arterioplasty [68, 69] (Fig. 18.9). Lung perfusion defects may be identified on dual-energy CT in patients with pulmonary arterial hypertension and pulmonary embolism [22, 70, 71].

In pulmonary artery sling, an aberrant left pulmonary artery arises from the proximal right pulmonary artery, courses between the trachea and the esophagus, and extends to the left pulmonary hilum. In addition to this anomalous course of the left pulmonary artery, cardiac CT can show associated airway anomalies, such as tracheal bronchus, bridging bronchus, congenital tracheal stenosis, and tracheomalacia [72–75]. Rarely, one of the two pulmonary arteries arises aberrantly from the ascending aorta and the other arises normally from the main pulmonary artery. Anomalous origin of the right pulmonary artery is far more frequent than the left one.

Pulmonary Vein

A part of (partial anomalous pulmonary venous return, PAPVR) or all (total anomalous pulmonary venous return, TAPVR) pulmonary veins may show anomalous drainage into a systemic vein, the right atrium, the coronary sinus, or the portal vein [76–79]. Exact sites of drainage and obstruction in TAPVR or PAPVR should be accurately identified before surgery, which can be better demonstrated on cardiac CT than on echocardiography (Figs. 18.10 and 18.11). TAPVR is classified as supracardiac (50 %), cardiac (25 %), infracardiac (20 %), or mixed (5 %) type according to anomalous drain sites. Infracardiac type is almost always obstructive due to an extrinsic narrowing by the diaphragm or pulmonary venous drainage through the hepatic sinusoids. Right-sided PAPVR is frequently associated with the sinus venous type of ASD [80] (Fig. 18.11). In addition, PAPVR is a component of scimitar syndrome and horseshoe lung is rarely associated with scimitar syndrome [81, 82].

Congenital pulmonary vein stenosis and hypoplasia/atresia may involve individual or multiple pulmonary veins [77]. The abnormalities may be focal or diffuse and unilateral or bilateral. Anatomic details of these abnormalities can be more accurately and promptly evaluated with cardiac CT than with echocardiography, and cardiac CT is, therefore, a viable alternative for invasive conventional catheter pulmonary venography [83, 84].

Systemic Vein

Persistent left SVC is frequently seen in patients with congenital heart disease [85]. A small or

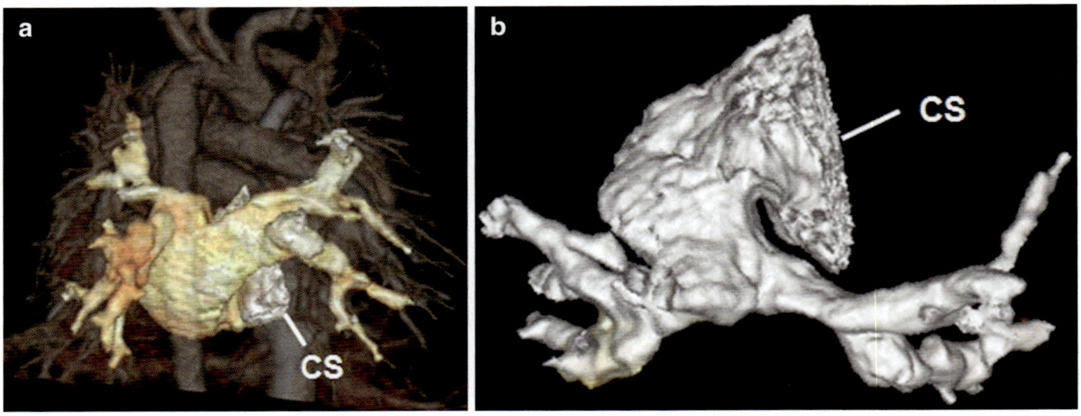

Fig. 18.10 Total anomalous pulmonary venous return (TAPVR). Volume-rendered CT image with a posterior view (**a**) and an inferior view (**b**) shows a cardiac type of TAPVR in which all pulmonary veins anomalously drain into the dilated coronary sinus (*CS*)

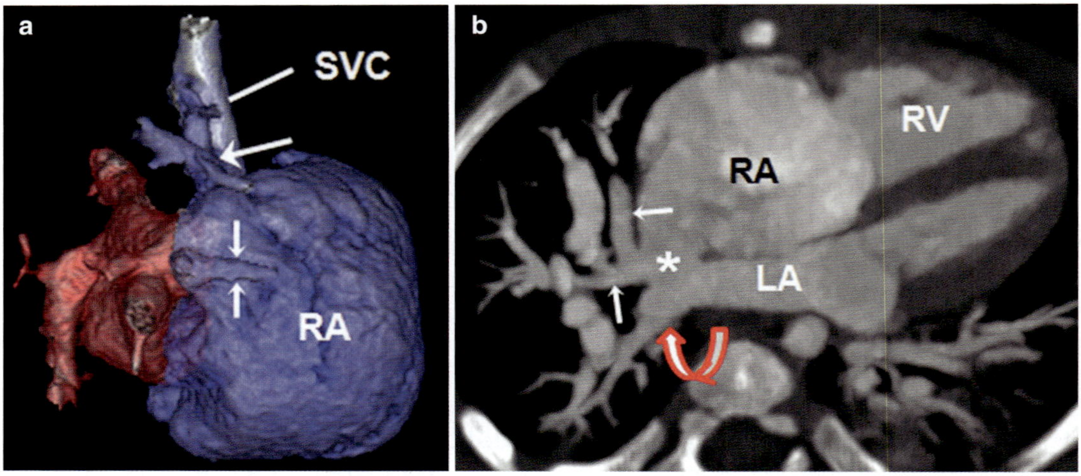

Fig. 18.11 Partial anomalous pulmonary venous return (PAPVR) and the sinus venous type of atrial septal defect (ASD). (**a**) Volume-rendered CT image with a right lateral view shows the right upper lobe vein (*long arrow*) and the right middle lobe vein (*short arrows*) anomalously draining into the superior vena cava (*SVC*) and the dilated right atrium (*RA*), respectively. (**b**) Four-chamber CT image reveals the sinus venous ASD (*asterisk*). The right middle lobe vein (*arrows*) anomalously drains into the RA, while the right lower pulmonary vein (*curved arrow*) normally drains into the left atrium (*LA*). *RV* right ventricle

large bridging vein is present between bilateral SVC in approximately 30 % of cases. In about 90 % of cases, a persistent left SVC drains into the right atrium via the dilated coronary sinus [86]. Less frequent drain sites include the inferior vena cava (IVC), hepatic vein, and left atrium. Recognition of a left SVC is clinically relevant when a procedure requiring upper limb venous access or cavopulmonary connection is planned. Left SVC drainage into the left atrium is almost always associated with other congenital anomalies. In left atrial isomerism, a left SVC often drains into the roof of the left atrium. The levoatriocardinal vein is a rare, persistent venous connection between the left atrium and systemic vein and often associated with left-sided obstructive lesions, such as CoA, hypoplastic left heart syndrome, congenial mitral stenosis, and cor

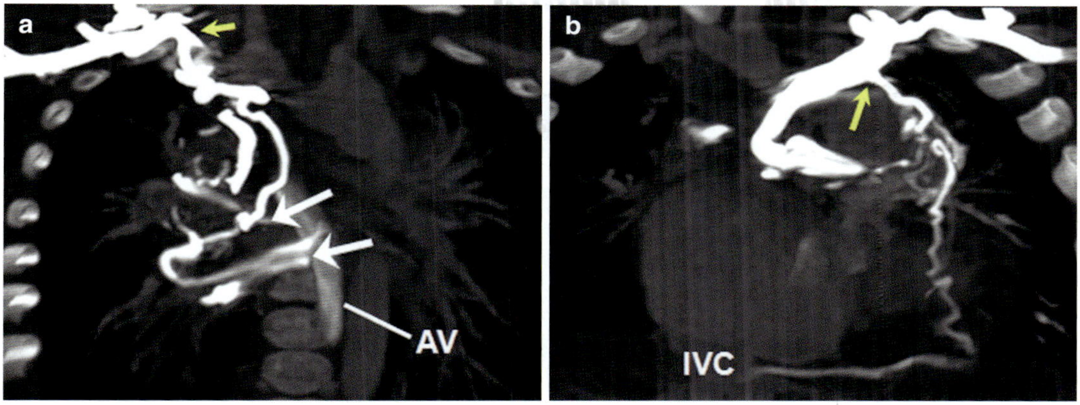

Fig. 18.12 Collateral veins developed after Fontan operation. (**a**) Coronal maximum intensity projection (MIP) CT image shows systemic-to-pulmonary venous collaterals between the right brachiocephalic vein (*short yellow arrow*) and the right pulmonary veins (*long arrows*). The dilated azygos vein (*AV*) is also noted. (**b**) Coronal MIP CT image reveals the systemic-to-systemic venous collaterals by an enlarged pericardiacophrenic vein extending from the left brachiocephalic vein (*arrow*) to the inferior vena cava (*IVC*) and a systemic-to-pulmonary venous collateral between the left brachiocephalic vein (*arrow*) and the left superior pulmonary vein

triatriatum [2]. Subaortic left innominate vein is more frequently seen in the right aortic arch, underdeveloped pulmonary artery, and abnormal elongation of the aortic arch [87, 88]. This anomalous vein can be clearly identified on cardiac CT although it has no clinical significance.

IVC interruption with azygos continuation is commonly associated with left atrial isomerism, whereas juxtaposition of the IVC and abdominal aorta is frequently seen in right atrial isomerism [2]. Separate hepatic venous drainage into the atrium may make Fontan completion difficult in patients with functional single ventricle (FSV). In patients with FSV, cavopulmonary connections are surgically created. Homogeneous vascular enhancement in Fontan pathway is difficult to be achieved on cardiac CT due to preferential cavopulmonary blood flow [5, 6, 89–91]. After Fontan procedure, systemic vein-to-pulmonary vein and systemic vein-to-systemic vein collaterals are often seen on cardiac CT [92] (Fig. 18.12).

Airways

Airway anomalies are often associated with congenital heart disease. Among them, the intimate relationship between congenital tracheal stenosis and pulmonary artery sling is described as the so-called sling-ring complex. Congenital tracheal stenosis also is frequently attributed to respiratory difficulty, difficult intubation, and postoperative ventilator weaning failure in children with congenital heart disease. In addition to airway anomalies, CT also is invaluable for evaluating extrinsic vascular compression of the central airways, most commonly the left main bronchus, in patients with congenital heart disease [8, 93–95]. CT is also useful to monitor the effects of surgical treatments for vascular airway compression, such as aortopexy and anterior translocation of the right pulmonary artery (Fig. 18.13). Traumatic placement of an endotracheal tube may cause an iatrogenic subglottic tracheal narrowing. Long-standing and extrinsic airway compression by dilated cardiovascular structures, endotracheal tube, or mediastinal lymphadenopathy may result in tracheobronchomalacia that can be assessed with cine CT or 4D airway CT as described in the previous section [5, 6, 44, 55, 56].

To determine atrial situs, the relationship of the upper lobar bronchus and the pulmonary artery can be assessed on cardiac CT [8]. The upper lobar bronchi are bilaterally eparterial in right isomerism, whereas they are bilaterally hyparterial in left isomerism (Fig. 18.14).

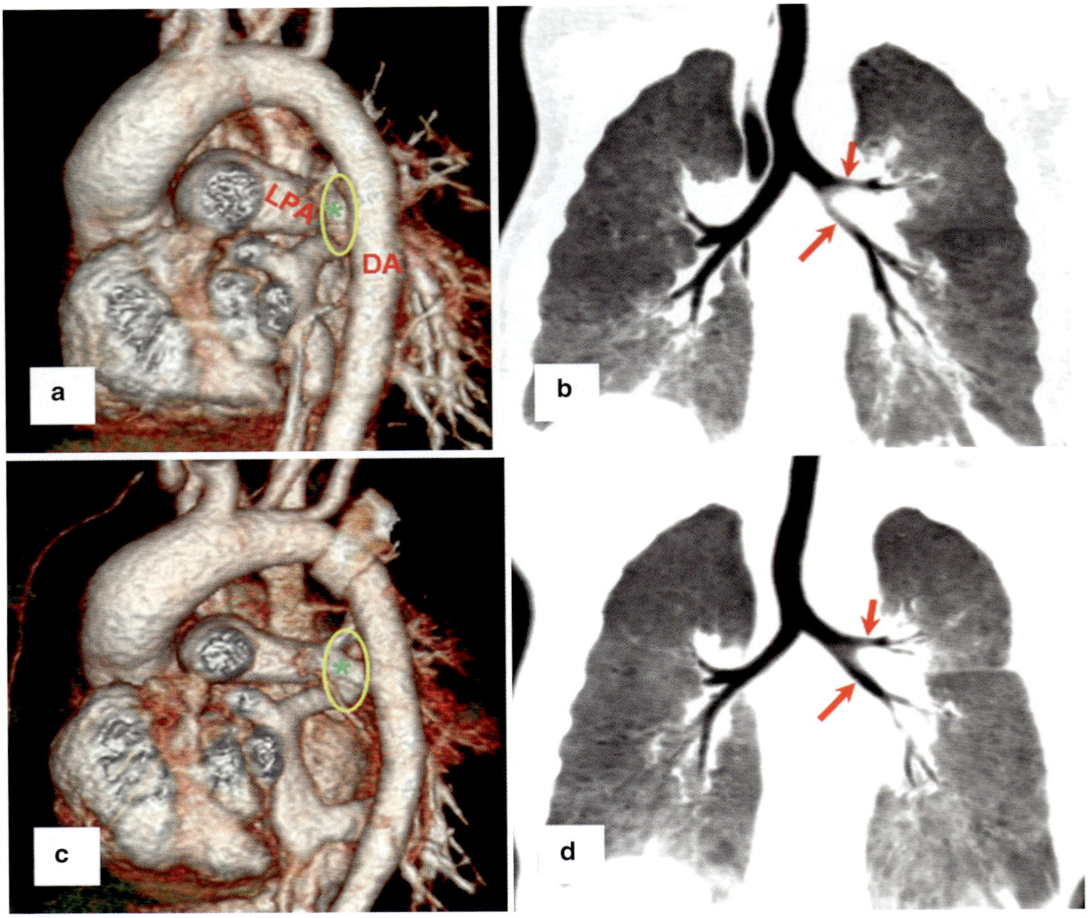

Fig. 18.13 A 4-month-old infant with complex congenital heart disease. (**a**) Volume-rendered CT image with an aortic arch view shows that potential space (*asterisk*) for the left bronchi between the left pulmonary artery (*LPA*) and the descending aorta (*DA*) is narrow. (**b**) Coronal minimum intensity projection (MinIP) CT image reveals narrowing (*arrows*) of the left bronchi. Of note, the branching pattern of the bronchial tree is situs inversus. (**c**) Volume-rendered CT image with an aortic arch view performed after posterior aortopexy demonstrates that the space (*asterisk*) for the left bronchi becomes considerably widened. (**d**) Coronal MinIP CT image performed after posterior aortopexy shows that the narrowing (*arrows*) of the left bronchi is improved

Coronary Arteries

In addition to hemodynamically significant coronary artery anomalies, trivial anomalies, such as high takeoff, and certain coronary artery anatomy, particularly in TOF and transposition of the great arteries (TGA), may be clinically very important in patients with congenital heart disease [13, 96]. Therefore, presurgical recognition of such anomaly or anatomy on cardiac CT may prevent coronary artery-related, postsurgical complications. In addition to unfavorable coronary artery anatomy, commissural malalignment of aortic-pulmonary sinus often seen up to 46 % in complete TGA may require alterative procedures for coronary artery transfer during arterial switch operation to avoid torsion or stretching of coronary arteries [97]. After arterial switch operation, cardiac CT may be used to detect potential stenosis (3–8 % of patients) of the transferred coronary arteries [13, 98]. Cardiac CT may be used to assess coronary artery abnormalities in Williams syndrome, such as dilated coronary arteries and coronary osteal stenosis [99].

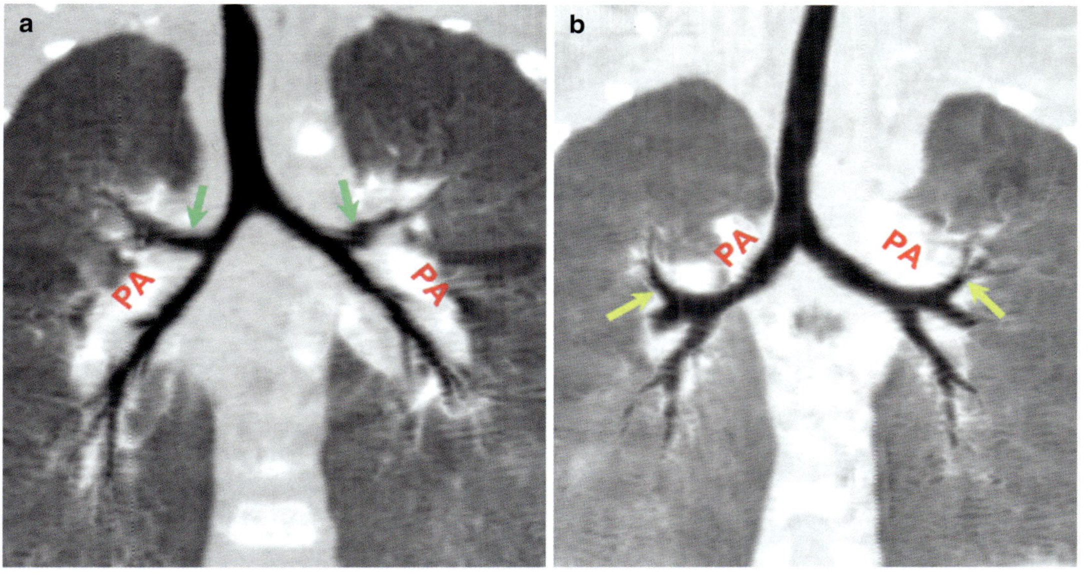

Fig. 18.14 The relationship of the upper lobar bronchus and the pulmonary artery (*PA*) in atrial isomerism. (**a**) In right atrial isomerism, coronal maximum intensity projection (MIP) minimum intensity projection (MinIP) CT image shows the bilaterally eparterial upper lobar bronchi (*arrows*). (**b**) In contrast, the bilaterally hyparterial upper lobar bronchi (*arrows*) are shown in left atrial isomerism

Cardiac Defects

Recent technical developments of cardiac CT enable us to evaluate conotruncal and intracardiac structures accurately without cardiac pulsation artifacts [5, 6, 44]. Therefore, clinical applications of cardiac CT in assessing conotruncal and intracardiac defects largely remain to be determined.

Anatomic features of the anomalies involving the arterial trunks, such as truncus arteriosus and aortopulmonary window, can be evaluated with cardiac CT [1–4, 8]. Truncus arteriosus is a single arterial trunk arising from the ventricles via a single semilunar valve (truncal valve) and classified as three types according to the origin of the pulmonary artery and the distance between the two origins (Fig. 18.15). Aortopulmonary window is an abnormal communication between the ascending aorta and the pulmonary trunk in the presence of separate aortic and pulmonary valves and classified as proximal, distal, or total, depending on its location.

The pulmonary trunk normally lies anterior and the left of the ascending aorta. The ascending aorta is located anterior and right (D-malposition) or left (L-malposition) to the pulmonary trunk in malposition of the great arteries, which is commonly seen in double outlet right ventricle (DORV) and TGA [7]. D-malposition of the great arteries is common in complete TGA, whereas L-malposition is frequently seen in congenitally corrected TGA. Side-by-side relationship of the great arteries in complete TGA is associated with increased incidence of unusual coronary artery patterns with high operative risks [13]. These relationships of the great arteries can be accurately evaluated with cardiac CT.

The semilunar valve is classified as the unicuspid, bicuspid, tricuspid, or quadricuspid valve, according to the number of valvular leaflets [7]. Semilunar valvular stenosis may be seen as thickening and doming of the valve on cardiac CT. On the other hand, semilunar valvular insufficiency may be seen as incomplete diastolic coaptation on cardiac CT. The semilunar valve may show membranous valvular atresia in pulmonary atresia and aortic atresia.

Dynamic morphology of ventricular outflow tract obstruction in various congenital heart

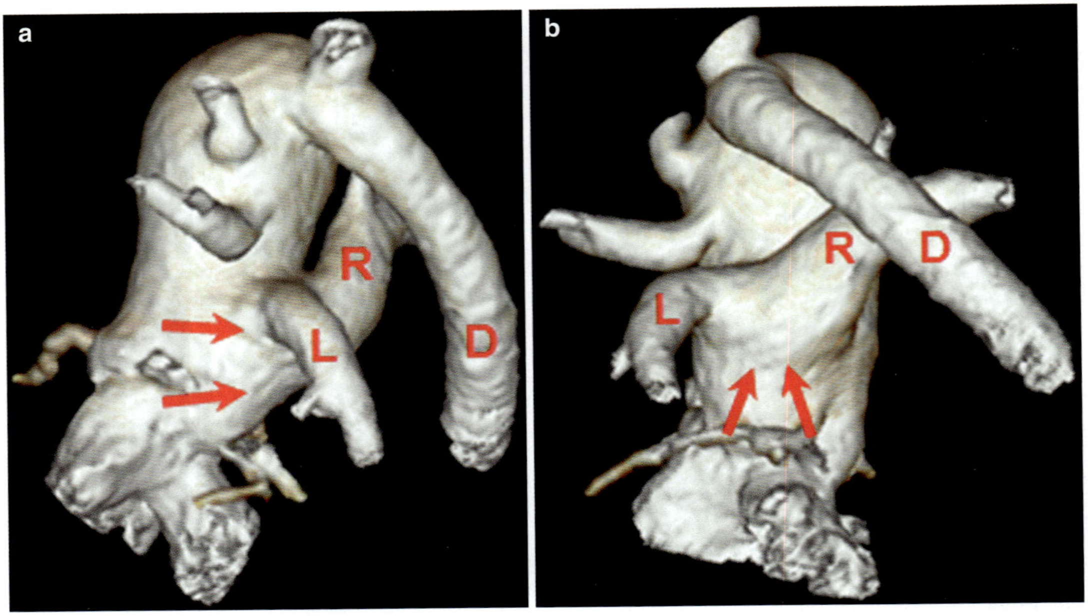

Fig. 18.15 Truncus arteriosus. Volume-rendered CT image with a left lateral view (**a**) and a posterior view (**b**) shows truncus arteriosus type 1 in which a single pulmonary trunk originates from the left lateral aspect of the common trunk (*arrows*). *L* left pulmonary artery, *R* right pulmonary artery, *D* descending aorta

diseases including TOF can be characterized by multiphase ECG-synchronized cardiac CT [5, 6, 44] (Fig. 18.16). Aneurysmal dilatation of the right ventricular outflow tract is often developed after total correction of TOF particularly using a transannular patch technique. In pulmonary atresia, CT can demonstrate the dimension of the right ventricular infundibulum as well as the distance between the infundibulum and the proximal end of the atretic pulmonary trunk, which may be important for surgical planning. Anatomic features and function of cardiac chambers also can be assessed by multiphase ECG-synchronized cardiac CT. As a result, ventricular enlargement and hypertrophy, ventricle function, and ventricle volumetry can be evaluated with CT. CT ventricle volumetry may be used to determine the optimal timing of pulmonary valve replacement in repaired TOF patients and to predict the feasibility of biventricular repair in patients with a marginally small ventricle [100]. In addition, left ventricular noncompaction, isolated or often associated with congenital heart disease, can be depicted on cardiac CT [101, 102]. Atrial situs can be determined on cardiac CT by the extent of the pectinate muscles of the atrial appendages [7]. The pectinate muscles extend to the corresponding atrioventricular junction in the right atrial appendage, whereas they show a limited extent in the left atrial appendage. In addition to the pectinate muscles, the systemic and pulmonary venoatrial connections and the crista terminalis may be used as landmarks for determining the atrial situs. A membranous obstruction in the left atrium, such as cor triatriatum (sinister) or supramitral ring, can be identified and measured on cardiac CT [103]. To differentiate these two entities, the connections of the left atrial appendage to the left atrium proper should be evaluated: its connection to the distal cavity in cor triatriatum and its connection to the proximal cavity in supramitral ring. Cor triatriatum may be difficult to be distinguished from bowed septum primum in infants with TAPVR [104].

The septum of the heart consists of three components: the interatrial, atrioventricular, and interventricular septa [7]. A defect in the interatrial or interventricular septum results in ASD or VSD. On the other hand, atrioventricular septal defect (AVSD) is a defect in the atrioventricular

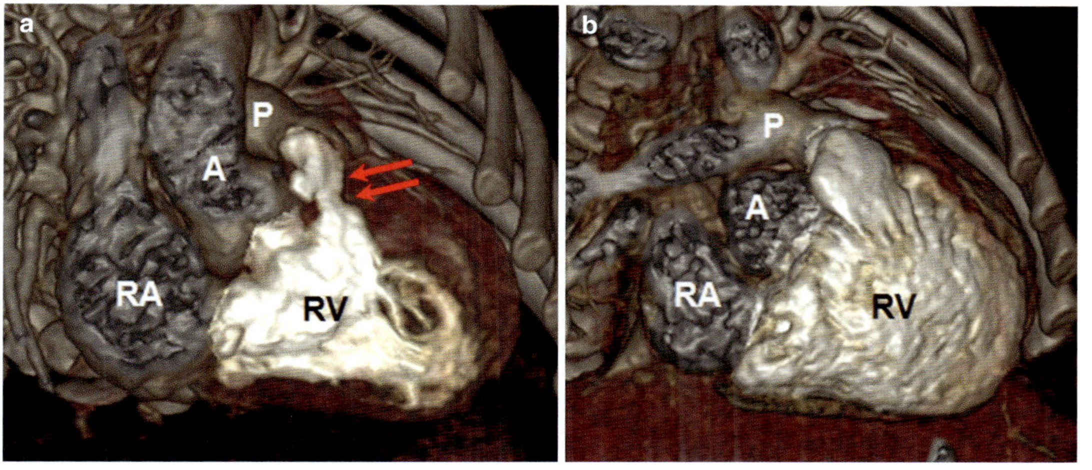

Fig. 18.16 Tetralogy of Fallot. Volume-rendered CT images with a right anterior oblique view obtained at end systole (**a**) and end diastole (**b**) demonstrate a dynamic infundibular narrowing (*arrows*). *RA* the right atrium, *RV* the right ventricle, *P* pulmonary trunk, *A* ascending aorta

septum variably involving the adjacent atrial and ventricular septa (usually the inlet portion of the interventricular septum). Size, location, and type of these septal defects can be evaluated with cardiac CT, especially by using an en face view. However, the diagnosis of the secundum ASD should be carefully made at cardiac CT since the fossa ovalis may be too thin to be identified on cardiac CT. In VSD, the so-called malalignment defect due to anterior or posterior deviation of the conal septum may be seen on cardiac CT. Furthermore, an aneurysm-like pouch formed by the adhesion of the tricuspid valve leaflet to the rim of a perimembranous defect, limiting actual shunt flow, may be seen on cardiac CT.

The atrioventricular valve may show atresia, stenosis, regurgitation, or various kinds of dysplasia. Tricuspid atresia may be classified into two major types: the more common type showing the absent right atrioventricular connection filled by areolar sulcus tissue and the rarer type showing imperforate tricuspid valve [8]. The right ventricle in a patient with tricuspid atresia is opacified via a bulboventricular foramen or ventriculo-coronary arterial communications (VCAC) on cardiac CT. Ebstein anomaly is defined as apical displacement of the attachment of the tricuspid, almost always septal and posterior, leaflets from the atrioventricular junction [8]. The atrialized and functioning right ventricle can be measured by cardiac CT [105]. In AVSD, there is an abnormal arrangement of the atrioventricular valve leaflets, consisting of anterior and posterior bridging leaflets, right and left mural leaflets, and an anterosuperior leaflet.

Discordant ventriculoarterial connection, i.e., the ascending aorta from the morphologic right ventricle and the pulmonary trunk from the morphologic left ventricle, is seen in complete or congenitally corrected TGA. In congenitally corrected TGA, atrioventricular connection is also discordant [106]. In DORV, both great arteries are connected to the morphologic right ventricle [107]. A great artery is regarded as being connected to a ventricle when more than half of its semilunar valve is connected to that ventricle, the so-called 50 % rule. Cardiac CT helps characterize anatomic variants of DORV resulting in various hemodynamic consequences clinically mimicking simple VSD, TOF, and complete TGA.

Conclusion

Recent technical developments allow cardiac CT to be used as an important diagnostic imaging modality in patients with congenital heart disease. Further studies are necessary to validate potential clinical implications of cardiac CT in evaluating cardiac defects.

Coupled with optimized imaging techniques of cardiac CT, evolving clinical applications of cardiac CT should be enthusiastically integrated to develop finest diagnostic algorithms for patients with congenital heart disease.

References

1. Goo HW, Park IS, Ko JK, et al. CT of congenital heart disease: normal anatomy and typical pathological conditions. Radiographics. 2003;23:S147–65.
2. Goo HW, Park IS, Ko JK, et al. Computed tomography for the diagnosis of congenital heart disease in pediatric and adult patients. Int J Cardiovasc Imaging. 2005;21:347–65.
3. Leschka S, Oechslin E, Husmann L, et al. Pre- and postoperative evaluation of congenital heart disease in children and adults with 64-section CT. Radiographics. 2007;27:829–46.
4. Sena L, Goo HW. Computed tomography in congenital heart disease. In: Donoghue V, editor. Radiological imaging of the neonatal chest. 2nd ed. Berlin: Springer; 2008. p. 319–46.
5. Goo HW. State-of-the-art CT, imaging techniques for congenital heart disease. Korean J Radiol. 2010;11:4–18.
6. Goo HW. Cardiac MDCT in children: CT technology overview and interpretation. Radiol Clin North Am. 2011;49:997–1010.
7. Goo HW. CT in pediatric heart disease. In: Saremi F, Achenbach S, Arbustini E, Narula J, editors. Revisiting cardiac anatomy: a computed-tomography-based atlas and reference. Oxford: Blackwell; 2011. p. 76–84.
8. Goo HW. Congenital heart disease in the pediatric population. In: Abramson S, editor. The complete guide to cardiac CT. New York: McGraw-Hill; 2012. p. 503–35.
9. Petersilka M, Bruder H, Krauss B, et al. Technical principles of dual source CT. Eur J Radiol. 2008; 68:362–8.
10. Nie P, Wang X, Cheng Z, et al. Accuracy, image quality and radiation dose comparison of high-pitch spiral and sequential acquisition on 128-slice dual-source CT angiography in children with congenital heart disease. Eur Radiol. 2012;22:2057–66.
11. Goo HW, Park IS, Ko JK, et al. Visibility of the origin and proximal course of coronary arteries on non-ECG-gated heart CT in patients with congenital heart disease. Pediatr Radiol. 2005;35:792–8.
12. Tsai IC, Lee T, Chen MC, et al. Visualization of neonatal coronary arteries on multidetector row CT: ECG-gated versus non-ECG-gated technique. Pediatr Radiol. 2007;37:818–25.
13. Goo HW, Seo DM, Yun TJ, et al. Coronary artery anomalies and clinically important anatomy in patients with congenital heart disease. Pediatr Radiol. 2009;39:265–73.
14. Ben Saad M, Rohnean A, Sigal-Cinqualbre A, Adler G, Paul JF. Evaluation of image quality and radiation dose of thoracic and coronary dual-source CT in 110 infants with congenital heart disease. Pediatr Radiol. 2009;39:668–76.
15. Goo HW, Yang DH. Coronary artery visibility in free-breathing young children with congenital heart disease on cardiac 64-slice CT: dual-source ECG-triggered sequential scan vs. single-source non-ECG-synchronized spiral scan. Pediatr Radiol. 2010;40: 1670–80.
16. Kim C, Goo HW, Yu JJ, Yun TJ. Coronary sinus ostial atresia with persistent left superior vena cava demonstrated on cardiac CT in an infant with a functional single ventricle. Pediatr Radiol. 2012;42:761–3.
17. Shin JH, Goo HW. Tracheomalacia in infants and children: detection by free-breathing cine CT [abstract VP32-11]. In: Program in brief of the 96th scientific assembly and annual meeting of Radiological Society of North America, Chicago, 2010. p. 164.
18. Goo HW, Kim HJ. Detection of air trapping on inspiratory and expiratory phase images obtained by 0.3-second cine CT in the lungs of free-breathing young children. AJR Am J Roentgenol. 2006;187: 1019–23.
19. Ha HI, Goo HW, Seo JB, et al. Effects of high-resolution CT of the lung using partial versus full reconstruction on motion artifacts and image noise. AJR Am J Roentgenol. 2006;187:618–22.
20. Greenberg SB. Dynamic pulmonary CT in children. AJR Am J Roentgenol. 2012;199:435–40.
21. Johnson TR, Krauss B, Sedlmair M, et al. Material differentiation by dual energy CT: initial experience. Eur Radiol. 2007;17:1510–7.
22. Goo HW. Initial experience of dual-energy lung perfusion CT using a dual-source CT system in children. Pediatr Radiol. 2010;40:1536–44.
23. Chae EJ, Seo JB, Goo HW, et al. Xenon ventilation CT with a dual-energy technique of dual-source CT: initial experience. Radiology. 2008;248:615–24.
24. Goo HW, Chae EJ, Seo JB, et al. Xenon ventilation CT using a dual-source dual-energy technique: dynamic ventilation abnormality in a child with bronchial atresia. Pediatr Radiol. 2008;38:1113–6.
25. Goo HW, Yang DH, Hong SJ, et al. Xenon ventilation CT using dual-source and dual-energy technique in children with bronchiolitis obliterans: correlation of xenon and CT density values with pulmonary function test results. Pediatr Radiol. 2010;40:1490–7.
26. Goo HW, Yang DH, Kim N, et al. Collateral ventilation to congenital hyperlucent lung lesions assessed on xenon-enhanced dynamic dual-energy CT: an initial experience. Korean J Radiol. 2011;12:25–33.
27. Goo HW, Yu J. Redistributed regional ventilation after the administration of a bronchodilator demonstrated on xenon-inhaled dual-energy CT in a patient with asthma. Korean J Radiol. 2011;12:386–9.

28. Zhang LJ, Wang ZJ, Zhou CS, et al. Evaluation of pulmonary embolism in pediatric patients with nephrotic syndrome with dual energy CT pulmonary angiography. Acad Radiol. 2012;19:341–8.
29. Geyer LL, Scherr M, Körner M, et al. Imaging of acute pulmonary embolism using dual energy CT system with rapid kVp switching: initial results. Eur J Radiol. 2012;81:3711–8.
30. Goo HW CT radiation dose optimization and estimation: an update for radiologists. Korean J Radiol. 2012;13:1–11.
31. Goo HW. Pediatric CT: understanding of radiation dose and optimization of imaging techniques. J Korean Radiol Soc. 2005;52:1–5.
32. Yang DH, Goo HW. Pediatric 16-slice CT protocols: radiation dose and image quality. J Korean Radiol Soc. 2008;59:333–47.
33. Goo HW. Individualized volume CT dose index determined by cross-sectional area and mean density of the body to achieve uniform image noise of contrast-enhanced pediatric chest CT obtained at variable kV levels and with combined tube current modulation. Pediatr Radiol. 2011;41:839–47.
34. Goo HW, Suh DS. Tube current reduction in pediatric non-ECG-gated heart CT by combined tube current modulation. Pediatr Radiol. 2006;36:344–51.
35. Lee CH, Goo JM, Ye HJ, et al. Radiation dose modulation techniques in the multidetector CT era: from basics to practice. Radiographics. 2008;28:1451–9.
36. Goo HW, Suh DS. The influences of tube voltage and scan direction on combined tube current modulation: a phantom study. Pediatr Radiol. 2006;36:833–40.
37. Leschka S, Stolzmann P, Schmid FT, et al. Low kilovoltage cardiac dual-source CT: attenuation, noise, and radiation dose. Eur Radiol. 2008;18:1809–17.
38. Weustink AC, Mollet NR, Pugliese F, et al. Optimal electrocardiographic pulsing windows and heart rate: effect on image quality and radiation exposure at dual-source coronary CT angiography. Radiology. 2008;248:792–8.
39. McCollough CH, Primak AN, Saba O, et al. Dose performance of a 64-channel dual-source CT scanner. Radiology. 2007;243:775–84.
40. Tzedakis A, Damilakis J, Perisinakis K, et al. Influence of z overscanning on normalized effective doses calculated for pediatric patients undergoing multidetector CT examinations. Med Phys. 2007;34:1163–75.
41. Deak PD, Langner O, Leil M, et al. Effects of adaptive section collimation on patient radiation dose in multisection spiral CT. Radiology. 2009;252:140–7.
42. Bittencourt MS, Schmidt B, Seltmann M, et al. Iterative reconstruction in image space (IRIS) in cardiac computed tomography: initial experience. Int J Cardiovasc Imaging. 2011;27:1081–7.
43. Han BK, Grant KL, Garberich R, et al. Assessment of an iterative reconstruction algorithm (SAFIRE) on image quality in pediatric cardiac CT datasets. J Cardiovasc Comput Tomogr. 2012;6:200–4.
44. Goo HW. Current trends in cardiac CT in children. Acta Radiol. 2012. doi:10.1258/ar.2012.120452.
45. Hu XH, Huang GY, Pa M, et al. Multidetector CT angiography and 3D reconstruction in young children with coarctation of the aorta. Pediatr Cardiol. 2008;29:726–31.
46. Yang DH, Goo HW, Seo DM, et al. Multislice CT angiography of interrupted aortic arch. Pediatr Radiol. 2008;38:89–100.
47. Ha HI, Seo JB, Lee SH, et al. Imaging of Marfan syndrome: multisystemic manifestations. Radiographics. 2007;27:989–1004.
48. Kalra VB, Gilbert JW, Malhotra A. Loeys-Dietz syndrome: cardiovascular, neuroradiological and musculoskeletal imaging findings. Pediatr Radiol. 2011;41:1495–504.
49. Kalfa D, Gronier C, Ly M, et al. Giant aortic aneurysm in an infant with arterial tortuosity syndrome. Ann Thorac Surg. 2012;94:e51.
50. Kim YS, Goo HW, Jhang WK, et al. Twelve years of experience with vascular ring surgery. Korean J Thorac Cardiovasc Surg. 2009;42:749–56.
51. Dillman JR, Attili AK, Agarwal PP, et al. Common and uncommon vascular rings and slings: a multimodality review. Pediatr Radiol. 2011;41:1440–54.
52. Schlesinger AE, Krishnamurthy R, Sena LM, et al. Incomplete double aortic arch with atresia of the distal left arch: distinctive imaging appearance. AJR Am J Roentgenol. 2005;184:1634–9.
53. Hong GS, Goo HW, Song JW. Prevalence of ligamentum arteriosum calcification on multi-section spiral CT and digital radiography. Int J Cardiovasc Imaging. 2012;28 Suppl 1:61–7.
54. Fleck RJ, Pacharn P, Fricke BL, et al. Imaging findings in pediatric patients with persistent airway symptoms after surgery for double aortic arch. AJR Am J Roentgenol. 2002;178:1275–9.
55. Goo HW. Evaluation of the airways in patients with congenital heart disease using multislice CT. J Korean Pediatr Cardiol Soc. 2004;8:37–43.
56. Lee EY, Zurakowski D, Waltz DA, et al. MDCT evaluation of the prevalence of tracheomalacia in children with mediastinal aortic vascular anomalies. J Thorac Imaging. 2008;23:258–65.
57. Philip S, Chen SY, Wu MH, et al. Retroesophageal aortic arch: diagnostic and therapeutic implications of a rare vascular ring. Int J Cardiol. 2001;79:133–41.
58. Song J, Kim WH, Kim H, et al. Repair of coarctation in right circumflex retroesophageal arch. Ann Thorac Surg. 2009;87:307–9.
59. Scott DJ, Campbell DN, Clarke DR, et al. Twenty-year surgical experience with congenital supravalvular aortic stenosis. Ann Thorac Surg. 2009;87:1501–7.
60. Kimura-Hayama ET, Melendez G, Mendizabal AL, et al. Uncommon congenital and acquired aortic diseases: role of multidetector CT angiography. Radiographics. 2010;30:79–98.
61. Ko SM, Song MG, Hwang HK. Bicuspid aortic valve: spectrum of imaging findings at cardiac MDCT and

cardiovascular MRI. AJR Am J Roentgenol. 2012; 198:89–97.
62. Wang XM, Wu LB, Sun C, et al. Clinical application of 64-slice spiral CT in the diagnosis of the tetralogy of Fallot. Eur J Radiol. 2007;64:296–301.
63. Rajeshkannan R, Moorthy S, Sreekumar KP, et al. Role of 64-MDCT in evaluation of pulmonary atresia with ventricular septal defect. AJR Am J Roentgenol. 2010;194:110–8.
64. Lin MT, Wang JK, Chen YS, et al. Detection of pulmonary arterial morphology in tetralogy of Fallot with pulmonary atresia by computed tomography: 12 years of experience. Eur J Pediatr. 2012;171:579–86.
65. Park JH, Kim HS, Jin GY, et al. Demonstration of peripheral pulmonary stenosis and supravalvular aortic stenosis by different cardiac imaging modalities in a patient with Williams syndrome – usefulness of noninvasive imaging studies. Int J Cardiol. 2008;128:e95–7.
66. Monge MC, Mainwaring RD, Sheikh AY. Surgical reconstruction of peripheral pulmonary artery stenosis in Williams and Alagille syndromes. J Thorac Cardiovasc Surg. 2012. doi:10.1016/j.jtcvs.2012.09.102. 2013;145: 476–81
67. Greil GF, Schoebinger M, Kuettner A, et al. Imaging of aortopulmonary collateral arteries with high-resolution multidetector CT. Pediatr Radiol. 2006;36: 502–9.
68. Taragin BH, Berdon WE, Printz B. MRI assessment of bronchial compression in absent pulmonary valve syndrome and review of the syndrome. Pediatr Radiol. 2006;36:71–5.
69. Brown JW, Ruzmetov M, Vijay P, et al. Surgical treatment of absent pulmonary valve syndrome associated with bronchial obstruction. Ann Thorac Surg. 2006;82:2221–6.
70. Kang MJ, Park CM, Lee CH, et al. Dual-energy CT: clinical applications in various pulmonary diseases. Radiographics. 2010;30:685–98.
71. Kim BH, Seo JB, Chae EJ, et al. Analysis of perfusion defects by causes other than acute pulmonary thromboembolism on contrast-enhanced dual-energy CT in consecutive 537 patients. Eur J Radiol. 2012;81:e647–52.
72. Lee KH, Yoon CS, Ko C, et al. Use of imaging for assessing anatomical relationships of tracheobronchial anomalies associated with left pulmonary artery sling. Pediatr Radiol. 2001;31:269–78.
73. du Plessis AM, Andronikou S, Goussard P. Bridging bronchus and sling left pulmonary artery: a rare entity demonstrated by coronal CT with 3-D rendering display and minimal-intensity projections. Pediatr Radiol. 2008;38:1024–6.
74. Calcagni G, Brunelle F, Vouhe P, et al. CT demonstration of "chicken trachea" resulting from complete cartilaginous rings of the trachea in ring-sling complex. Pediatr Radiol. 2008;38:798–800.
75. Zhong YM, Jaffe RB, Zhu M, et al. CT assessment of tracheobronchial anomaly in left pulmonary artery sling. Pediatr Radiol. 2010;40:1755–62.
76. Vyas HV, Greenberg SG, Krishnamurthy R. MR imaging and CT evaluation of congenital pulmonary vein abnormalities in neonates and infants. Radiographics. 2012;32:87–98.
77. Dillman JR, Yarram SG, Hernandez RJ. Imaging of pulmonary venous developmental anomalies. AJR Am J Roentgenol. 2009;192:1272–85.
78. Kim TH, Kim YM, Suh CH, et al. Helical CT angiography and three-dimensional reconstruction of total anomalous pulmonary venous connections in neonates and infants. AJR Am J Roentgenol. 2000;175: 1381–6.
79. Oh KH, Choo KS, Lim SJ, et al. Multidetector CT evaluation of total anomalous pulmonary venous connections: comparison with echocardiography. Pediatr Radiol. 2009;39:950–4.
80. Otsuka M, Itoh A, Haze K. Sinus venosus type of atrial septal defect with partial anomalous pulmonary venous return evaluated by multislice CT. Heart. 2004;90:901.
81. Konen E, Raviv-Zilka L, Cohen RA, et al. Congenital pulmonary venolobar syndrome: spectrum of helical CT findings with emphasis on computerized reformatting. Radiographics. 2003;23:1175–84.
82. Goo HW, Kim YH, Ko JK, et al. Horseshoe lung: useful angiographic and bronchographic images using multidetector-row spiral CT in two infants. Pediatr Radiol. 2002;32:529–32.
83. Ou P, Marini D, Celermajer DS, et al. Non-invasive assessment of congenital pulmonary vein stenosis in children using cardiac-non-gated CT with 64-slice technology. Eur J Radiol. 2009;70:595–9.
84. Mataciunas M, Gumbiene L, Cibiras S, et al. CT angiography of mildly symptomatic, isolated, unilateral right pulmonary vein atresia. Pediatr Radiol. 2009;30:1087–90.
85. Irwin RB, Greaves M, Schmitt M. Left superior vena cava: revisited. Eur Heart J Cardiovasc Imaging. 2012;13:284–91.
86. Fang CC, Jao YT, Han SC, et al. Persistent left superior vena cava: multi-slice CT images and report of a case. Int J Cardiol. 2007;121:112–4.
87. Kim SH, Chung JW, Im JG, et al. Subaortic left innominate vein: radiologic findings and consideration of embryogenesis. J Thorac Imaging. 1999;14: 142–6.
88. Chen SJ, Liu KL, Chen HY, et al. Anomalous brachiocephalic vein: CT, embryology, and clinical implications. AJR Am J Roentgenol. 2005;184:1235–40.
89. Greenberg SB, Bhutta ST. A dual contrast injection technique for multidetector computed tomography angiography of Fontan procedures. Int J Cardiovasc Imaging. 2008;24:345–8.
90. Prabhu SP, Mahmood S, Sena L, et al. MDCT evaluation of pulmonary embolism in children and young adults following a lateral tunnel Fontan procedure: optimizing contrast-enhancement techniques. Pediatr Radiol. 2009;39:938–44.

91. Goo HW, Yang DH, Park IS, et al. Time-resolved three-dimensional contrast-enhanced magnetic resonance angiography in patients who have undergone a Fontan operation or bidirectional cavopulmonary connection: initial experience. J Magn Reson Imaging. 2007;25:727–36.
92. Goo HW. Haemodynamic findings on cardiac CT in children with congenital heart disease. Pediatr Radiol. 2011;41:250–61.
93. Kim YM, Yoo SJ, Kim TH, et al. Three-dimensional computed tomography in children with compression of the central airways complicating congenital heart disease. Cardiol Young. 2002;12:44–50.
94. Choo KS, Lee HD, Ban JE, et al. Evaluation of obstructive airway lesions in complex congenital heart disease using composite volume-rendered images from multislice CT. Pediatr Radiol. 2006;36: 219–23.
95. Jhang WK, Park JJ, Seo DM, et al. Perioperative evaluation of airways in patients with arch obstruction and intracardiac defects. Ann Thorac Surg. 2008;85:1753–8.
96. Tsai WL, Wei HJ, Tsai IC. High-take-off coronary artery: a haemodynamically minor, but surgically important coronary anomaly. Pediatr Radiol. 2010;40: 232–3.
97. Kim SJ, Kim WH, Lim C, et al. Commissural malalignment of aortic-pulmonary sinus in complete transposition of great arteries. Ann Thorac Surg. 2003;76:1906–10.
98. Ou P, Mousseaux E, Azarine A, et al. Detection of coronary complications after the arterial switch operation for transposition of the great arteries: first experience with multislice computed tomography in children. J Thorac Cardiovasc Surg. 2006;131: 639–43
99. Ergul Y, Nisli K, Kayserili H, et al. Evaluation of coronary artery abnormalities in Williams syndrome patients using myocardial perfusion scintigraphy and CT angiography. Cardiol J. 2012;19:301–8.
100. Kim HJ, Goo HW, Park SH, et al. Left ventricle volume measured by cardiac CT in an infant with a small left ventricle: a new and accurate method in determining uni- or biventricular repair. Pediatr Radiol. 2012. doi:10.1007/00247-012-2464-5. 2013; 43:243–6
101. Goo HW, Park IS. Left ventricular noncompaction in an infant: use of non-ECG-gated cardiac CT. Pediatr Radiol. 2007;37:217–20.
102. Melendez-Ramirez G, Castillo-Castellon F, Espinola-Zavaleta N, et al. Left ventricular noncompaction: a proposal of new diagnostic criteria by multidetector computed tomography. J Cardiovasc Comput Tomogr. 2012;6:346–54.
103. Shan SJ, Johnson PT, Fishman EK. Asymptomatic cor triatriatum: utility of 64-slice multidetector computed tomography with 3-dimensional volume rendering. J Comput Assist Tomogr. 2009;33: 779–81.
104. Gonzalez-Ramirez N, Castillo-Castellon F, Kimura-Hayama E. Cor triatriatum sinister versus bowed septum primum in an infant with total anomalous pulmonary venous connection: a difficult imaging distinction. Pediatr Radiol. 2012;42:1254–8.
105. Chauvaud SM, Hernigou AC, Mousseaux ER, et al. Ventricular volumes in Ebstein's anomaly: x-ray multislice computed tomography before and after surgery. Ann Thorac Surg. 2006;81:1443–9.
106. Lembcke A, Koch C, Dohmen PM, et al. Electrocardiographic-gated multislice computed tomography for visualization of cardiac morphology in congenitally corrected transposition of the great arteries. J Comput Assist Tomogr. 2005;29: 234–7.
107. Chen SJ, Lin MT, Liu KL, et al. Usefulness of 3D reconstructed computed tomography imaging for double outlet right ventricle. J Formos Med Assoc. 2008;107:371–80.

Surgical Considerations in Adult Patients with Congenital Heart Disease

19

Sameh M. Said, Harold M. Burkhart, and Joseph A. Dearani

The number of adults with congenital heart disease (CHD) has dramatically increased over the past decades. It is estimated that more than a million adults with CHD are in the United States alone [1] and it is expected that this number will continue to grow as the population increases. This is secondary to the significant improvement in cardiac surgery and perioperative care. Now, at least 95 % of newborns with CHD will survive to adulthood [2]; however, despite this improvement, residual or recurrent lesions may progress over years and decades resulting in an increase in the need for reoperation. Valve procedures are the most common, and many patients may require numerous surgical procedures or interventions over a lifetime. This chapter will review the surgical issues associated with reoperation in adults with CHD and discuss the role of available imaging modalities in the perioperative management of this growing patient population.

Adults with Congenital Heart Disease

Two different groups of adult patients fall into this category: the first group, which is the majority, includes those who will need reoperation to fix residual or recurrent defects or treat long-term complications (e.g., valve deterioration) and the second group includes those with previously undetected CHD who present for the first time in adulthood. Despite the term "total correction," there are very few lesions that are truly corrected for a lifetime without the need for further intervention. One example could include the ligated and divided patent ductus arteriosus [2]. The majority of many other patients with CHD are at risk of needing late intervention or repeat operation. Surgical repairs of most anomalies are therefore considered palliative. Most reoperations in these patients are related to valve dysfunction, residual or recurrent intracardiac defects, or arrhythmias.

Several factors are important and contribute to perioperative mortality with repeat operations. Some of these factors are older age, female sex, preoperative organ system dysfunction, preoperative renal failure, prior history of stroke, and obesity [3]. Additional factors have been identified by Park et al. [4] included previous radiation, preoperative heart failure or cardiogenic shock, previous coronary artery bypass grafts, and emergency status. The resternotomy mortality increases dramatically from 6.5 % with no injury to 25 % when significant hemorrhage is encountered secondary to the inadvertent cardiotomy.

S.M. Said, MD • H.M. Burkhart, MD
J.A. Dearani, MD (✉)
Division of Cardiovascular Surgery, Mayo Clinic, 200 First Street, SW, Rochester, MN 55905, USA
e-mail: jdearani@mayo.edu

F. Saremi (ed.), *Cardiac CT and MR for Adult Congenital Heart Disease*,
DOI 10.1007/978-1-4614-8875-0_19, © Springer Science+Business Media New York 2014

Technical Considerations and Pitfalls During Reoperation

Prior to reoperation, the surgeon should assess the overall risks of mortality and morbidity and discuss all available options and alternatives with the patient. Communication with the cardiology, anesthesia, perfusion, and operating room team members is essential to success during these challenging procedures. The following is our strategy:

- Peripheral cannulation of femoral or axillary vessels if repeat sternotomy will be associated with injury to cardiac or great vessel (e.g., aorta, conduit, innominate vein) structures. This is determined by preoperative evaluation of cross-sectional images and the close relationship of these structures to the posterior sternum. The advent of percutaneous techniques of cannulation facilitate right internal jugular and groin cannulation with almost no need for an incision in the case of emergency (Fig. 19.1a–d); however, we prefer cutdown exposure of groin vessels so that repair can be accomplished under direct vision.
- Currently, we use a percutaneous cannula placed into the right internal jugular vein and

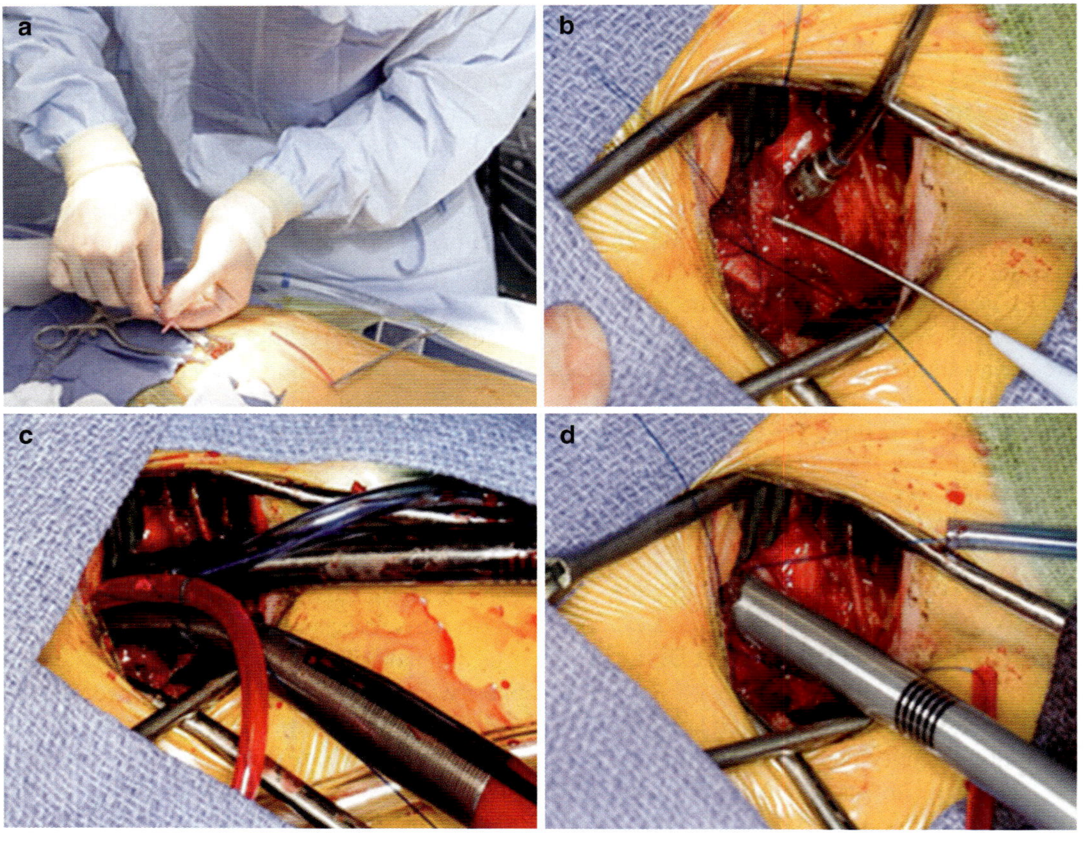

Fig. 19.1 Intraoperative photographs showing the cutdown technique of femoral cannulation in preparation for cardiopulmonary bypass prior to redo sternotomy. (**a**) Small groin incision is performed to expose the femoral vessels and Seldinger technique using a guidewire is performed with purse-string sutures on the vessels. (**b**) The puncture site is then dilated over the guidewire prior to insertion of the cannula. (**c**) The femoral arterial and (**d**) femoral venous cannulae are inserted and secured in place with the final position of the venous cannula confirmed using intraoperative transesophageal echocardiography. When the femoral artery is noted to be small, a chimney graft is sewn end-to-side to the femoral artery. One or both groins can be cannulated based on vascular anatomy. Frequent postoperative examination of distal pulses and extremity perfusion are essential to identify potential compartment syndrome

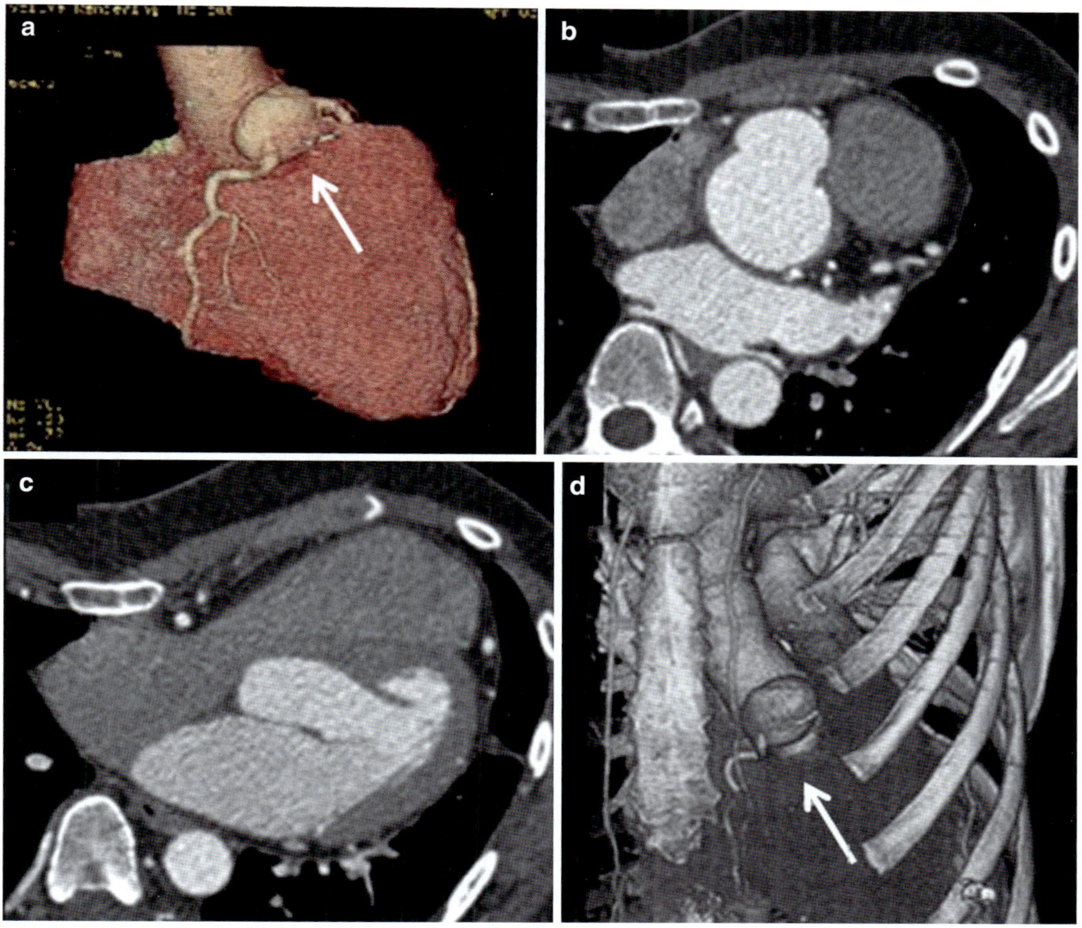

Fig. 19.2 Preoperative cross-sectional imaging with 3-D reconstruction are of paramount importance in reoperations. (**a**) 3-D reconstruction showing a right coronary artery aneurysm (*arrow*); (**b**, **c**) the same patient also has a severe pectus deformity with the mediastinal structures displaced into the left hemithorax; (**d**) 3-D reformat showing the relationship of the leftward position of the right coronary artery aneurysm (*arrow*) to the sternum

advance it into the superior vena cava for additional venous return.

- Vacuum-assisted venous drainage is used selectively and is avoided if there are any residual intracardiac shunts so that if injury occurs to a cardiac structure (usually right-sided) during dissection, air embolism is avoided.
- Certain situations may necessitate initiation of cardiopulmonary bypass (CPB) before sternotomy, and this is determined by the relationship of mediastinal structures to the sternum and chest wall (Fig. 19.2) and the number of previous sternotomies.
- The use of pericardial substitute (e.g., Gore-Tex pericardial membrane) may be considered if additional reoperation(s) is expected in order to minimize or reduce the risk of cardiac injury; however, their use has been controversial [5, 6]. A previous report from our institution identified that the incidence of injury is reduced if the native pericardium was approximated during the prior surgical procedure [4].
- The initiation of CPB prior to resternotomy does not necessarily protect the right ventricle (RV) from injury; however, it provides a decompressed right heart and creates a controllable situation and minimizes the

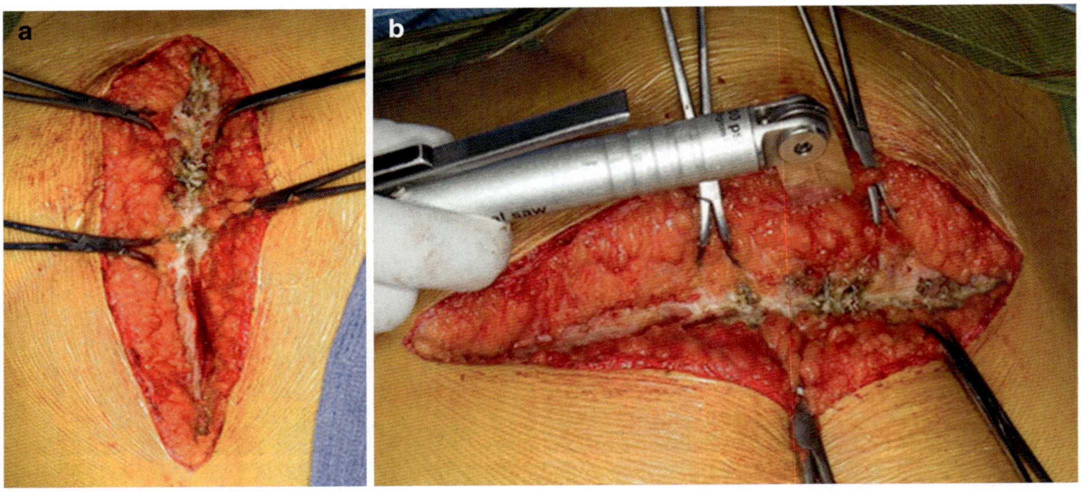

Fig. 19.3 Intraoperative photos demonstrating our technique of resternotomy: (**a**) towel clips are used on either side of the sternum to elevate the corresponding half during the resternotomy; (**b**) the microsagittal saw is preferred during redo sternotomy due to its ease of handling. In general, we use the saw for division of the anterior sternal table and heavy blunt scissors to divide the posterior table

amount of blood loss if injury occurs and facilitates dissection. This is particularly helpful when there is significant right heart enlargement or there are elevated right-sided pressures.

- Although CPB can facilitate a safe resternotomy, it does result in longer CPB times, which has been shown to increase mortality and morbidity. As a result, the operation should be orchestrated so that the CPB time is as short, but safe, as possible. This can be accomplished by using peripheral CPB to facilitate resternotomy, then separating from CPB after sternal division to complete the mediastinal dissection whenever possible. In some situations, the dissection may be facilitated if the heart is maintained decompressed while on CPB; the decision to perform the dissection on or off bypass is individualized.
- Controversy exists regarding the need to remove the previously placed sternal wires or to retain them in place during the actual sawing of the sternum (Fig. 19.3a). There is no conclusive evidence that cardiac injury is decreased with keeping them intact; the decision is generally based on surgeon preference.
- We use the air-driven microsagittal saw (Fig. 19.3b) during repeat sternotomy and divide the anterior sternal table with the saw followed by careful division of the posterior table with a heavy scissors under direct vision with the help of Volkmann retractors that elevate the two halves of the sternum (Fig. 19.4a). The microsagittal saw has the advantage of precise perpendicular division of the sternum, with relatively easy control of the depth of blade penetration and the ability to feel the posterior sternal table [7].
- The heart and great vessels should be gently released in a stepwise fashion from the back of the sternum with combination scissors and low-energy electrocautery to allow safe separation of the two sternal halves and safe placement of the sternal retractor later on (Fig. 19.4b). We intentionally enter each pleural space so that the mediastinum falls away from the chest wall.
- Limiting dissection only to the necessary areas of the intended procedure is an important consideration as it decreases the risk of injury to cardiac structures and results in less bleeding from dissected areas at the end of the procedure.

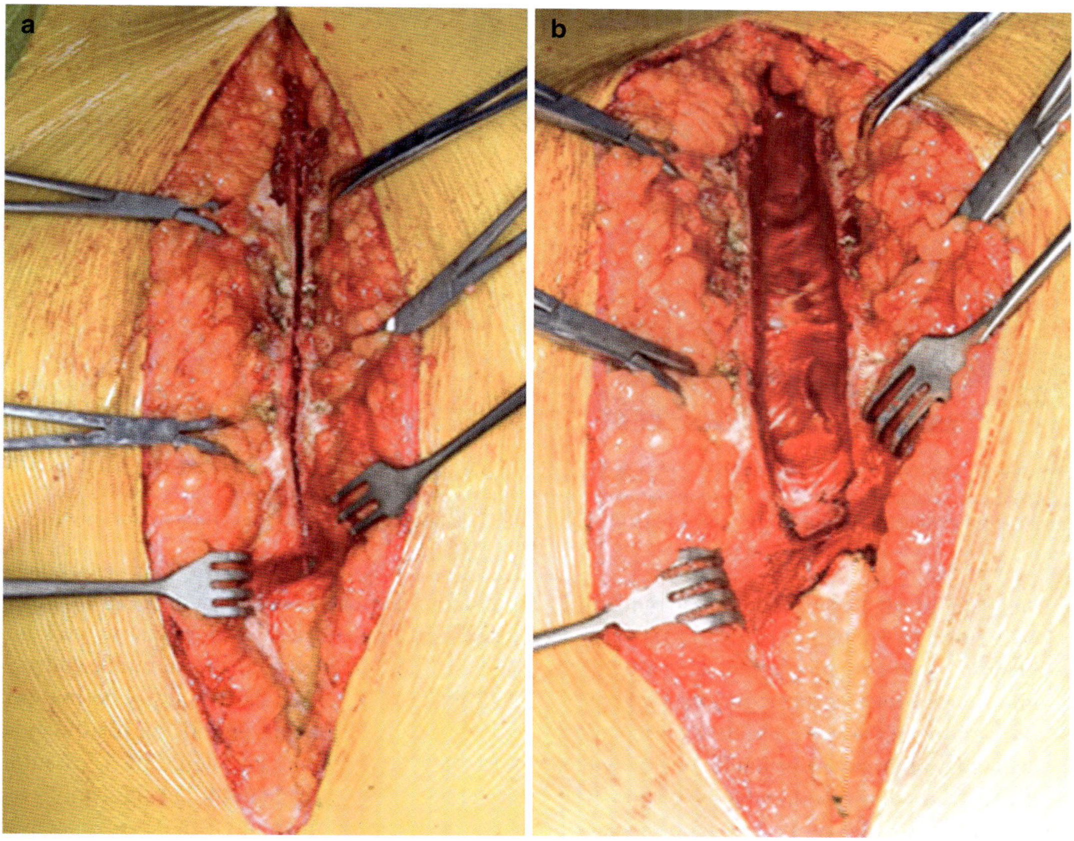

Fig. 19.4 Intraoperative photos demonstrating our preferred technique of resternotomy: (**a**) The anterior table of the sternum is divided with the microsagittal saw, and then with the help of Volkmann retractors, the posterior table is divided with the scissors under vision; (**b**) after dividing the posterior sternal table, the mediastinal structures are dissected and released carefully from the sternum using low-energy electrocautery and scissors. Each hemithorax is entered so the mediastinum falls away from the chest wall allowing sternal separation without tearing of upper mediastinal or cardiac structures

Role of Echocardiography

Echocardiography plays a significant role in the preoperative preparation for cardiac surgery, for both primary and repeat operations. It provides an accurate diagnosis, details about valve anatomy, the presence of septal defects, outflow tract anatomy, chamber dilatation or hypertrophy, and ventricular function. Preoperative transthoracic echocardiography and intraoperative transesophageal echocardiography are used routinely. Specific issues essential in the planning of a reoperation are outlined below:

- It is important to identify an intracardiac shunt (atrial or ventricular level) as there is a risk of air embolism if inadvertent cardiotomy occurs while the heart is decompressed on cardiopulmonary bypass. When a septal defect is present, we maintain a positive central venous pressure of at least 5 mmHg to avoid air entry into the right heart with subsequent systemic embolization across the shunt. An aortic tack vent is used routinely and the bed is maintained in Trendelenburg position and the operative field is flooded with carbon dioxide. If the laceration involves a left-sided structure, aorta or pulmonary venous atrium, then CPB and deep hypothermia may become necessary to facilitate resternotomy.

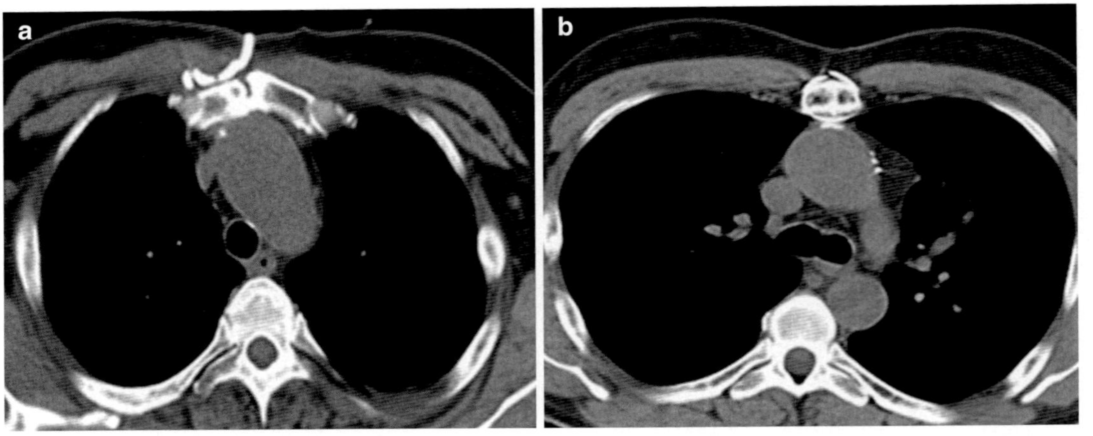

Fig. 19.5 The value of preoperative cross-sectional images in demonstrating the relationship of the mediastinal structures to the underside of the sternum. In this particular case, the ascending aorta (**a**) and the aortic arch (**b**) are eroding into the sternum. Knowledge of this preoperatively is essential when planning redo sternotomy

- Analysis of all intracardiac valve function is essential, but evaluation of the aortic valve to identify aortic regurgitation is particularly important. When aortic regurgitation is present, venting of the left ventricle is critical in the event that ventricular fibrillation occurs (which is expected with hypothermic bypass) in order to avoid distention of the left ventricle and its deleterious effects on ventricular function.
- Intraoperative transesophageal echocardiography also provides guidance for peripheral cannulation and ensures proper positioning of both arterial and venous cannulae; it helps in evaluating collapse of the cardiac chambers after initiation of peripheral CPB, provides a continuous evaluation to the contractile status and distension of the ventricle(s), and guides the de-airing process at the conclusion of bypass.

Role of Cross-Sectional Imaging Computed Tomography (CT) Scan

The relationship and position of cardiac structures (chambers and great vessels) to each other and to the chest wall is essential when planning reoperation. Anatomic landmarks especially coronary arteries may be obscured, and an extracardiac conduit or dilated ascending aorta may become very close or even adherent to the undersurface of the sternum or chest wall (Fig. 19.5). In advanced cases, imaging of these anatomic structures has demonstrated erosion into the sternum, and this significantly increases the risk of resternotomy. Cross-sectional imaging provides a road map of these important anatomic findings that is essential in the preoperative evaluation. The indications for CT scan or MR imaging include a congenital diagnosis and prior surgery; information about great vessel anatomy (dilatation, stenosis, etc.) is particularly helpful. Advantages and disadvantages of CT vs MR are beyond the scope of this chapter and described elsewhere in this textbook. In general, MR is preferred when feasible since the exposure to radiation is reduced and the need for multiple studies over a lifetime is common in the patient population. The recent introduction of three-dimensional reconstructions is also invaluable in redo surgery as it provides the surgeon with an anatomic model of the heart and mediastinal structures, their relation to the sternum, location of extracardiac conduits, and anomalous course of major coronary arteries, and facilitates operative planning (Fig. 19.6).

Magnetic Resonance Imaging (MRI)

While MR imaging also provides excellent cross-sectional imaging similar to CT scanning, MR

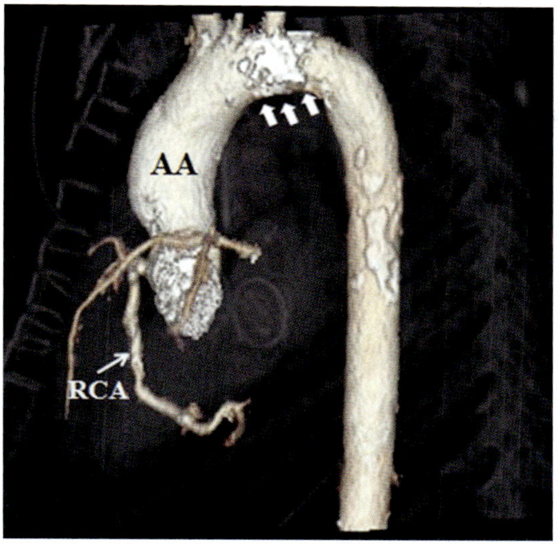

Fig. 19.6 CT with 3-D reconstruction showing dilated ascending aorta (*AA*) above the sinutubular junction, location of the major coronary arteries in relation to the sternum, and the degree of calcification in the aortic arch (*white arrows*) and to a lesser degree in the ascending and descending aorta. *RCA* right coronary artery

imaging is particularly helpful at providing additional information about cardiac chamber size and ventricular function. Decreased myocardial function has been one of the independent risk factors of perioperative mortality and overall outcome in many studies [8]. MRI plays an important role in evaluation of the right ventricular function which is difficult to evaluate by echocardiography with accuracy.

MRI is increasingly used in all types of patients with cardiac disease, including those with Ebstein malformation and other forms of congenital tricuspid regurgitation (TR) and right-sided disease (e.g., tetralogy of Fallot). Functional assessment can be made including quantitative measurement of left and right ventricular size and function (Fig. 19.7). At present, we rely on echocardiography (2- and 3-D) for detailed evaluation of valve anatomy (ventricular size and function to a lesser extent) and MRI for detailed assessment of right and left ventricular dimensions and function.

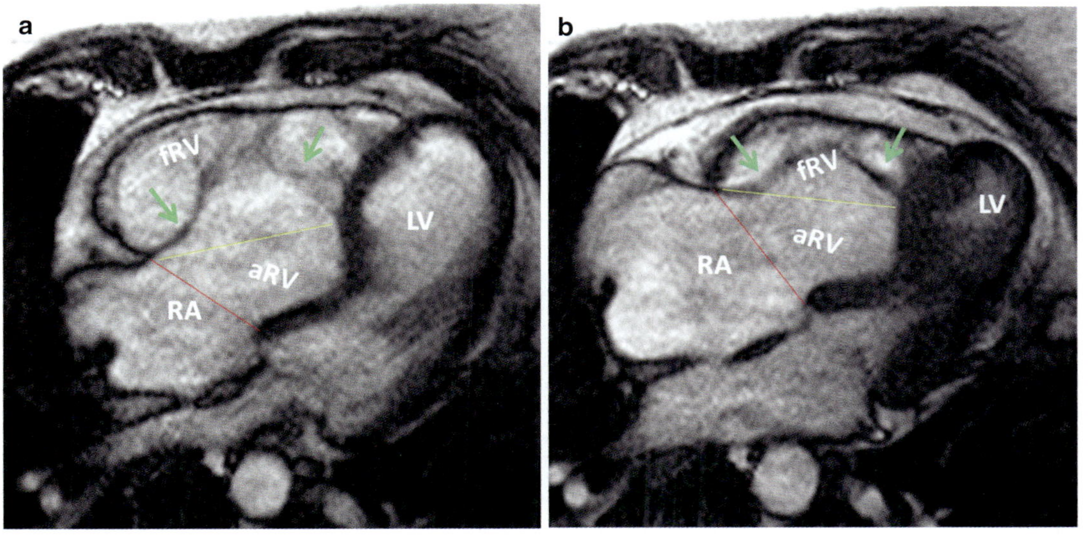

Fig. 19.7 Measurements of right ventricular volumes in Ebstein by MRI. Steady-state free-precession (SSFP) axial MR images in end-diastole (**a**) and end-systole (**b**) are shown. Tricuspid leaflets are shown by *green arrows*. The border between functional right ventricle (*fRV*) and atrialized right ventricle (*aRV*) is demarcated by *yellow lines* connecting the free wall attachment of the anterior tricuspid leaflet and septal attachment of the apically displaced septal leaflet. The border between the aRV and the right atrium (*RA*) is shown by red lines connecting the free wall attachment of the anterior tricuspid leaflet and the point of presumed normal attachment of the septal tricuspid valve leaflet. Measurements are obtained in end-diastole (**a**) and end-systole (**b**). The severity of clinical disease is thought to be inversely correlated to the size of the functional RV (fRV). In adults with unrepaired Ebstein anomaly, aRV volume is independently related to exercise test capacity and may express severity of disease [8]. *LV* left ventricle (Courtesy of Farhood Saremi MD. University of Southern California)

Role of Cardiac Catheterization

Cardiac catheterization is used selectively in the preoperative testing for adults with CHD prior to reoperation. Its role is mostly related to hemodynamic assessment in selected situations. However, cardiac catheterization can also play a supplemental role in imaging, e.g., great vessel anatomy, pulmonary artery, and coronary anatomy. Knowledge of coronary artery anatomy and distribution and the presence of acquired lesions are critical when planning resternotomy and the potential need for bypass grafting. Patients who had prior repair of tetralogy of Fallot with or without RV-to-pulmonary artery (PA) conduit may require reoperation for pulmonary valve or conduit replacement. Limited ventriculotomy may be necessary during pulmonary valve replacement or right ventricular outflow tract (RVOT) reconstruction. Accurate placement of this incision is of paramount importance to avoid injury to important coronary artery branches that may be crossing the RVOT (e.g., anomalous origin of left anterior descending branch from the right coronary artery) and this can be clearly delineated from preoperative cardiac catheterization or CT cross-sectional images as well (Fig. 19.8).

Alternate Cannulation Sites and Peripheral Access Evaluation: Role of Ultrasonography

Patients with CHD frequently require repeat operations over a lifetime. As the number of sternotomies increases, the risk of cardiac injury increases as well. Peripheral vascular access may be compromised and limited from multiple prior cardiac procedures including open-heart surgery with perioperative invasive monitoring, cardiac catheterization(s), electrophysiology procedure(s), and/or pacemaker insertion. This may lead to scarring, stenosis, and obstruction of peripheral arterial and venous structures in the neck and groin, or they may be at risk for pseudoaneurysm, arteriovenous fistulae, or other complications associated with any of these procedures. Since peripheral cannulation for cardiopulmonary bypass becomes

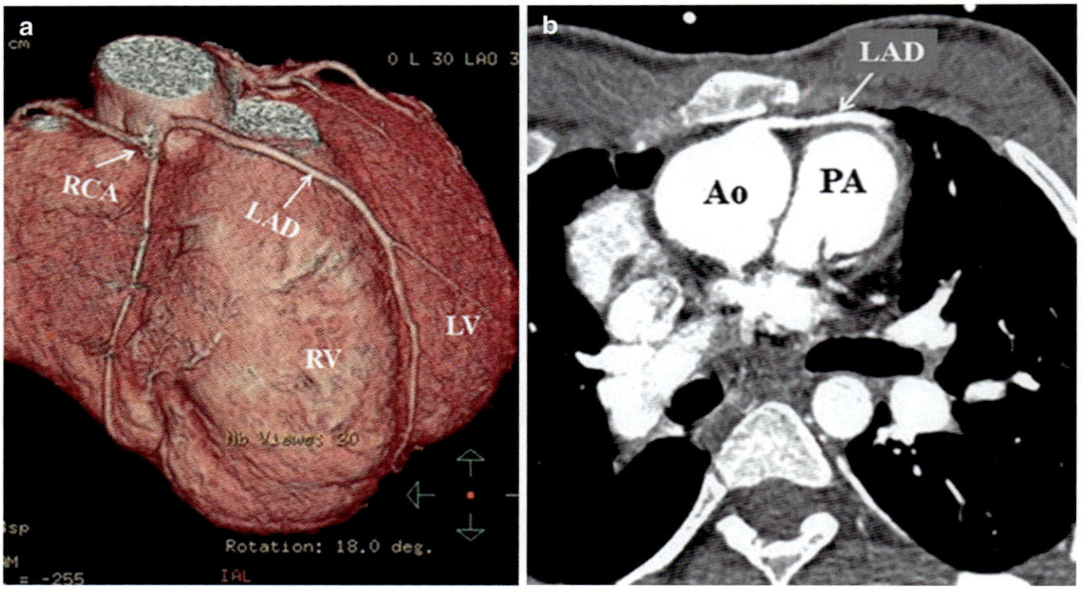

Fig. 19.8 Computed tomography scan with 3-D reconstruction (**a**) showing: anomalous origin of the left anterior descending artery (*LAD*) from the right coronary artery (*RCA*) crossing the right ventricular outflow tract in a patient with tetralogy of Fallot. Corresponding cross-sectional image (**b**) shows its close proximity to the sternum. *RV* right ventricle, *LV* left ventricle, *Ao* aorta, *PA* pulmonary artery

a strategic alternative and facilitates initiation of bypass prior to a hazardous resternotomy, knowledge of the peripheral vessel patency (groin and neck) is essential during the preop workup.

Preoperative evaluation of peripheral vasculature using ultrasonography is very important during the preoperative evaluation as it will change the plan with regard to cannulation. Peripheral arterial options include femoral or axillary artery; occasionally the innominate or carotid artery is considered in young children. Peripheral venous options include femoral and right internal jugular vein with advancement of the cannula into the right atrium via the superior or inferior vena cava. The decision to expose or cannulate the peripheral vessels and the timing of initiation of CPB before sternotomy is individualized, and preoperative imaging aids in this decision making.

The following alternative cannulation sites may be considered if there is a high risk of cardiac injury during the sternotomy:

- Femoral artery or vein vessels
- Iliac artery or vein vessels
- Axillary artery
- Carotid artery (usually right)
- Innominate artery
- Internal jugular vein (usually right)
- Right atrium or ascending aorta (via right thoracotomy)
- Left ventricular apex (via left thoracotomy)
- Pulmonary artery (via left thoracotomy)
- Abdominal aorta

Specific Pathology

The following lesions are examples of how preoperative imaging plays a critical role in guiding the surgeon during reoperation and minimizing the risks associated with resternotomy.

Tetralogy of Fallot/Pulmonary Atresia

Patients who had prior tetralogy of Fallot (TOF) or pulmonary atresia with ventricular septal defect (PA/VSD) repair using an extracardiac conduit, the conduit usually lies to the left of the midline and the aorta may be dilated (as is the case with all conotruncal anomalies) and they may be in close proximity to the back of the sternum (see Fig. 19.8).

Coronary artery anomalies are not uncommon and determination of the location of major coronary arterial branches (i.e., anomalous left anterior descending from the right coronary artery) is important during reoperation (Fig. 19.8). Anomalous vessels can be vulnerable during sternal reentry or at the time of any ventricular incisions that may be needed for a given procedure.

Truncus Arteriosus/Transposition of the Great Arteries

The Rastelli procedure (VSD closure with RV-PA conduit placement) has been the most common procedure to treat transposition with VSD and pulmonary stenosis. The position of the RV-to-PA conduit can be located to the left or right of the ascending aorta. Either way, the conduit commonly lies in a midline position and very close to the back of the sternum or even eroding into it.

Ross Procedure

This group of patients may have aneurysmal dilatation of the proximal aortic root – the pulmonary autograft (neoaorta). It is not uncommon for this proximal dilated segment of aorta to be abutting the sternum (Fig. 19.9). In addition, the right coronary artery button origin is often high on this dilated proximal segment of aorta and can also be abutting the back of the sternum and be at risk with resternotomy. This emphasizes the importance of cross-sectional imaging in any patient with previous aortic root surgery. Reoperation after the Ross procedure is almost inevitable for most patients and the most common indications are the following:

- Pulmonary homograft (or RV-PA conduit) structural degeneration
- Autograft (neoaorta) valve regurgitation

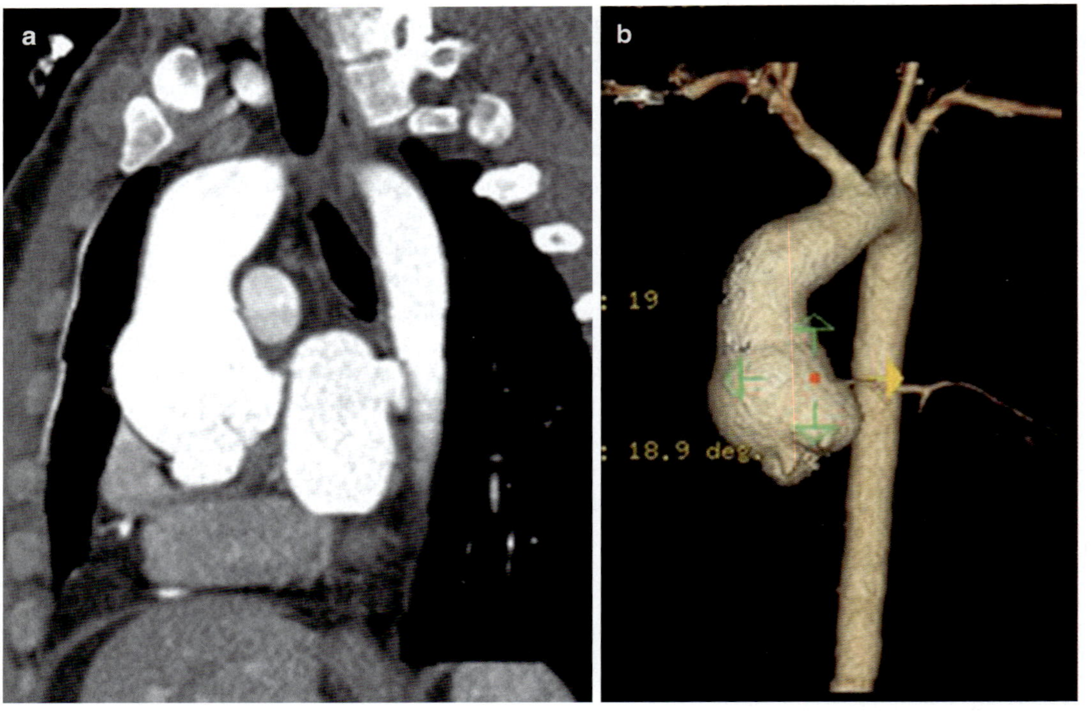

Fig. 19.9 Sagittal CT angiogram (**a**) with 3-D reconstruction (**b**) in a patient who had undergone the Ross procedure. The proximal ascending aorta – the neoaortic root (pulmonary autograft) – is dilated, and the abrupt cutoff in the mid-ascending aorta is the location of the distal suture line from the autograft to the native ascending aorta

- Autograft dilatation
- Concomitant tricuspid or mitral valve regurgitation
- Coronary artery abnormalities (usually button or proximal segments)

Functional Single Ventricle

Imaging of cardiac structures and great vessel anatomy as well as hemodynamic assessment is essential in patients with a Fontan circulation being considered for reoperation. Important anatomy includes the Fontan pathways, pulmonary venous pathways, systemic ventricular outflow tract, valvar function and ventricular dimension, presence of hypertrophy or dilatation, and ventricular function (systolic and diastolic). In addition, information about residual intracardiac shunts and collateralization is needed. Depending upon the type of connection, a dilated right atrium in the setting of an atriopulmonary connection may be adherent to the underside of the sternum and susceptible to injury.

Ebstein Malformation

Severe right-sided enlargement (atrium and ventricle) is the rule with this diagnosis Fig. 19.10). A right ventricular myopathy is always present in combination with tricuspid regurgitation. Echocardiography plays an important role in analysis of tricuspid valve anatomy and MR or CT imaging in right ventricular size and function. In MR assessment of the RV function, axial imaging appears to provide more reproducible data than standard short-axis views [8]. Cardiac catheterization is performed selectively to ascertain right- and left-sided filling pressures if consideration is being given to applying the bidirectional cavopulmonary anastomosis.

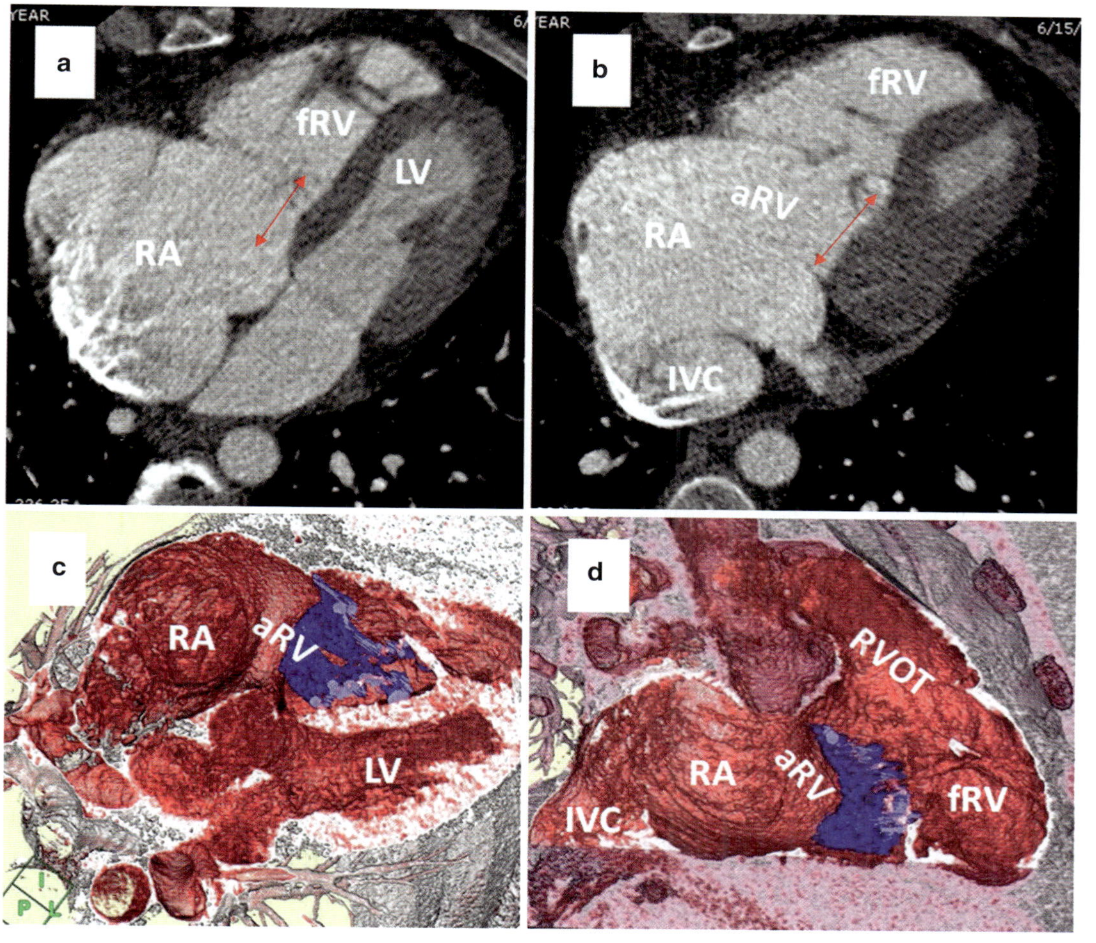

Fig. 19.10 (**a**, **b**) Axial images of computed tomography angiography showing a markedly dilated right atrium and right ventricle in relation to the underside of the sternum; this is a common finding in patients with Ebstein malformation presenting for late reoperation. Magnitude of apical displacement of the septal tricuspid valve is shown by *red arrows* which is an indicator of disease severity. (**c**, **d**) Are color-coded CT in the same patient in four-chamber (**c**) and right ventricle outflow tract (**d**) views. Tricuspid valve is shown in blue. *aRV* atrialized right ventricle, *fRV* functional right ventricle, *RV* right ventricle, *RVOT* right ventricle outflow tract, *LV* left ventricle, *IVC* inferior vena cava (Courtesy of Farhood Saremi MD. University of Southern California)

Residual Intracardiac Shunts

The importance of identifying residual or recurrent atrial or ventricular septal defects is paramount during resternotomy as there can be an increased risk of systemic air embolism if precautions are not applied with the conduct of cardiopulmonary bypass during resternotomy and inadvertent cardiotomy occurs.

Prior Homografts

Homografts have been utilized in the CHD population for decades. They have been used mostly for RV-to-PA conduit reconstruction and to a lesser extent in the aortic root position. At present, homografts are commonly used in the neonate and infant for right-sided reconstructions. In the adult population, homograft tissue

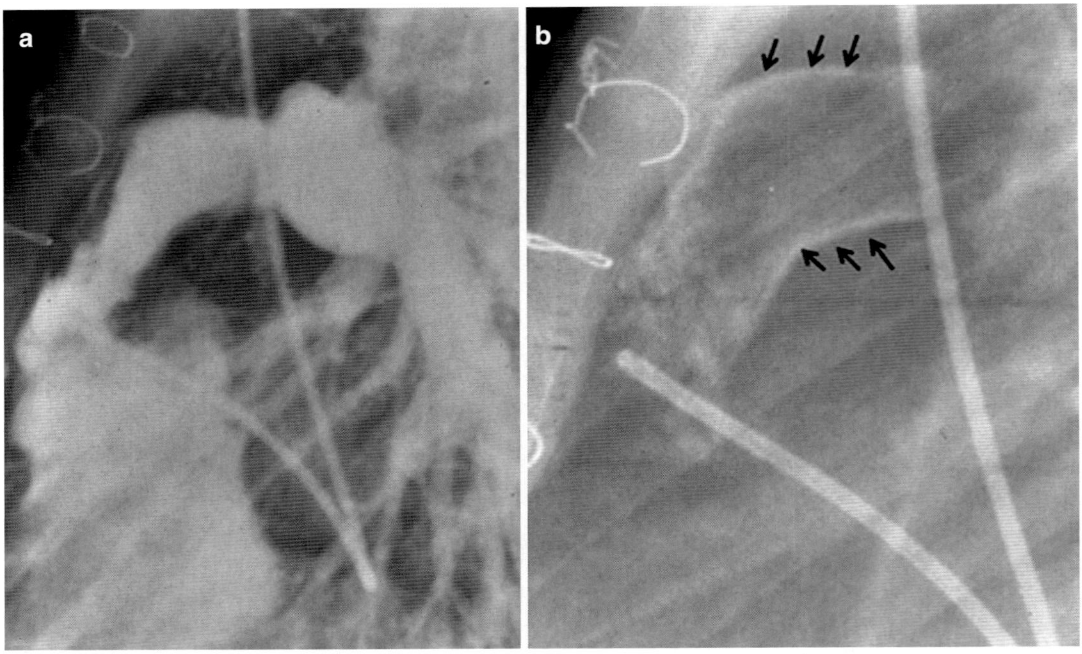

Fig. 19.11 Lateral views of chest angiogram (**a**) and plain X-ray (**b**) in a patient with a prior homograft right ventricle-to-pulmonary artery conduit who had undergone a Rastelli procedure for transposition of the great arteries with pulmonary stenosis and ventricular septal defect. The extensive degree of calcification (*black arrows*) and erosion into the posterior sternum is clearly evident

is commonly used in the setting of active valvar endocarditis (aortic or pulmonary valve/conduit). Homograft tissue is very vulnerable to calcification, often circumferential calcification, which can complicate the conduct of the operation. Preoperative radiographs (Fig. 19.11) and cross-sectional imaging are useful in identifying the position of the homograft and its relation to the underside of the sternum. It also shows the extent of homograft calcification and location of the aorta and right coronary artery and prepares the surgeon for the expected difficulty and risks during reoperation. It is important to look for the extent of previous homograft replacement from preoperative CT scan as this may change the plan of the operation. Peripheral cannulation may be considered if the distal anastomosis of the homograft extends to the base of the innominate artery or if it has been used as a hemiarch technique as extensive calcification in these areas may interfere with proper cannula placement or aortic cross-clamp application.

Tricuspid Valve Regurgitation

Tricuspid valve (TV) regurgitation has been considered as a relatively benign lesion for a long time; however recent data suggest that irrespective of the pulmonary artery pressure or left ventricular ejection fraction, TR has a negative impact on survival [9]. Severe TR starts a vicious circle of chronic right ventricular volume overload and right ventricular dilatation and dysfunction which results in right heart failure. Correction of TR in a timely fashion preserves right ventricular function and interrupts this circle; however, optimal timing has been controversial, but it is generally recommended before the onset of right ventricular dysfunction, even in asymptomatic patients [10, 11]. From our experience we consider the following as indications for TV surgery: presence of symptoms or cyanosis (occurs in the presence of atrial septal defect), decreased exercise tolerance, progressive cardiomegaly on chest X-ray, progressive right ventricular dilatation or reduction of right ventricular systolic function by echocardiography, and the occurrence or progression of atrial or ventricular arrhythmias. Progression of TR is also taken into consideration for timing of intervention for pulmonary valve replacement (PVR). In general we repair TR when the degree of TR is moderate or more at the time of operation for another reason, PVR being most common.

The decision for TV intervention should be made based on preoperative outpatient echocardiography and not the intraoperative echocardiography because of the different (more favorable) hemodynamics under the conditions of general anesthesia.

Pacemaker-Induced Tricuspid Valve Regurgitation

There is increased use of permanent pacemaker (PPM) and implantable cardioverter-defibrillators (ICD) in adults with CHD as a result of atrial or ventricular arrhythmias which are common late sequelae of many CHD pathologies [12]. Different mechanisms of TR were reported among our experience [13]: (1) leaflet perforation by the lead, (2) lead entanglement of the TV apparatus, (3) lead impingement of the TV leaflets, and (4) lead adherence to the TV (Fig. 19.12a–c). In our experience, we analyzed the records of 571 consecutive patients with congenital (non-Ebstein) TR who underwent TV operation for severe TR. Twenty-five patients (4 %) had severe TR secondary to PPM or ICD lead placement. TV replacement was performed in 14 patients (56 %), while it was repaired in the remaining 11 patients (44 %).

Hypoplastic Left Heart Syndrome

Hypoplastic left heart syndrome (HLHS) is a spectrum of malformation that share in common the inability of the left-sided structures to support the systemic circulation. It includes a variety of lesions ranging from aortic atresia or stenosis with or without mitral atresia or stenosis; the left ventricle is always hypoplastic (Fig. 19.13). Typically, the surgical management of patients with HLHS involves three-staged palliation procedures starting with the Norwood stage I and ends with the completion Fontan procedure. Surgical outcomes have been improved remarkably in the current era; however reoperation or late intervention is inevitable for the majority. Recurrent aortic arch obstruction is one example of an issue that appears after stage I Norwood and it ranges from 9 to 37 % [14]; it is very deleterious to the single ventricle as it will lead to significant systemic ventricular dysfunction and even mortality. In addition, the following are

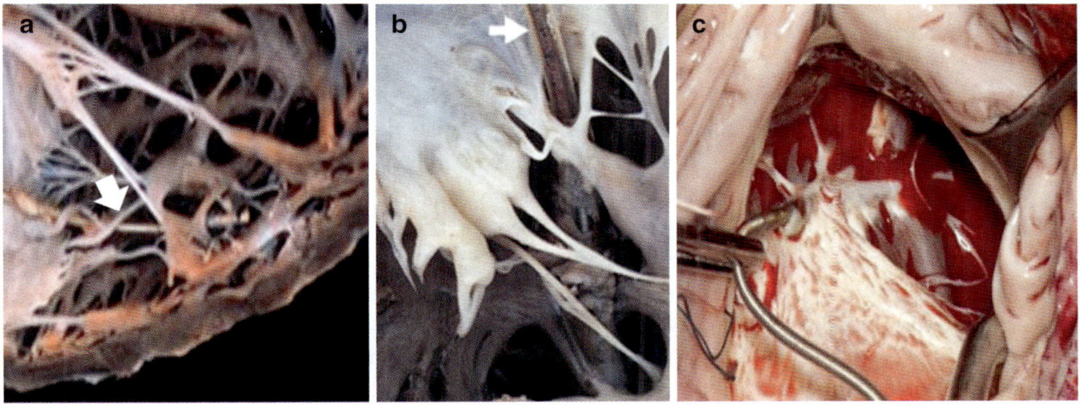

Fig. 19.12 Pathologic specimens (**a**, **b**) showing entanglement of the pacemaker lead (*arrows*) with the subvalvar apparatus of the tricuspid valve. (**c**) Intraoperative photograph showing perforation of the septal leaflet and entanglement of the tricuspid subvalvar apparatus adjacent to the anteroseptal commissure with the pacemaker or internal cardioverter-defibrillator lead

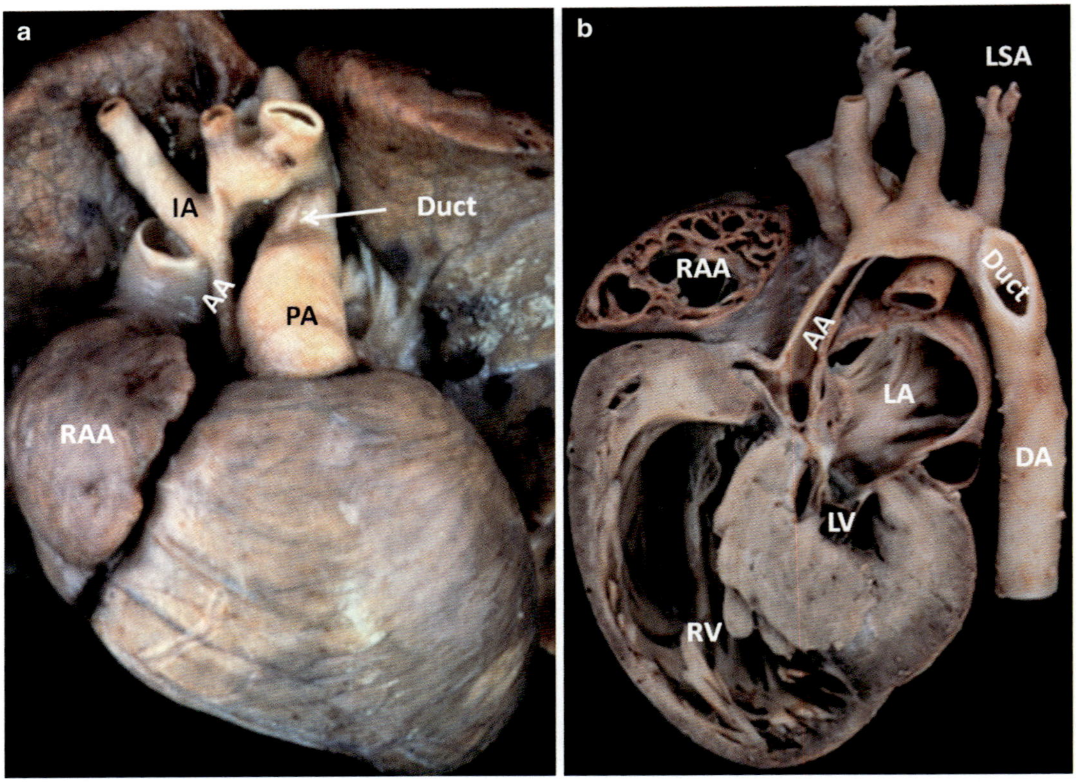

Fig. 19.13 (**a**, **b**) Pathologic specimens showing the characteristic features of hypoplastic left heart syndrome: hypoplastic aortic arch, hypoplastic left ventricle (*LV*), and diminutive ascending aorta (*AA*). *DA* descending aorta, *LSA* left subclavian artery, *LA* left atrium, *IA* innominate artery, *RV* right ventricle, *RAA* right atrial appendage

some of the issues that arise in adults who have undergone completion Fontan for HLHS:

Fontan Conversion and Arrhythmia Surgery

Those who are faced with failing Fontan circulation may be considered for Fontan conversion which entails conversion of prior atriopulmonary Fontan (Fig. 19.14) to total extracardiac cavopulmonary connection (Fig. 19.15), arrhythmia surgery, treating any concomitant systemic atrioventricular valve dysfunction, and relieving any obstruction in the Fontan pathway [15].

Neoaortic Root Aneurysm After Fontan Completion

This is similar to what can happen after Ross procedure when including the native pulmonary root in the reconstruction of the neoaorta at the time of Norwood and subsequent exposure of the pulmonary valve and root to systemic arterial pressure [16]. Valve-sparing aortic root replacement represents a reasonable option in these patients.

Transplantation

Those patients who underwent cardiac transplantation as their initial or intermediate treatment step can still present late with issues related to aortic coarctation or aneurysmal enlargement of the neoaorta that may require late intervention [17].

Percutaneous Interventions

Pulmonary Valve Replacement

PVR is one of the most common procedures performed in adults with CHD [18]. It is usually

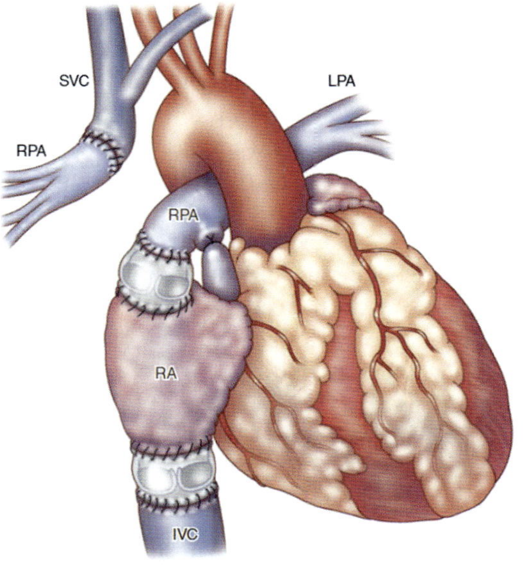

Fig. 19.14 Illustration showing the original Fontan procedure that included an end-to-side anastomosis of the distal end of right pulmonary artery (*RPA*) to superior vena cava (*SVC*) (classic Glenn anastomosis); end-to-end anastomosis of right atrial appendage (*RAA*) to proximal end of RPA by means of an aortic valved homograft; closure of atrial septal defect; insertion of a pulmonary valved homograft at the inferior vena cava (*IVC*) to right atrium (*RA*) junction; and ligation of main pulmonary artery

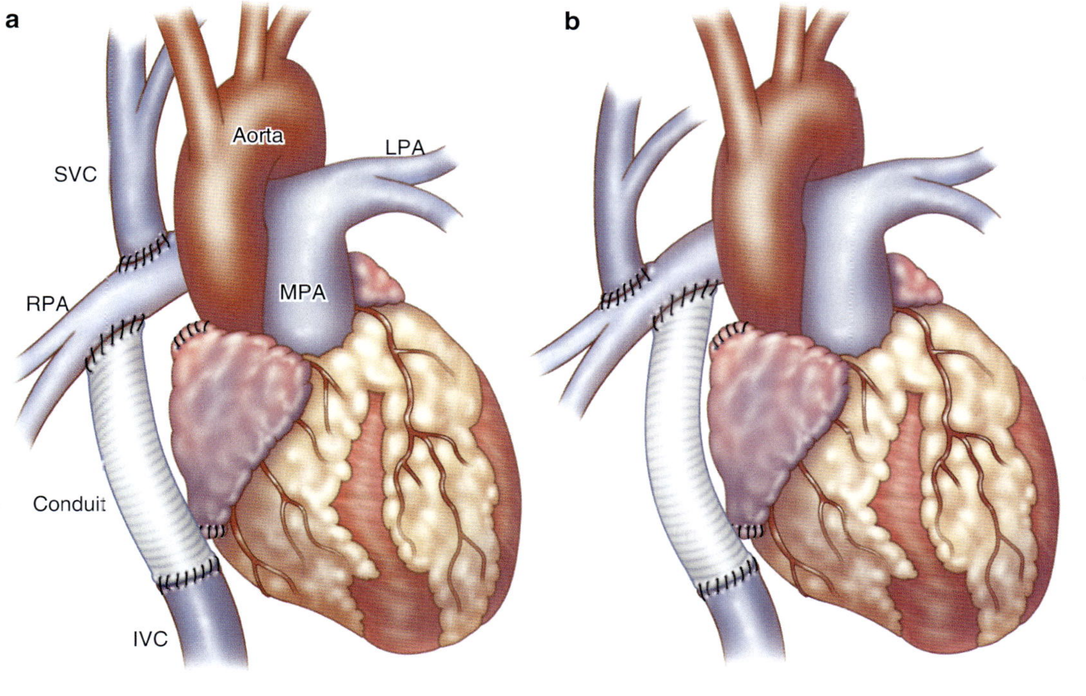

Fig. 19.15 (**a**, **b**) Extracardiac conduit-modified Fontan procedure as popularized by Marcelletti in 1990. This technique includes a bidirectional superior cavopulmonary anastomosis and placement of a synthetic graft between the inferior vena cava and the right pulmonary artery (total cavopulmonary connection). The location of the distal anastomosis between the extracardiac conduit graft and the right pulmonary artery can be to the right (**a**; Puga) or to the left (**b**; Marcelletti) of the bidirectional superior cavopulmonary anastomosis

performed for free PR that resulted from RVOT reconstruction during prior repair of tetralogy of Fallot. The etiology can be regurgitation or stenosis in the setting of a conduit for pulmonary atresia, transposition of great arteries with pulmonary stenosis, or truncus arteriosus. Reoperation is a common pathway for all these different pathologies and it is not uncommon for many to require multiple PVR during their lifetime. Transcatheter techniques have emerged as a reasonable alternative for patients who require repeat operations or those who are at high risk for reoperation. The indications and the timing for PVR have been somewhat controversial. However, the general trend is earlier intervention to avoid the deleterious effects of volume overload with subsequent right ventricular enlargement and dysfunction [19]. PVR may also be considered in the presence of RVOT obstruction due to previous conduit valve/biologic valve structural degeneration with a peak gradient >50 mmHg. Other indications may include reduced exercise capacity, increased right ventricular end-diastolic dimension, or concomitant moderate or severe TR [20]. Percutaneous PVR was first described by Bonhoeffer et al. [21] and consisted of bovine jugular venous valve that was sutured to the wall of a balloon expandable stent. A modified version of the initial device (the Melody valve; Medtronic Inc) is currently approved and is in use with good short-term results and successful relief of RVOT gradient and correction of pulmonary valve regurgitation [22].

Hybrid Strategy

Branch Pulmonary Artery Stenting

Branch pulmonary artery stenosis is frequently treated with percutaneous stenting techniques [23]. This approach may be challenging in the presence of concomitant RVOT obstruction and, therefore, the hybrid approach where deployment of these stents will be more technically feasible, provides an alternative approach [24, 25], (Figs. 19.16 and 19.17). Intraoperative branch PA stenting may also be considered as a rescue procedure following complications of the percutaneous approach. The traditional repair technique of branch PA stenosis has been patch arterioplasty, but this may not be possible in all cases. Repeat operations with extensive scarring or distally located stenosis can make surgical repair difficult and time consuming. The increased cardiopulmonary bypass time and subsequent duration of surgery can be minimized with the hybrid approach [26]. Endovascular stenting may also provide a structural support to the repaired PA and decrease the chance of compression by surrounding structures. We have published our experience with such strategy in 24 patients between 1997 and 2006 [27]. The median age was 15

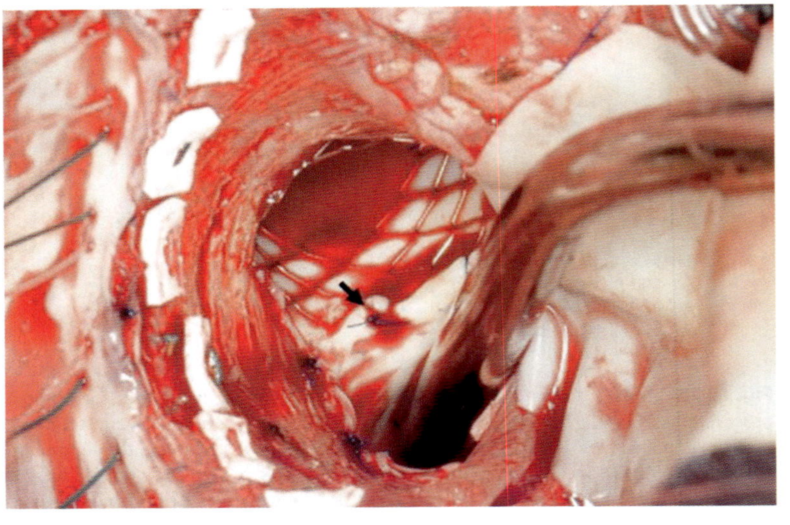

Fig. 19.16 Intraoperative photograph of a combined pulmonary valve replacement and right pulmonary artery stenting. The proximal end of the stent is flared and sutured (*arrow*) close to the pulmonary bifurcation. The bovine pericardial roof is seen on the right and the suction catheter is in the left pulmonary artery

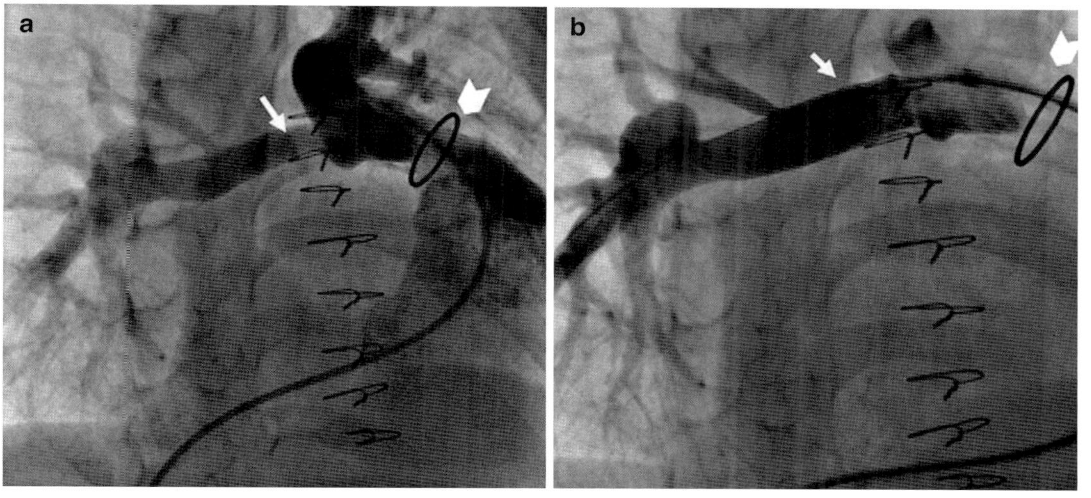

Fig. 19.17 Cardiac catheterization showing; (**a**) Percutaneous treatment of proximal right pulmonary artery stenosis (*thin arrow*) with severe right ventricle-to-pulmonary artery conduit valve (*wide arrowhead*) regurgitation. (**b**) The appropriately placed stent in the proximal right pulmonary artery (*thin arrow*)

years and a total of 27 stents were deployed, most commonly in the left PA (13 stents). The most common diagnoses were pulmonary atresia with septal defect and TOF. This was almost always done with RVOT reconstruction or pulmonary valve replacement. Two procedures were done as rescue procedures following complications (stent migration and catheter impaction) of percutaneous approaches. There was no early mortality or pulmonary artery tear, dissection, or stent thrombosis.

In these cases, preoperative imaging studies are important for surgical planning. Cardiac catheterization, CT scan, or MRI will allow determination of the appropriate stent length, stent position to avoid side-branch "jailing," and the appropriate stent diameter to achieve complete relief of the branch PA stenosis without overdilatation of the distal PA branch.

Pulmonary Venous Baffle Obstruction After Prior Atrial Switch

Although the current standard treatment for transposition of the great arteries is the arterial switch operation, the atrial switch is still performed as part of the "double-switch" operation for congenitally corrected transposition [28], and there are many late survivors of the atrial switch for transposition from the early era of cardiac surgery. Pulmonary venous pathway baffle obstruction is a potential late complication following the atrial switch operation. Treatment of such sequelae is very challenging and gaining peripheral access to the pulmonary venous baffle/pathway is also very difficult. While only case reports exist in the literature for approaches to pulmonary venous baffle obstruction, there are also only a few reports of the use of interventional catheterization techniques to relieve *systemic* venous baffle obstruction [29, 30]. We reported our experience with such approach in a 28-year-old female who underwent an atrial switch procedure at 11 months of age and presented with late pulmonary venous pathway baffle obstruction [31]. Preoperative transthoracic echocardiography revealed a mean gradient of 14 mmHg across the pulmonary venous pathway (Fig. 19.18a). A mini right thoracotomy was performed, and a purse-string suture was placed on the right atrial free wall, and a sheath was advanced allowing a stent to be deployed. The intraoperative gradient dropped to 4 mmHg after stent deployment. One year later, follow-up echocardiography revealed a widely patent stent (Fig. 19.18b). The same technique was repeated in two other patients from our institution with similar success.

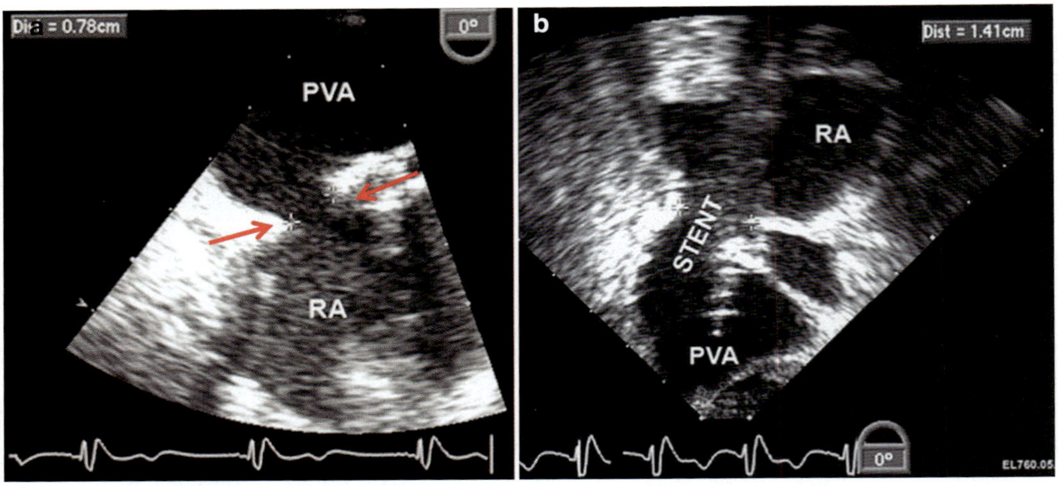

Fig. 19.18 (**a**) Two-dimensional transesophageal echocardiography during a hybrid procedure demonstrates severe stenosis (0.78 cm) of the pathway (between *arrows*) between the pulmonary venous atrium (*PVA*) and the native right atrium (*RA*) in a patient that had undergone an atrial switch procedure. (**b**) Following placement of a stent across the stenosis. Pulmonary venous pathway diameter now equals 1.41 cm after stent deployment

Several advantages to this technique are worth mentioning. The operation is performed via a small incision with adequate exposure to the right atrial wall. It provides direct access to the area of obstruction thereby avoiding the difficulty that is usually encountered with the percutaneous approaches. Other advantages include the avoidance of CPB and the risks associated with repeat sternotomy.

Mayo Clinic Experience

We reviewed our experience with 984 adult patients (495 male) with CHD who underwent reoperation between January 1993 and December 2007 [32]. The mean age at reoperation was 36.4 years. The most common diagnoses were conotruncal anomaly, 361 (37 %); Ebstein/tricuspid valve, 174 (18 %); pulmonary stenosis/right ventricular outflow tract obstruction, 92 (9 %); single ventricle, 71 (7 %); atrioventricular septal defect, 64 (7 %); subaortic stenosis, 62 (6 %); aortic arch abnormalities, 23 (2 %); and anomalous pulmonary veins, 21 (2 %). The overall mortality was 3.6 %. Repeat sternotomy with the potential risk of cardiac injury conferred an increased mortality of 6 %. The following factors were independent predictors of cardiac injury: single-ventricle diagnosis and increased number of prior sternotomies. It was also noticed that with increase time from previous sternotomy, there is a decrease incidence of cardiac injury. Predictors of perioperative mortality included urgency of the operation, single-ventricle diagnosis, and longer bypass time.

Summary

In summary, adults with CHD are subject to repeat reoperations and complex procedures. Thoughtful surgical planning and proper preoperative imaging are critical to a safe, successful operation.

References

1. Hoffman JI, Kaplan S, Liberthson RR. Prevalence of congenital heart disease. Am Heart J. 2004;147:425–39.
2. Warnes CA. The adult with congenital heart disease: born to be bad? J Am Coll Cardiol. 2005;46:1–8.
3. Christenson JT, Schmziger M, Simmat F. Reoperative coronary artery bypass. Risk factors for early mortality and late survival. Eur J Cardiothorac Surg. 1997;1:129–33.

4. Park CB, Suri RM, Burkhart HM, Greason KL, Dearani JA, Schaff HV, Sundt 3rd TM. Identifying patients at particular risk of injury during repeat sternotomy: analysis of 2555 cardiac reoperations. J Thorac Cardiovasc Surg. 2010;140(5):1028–35.
5. Walther T, Rastan A, Dähnert I, et al. A novel adhesion barrier facilitates reoperations in complex congenital cardiac surgery. J Thorac Cardiovasc Surg. 2005;129:359–63.
6. Kirshbom PM, Myung RJ, Simsic JM, et al. One thousand repeat sternotomies for congenital cardiac surgery: risk factors for reentry injury. Ann Thorac Surg. 2009;88:158–61.
7. Akl BF, Pert SB, Wernly JA. Use of a sagittal oscillating saw for repeat sternotomy: a safer and simpler technique. Ann Thorac Surg. 1984;38:646–7.
8. Yalonetsky S, Tobler D, Greutmann M, et al. Cardiac magnetic resonance imaging and the assessment of ebstein anomaly in adults. Am J Cardiol. 2011;107(5):767–73.
9. Koelling TM, Aaronson KD, Cody RJ, et al. Prognostic significance of mitral regurgitation and tricuspid regurgitation in patients with left ventricular systolic dysfunction. Am Heart J. 2002;144:524–9.
10. Lee JW, Song JM, Park JP, et al. Long-term prognosis of isolated significant tricuspid regurgitation. Circ J. 2010;74:375–80.
11. Shibata Y, Sato M, Chanda J, et al. Isolated tricuspid regurgitation due to atypical morphology of anterior-posterior leaflets in an adult: a case report and review of the literature. J Cardiovasc Surg. 1999;40:527–30.
12. Said SM, Burkhart HM, Dearani JA. Surgical management of congenital (non-Ebstein) tricuspid valve regurgitation. Semin Thorac Cardiovasc Surg Pediatr Card Surg Annu. 2012;15(1):46–60.
13. Lin G, Nishimura RA, Connolly HM, et al. Severe symptomatic tricuspid valve regurgitation due to permanent pacemaker or implantable cardioverter-defibrillator leads. J Am Coll Cardiol. 2005;45:1672–5.
14. Ishino K, Stumper O, De Giovanni JJ, et al. The modified Norwood procedure for hypoplastic left heart syndrome: early to intermediate results of 120 patients with particular reference to aortic arch repair. J Thorac Cardiovasc Surg. 1999;117:920–30.
15. Said SM, Burkhart HM, Dearani JA. Fontan connections: past, present, and future. World J Pediatr Cong Heart Surg. 2012;32:171–82.
16. Laudito A, Brook MM, Suleman S, et al. The Ross procedure in children and young adults: a word of caution. J Thorac Cardiovasc Surg. 2001;122:147–53.
17. Said SM, Dearani JA, Silversides CK, et al. Longer-term issues for young adults with hypoplastic left heart syndrome: contraception, pregnancy, transition, transfer, counseling, and re-operation. Cardiol Young. 2011;21 Suppl 2:93–100.
18. Dore A, Glancy DL, Stone S, Menashe VD, Somerville J. Cardiac surgery for grown-up congenital heart patients: survey of 307 consecutive operations from 1991–1994. Am J Cardiol. 1997;80:906–13.
19. Perloff JK, Natterson PD. Atrial aarhythmias in adults after repair of teratlogy of Fallot. Ann Thorac Surg. 1995;91:2118–9.
20. Warnes CA, Williams RG, Bashore TM, Child JS, Connolly HM, Dearani JA, et al. ACC/AHA 2008 Guidelines for the management of adults with congenital heart disease: a report of the American College of Cardiology/American Heart Association Task Force on Practice Guidelines (writing committee to develop guidelines on the management of adults with congenital heart disease). Circulation. 2008;118:2395–451.
21. Bonhoeffer P, Boudjemline Y, Saliba Z, et al. Percutaneous replacement of pulmonary valve in a right ventricle to pulmonary artery prosthetic conduit with valve dysfunction. Lancet. 2000;356:1403–5.
22. McElhinney DB, Hellebrand WE, Zahn EM, et al. Short- and medium-term outcomes after transcatheter pulmonary valve placement in the expanded multicenter US Melody valve trial. Circulation. 2010;122:507–16.
23. Bergersen L, Lock JE. What is the current option of first choice for treatment of pulmonary arterial stenosis? Cardiol Young. 2006;16(4):329–38.
24. Ing FF. Delivery of stents to target lesions: techniques of intraoperative stent implantation and intraoperative angiograms. Pediatr Cardiol. 2005;26(3):260–6.
25. Shaffer KM, Mullins CE, Grifka RG, O'Laughlin MP, McMahon W, Ing FF, Nihill MR. Intravascular stents in congenital heart disease: short- and long-term results from a large single-center experience. J Am Coll Cardiol. 1998;31(3):661–7.
26. Bacha EA, Marshall AC, McElhinney DB, del Nido PJ. Hybrid pediatric cardiac surgery. Pediatr Cardiol. 2005;26(4):315–22.
27. Menon SC, Cetta F, Dearani JA, Burkhart HM, Cabalka AK, Hagler DJ. Hybrid intraoperative pulmonary artery stent placement for congenital heart disease. Am J Cardiol. 2008;102:1737–41.
28. Koh M, Yagihara T, Uemura H, et al. Intermediate results of the double-switch operations for atrioventricular discordance. Ann Thorac Surg. 2006;81:671–7.
29. Dragulescu A, Sidibe N, Aubert F, Fraisse A. Successful use of covered stent to treat superior systemic baffle obstruction and leak after atrial switch procedure. Pediatr Cardiol. 2008;29:954–6.
30. Ebeid MR, Gaymes CH, McMullan MR, Shores JC, Smith JC, Joransen JA. Catheter management of occluded superior baffle after atrial switch procedures for transposition of great vessels. Am J Cardiol. 2005;95:782–6.
31. Sareyyupoglu B, Burkhart HM, Hagler DJ, Dearani JA, Cabalka A, Cetta F, Schaff HV. Hybrid approach to repair of pulmonary venous baffle obstruction after atrial switch operation. Ann Thorac Surg. 2009;88(5):1710–1.
32. Holst KA, Dearani JA, Burkhart HM, Connolly HM, Warnes CA, Li Z, Schaff HV. Risk factors and early outcomes of multiple reoperations in adults with congenital heart disease. Ann Thorac Surg. 2011;92:122–30.

MRI in Repaired Congenital Heart Disease

20

Julia Geiger and Michael Markl

Congenital heart disease (CHD) represents the most common form of birth defects and is the leading cause of birth defect-related deaths [1, 2]. Current data suggest that the total incidence for nonchromosomal CHD in the USA is 12 per 1,000 births [2]. An estimated 6 % of these babies die before the age of 1 year [3, 4]. As treatment of CHD has improved, there is a need for regular diagnostic follow-up in this growing population across all age ranges [5, 6]. Expert guidelines for the definition of care have been developed but are based on limited data, and there is an ongoing debate about indications for surgery or re-intervention and longitudinal evaluation [7, 8]. It is therefore crucial to establish efficient methods for the diagnosis, therapy planning, and post-interventional monitoring of CHD in order to provide biomarkers for long-term outcome and longitudinal care.

The main needs in CHD are successful early treatment and ongoing care for affected children and adults. Transthoracic and transesophageal echocardiography (TTE and TEE) are readily available imaging options and are the primary modalities for managing patients with CHD [9, 10]. The major limitation of TTE and TEE is their inability to sufficiently visualize the pulmonary arteries and veins beyond the hilus. In addition, TTE and TEE are limited in their ability to accurately quantify ventricular volumes and blood flow parameters. As patients grow older, acoustic windows often become more restrictive and further limit the diagnostic role of echocardiography. More complete anatomic and functional assessment can be performed with catheter-based angiography [11], computed tomographic angiography (CTA) [12, 13], or magnetic resonance imaging (MRI) [7, 14–16]. Due to radiation concerns, particularly in the pediatric patient population, cardiac catheterization and CT should only be considered as modalities of second choice [17]. For many years, the assessment of the left ventricle was emphasized in diagnosis of CHD. However, the importance of studying the vastly different morphology and function of the right ventricle has recently been recognized [18]. Imaging protocols adapted to the right heart have been developed to evaluate morphologic changes [19–21].

In recent years, cardiovascular MRI has gained increasing relevance for evaluation of right and left ventricular structure and function and is used as a standard tool in the assessment of repaired CHD next to echocardiography [22]. In this context, MRI can provide standardized quantification of peak velocities, volumetric blood flow, or retrograde fraction to evaluate valve insufficiency. For the assessment of ventricular

J. Geiger, MD (✉)
Department of Radiology, Medical Physics, University Hospital Freiburg, Hugstetter Str. 55, 79106 Freiburg, Germany
e-mail: julia.geiger@uniklinik-freiburg.de

M. Markl, PhD
Department of Radiology and Biomedical Engineering, Northwestern University, 737 N. Michigan Avenue Suite 1600, Chicago, IL, 60611, USA
e-mail: mmarkl@northwestern.edu

F. Saremi (ed.), *Cardiac CT and MR for Adult Congenital Heart Disease*,
DOI 10.1007/978-1-4614-8875-0_20,

volumes, MRI is considered the gold standard [23, 24]. In addition, cardiac MRI permits the evaluation of the thoracic anatomy, global and regional cardiac function, blood flow in the great vessels, and myocardial viability within one examination. Recently introduced flow-sensitive MRI techniques with full volumetric coverage and encoding of all three principal directions of blood flow [often termed 4-dimensional (4D) flow MRI] can provide information on 3D hemodynamics of the heart and surrounding vessels.

As surgical techniques have improved, patients with CHD are being followed into their fourth and fifth decades of life, such that there are now more adults with CHD than children. In fact, the number of adults with CHD in the USA now exceeds more than 1,000,000 patients, and epidemiologists anticipate that 1 in 150 young adults are expected to have some form of CHD in the next decade. Such patients will require frequent diagnostic testing in order to plan surgical repair, assess preoperative risk, and/or survey for important long-term complications. Since the diagnostic questions of this patient population are different from the typical cardiac disease patient in adulthood [25], it is essential that radiologists have an understanding of the pathophysiology of common forms of CHD and a good knowledge of the typical postsurgical anatomy as well as mid- and long-term complications.

In the following chapter we focus on the application of MRI to the most common repaired CHD one will face in routine diagnostics: patients after repair of tetralogy of Fallot (TOF), transposition of the great arteries (TGA), and heart defects leading to single-ventricle physiology and Fontan procedure.

Magnetic Resonance Imaging

Cardiovascular MRI has undergone substantial advances over the last decade. A typical imaging protocol for the diagnostic workup of CHD patients is shown in Fig. 20.1. After initial localizer scans, the data acquisition work flow includes the assessment of cardiac function with multiple ECG synchronized 2D time-resolved (CINE) pulse sequences that cover the heart in different orientations and in multiple contiguous slices.

Images are obtained during suspended respiration in order to avoid artifact from respiratory motion. Vascular anatomy is assessed with a 3D contrast-enhanced MR angiogram (MRA). For

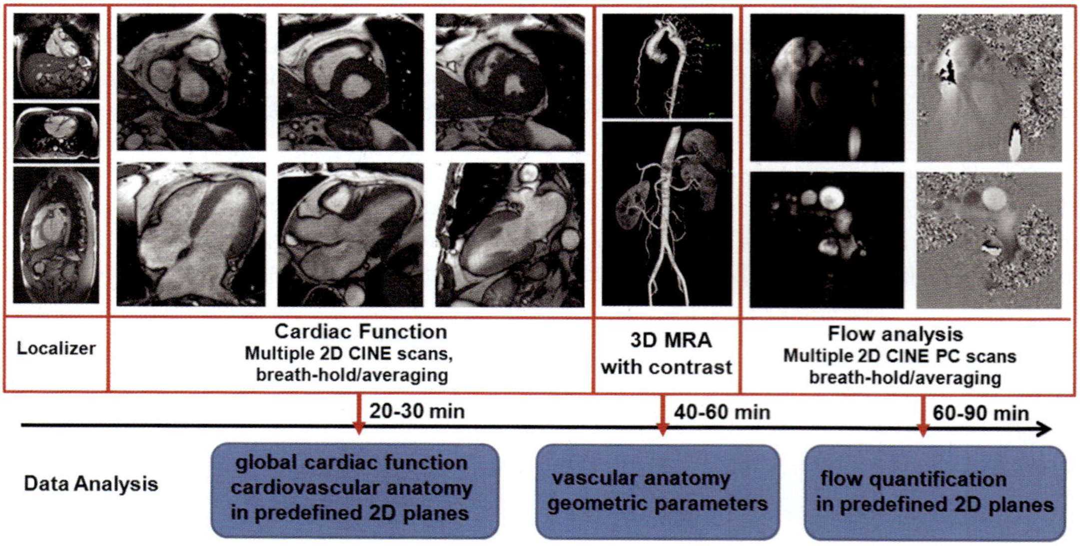

Fig. 20.1 Work flow of standard congenital heart disease MRI. Dark-blood or bright-blood sequences may be included for further anatomic assessment. Delayed post contrast images can be obtained at the end if necessary. *2D* two dimensional, *3D* three dimensional, *MRA* MR angiography, *PC* phase contrast

the purposes of hemodynamic analysis in patients with CHD, multiple 2D CINE phase-contrast (PC) images are used to provide maps of the through-plane velocity of blood. CHD exams typically require multiple acquisitions which, due to the complex cardiovascular geometry, are difficult to localize and may have to be repeated several times. As a result, CHD exams require many more MR measurements compared to patients with less complex pathologies and can be up to 60–90 min in duration [26]. To ensure robust image quality for cardiovascular MRI, a dedicated phased-array cardiac coil (typically 12–32 channels) should be used.

The majority of the cardiovascular MRI protocols established for adult acquired heart disease focus on the evaluation of impaired global function, perfusion, and viability of the left ventricle that are associated with myocardial infarction and myocarditis or aortic valve disease. In patients after repair for CHD, however, the right heart is often affected either due to progressive overload as a consequence of pulmonary regurgitation or due to its function as systemic ventricle [21]. MRI-based assessment of the right ventricle is more challenging and should be adapted to the individual heart defect and type of surgical repair. Moreover, for pediatric cardiac MRI exams, it is important to adjust image parameters to the faster heart rate and smaller size of children [14]. Younger children have to be examined in sedation or during anesthesia. Therefore, sequences with diaphragm navigation are important.

In general, a CHD MRI protocol consists of four groups of acquisition techniques to obtain information on the anatomy and function of the heart and surrounding vessels:

1. Anatomic/morphologic imaging
2. Dynamic imaging: ventricular and valve function
3. Blood flow quantification
4. 3D angiography

1. Anatomic assessment is typically based on bright-blood imaging using fast gradient echo and balanced steady-state free precession (SSFP) sequences in the three standard anatomic dimensions [27]. These sequences have an inherently high myocardial-to-blood-contrast and can be performed during breath-held imaging [28]. Alternatively, black-blood pulse sequences (T1- or T2-weighted fast spin echo, T2-weighted HASTE) can be applied. More recently introduced respiratory- and ECG-gated 3D SSFP pulse sequences provide high image quality and have the advantage to obtain an isotropic volumetric data set which can be reformatted in multiplanar directions [29]. Stents often lead to artifacts which tend to be more pronounced in SSFP than in T1 TSE sequences (Fig. 20.2).

2. ECG-gated and time-resolved 2D (CINE) SSFP sequences are used for dynamic imaging of cardiac function in the standard short-axis, long-axis 4-chamber/2-chamber/3-chamber, and axial transverse views. Additional orientations such as the right ventricular outflow tract (RVOT) or coronal may be acquired depending on the specific heart defect [30]. In addition to the assessment of ventricular motion over the heart cycle, CINE MRI can be employed to evaluate systolic and diastolic valve movements and detect valve or conduit stenosis and insufficiency. 2D CINE images covering the heart ("short-axis stack" sections from base to apex) are used for the quantification of global cardiac function (stroke volume, ejection fraction) as well as ventricular mass and volumes. The summation disc method for ventricular volume calculation and ejection fraction is considered the clinical reference standard [31, 32]. Cardiovascular MR measurements show good interobserver variability and high reproducibility [33–35], and there are several studies which provide age- and gender-specific reference values for right ventricular volumes for adults [36] and pediatric patients [37, 38]. The right ventricle differs from the left ventricle in its geometric shape but also in the more trabeculated myocardium and thinner wall. Due to its complex geometry, image acquisition of multi-slice 2D CINE MRI in axial orientation has been suggested as the method of choice by a number of groups [39, 40] (Fig. 20.3).

3. For the assessment of aortic and pulmonary valve disease or intracardiac shunts, 2D CINE phase-contrast (PC) MRI with through-plane velocity encoding is applied [41]. This technique allows quantifying blood flow (net flow,

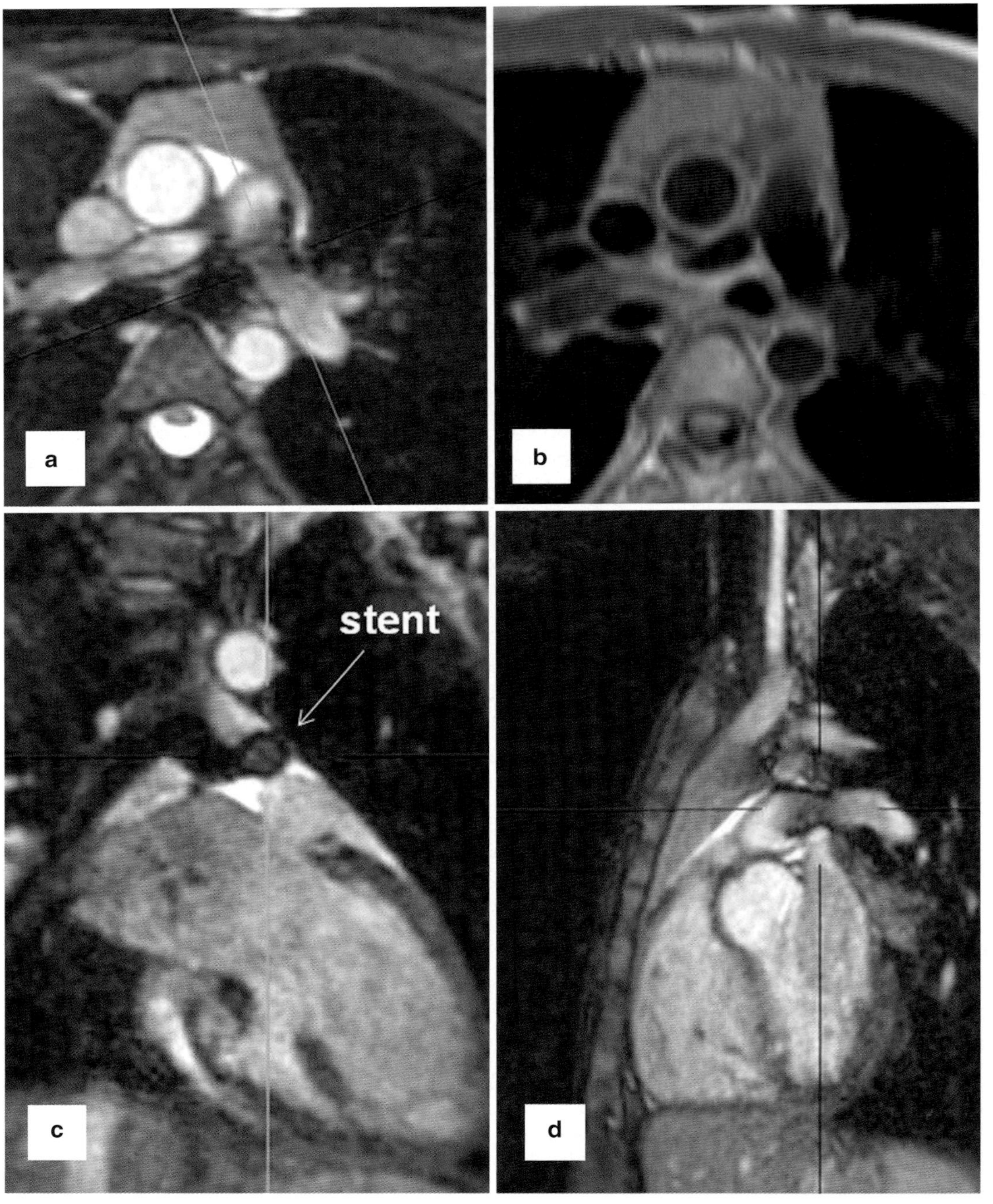

Fig. 20.2 Balanced steady-state free precession sequence with multi-planar reformations (MPR) in a patient with stent implantation in hypoplastic left pulmonary artery. (**a**) Axial, (**c**) coronal, (**d**) sagittal. (**b**) Axial dark-blood fast spin echo T1-weighted image at the level of the stent

peak velocity, regurgitant fraction) to evaluate vessel, valve or conduit stenosis or intracardiac shunts (Fig. 20.4). Using the simplified Bernoulli equation, the pressure gradient over a stenosis can be estimated. Similar to direct trans-stenotic pressure measurements invasively acquired by

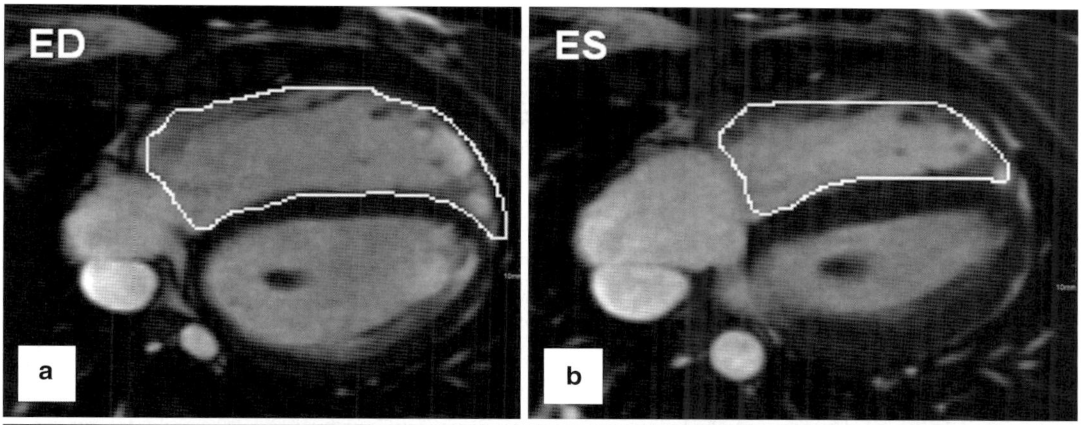

Right Ventricle - Normalized

Cardiac Function			Normal Range (F) (MRI)	Units
End Diastolic Volume	EDV	157.1	48.00 ... 87.00	ml/m^2
End Systolic Volume	ESV	73.7	11.01 ... 27.60	ml/m^2
Stroke Volume	SV	83.4	27.00 ... 57.00	ml/m^2
Cardiac Index	CI	5.34	1.75 ... 3.80	l/min/m^2
Myocardial Mass (at ED)		----	----	g/m^2
Myocardial Mass (Avg)		----	----	g/m^2
Filling and Ejection Data				
Peak Ejection Rate		----	n.a.	EDV/sec
Peak Filling Rate		----	n.a.	EDV/sec

c

* normalized to patient surface area 1.7 m^2

Fig. 20.3 Volumetry of the right ventricle based on axial (transversal) cine-balanced steady-state free precession sequence images. (**a**) *ED* end diastole. (**b**) *ES* end systole. (**c**) Table shows an example for normalized to body surface area cardiac parameters for a female 14-year-old patient with enlarged right ventricle after surgery for tetralogy of Fallot

catheter or echocardiography, pressure gradients can be estimated following the modified Bernoulli equation $\Delta P = 4(v^2)$. A further clinical application of 2D CINE PC MRI is the evaluation of shunting, which is indicative of septal defects allowing blood transfer from the arterial to the venous system or vice versa (from the system with the higher to the lower pressure). To quantify shunt volume, two flow measurements are performed. 2D CINE PC MRI in the ascending aorta and in the pulmonary artery is used to quantify the left and right ventricular stroke volumes, QS and QP, respectively. The ratio of QP/QS represents the direction of shunt and the shunt volume. For QP/QS = 1, no shunt is present; if QP/QS > 1, a shunt from the aortic circulation to the pulmonary circulation is present and vice versa for QP/QS < 1.

2D CINE PC MRI is a valid technique that can easily be performed in simple vessel geometries. For complex anatomic situations after the repair of a congenital heart defect, however, flow measurements in multiple 2D planes are often

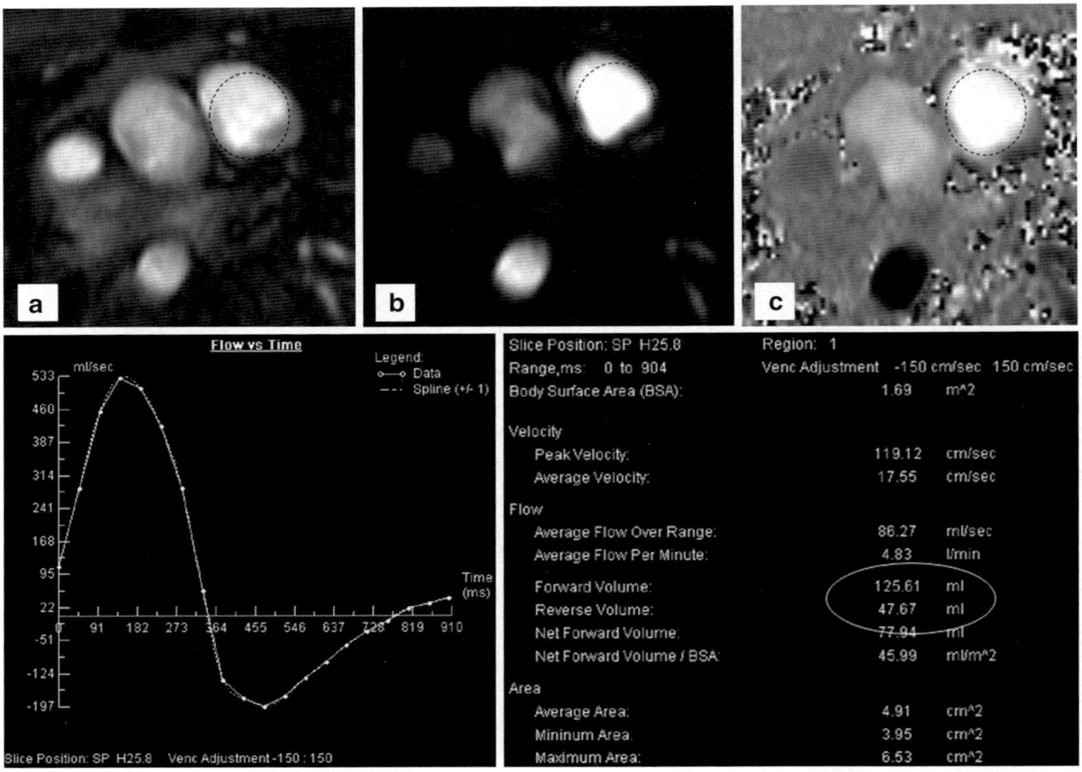

Fig. 20.4 Two-dimensional phase-contrast imaging with region of interest (*dotted circles*) in the pulmonary trunk: (**a**) Cine, (**b**) magnitude, and (**c**) phase-encoding image of a patient with relevant pulmonary reflux. Flow-time curve reveals retrograde flow below the *x*-axis. Table shows quantitative data with a regurgitation fraction of about 38 %

needed to capture the complex hemodynamic situation. This can be a rather challenging task, even for experienced technicians and radiologists. Measurements often have to be repeated due to incorrect velocity encoding or placement and angulation of imaging planes.

4. Gadolinium contrast-enhanced MR angiography (CE MRA) often reveals more detailed anatomic information of the surrounding vessels compared to the standard anatomic sequences and can depict aortopulmonary collaterals. CE MRA can be performed as a high spatial resolution angiography which can depict, for example, small collateral vessels in aortic coarctation (Fig. 20.5). In other cases the use of time-resolved MRA is preferred which allows to depict the dynamics of the passage of the injected contrast medium through the different cardiac compartments and vessels to simultaneous assess the pulmonary arteries, aorta, and shunts [42, 43] (Fig. 20.6). Additional late-enhancement imaging for viability imaging may be considered to evaluate potential left or right ventricular fibrosis or scars due to coronary insufficiency.

Traditionally, MR imaging of flow using PC sequence is accomplished by using methods that resolve single-directional flow in two spatial dimensions of an individual slice. More recently, 3D spatial encoding combined with three-directional velocity encoded PC MRI (4D flow MRI) has drawn increased attention. 4D flow MRI offers the ability to measure and to visualize the temporal evolution of complex blood flow patterns within an acquired 3D volume. 4D flow MRI has become a valuable method for the comprehensive assessment of 3D cardiovascular hemodynamics within a wide range of applications [44–50]. Using 4D flow MRI, pathological blood flow patterns in

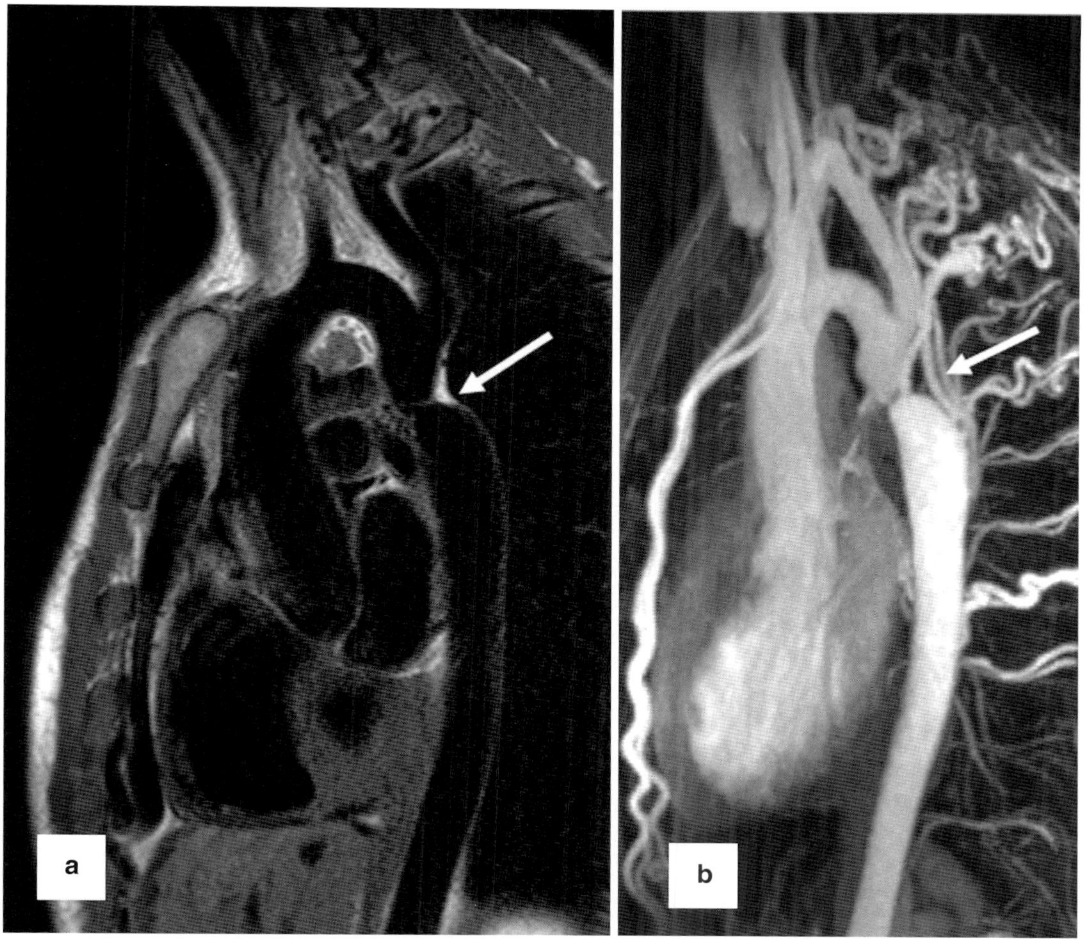

Fig. 20.5 (**a**) Dark-blood T2 pulse sequence reveals aortic coarctation (*arrow*). (**b**) High spatial resolution contrast-enhanced MR angiography for depiction of multiple collateral arteries (intercostal and internal mammary) in (*arrow*) aortic coarctation

the aorta caused by aortic valve disease or aortic coarctation or in patients with Marfan syndrome have been evaluated in comparison with normal aortic hemodynamics [51–55]. Correlations between morphologic changes and flow alterations as well as the development of aneurysms and abnormal wall shear stress were examined [52, 56–58]. The 4D flow MRI acquisition scan can be prescribed as a single 3D volumetric acquisition covering the whole mediastinal cardiovascular system and therefore has several advantages in comparison with multiple 2D PC MRI: (1) All vessels of interest are scanned within on a single measurement, (2) pre- and post-processing tools allow investigation of blood flow at any location in the vessel of interest at every time point during the heart cycle, and (3) 3D visualization of complex blood flow patterns.

Since the acquisition of volumetric data requires considerably longer total scan times (up to 20 min) compared to traditional 2D CINE PC MRI, exams can no longer be performed during a breath hold. Patient breathing can cause data inconsistencies that result in image ghosting and blurring. Therefore, respiratory gating is usually applied to minimize artifacts. Most widely available approaches include bellows reading or navigator gating of the diaphragm

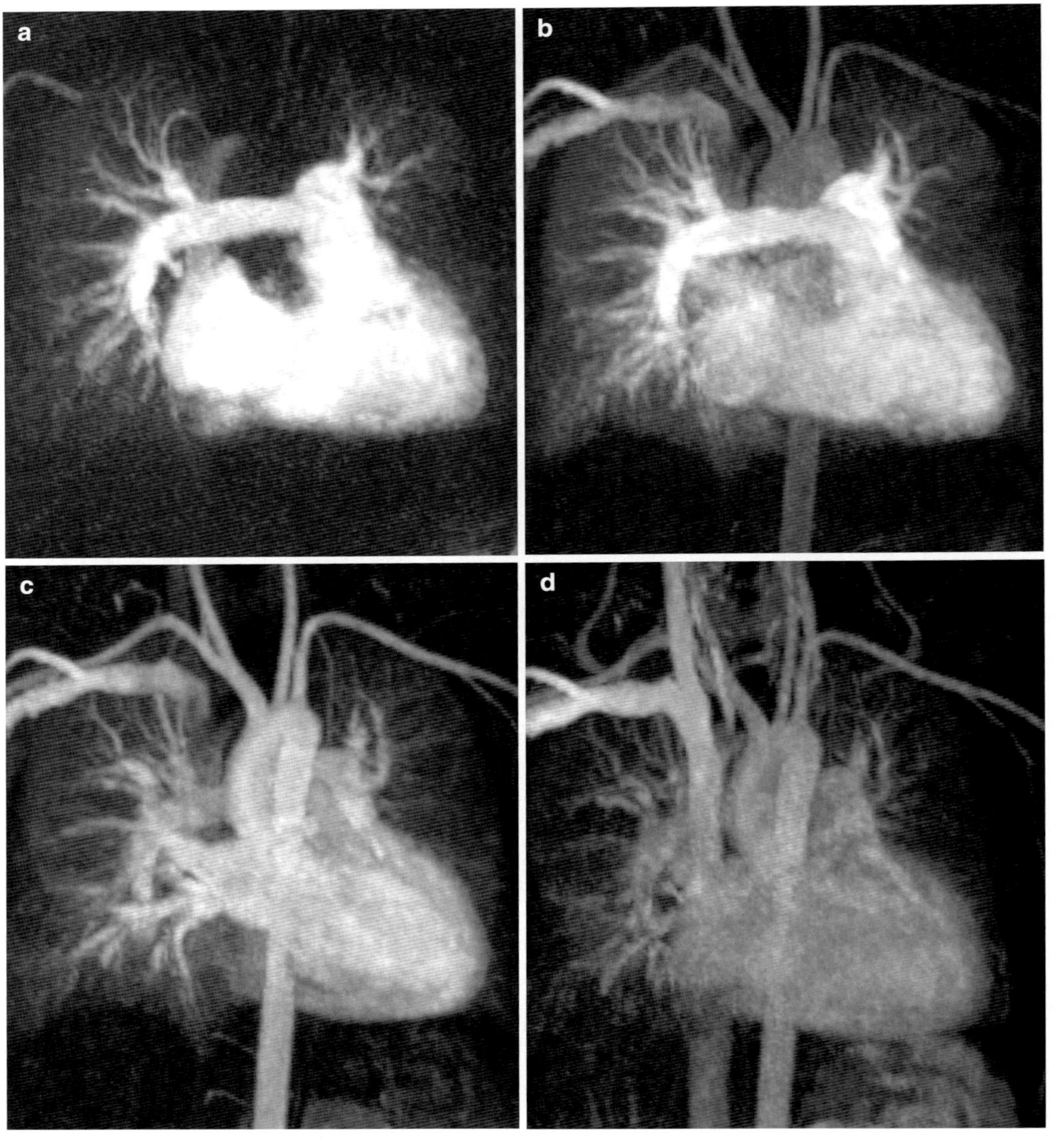

Fig. 20.6 Time-resolved contrast-enhanced MR angiography in a patient with repaired tetralogy of Fallot at four different time steps: (**a**) At 25 s after gadolinium injection, (**b**) at 30 s, (**c**) at 35 s, (**d**) at 46 s. (**a**) The right atrium, ventricle, and pulmonary arteries are equally enhanced. (**b**) Enhancement of the right heart, pulmonary arteries, and veins; beginning enhancement of the aorta and supra-aortic branches. (**c**) Persisting pulmonary vessel enhancement which does not interfere with the left ventricle and sharp aortic enhancement. (**d**) Residual contrast medium in the heart, pulmonary vessels, and aorta in the venous phase due to prolongated contrast-medium injection

movements. Overall scan time depends on heart rate and efficiency of respiration control and takes about 5–10 min for a volume covering the thoracic aorta and 10–20 min for whole-heart acquisitions.

To subsequently analyze the flow data by quantitative means and visualization of complex, three-directional blood flow patterns various tools have been proposed. The complex nature of the 4D flow MRI data (three spatial dimension, three velocity directions, and time within the cardiac cycles) imposes the challenge to translate the multidimensional information into images that can clearly depict the underlying anatomic and functional information. The combination of angiographic data (3D PC MRA) and 3D blood flow visualization, which can both be derived from the 4D flow data, can be powerful tools to efficiently display vascular anatomy and blood flow in 3D and over time.

There are different methods for the visualization of three-directional blood flow including 3D streamlines, time-resolved 3D pathlines, and 2D vector graphs. Vector graph displays the magnitude and direction of blood velocity within a specific voxel, encompassing all three measured velocity directions; 3D streamlines are used to describe an instantaneous path tangent to the velocity vectors at a specific point in time and provide an overview over flow field patterns at a specific point within the cardiac cycle. Time-resolved pathlines can be considered massless particles that display the temporal evolution of the blood flow velocity data over one or multiple heartbeats. Both streamlines and pathlines can be color-coded according to the flow velocity magnitude which allows a clear visualization of the velocity distribution within the cardiac chambers and vessels. Alternatively, traces can be color-coded according to their vascular origin to identify complex flow pathways in complex cases of CHD (Fig. 20.7).

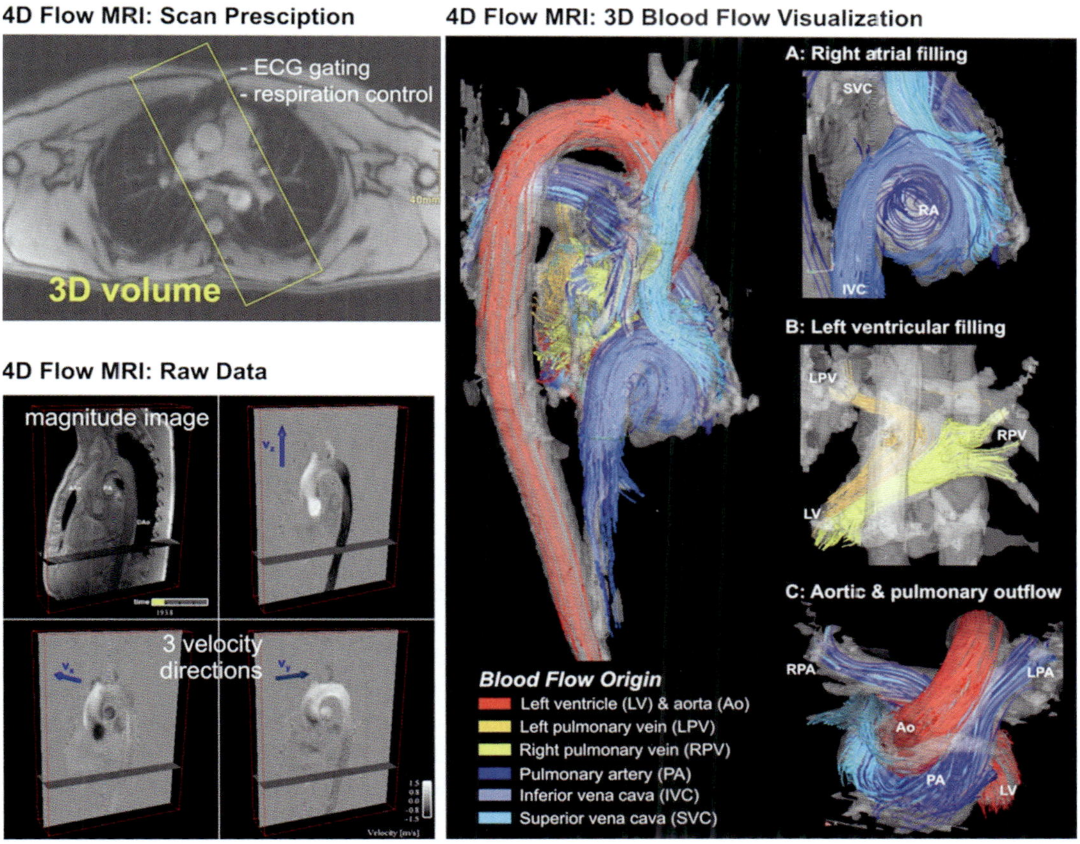

Fig. 20.7 Four-dimensional (*4D*) flow MRI data acquisition: Measurements are synchronized with the ECG cycle and the resulting raw data comprise information along all three spatial dimensions, three velocity directions, and time in the cardiac cycle. 3D blood flow visualization of the heart and large vessels using streamlines show the large-scale intracavity flow structures in ventricular systole and diastole in a healthy volunteer. *Color* coding is based on the streamline origin

Since 4D flow MRI data reflect the true underlying time-resolved blood flow velocity vector field, it is possible to perform quantitative analysis of the measured blood flow. Previous studies have demonstrated close agreement for flow derived from standard time-resolved 2D and 4D data [59, 60].

The aforementioned advantages play a key role for the use of 4D MRI technique in repaired CHD, particularly for the evaluation of the pulmonary arteries and the low-pressure system which is affected more frequently in this patient cohort than in adults with acquired valve or heart diseases.

Tetralogy of Fallot After Repair

Tetralogy of Fallot (TOF), the most common cyanotic congenital heart defect, accounts for about 5–10 % of all congenital heart diseases [61, 62]. Based on the main defects of this relatively common CHD (pulmonary stenosis, ventricular septal defect (VSD), overriding aorta, and hypertrophy of the right ventricle), these patients usually undergo corrective surgery in their first year of life. Advances in diagnosis, surgical techniques, and postoperative treatment have led to an increasing number of patients reaching adulthood [63] and a high survival rate of almost 90 % at 30 years [64].

Surgical treatment for TOF consists of the closure of the VSD and reconstruction of the RVOT [65]. Despite the great progress of surgical management, the majority of adult patients are burdened with functional abnormalities which can usually be tolerated well until adolescence [66]. Different surgical techniques have been used for RVOT reconstruction: homograft, transannular patch, or a valve-preserving technique. Despite the success of these interventional techniques, restenosis or aneurysm formation of the pulmonary outflow tract can complicate the patients' mid- and long-term outcome [67, 68]. Pulmonary valve insufficiency with consecutive right ventricular volume overload is the most common and serious postoperative long-term complication in more than 70 % of TOF patients after repair [69, 70]. Progressive right ventricular dilatation or reduced ventricular function is an indicator of the need for valve replacement [71, 72].

MRI is superior to echocardiography for the evaluation of pulmonary artery stenosis, for detecting and quantifying pulmonary valve insufficiency, for assessing right ventricle volume, and for monitoring progression of pulmonary regurgitation and right ventricular dilatation [22, 24, 73]. The role of MRI as the preferred noninvasive imaging modality in patients with repaired TOF has gained international acceptance [66].

Standard MRI protocols based on ECG-gated SSFP sequences provide anatomic and volumetric information. Typically, the right ventricle is dilated and has a thickened trabecular wall. In the 4-chamber view, the interventricular septum is shifted backward to a horizontal position. Proximal stenosis of the left pulmonary artery (LPA) can often be observed on anatomic images, occasionally in association with poststenotic ectasia or in conjunction with hypoplastic LPA (Fig. 20.8). Time-resolved contrast-enhanced MRA can provide information on abnormal lung perfusion by depicting asymmetric contrast-medium distribution to both lungs (Fig. 20.8). MRA can additionally help to detect abnormalities of the aorta and supra-aortic arteries. In this context, post-processing of the MRA data to generate 3D surface-rendered or maximum intensity projection (MIP) images can often provide an improved 3D impression of the aortic and pulmonary vasculature (Fig. 20.9).

2D CINE MRI in oblique sagittal orientation to depict the RVOT should be acquired in addition to basic 4- and 2-chamber views. By viewing 2D CINE images dynamically over the cardiac cycle, jet flow phenomena or flow turbulences caused by valve stenosis or insufficiency can be observed in the pulmonary outflow tract and pulmonary arteries of repaired TOF patients (Fig. 20.10). To quantify aortic and pulmonary blood flow and the degree of valve regurgitation, 2D PC MRI is used. Postsurgical anatomy often complicates 2D PC MRI planning, and RVOT 2D CINE images can facilitate the exact placement of the 2D PC plane in the main pulmonary artery.

For the assessment of ventricular volumes and global cardiac function, 2D CINE SSFP planes in

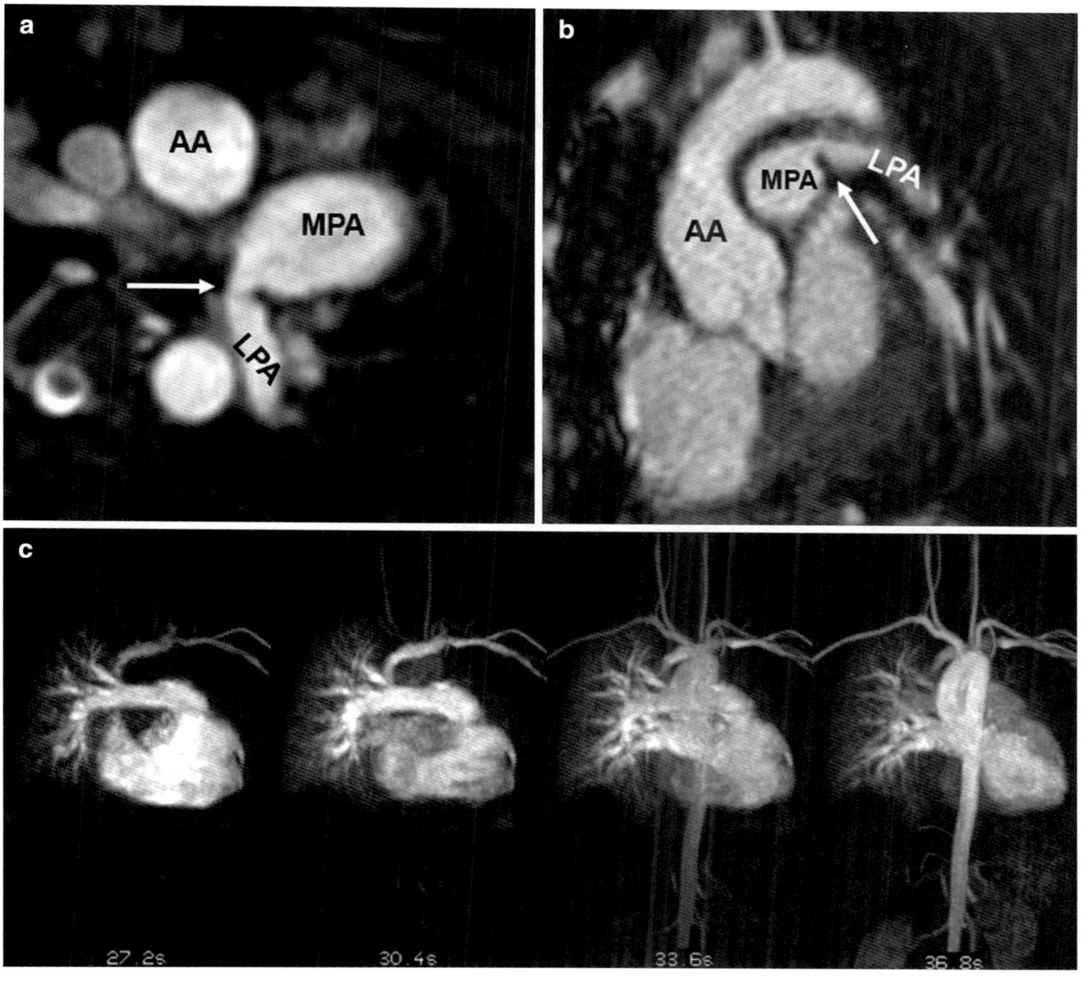

Fig. 20.8 (**a**) Axial and (**b**) sagittal balanced steady-state free precession (SSFP) images show high-grade proximal left pulmonary artery (*LPA*) stenosis in a Fallot patient (*arrows*); the poststenotic LPA is hypoplastic. (**c**) Time-resolved MR angiographies at four different time steps show markedly delayed and reduced contrast-medium filling of the LPA and peripheric lung vessels. *AA* ascending aorta, *MPA* main pulmonary artery

the ventricular short axis, which is preferred for biventricular volumetry, or in the axial plane should be performed. Both views allow for visual evaluation of regional wall motion abnormalities and ventricular asynchrony in contraction and relaxation.

This standard MRI protocol described above provides a broad overview over anatomy and function of the repaired heart after TOF but does not provide detailed information on potential right heart flow alterations associated with post-repair TOF. Since altered hemodynamics can result in right ventricular dilatation and thus at risk for sudden death and tachyarrhythmias [74], it is vital to obtain a better understanding of in vivo 3D flow patterns in TOF patients.

4D flow MRI pilot studies have shown that color-coded visualization by streamlines or particle traces can demonstrate increased peak velocity in the pulmonary trunk of TOF patients compared to normal controls. Higher flow velocity was frequently observed even in the absence of residual or restenosis of the RVOT (Fig. 20.11). Blood flow distribution to the right and left lung can easily be appreciated and

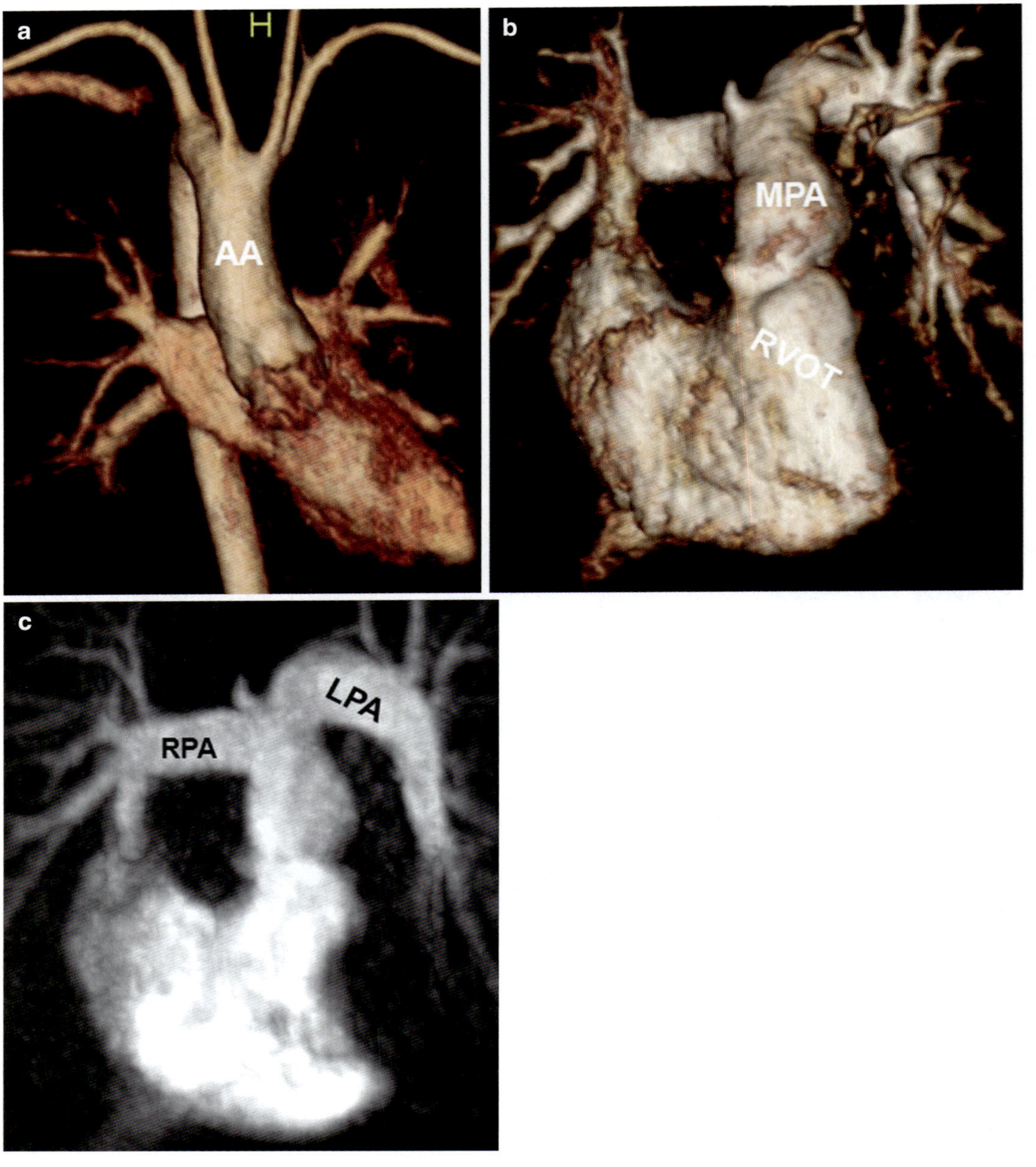

Fig. 20.9 Tetralogy of Fallot. (**a**) Volume-rendered anterior view of the systemic circulation shows a right aortic arch. Volume-rendered (**b**) and maximum intensity projection (**c**) images of the pulmonic circulation show ectatic right ventricular outflow tract (*RVOT*) and the pulmonary arteries with a curved shape of the left pulmonary artery (*LPA*). *AA* ascending aorta, *RPA* right pulmonary artery, *MPA* main pulmonary artery

measured by 4D MRI leading to an assessment of potential abnormal flow ratios (Fig. 20.12). In addition, 4D flow MRI can visualize diastolic retrograde flow in the pulmonary arteries and the RVOT (Figs. 20.11 and 20.12). A more precise assessment of pulmonary regurgitation is obtained by quantitative measurements. Accurate positioning of planes for regional flow quantification can be challenging in standard 2D phase-contrast imaging, particularly in TOF where the left pulmonary artery is often angulated or hypoplastic. Incorrect plane placement cannot be corrected after 2D data acquisition whereas the 4D data allow retrospectively for correct quantification of the regurgitation fraction. Feasibility studies depicted flow disturbances in the pulmonary trunk in terms of vortices or increased helical flow patterns which may be associated with pulmonary artery dilatation (Fig. 20.13). This observation has already been made in previous 4D flow MRI studies of the aorta showing that abnormal flow patterns and vortices contribute to ineffective vascular flow [56, 57, 75]. Similarly, pulmonary trunk abnormalities may influence the development of regurgitation and hemodynamic alterations. These observations in small patient

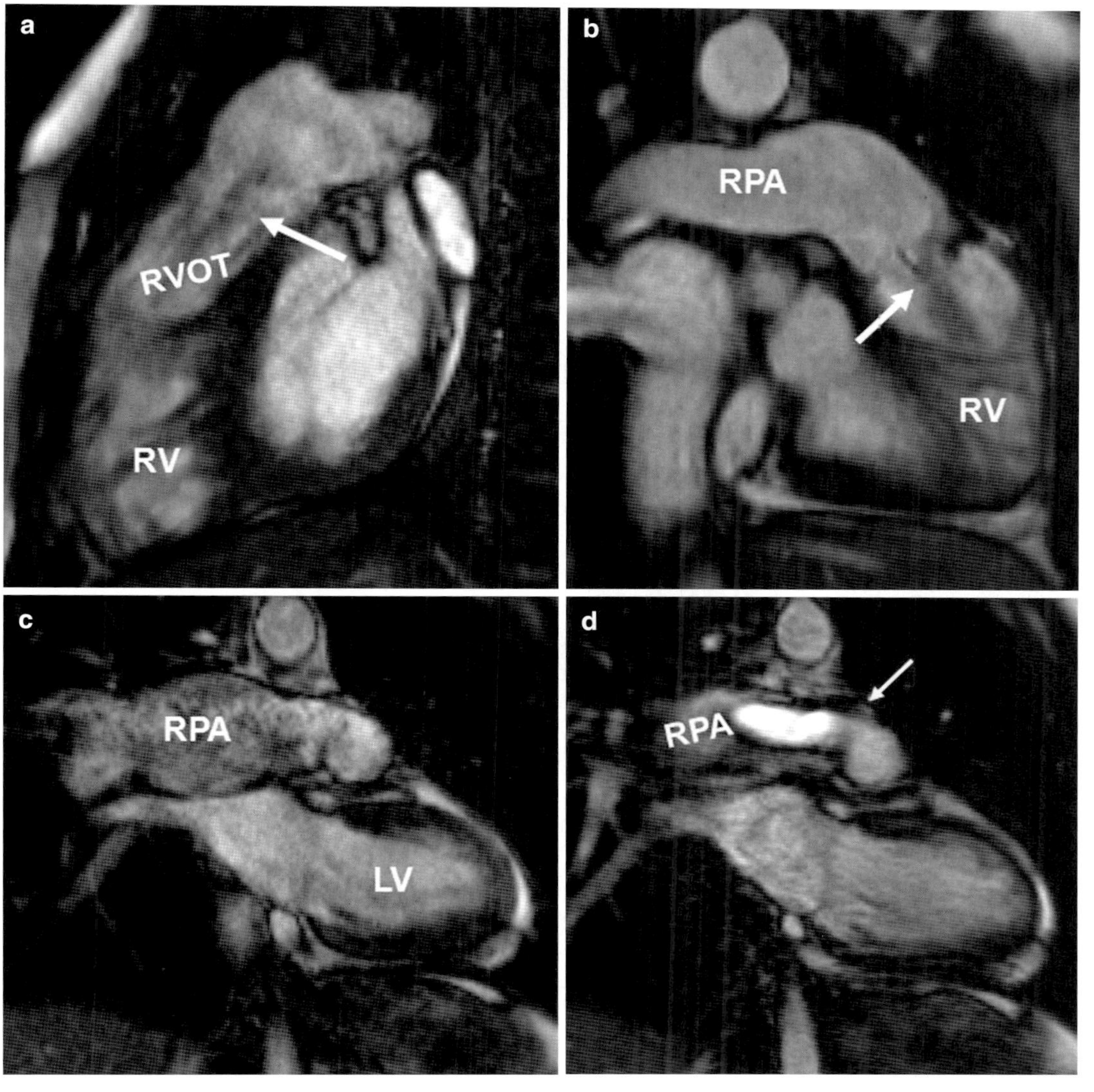

Fig. 20.10 (**a**) Sagittal and (**b**) oblique coronal balanced steady-state free precession (SSFP) images in two patients with tetralogy of Fallot depict ectatic right ventricular outflow tract (*RVOT*) with a low signal jet in diastole due to pulmonary valve insufficiency (*arrows*). Ectasia of the pulmonary trunk distal the valve is seen in both cases and the right pulmonary artery (*RPA*) dilatation is seen in the second case. (**c**, **d**). Coronal CINE SSFP images show signal alterations in the aneurysmatic RPA in (c) and a systolic high-velocity flow jet (*arrow*) in the RPA in (d). *RV* right ventricle, *LV* left ventricle

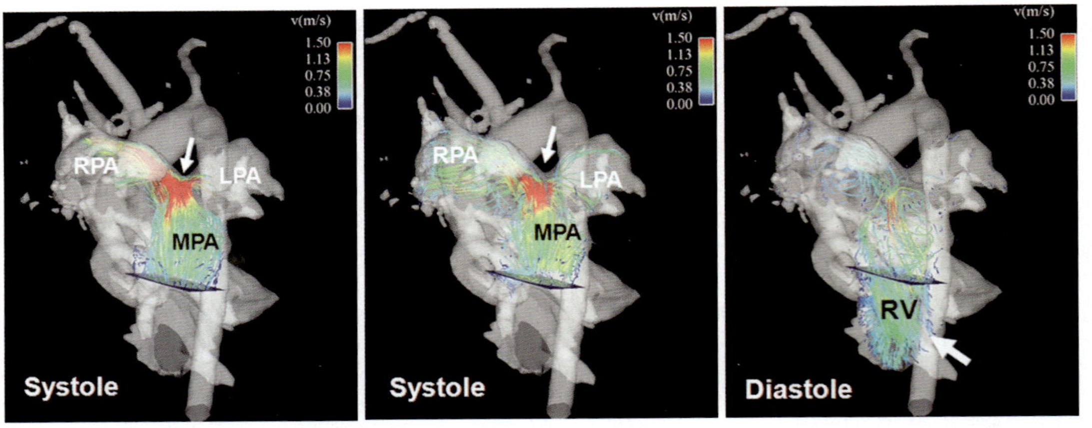

Fig. 20.11 Four-dimensional flow visualization by color-coded particle traces depicts high flow velocity above 1.5 m/s in the main pulmonary artery (*MPA*) and right pulmonary artery (*RPA*), particularly at the bifurcation during systole (*arrow*). There is a noticeably asymmetric flow distribution to the RPA and left pulmonary artery (*LPA*) although there is no vessel stenosis. Remarkable pulmonary reflux into the right ventricle (*RV*) can be visualized during diastole (*arrow*)

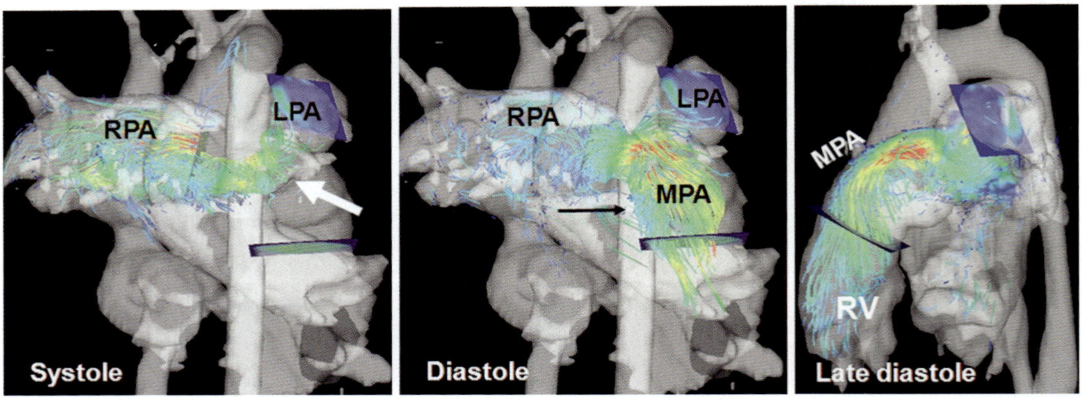

Fig. 20.12 Four-dimensional (4D) flow visualization of insufficient flow hemodynamics: particle traces emitted from a plane in the right pulmonary artery (*RPA*) flow partially backward to the left pulmonary artery (*LPA*) in late systole (*arrow*) showing strong helical flow patterns, which marked reflux to the main pulmonary artery (*MPA*) and into the right ventricle (*RV*) during the entire diastole

cohorts are promising as 4D flow MRI may help to understand pathophysiological considerations of altered hemodynamics in TOF patients.

Transposition of the Great Arteries After Arterial Switch Repair

Transposition of the great arteries (TGA) is a cyanotic congenital heart defect characterized by ventriculoarterial discordance with the aorta originating from the right ventricle and the pulmonary artery from the left ventricle [76]. Initial surgical interventions by Senning and modification by Mustard (atrial switch procedures) left the right ventricle acting as the systemic ventricle [77, 78]. In this procedure, intra-atrial baffles were used to direct the blood to the corresponding ventricle, resulting in a physiological but not anatomic repair [79]. This condition gives rise to complications such as arrhythmia, progressive ventricular dysfunction, and heart failure [80, 81]. Subsequently, the treatment for TGA has been modified and is nowadays based on

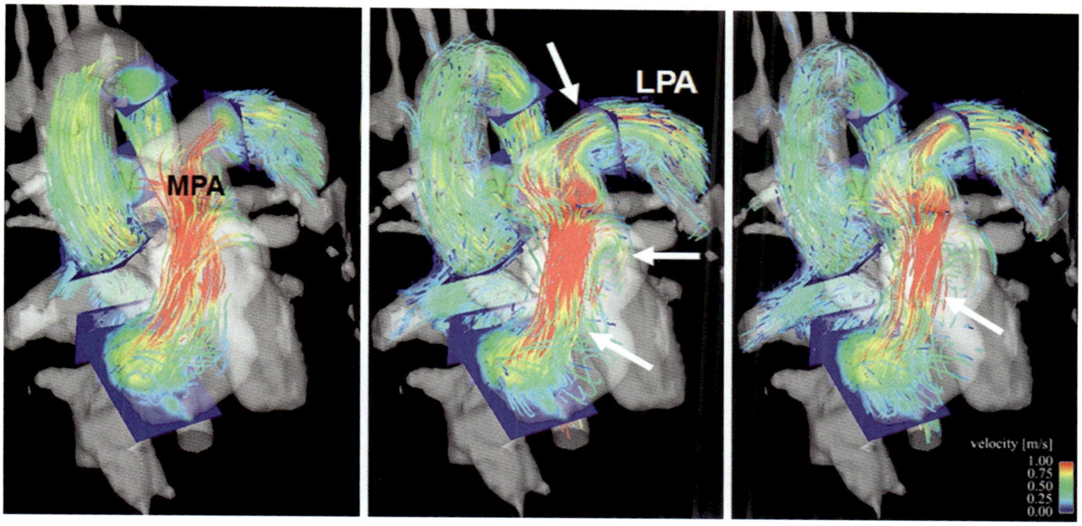

Fig. 20.13 Four-dimensional particle traces flow visualization of the right ventricular outflow tract (RVOT) at three different time points during systole. High flow velocity in the ectatic RVOT with helical and vortical flow disturbances (*arrows*), additional vortex in the left pulmonary artery (*LPA*) (*arrows*). *MPA* main pulmonary artery

the arterial switch procedure during the neonatal period (Jatene principle) which involves a surgical correction of the arterial displacement [82]. The arterial switch operation consists of transection of the aorta and the main pulmonary artery at their roots to correct the ventriculoarterial discordance with transfer of the coronary arteries to the neoaortic root (Fig. 20.14).

In the typical postoperative Lecompte position, the pulmonary trunk is located anterior to the ascending aorta and the pulmonary arteries embrace the ascending aorta [83]. In some cases, e.g., in case of associate defects such as VSDs, the classical Lecompte position cannot be accomplished and the left pulmonary artery is routed posterior to the ascending aorta (Fig. 20.15).

Most common midterm and long-term complications include stenosis of the right ventricular outflow tract and the pulmonary arteries, coronary artery stenosis, aortic root dilatation, or valve insufficiency [84–88]. A recent study by Kempny and coworkers reported that coronary complications and aortic valve dysfunctions are rare. In contrast, RVOT obstructions or pulmonary valve insufficiencies were more frequently observed and lead to re-intervention [89]. Therefore, regular follow-up by echocardiography and MRI is mandatory to monitor ventricular size and function and to identify vessel stenosis or valve insufficiency needing intervention [90]. Echocardiography is challenging for older children due to the limited acoustic window by the postsurgically retrosternal location of the pulmonary trunk and the pulmonary arteries [91]. The complex postsurgical cardiovascular geometry requires multi-planar acquisitions as either dark-blood T2 HASTE or bright-blood SSFP MRI to completely capture the altered anatomy and detect a potential RVOT stenosis (Fig. 20.16) [92–95]. In analogy to the follow-up of Fallot patients, the use of 3D SSFP sequences with free-breathing and full volumetric coverage can facilitate the assessment of the complex cardiac anatomy and the measurement of vessel diameters [96].

Time-resolved CE MRA is most useful for the assessment of the extracardiac anatomy. It has the potential to demonstrate segmental pulmonary artery stenosis or morphologic alterations of the pulmonary trunk and the aortic root (Fig. 20.16). Because of the subsequent contrast filling of the different cardiac compartments, a detailed depiction of the vessels is warranted without interfering overlay by venous structures or suboptimal timing in contrast-medium arrival time using standard 3D MRA. In addition, information on the dynamics

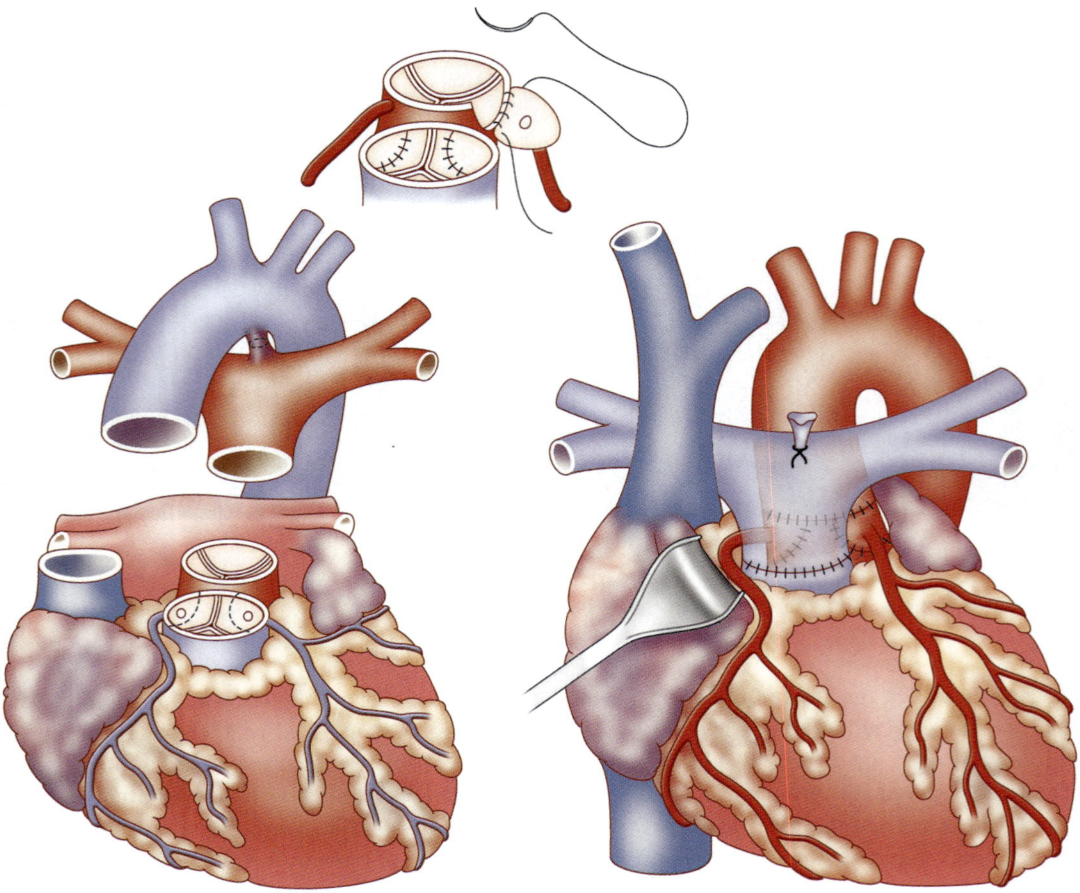

Fig. 20.14 Outline of arterial switch procedure in transposition of the great arteries

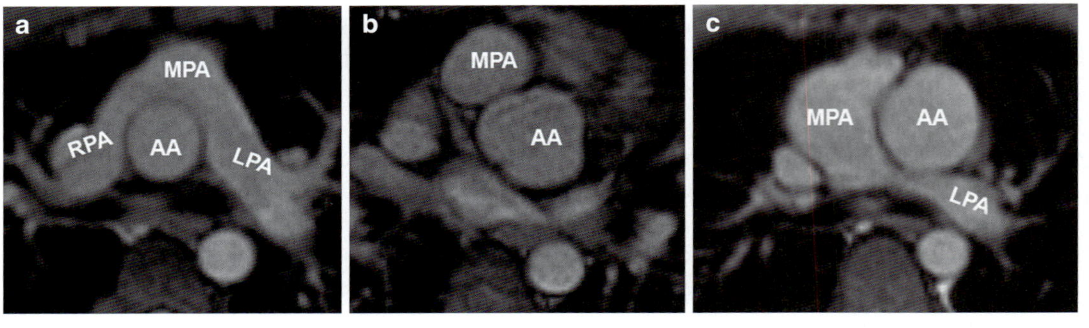

Fig. 20.15 (**a**) Axial image of balanced steady-state free precession (SSFP) sequence in a patient with transposition of the great arteries (TGA) after arterial switch procedure reveals the "typical" postsurgical anatomy with anterior main pulmonary artery (*MPA*) location and Lecompte position of the pulmonary arteries. (**b**) Axial SSFP image in another patient shows the MPA located right anterior in relation to the ascending aorta (*AA*) which has an ectatic root. (**c**) Axial SSFP slice demonstrates an ectatic MPA and an atypical course of the left pulmonary artery (*LPA*) dorsal the AA. *RPA* right pulmonary artery

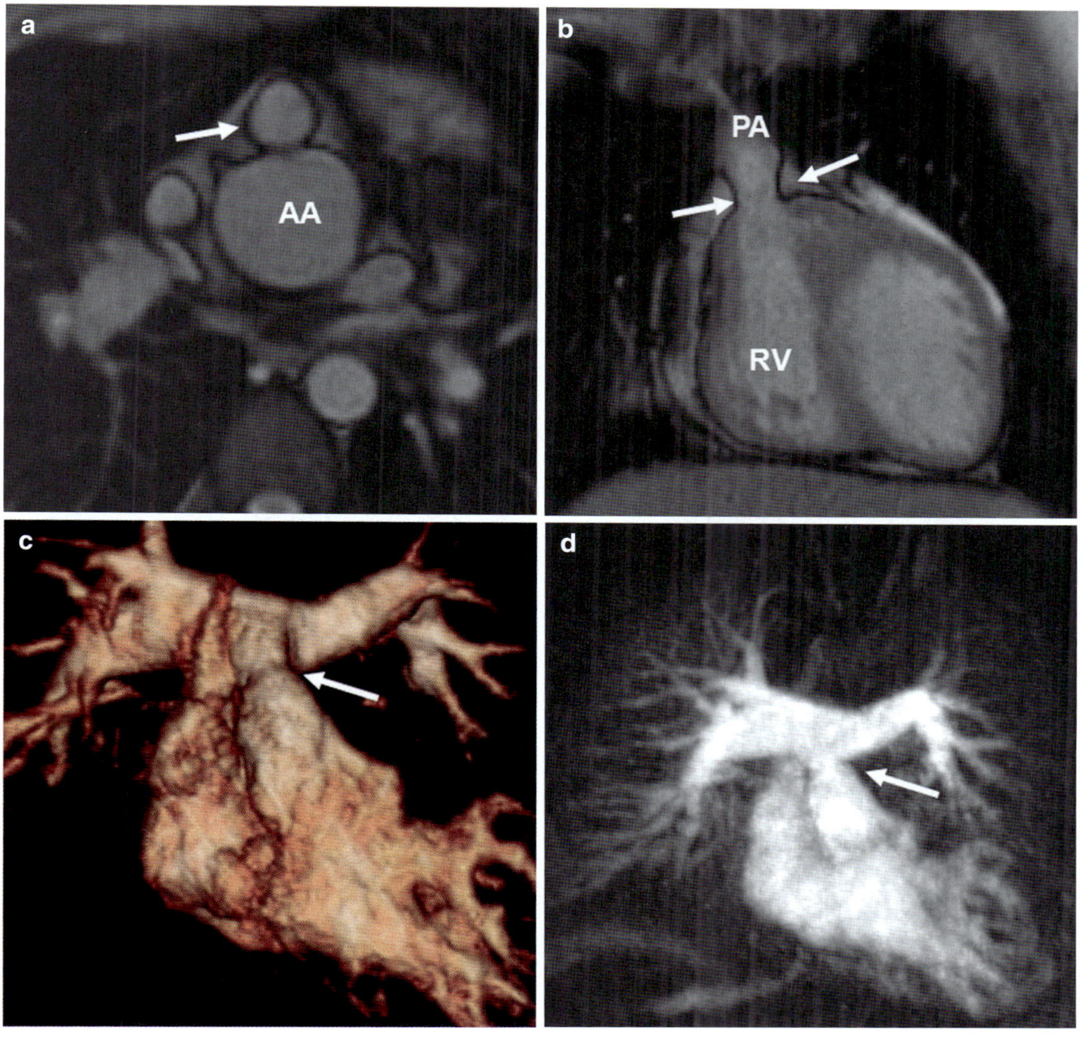

Fig. 20.16 (**a**) Axial and (**b**) coronal balanced steady-state free precession (SSFP) images show valvular pulmonary stenosis (*arrows*) and aortic root dilatation after arterial switch. (**c**) Volume-rendered and (**d**) maximum intensity projection images of another patient with a moderate supravalvular pulmonary artery stenosis (*arrow*) but no pulmonary valve stenosis and with regular symmetric contrast enhancement of both lungs *AA* ascending aorta, *RV* right ventricle, *PA* pulmonary artery

of the passage in the contrast agent through the cardiovascular system can be used to detect symmetric or delayed perfusion of the right and left pulmonary system (Fig. 20.17).

For the evaluation of ventricular function, a series of 2D CINE SSFP images is obtained in standard planes (4-chamber, 2-chamber, short-axis stack) and for the RVOT and LVOT. Similar to Fallot patients, an axial image stack may be used to assess the right ventricular volume. For flow quantification to evaluate valve insufficiency and residual shunts, 2D PC MRI is performed at the level of the ascending aorta and main pulmonary artery [97]. Blood flow in the pulmonary arteries can also be evaluated with 2D CINE PC MRI to investigate pulmonary stenosis arising from morphologic vessel lumen changes during the heart cycle [91].

Viability studies should be performed in suspicion of coronary artery stenosis or occlusion; infarction as a consequence of coronary artery

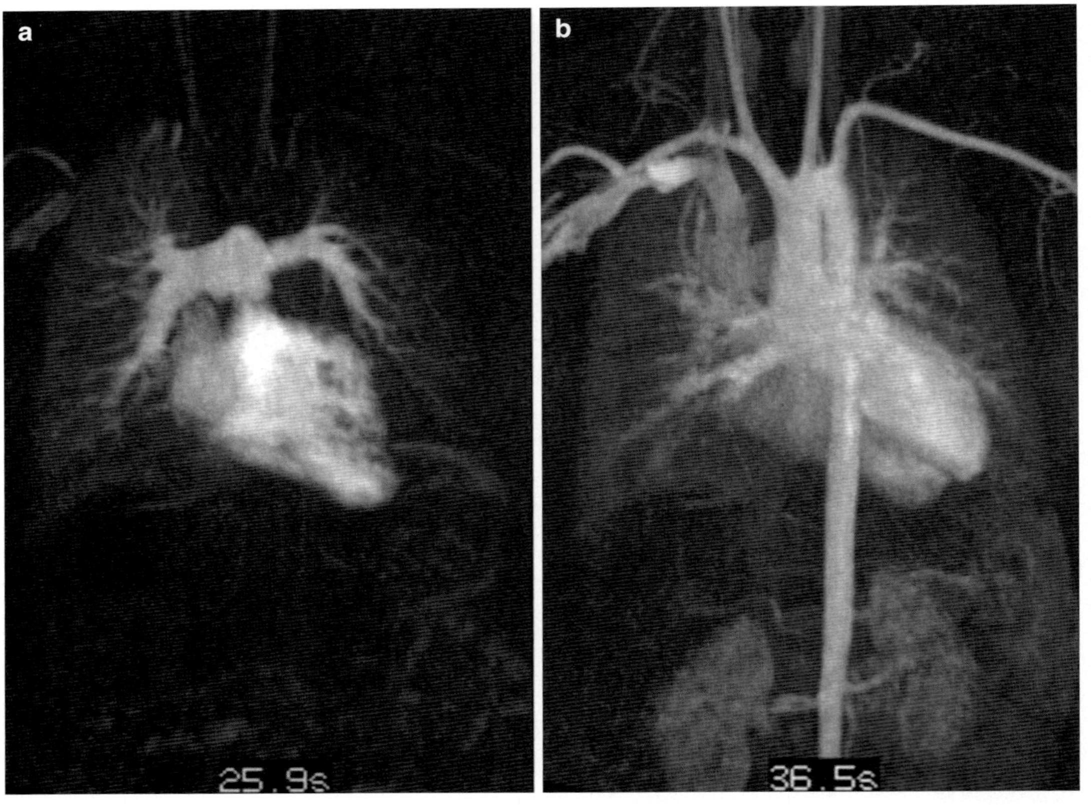

Fig. 20.17 Transposition of the great arteries (TGA) after arterial switch procedure. Time-resolved contrast-enhanced MR angiography at two different time steps. (**a**) Pulmonary contrast filling reveals asymmetric and delayed contrast enhancement of the left lung. (**b**) Aortic enhancement with slight venous overlay by pulmonary veins and capillary vessels

occlusion may be detected in late-enhancement images of myocardium. Thinly sliced MPR-capable 3D SSFP MRI performed in end diastole covering the aortic and pulmonary root can depict the exact course of the proximal coronary arteries, e.g., to aid re-intervention surgery.

The advantages of 4D MRI for evaluation of TGA patients after switch procedure are similar to those of the Fallot patients. The location of peak velocities in the pulmonary trunk and pulmonary arteries can easily be identified using 3D flow visualization. Retrospective flow quantification at these locations can provide a more accurate assessment of peak velocities compared to 2D PC methods [59]. Initial feasibility studies have shown that TGA patients have increased flow disturbances in the pulmonary trunk and pulmonary arteries in comparison with healthy persons. Helical flow patterns were frequently seen in the left pulmonary artery (Fig. 20.18). The flow alterations could be subject to geometric properties as they are dependent on the location of the pulmonary trunk in relation to the ascending aorta. A straight anterior MPA position may provoke more flow disturbances than a slight laterally shifted MPA (Fig. 20.18).

Although aortic insufficiency is usually mild to moderate, it is well known that the aortic root is often dilated in TGA patients [98, 99]. These observations might be related to the helical flow patterns in the ascending aorta that have been observed in a preliminary study (Fig. 20.19).

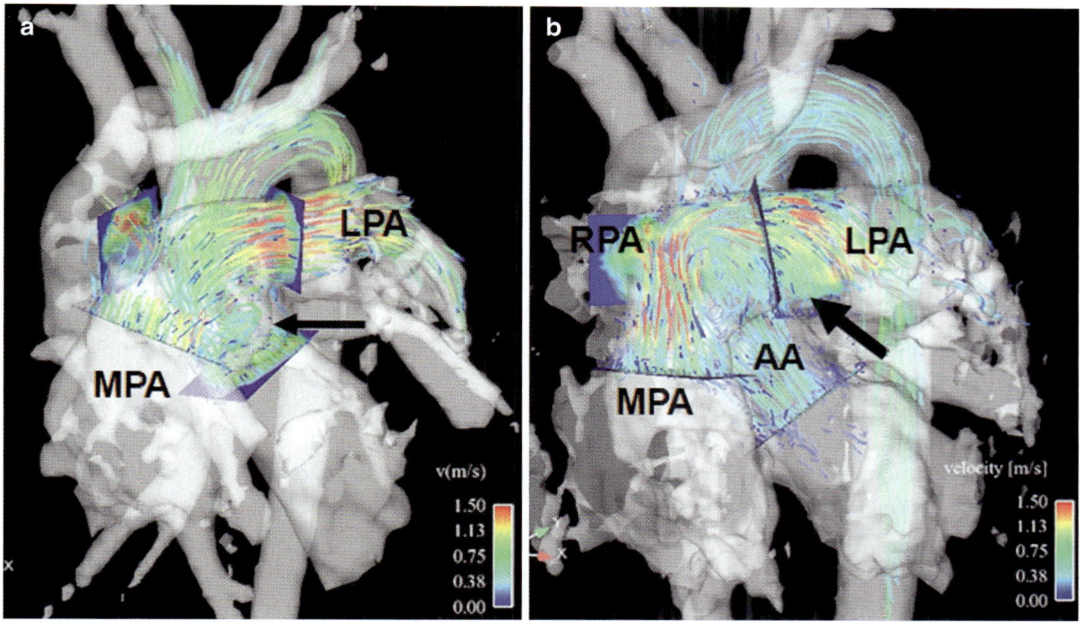

Fig. 20.18 (**a**) Particle traces visualization shows vortex located at the left ectatic side of the main pulmonary artery (*MPA*) (*arrow*) and increased flow velocity in both pulmonary arteries. (**b**) Vortex formation in the proximal left pulmonary artery (*LPA*) (*arrow*) and helical flow in the LPA can be observed by four-dimensional flow visualization

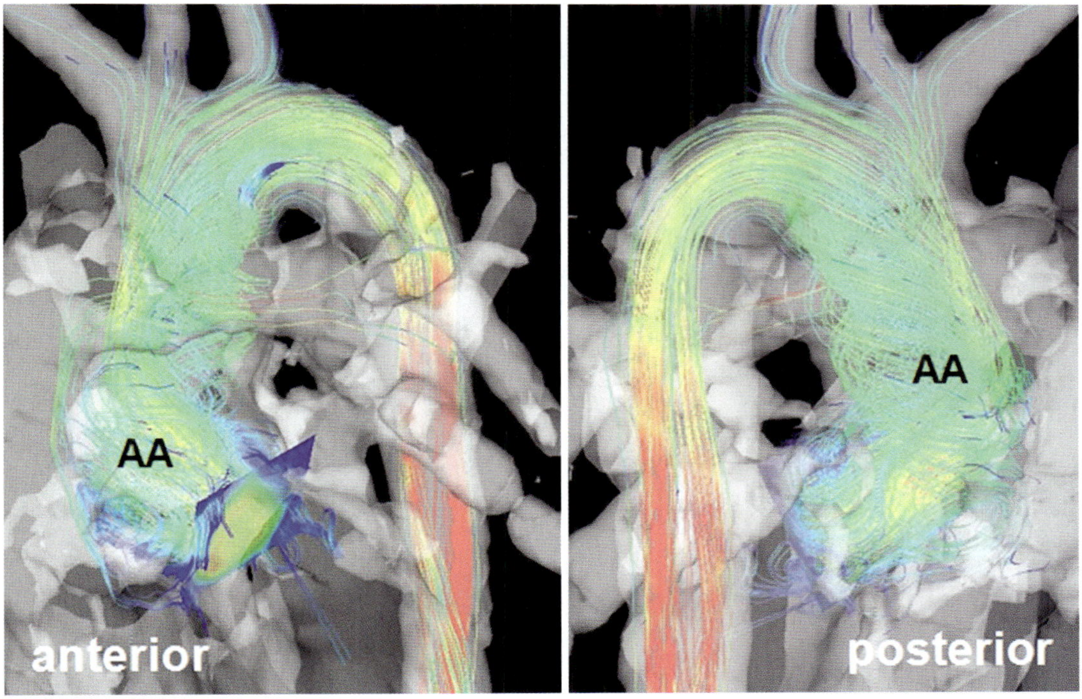

Fig. 20.19 Helical flow patterns in the ascending aorta (*AA*) visualized by streamlines (anterior and posterior view)

Total Cavopulmonary Connection/ Fontan

Hypoplastic left or right heart syndrome is one of the most severe forms of congenital heart disease. The hypogenesis of one ventricle typically requires multiple surgical interventions to construct a single-ventricle physiology. This involves the venous return being routed directly to the lungs, while the remaining intact ventricle provides the systemic circulation. Initially, the Glenn procedure routed the superior caval venous return to the pulmonary arteries. With the addition of the Fontan completion surgery, the inferior caval venous return is also connected to the pulmonary arteries.

The total cavopulmonary connection (TCPC), a variation of the traditional Fontan procedure, is the surgical method of choice for the palliation of a number of CHD which can be summarized as single-ventricle defects [100, 101]. These CHDs comprise hypoplastic left heart syndrome (HLHS), double inlet left ventricle (DILV), double outlet right ventricle (DORV), pulmonary atresia with hypoplastic right ventricle, and tricuspidal atresia. While pulmonary arteries were directly connected to the right atrium in the past, there are two main different modifications of the original Fontan procedure: the lateral intracardiac tunnel with or without fenestration and the extracardiac conduit [102] (Fig. 20.20).

In HLHS, three steps called Norwood procedure have to be performed to achieve the separation of systemic and pulmonary circulation [103]: The initial stage performed in the first days of life ensures unobstructed systemic flow by creating a common outflow between the aortic root and the pulmonary valve called Damus-Kaye-Stansel anastomosis and reconstruction of the hypoplastic aortic arch. At this stage the intervention is completed by excision of the atrial septum and a modified Blalock-Taussig (BT) shunt from one of the subclavian arteries to the pulmonary arteries. In the second step, the BT shunt is eliminated and a connection from the superior vena cava (SVC) to the right pulmonary artery is established which is usually performed as a bidirectional Glenn anastomosis nowadays. For completion of the Fontan circulation, blood from the inferior vena cava (IVC) is directed to the right pulmonary artery via a tunnel or conduit.

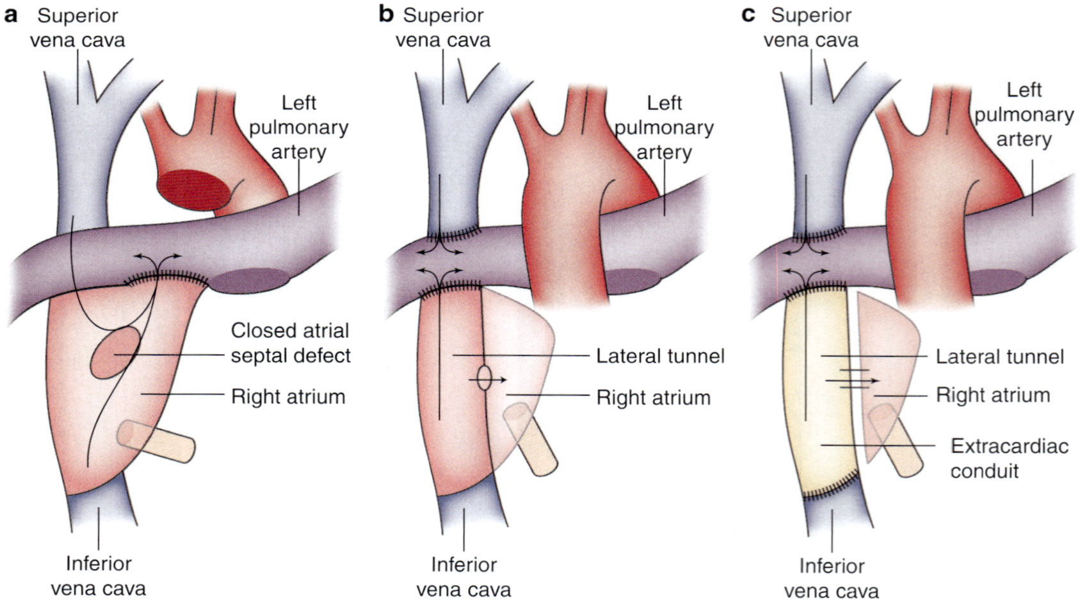

Fig. 20.20 Different types of total cavopulmonary connection. (**a**) The pulmonary arteries are connected to the right atrium in the original Fontan procedure. (**b**) One modification is the lateral intraatrial tunnel which leads the blood from the inferior vena cava (IVC) to the right pulmonary artery. (**c**) Another modification represents the extracardiac conduit which diverts the blood from the IVC to the pulmonary arteries

Survival rates have significantly improved with a reported 20-year survival of about 85 % [104]. Despite the success of the surgical procedure, limitations remain. For example, it is unclear why some patients develop "failing Fontan physiology" early in life while others remain asymptomatic into their 20s and 30s. The Fontan circulation is a palliative procedure which results in altered anatomic and physiological consequences with an increased risk of inefficient flow dynamics. Sequelae include cardiac and extracardiac complications such as atrial arrhythmia, thromboembolic complications, and subsequent failing which can lead to increased pressure in the IVC, cardiac cirrhosis, and portal hypertension [105, 106]. Due to a maldistribution of hepatic factors to the pulmonary circulation, pulmonary arteriovenous malformations can develop, causing progressive hypoxia [107]. Another limitation is the impaired increase in exercise capacity through the passive flowing blood in the TCPC pathway [108–110]. Rare, but serious, life-threatening consequences involving the lymphatic system with protein-loss enteropathy, pleural effusions, and plastic bronchitis have also been reported [111].

Cardiac MRI in single-ventricle patients includes a detailed depiction of the cardiovascular anatomy based on multi-planar anatomic imaging as well as 2D CINE and 2D PC MRI for the evaluation of the single ventricle and valvular function and the flow through the cavopulmonary anastomoses. In this context, 2D CINE SSFP images in different orientations are performed to assess ventricular function and the patency of the Fontan pathway. Isotropic 3D SSFP imaging is helpful to evaluate the complex anatomy and to rule out anastomosis or pulmonary artery stenoses (Fig. 20.21). In addition, dilatation of the intracardiac tunnel or the right atrium in Fontan patients can occur and may result in lung vein compression and risk of swirling blood flow in the enlarged atrium which delays flow to the lungs and facilitates thrombus formation (Fig. 20.21). Image interpretation due to artifacts may be limited in the presence of foreign material, e.g., after coiling of collateral vessels or after stent implantation. Infrequent stent complications may result in compression of adjacent structures, e.g., the bronchi or other vessels (Fig. 20.21). CE MRA can assist in the evaluation of the aorta, the pulmonary arteries, and veins, particularly for the evaluation of a residual hypoplastic arch after reconstruction, recoarctation (Fig. 20.22), pulmonary arteriovenous malformations, or aortopulmonary collaterals. Depending on the site of contrast-medium injection during the time-resolved MRA, there might be asymmetric filling to the right pulmonary artery via the SVC, whereas the left pulmonary artery may be filled later after the diluted contrast medium returns via the IVC to the pulmonary arteries.

The anatomy in single-ventricle patients can vary considerably between patients since the disease is often associated with other vascular anomalies or situs ambiguous or inversus. A detailed patient history of previous operations and the discussion with the referring clinician are thus of high importance for optimal planning of the MRI exam and image interpretation.

PC MRI can be employed to quantify the cardiac output and the differential pulmonary blood flow to the right and left pulmonary arteries. A previous study has shown that the measurement of total flow in the pulmonary veins is the most reliable measurement of pulmonary flow [79]. For a complete quantitative flow assessment, imaging planes should be placed in the ascending and descending aorta, the SVC and IVC, as well as in all four pulmonary veins.

The hemodynamic conditions in this patient group have been studied extensively with the aim to define the optimal surgical strategy for non-disturbed flow dynamics. Various studies with different MRI techniques, computer-based models, and radionuclide washout have investigated the blood flow distribution from the superior and inferior vena cava (SVC/IVC) to the pulmonary arteries [112–120]. 4D flow MRI has become a valuable technique to identify, visualize, and quantify in vivo blood flow and has shown variable flow patterns independently of geometric characteristics [121–124]. In this context, the benefit of the

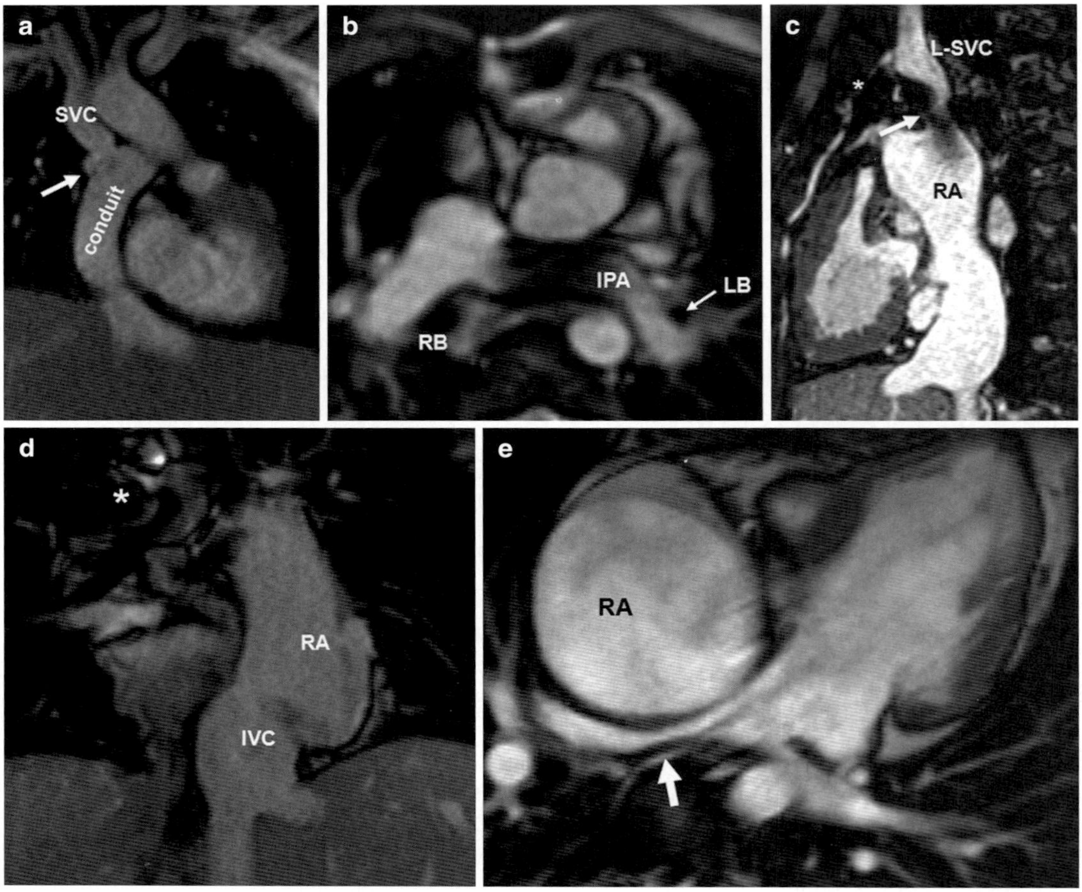

Fig. 20.21 (**a**) Coronal balanced steady-state free precession (SSFP) image of the total cavopulmonary connection (TCPC) with extracardiac Gore-tex conduit with moderate proximal right pulmonary stenosis (RPA) stenosis (*arrow*) in a patient with abdominal situs ambiguus. (**b**) Axial SSFP image reveals severe left bronchus (*LB*) compression due to stent in left pulmonary artery (LPA). The bronchus lumen can be appreciated more distally (*arrow*). The right bronchus (*RB*) appear normal in caliber. (**c**) Sagittal SSFP image shows a stenosis of the upper anastomosis with persisting left superior vena cava (*L-SVC*) (*arrow*). This patient has right atrial isomerism with heterotaxia, same patient as in (**d**) coronal SSFP image, status post Fontan procedure in which the right atrium (*RA*) was connected to the pulmonary arteries. Note dilated RA. Artifacts due to occlusion of the right SVC which is marked by (*). (**e**) Axial CINE SSFP image in another patient with prior Fontan procedure depicts massive right atrial dilatation compressing the right pulmonary vein (*arrow*). *IVC* inferior vena cava

4D velocity acquisition method is its capacity to obtain a comprehensive evaluation of the 3D whole-heart hemodynamics. Based on 3D flow connectivity mapping, the distribution of the SVC and IVC blood flow to the pulmonary arteries can be evaluated (Figs. 20.23 and 20.24). In addition, 4D flow MRI allows for a complete quantitative assessment of the blood flow in different cardiovascular compartments. Therefore, 4D MRI has the potential to improve postoperative evaluation of ineffective hemodynamics which may contribute to understanding of the failing Fontan.

Summary

MRI is superior to echocardiography in many respects for imaging of different kinds of CHD after repair. CHD patients are often confronted

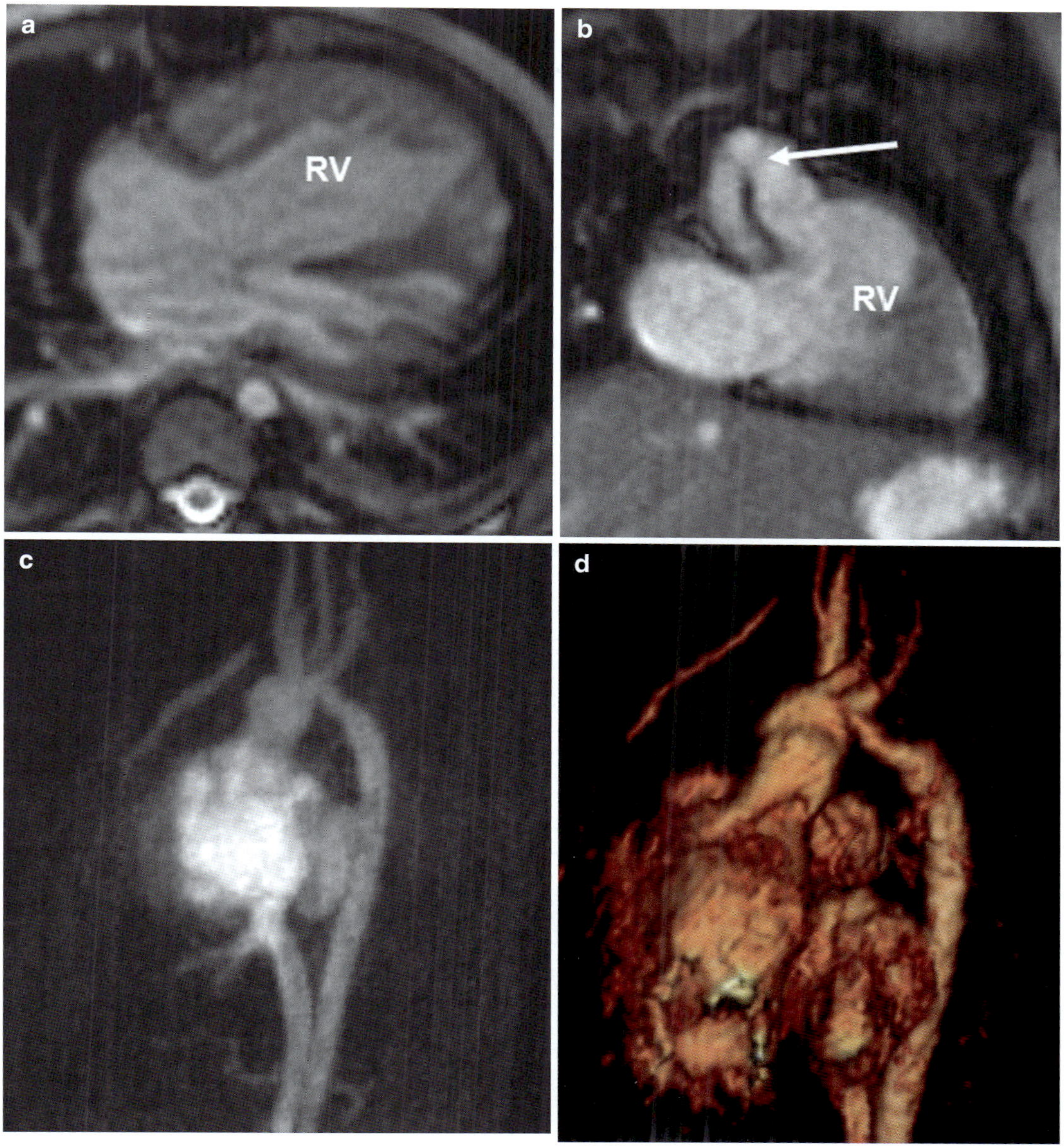

Fig. 20.22 (**a**) Axial balanced steady-state free precession (SSFP) image in a patient with hypoplastic left heart syndrome after Norwood step 2 depicts prominent right ventricle (*RV*) which acts as the systemic ventricle. (**b**) Coronal SSFP image of the Damus-Kaye-Stansel (DKS) anastomosis (*arrow*). (**c**) Maximum intensity projection and (**d**) three-dimensional volume-rendered reconstruction of MR angiography reveal DKS anastomosis and the hypoplastic aortic arch of the same patient

with postoperative long-term sequelae which might reduce life expectancy and need reintervention. Therefore, the advantages of MRI diagnostics for depiction and recognition of eventual cardiovascular problems make MRI indispensable. Using additional 4D MR flow analysis, the complexity of vascular hemodynamics and its influence on morphology and function may be investigated more precisely than is possible using any other imaging tool.

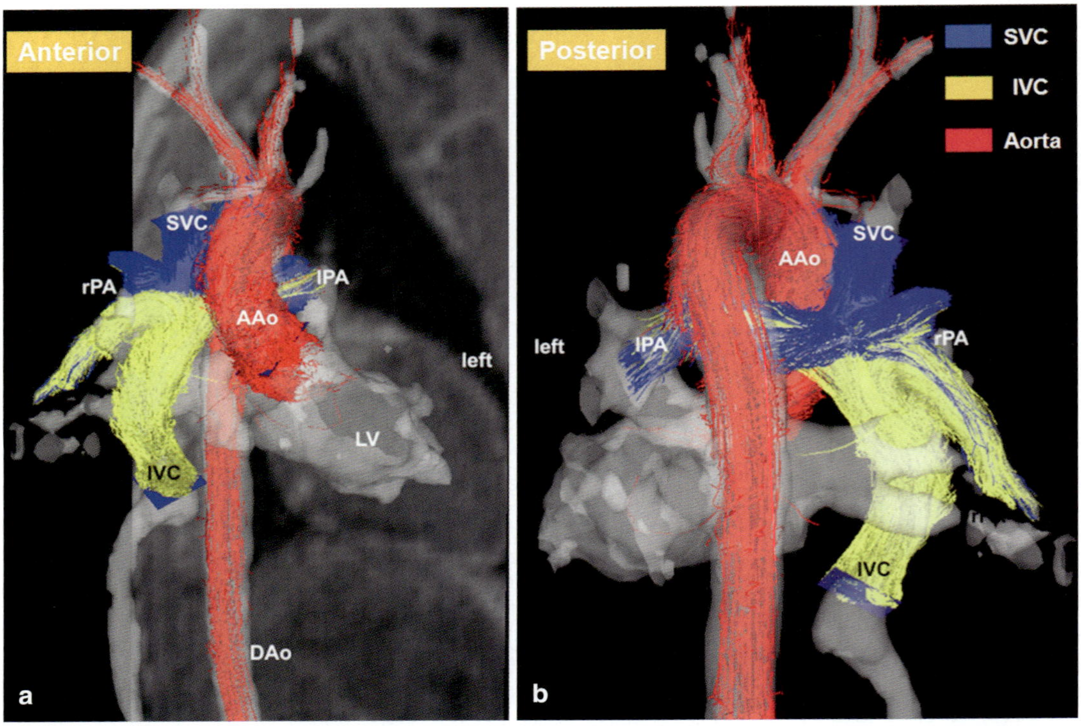

Fig. 20.23 Three-dimensional blood flow visualization of a patient after total cavopulmonary connection (TCPC) with *color-coded streamlines* based on streamline vessel origin reveals the blood flow distribution of blood from the superior and inferior caval veins (SVC, IVC) to the pulmonary arteries. *AAo* ascending aorta, *DAo* descending aorta, *RPA* right pulmonary artery, *LPA* left pulmonary artery, *IVC* inferior vena cava, *LV* left ventricle, *SVC* superior vena cava. (**a**) anterior view, (**b**) posterior view

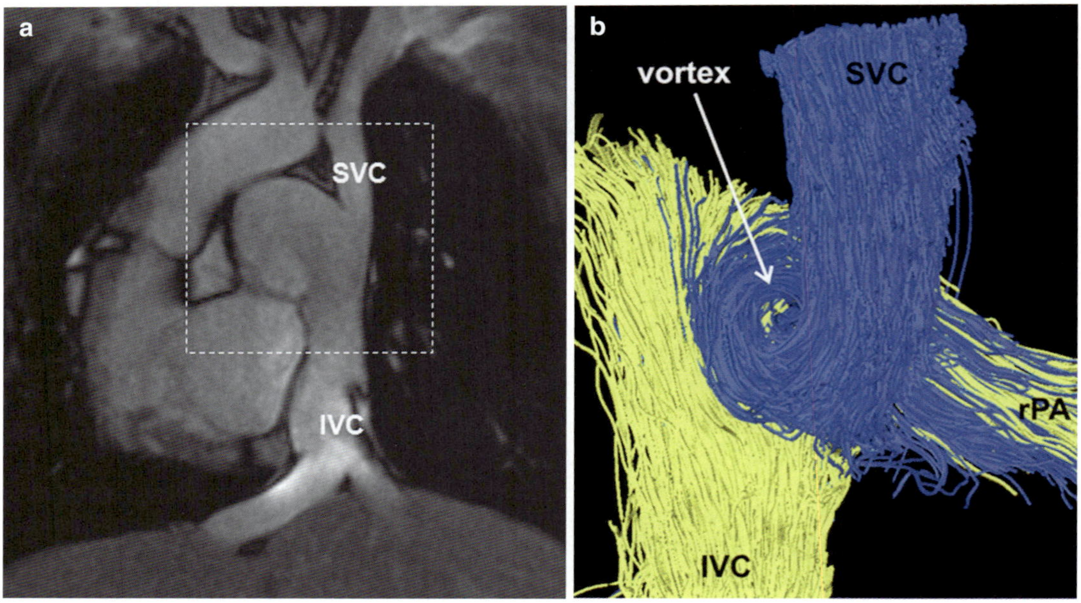

Fig. 20.24 (**a**) Coronal balanced steady-state free precession (SSFP) of a patient after total cavopulmonary connection (TCPC) with development of a dilated anastomosis. (**b**) *Color-coded streamline* visualization (*blue* representing blood from the SVC, *yellow* blood from the IVC) shows a large vortex formation in the ectatic segment. *IVC* inferior vena cava, *RPA* right pulmonary artery, *SVC* superior vena cava

References

1. Talner CN et al. Report of the New England Regional Infant Cardiac Program, by Donald C. Fyler, MD, Pediatrics, 1980;65(suppl):375–461. Pediatrics. 1998; 102:258–9.
2. Roger VL, Go AS, Lloyd-Jones DM, Adams RJ, Berry JD, Brown TM, Carnethon MR, Dai S, de Simone G, Ford ES, Fox CS, Fullerton HJ, Gillespie C, Greenlund KJ, Hailpern SM, Heit JA, Ho PM, Howard VJ, Kissela BM, Kittner SJ, Lackland DT, Lichtman JH, Lisabeth LD, Makuc DM, Marcus GM, Marelli A, Matchar DB, McDermott MM, Meigs JB, Moy CS, Mozaffarian D, Mussolino ME, Nichol G, Paynter NP, Rosamond WD, Sorlie PD, Stafford RS, Turan TN, Turner MB, Wong ND, Wylie-Rosett J. Heart disease and stroke statistics–2011 update: a report from the American Heart Association. Circulation. 2011;123:e18–209.
3. Hoffman JI, Kaplan S. The incidence of congenital heart disease. J Am Coll Cardiol. 2002;39:1890–900.
4. Hoffman JI, Kaplan S, Liberthson RR. Prevalence of congenital heart disease. Am Heart J. 2004;147:425–39.
5. Khairy P, Ionescu-Ittu R, Mackie AS, Abrahamowicz M, Pilote L, Marelli AJ. Changing mortality in congenital heart disease. J Am Coll Cardiol. 2010;56:1149–57.
6. Marelli AJ, Mackie AS, Ionescu-Ittu R, Rahme E, Pilote L. Congenital heart disease in the general population: changing prevalence and age distribution. Circulation. 2007;115:163–72.
7. Warnes CA, Williams RG, Bashore TM, Child JS, Connolly HM, Dearani JA, del Nido P, Fasules JW, Graham Jr TP, Hijazi ZM, Hunt SA, King ME, Landzberg MJ, Miner PD, Radford MJ, Walsh EP, Webb GD, Smith Jr SC, Jacobs AK, Adams CD, Anderson JL, Antman EM, Buller CE, Creager MA, Ettinger SM, Halperin JL, Krumholz HM, Kushner FG, Lytle BW, Nishimura RA, Page RL, Riegel B, Tarkington LG, Yancy CW. ACC/AHA 2008 guidelines for the management of adults with congenital heart disease: a report of the American College of Cardiology/American Heart Association Task Force on practice guidelines (Writing Committee to Develop Guidelines on the Management of Adults with Congenital Heart Disease). Developed in Collaboration with the American Society of Echocardiography, Heart Rhythm Society, International Society for Adult Congenital Heart Disease, Society for Cardiovascular Angiography and Interventions, and Society of Thoracic Surgeons. J Am Coll Cardiol. 2008;52: e1–121.
8. Sable C, Foster E, Uzark K, Bjornsen K, Canobbio MM, Connolly HM, Graham TP, Gurvitz MZ, Kovacs A, Meadows AK, Reid GJ, Reiss JG, Rosenbaum KN, Sagerman PJ, Saidi A, Schonberg R, Shah S, Tong E, Williams RG. Best practices in managing transition to adulthood for adolescents with congenital heart disease: the transition process and medical and psychosocial issues: a scientific statement from the American Heart Association. Circulation. 2011;123:1454–85.
9. Marelli AJ, Child JS, Perloff JK. Transesophageal echocardiography in congenital heart disease in the adult. Cardiol Clin. 1993;11:505–20.
10. Weintraub R, Shiota T, Elkadi T, Golebiovski P, Zhang J, Rothman A, Ritter SB, Sahn DJ. Transesophageal echocardiography in infants and children with congenital heart disease. Circulation. 1992;86:711–22.
11. McLaughlin P, Benson L, Horlick E. The role of cardiac catheterization in adult congenital heart disease. Cardiol Clin. 2006;24:531–56, v.
12. Hughes Jr D, Siegel MJ. Computed tomography of adult congenital heart disease. Radiol Clin North Am. 2010;48:817–35.
13. Cook SC, Raman SV. Multidetector computed tomography in the adolescent and young adult with congenital heart disease. J Cardiovasc Comput Tomogr. 2008;2:36–49.
14. Kellenberger CJ, Yoo SJ, Buchel ER. Cardiovascular MR imaging in neonates and infants with congenital heart disease. Radiographics. 2007;27:5–18.
15. Chung T. Assessment of cardiovascular anatomy in patients with congenital heart disease by magnetic resonance imaging. Pediatr Cardiol. 2000;21:18–26.
16. Krishnamurthy R. The role of MRI and CT in congenital heart disease. Pediatr Radiol. 2009;39 Suppl 2:S196–204.
17. Achenbach S, Barkhausen J, Beer M, Beerbaum P, Dill T, Eichhorn J, Fratz S, Gutberlet M, Hoffmann M, Huber A, Hunold P, Klein C, Krombach G, Kreitner KF, Kühne T, Lotz J, Maintz D, Mahrholdt H, Merkle N, Messroghli D, Miller S, Paetsch I, Radke P, Steen H, Thiele H, Sarikouch S, Fischbach R. Consensus recommendations of the German Radiology Society (DRG), the German Cardiac Society (DGK) and the German Society for Pediatric Cardiology (DGPK) on the use of cardiac imaging with computed tomography and magnetic resonance imaging. Rofo. 2012;184:345–68 [Article in German].
18. Haddad F, Hunt SA, Rosenthal DN, Murphy DJ. Right ventricular function in cardiovascular disease, I: anatomy, physiology, aging, and functional assessment of the right ventricle. Circulation. 2008;117: 1436–48.
19. Haddad F, Doyle R, Murphy DJ, Hunt SA. Right ventricular function in cardiovascular disease, part II: pathophysiology, clinical importance, and management of right ventricular failure. Circulation. 2008;117:1717–31.
20. Davlouros PA, Niwa K, Webb G, Gatzoulis MA. The right ventricle in congenital heart disease. Heart. 2006;92 Suppl 1:i27–38.
21. Babar JL, Jones RG, Hudsmith L, Steeds R, Guest P. Application of MR imaging in assessment and follow-up of congenital heart disease in adults. Radiographics. 2010;30(4):1145.
22. Kilner PJ, Geva T, Kaemmerer H, Trindade P, Schwitter J, Webb G. Recommendations for cardiovascular magnetic resonances in adults with congenital heart disease from the respective working groups of the European Society of Cardiology. Eur Heart J. 2010;31:794–805.

23. Pennell DJ, Sechtem UP, Higgins CB, Manning WJ, Pohost GM, Rademakers FE, van Rossum AC, Shaw LJ, Yucel EL. Clinical indications for cardiovascular magnetic resonance (CMR): Consensus Panel report. Eur Heart J. 2004;25:1940–65.
24. Norton KI, Tong C, Glass RB, Nielsen JC. Cardiac MR imaging assessment following tetralogy of Fallot repair. Radiographics. 2006;26:197–211.
25. Warnes CA. Adult congenital heart disease. Importance of the right ventricle. J Am Coll Cardiol. 2009;54:1903–10.
26. Ntsinjana HN, Hughes ML, Taylor AM. The role of cardiovascular magnetic resonance in pediatric congenital heart disease. J Cardiovasc Magn Reson. 2011;13:51.
27. Valsangiacomo Buechel ER, Mertens L. Imaging the right heart: the use of integrated multimodality imaging. Eur Heart J. 2012;33:949–60.
28. Scheffler K, Lehnhardt S. Principles and applications of balanced SSFP techniques. Eur Radiol. 2003;13:2409–18.
29. Krishnam MS, Tomasian A, Malik S, Desphande V, Laub G, Riehm SG. Image quality and diagnostic accuracy of unenhanced SSFP MR angiography compared with conventional contrast-enhanced MR angiography for the assessment of thoracic aortic diseases. Eur Radiol. 2010;20:1311–20.
30. Plein S, Bloomer TN, Ridgway JP, Jones TR, Bainbridge GJ, Sivananthan MU. Steady-state free precession magnetic resonance imaging of the heart: comparison with segmented k-space gradient-echo imaging. J Magn Reson Imaging. 2001;14:230–6.
31. Longmore DB, Klipstein RH, Underwood SR, Firmin DN, Hounsfield GN, Watanabe M, Bland C, Fox K, Poole-Wilson PA, Rees RS, et al. Dimensional accuracy in magnetic resonance in studies of the heart. Lancet. 1985;1:1360–4.
32. Rehr RB, Malloy CR, Filipchuk NG, Peshock RM. Left ventricular volumes measured by MR imaging. Radiology. 1985;156:717–9.
33. Groethues F, Moon J, Bellenger N, Smith G, Klein H, Pennell D. Interstudy reproducibility of right ventricular volumes, function, and mass with cardiovascular magnetic resonance. Am Heart J. 2004;147:218–23.
34. Sarikouch S, Peters B, Gutberlet M, Leisman B, Kelter-Kloepping A, Koerperich H, Kuehne T, Beerbaum P. Sex-specific pediatric-percentiles for ventricular size and mass as reference values for cardiac MRI/clinical perspective. Circulation. 2010;3:65–76.
35. Clarke CJ, Gurka M, Norton PT, Kramer CM, Hoyer AW. Assessment of the accuracy and reproducibility of RV volume measurements by CMR in congenital heart disease. JACC Cardiovasc Imaging. 2012;5:28–37.
36. Maceira A, Prasad S, Khan M, Pennell D. Reference right ventricular systolic and diastolic function normalized to age, gender and body surface area from steady-state free precession cardiovascular magnetic resonance. Eur Heart J. 2006;27:2879–88.
37. Buechel E, Kaiser T, Jackson C, Schmitz A, Kellenberger C. Normal right- and left ventricular volumes and myocardial mass in children measured by steady state free precession cardiovascular magnetic resonance. J Cardiovasc Magn Reson. 2009;11:19.
38. Robbers-Visser D, Boersma E, Helbing WA. Normal biventricular function, volumes, and mass in children aged 8 to 17 years. J Magn Reson Imaging. 2009;29:552–9.
39. Alfakih K, Plein S, Bloomer T, Jones T, Ridgway J, Sivananthan M. Comparison of right ventricular volume measurements between axial and short axis orientation using steady-state free precession magnetic resonance imaging. J Magn Reson Imaging. 2003;18:25–32.
40. Fratz S, Schuhbaeck A, Buchner C, Busch R, Meierhofer C, Martinoff S, Hess J, Stern H. Comparison of accuracy of axial slices versus short-axis slices for measuring ventricular volumes by cardiac magnetic resonance in patients with corrected tetralogy of Fallot. Am J Cardiol. 2009;103:1764–9.
41. Rebergen SA, van der Wall EE, Doornbos J, de Roos A. Magnetic resonance measurement of velocity and flow: technique, validation, and cardiovascular applications. Am Heart J. 1993;126:1439–56.
42. Mohrs OK, Petersen S, Voigtlaender T, et al. Time-resolved contrast-enhanced MR angiography of the thorax in adults with congenital heart disease. Am J Roentgenol. 2006;187:1107–14.
43. Cornfeld D, Mojibian H. Clinical uses of time-resolved imaging in the body and peripheral vascular system. Am J Roentgenol. 2009;193:W546–57.
44. Bogren HG, Mohiaddin RH, Yang GZ, Kilner PJ, Firmin DN. Magnetic resonance velocity vector mapping of blood flow in thoracic aortic aneurysms and grafts. J Thorac Cardiovasc Surg. 1995;110(3):704–14.
45. Markl M, Draney MT, Hope MD, Levin JM, Chan FP, Alley MT, Pelc NJ, Herfkens RJ. Time-resolved 3-dimensional velocity mapping in the thoracic aorta: visualization of 3-directional blood flow patterns in healthy volunteers and patients. J Comput Assist Tomogr. 2004;28:459–68.
46. Hope TA, Markl M, Wigstrom L, Alley MT, Miller DC, Herfkens RJ. Comparison of flow patterns in ascending aortic aneurysms and volunteers using four-dimensional magnetic resonance velocity mapping. J Magn Reson Imaging. 2007;26(6):1471–9.
47. Bogren HG, Buonocore MH, Valente RJ. Four-dimensional magnetic resonance velocity mapping of blood flow patterns in the aorta in patients with atherosclerotic coronary artery disease compared to age-matched normal subjects. J Magn Reson Imaging. 2004;19:417–27.
48. Markl M, Wegent F, Zech T, Bauer S, Strecker C, Schumacher M, Weiller C, Hennig J, Harloff A. In vivo wall shear stress distribution in the carotid artery: effect of bifurcation geometry, internal carotid artery stenosis, and recanalization therapy. Circ Cardiovasc Imaging. 2010;3:647–55.
49. Kvitting JP, Ebbers T, Wigström L, Engvall J, Olin CL, Bolger AF. Flow patterns in the aortic root and the aorta studied with time-resolved, 3-dimensional, phase-contrast magnetic resonance imaging: implica-

tions for aortic valve-sparing surgery. J Thorac Cardiovasc Surg. 2004;127(6):1602–7.
50. Markl M, Draney M, Miller DC, Levin JM, Williamson EE, Pelc NJ, Liang DH, Herfkens RJ. Time-resolved three-dimensional magnetic resonance velocity mapping of aortic flow in healthy volunteers and patients after valve-sparing aortic root replacement. J Thorac Cardiovasc Surg. 2005;130(2):456–63.
51. Barker AJ, Lanning C, Shandas R. Quantification of hemodynamic wall shear stress in patients with bicuspid aortic valve using phase-contrast MRI. Ann Biomed Eng. 2010;38:788–800.
52. Frydrychowicz A, Arnold R, Hirtler D, Schlensak C, Stalder AF, Hennig J, Langer M, Markl M. Multidirectional flow analysis by cardiovascular magnetic resonance in aneurysm development following repair of aortic coarctation. J Cardiovasc Magn Reson. 2008;10(1):30.
53. Hope MD, Meadows AK, Hope TA, Ordovas KG, Saloner D, Reddy GP, Alley MT, Higgins CB. Clinical evaluation of aortic coarctation with 4D flow MR Imaging. J Magn Reson Imaging. 2010;31(3): 711–8.
54. Frydrychowicz A, Markl M, Hirtler D, Harloff A, Schlensak C, Geiger J, Stiller B, Arnold R. Aortic hemodynamics in patients with and without repair of aortic coarctation: in vivo analysis by 4D flow-sensitive magnetic resonance imaging. Invest Radiol. 2011;46(5):317–25.
55. Geiger J, Markl M, Herzer L, Hirtler D, Loeffelbein F, Stiller B, Langer M, Arnold R. Aortic flow patterns in patients with Marfan syndrome assessed by flow-sensitive 4D MRI. J Magn Reson Imaging. 2012;35(3):594–600.
56. Hope MD, Hope TA, Crook SES, Ordovas KG, Urbania TH, Alley MT, Higgins CB. 4D flow CMR in assessment of valve-related ascending aortic disease. JACC Cardiovasc Imaging. 2011;4(7):781–7.
57. Frydrychowicz A, Berger A, Russe MF, Stalder AF, Harloff A, Dittrich S, Hennig J, Langer M, Markl M. Time-resolved magnetic resonance angiography and flow-sensitive 4-dimensional magnetic resonance imaging at 3 Tesla for blood flow and wall shear stress analysis. J Thorac Cardiovasc Surg. 2008;136(2):400–7.
58. Frydrychowicz A, Stalder AF, Russe MF, Bock J, Bauer S, Harloff A, Berger A, Langer M, Hennig J, Markl M. Three-dimensional analysis of segmental wall shear stress in the aorta by flow-sensitive four-dimensional-MRI. J Magn Reson Imaging. 2009;30(1):77–84.
59. Stalder AF, Russe MF, Frydrychowicz A, Bock J, Hennig J, Markl M. Quantitative 2D and 3D phase contrast MRI: optimized analysis of blood flow and vessel wall parameters. Magn Reson Med. 2008;60: 1218–31.
60. Nordmeyer S, Riesenkampff E, Crelier G, et al. Flow-sensitive four-dimensional cine magnetic resonance imaging for offline blood flow quantification in multiple vessels: a validation study. J Magn Reson Imaging. 2010;32(3):677–83.
61. Gatzoulis MA. Tetralogy of Fallot. In: Gatzoulis M, Webb G, Daubeney P, editors. Diagnosis and management of adult congenital heart disease. London: Elsevier; 2003. p. 315–26.
62. Therrien J, Webb G. Clinical update on adults with congenital heart disease. Lancet. 2003;362:1305–13.
63. Apitz C, Webb GD, Redington AN. Tetralogy of Fallot. Lancet. 2009;274:1462–71.
64. Murphy JG, Gersh BJ, Mair DD, et al. Long-term outcome in patients undergoing surgical repair of tetralogy of Fallot. N Engl J Med. 1993;329:593–9.
65. Lillehei CW, Varco RL, Cohen M, et al. The first open heart repairs of ventricular septal defect, atrioventricular communis and tetralogy of Fallot using extracorporeal circulation by cross-circulation: a 30-year follow-up. Ann Thorac Surg. 1986;41:4–21.
66. Geva T. Repaired tetralogy of Fallot: the roles of cardiovascular magnetic resonance in evaluating pathophysiology and for pulmonary valve replacement decision support. J Cardiovasc Magn Reson. 2011;13:9.
67. Davlouros PA, Kilner PJ, Hornung TS, Li W, Francis JM, Moon JCC, Smith GC, Tat T, Pennell DJ, Gatzoulis MA. Right ventricular function in adults with repaired tetralogy of Fallot assessed with cardiovascular magnetic resonance imaging: detrimental role of right ventricular outflow aneurysms or akinesia and adverse right-to-left ventricular interaction. J Am Coll Cardiol. 2002;40:2044–52.
68. Ammash NM, Dearani JA, Burkhart HM, Connolly HM. Pulmonary regurgitation after tetralogy of Fallot repair: clinical features, sequelae, and timing of pulmonary valve replacement. Congenit Heart Dis. 2007;2:386–403.
69. Huehnergarth KV, Gurvitz M, Stout KK, Otto CM. Repaired tetralogy of Fallot in the adult: monitoring and management. Heart. 2008;94:1663–9.
70. Frigiola A, Redington AN Cullen S, Vogel M. Pulmonary regurgitation is an important determinant of right ventricular contractile dysfunction in patients with surgically repaired tetralogy of Fallot. Circulation. 2004;110:II153–7.
71. Therrien J, Provost Y, Merchant N, Williams W, Colman J, Webb G. Optimal timing for pulmonary valve replacement in adults after tetralogy of Fallot repair. Am J Cardiol. 2005;95:779–82.
72. Adamson L, Vohra HA, Haw MP. Does pulmonary valve replacement post repair of tetralogy of Fallot improve right ventricular function? Interact Cardiovasc Thorac Surg. 2009;9(3):520–7. Epub 2009 Jun 30.
73. Boechat MI, Ratib O, Williams PL, Gomes AS, Child JS, Allada V. Cardiac MR imaging and MR angiography for assessment of complex tetralogy of Fallot and pulmonary atresia. Radiographics. 2005;25:1535–46.
74. Gatzoulis MA, Balaji S, Webber SA, Liu SC, Hokanson JS, Poile C, Rosenthal M, Nakazawa M, Moller JH, Gillette PC, Webb GD, Redington AN. Risk factors for arrhythmia and sudden cardiac death late after repair of tetralogy of Fallot: a multicentre study. Lancet. 2000;356:975–81.

75. Hope MD, Hope TA, Meadows AK, Ordovas KG, Urbania TH, Alley MT, Higgins CB. Bicuspid aortic valve: four-dimensional MR evaluation of ascending aortic systolic flow patterns. Radiology. 2010;255(1): 53–61.
76. Martins P, Castela E. Transposition of the great arteries. Orphanet J Rare Dis. 2008;3:27.
77. Senning A. Surgical correction of transposition of the great vessels. Surgery. 1959;45:966–80.
78. Mustard WT, Keith JD, Trusler GA, Fowler R, Kidd L. The surgical management of transposition of the great vessels. J Thorac Cardiovasc Surg. 1964;48:953–8.
79. Lu JC, Dorfman AL, Attili AK, Ghadimi Mahani M, Dillman JR, Agarwal PP. Evaluation with cardiovascular MR imaging of baffles and conduits used in palliation or repair of congenital heart disease. Radiographics. 2012;32(3):E107–27.
80. Khairy P, Landzberg MJ, Lambert J, O'Donnell CP. Long-term outcomes after the atrial switch for surgical correction of transposition: a meta-analysis comparing the Mustard and Senning procedures. Cardiol Young. 2004;14:284–92.
81. Roos-Hesselink JW, Meijboom FJ, Spitaels SE, et al. Decline in ventricular function and clinical condition after mustard repair for transposition of the great arteries (a prospective study of 22–29 years). Eur Heart J. 2004;25:1264–70.
82. Jatene AD, Fontes VF, Paulista PP, Souza LC, Neger F, Galantier M, Sousa JE. Anatomic correction of transposition of the great vessels. J Thorac Cardiovasc Surg. 1976;72(3):364–70.
83. Lecompte Y, Zannini L, Hazan E, Jarreau MM, Bex JP, Tu TV, Neveux JY. Anatomic correction of transposition of the great arteries. J Thorac Cardiovasc Surg. 1981;82(4):629–31.
84. Massin MM, Nitsch GB, Däbritz S, Seghave MC, Messmer BJ, von Bernuth G. Growth of pulmonary artery after arterial switch operation for simple transposition of the great arteries. Eur J Pediatr. 1998;157(2):95–100.
85. McMahon CJ, Ravekes WJ, O'Brian Smith E, et al. Risk factors for neo-aortic root enlargement and aortic regurgitation following arterial switch operation. Pediatr Cardiol. 2004;25:329–35.
86. Hutter PA, Kreb DL, Mantel SF, Hitchcock JF, Meijboom EJ, Bennink GB. Twenty-five years' experience with arterial switch operation. J Thorac Cardiovasc Surg. 2002;124:790–7.
87. De Koning WB, van Osch-Grevers M, Ten Harkel AD, van Domburg RT, Spijkerboer AW, Utens EM, Bogers AJ, Helbing WA. Follow-up outcomes 10 years after arterial switch operation for transposition of the great arteries: comparison of cardiological health status and health-related quality of life to those of the a normal reference population. Eur J Pediatr. 2008;167(9):995–1004.
88. Fricke TA, d'Udekem Y, Richardson M, Thuys C, Dronavalli M, Ramsay J, Wheaton G, Grigg LE, Brizard CP, Konstantinov IE. Outcomes of the arterial switch operation for transposition of the great arteries: 25 years of experience. Ann Thorac Surg. 2012;94(1):139–45.
89. Kempny A, Wustmann K, Borgia F, Dimopoulos K, Uebing A, Li W, Chen SS, Piorkowski A, Radley-Smith R, Yakoub MH, Gatzouilis MA, Shore DF, Swan L, Diller GP. Outcome in adult patients after arterial switch operation for transposition of the great arteries. Int J Cardiol. 2013;167(6):2588–93.
90. Warnes CA. Transposition of the great arteries. Circulation. 2006;114:2699–709.
91. Gutberlet M, Boeckel T, Hosten N, et al. Arterial switch procedure for D-transposition of the great arteries: quantitative midterm evaluation of hemodynamic changes with cine MR imaging and phase-shift velocity mapping-initial experience. Radiology. 2000;214:467–75.
92. Blakenberg F, Rhee J, Hardy C, Helton G, Higgins SS, Higgins CB. MRI vs echocardiography in the evaluation of the Jatene procedure. J Comput Assist Tomogr. 1994;18:749–54.
93. Hardy CE, Helton GJ, Kondo C, Higgins SS, Young NJ, Higgins CB. Usefulness of magnetic resonance imaging for evaluating great-vessel anatomy after arterial switch operation for D-transposition of the great arteries. Am Heart J. 1994;128:326–3323.
94. Cohen MD, Johnson T, Ramrakhiani S. MRI of surgical repair of transposition of the great arteries. Am J Roentgenol. 2010;191:250–60.
95. Weiss F, Habermann CR, Lilje C, Nimz M, Rasek V, Dallmeyer J, Stork A, Graesnner J, Weil J, Adam G. MRT der Pulmonalarterien bei Kindern nach arterieller Switch-Operation (ASO) bei Transposition der großen Gefäße (d-TGA). Fortschr Röntgenstr. 2005;177:849–55.
96. Sørensen TS, Körperich H, Greil GF, et al. Operator-independent isotropic three-dimensional magnetic resonance imaging for morphology in congenital heart disease: a validation study. Circulation. 2004;110(2):163–9.
97. Beerbaum P, Körperich H, Barth P, Esdorn H, Gieseke J, Meyer H. Noninvasive quantification of left-to-right shunt in pediatric patients: phase-contrast cine magnetic resonance imaging compared with invasive oximetry. Circulation. 2001;103(20): 2476–82.
98. Schwartz ML, Gauvreau K, del Nido P, Mayer J, Colan SD. Long-term predictors of aortic root dilatation and aortic regurgitation after arterial switch operation. Circulation. 2004;110:128–32.
99. Losay J, Touchot A, Capderou A, Piot JD, Belli E, Planché C, Serraf A. Aortic valve regurgitation after arterial switch operation for transposition of the great arteries: incidence, risk factors, and outcome. J Am Coll Cardiol. 2006;47(10):2057–62.
100. Fontan F, Baudet E. Surgical repair of tricuspid atresia. Thorax. 1971;26:240–8.
101. De Laval MR, Kilner P, Gewillig M, Bull C. Total cavopulmonary connection: a logical alternative to atriopulmonary connection for complex Fontan operations. J Thorac Cardiovasc Surg. 1988;96:682–95.
102. Fredenburg TB, Johnson TR, Cohen MD. The Fontan procedure: anatomy, complications and manifestations of failure. Radiographics. 2011;31:453–63.

103. Norwood WI, Kirklin JK, Sanders SP. Hypoplastic left heart syndrome: experience with palliative surgery. Am J Cardiol. 1980;45:87–91.
104. d'Udekam Y, Ivengar AJ, Cochrane AD, Grigg LE, Ramsay JM, Wheaton GR, Penny DJ, Brizard CP. The Fontan procedure: contemporary techniques have improved long-term outcomes. Circulation. 2007;116:I157–64.
105. O'Donnell CP, Landzberg MJ. The 'failing' Fontan circulation. Prog Pediatr Cardiol. 2002;16:105–14.
106. Khairy P, Fernandes MS, John J, Mayer E, Triedman JK, Walsh EP, Lock JE, Landzberg MJ. Long-term survival, modes of death, and predictors of mortality in patients with Fontan surgery. Circulation. 2008;117:85–92.
107. Duncon B, Desai S. Pulmonary arteriovenous malformations after cavopulmonary anastomosis. Ann Thorac Surg. 2003;76:1759–66.
108. Rosenthal M, Bush A, Deanfield AJ, Redington A. Comparison of cardiopulmonary adaptation during exercise in children after the atriopulmonary and total cavopulmonary connection Fontan procedures. Circulation. 1995;91:372–8.
109. Sundareswaran KS, Pekkan K, Dasi LP, Whitehead K, Sharma S, Kanter K, Fogel M, Yoganathan AP. The total cavopulmonary connection resistance: a significant impact on single ventricle hemodynamics at rest and exercise. Am J Physiol Heart Circ Physiol. 2008;295:H2427–35.
110. Whitehead KK, Pekkan K, Kitajima HD, Paridon SM, Yoganathan AP, Fogel MA. Nonlinear power loss during exercise in single-ventricle patients after the Fontan: Insights from computational fluid dynamics. Circulation. 2007;116:I165–71.
111. Khanna G, Bhalla S, Krishnamurthy R, Canter C. Extracardiac complications of the Fontan circuit. Pediatr Radiol. 2012;42:233–41.
112. Be'eri E, Maier SE, Landzberg MJ, Chung T, Geva T. In vivo evaluation of Fontan pathway flow dynamics by multidimensional phase-velocity magnetic resonance imaging. Circulation. 1998;98(25):2873–82.
113. Fogel MA, Weinberg PM, Rychik J, Hubbard A, Jacobs M, Spray TL, Haselgrove J. Caval contribution to flow in the branch pulmonary arteries of Fontan patients with a novel application of magnetic resonance presaturation pulse. Circulation. 1999;99(9):1215–21.
114. Fratz S, Hess J, Schwaiger M, Martinoff S, Stern HC. More accurate quantification of pulmonary blood flow by magnetic resonance imaging than by lung perfusion scintigraphy in patients with Fontan circulation. Circulation. 2002;106(12):1510–3.
115. Gutberlet M, Hosten N, Abdul-Khaliq H, Rechter S, Vojtovic P, Oellinger H, Ehrenstein T, Vogel M, Alexi-Meshkishvili V, Hetzer R, Felix R, 6. The value of magnetic resonance tomography (MRT) for evaluating ventricular and anastomotic functions in patients with an extra- or intracardiac total cavopulmonary connection (TCPC)-modified Fontan operation [Article in German]. Rofo. 1999; 171:431–41.
116. Tayama M, Hirata N, Matsushita T, Sano T, Fukushima N, Sawa Y, Nishimura T, Matsuda H. Pulmonary blood flow distribution after the total cavopulmonary connection for complex cardiac anomalies. Heart Vessels. 1999,14(3):154–60.
117. DeGroff CG, Carlton JD, Weinberg CE, Ellison MC, Shandas R, Valdes-Cruz L. Effect of vessel size on the flow efficiency of the total cavopulmonary connection: in vitro studies. Pediatr Cardiol. 2002;23(2):171–7.
118. DeGroff C, Birnbaum B, Shandas R, Orlando W, Hertzberg J. Computational simulations of the total cavo-pulmonary connection: insights in optimizing numerical solutions. Med Eng Phys. 2005; 27(2):135–46.
119. Khunatorn Y, Mahalingam S, DeGroff CG, Shandas R. Influence of connection geometry and SVC-IVC flow rate ratio on flow structures within the total cavopulmonary connection: a numerical study. J Biomech Eng. 2002;124(4):364–77.
120. Dasi LP, Whitehead K, Pekkan K, de Zelicourt D, Sundereswaran K, Kanter K, Fogel MA, Yoganathan AP. Pulmonary hepatic flow distribution in total cavopulmonary connections: extracardiac versus intracardiac. J Thorac Cardiovasc Surg. 2011; 141:207–14.
121. Markl M, Geiger J, Kilner PJ, Föll D, Stiller B, Beyersdorf F, Arnold R, Frydrychowicz A. Time-resolved three-dimensional magnetic resonance velocity mapping of cardiovascular flow paths in volunteers and patients with Fontan circulation. Eur J Cardiothorac Surg. 2011;39(2):206–12.
122. Frydrychowicz A, Arnold R, Harloff A, Schlensak C, Hennig J, Langer M, Markl M. In vivo 3-dimensional flow connectivity mapping after extracardiac total cavopulmonary connection. Circulation. 2008;118:16–7.
123. Valverde I, Nordmeyer S, Uribe S, Greil G, Berger F, Kuehne T, Beerbaum P. Systemic-to-pulmonary collateral flow in patients with palliated univentricular heart physiology: measurement using cardiovascular magnetic resonance 4D velocity acquisition. J Cardiovasc Magn Reson. 2012;14:25.
124. Bächler P, Valverde I, Uribe S. Quantification of caval flow contribution to the lungs in vivo after total cavopulmonary connection with 4-dimensional flow magnetic resonance imaging. J Thorac Cardiovasc Surg. 2012;143:742–3.

Cardiac CT and MR Evaluation of the Adult Fontan Patient

21

Tiffanie R. Johnson, Margaret M. Samyn, and Laureen Sena

Congenital heart disease resulting in single ventricular physiology includes many diverse diagnoses (Table 21.1). Optimal palliation for such patients requires that the ventricle act as the systemic pump and that a secure source of pulmonary blood flow is created. Unobstructed flow to the systemic and pulmonary circulations is the goal; optimally, widely patent aortic anatomy and branch pulmonary arteries are desirable.

Due to complex anatomy and hemodynamics, any single ventricle patient with Fontan palliation requires continued meticulous medical surveillance. A critical component of this care involves advanced cardiac imaging. A multimodality imaging approach for the Fontan patient is best performed at a center with expertise in adult congenital heart disease and in-depth knowledge regarding the advantages and disadvantages of each imaging technique. Cardiac magnetic resonance (CMR) imaging and multidetector cardiac computed tomography (MDCT) are the noninvasive, advanced cardiac imaging techniques presented here.

The Fontan Procedure

Genesis for single ventricle palliation came with animal studies conducted by Rodbard in 1948, who for the first time successfully bypassed the canine right ventricle by anastomosing the right atrial appendage to the proximally ligated main pulmonary artery [1]. An innovative technique, the cavopulmonary shunt, was first performed by William Glenn in North America on a dog (1954) and shortly thereafter in a patient (1957). It became the standard at several institutions, paving the way for the Fontan palliation for single ventricle patients [2].

Table 21.1 Common heart defects resulting in single ventricle physiology

RV morphology	LV morphology	RV or LV morphology
Hypoplastic left heart syndrome (HLHS)	Tricuspid atresia	Unbalanced AV canal defect
Complex double-outlet right ventricle	Pulmonary atresia	Straddling or crisscross AV valve connections
	Double-inlet left ventricle	Heterotaxy
	Severe Ebstein's anomaly	

AV atrioventricular

T.R. Johnson, MD, FAAP, FACC (✉)
Section of Pediatric Cardiology, Riley Hospital for Children, Indiana University, 705 Riley Hospital Drive, Riley Research Rm 127, Indianapolis, IN 46202-5225, USA
e-mail: tifjohns@iu.edu

M.M. Samyn, MD, FAAP, FACC
Pediatric Cardiology, The Herma Heart Center, Children's Hospital of Wisconsin, Medical College of Wisconsin, 9000 West Wisconsin Avenue, Milwaukee, WI, 53226, USA
e-mail: msamyn@chw.org

L. Sena, MD
Department of Radiology, Boston Children's Hospital. Harvard Medical School, 300 Longwood Ave, Boston, MA 02115, USA
e-mail: laureen.sena@childrens.harvard.edu

F. Saremi (ed.), *Cardiac CT and MR for Adult Congenital Heart Disease*, DOI 10.1007/978-1-4614-8875-0_21,

The Fontan operation was first described in 1971 as a physiologic corrective surgical procedure for patients with tricuspid atresia [3]. In this original description of the Fontan operation, full oxygenation of blood before returning to the left heart was achieved by direction of systemic venous return to the pulmonary arteries and closing the atrial septal defect (Fig. 21.1a, b).

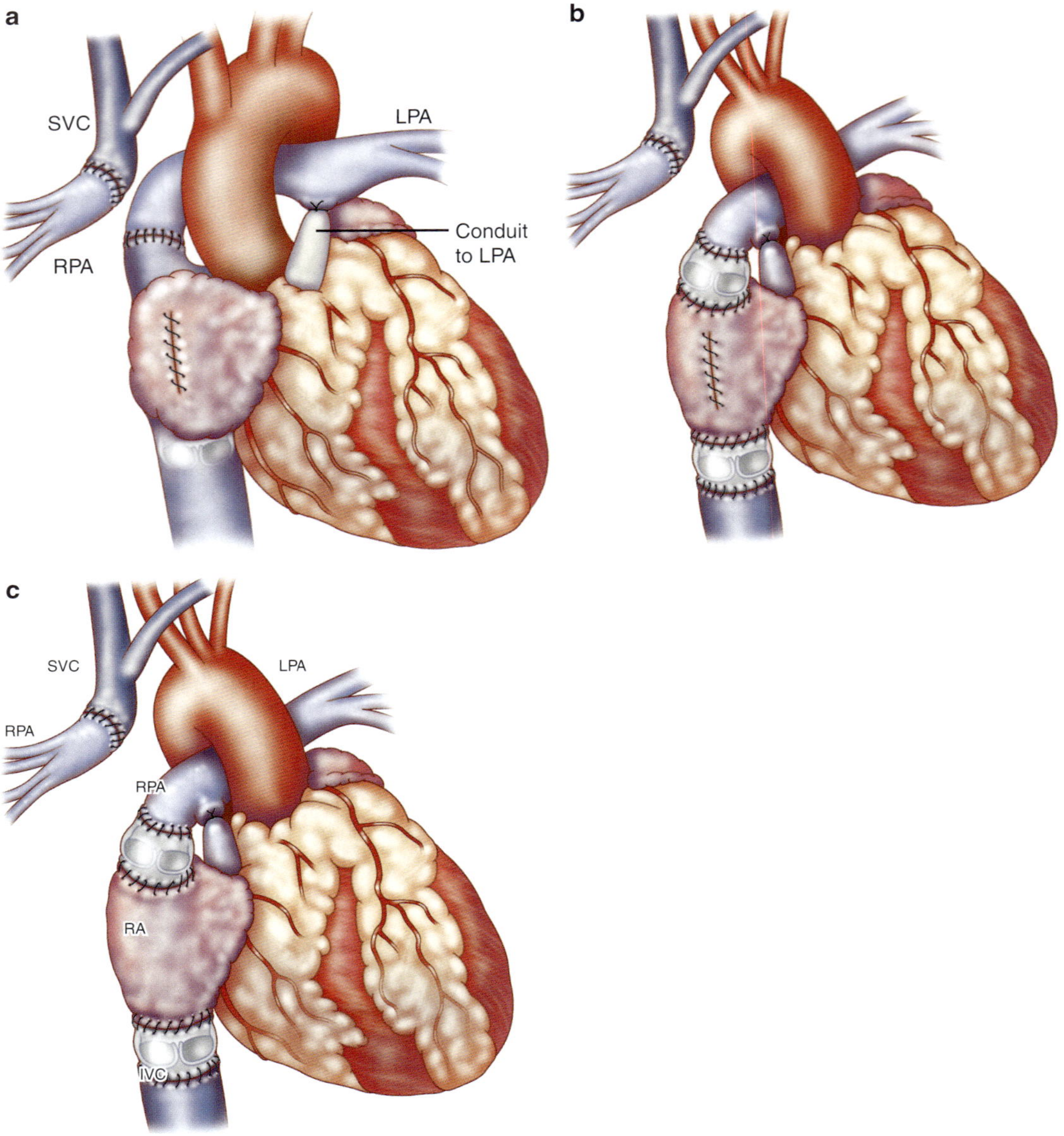

Fig. 21.1 (**a**, **b**) Original Fontan operation: the pulmonary artery (*PA*) is ligated at its connection to the ventricle. (**c**) The superior vena cava (*SVC*) is disconnected from the right atrium (*RA*) and anastomosed to the disconnected right pulmonary artery (*RPA*) (Glenn procedure). The RA appendage was attached to the left PA (*LPA*) to direct blood to the left lung directly (**a**) or via an aortic valve homograft (**b**). A pulmonary valve homograft is inserted into the inferior vena cava (*IVC*) and the atrial septal defect is closed (Reproduced with permission from Fontan and Baudet [3]). (**d**) Kreutzer modification: Anterior connection of the RA appendage to the *PA* is performed with the patient's own pulmonary valve or a nonvalved Dacron tube. (**e**) Björk modification: *RA* to right ventricle outflow tract anastomosis with a pericardial patch or valved conduit

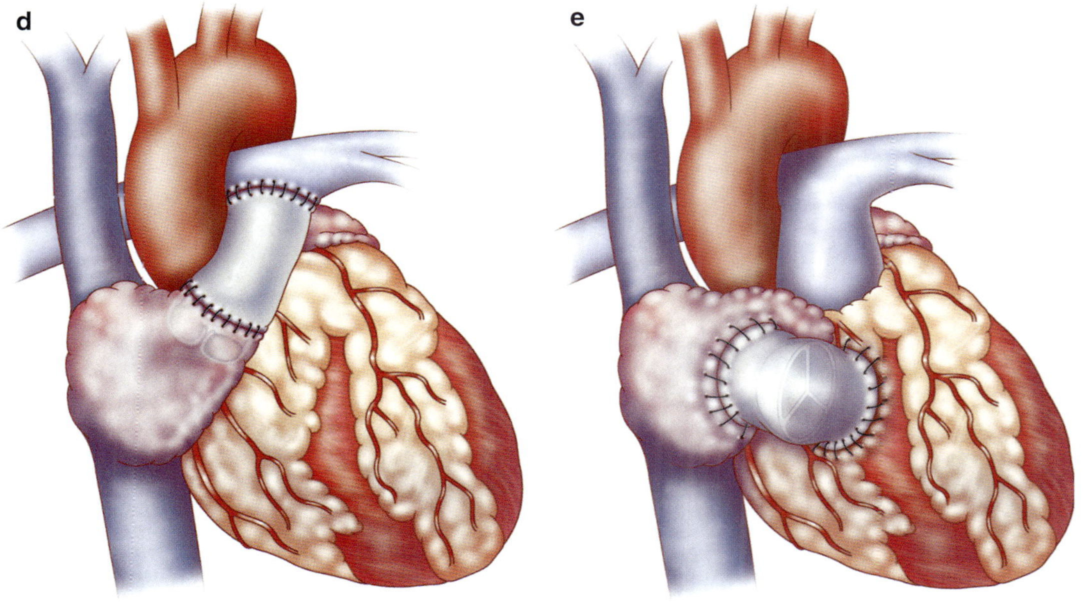

Fig. 21.1 (continued)

Since its original description, there have been several modifications to the Fontan procedure, which has been applied to many types of congenital heart disease resulting in single ventricle physiology, regardless of whether cyanosis or pulmonary overcirculation existed initially [4, 5]. In 1973, Kreutzer described maintenance of branch pulmonary artery continuity by direct anterior connection of the right atrial appendage (RAA) to the main pulmonary artery with omission of the Glenn procedure and without a pulmonary valve homograft at the inferior vena cava-right atrium (IVC-RA) junction (Fig. 21.1c). A fenestration was also placed in the atrial septum [6]. Later, Kreutzer performed the posterior atriopulmonary anastomosis, a technique he believed was superior to the anterior anastomosis for reduced patient mortality [7]. The Björk modification incorporated a right atrial to right ventricular anastomosis in tricuspid atresia for potential use of the hypoplastic right ventricle (RV) as a pumping chamber [8] (see Fig. 21.1d). The success of these early procedures has been recognized as one of the major historic advances in surgical treatment for patients with varying types of univentricular heart defects [5, 9]. As these first reports included multiple variations, the term "classic Fontan" is not specific enough, and deviations will be seen in the literature. Thus, it is important to understand the variety of surgical procedures that can be found in adults with single ventricle physiology who have undergone surgical palliation as young children.

With the Fontan palliation performed in a manner incorporating the anastomosis of the right atrial appendage to the pulmonary artery, long-term complications in many have included significant right atrial dilation along with atrial arrhythmias and/or atrial thrombus formation, often accompanied by ventricular dysfunction and worsening cyanosis, among other issues [10, 11] (Fig. 21.2). In an attempt to address complications encountered in the early Fontan techniques, more recent modifications have included the total cavopulmonary connection reported by de Leval in 1988 [12]. He anastomosed the SVC to the right pulmonary artery (RPA) and created an intra-atrial tunnel formed from the posterior atrial wall and a prosthetic patch, with or without a fenestration, spanning the pathway from the inferior vena cava (IVC) to the SVC-RA junction (Fig. 21.3). As reported

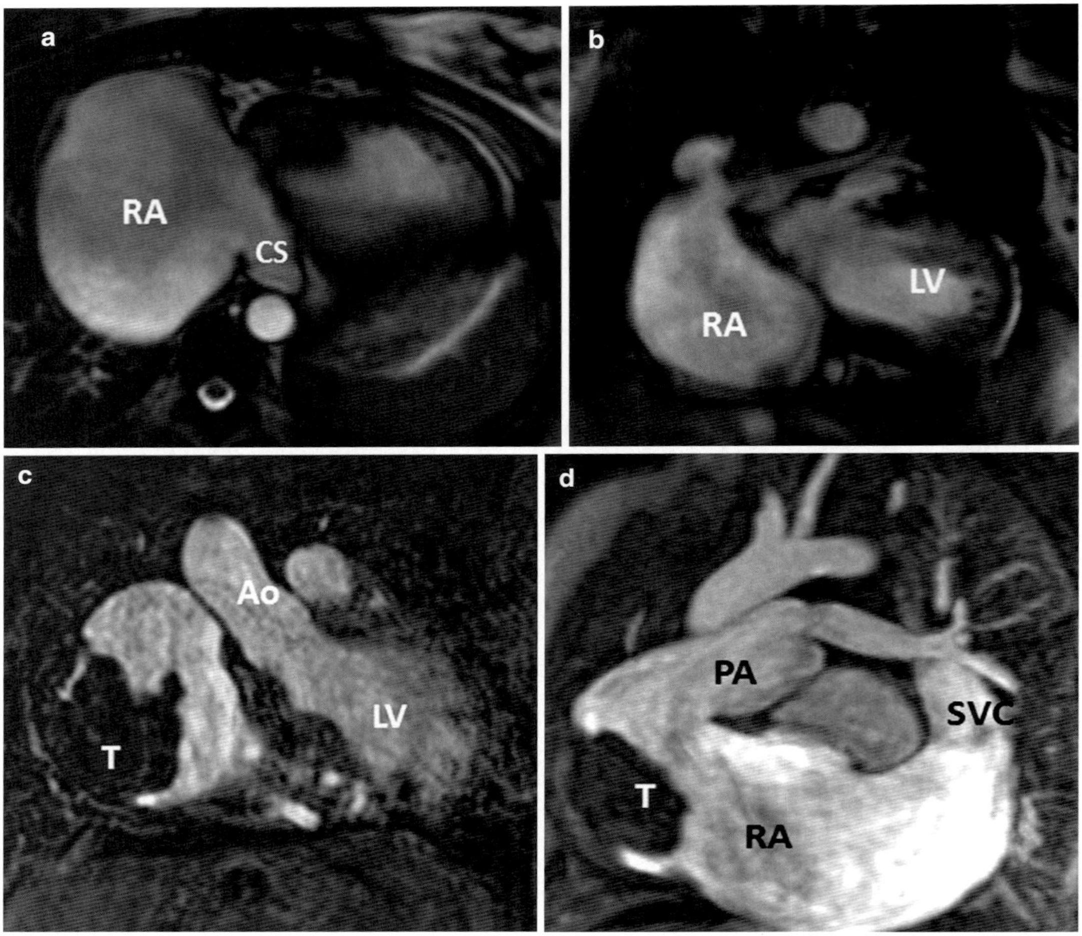

Fig. 21.2 (**a**, **b**) A 34-year-old female with tricuspid atresia and history of right Glenn and left Blalock-Taussig shunt as a young child; at age 24 years pulmonary artery (*PA*) continuity was reestablished along with connection of the right atrium (*RA*) appendage to the *PA*. Cardiac MR (*CMR*) steady-state free precession, bright., Rady Children's, San Diego, CA. blood images in axial (**a**) and oblique coronal (**b**) orientations demonstrate a severely dilated *RA* and a dilated coronary sinus. (**c**, **d**) A 26-year-old male with tricuspid atresia, atriopulmonary Fontan at age 8 years, severely dilated *RA*, recurrent atrial arrhythmias at age 19 years, treated with amiodarone and warfarin and required electrical cardioversion at age 24 and 25 years, presented for cardiac MR due to fatigue, shortness of breath, and oxygen saturation in the upper 80s and a large *RA* thrombus (*T*) was found. Steady-state free precession, bright-blood images in (**c**) coronal and (**d**) oblique sagittal orientations. *CS* coronary sinus, *LV* left ventricle, *Ao* aorta, *SVC* superior vena cava (Courtesy of Beth Printz, M.D)

in 1990, Marcelletti promoted the extracardiac Fontan, which consisted of a caval conduit entirely outside the atrium from the IVC to the pulmonary artery [13]. The intra-atrial baffle was first described by the Mayo Clinic group and proved useful for patients with anomalous venous drainage [4] (Fig. 21.4). These caval connection modifications have decreased the incidence of complications related to the enlarged right atrium [10, 12, 14].

Completion of the Fontan procedure has now became a two-stage endeavor; first the hemi-Fontan or bidirectional Glenn operation connects the SVC to the branch pulmonary arteries, followed by connection of the IVC via the caval conduit to the branch pulmonary arteries, usually within 2–3 years [15]. In heterotaxy patients with azygous continuation of the IVC to the SVC, the Kawashima procedure [16] is commonly performed to connect the

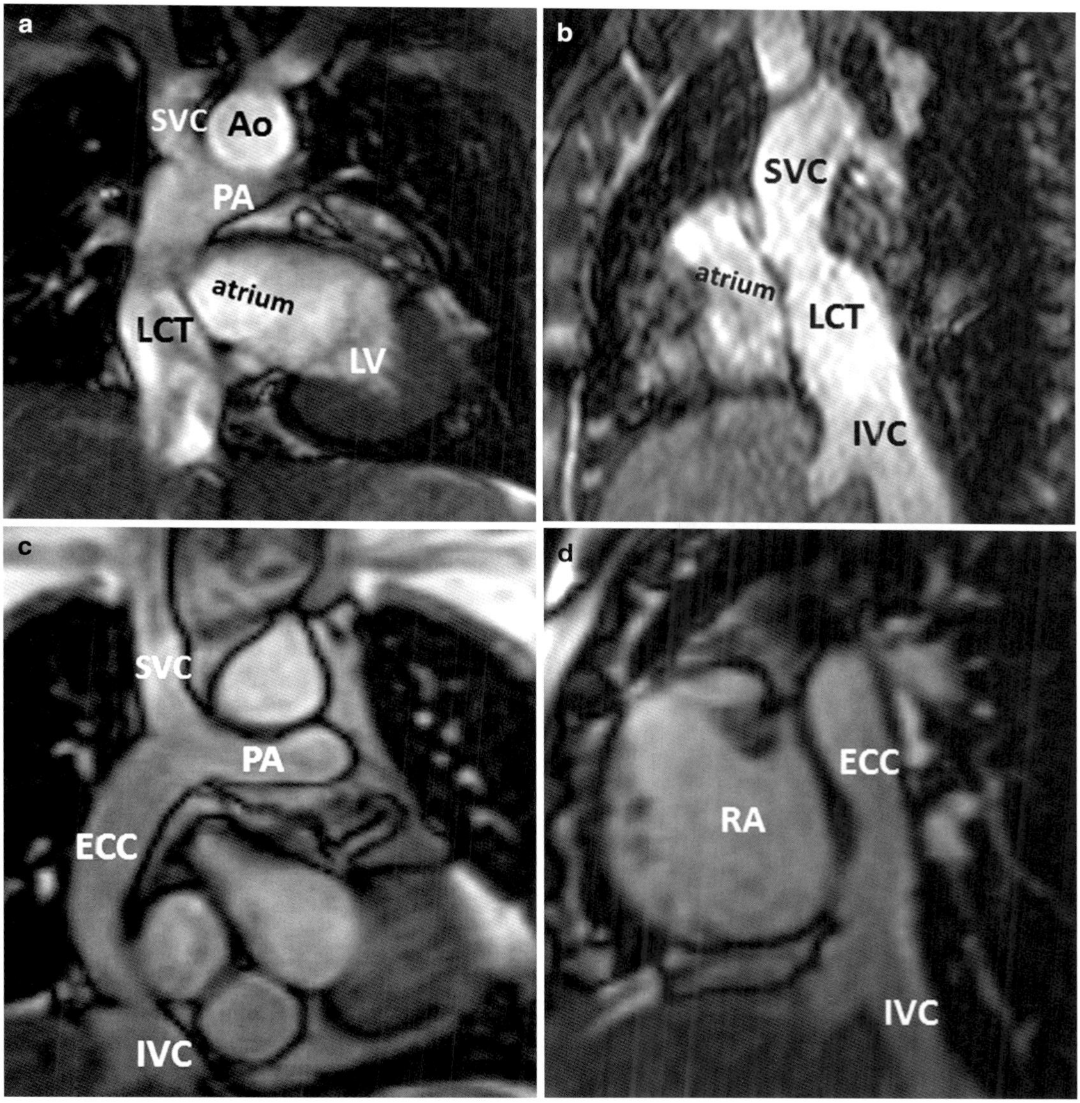

Fig. 21.3 Modified Fontan procedure with total cavopulmonary connections. (**a**, **b**) fenestrated lateral caval/intra-atrial tunnel. Oblique coronal (**a**) and sagittal (**b**) steady-state free precession, bright-blood CMR images of a 16-year-old female with double-inlet left ventricle (*LV*) with a fenestrated lateral caval tunnel constructed from prosthetic material and the lateral wall of the right atrium (*RA*). (**c**, **d**) Non-fenestrated extracardiac conduit connection. Oblique coronal (**c**) and sagittal (**d**) steady-state free precession, bright-blood MR images of a 27-year-old female with pulmonary atresia, hypoplastic right ventricle, after conversion from atriopulmonary Fontan connection to a non-fenestrated extracardiac Fontan conduit (*LCT* lateral caval tunnel, *PA* pulmonary artery, *Ao* aorta, *ECC* extracardiac conduit, *SVC* superior vena cava, *IVC* inferior vena cava)

SVC to the pulmonary artery, and later the hepatic veins are joined to the pulmonary circulation, preventing the development of pulmonary arteriovenous malformations [17, 18] (Fig. 21.5).

While over the years, there have been improved clinical outcomes immediately postoperative and improved patient prognosis and survival into adulthood [12, 19, 20], complications and hemodynamic problems continue to be seen

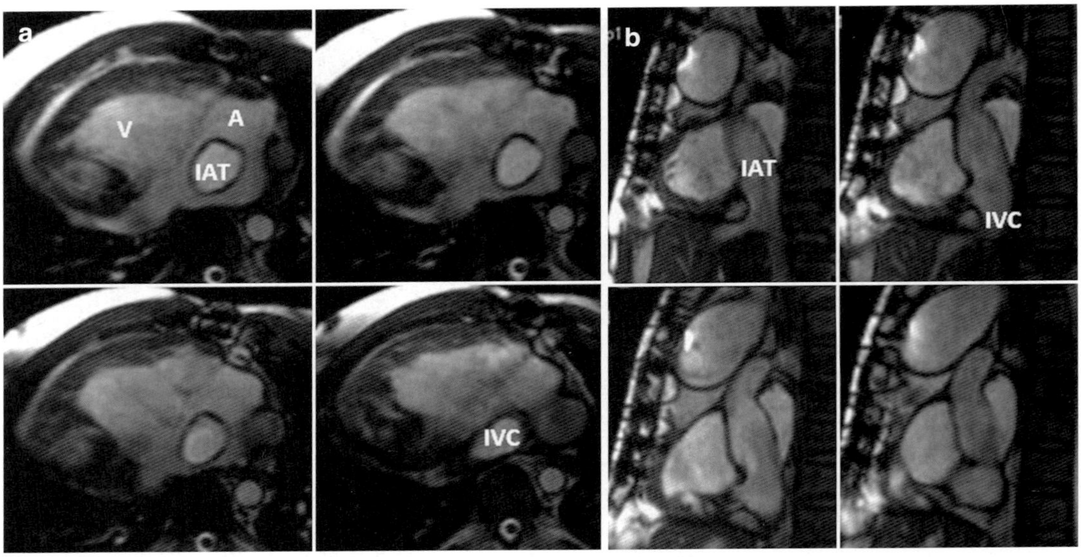

Fig. 21.4 Modified Fontan procedure with total cavopulmonary connections. Oblique axial (**a**) and sagittal (**b**) steady-state free precession, bright-blood cardiac MR images of a 29-year-old male with dextrocardia, pulmonary atresia, unbalanced atrioventricular canal with bidirectional Glenn, and intra-atrial tunnel. *IAT* intra-atrial tunnel, *IVC* inferior vena cava

in the Fontan patient with single ventricle physiology [21, 22]. These include pleural effusions, thromboembolism, atrial dilation and dysrhythmias, conduit stenosis and dilation, exercise intolerance, ventricular failure, pulmonary arteriovenous malformations, aortopulmonary collaterals, venovenous collaterals, protein-losing enteropathy, and plastic bronchitis [11, 14]. Many older patients have experienced relief of symptoms with conversion of their original Fontan atriopulmonary connection to a lateral atrial tunnel or extracardiac conduit, often in conjunction with atrial reduction and/or a Maze procedure to address atrial arrhythmias [10].

Approach to MDCT for the Patient with Fontan Palliation

It is generally preferable to use echocardiography and/or CMR as a first approach to obtain adequate morphologic and functional information when imaging Fontan patients. As echocardiography becomes more difficult in older and larger patients who have had multiple chest surgeries, CMR assumes an important role in noninvasive evaluation of Fontan patients for serial follow-up to assess patency of the systemic venous to pulmonary artery pathways, ventricular function, and flow quantification. MDCT is most often utilized if evaluation of the postoperative vascular morphology is limited on MRI because of susceptibility artifacts from indwelling ferromagnetic materials such as stents, coils, and occlusion devices. Major artifact from vascular occlusion coils obscuring the heart and vasculature can be seen in up to 36 % of Fontan patients [23] (Fig. 21.6). MDCT can be used as an alternative imaging method in patients with indwelling pacemakers and retained pacing wires, which remain as contraindications for CMR. MDCT angiography can provide accurate imaging of the extracardiac vasculature that is comparable to MRI with shorter procedure times and less need for sedation and general anesthesia [24]. MDCT acquisitions with ECG gating or triggering can assess intracardiac and coronary morphology and ventricular function. A significant limitation of using MDCT to evaluate Fontan patients is its current inability to provide flow information to quantify valvular regurgitation, pulmonary and systemic blood flow, and aortopulmonary

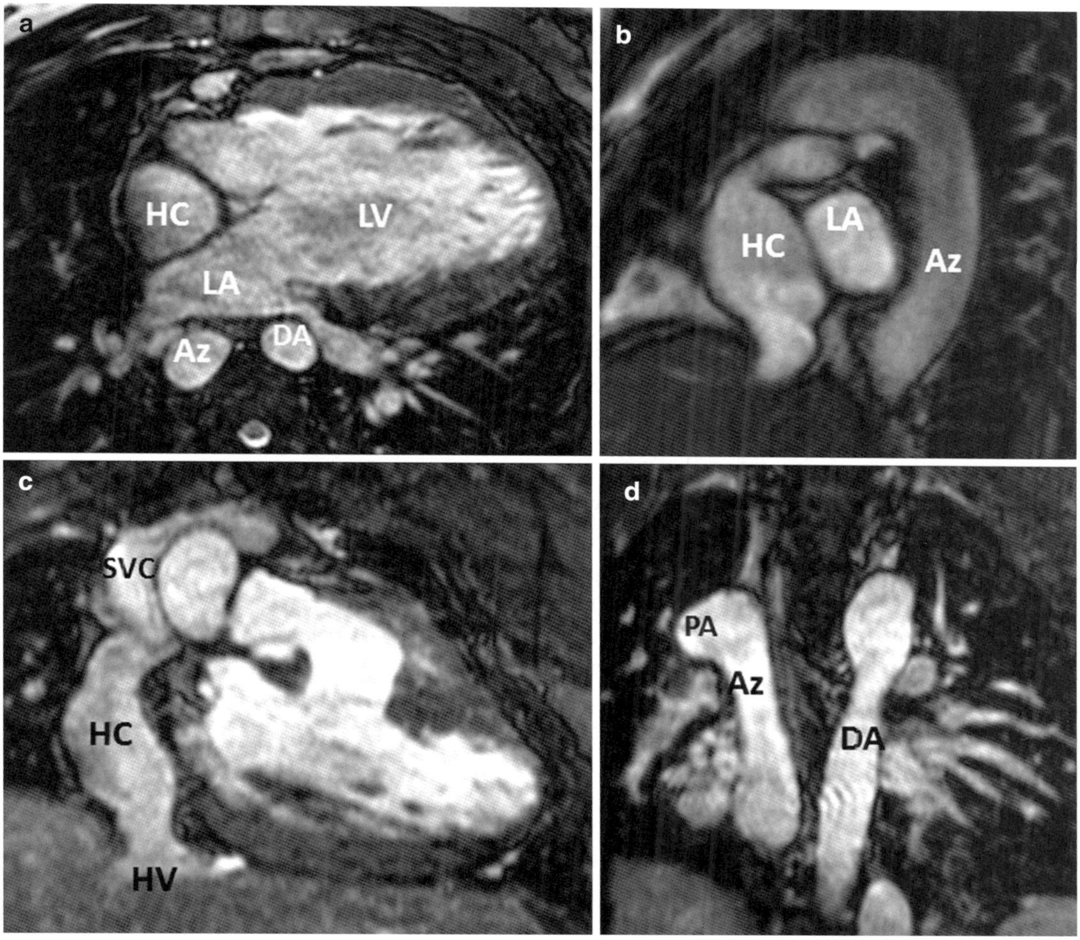

Fig. 21.5 Images from a 3D steady-state free precession, bright-blood acquisition using ECG gating and respiratory (diaphragm) triggering. A 19-year-old male with double-inlet left ventricle (*LV*), l-transposition, azygous (*Az*) continuation of inferior vena cava (*IVC*), aortic coarctation after coarctation repair at age 8 days, Kawashima procedure at age 20 months, and completion of Fontan procedure at age 3 years with intra-atrial patch tunnel of the hepatic veins (*HV*) to right pulmonary artery (PA). (**a**) Axial, (**b**) oblique sagittal, (**c**) anterior coronal, and (**d**) posterior coronal orientations demonstrating hepatic conduit (*HC*) to the right *PA*, azygous continuation of the *IVC* and the descending aorta. *LA* left atrium

collaterals. Therefore, it is preferable to use CMR as opposed to MDCT if there are no contraindications or artifacts on CMR.

Technical Considerations

Cardiovascular imaging using current MDCT technology applies fast tube rotation times to decrease cardiovascular motion artifacts and routinely produces images with sub-mm isotropic spatial resolution. Increased emphasis on radiation dose reduction with improved scanner design over the past 10 years has significantly reduced patient doses with MDCT imaging [25]. Of the many factors that can affect radiation dose, the most important for reducing radiation exposure are to use techniques that adjust the tube current according to the weight of the patient [26], automatic tube current modulation to automatically adjust the tube current based on the size, shape and density of the body part being

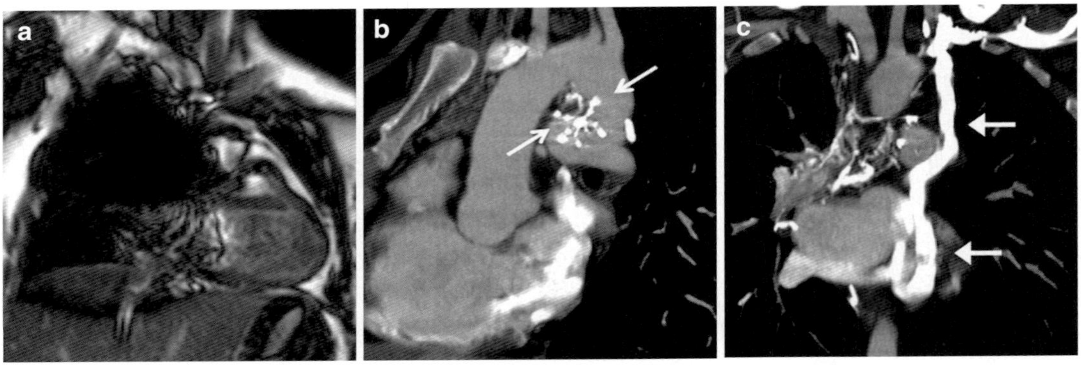

Fig. 21.6 Fontan patient presenting with cyanosis. This patient has a history of prior occlusion of a PDA with a Clamshell device (*arrows* in **b**) which resulted in a large artifact obscuring most of the mediastinum on MRI (**a**) but caused very little artifact on subsequent CT (**b**) sagittal oblique image). A coronal reformatted CT (**c**) reveals the source of the cyanosis to be a large systemic to pulmonary venous collateral (*arrows*) from the left innominate vein to the left-sided pulmonary veins

scanned [27], and fast gantry rotation times [28, 29]. In the past few years, iterative reconstruction of CT images has made a substantial impact on lowering patient doses, in addition to improving image quality by reducing image noise due to streak artifacts from calcification and metallic artifacts [30–33].

Higher patient doses are generally associated with ECG-gated acquisitions which are not needed for routine angiography of the thoracic vasculature. ECG gating is necessary for evaluation of the aortic root and ascending aortic dimensions, coronary arteries, and ventricular function, and therefore, cardiac MDCT angiography with ECG-gated acquisitions should be restricted to these applications. Retrospective ECG gating is used to obtain images throughout the entire cardiac cycle for quantification of ventricular function, wall motion, and motion of valves [34], and the measurement of ventricular volumes, mass, and function has shown good correlation with measurements from CMR [35]. Retrospective ECG gating delivers a relatively high radiation dose because the x-ray tube is on throughout the cardiac cycle to acquire imaging data, and reconstructing multiple phases requires oversampling of image data and results in longer scan times. When imaging the aorta and coronary arteries, radiation doses can be substantially reduced by using prospective ECG triggering instead of retrospective ECG gating. With prospective ECG triggering, scanning is initiated at a predefined moment in the cardiac cycle from the QRS complex, usually in diastole. This technique delivers a low radiation dose because the x-ray tube is only turned on during a predefined portion of the cardiac cycle [36]. MDCT scanners with 320 detector rows (volumetric scanners) or second-generation dual-source scanners have become available with faster scanning so that sedation and breath holding are no longer necessary [37], and gated acquisitions for assessment of the heart and coronary arteries have significantly improved temporal resolution and allowed substantial reduction in radiation doses [38–40].

An important consideration when performing MDCT angiography of Fontan patients is the timing of the contrast injection and initiation of scanning [41]. Because the flow through the Fontan circulation is passive from the systemic venous system to the pulmonary arteries, homogeneous enhancement of the Fontan pathway cannot be obtained until the venous phase of contrast administration is reached. A common error is to commence scanning a Fontan patient with a standard protocol for routine pulmonary MDCT angiography when the pulmonary arteries just begin to be opacified. Scanning this early will result in inhomogeneous enhancement of the Fontan pathway (Fig. 21.7). There are several options for timing the contrast administration and scanning depending on the information that is needed from the examination and the intravenous access that

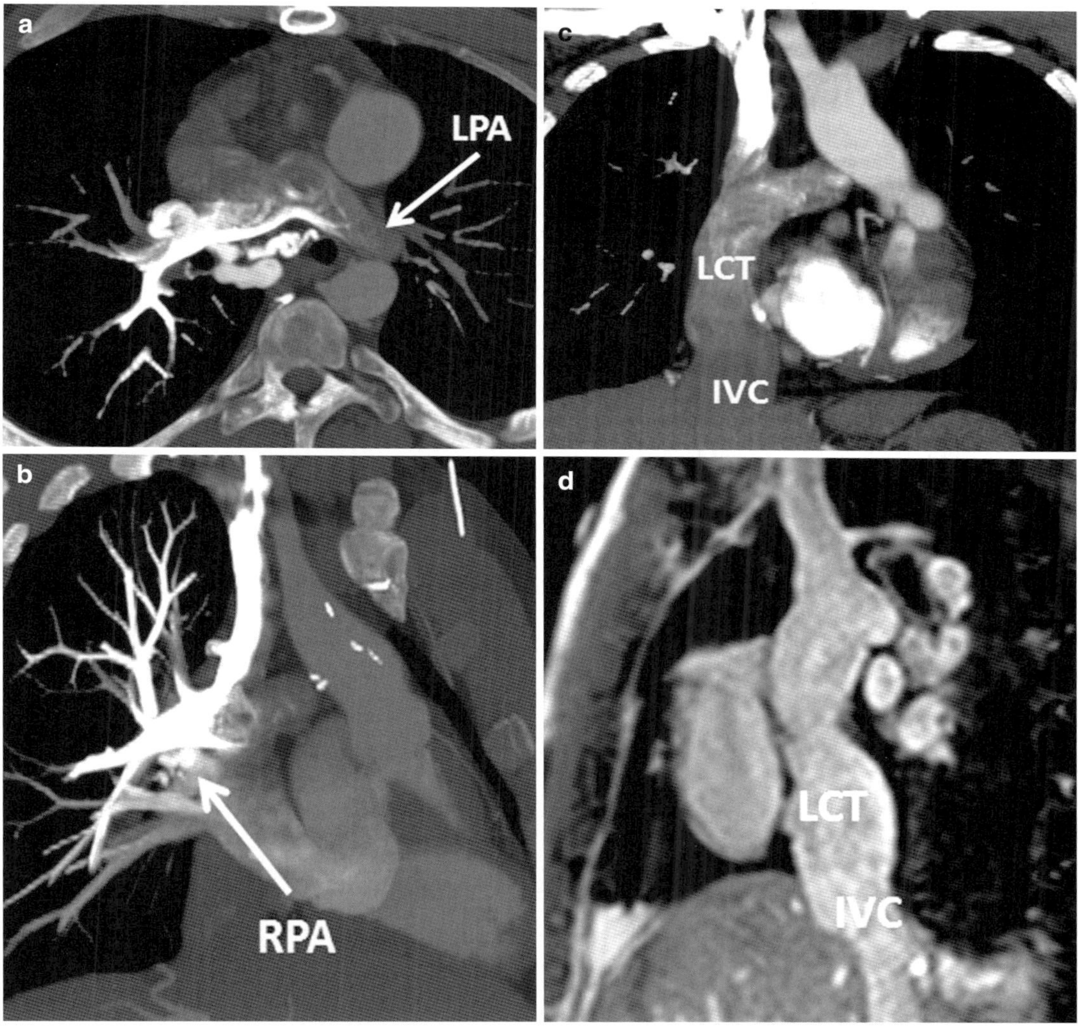

Fig. 21.7 Example of inhomogeneous opacification of the Fontan circulation on CT. Patient with congenitally corrected transposition of the great arteries (TGA) and straddling tricuspid valve status post lateral tunnel Fontan presented with chest pain and concern for pulmonary embolism. Scanning was initiated during bolus tracking when the contrast had just started to enhance the pulmonary arteries, resulting in inhomogeneous opacification of the central pulmonary arteries (oblique axial image **a**) and preferential enhancement of the right pulmonary artery (*RPA*) from an upper extremity injection (oblique coronal image **b**). The lateral conduit tunnel (*LCT*) from the inferior vena cava (*IVC*) to the *RPA* (coronal image, **c**) has unopacified blood from the *IVC* simulating extensive filling defect from thrombus. (**d**) An oblique sagittal steady-state free precession image from a subsequent MRI shows a patent *LCT* with no intraluminal thrombus. *LPA* left pulmonary artery

can be established. Imaging to assess the Fontan pathway and pulmonary artery patency and possible thrombus requires homogeneous opacification which can be obtained with administering contrast via an upper or lower extremity IV and scanning at 50–70 s. Bolus tracking of the IVC for an upper extremity injection and bolus tracking of the SVC for a lower extremity injection can be used, but care must be taken to delay the initiation of the bolus tracking during the contrast injection in order to keep the radiation dose low. Based on this author's experience, a 60-s scan delay routinely provides adequate contrast opacification of all of the intrathoracic vasculature with only

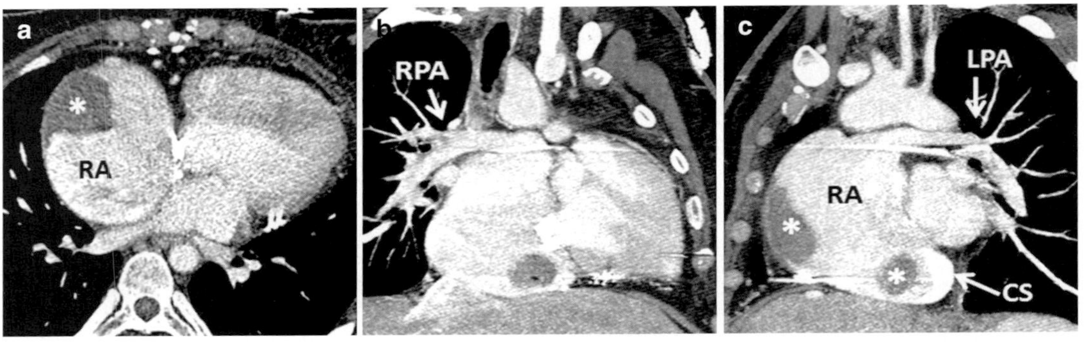

Fig. 21.8 Status post Fontan with right atrial appendage to pulmonary artery anastomosis for double-inlet/double-outlet right ventricle and pacemaker insertion for complete heart block. CT requested prior to catheter ablation of persistent atrial flutter. Axial (**a**) and oblique coronal (**b**, **c**) images acquired with delayed scanning approximately 1 min following contrast injection show a severely dilated right atrium (*RA*) with extensive intraluminal thrombus (*asterisks*). The central pulmonary arteries are homogeneously opacified with no evidence of pulmonary embolism. *LPA* left pulmonary artery, *CS* coronary sinus, *RPA* right pulmonary artery

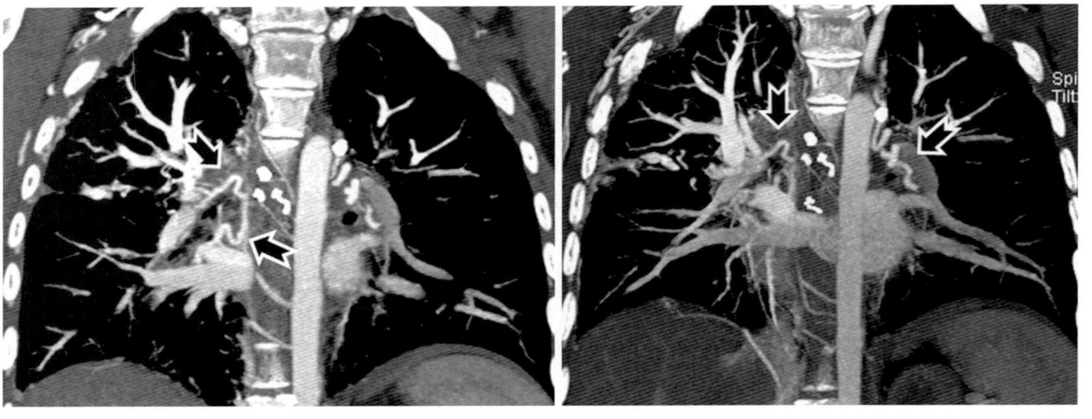

Fig. 21.9 Aortopulmonary collaterals in a patient presenting with hemoptysis status post lateral tunnel Fontan for mitral atresia. Despite extensive prior efforts at coil occlusion of multiple aortopulmonary collaterals, arterial phase CT scanning (coronal maximum intensity projection images) shows recurrent or residual collaterals extending into pulmonary veins on both sides (*arrows*)

minor inhomogeneity (Fig. 21.8). Others have found that waiting until 3 min after contrast administration provides the most homogeneous contrast opacification [42], but this is at the expense of overall reduction of contrast density, which can make image interpretation difficult, especially if low radiation dose protocols are utilized. Another option is to administer contrast with simultaneous injections of the upper and lower extremity, which allows denser opacification of the entire Fontan circulation but can be difficult if there is poor IV access. For detection of aortopulmonary collaterals, which can be a source of life-threatening hemoptysis, an earlier arterial phase scan for dense opacification of the aorta is required (Fig. 21.9).

Imaging of Fontan patients with MDCT as an alternative to CMR could be considered in the following situations: patients with acute decompensation and suspected thrombus in the Fontan circulation and pulmonary embolism (Fig. 21.8) and suspected airway compromise in patients who have persistent respiratory symptoms, as with plastic bronchitis [43] (Fig. 21.10) or prolonged

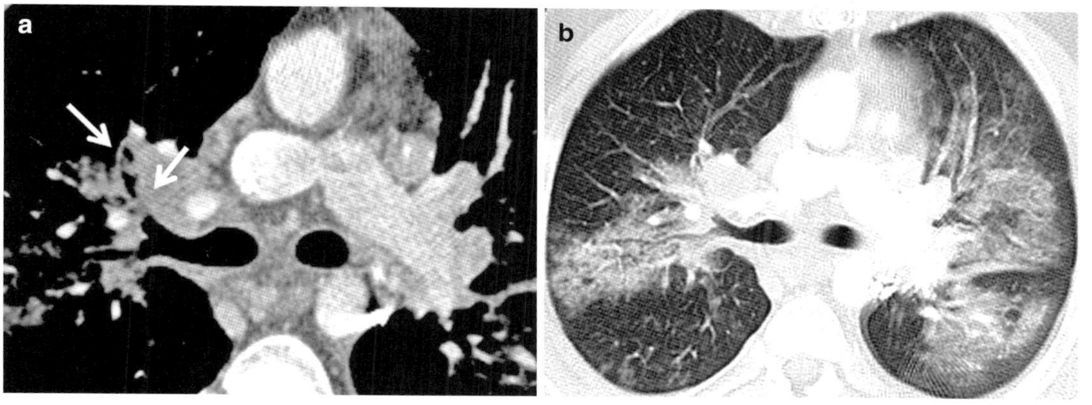

Fig. 21.10 Plastic bronchitis status post fenestrated Fontan for double-outlet right ventricle (*DORV*) and pacemaker insertion for sick sinus syndrome. Axial CT images with mediastinal (**a**) and lung windows (**b**) show filling defects within the right upper lobe bronchus (*arrows* in **a**) consistent with bronchial casts associated with extensive areas of lobar consolidation within the lungs (**b**)

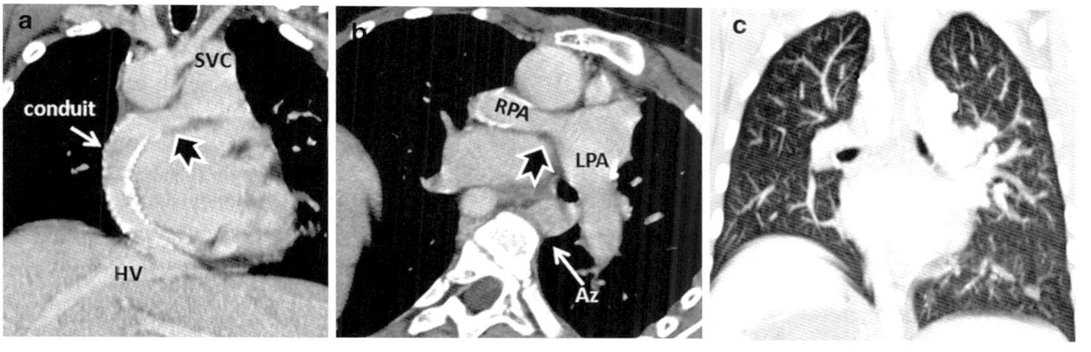

Fig. 21.11 Pulmonary arteriovenous communications causing cyanosis developed in a patient with heterotaxy, double-outlet right ventricle and interrupted inferior vena cava with left azygous (*AZ*) continuation status post Kawashima with left superior vena cava (*SVC*) to left pulmonary artery (*LPA*) anastomosis and an extracardiac conduit to baffle the hepatic veins (*HV*) to the pulmonary arteries. (**a**, **b**) Narrowing of the intrapulmonary artery confluence (*arrows*) results in preferential flow of the hepatic venous blood through the conduit to the right pulmonary artery (*RPA*). (**c**) Diffuse increased peripheral vascularity is present throughout the left lung as compared with the right consistent with multiple pulmonary arteriovenous communications

requirement for mechanical ventilation in the early postoperative period [44] and for reliable visualization of the vascular lumen inside stents to provide an accurate noninvasive assessment of stent patency [45]. MDCT can be used to detect sources of cyanosis such as systemic to pulmonary venous collaterals (Fig. 21.6) or pulmonary arteriovenous malformations (AVMs). Pulmonary AVMs can develop in patients who have a Glenn or Fontan circulation that results in a relative lack of hepatic venous blood being able to reach the pulmonary circulation. There is also increased incidence of pulmonary AVMs in heterotaxy patients with interrupted IVC and azygous continuation who have had the Kawashima operation (bidirectional cavopulmonary connections in the setting of azygous continuation of an interrupted IVC to the SVC) if the hepatic venous blood is not incorporated into the pulmonary circulation. Pulmonary AVMs may also develop if the hepatic venous blood is asymmetrically distributed to the pulmonary arteries (Fig. 21.11). Pulmonary AVMs tend to be very small and diffuse and are more readily visualized on MDCT if they are unilateral [46].

Approach to Cardiac MRI for the Adult Fontan Patient

While echocardiography remains in the forefront for cardiac imaging due to its accessibility, in recent years, value has been seen with the additional information obtained from CMR [47]. Clinical assessment of the single ventricle patient requires working knowledge of the complex anatomy and is best undertaken after review of all pertinent clinical data (including operative report, clinical history, recent chest x-ray, recent catheterization, and echocardiographic data) so that there is a clear understanding of the question(s) to be answered. While the CMR study should be complete, including not only anatomic definition and standard volumetric and flow data acquisition, features obtained with CMR can be tailored to answer pertinent clinical concerns (Table 21.2).

MR views should include not only the Fontan circuit but also the Glenn anastomosis and branch pulmonary arteries, the atrial septal defect, the atrioventricular valve(s), aorta (or neo-aorta), aortic arch, pulmonary venous and systemic venous drainage, coronaries, and aortopulmonary collaterals. Interventional procedures with device placement, such as for fenestration closure (Fig. 21.12) and stenting of arteries (Fig. 21.13), must be considered in choosing the optimal

Table 21.2 Key cardiac MR assessments in Fontan patients

Clinical issue	Focus of CMR assessment
Hepatomegaly	Baffle patency
Ascites/protein-losing enteropathy	Atrioventricular valvular regurgitation/stenosis
Superior vena cava syndrome	Myocardial function/ischemia
Hypoxia	Fenestration patency/baffle leak/Qp:Qs
	Branch pulmonary arterial flow
	Venovenous collaterals
Decreased cardiac output	Myocardial function/ischemia
	Valvular regurgitation (atrioventricular valve/aorta)
	Residual arch obstruction
Stroke	Thrombus
Arrhythmia	Valvular regurgitation/stenosis
	Atrial and ventricular size
	Myocardial function/fibrosis

Qp pulmonary flow, *Qs* systemic flow

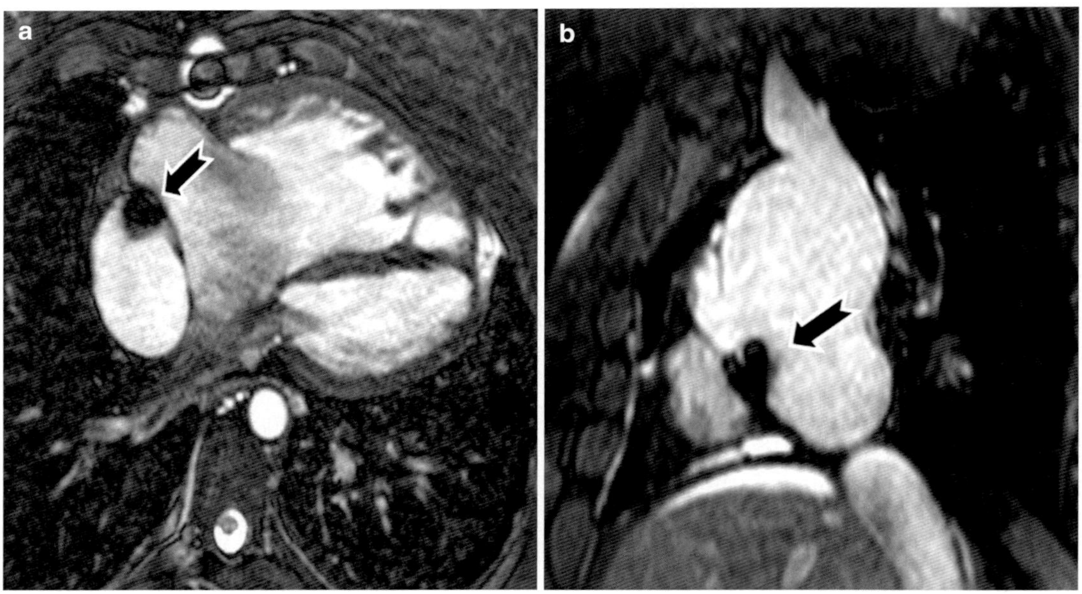

Fig. 21.12 A 20-year-old with double-outlet right ventricle, d-transposition of the great arteries, pulmonary atresia status post right atrium to pulmonary artery Fontan, and fenestration device closure (*black arrows*). Cardiac MR steady-state free precession/bright-blood images in axial (**a**) and sagittal (**b**) projections

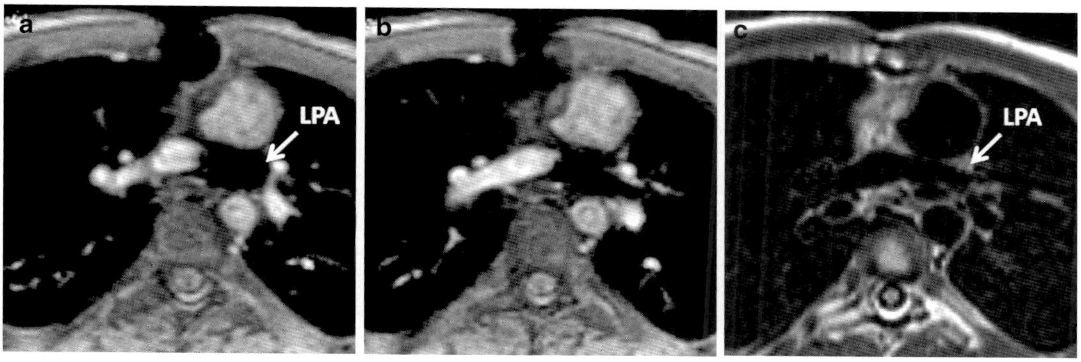

Fig. 21.13 Patient with Fontan and left pulmonary artery (LPA) stenosis with placement of stent in LPA. (**a**, **b**) CMR steady-state free precession (*SSFP*) bright-blood images show artifact from stent (*arrows*). Also note sternal wire artifact in SSFP images. (**c**) Dark blood image allows better visualization of *LPA* (E-*white arrow*). Dark blood sequence is usually fast spin echo which makes it less sensitive to local field inhomogeneity

Table 21.3 CMR single ventricle imaging protocol

Imaging sequence	Potential issues
True FISP/SSFP or fast spin echo: 3D or multiplanar	3D acquisition is time-consuming; dark blood images may fail to fully suppress sluggish flow: ?
Cine SSFP: 2Ch, 4Ch, SA, select planes including coronal and sagittal Fontan baffle, branch PA flow as indicated	Artifact from turbulent flow may be addressed with use of gradient echo (GRE)
Cine GRE: as needed for less artifact	Time-consuming scan
First-pass perfusion: 3 slices SA, 1 slice 4Ch (optional)	Gadolinium injection, timing, limited slice acquisition
MRA	Gadolinium injection, timing Spatial vs. time-resolved acquisition
VENC PC cine (during 10-min delay)	Estimate flow velocity from ECHO or knowledge of normal velocities
Cross sections: IVC, SVC, DA, RPA and LPA, Aorta, PV Parallel Fontan, SVC, IVC	Acquisition planes may be difficult for PV
Delayed enhancement: same slices as first pass, plus 2Ch, 4Ch, SA	Timing and selection of correct time of inversion important

SSFP steady-state free precession, *PA* pulmonary artery, *Ch* chamber, *SA* short axis, *IVC* inferior vena cava, *SVC* superior vena cava, *DA* descending aorta, *RPA* right pulmonary artery, *LPA* left pulmonary artery, *PV* pulmonary veins, *VENC PC* velocity-encoded phase contrast

sequence of imaging to acquire data desired from the CMR exam. Artifacts may completely obscure the anatomy in question with some acquisitions and not others. Some metal creates large artifact, while others only result in a local artifact (Figs. 21.6 and 21.13). In addition, definition of the myocardial mass and the relationship of the single ventricle to the vasculature are of paramount importance. This can all be achieved with a standard protocol (Table 21.3), but for best results requires that the CMR clinician be present at the scanner during imaging to adjust imaging planes and method of image acquisition.

Besides anatomic definition, CMR offers the ability to assess myocardial function in a quantitative fashion, whether the patient has a morphologic right or left ventricle as the dominant single ventricle. Quantification techniques, using commercially available post-processing software, have been described elsewhere [48, 49]. Qualitative regional wall motion assessment can be undertaken with emerging novel research to

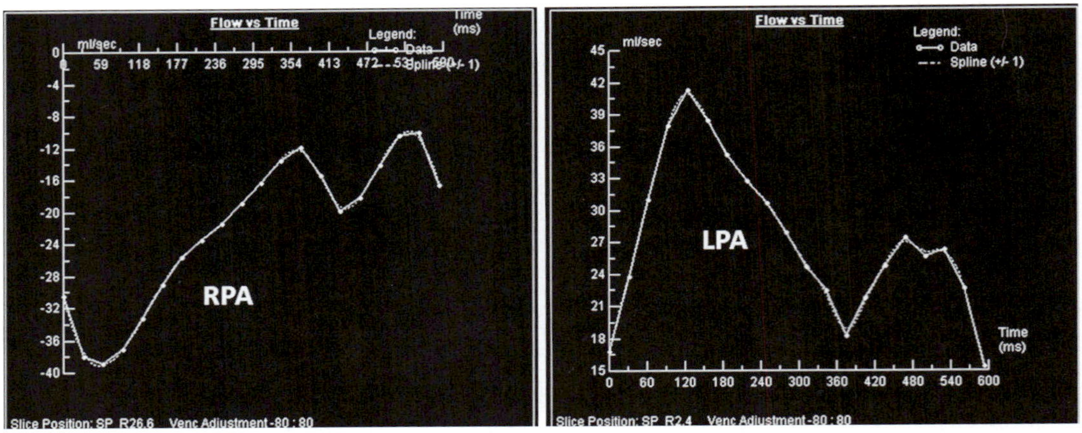

Fig. 21.14 Flow versus time curves of the pulmonary arteries. Flows in the right pulmonary artery (*RPA*) and left pulmonary artery (*LPA*) are measured separately to determine differential pulmonary artery flow. In Fontan patients, velocity encoding settings are usually lower with expected venous flow patterns

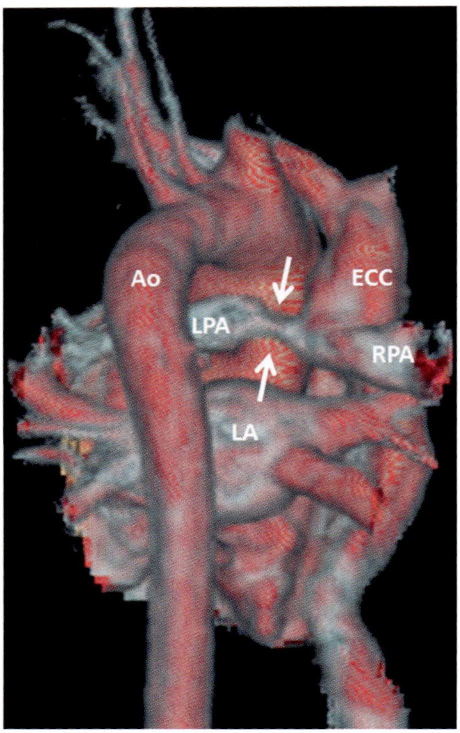

Fig. 21.15 Posterior view of 3D volume rendering of extracardiac Fontan patient with narrow central pulmonary artery region (between *arrows*). *Ao* aorta, *LPA* left pulmonary artery, *RPA* right pulmonary artery, *ECC* extracardiac conduit, *LA* left atrium

quantify regional wall stress and strain by CMR which may allow a better understanding of ventricular failure long term [50].

CMR assessment of blood flow for the patient after Fontan palliation requires a systematic approach, so as to derive maximal benefit from scanning (see Chap. 23 for details). In addition to determining the degree of atrioventricular valve and aortic (or neo-aortic) valve regurgitation with standard flow methods described elsewhere in this text, CMR allows quantification of differential pulmonary flow (Figs. 21.14 and 21.15) and estimation of aortopulmonary collateral (APC) blood flow [51, 52]. The latter can be achieved in the Fontan circulation by one of the methods described by Grosse-Wortmann et al with fair agreement between the two methods ($r = 0.73$):

Method A: APC flow = Total pulmonary vein flow − right + left pulmonary artery flow

Method B: APC flow = Ascending aorta flow − Descending aorta at the diaphragm + superior venacava flow

APC flow volume fraction is the ratio of APC flow to the total pulmonary vein flow.

Finally, gadolinium contrast can be used in several ways to evaluate the patient presenting with Fontan physiology. It may be given as a single bolus to capture a magnetic resonance angiogram

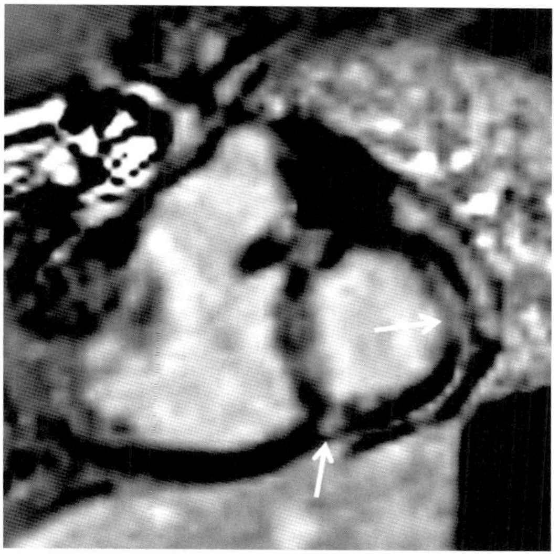

Fig. 21.16 A 13-year-old with history of double-outlet right ventricle, hypoplastic left ventricle (*LV*), combined ventricular function of 33 %, and fibrosis detected in portions of the LV (*arrows*). MR (phase-sensitive inversion recovery, steady-state free precession) demonstrates myocardial delayed enhancement 10 min after gadolinium administration

(MRA) that allows a three-dimensional reconstruction of anatomy to be rendered. This often allows enhanced appreciation of anatomic issues, such as aortic root dilation, branch pulmonary artery compression, location of systemic and pulmonary veins relative to the Fontan circuit (see Fig. 21.14). Alternatively, some of the gadolinium contrast may be used for perfusion imaging at rest or after pharmacologic stress. Techniques are described elsewhere in this book. Understanding the presence, location, and extent of delayed enhancement may better allow the clinician to understand why ventricular failure or rhythm abnormalities may have ensued. Myocardial fibrosis (Fig. 21.16), detected by CMR as late gadolinium enhancement, has been associated with adverse myocardial mechanics and ventricular tachycardia [53].

Conclusion

Over the past four decades, the Fontan procedure has undergone multiple adaptations and has been applied in numerous patients who have complex congenital cardiac defects with single ventricle physiology. Each modification was developed and applied in an attempt to decrease complications related to the original Fontan procedure, with the hope of improving patient survival and quality of life. However, long-term clinical deterioration continues to occur due to high central venous pressure, chronic low cardiac output, and ventricular dysfunction. The advanced imaging techniques of MDCT and CMR assist providers in making critical clinical decisions as they care for these complex patients into adulthood.

References

1. Castaneda AR. From Glenn to Fontan. A continuing evolution. Circulation. 1992;86:II80–4.
2. Trusler GA, Williams WG, Cohen AJ, et al. William Glenn lecture. The cavopulmonary shunt. Evolution of a concept. Circulation. 1990;82:IV131–8.
3. Fontan F, Baudet E. Surgical repair of tricuspid atresia. Thorax. 1971;26:240–8.
4. Reul GJ, Gregoric ID. Recent modifications of the Fontan procedure for complex congenital heart disease. Tex Heart Inst J. 1992;19:223–31.
5. Said SM, Burkhart HM, Dearani JA. The Fontan connections: past, present, and future. World J Pediatr Congenit Heart Surg. 2012;3:171–82.
6. Kreutzer G, Galindez E, Bono H, De Palma C, Laura JP. An operation for the correction of tricuspid atresia. J Thorac Cardiovasc Surg. 1973;66:613–21.
7. Kreutzer GO, Vargas FJ, Schlichter AJ, et al. Atriopulmonary anastomosis. J Thorac Cardiovasc Surg. 1982;83:427–36.
8. Bjork VO, Olin CL, Bjarke BB, Thoren CA. Right atrial-right ventricular anastomosis for correction of tricuspid atresia. J Thorac Cardiovasc Surg. 1979;77:452–8.
9. Cowgill LD. The Fontan procedure: a historical review. Ann Thorac Surg. 1991;51:1026–30.
10. Mavroudis C, Backer CL, Deal BJ, Johnsrude C, Strasburger J. Total cavopulmonary conversion and maze procedure for patients with failure of the Fontan operation. J Thorac Cardiovasc Surg. 2001;122:863–71.
11. Fredenburg TB, Johnson TR, Cohen MD. The Fontan procedure: anatomy, complications, and manifestations of failure. Radiographics. 2011;31:453–63.
12. de Leval MR, Kilner P, Gewillig M, Bull C. Total cavopulmonary connection: a logical alternative to atriopulmonary connection for complex Fontan operations. Experimental studies and early clinical experience. J Thorac Cardiovasc Surg. 1988;96:682–95.
13. Marcelletti C, Corno A, Giannico S, Marino B. Inferior vena cava-pulmonary artery extracardiac conduit. A new form of right heart bypass. J Thorac Cardiovasc Surg. 1990;100:228–32.

14. Rogers LS, Glatz AC, Ravishankar C, et al. 18 years of the Fontan operation at a single institution: results from 771 consecutive patients. J Am Coll Cardiol. 2012;60:1018–25.
15. Norwood WI, Jacobs ML. Fontan's procedure in two stages. Am J Surg. 1993;166:548–51.
16. Kawashima Y, Kitamura S, Matsuda H, Shimazaki Y, Nakano S, Hirose H. Total cavopulmonary shunt operation in complex cardiac anomalies. A new operation. J Thorac Cardiovasc Surg. 1984;87:74–81.
17. Srivastava D, Preminger T, Lock JE, et al. Hepatic venous blood and the development of pulmonary arteriovenous malformations in congenital heart disease. Circulation. 1995;92:1217–22.
18. McElhinney DB, Kreutzer J, Lang P, Mayer Jr JE, del Nido PJ, Lock JE. Incorporation of the hepatic veins into the cavopulmonary circulation in patients with heterotaxy and pulmonary arteriovenous malformations after a Kawashima procedure. Ann Thorac Surg. 2005;80:1597–603.
19. Bradley SM, Mosca RS, Hennein HA, Crowley DC, Kulik TJ, Bove EL. Bidirectional superior cavopulmonary connection in young infants. Circulation. 1996;94:II5–11.
20. Lemler MS, Scott WA, Leonard SR, Stromberg D, Ramaciotti C. Fenestration improves clinical outcome of the fontan procedure: a prospective, randomized study. Circulation. 2002;105:207–12.
21. Rychik J, Goldberg D, Dodds K. Long-term results and consequences of single ventricle palliation. Prog Pediatr Cardiol. 2010;29:19–23.
22. Rychik J. Forty years of the Fontan operation: a failed strategy. Semin Thorac Cardiovasc Surg Pediatr Card Surg Annu. 2010;13:96–100.
23. Garg R, Powell AJ, Sena L, Marshall AC, Geva T. Effects of metallic implants on magnetic resonance imaging evaluation of Fontan palliation. Am J Cardiol. 2005;95:688–91.
24. Lambert V, Sigal-Cinqualbre A, Belli E, et al. Preoperative and postoperative evaluation of airways compression in pediatric patients with 3-dimensional multislice computed tomographic scanning: effect on surgical management. J Thorac Cardiovasc Surg. 2005;129:1111–8.
25. McCollough CH, Chen GH, Kalender W, et al. Achieving routine submillisievert CT scanning: report from the summit on management of radiation dose in CT. Radiology. 2012;264:567–80.
26. Donnelly LF, Emery KH, Brody AS, et al. Minimizing radiation dose for pediatric body applications of single-detector helical CT: strategies at a large Children's Hospital. AJR Am J Roentgenol. 2001;176: 303–6.
27. Kalra MK, Maher MM, Toth TL, et al. Strategies for CT radiation dose optimization. Radiology. 2004;230: 619–28.
28. Frush DP. Strategies of dose reduction. Pediatr Radiol. 2002;32:293–7.
29. Lell MM, May M, Deak P, et al. High-pitch spiral computed tomography: effect on image quality and radiation dose in pediatric chest computed tomography. Invest Radiol. 2011;46:116–23.
30. Renker M, Ramachandra A, Schoepf UJ, et al. Iterative image reconstruction techniques: applications for cardiac CT. J Cardiovasc Comput Tomogr. 2011;5:225–30.
31. Han BK, Grant KL, Garberich R, Sedlmair M, Lindberg J, Lesser JR. Assessment of an iterative reconstruction algorithm (SAFIRE) on image quality in pediatric cardiac CT datasets. J Cardiovasc Comput Tomogr. 2012;6:200–4.
32. Nelson RC, Feuerlein S, Boll DT. New iterative reconstruction techniques for cardiovascular computed tomography: how do they work, and what are the advantages and disadvantages? J Cardiovasc Comput Tomogr. 2011;5:286–92.
33. Mieville FA, Gudinchet F, Rizzo E, et al. Paediatric cardiac CT examinations: impact of the iterative reconstruction method ASIR on image quality–preliminary findings. Pediatr Radiol. 2011;41: 1154–64.
34. Flohr T, Prokop M, Becker C, et al. A retrospectively ECG-gated multislice spiral CT scan and reconstruction technique with suppression of heart pulsation artifacts for cardio-thoracic imaging with extended volume coverage. Eur Radiol. 2002;12: 1497–503.
35. Takx RA, Moscariello A, Schoepf UJ, et al. Quantification of left and right ventricular function and myocardial mass: comparison of low-radiation dose 2nd generation dual-source CT and cardiac MRI. Eur J Radiol. 2012;81:e598–604.
36. Kim HY, Lee JW, Hong YJ, et al. Dual-source coronary CT angiography in patients with high heart rates using a prospectively ECG-triggered axial mode at end-systole. Int J Cardiovasc Imaging. 2012;28 (Suppl 2):101–7.
37. Baumueller S, Alkadhi H, Stolzmann P, et al. Computed tomography of the lung in the high-pitch mode: is breath holding still required? Invest Radiol. 2011;46:240–5.
38. Han BK, Lindberg J, Overman D, Schwartz RS, Grant K, Lesser JR. Safety and accuracy of dual-source coronary computed tomography angiography in the pediatric population. J Cardiovasc Comput Tomogr. 2012;6:252–9.
39. Fink C, Krissak R, Henzler T, et al. Radiation dose at coronary CT angiography: second-generation dual-source CT versus single-source 64-MDCT and first-generation dual-source CT. AJR Am J Roentgenol. 2011;196:W550–7.
40. Paul JF, Rohnean A, Elfassy E, Sigal-Cinqualbre A. Radiation dose for thoracic and coronary step-and-shoot CT using a 128-slice dual-source machine in infants and small children with congenital heart disease. Pediatr Radiol. 2011;41:244–9.
41. Prabhu SP, Mahmood S, Sena L, Lee EY. MDCT evaluation of pulmonary embolism in children and young adults following a lateral tunnel Fontan procedure: optimizing contrast-enhancement techniques. Pediatr Radiol. 2009;39:938–44.

42. Park EA, Lee W, Chung SY, Yin YH, Chung JW, Park JH. Optimal scan timing and intravenous route for contrast-enhanced computed tomography in patients after Fontan operation. J Comput Assist Tomogr. 2010;34:75–81.
43. Goo HW, Jhang WK, Kim YH, et al. CT findings of plastic bronchitis in children after a Fontan operation. Pediatr Radiol. 2008;38:989–93.
44. Kim YM, Yoo SJ, Kim TH, et al. Three-dimensional computed tomography in children with compression of the central airways complicating congenital heart disease. Cardiol Young. 2002;12:44–50.
45. Eichhorn JG, Long FR, Hill SL, et al. Assessment of in-stent stenosis in small children with congenital heart disease using multi-detector computed tomography: a validation study. Catheter Cardiovasc Interv. 2006;68:11–20.
46. Choi YH, Lee W, Cheon JE, et al. CT findings in unilateral hepatopulmonary syndrome after the Fontan operation. Pediatr Radiol. 2009;39:336–42.
47. Babu-Narayan SV, Kilner PJ, Gatzoulis MA. When to order cardiovascular magnetic resonance in adults with congenital heart disease. Curr Cardiol Rep. 2003;5:324–30.
48. Alfakih K, Thiele H, Plein S, Bainbridge GJ, Ridgway JP, Sivananthan MU. Comparison of right ventricular volume measurement between segmented k-space gradient-echo and steady-state free precession magnetic resonance imaging. J Magn Reson Imaging. 2002;16:253–8.
49. Robbers-Visser D, Boersma E, Helbing WA. Normal biventricular function, volumes, and mass in children aged 8 to 17 years. J Magn Reson Imaging. 2009;29:552–9.
50. Hor KN, Gottliebson WM, Carson C, et al. Comparison of magnetic resonance feature tracking for strain calculation with harmonic phase imaging analysis. JACC Cardiovasc Imaging. 2010;3:144–51.
51. Grosse-Wortmann L, Al-Otay A, Yoo SJ. Aortopulmonary collaterals after bidirectional cavopulmonary connection or Fontan completion: quantification with MRI. Circ Cardiovasc Imaging. 2009;2:219–25.
52. Whitehead KK, Gillespie MJ, Harris MA, Fogel MA, Rome JJ. Noninvasive quantification of systemic-to-pulmonary collateral flow: a major source of inefficiency in patients with superior cavopulmonary connections. Circ Cardiovasc Imaging. 2009;2:405–11.
53. Rathod RH, Prakash A, Powell AJ, Geva T. Myocardial fibrosis identified by cardiac magnetic resonance late gadolinium enhancement is associated with adverse ventricular mechanics and ventricular tachycardia late after Fontan operation. J Am Coll Cardiol. 2010;55:1721–8.

Transcatheter Interventions in Adult Congenital Heart Disease

22

Damien Kenny, John Hibbeln, and Ziyad M. Hijazi

Recent reports have suggested that the number of adults with congenital heart disease (CHD) has surpassed pediatric numbers and that approximately 1 in 150 adults has some form of CHD [1, 2]. Significant rates of intervention and re-intervention are required in this cohort of patients with one report demonstrating 20 % of young adults with CHD requiring cardiovascular surgery [3]. Increasingly, transcatheter alternatives to surgery exist in this population particularly in the field of transcatheter pulmonary valve replacement (tPVR), and recommendations for catheter intervention in adults with CHD have been published in the context of overall care of these patients [2].

Case complexity will vary according to the underlying diagnosis ranging from more straightforward interventions such as atrial septal defect closure to complex stenting interventions for interatrial baffle leak in patients following atrial switch surgery for transposition of the great arteries. Many of the more complex patients may have had multiple previous interventions, and detailed review of previous data as well as sensible use of pre-procedural imaging techniques including cardiac CT and MRI is essential. This chapter will outline some of the procedural techniques and the diagnostic imaging tools used to optimize patient selection and procedural success. Outcome data where available will also be discussed in relation to the range of transcatheter interventions seen in this patient group.

Preparation

Preparation is key to a successful intervention. Patient records are often voluminous and may span over two to three decades. Data, particularly regarding surgical interventions, may be sparse or conflicting. Comorbidities often significantly complicate the procedure, and challenging vascular access if not appreciated prior to the intervention may significantly disrupt the optimal approach. Review of prior imaging is vital. Collaboration with cardiovascular radiology colleagues including review of pre-procedural specialized imaging may determine success or failure of the procedure and may also highlight other previously undiagnosed lesions (Fig. 22.1).

D. Kenny, MD, MRCPCH (✉)
Rush Center for Congenital and Structural Heart Disease, Rush University Medical Center, 1653 West Congress Parkway, Chicago, IL 60612, USA
e-mail: damien_kenny@rush.edu

J. Hibbeln, MD, FACR
Department of Radiology, Rush University Medical Center, 1653 West Congress Parkway, Chicago, IL 60612, USA

Z.M. Hijazi, MD, MPH, FSCAI
Rush Center for Congenital and Structural Heart Disease, Rush University Medical Center, 1653 West Congress Parkway, Chicago, IL 60612, USA
e-mail: zhijazi@rush.edu

F. Saremi (ed.), *Cardiac CT and MR for Adult Congenital Heart Disease*,
DOI 10.1007/978-1-4614-8875-0_22, © Springer Science+Business Media New York 2014

Careful attention should be given to the type of anesthesia required and access to a high-risk preanesthesia clinic is helpful. Decision regarding the type of anesthesia may reflect the complexity of the intervention or the need for and type of intraprocedural imaging (intracardiac vs transesophageal echocardiography). In simpler cases or those who are high-risk patients, general anesthesia may be avoided with the use of intracardiac echocardiography (ICE). ICE provides detailed images of all intracardiac structures including the pulmonary valve following transcatheter pulmonary valve replacement when residual catheters across the valve required for angiography may exaggerate the degree of pulmonary incompetence (Fig. 22.2).

Collaboration between pediatric and coronary interventionalists should be encouraged as varying experiences bring fresh perspective particularly in the setting of coronary artery work with coronary artery fistulae, when the need for rapid intervention to the coronary artery may be required (Fig. 22.3). Honesty is required regarding level of comfort with each specific procedure, and expectation and pride should never impact upon optimal patient care.

Thus the adult congenital interventionalist is often required to be the coordinator for a number of subspecialists to focus detailed imaging review and collaborate with colleagues who provide specialist input so as to optimize outcomes from complex and varied interventions.

Defect and Vascular Occlusion

Transcatheter Atrial Septal Defect Closure

Atrial septal defect (ASD) accounts for 25–30 % of congenital heart defects that are diagnosed in adulthood. Clinical guidelines for closure in adults are published [2] and class one indications (*level of evidence B*) support closure in the presence of right atrial and right ventricular enlargement with or without symptoms. The presence or absence of symptoms has clinical relevance to outcomes, although most long-term follow-up studies evaluate surgical closure. Historical data indicate that outcomes after ASD closure in symptomatic adults <25 years old are similar to age-matched controls; however, patients >40 years old undergoing closure have lower survival than controls [4]. That said, closure in

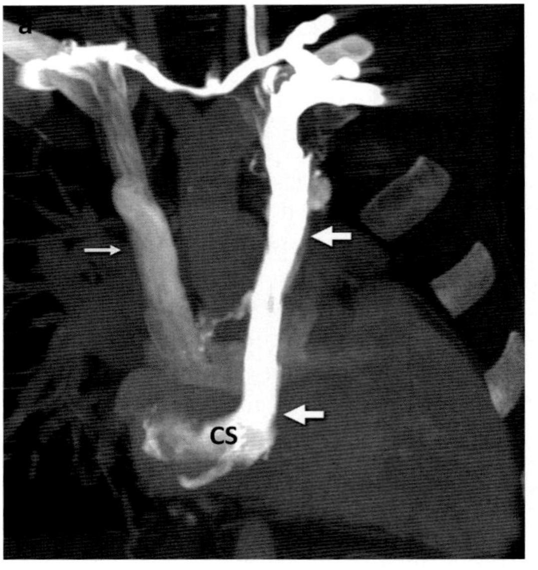

Fig. 22.1 (**a**) CTA from a patient with a Mustard procedure for transposition of the great arteries. There is a large left-sided SVC, which drains to the coronary sinus (*thick arrows*). The right-sided SVC (*thin arrow*) is baffled to the subpulmonic (morphological left) ventricle. The coronary sinus (*CS*) has been incorporated into the pulmonary venous side of the baffle (systemic atrium), giving rise to a right-to-left shunt (**b**) Series of transesophageal echocardiography images in the same patient. (*A*) Demonstrates a 4-chamber view with systemic right superior vena cava flow baffled (*white arrow*) to the left (subpulmonic) ventricle (*LV*). The pulmonary venous atrium is indicated by the *asterisk* (*). (*B*) Bubble contrast injection in the left arm demonstrates preferential filling of the pulmonary venous atrium and right (subaortic) ventricle (*RV*) consistent with right-to-left shunt. (*C*) Demonstrates the Amplatzer duct occluder in position in the left SVC (*dashed arrow*). (*D*) Repeat bubble contrast injection in the left arm with no further filling of the pulmonary venous circuit/RV indicating abolition of the right-to-left shunt. (**c**) Series of angiographic images outlining the angiographic findings. (*A*) Left SVC draining to the systemic venous atrium. (*B*) Balloon occlusion of the left SVC with subsequent venous drainage to the right SVC. (*C*) Final angiogram following release of the Amplatzer duct occluder

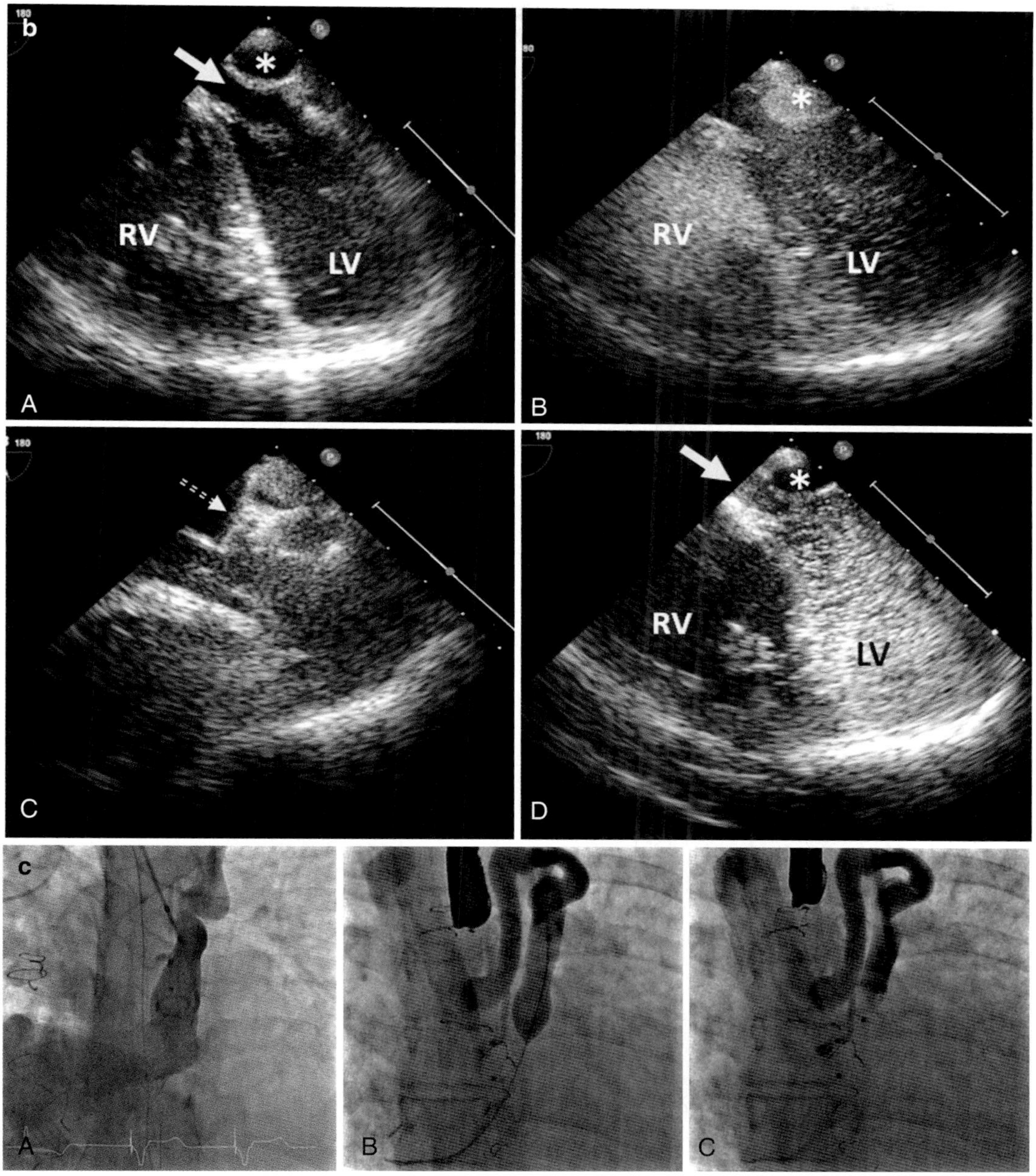

Fig. 22.1 (continued)

symptomatic adults >40 years still provides a survival advantage [4, 5]. In contrast closure in asymptomatic adults reduces morbidity but not mortality [6].

Randomized comparisons of transcatheter and surgical closure of ASDs are lacking; however, a non-randomized comparison of 596 patients undergoing ASD closure (442 surgical and 154 transcatheter) revealed a periprocedural complication rate of 7 % in the transcatheter group versus 24 % in the surgical group. This has been corroborated in older patients, most

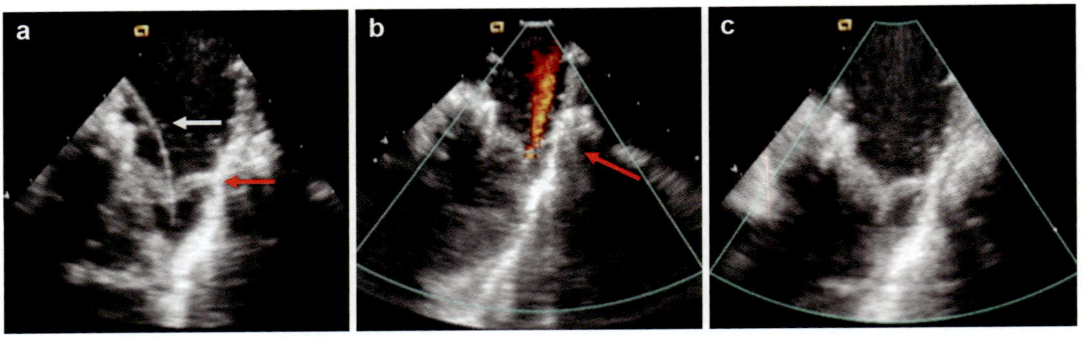

Fig. 22.2 Series of intracardiac echocardiogram images following transcatheter pulmonary valve replacement. (**a**) Following valve deployment (*red arrow*), there is a wire (*white arrow*) still across the valve. (**b**) Mild pulmonary valve regurgitation (*red arrow*) is seen as a consequence of the wire distorting the valve. This was also seen on angiography with the catheter across the valve. (**c**) Once the wire is removed, the ICE images clearly demonstrate no appreciable pulmonary regurgitation

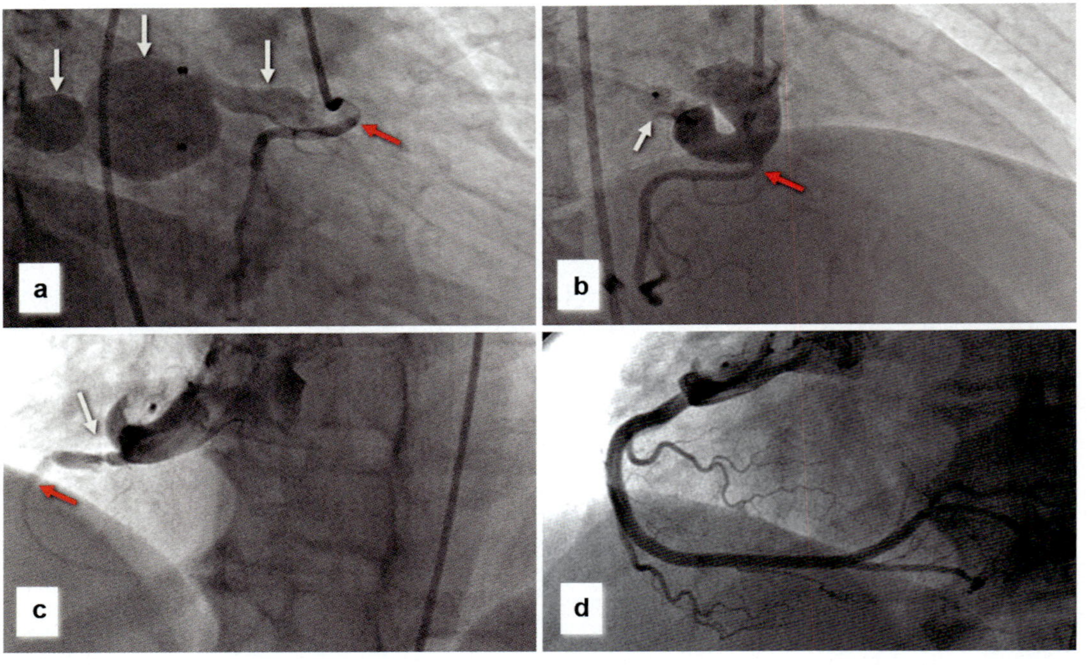

Fig. 22.3 (**a**) Right coronary angiogram demonstrating large bilobed coronary artery fistula (*white arrows*) originating from the proximal right coronary artery (*RCA*) (*red arrow*) and draining to the right atrium (*white arrow*). (**b**) Following deployment of an Amplatzer muscular occluder (*white arrow*), there is no residual distal flow to the fistula and the RCA fills well (*red arrow*). (**c**) ST elevation was noted on a routine post-procedural ECG with repeat right coronary angiography demonstrating a discrete narrowing in the RCA (probable intimal flap – *white, arrow*) with severely attenuated distal filling (*red arrow*). (**d**) Final RCA angiogram following implantation of three coronary stents demonstrates excellent rehabilitation of the RCA

recently in a report evaluating clinical outcomes after device (81 %) or surgical (19 %) ASD closure in 67 patients with a mean age at closure of 68 years [7]. At follow-up of 3.3 years, right ventricular end-diastolic dimensions, right ventricular function, and New York Heart Association functional class showed significant improvement in both groups; however, major complications were higher for the surgical group (23 % vs 7 %). Major procedural complications during/following transcatheter closure included device embolization and atrial erosion with a large contemporary multi-institutional report revealing a major adverse event rate of 1.1 % [8]. A large database analysis demonstrated a risk of device embolization of approximately 0.6 % [9]. Percutaneous retrieval is often possible; however if surgical retrieval is required, the mortality rate for the procedure increases to approximately 2 % [10]. The exact mechanisms leading to atrial erosion are unclear; however, device oversizing and inadequate anterosuperior rims have been implicated with an overall reported incidence with the Amplatzer septal occluder (St Jude Medical, St Paul, MN) between 0.1 and 0.2 % [11]. CT imaging has been used in this setting to evaluate particularly larger device position in relation to the surrounding cardiac structures [12] and has been useful in less clear-cut cases to determine if one of the discs of the ASD device has migrated from within the atrium (Fig. 22.4). Erosion has not been reported with the only other FDA-approved device for ASD closure, the Gore septal occluder (Gore and Associates, Flagstaff, AZ); however, device fracture rates of up to 7 % have been seen especially with the largest (35 mm) occluder. Future endeavors are likely to concentrate on biodegradable implants; however, although initial clinical experience with a predominantly bioabsorbable device was promising [13], this has not reached widespread acceptance as yet.

Transcatheter Ventricular Septal Defect Closure

Most clinically relevant VSDs are closed in childhood; however, hemodynamically, significant shunts [defined as a Qp/Qs >1.5:1 in adults [2]] may be only become clinically relevant in early adulthood. Reports outlining transcatheter closure exclusively in adults have been published [14, 15]. Indications for closure (Table 22.1) in these studies included symptoms and/or ventricular dilatation in 40–60 % of patients. Other common indications included pulmonary hypertension and endocarditis. Aortic valve prolapse leading to aortic regurgitation may be seen with small subaortic VSDs secondary to the Venturi effect in essence "sucking," most commonly, the right coronary cusp inferiorly towards the VSD, and surgery is usually preferred in these instances as device placement may impinge upon the aortic leaflets worsening the aortic regurgitation. Transcatheter closure of perimembranous defects has been halted in the USA due to significant concerns regarding complete heart block [approximately 5 % in the European registry series [16] and 3 % in the US trial [17]] following device placement. Recovery of atrioventricular block has been reported with early treatment with steroid [18] or early surgical removal of the membranous occluder [19]; comparable rates of complete heart block following surgical closure in younger patients have been reported at less than 1 % [20]. Newer devices are being evaluated with design modifications to reduce radial force on the conduction tissue and potential for heart block. Overall, reported complication rates have varied ranging from 6.5 % in the European registry [16] to 10.7 % in the US perimembranous registry including device embolization, cardiac perforation, stroke, and two deaths [17]. Exclusion criteria have also been cited and include inadequate distance for device placement (usually 4 mm) between the VSDs and either the atrioventricular or semilunar valves, active sepsis, or pulmonary vascular resistance >7 indexed Wood units.

Persistent Ductus Arteriosus

There are closure-related issues in regard to the persistent arterial duct specific to the adult population including calcification of ductal tissue and an increased likelihood of pulmonary hypertension [21]. Change in the orientation of the arterial duct with age may lead to a more horizontal entry into the pulmonary artery and this may also have implications for transcatheter approach and device choice. The most widely reported device

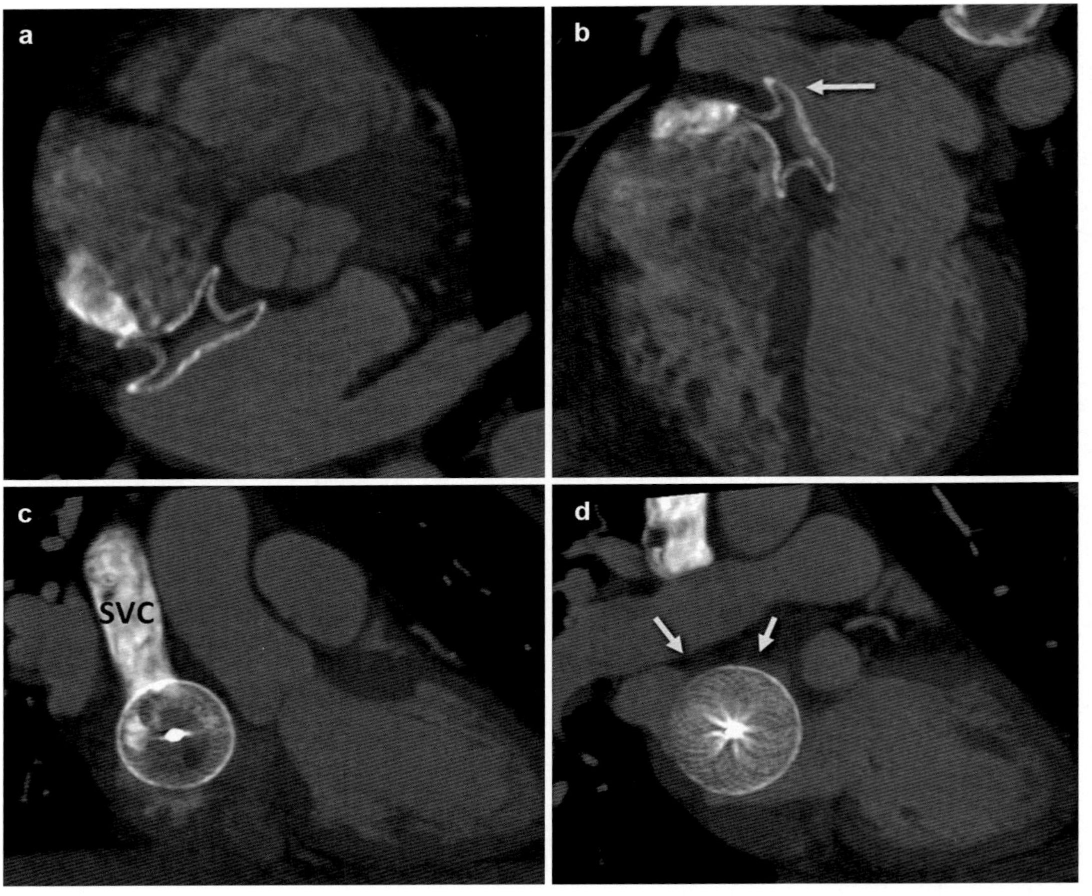

Fig. 22.4 Series of CT images in an older patient who underwent transcatheter ASD closure with an Amplatzer septal occluder. There was a small pericardial effusion by echocardiography the day following defect closure, and CT was performed to evaluate the position of the device in relation to the other cardiac structures. (**a**) Axial CT maximal intensity projection (MIP) image demonstrates the occluder device in place approaching the aorta posterolaterally; with no evidence, it has moved beyond the borders of the atrial wall. (**b**) Four-chamber view demonstrating the relationship of the device to the right upper pulmonary vein (*white arrow*). (**c**) Demonstrates en face view of the right atrial disc and its relationship to the aorta. There is contrast in the superior vena cava (*SVC*) superiorly. (**d**) Same projection demonstrates the relationship of the left atrial disc to the roof of the atrium (*arrows*)

is the Amplatzer duct occluder (St Jude Medical); however, the symmetrical design of the Amplatzer muscular occluder may be more appropriate particularly when there is concern regarding pulmonary hypertension [21]. Closure rates are well over 90 % with low procedural morbidity [22].

Coronary Artery Fistulae

Congenital coronary artery fistulae are rare with a reported incidence of approximately 0.5 %. Most are small, have no clinical implication, and may regress spontaneously; however, larger fistulae may lead to significant left-to-right shunting and symptoms in adult life. Pre-procedural advanced imaging may be beneficial in determining the degree and extent of coronary dilation assisting with procedural planning and supporting decision making (Fig. 22.5). Both surgical and transcatheter closure have been described. Concerns regarding propagation of clot and acute myocardial infarction exist following device closure. A recent follow-up report of 76 patients over 50 years of age, assessing both transcatheter ($n=44$) and surgical management, demonstrated major

Table 22.1 Indications for interventional procedures

Intervention	Indication
Transcatheter VSD closure	Qp/Qs ≥2.0 and clinical evidence of LV volume overload (class I) Qp/Qs >1.5 with pulmonary artery pressure less than two thirds of systemic pressure and PVR less than two thirds of systemic vascular resistance (class IIa) Device closure is a class IIb recommendation [2]
Balloon pulmonary valvuloplasty	Symptoms or asymptomatic with peak Doppler gradient >60 mmHg/mean Doppler gradient >40 mmHg
Balloon aortic valvuloplasty	Symptoms and peak-to-peak gradient catheter gradient >50 mmHg. Asymptomatic patient: peak-to-peak gradient catheter gradient >60 mmHg
Balloon angioplasty/stenting for CoA	Transcatheter systolic coarctation gradient of >20 mmHg or <20 mmHg in the presence of significant collateral vessels and suitable angiographic anatomy, irrespective of patient age, as well as in patients with univentricular heart or with significant ventricular dysfunction
Pulmonary artery stenting	Gradient >20 mmHg across the stenosis area, elevation of the RV or proximal main pulmonary artery pressure to greater than one half to two thirds of systemic pressure, or relative flow discrepancy between the two lungs of 35 %/65 % or worse

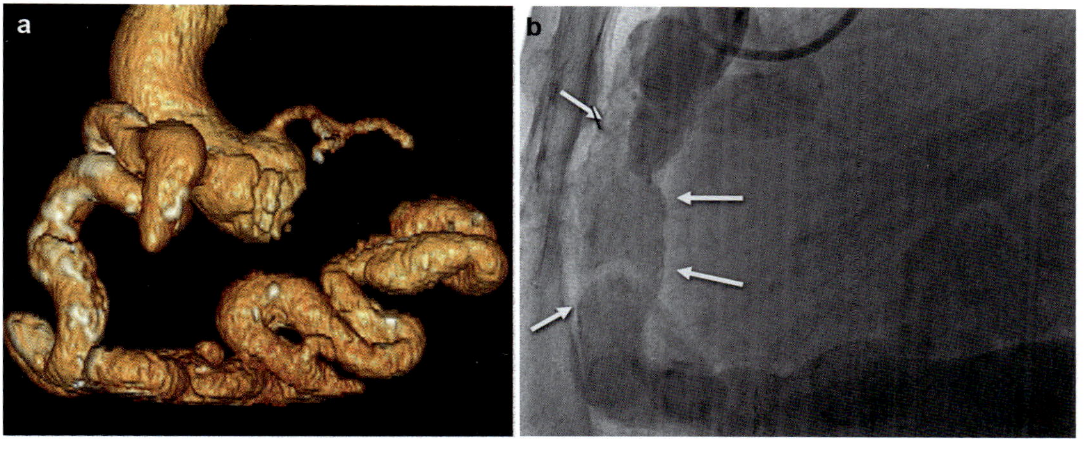

Fig. 22.5 (**a**) Volume-rendered CT coronary angiogram from a 66-year-old with high output congestive heart failure. There is a large dilated, calcified, and tortuous RCA. (**b**) RCA angiography confirmed the large dilated RCA (*white arrows*), and due to concomitant left coronary artery disease, he underwent surgical bypass grafting along with tricuspid valve repair. The CT images were extremely useful in guiding the decision making regarding optimal therapy in this patient

complications in 15 % of patients, the majority of these being myocardial infarction [23]. This series did not carry out adequate serial imaging of the coronary arteries and it may be that more subtle abnormalities remain undetected. Predictors of adverse outcomes included drainage to the coronary sinus, older age at diagnosis, systemic hypertension, and hyperlipidemia. Collaboration with coronary interventionalists may be advised as acute coronary complications may occur (Fig. 22.3). We advocate CT imaging as a tool to follow these patients. Attention to the coronary arteries is extremely important since many of these patients post closure of the fistulae may have abnormal coronary arteries.

Ruptured Sinus of Valsalva Aneurysms

Sinuses of Valsalva aneurysms (SoVA) are rare however are prone to rupture usually in adult life and lead to significant mortality within 2–4 years. Congenital SoVAs arise due to a deficiency of elastic fibers in the aortic media leading to progressive dilatation over time. The right sinus of Valsalva is affected in up to 85 % of cases with the left sinus almost never affected. Usually the rupture occurs into the right atrium or ventricle leading to significant left-to-right shunt and congestive cardiac failure. Although historically surgery was the mainstay of treatment, transcatheter closure has established itself as a less-invasive alternative. Most reported cases to date have described use of the Amplatzer duct occluder (St Jude Medical) [24, 25]. Although most reports are limited to small numbers, successful occlusion with clinical improvement has been achieved in over 90 % of cases [24, 25]. Longer-term outcomes are as yet unknown.

Other Lesions

In patients with inadequate pulmonary blood flow (i.e., tetralogy of Fallot), aortopulmonary collaterals may develop, leading to left-to-right shunting and/or hemoptysis. Coil occlusion has been reported successfully for many years with good occlusion and low complication rates. In patients with chronic hypoxemia however, these lesions may be complex and progressive and coiling may in fact limit distal access to further developing lesions. More recently deployment of microspheres and copolymers of ethylene vinyl alcohol have been reported [26], providing a more complete distal occlusion of all branching vessels.

Intrapulmonary arteriovenous malformations (AVMs) leading to hypoxemia or risk of systemic embolization may occur as an isolated congenital malformation or as part of a systemic syndrome (Osler-Weber-Rendu syndrome). Successful transcatheter occlusion has been reported [27]. More diffuse micro-AVMs may be seen in patients with complex congenital palliative surgeries where hepatic blood flow is excluded from the pulmonary microvasculature, thought to occur secondary to an as yet unidentified "hepatic factor." These AVMs are usually not amenable to transcatheter treatment but may regress with restoration of hepatic venous blood flow to the pulmonary circuit.

Other collateral vessels encountered in patients with congenital heart disease include large venovenous collaterals in the setting of a single-ventricle circulation, particularly recanalization of a left superior vena cava in patients with a superior cavo-pulmonary anastomosis or total cavo-pulmonary connection. Device occlusion has also been described for fenestrated inferior cavo-pulmonary connections, surgically created to decompress the pulmonary vascular bed in patients with marginal pulmonary vascular resistance in the setting of single-ventricle palliation, with good success. Test occlusion is usually carried out prior to definitive device closure to ensure cardiac output is not significantly compromised [28].

Angioplasty and Valvuloplasty

Balloon Pulmonary Valvuloplasty

Pulmonary valvuloplasty for congenital pulmonary valve stenosis has demonstrated excellent outcomes with low complication rates over the past 30 years. Indications in the adult population include a peak instantaneous Doppler gradient >60 mmHg (mean >40 mmHg); however, intervention at lower gradients may be acceptable in the presence of symptoms [2]. Balloon-to-annulus ratios of up to 1.4:1 have been recommended in the past; however, due to development of moderate to severe pulmonary insufficiency in younger patients, a more conservative approach has been advocated [balloon/annulus ratio of 1.2:1]. With larger annulus diameters in adults, a double-balloon technique may be required to achieve effective dilation of the valve. Long-term follow-up data is available in adults [29]. Significant decreases in peak pulmonary gradients were achieved in 90 adults with congenital pulmonary valvular stenosis undergoing balloon dilation, with regression in pulmonary infundibular stenosis and tricuspid regurgitation over time, following decompression of the right ventricle. Thirty percent of the cohort developed mild pulmonary regurgitation; however, this was nonprogressive in all but two cases which is less than the majority of reported cases following surgical valvotomy. Balloon dilation has also been employed in younger patients for both subvalvular and supravalvular stenoses; however, responses to treatment in this setting have been less encouraging.

Balloon Aortic Valvuloplasty

Congenital valvular aortic stenosis accounts for approximately 5 % of congenital heart defects and may be associated with genetic defects such as Turner's syndrome. In milder cases progression of stenosis may occur through childhood with one study demonstrating 17 % of children requiring intervention at a median age of 10.5 years, following initial diagnosis at a median age of 2 years [30]. Indications for intervention are outlined in Table 22.1. The standard approach in older patients has been retrograde via a transfemoral approach. However reports in adults have suggested that crossing the aortic valve in the same direction as blood flow (via a transeptal venous approach) may reduce the risk of valve leaflet perforation and leaflet avulsion during inflation, thus limiting some of the major precipitants for significant aortic valve damage during valvuloplasty [31]. Rapid ventricular pacing has been introduced to maximize balloon stability during inflation. Balloon/annulus ratios of 0.9–1.0:1 are recommended with larger ratios associated with increased post-procedural aortic regurgitation [32]; however, some reports suggest that progression of aortic regurgitation may occur over time irrespective of the initial balloon size used and may be related to valve morphology [33]. The above reports underlie the fact that, despite advances in balloon design and operator experience, it is difficult to predict the response of each individual valve to valvuloplasty even within recommended balloon/annulus ratios. Major complications in both children and adults include acute arterial complications with retrograde approach and the development of aortic regurgitation. In the largest follow-up study in the USA evaluating 509 patients with congenital aortic stenosis over a median follow-up of 9.3 years, mean survival free from any aortic valve re-intervention at 5 years was 72 %, at 10 years 54 %, and at 20 years 27 % [34]. Just less than 50 % of patients required an aortic valve replacement at 20 years follow-up. Using multivariate analysis, lower post-dilatation gradient and lower grade of aortic regurgitation were associated with longer freedom from aortic valve replacement. However even mild post-procedural rates of aortic regurgitation were associated with the need for aortic valve replacement, suggesting that aortic regurgitation as discussed above may worsen with time.

Balloon dilation has also been used for congenital supravalvular aortic stenosis often seen in association with William's syndrome; however, this approach has failed to become a mainstream therapy. More positive outcomes have been described recently with balloon dilatation of congenital subaortic stenosis [35]. In 76 patients with an isolated thin discrete subaortic membrane and mean age of treatment of 19 years, the mean subvalvular gradient reduced from 70 to 18 mmHg with 77 % of patients, demonstrating sustained relief at mean follow-up of 16 years.

Mitral Valvuloplasty

Balloon mitral valvuloplasty has been described for congenital mitral stenosis but there are limited reports in adults. The general perception is that this will respond less well to balloon therapy than rheumatic mitral stenosis. The Boston group described their experience with balloon mitral valvuloplasty in 64 of 108 children undergoing intervention for severe congenital mitral valve stenosis [36]. Valvuloplasty decreased the mean mitral gradient by 38 % and however was complicated by significant mitral regurgitation in 28 %. Survival free from failure of biventricular repair or mitral valve replacement was 55 % at 5 years. Patients with a supramitral ring were less likely to respond to valvuloplasty.

Stenting

Coarctation of the Aorta

Balloon angioplasty for coarctation was first reported in 1982, and although medium-term outcome studies showed good initial relief of stenosis, high rates of re-coarctation and aneurysm formation (35 %) were reported [37]. Hence stent implantation is now the preferred intervention for coarctation in adults with persistent relief of stenosis and lower incidence of aneurysm formation compared to balloon angioplasty or surgery [38]. Guidelines have been published for transcatheter treatment of both native and recurrent coarctation [2] (Table 22.1). Both ballooning and stenting are indicated when there is a transcoarctation gradient of >20 mmHg at the time of catheterization although intervention may be warranted with less-severe gradients if there is systemic hypertension with anatomical narrowing or presence of collateral vessels or elevated LVEDP [2].

Covered stents (both balloon expandable and self-expanding) offer the advantage of excluding any stretch-induced wall trauma from the endoluminal aspect of the aorta particularly in the catastrophic event of aortic rupture, which is a significant concern in older patients [39]. These stents are not currently approved for use in patients with CoA in the USA, and therefore novel approaches of applying a Gore-Tex covering to a bare metal stent have been reported to counter this [40]. Both pre- and post-procedural imaging may be useful in predicting anatomical subtypes and evaluating the aortic response to stenting (Fig. 22.6).

Post-stenting, patients have demonstrated midterm left ventricular mass regression and long-axis function improvement and amelioration in central aortic function with associated reduction of daytime ambulatory systolic blood pressure. Follow-up with CT examination suggests that overall aneurysm rate is low (1–2 %) [41]; however, other reports have variable results.

Pulmonary Artery Stenting

Peripheral pulmonary artery stenosis has been reported in patients with tetralogy of Fallot repair, following arterial switch operation for transposition of the great arteries, and as a consequence of surgery involving the pulmonary arteries in patients with univentricular circulation. Pulmonary artery narrowing in this setting may lead to increased afterload on the subpulmonary ventricle and may

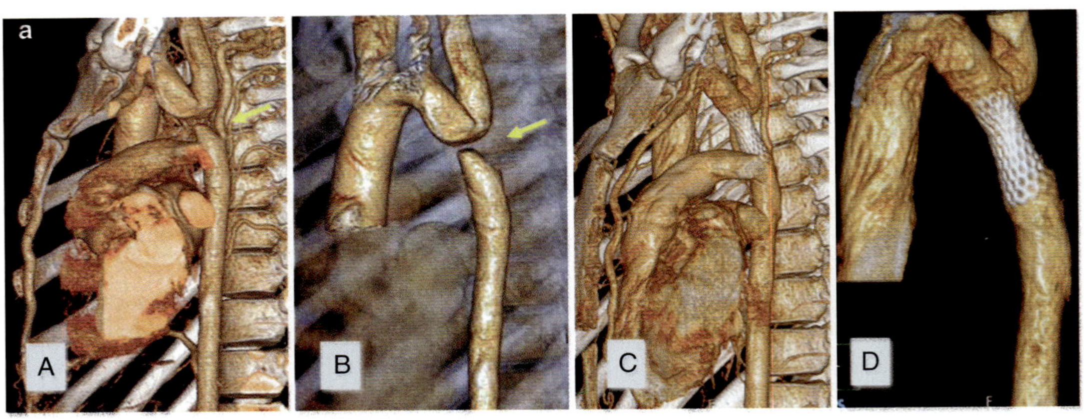

Fig. 22.6 (**a**) (*A, B*) Volume-rendered 3-D CTA of the aortic arch in a right posterior oblique projection demonstrating acquired atresia of the aortic arch (*Yellow arrows*). (*C, D*) Reconstructed 3-D CTA imaging of the aorta in a similar projection following deployment of a self-fabricated covered stent across the atretic aorta (**b**) Series of angiographic images outlining the procedural approach. (*A–D*) Initial angiograms demonstrate the atretic portion as indicated by the *white arrow*. (*E–G*) Crossing the atretic aorta with a needle (*E*), wire (*F*), and catheter (*G*) (indicated by the *white arrows*) to establish continuity with the arch from below. (*H–M*) Delivery and deployment of the balloon-expandable covered stent (*white arrows*) across the punctured aorta from below. (*N*) Final angiogram demonstrating a confluent descending thoracic aorta with no aneurysm formation. The stent was intentionally not inflated to a maximum size due to concerns regarding aortic damage, and the patient was scheduled for an elective redilation of the stent, which was well tolerated

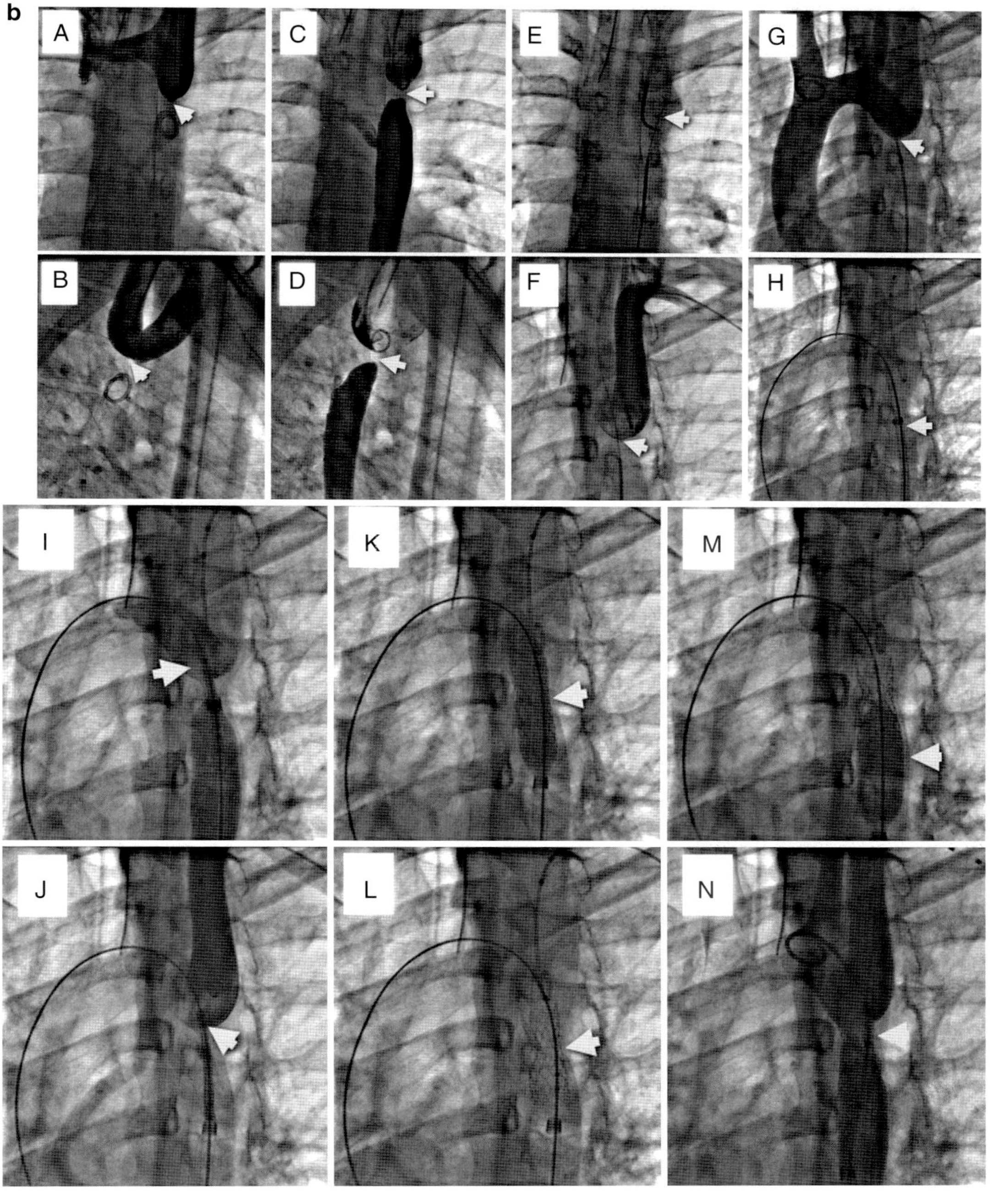

Fig. 22.6 (continued)

exacerbate preexisting lesions such as pulmonary incompetence particularly in the setting of tetralogy of Fallot, and thus aggressive management is indicated. Stent implantation is generally preferable to balloon dilation in older patients. Indications for intervention are outlined in Table 22.1. In many cases multiple unilateral or bilateral stenting may be required. Stent embolization may be a concern

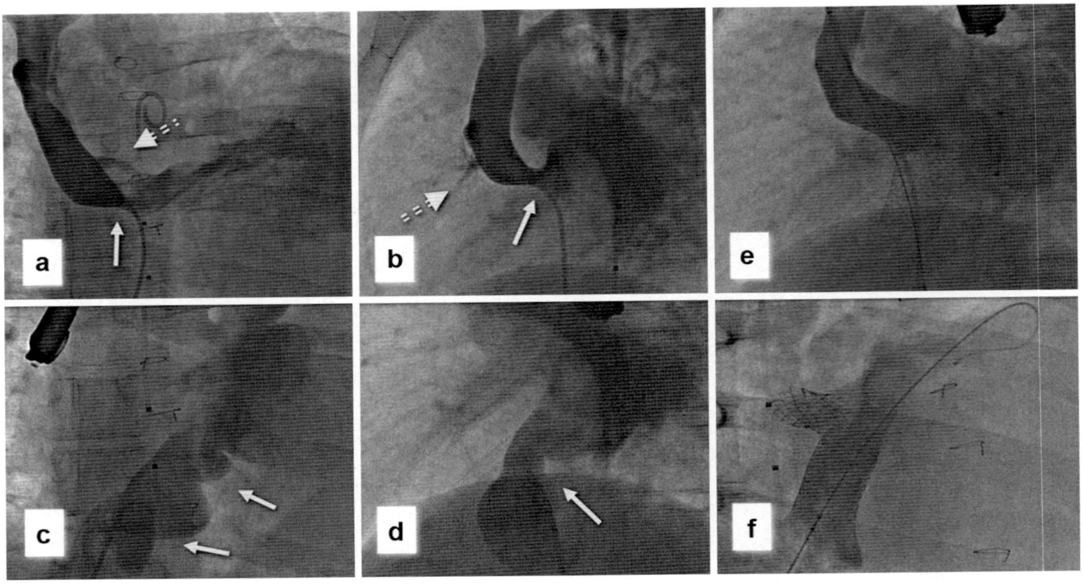

Fig. 22.7 Series of angiographic images of a superior and inferior systemic venous baffle stenosis along with a superior baffle leak in a patient with a Mustard procedure for transposition of the great vessels. (**a**, **b**) Biplane angiographic images demonstrating the baffle stenosis (*thin arrows*) and baffle leak (*dashed arrows*) in the superior baffle. (**c**, **d**) Biplane angiographic images demonstrating multiple levels of baffle obstruction (*white arrows*) in the inferior baffle. (**e**) Angiographic image of the superior venous baffle following implantation of a covered stent with no residual stenosis or baffle leak. (**f**) Angiographic image of the inferior baffle with resolution of the previously seen inferior baffle stenosis

in older patients particularly those with pulmonary regurgitation [42]. Intimal stent ingrowth may occur more frequently with larger stent/pulmonary artery narrowing ratios.

Intracardiac Baffle Stenting and Other Stenting Procedures

The incidence of baffle leak with or without stenosis following atrial redirection surgery for transposition of the great arteries has been reported as high as 35 % [43, 44]. Both device occlusion and covered stenting (Fig. 22.7) have been described to treat baffle leak with covered stent preferred if baffle stenosis is present [44]. The procedure is effective, leading to significant improvements in oxygen saturations and reduction in hemoglobin concentrations [44].

Stenting has also been described in the setting of congenital pulmonary vein stenosis although intimal ingrowth/restenosis rates are high. Left ventricular outflow tract stenting in patients with congenital heart disease has also been reported, but high stent fracture rates (>40 %) leading to recurrent obstruction have prevented mainstream acceptance [45].

Transcatheter Valve Replacement

Transcatheter Pulmonary Valve Replacement

Transcatheter pulmonary valve replacement (tPVR) has evolved into a viable, less-invasive alternative to surgical conduit replacement. Pre-procedural imaging with cardiac MR has redefined indications for re-intervention with most centers accepting right ventricular end-diastolic volumes >150 ml/m^2, pulmonary regurgitant fractions of >40 %, and right ventricular ejection fractions of <40 % as markers for intervention in the setting of dominant regurgitant

Table 22.2 Published inclusion criteria for clinical trials with both the Melody and SAPIEN valves :

Inclusion criteria (Melody) [48]	Inclusion criteria (Edwards) [49]
Age ≥5 years	Weight >35 kg
Weight ≥30 kg	In situ conduit ≥16 mm and ≤24 mm
Original conduit diameter ≥16 mm	*Dysfunctional RV-PA conduit ≥3+ PR(TTE) or PRF ≥ 40 %(MRI) ± stenosis*
Echocardiographic RVOT conduit dysfunction:	
Patients classified as NYHA class II, III, or IV	
Doppler mean gradient ≥35 mmHg or ≥ moderate PR	
Patients classified as NYHA class I	
Doppler mean gradient ≥40 mmHg or severe PR associated with TV annulus z-score ≥2 or RVFS <40 %	

lesions. Direct comparisons with surgical implants evaluating functionality and durability are lacking; however, short- to medium-term outcomes for tPVR are excellent with low morbidity and low valve failure rates. Initial stent fracture rates of 30 % with the Melody valve (Medtronic Inc, Minneapolis, MN) [46] have been reduced to as low as 5 % with aggressive pre-stenting of the right ventricular outflow tract (RVOT) [47]. Indications for the procedure are evolving and have mostly been guided by two clinical trials in the USA [48, 49] but include significant conduit stenosis, regurgitation, or both (Table 22.2). Two valve systems are currently available: the Medtronic Melody valve as mentioned above and the Edwards SAPIEN valve (Edwards Lifesciences, Irvine, CA). In the US clinical trial evaluating 1-year follow-up with the Melody valve, the median peak RVOT gradient was reduced from 37 to 12 mmHg [48]. Pulmonary regurgitant fraction was reduced from mean of 24.8–2.8 % post valve implantation. Although stent fracture rates were 21 %, freedom from valve dysfunction or need for re-intervention was 93.5 % with higher RVOT gradient and younger age at implantation associated with shorter freedom from re-intervention. Similar gradient reductions and valvular competency have been reported for the Edwards SAPIEN valve at 6-month follow-up with no stent fractures noted [49]. Stent migration was seen in three patients (8.8 %) with two of them requiring surgery. Other reported complications encountered during tPVR include conduit rupture, coronary artery compression, and pulmonary hemorrhage. Follow-up CT imaging through evaluation of the expansion ratio of the stented valve may predict need for re-intervention (data presented in abstract format) (Fig. 22.8).

Efforts are ongoing to widen the applicability of this technology, particularly to the significant number of patients with dilated native RVOTs, and early experience with a self-expanding valve model has been reported [50]. Challenges exist with this endeavor, customizing a single valve to the wide variability of RVOT morphology seen throughout the cardiac cycle. Other concerns relating to cost-effectiveness of tPVR in comparison to surgical valve replacement have been raised, and it is likely that this issue will need to be addressed before this approach achieves widespread acceptance particularly in developing economies.

Transcatheter Tricuspid Valve Replacement

With the evolution of tPVR, stented valves have been deployed across dysfunctional tricuspid valve tissue prostheses. This approach was reported in 15 patients using the Medtronic Melody valve with reduction in mean tricuspid gradient from 12.9 to 3.9 mmHg with all patients having mild tricuspid regurgitation or less [51]. One patient required a pacemaker due to complete heart block. Reports using the Edwards SAPIEN valve for this indication have also been published. Concerns have since been raised regarding early valve failure with this approach [52].

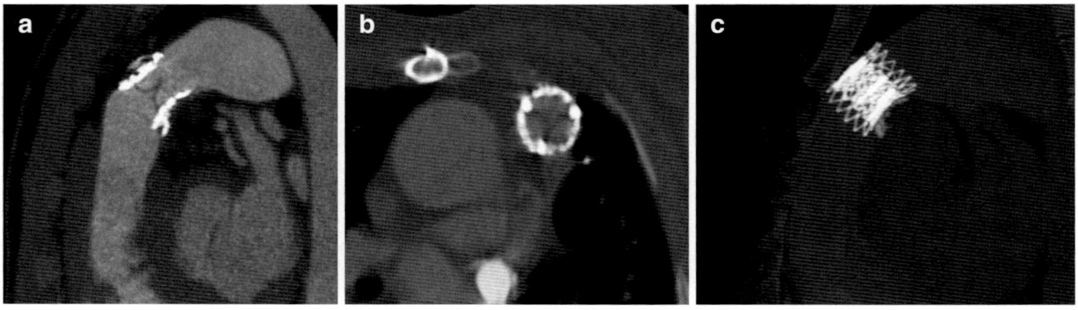

Fig. 22.8 Series of thick and thin slab maximal intensity projection (MIP) CT images following transcatheter pulmonary valve replacement. (**a**) Demonstrates a sagittal view of the stented valve with the valve leaflets clearly seen within the stent. There is no aneurysm formation noted. (**b**) Axial or short-axis view of the valve with again the trileaflet nature of the stented valve clearly seen and the circular deployment of the stent. (**c**) Thick-MIP image of the valve stent demonstrating no stent fracture. Detailed measurements of the valve and stent diameters can be made from these images to evaluate circularity and eccentricity of the stent valve complex. More asymmetrical valves have an association with increasing valve stenosis and may be predictive of those requiring valve replacement [53]

Summary

In conclusion there are more adults than children now living with congenital heart disease. These patients often have complex anatomical lesions that give rise to hemodynamic and clinical challenges and these are increasing investigated and treated with transcatheter therapies. This chapter outlined the lesions and transcatheter treatments available.

References

1. Marelli AJ, Mackie AS, Ionescu-Ittu R, et al. Congenital heart disease in the general population: changing prevalence and age distribution. Circulation. 2007;115:163–72.
2. Warnes CA, Williams RG, Bashore TM, et al. ACC/AHA 2008 guidelines for the management of adults with congenital heart disease: a report of the American College of Cardiology/American Heart Association Task Force on Practice Guidelines. Circulation. 2008;118:2395–451.
3. Zomer AC, Verheugt CL, Vaartjes I, et al. Surgery in adults with congenital heart disease. Circulation. 2011;124:2195–201.
4. Murphy JG, Gersh BJ, McGoon MD, et al. Long-term outcome after surgical repair of isolated atrial septal defect: follow-up at 27 to 32 years. N Engl J Med. 1990;323:1645–50.
5. Horvath KA, Burke RP, Collins Jr JJ, Cohn LH. Surgical treatment of adult atrial septal defect: early and long-term results. J Am Coll Cardiol. 1992;20:1156–9.
6. Attie F, Rosas M, Granados N, Zabal C, Buendia A, Calderon J. Surgical treatment for secundum atrial septal defect in patients >40 years old: a randomized clinical trial. J Am Coll Cardiol. 2001;38: 2035–42.
7. Hanninen M, Kmet A, Taylor DA, Ross DB, Rebeyka I, Vonder Muhll IF. Atrial septal defect closure in the elderly is associated with excellent quality of life, functional improvement, and ventricular remodelling. Can J Cardiol. 2011;27:698–704.
8. Everett AD, Jennings J, Sibinga E, et al. Community use of the amplatzer atrial septal defect occluder: results of the multicenter MAGIC atrial septal defect study. Pediatr Cardiol. 2009;30: 240–7.
9. Delaney JW, Li JS, Rhodes JF. Major complications associated with transcatheter atrial septal occluder implantation: a review of the medical literature and the manufacturer and user facility device experience (MAUDE) database. Congenit Heart Dis. 2007;2:256–64.
10. DiBardino DJ, McElhinney DB, Kaza AK, Mayer Jr JE. Analysis of the US Food and Drug Administration Manufacturer and User Facility Device Experience database for adverse events involving Amplatzer septal occluder devices and comparison with the Society of Thoracic Surgery congenital cardiac surgery database. J Thorac Cardiovasc Surg. 2009;137: 1334–41.
11. Diab K, Kenny D, Hijazi ZM. Erosions, erosions, and erosions! Device closure of atrial septal defects: how safe is safe? Catheter Cardiovasc Interv. 2012;80:168–74.
12. Marini D, Ou P, Boudjemline Y, Kenny D, Bonnet D, Agnoletti G. Midterm results of percutaneous closure of very large atrial septal defects in children: role of multislice computed tomography. EuroIntervention. 2012;7:1317–25.

13. Mullen MJ, Hildick-Smith D, De Giovanni JV, et al. BioSTAR Evaluation STudy (BEST): a prospective, multicenter, phase I clinical trial to evaluate the feasibility, efficacy, and safety of the BioSTAR bioabsorbable septal repair implant for the closure of atrial-level shunts. Circulation. 2006;114:1962–7.
14. Chessa M, Butera G, Negura D, et al. Transcatheter closure of congenital ventricular septal defects in adult: mid-term results and complications. Int J Cardiol. 2009;133:70–3.
15. Al-Kashkari W, Balan P, Kavinsky CJ, et al. Percutaneous device closure of congenital & iatrogenic ventricular septal defects in adult patients. Catheter Cardiovasc Interv. 2011;77:260–7.
16. Carminati M, Butera G, Chessa M, Investigators of the European VSD Registry. Transcatheter closure of congenital ventricular septal defects: results of the European Registry. Eur Heart J. 2007;28:2361–8.
17. Fu YC, Bass J, Amin Z, et al. Transcatheter closure of perimembranous ventricular septal defects using the new Amplatzer membranous VSD occluder: results of the U.S. phase I trial. J Am Coll Cardiol. 2006; 47:319–25.
18. Walsh MA, Bialkowski J, Szkutnik M, et al. Atrioventricular block after transcatheter closure of perimembranous ventricular septal defects. Heart. 2006;92:1295–7.
19. Ovaert C, Dragulescu A, Sluysmans T, et al. Early surgical removal of membranous ventricular septal occluder might allow recovery of atrio-ventricular block. Pediatr Cardiol. 2008;29:971–5.
20. Tucker EM, Pyles LA, Bass JL, Moller JH. Permanent pacemaker for atrioventricular conduction block after operative repair of perimembranous ventricular septal defect. J Am Coll Cardiol. 2007;50: 1196–2000.
21. Yan C, Zhao S, Jiang S, et al. Transcatheter closure of patent ductus arteriosus with severe pulmonary arterial hypertension in adults. Heart. 2007;93:514–8.
22. Lee CH, Leung YL, Kwong NP, et al. Transcatheter closure of patent ductus arteriosus in Chinese adults: immediate and long-term results. J Invasive Cardiol. 2003;15:26–30.
23. Valente AM, Lock JE, Gauvreau K, et al. Predictors of long-term adverse outcomes in patients with congenital coronary artery fistulae. Circ Cardiovasc Interv. 2010;3:134–9.
24. Fedson S, Jolly N, Lang RM, Hijazi ZM. Percutaneous closure of a ruptured sinus of Valsalva aneurysm using the Amplatzer Duct Occluder. Cathether Cardiovasc Interv. 2003;58:406–11.
25. Sivadasanpillai H, Valaparambil A, Sivasubramonian S. Percutaneous closure of ruptured sinus of Valsalva aneurysms: intermediate term follow-up results. EuroIntervention. 2010;6:214–9.
26. Bommart S, Bourdin A, Giroux MF, et al. Transarterial ethylene vinyl alcohol copolymer visualization and penetration after embolization of life threatening hemoptysis: technical and clinical outcomes. Cardiovasc Intervent Radiol. 2012;35:668–75.
27. Tabori NE, Love BA. Transcatheter occlusion of pulmonary arteriovenous malformations using the Amplatzer Vascular Plug II. Catheter Cardiovasc Interv. 2008;71:940–3.
28. Hijazi ZM, Fahey JT, Kleinman CS, Kopf GS, Hellenbrand WE. Hemodynamic evaluation before and after closure of fenestrated Fontan. An acute study of changes in oxygen delivery. Circulation. 1992;86:196–202.
29. Fawzy ME, Hassan W, Fadel BM, et al. Long-term results (up to 17 years) of pulmonary balloon valvuloplasty in adults and its effects on concomitant severe infundibular stenosis and tricuspid regurgitation. Am Heart J. 2007;153:433–8.
30. Kitchiner D, Jackson M, Walsh K, Peart I, Arnold R. The progression of mild congenital aortic valve stenosis from childhood into adult life. Int J Cardiol. 1993;42:217–23.
31. Cubeddu RJ, Jneid H, Don CW, et al. Retrograde versus antegrade aortic balloon valvuloplasty: immediate, short- and long-term outcomes at 2 years. Catheter Cardiovasc Interv. 2009;74:255–31.
32. McCrindle BW. Independent predictors of immediate results of percutaneous balloon aortic valvotomy in children. Valvuloplasty and Angioplasty of Congenital Anomalies (VACA) Registry Investigators. Am J Cardiol. 1996;77:286–93.
33. Balmer C, Beghetti M, Fasnacht M, Friedli B, Arbenz U. Balloon aortic valvoplasty in paediatric patients: progressive aortic regurgitation is common. Heart. 2004;90:77–81.
34. Brown DW, Dipilato AE, Chong EC, Lock JE, McElhinney DB. Aortic valve reinterventions after balloon aortic valvuloplasty for congenital aortic stenosis intermediate and late follow-up. J Am Coll Cardiol. 2010;56:1740–9.
35. de Lezo JS, Romero M, Segura J, et al. Long-term outcome of patients with isolated thin discrete subaortic stenosis treated by balloon dilation: a 25-year study. Circulation. 2011;124:1461–8.
36. McElhinney DB, Sherwood MC, Keane JF, del Nido PJ, Almond CS, Lock JE. Current management of severe congenital mitral stenosis: outcomes of transcatheter and surgical therapy in 108 infants and children. Circulation. 2005;112:707–14.
37. Cowley CG, Orsmond GS, Feola P, McQuillan L, Shaddy RE. Long-term, randomized comparison of balloon angioplasty and surgery for native coarctation of the aorta in childhood. Circulation. 2005;111: 3453–6.
38. Forbes TJ, Kim DW, Du W, CCISC Investigators, et al. Comparison of surgical, stent, and balloon angioplasty treatment of native coarctation of the aorta an observational study by the CCISC (Congenital Cardiovascular Interventional Study Consortium). J Am Coll Cardiol. 2011;58:2664–74.
39. Forbes TJ, Garekar S, Amin Z, Congenital Cardiovascular Interventional Study Consortium (CCISC). Procedural results and acute complications in stenting native and recurrent coarctation of the aorta

in patients over 4 years of age: a multi-institutional study. Catheter Cardiovasc Interv. 2007;70:276–85.
40. Kenny D, Cao QL, Kavinsky C, Hijazi ZM. Innovative resource utilization to fashion individualized covered stents in the setting of aortic coarctation. Catheter Cardiovasc Interv. 2011;78:413–8.
41. Chakrabarti S, Kenny D, Morgan G, et al. Balloon expandable stent implantation for native and recurrent coarctation of the aorta–prospective computed tomography assessment of stent integrity, aneurysm formation and stenosis relief. Heart. 2010;96: 1212–6.
42. Kenny D, Amin Z, Slyder S, Hijazi ZM. Medium-term outcomes for peripheral pulmonary artery stenting in adults with congenital heart disease. J Interv Cardiol. 2011;24:373–7.
43. Helbing WA, Hansen B, Ottenkamp J, et al. Long-term results of atrial correction for transposition of the great arteries. Comparison of Mustard and Senning operations. J Thorac Cardiovasc Surg. 1994;108: 363–72.
44. Bentham J, English K, Hares D, Gibbs J, Thomson J. Effect of transcatheter closure of baffle leaks following senning or mustard atrial redirection surgery on oxygen saturations and polycythaemia. Am J Cardiol. 2012;110:1046–50.
45. Porras D, McElhinney DB, Del Nido P, Lock JE, Meadows J, Marshall AC. Clinical and stent-related outcomes after transcatheter or operative placement of bare-metal stents in the ventricular septum or subvalvar systemic outflow tract. Circ Cardiovasc Interv. 2012;5:570–81.
46. Nordmeyer J, Lurz P, Khambadkone S, et al. Prestenting with a bare metal stent before percutaneous pulmonary valve implantation: acute and 1-year outcomes. Heart. 2011;97:118–23.
47. Eicken A, Ewert P, Hager A, et al. Percutaneous pulmonary valve implantation: two-c3ntre experience with more than 100 patients. Eur Heart J. 2011;32: 1260–5.
48. McElhinney DB, Hellenbrand WE, Zahn EM, et al. Short- and medium-term outcomes after transcatheter pulmonary valve placement in the expanded multicenter US melody valve trial. Circulation. 2010;122: 507–16.
49. Kenny D, Hijazi ZM, Kar S, et al. Percutaneous implantation of the Edwards SAPIEN transcatheter heart valve for conduit failure in the pulmonary position: early phase 1 results from an international multicenter clinical trial. J Am Coll Cardiol. 2011;58:594–8.
50. Schievano S, Taylor AM, Capelli C, et al. First-in-man implantation of a novel percutaneous valve: a new approach to medical device development. EuroIntervention. 2010;5:745–50.
51. Roberts PA, Boudjemline Y, Cheatham JP, et al. Percutaneous tricuspid valve replacement in congenital and acquired heart disease. J Am Coll Cardiol. 2011;58:117–2.
52. Bentham JR, Qureshi S, Eicken A, Gibbs JL, Ballard G, Thomson JDR. Early percutaneous valve failure within bioprosthetic tricuspid tissue valve replacements. Catheter Cardiovasc Interv. 2013;82(3): 428–35.
53. Ghawi H et al. Presented at PICS 2013, Miami, FL

Virtual Surgery in Congenital Heart Disease

23

Thomas Sangild Sørensen, Jesper Mosegaard, Stefan Kislinskiy, and Gerald F. Greil

Teaching, diagnosing, and planning of therapy in patients with complex structural cardiovascular heart disease require profound understanding of the three-dimensional (3D) nature of cardiovascular structures in these patients. To obtain such understanding, modern imaging modalities provide high-resolution two-dimensional (2D), three-dimensional (3D), and sometimes even time-resolved 3D imaging of the cardiovascular anatomy of the chest. When 3D structures need to be understood based on 2D images, a 3D model is a very helpful tool to visualize and to understand the often complex 3D structures [1].

T.S. Sørensen, PhD
Department of Clinical Medicine and Department of Computer Science, Aarhus University, Åbogade 34, Building 5341, Aarhus 8200, Denmark
e-mail: sangild@cs.au.dk

J. Mosegaard, PhD
Computer Graphics Lab, The Alexandra Institute Ltd., Åbogade 34, Århus N. 8200, Denmark
e-mail: jesper.mosegaard@alexandra.dk

S. Kislinskiy, MSc
Division of Medical and Biological Informatics, German Cancer Research Center (DKFZ), Im Neuenheimer Feld 280, Heidelberg 69120, Germany
e-mail: s.kislinskiy@dkfz.de

G.F. Greil, MD, PhD (✉)
Division of Imaging Sciences and Biomedical Engineering, Department of Pediatric Cardioloy, Guy's and St. Thomas' Hospital/Evelina Children's Hospital, The Rayne Institute, King's College London, 4th Floor Lambeth Wing St. Thomas' Hospital, London SE1 7EH, UK
e-mail: gerald.greil@kcl.ac.uk

In combination with the availability of virtual models of congenital heart disease (CHD), techniques for computer-based simulation of cardiac interventions have enabled early clinical exploration of the emerging concept of virtual surgery [2, 3]. This chapter serves as an introduction to virtual surgery for patient-specific preoperative planning and teaching of cardiovascular anatomy and interventions for clinicians. The chapter is mainly based on the discussion of a few examples. An overview of the underlying imaging and data-processing techniques is provided.

Figure 23.1 depicts the generic setup. Using computer-simulation techniques the user can rotate and investigate the cardiac anatomy. Two haptic devices provide both positional and rotational freedom during interaction as well as force feedback. The heart of the virtual patient is a reconstruction based on a 3D scan, in this case from magnetic resonance imaging. In Figure 23.2 the ventricular portion of the heart is zoomed. A ventricular septal defect (VSD) is visualized from a surgeon's view. In the following paragraphs the simulation of structural cardiovascular disease for preoperative planning and surgical training is discussed.

Planning of interventions in patients with CHD, in particular surgical procedures, can be very difficult. Often surgical decisions are based on previous experience and therefore the result is very often operator dependent. Patient-specific virtual surgery simulation could improve the surgeon's or interventionalist's preoperative planning and training opportunities, therefore reducing the risk of cardiothoracic interventions

F. Saremi (ed.), *Cardiac CT and MR for Adult Congenital Heart Disease*,
DOI 10.1007/978-1-4614-8875-0_23, © Springer Science+Business Media New York 2014

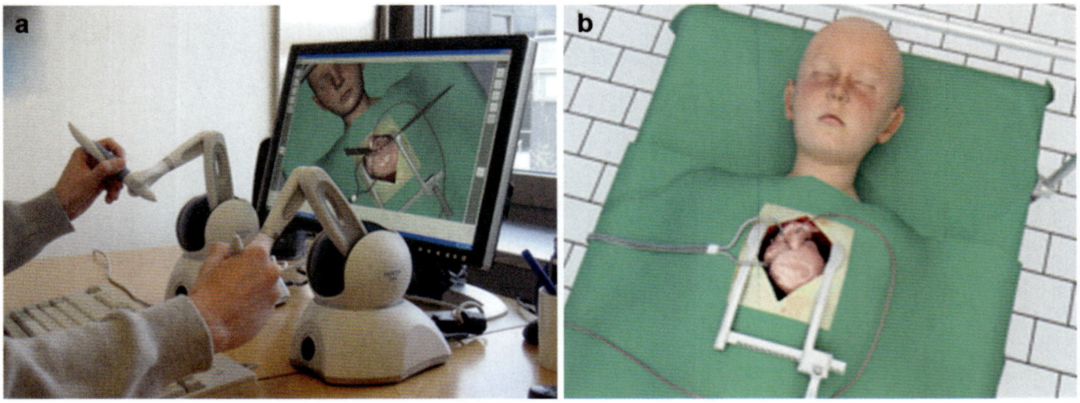

Fig. 23.1 Haptic devices for interactive manipulation of anatomical structures reconstructed from three-dimensional (3D) datasets. The operator can interactively rotate and dissect a virtual specimen to study the anatomy in detail. The corresponding forces are felt through the haptic devices (**a**). A virtual patient in the operating theatre, with a heart reconstructed from a 3D MRI dataset (**b**)

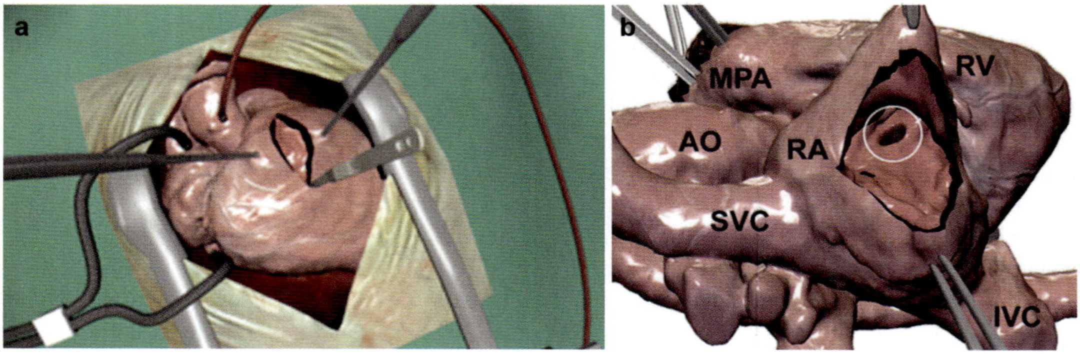

Fig. 23.2 Magnified view of the virtual patient from Fig. 23.1 in a full rendering of the surgical setting (**a**). Only the heart is visualized in (**b**) depicting a ventricular septal defect (VSD, *circle*). The heart was reconstructed from a 3D MRI dataset. It can be manipulated by lifting, rotation, dissection, insertion of a virtual patch, etc. using the devices displayed in Fig. 23.1. The corresponding forces to the virtual manipulations, such as performing a myocardial incision and traction of myocardial tissue using a forceps, are transmitted to the user via the haptic devices (Fig. 23.1a). *AO* aorta, *IVC* inferior vena cava, *MPA* main pulmonary artery, *RA* right atrium, *RV* right ventricle, *SVC* superior vena cava

and improve outcome. Using simulation, the optimal interventional strategy can be planned in advance and different approaches can be discussed with colleagues from other institutions with different grades of experience. The 3D model is a useful communication tool that enables the pediatric cardiac surgeon or interventionalist to discuss interventional strategies. Instead of discussing treatment options purely based on 2D imaging and 3D renderings of the extracardiac anatomy, patient-specific virtual surgery provides the surgeon with a useful tool to communicate the surgical view of the intra- and extracardiac morphology and allows testing of different strategies to repair a cardiovascular defect.

So far heart specimens were essential to understand the various complex pathologies in patients with congenital heart disease. Studies in the pathology laboratory are only possible in a few institutions worldwide, and the number of these rare specimens is very limited. A combination of virtual and physical reproduction of anatomical specimens in conjunction with demonstration of modern imaging techniques could be ideal for

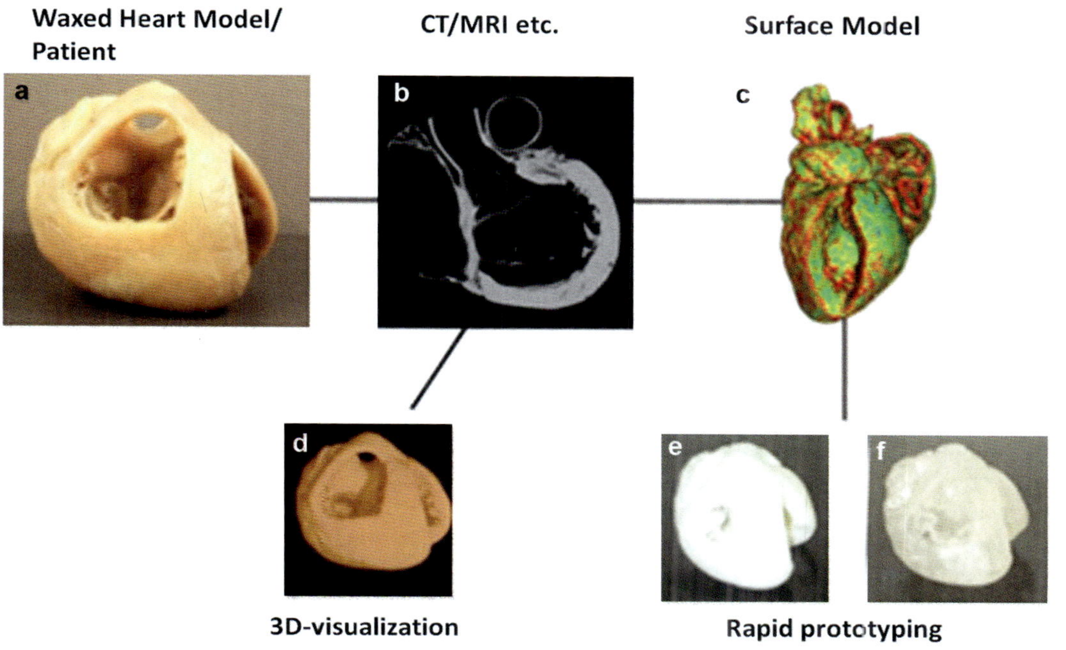

Fig. 23.3 A schematic overview of the production process from a specimen (**a**) via imaging (**b**) to virtual reconstruction (**d**) and physical reproduction using rapid prototyping (**e**, **f**) after creation of a STL file (**c**). Computed tomography was used as the imaging modality in this example, but other 3D imaging techniques can be used in the production process as well

training in the clinical environment. As outlined in Fig. 23.3, virtual reconstruction and physical reproduction using rapid prototyping is a very interesting concept in this respect. Virtual cardiotomy could be a cost-effective supplementary technique to rapid prototyping. Different types of incisions and interventional procedures can be tested and demonstrated independently of the level of experience of the operator and without any risk for the patient. As the models are patient specific, personalized treatment strategies can be developed using this technology.

From Imaging to 3D Modeling

As a prerequisite of virtual surgery, three steps are required:

1. Image acquisition
2. Image segmentation
3. Three-dimensional modeling

A visual illustration of these three steps is provided in Fig. 23.3 and a dedicated section for each step is provided below. The description is intended as an overview of one possible approach to obtain a model suitable for virtual surgery.

It is important to understand that each of these steps is some kind of interpretation of the image data and therefore some errors may be introduced in comparison to the original anatomical structure. These errors can be minimized by improved image quality, e.g., by raising image resolution and improving contrast. In case of virtual surgery, which is performed to predict exact results of a surgical procedure, these errors must be considered when evaluating surgical outcome. Because of this surgeons and interventionalists should be critical of simulation results and be prepared for variations during the actual procedure.

Image Acquisition

The initial step towards obtaining an accurate model for simulation of virtual surgery is acquisition of an image dataset with high resolution and contrast for optimal 3D modeling of the morphology of the congenital heart defect. Frequently an end-diastolic scan is preferred from a surgeon's point of view, as it is closest to the state of the heart on the heart-lung machine [4]. However, the dynamic component of a beating heart is not displayed with this approach. Novel 3D techniques allow acquisition of at least two cardiac phases within one cardiac cycle (end systole and mid diastole) [5]. A complete time-resolved dataset of the cardiac cycle would be ideal [6]. Each individual phase could then be segmented and the results of an intervention could be modeled on a beating heart model.

The present chapter focuses on the concept of virtual interventions in open-heart surgery. Therefore it is assumed that a single-phase three-dimensional (3D) scan in end diastole should be sufficient. Currently multidetector computed tomography (MDCT) or magnetic resonance imaging (MRI) is used for a 3D virtual surgery dataset. MRI as a radiation-free and noninvasive method is most commonly used in patients with CHD in clinical routine. Therefore our examples in this book chapter are based on MRI datasets.

3D MRI

A range of publications is dedicated to 3D MRI. Early research focused on delineating the vasculature structures using contrast-enhanced imaging [7, 8]. As data are usually acquired within one breath hold, ECG triggering is not used to shorten data acquisition time. Therefore intracardiac structures are not imaged adequately. Respiratory-gated and ECG-triggered sequences allow the acquisition of whole-heart MRI datasets suitable for segmental morphological analysis [5, 9]. It was initially evaluated in adolescents and adults with congenital heart disease [4]. After further technical developments, now intracardiac structures in infants and children can be imaged and used for 3D modeling [5, 10]. Recently new intravascular contrast agents have enabled contrast-enhanced imaging triggered to the cardiac cycle. These improvements enable 3D MRI to be acquired in all age groups in clinically acceptable time frames [11, 12]. Figure 23.4a illustrates the current standard image quality obtainable for the dataset underlying the 3D reconstruction demonstrated in Figs. 23.1 and 23.2.

Image Segmentation

Tissue and blood pool need to be segmented to create suitable models for virtual surgery. With the current sequences used, the vessel walls are indistinguishable from the blood lumen and surrounding tissue. Therefore the myocardium and blood pool are segmented. Vessel walls are created by software unless the blood pool is already bordered by the myocardium.

It is out of the scope of this chapter to discuss various segmentation algorithms. For the present work a marker-based segmentation algorithm was applied [1]. The user inserts a number of colored markers in the blood pool, myocardium, and background, respectively. One color is dedicated for each category. From this input the software

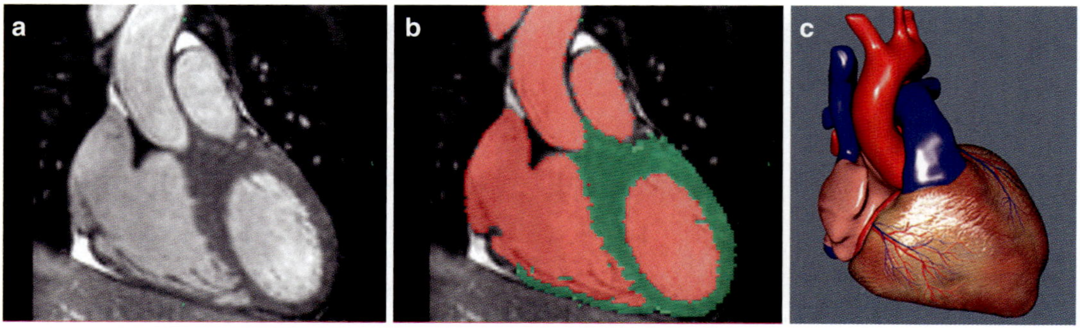

Fig. 23.4 A three-step process to create a model for virtual surgery is shown: 3D imaging (**a**), semiautomatic segmentation (**b**), and 3D reconstruction of a virtual model for visualization and simulation (**c**)

computes and visualizes a corresponding segmentation in real time. This procedure can be carried out in just a few minutes, assuming a reasonable image quality has been obtained. Unfortunately it is usually more time consuming to subsequently verify and manually correct residual segmentation errors. A previous study showed that about 1 h for segmentation was required for a suitable model for surgical simulation [3]. Improvements of segmentation software, image contrast, and resolution will reduce the time for creating models for virtual surgery. Figure 23.4b shows a segmented slice corresponding to the non-segmented slice seen on the left (Fig. 23.4a). With this software the segmentation is done in 3D and *not* slice by slice to reduce the time for preparation of the virtual surgery model. The blood pool is colored in red and the myocardium in green (Fig. 23.4b).

3D Modeling

Proceeding to the 3D modeling step, two scenarios should be distinguished:

- Patient-specific preoperative planning
- Generic modeling for training and teaching

A brief section is dedicated to each scenario outlined below. The simulation of realistic tissue deformation behavior in response to surgical tools is required for both scenarios. This needs to be interactive and in real time. Haptic feedback from freely movable tools in 3D is preferred (Fig. 23.1a). A fundamental requirement of virtual surgery is the possibility of making arbitrary tissue incisions. The underlying technical foundation to the system discussed below has been published [13].

Patient-Specific Modeling

Once the segmentation of the morphological scan has been completed, it can be exported into the simulator, which automatically sets up a simulation environment such as the one depicted in Figs. 23.1 and 23.2. In the next section the applicability of the system will be discussed.

It might be necessary to preprocess the data structure of a 3D model, i.e., the mesh, to achieve reliable results from the simulation or to speed up the simulation itself for real-time purposes. Preprocessing ranges from reducing overly sampled parts of a 3D model to completely resampling a raw, initially highly sampled model. Even during a simulation 3D models have to adapt to their meshes, e.g., to allow for arbitrary incisions, in which case, the data structure has to be aligned along these incisions. This technical aspect is particularly important since automatic modifications of the data structure are the third source for errors referred to the original anatomical structure after image acquisition and segmentation.

Generic Modeling

To define a convincing new training or teaching environment, further processing is advisable. As a demonstration model we scanned a volunteer and constructed a 3D model of his heart and major vessels [2]. Some desired morphological defects were manually introduced, specifically two atrial septal defects (ASDs) and two ventricular septal defects (VSDs). An option of dynamically configuring whether these defects should all be present for a given simulation session was implemented. A graphical artist was employed to colorize the models and enhance their visual appearance. An example of such visual model enhancement is provided in Fig. 23.4c. The significant effort to create these realistic models is justified by their unlimited and universal use.

Virtual Surgery Examples

Preoperative Planning

Congenital heart disease often has complex intra- and extracardiac malformations, which need to be addressed individually by a specific surgical or interventional approach. The surgeon needs to be able to view all cardiovascular structures of interest to plan the incision and the operative strategy to achieve optimal results. There is further a need for the surgeon to interact with the dataset to try out different types of surgical techniques including the design of patches to produce optimal surgical results.

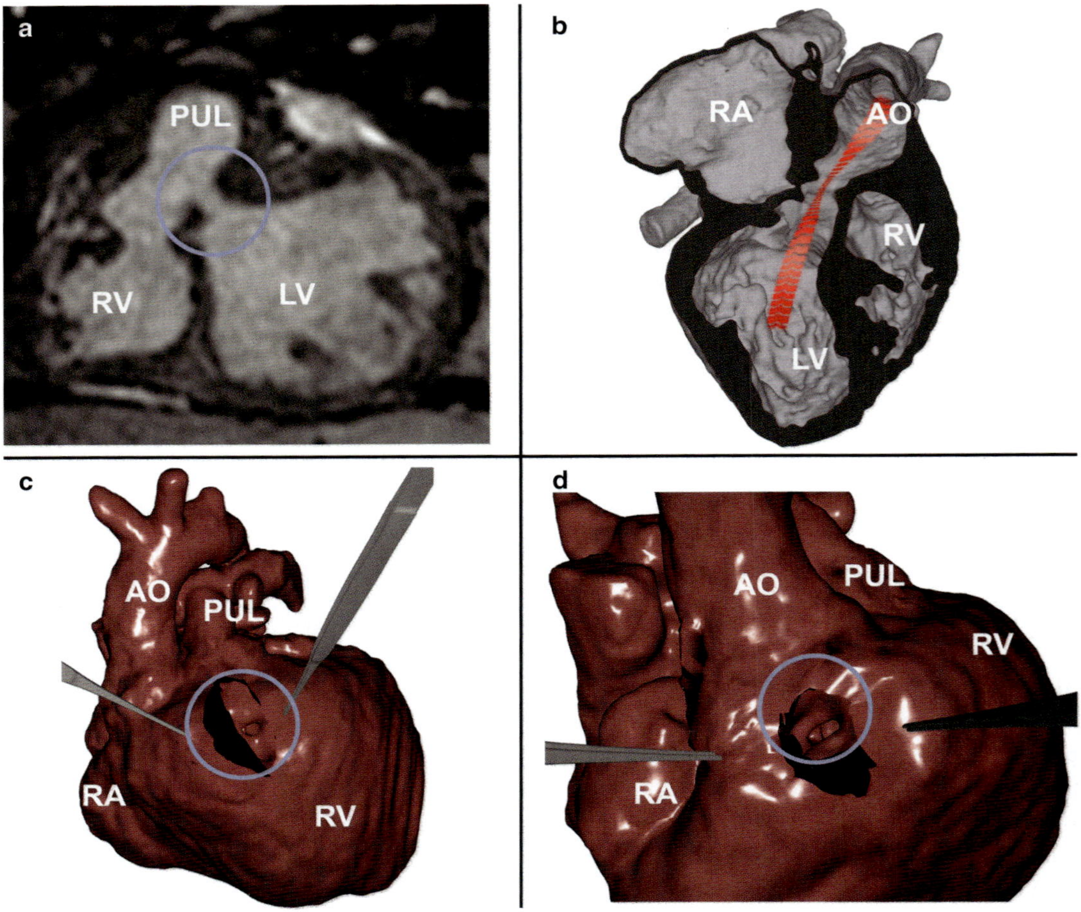

Fig. 23.5 Post-surgical 3D visualization and simulation from a MRI data set of a 10-year-old girl after an intraventricular repair of a double-outlet-right ventricle (*DORV*) is shown. The aorta was to the right of the pulmonary artery in a side-by-side position. Two baffle leakages and a narrow baffle pathway from the left ventricle to the aorta were imaged postoperatively. (**a**) Oblique slice from the 3D MRI data set depicting the larger sub-pulmonary baffle leakage (*circle*). (**b**) 3D visualization of the baffle pathway from the left ventricle to the aorta (*red arrow*). (**c**) An incision in the sub-pulmonary region reveals the exact 3D position of the larger residual baffle leakage (*circle*). (**d**) An incision in the sub-aortic region shows the narrow baffle pathway (*circle*) from the left ventricle to the aorta. *AO* aorta, *LV* left ventricle, *PUL* pulmonary artery, *RA* right atrium, *RV* right ventricle

Figures 23.5 and 23.6 provide two examples of virtual cardiotomy to illustrate what can be achieved using this tool. Figure 23.5 shows a patient with double-outlet right ventricle (DORV) after an intracardiac baffle repair connecting the left ventricle to the aorta and the right ventricle to the pulmonary artery. This is a challenging operation even for an experienced surgeon [14]. The 3D visualization and simulation tools were used to evaluate the post-surgical outcome. An oblique reformatting of the 3D MRI reveals a residual sub-pulmonary baffle leakage (Fig. 23.5a). The precise position of this baffle leakage is visualized with a virtual incision in the right ventricle (Fig. 23.5c). The passage of blood through the baffle is visualized in Fig. 23.5b, d. The red arrow (Fig. 23.5b) indicates the path through the baffle from the left ventricle to the aorta. The virtual incision (Fig. 23.5d) in the sub-aortic region demonstrates the narrow intraventricular pathway from the left ventricle to the aorta.

Figure 23.6 compares the operative situs of a patient with a VSD with the virtual model to prove the suitability but also the limitations of this tool.

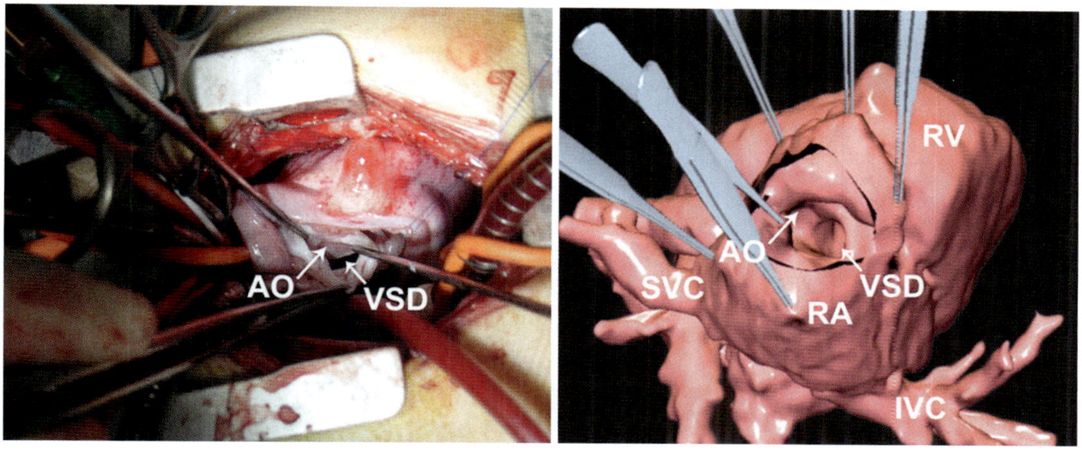

Fig. 23.6 Surgical image (*left*) and virtual cardiotomy (*right*) in a 1-year-old child with a ventricular septal defect. An incision in the right atrium gives access to the defect, which is located just below the aortic outflow tract. *IVC* inferior vena cava, *RA* right atrium, *RV* right ventricle, *SVC* superior vena cava, *VSD* ventricular septal defect

Predictive Simulation

In the context of cardiovascular surgery, predictive simulation is a recently emerging field. First examples regarding the extracardiac vasculature can be found in the literature [15, 16]. The challenge of predictive simulation systems is to behave as physically correct as possible to provide reliable previews of outcomes for different surgical approaches. This slight shift of focus entails several requirements and opportunities for such simulation systems. Rather than simulating surgical tools controlled in real time through haptic input devices for virtual operations, such a simulation system can be considered to be the tool itself.

A surgeon, already experienced in incising and suturing, is supposed to interact on a higher level with the software, e.g., by just indicating incisions or choosing incisions, which should be sutured automatically. Solely the result is of interest to be able to evaluate different approaches for an intervention. While the simple interaction is done in real time, e.g., by clicking on a static 3D model, the resulting deformations are simulated directly afterwards without strong real-time requirements. This allows the simulation to utilize very sophisticated mathematical models for accurately predicting the outcome or proposing optimal patch shapes for most promising results regarding blood flow for example.

Figure 23.7 shows an early prototype of a predictive simulation system for interventions in patients with malformed extracardiac vasculature [16]. Different approaches to correct a patient with coarctation of the aorta are simulated. In the future this may lead to better results in these patients as different surgical approaches can virtually be tested and the best result can be predicted. In this case the surgeon would then choose the technique providing the best result based on the recommendations of the modeling tool. It is very important that the physician who is actually performing the procedure makes the final decision.

Training and Teaching

How virtual surgery can support training, teaching, and clinical medicine and therefore improve patient outcome is outlined below. The approach for training and teaching has a different focus than the clinical setup, but many of the technical considerations are similar. Data can be acquired from heart specimens using high-resolution computed tomography to obtain optimal imaging results [17, 18]. Models can be post-processed by an artist to obtain most realistic results of the cardiac morphology, which needs to be demonstrated. Time for reconstructing these models is not as crucial as in the clinical setup, and many of

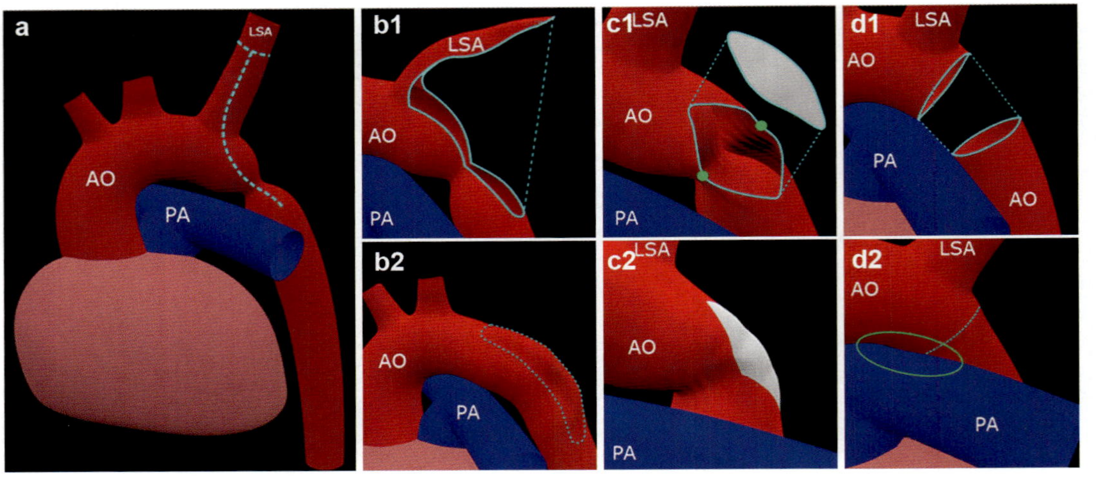

Fig. 23.7 A prototype for preoperative planning of surgery of coarctation of the aortic arch is shown (**a**). Deformations caused by different interventions are simulated: before and after a subclavian flap aortoplasty (**b**), patch aortoplasty (**c**), and an end-to-end anastomosis (**d**) (From Kislinskiy et al. [16] with permission)

the specimens used are more a template for a typical form of congenital heart disease rather than a very specific patient model.

For clinical purposes the heart of the patient needs to be imaged as precisely as possible prior to surgery. The time required for segmentation and preparing the model should be within reasonable time limits to make it applicable in a clinical setup in a cost-effective way. The models produced need to be evaluated regarding their reliability to depict the relevant structures of the intracardiac anatomy to enable optimal surgical results.

Because of further developments in imaging technology and computer hardware and software, it can be expected that this technology will be an essential part in teaching and training, research, and clinical medicine with the final goal to improve patient outcome.

References

1. Sorensen TS, Pedersen EM, Hansen OK, Sorensen K. Visualization of morphological details in congenitally malformed hearts: virtual three-dimensional reconstruction from magnetic resonance imaging. Cardiol Young. 2003;13:451–60.
2. Sorensen TS, Greil GF, Hansen OK, Mosegaard J. Surgical simulation–a new tool to evaluate surgical incisions in congenital heart disease? Interact Cardiovasc Thorac Surg. 2006;5:536–9.
3. Sorensen TS, Beerbaum P, Mosegaard J, Rasmusson A, Schaeffter T, Austin C, Razavi R, Greil GF. Virtual cardiotomy based on 3-D MRI for preoperative planning in congenital heart disease. Pediatr Radiol. 2008;38:1314–22.
4. Sorensen TS, Korperich H, Greil GF, Eichhorn J, Barth P, Meyer H, Pedersen EM, Beerbaum P. Operator-independent isotropic three-dimensional magnetic resonance imaging for morphology in congenital heart disease: a validation study. Circulation. 2004;110:163–9.
5. Hussain T, Lossnitzer D, Bellsham-Revell H, Valverde I, Beerbaum P, Razavi R, Bell AJ, Schaeffter T, Botnar RM, Uribe SA, Greil GF. Three-dimensional dual-phase whole-heart mr imaging: clinical implications for congenital heart disease. Radiology. 2012;263:547–54.
6. Uribe S, Tejos C, Razavi R, Schaeffter T. New respiratory gating technique for whole heart cine imaging: integration of a navigator slice in steady state free precession sequences. J Magn Reson Imaging. 2011;34:211–9.
7. Greil GF, Powell AJ, Gildein HP, Geva T. Gadolinium-enhanced three-dimensional magnetic resonance angiography of pulmonary and systemic venous anomalies. J Am Coll Cardiol. 2002;39:335–41.
8. Valsangiacomo ER, Levasseur S, McCrindle BW, MacDonald C, Smallhorn JF, Yoo SJ. Contrast-enhanced mr angiography of pulmonary venous abnormalities in children. Pediatr Radiol. 2003;33:92–8.
9. Sorensen TS, Beerbaum P, Korperich H, Pedersen EM. Three-dimensional, isotropic MRI: a unified approach to quantification and visualization in congenital heart disease. Int J Cardiovasc Imaging. 2005;21:283–92.
10. Tangcharoen T, Bell A, Hegde S, Hussain T, Beerbaum P, Schaeffter T, Razavi R, Botnar RM, Greil GF. Detection of coronary artery anomalies in infants and young children with congenital heart disease by using MR imaging. Radiology. 2011;259:240–7.

11. Makowski MR, Wiethoff AJ, Uribe S, Parish V, Botnar RM, Bell A, Kiesewetter C, Beerbaum P, Jansen CH, Razavi R, Schaeffter T, Greil GF. Congenital heart disease: cardiovascular MR imaging by using an intravascular blood pool contrast agent. Radiology. 2011;260:680–8.
12. Kozerke S, Tsao J, Razavi R, Boesiger P. Accelerating cardiac cine 3D imaging using k-t blast. Magn Reson Med. 2004;52:19–26.
13. Mosegaard J, Herborg P, Sorensen TS. A GPU accelerated spring mass system for surgical simulation. Stud Health Technol Inform. 2005;111:342–8.
14. Sorensen TS, Mosegaard J, Greil GF, Miller S, Seeger A, Hansen OK, Sieverding L. Images in cardiovascular medicine. Virtual cardiotomy for preoperative planning. Circulation. 2007;115:e312.
15. Li H, Leow WK, Chiu IS. Predictive simulation of bidirectional glenn shunt using a hybrid blood vessel model. Med Image Comput Comput Assist Interv Int Conf Med Image Comput Comput Assist Interv. 2009;12:266–74.
16. Kislinskiy S, Golembiovský T, Duriez C, Riesenkampff E, Kuehne T, Meinzer HP, Heimann T. Simulation of congenital heart defect corrective surgeries using thin shell elements. In: Wittek A, Miller K, Nielsen PMF, editors. Computational biomechanics for medicine – models, algorithms and implementation. New York, Heidelberg, Dordrecht, London: Springer; 2013:63–74.
17. Greil GF, Wolf I, Kuettner A, Fenchel M, Miller S, Martirosian P, Schick F, Oppitz M, Meinzer HP, Sieverding L. Stereolithographic reproduction of complex cardiac morphology based on high spatial resolution imaging. Clin Res Cardiol. 2007;96:176–85.
18. Greil GF, Kuettner A, Flohr T, Grasruck M, Sieverding L, Meinzer HP, Wolf I. High-resolution reconstruction of a waxed heart specimen with flat panel volume computed tomography and rapid prototyping. J Comput Assist Tomogr. 2007;31:444–8.

24 Aortic Arch Anomalies

Scott DeRoo, Jonathan R. Dillman, Philip Cascade, Richard G. Ohye, and Baskaran Sundaram

Congenital anomalies of the aortic arch represent a diverse set of malformations with a common embryologic origin and a wide array of clinical manifestations. Arch anomalies are noted in 1–10/1,000 live births and account for approximately 15–20 % of all congenital heart disease [1]. Presentation of aortic arch anomalies is highly variable with many patients remaining asymptomatic throughout life. When present, symptoms generally result from compression of surrounding mediastinal structures or associated intracardiac defects. Successful management of symptomatic arch anomalies often relies on surgical or endovascular intervention aimed at relieving compression or improving hemodynamics. In this review, we present several common aortic anomalies in correlation with their embryologic development and clinical features.

S. DeRoo, MD
Division of Cardiothoracic Surgery, Columbia University, New York, NY, USA

J.R. Dillman, MD
Department of Radiology, University of Michigan Health System, 1500 East Medical Center Drive, Ann Arbor, MI 48109, USA
e-mail: jonadill@med.umich.edu

P. Cascade, MD
Division of Cardiothoracic Radiology, Department of Radiology, University of Michigan Health System, Cardiovascular Center 5481, Ann Arbor, MI 48109, USA
e-mail: pcascade@med.umich.edu

R.G. Ohye, MD
Department of Cardiac Surgery, University of Michigan Health System, 1500 East Medical Center Drive, Ann Arbor, MI 48109, USA
e-mail: ohye@umich.edu

B. Sundaram, MBBS, MRCP, FRCR (✉)
Division of Cardiothoracic Radiology, Department of Radiology, University of Michigan Health System, Cardiovascular Center 5481, 1500 East Medical Center Drive, Ann Arbor, MI 48109, USA
e-mail: sundbask@umich.edu

Embryology of the Normal Aortic Arch

The majority of development of the adult aortic arch occurs between intrauterine weeks 4 and 7. Arch development proceeds through the branchial apparatus, which consists of paired dorsal and ventral aorta connected by six branchial segments or arches, numbered 1–6 from cephalad to caudad (Fig. 24.1a). Typically, arches one, two, and five involute completely. The third arches develop to form the common carotid arteries and proximal portion of the internal carotid arteries. The left fourth arch forms the portion of the aortic arch between the left common carotid and left subclavian arteries. A portion of the right fourth arch involutes between the right subclavian artery and descending aorta, with the remaining segment ultimately giving rise to the proximal portion of the right subclavian artery. The proximal portions of the right and left sixth arch form the proximal right and left pulmonary arteries, respectively. Typically, the distal sixth arch forms the ductus arteriosus on the left side and regresses completely on the right.

F. Saremi (ed.), *Cardiac CT and MR for Adult Congenital Heart Disease*,
DOI 10.1007/978-1-4614-8875-0_24, © Springer Science+Business Media New York 2014

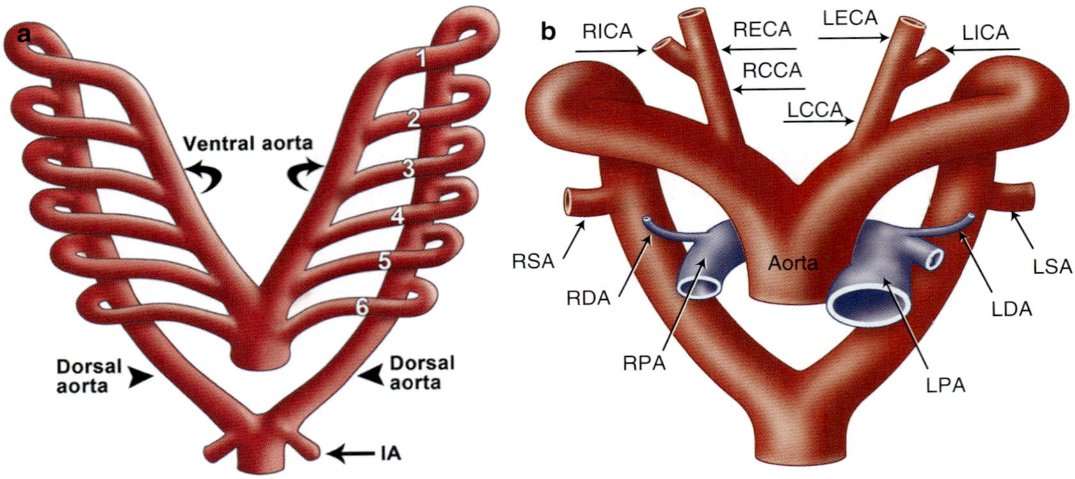

Fig. 24.1 (**a**) Diagram representing six paired branchial arches (numbers 1–6) and an intersegmental artery (*IA*). The arches connect paired dorsal and ventral aortae during development. (**b**) Schematic representation of the Edwards hypothetical double arch. Dual right- and left-sided aortic arches give rise to bilateral common carotid arteries and subclavian arteries as independent structures. The selective involution of arch segments gives rise to the final adult aortic arch and serves as a mechanism to explain several common arch anomalies. *LCCA* left common carotid artery, *LECA* left external carotid artery, *LICA* left internal carotid artery, *RCCA* right common carotid artery, *RECA* right external carotid artery, *RICA* right internal carotid artery, *LSA* left subclavian artery, *RSA* right subclavian artery, *LDA* left ductus arteriosus, *RDA* right ductus arteriosus, *LPA* left pulmonary artery, *RPA* right pulmonary artery, *MPA* main pulmonary artery

In order to conceptualize how specific perturbations in arch development affect aortic anatomy, it is helpful to rely on the Edwards hypothetical double arch concept (Fig. 24.1b). In this model the developing aorta is represented by dual right- and left-sided arches with ductus arteriosus on each side. Although development of the aortic arch proceeds such that this structure does not exist in its entirety at any one time, it has nonetheless proven helpful in showcasing the effect of interruptions to the developing aorta at specific locations.

Imaging of the Aortic Arch and Associated Structures

Chest Radiography and Echocardiography

Although limited in its ability to provide detailed anatomic information regarding the aorta and its associated vessels, there are several direct and indirect findings on chest radiography (CXR) that may raise the suspicion for an aortic arch anomaly. Evaluation of the position of the aortic knob and para-aortic stripe provides information as to whether the arch is left or right sided, as does the position of the descending aorta. Similarly, in infants and small children, a deviated trachea may serve an indirect sign of compression by an aortic arch opposite the side of deviation. Lateral CXR may suggest a vascular anomaly when there is obscuration of the retrotracheal lucency (an area commonly known as Raider's triangle) [2]. Along with CXR, echocardiography has been used as a first-line imaging modality to examine pediatric patients for suspected aortic arch anomalies. Echocardiography has the benefit of not utilizing ionizing radiation and the relative ease at which it can be performed at the bedside. However, it is challenging to visualize the entirety of the thoracic aorta, and patient habitus, operator skill, and available sonographic windows may limit the final images. Although at experienced centers echocardiography can be utilized to accurately diagnose vascular rings, local expertise may limit its role to the diagnosis of associated cardiac abnormalities. Rarely, aortic arch anomalies may also be diagnosed in utero through fetal echocardiography [3, 4].

Computed Tomography and Magnetic Resonance Imaging

The advent of ECG gating, multiple detectors and spiral imaging, and radiation dose reduction methods has recently revolutionized computed tomography (CT) imaging. Using these techniques, CT is capable of generating detailed anatomic images in a matter of seconds with isotropic submillimeter resolution that can be used to reconstruct images in any two-dimensional plane. Improvements in advanced post-processing methods utilizing maximum and minimum intensity projections, as well as three-dimensional models with surface and volume rendering methods, allow CT to play an important role in imaging aortic arch pathology. The speed, ease, access, and lack of sedation requirements make CT a reasonable imaging choice in both the adult and pediatric populations. However, CT imaging utilizes potentially carcinogenic ionizing radiation and often requires iodinated contrast agents that on occasion evoke anaphylactoid reactions (about 0.6–0.7/100 adult patients). Iodinated contrast agents are also known nephrotoxic agents, and it should be noted that unlike other imaging modalities such as MRI or echocardiography, CT cannot assess or quantify normal or abnormal blood flow and pattern. Overall, the risk of adverse events from CT scan is likely much lower than the expected benefit for the great majority of patients. The precise technique and scan parameters may depend on the specific CT machine and the type of study. Contrast-enhanced CT angiogram (CTA) is usually performed with thin collimation (0.5–1 mm) and multiplanar images are reconstructed as thin slices of around 1–2 mm. Typically, injection rates of 3–5 ml per second of intravenous iodinated contrast containing are used, through a peripheral intravenous cannula placed in the right upper extremity to minimize streak artifact from dense contrast material in the innominate veins. In most cases, the scan can be triggered by automated bolus tracking by placing the region of interest (ROI) in the aortic lumen, at an attenuation threshold of 150–180 Hounsfield units to achieve reliable aortic enhancement. Cardiac pulsation artifact mainly affects the aortic root in non-gated examinations. Electrocardiogram (ECG)-gated CT may be preferred for the assessment of the aortic root with minimal or no motion-related artifacts. Slowing the heart rate with β-blockers may also be helpful in improving image quality. The penalty of using ECG gating, especially in retrospective gating mode, is an increase in radiation dose.

In addition to morphological assessment, blood flow velocity mapping, directional flow assessment, and pressure gradient calculation are routinely performed in MRI. These examinations can be performed either with or without intravenous gadolinium-containing contrast material. Multiphasic postcontrast evaluation is also possible in MRI. However, drawbacks to MRI examinations include claustrophobia, incompatibility with metallic devices, renal impairment restricting the use of gadolinium (due to the potential for development of nephrogenic systemic fibrosis), and prolonged examination times requiring sedation or, particularly in children, general anesthesia. Relatively limited access, affordability, and expertise may also prohibit the routine use of MRI.

The decision to utilize CT vs. MRI or another imaging modality is made based on individual patient factors as well as institutional preference and expertise.

The Normal Aortic Arch

Typically the aorta originates just left of midline and ascends obliquely and slightly to the right before turning posteriorly and leftward to form the aortic arch. The aorta completes its course by then descending just left of midline adjacent to the anterior thoracic vertebral bodies, exiting the diaphragm through the aortic hiatus. After the coronary arteries, the first major vessel arising from the aortic arch is the brachiocephalic (innominate) artery, which bifurcates quickly to form the right subclavian and right common carotid arteries, followed by the origins of the left common carotid artery and left subclavian artery (Fig. 24.2a). On the right side the primitive ductus arteriosus involutes completely, while on the

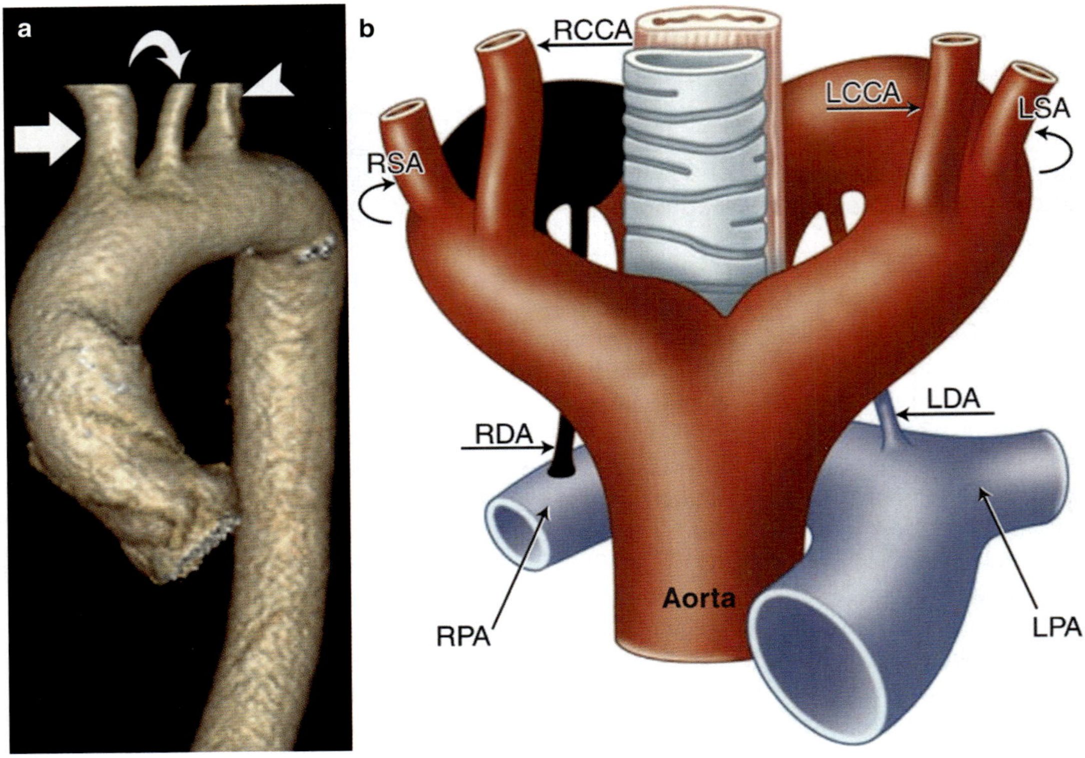

Fig. 24.2 (**a**) Normal aortic arch morphology. There are three normal great vessels emanating from the arch in the typical fashion: right brachiocephalic artery (*arrow*), left common carotid artery (*curved arrow*), and left subclavian artery (*arrow head*). (**b**) Schematic representation of the normal aortic arch via the Edwards hypothetical double arch concept. The area shaded in black undergoes involution resulting in the formation of the normal left-sided aortic arch. The right arch segment proximal to the area of involution forms the brachiocephalic trunk, and the persistent left arch segment forms the aortic arch and proximal descending aorta. Typically, the right ductus arteriosus undergoes involution leaving only the left aortic arch with left ductus arteriosus. *LCCA* left common carotid artery, *LSA* left subclavian artery, *RCCA* right common carotid artery, *RSA* right subclavian artery, *LDA* left ductus arteriosus, *RDA* right ductus arteriosus, *LPA* left pulmonary artery, *RPA* right pulmonary artery

left it persists to serve as a fetal bypass of the pulmonary vasculature. This typical branching pattern is eventually accomplished through interruption of the Edwards hypothetical double arch distal to the right subclavian artery (Fig. 24.2b).

Normal Variants in Aortic Arch Vessel Branching

Large case studies have demonstrated that this "normal" arch configuration exists in only approximately 65–75 % of the population [5–7]. The most common variant arch vessel branching pattern is the so-called "bovine" aortic arch.

Bovine Aortic Arch

The bovine aortic arch branching configuration occurs when the left common carotid artery is shifted leftward to share a common origin with the brachiocephalic trunk as opposed to arising directly from the aortic arch. Slightly less common is a variant of bovine aortic arch in which the left common carotid artery arises as a branch off the brachiocephalic trunk as opposed to sharing a common ostium [8]. The incidence of bovine aortic arch has been reported in the literature at approximately 15–27 %, with most large studies placing that estimate between 15 and 20 % [5–7]. Both bovine arch variants are generally asymptomatic.

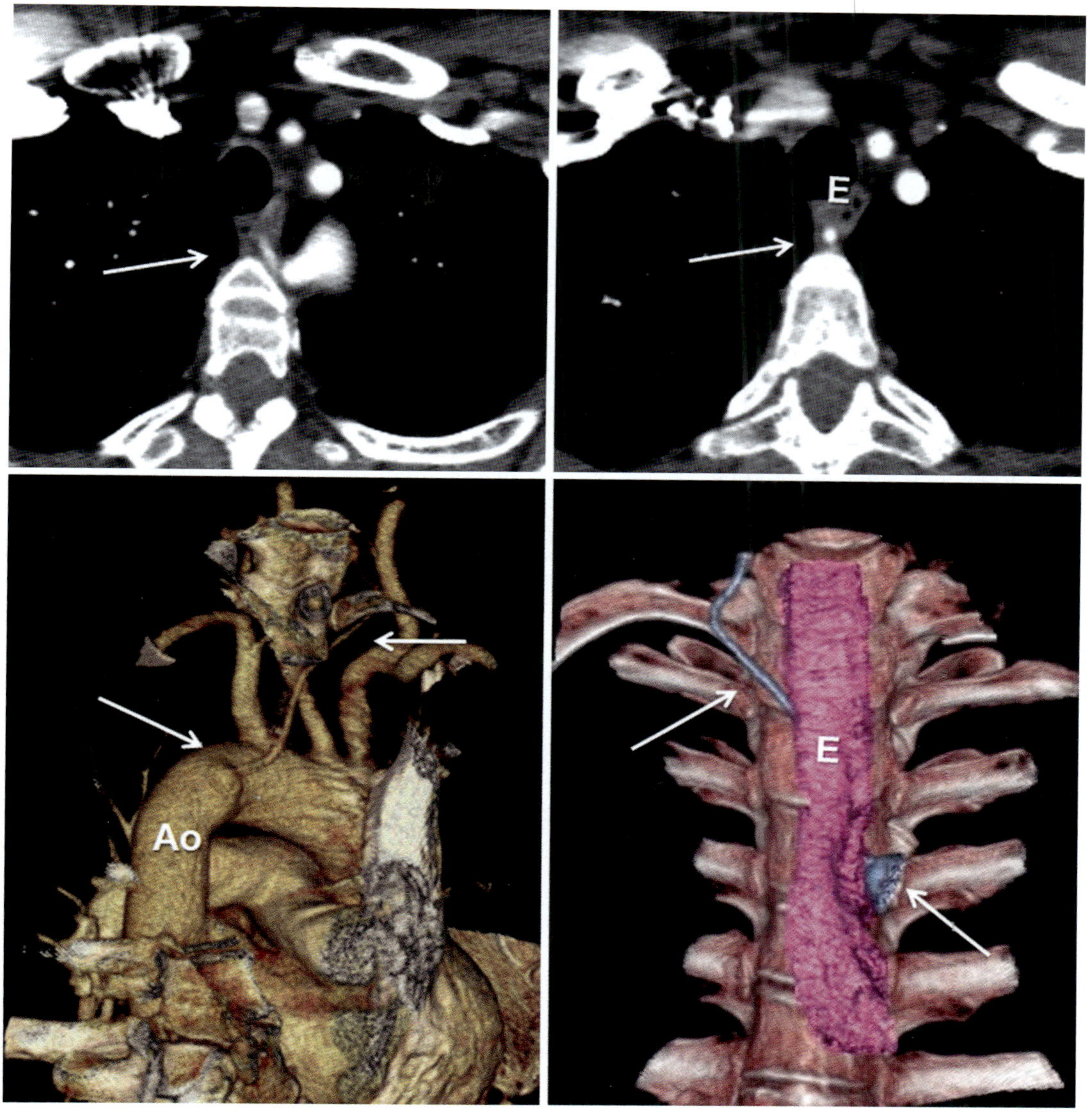

Fig. 24.3 Vertebral arteria lusoria (*arrows*). Aberrant origin of the left vertebral artery from distal aortic arch (*Ao*) shown in CT images. Note diverticular outpouching at its origin. The vessel travels obliquely behind the esophagus (*E*) and may be compressed between the esophagus and vertebra (Courtesy of Farhood Saremi MD, USC)

Aberrant Origin of Vertebral Artery

The left vertebral artery will occasionally arise not from the left subclavian artery, but instead will originate directly from the aortic arch. This arch variant is generally asymptomatic, with several studies observing this branching pattern in approximately 1–8 % of the study population [5, 9, 10]. With less frequency, the right vertebral artery may directly arise from the aortic arch. Aberrant origin of the right vertebral artery from the aorta distal to the origin of the left subclavian artery is very rare (Fig. 24.3). It courses behind the esophagus and may have a diverticulum at its origin (vertebral lusoria) [9].

Anomalous Brachiocephalic Trunk

In this condition the origin of the brachiocephalic artery is displaced just left of midline on the aortic arch. Historically, this condition has been thought to be a cause of respiratory symptoms in infants and young children; however, more recent studies have demonstrated that the brachiocephalic trunk arises left of the trachea in >95 % of newborns and that most infants and young children display some degree of asymptomatic tracheal indentation. Only when tracheal compression exceeds 50 % of the AP diameter is this condition considered potentially pathologic, although some patients may remain asymptomatic even at this degree of compression due to its dynamic nature. While tracheal deformity was believed to be primarily due to the variant brachiocephalic trunk origin, it is now thought to represent a functional anomaly primarily related to immature tracheal cartilage [11]. Most infants and children display few, if any, symptoms related to tracheal compression, although some may develop significant respiratory compromise. When symptoms are clinically significant, the condition is known as innominate artery compression syndrome.

Currently both CT and MRI are able to delineate the aortic arch anatomy as well as quantify the degree of tracheal compression. Unlike bronchoscopy, however, neither can easily visualize tracheal changes throughout the respiratory cycle. In contrast to cross-sectional imaging, bronchoscopy offers no additional relevant information, such as surrounding vascular anatomy or associated cardiac defects.

Symptomatic patients may be treated with surgical suspension of the brachiocephalic trunk to the posterior sternum via a procedure known as retrosternal innominate arteriopexy in order to provide symptomatic relief or reimplantation of the artery in an anatomically correct position on the aortic arch.

Anomalies of the Aortic Arch

Classification of Aortic Arch Anomalies

Aortic arch anomalies may be classified with the Edwards hypothetical double arch, with stratification based upon the point at which the hypothetical arch has been interrupted. Clinically, classification is most likely to proceed on the basis of anatomy and morphology, where the course of the aorta and arch vessels form the basis for classification. In this system, arch anomalies may be characterized as right or left sided, interrupted, double, or cervical, with additional classification based on the pattern of arch vessel branching. Further, anomalies may be characterized as symptomatic or asymptomatic. The majority of aortic arch malformations remain asymptomatic; however, certain anomalies may be symptomatic, commonly due to tracheobronchial or esophageal compression from a vascular ring and rarely due to a cerebral "steal" phenomenon where blood is shunted away from the cerebral vasculature to provide reconstituted flow to an isolated vessel.

Left Aortic Arch

The left aortic arch morphology is described earlier under "The Normal Aortic Arch."

When classified based on arch vessel branching, there are three configurations of major vessels that are seen with a left-sided aortic arch: normal, aberrant right subclavian artery, and isolated subclavian artery.

Aberrant Right Subclavian Artery

Pathology and Embryology

Aberrant right subclavian artery (ARSA) is the most common form of thoracic arterial anomaly with a prevalence of 0.4–2 % [12]. An ARSA is believed to be the result of complete involution of the right fourth pharyngeal arch and proximal right dorsal aorta, with the right seventh intersegmental artery giving rise to the right subclavian artery from a segment of persistent dorsal aorta. The aortic remnant often persists as a saccular diverticulum known as a Kommerell diverticulum, which in approximately 8 % of patients may become aneurysmal requiring surgical resection [13]. According to the Edwards hypothetical double arch model, the site of interruption occurs between the right common carotid and right subclavian arteries (Fig. 24.4). In order to reach the right upper extremity, the artery takes a right

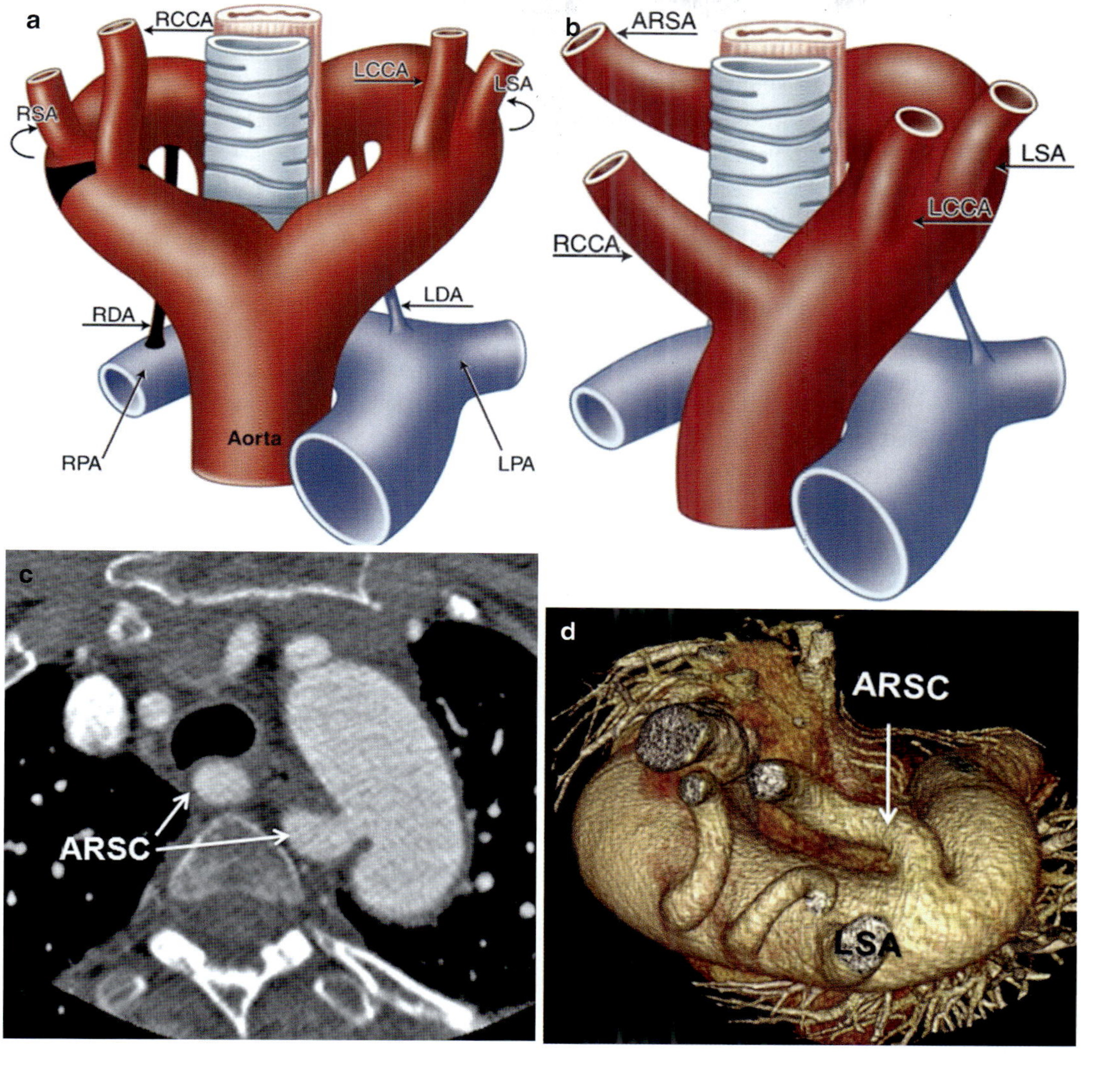

Fig. 24.4 (**a**, **b**) Schematic representation of the left aortic arch with aberrant right subclavian artery (ARSA). (**a**) The *black-shaded* area represents the break point in the Edwards hypothetical double arch. (**c**) Axial CT and (**d**) superior volume-rendered view of the aortic arch demonstrate ARSC coursing behind the esophagus. *LCCA* left common carotid artery, *LSA* left subclavian Artery, *RCCA* right common carotid artery, *RSA* right subclavian artery, *LDA* left ductus arteriosus, *RDA* right ductus arteriosus, *LPA* left pulmonary artery, *RPA* right pulmonary artery

superior oblique course passing behind the esophagus in the majority of cases; however, in rare cases it may pass between the esophagus and trachea or anterior to the trachea [14].

Associations

An ARSA occasionally occurs in conjunction with several intracardiac anomalies, the most common of which is tetralogy of Fallot. Among patients with tetralogy of Fallot, the incidence of ARSA is approximately 5–16 %, with rates slightly higher in patients with both tetralogy of Fallot and pulmonary atresia [15–17]. Other associated cardiac defects include left-sided obstructive lesions, atrioventricular canal defects, interrupted aortic arch, and coarctation of the aorta; however, these remain less commonly associated.

Clinical Symptoms

An ARSA is most commonly asymptomatic. Very rarely, infants and young children may develop dysphagia or respiratory symptoms resulting from tracheoesophageal compression. The presence of severe symptoms in a child suggests the presence of an additional lesion forming a complete vascular ring. Causes of this condition include a persistent double aortic arch, common origin of both carotid arteries, or right-sided ductus arteriosus.

Patients in their seventh and eighth decades may develop late dysphagia as the ARSA becomes stiffened and ectatic by atherosclerotic changes and compresses the posterior esophagus. Symptoms of tracheoesophageal compression due to an ARSA have been termed *dysphagia lusoria* ("prank of nature") [18].

Imaging

On frontal CXR the findings of an oblique edge or opacity extending to the right from the aortic knob, demonstration of the vessel through the lucency of the tracheal air column, or a mass effect at the medial right clavicular area suggest the presence of ARSA. On lateral CXR, obscuration of the retrotracheal opacity (Raider's triangle), aortic arch obscuration, and posterior tracheal imprint provide evidence for this condition but remain a poor means of definitive diagnosis [19].

In general most patients will be diagnosed with ARSA incidentally on cross-sectional imaging. Both CT and MRI will demonstrate a vessel emerging from the aortic arch distal to the left subclavian artery that course obliquely, right, and superiorly towards the right axilla (Fig. 24.4). Often slight tracheal or esophageal indentation, and rarely significant tracheoesophageal compression, may be appreciable on imaging.

Treatment

In cases of severe dysphagia, respiratory compromise, or aneurysmal dilation, surgery may be employed to reimplant the anomalous subclavian artery at a more favorable location. Often this is accomplished through a modified right carotid-subclavian artery bypass or reimplantation of the vessel at a more proximal arch position. Commonly, this is now accomplished via a two-stage hybrid procedure involving transcatheter occlusion of the origin of the ARSA followed by open carotid-subclavian bypass [20, 21].

Right Aortic Arch

Right aortic arch occurs when the aortic arch both originates and descends to the right of the vertebral bodies. The incidence of right aortic arch is approximately 0.1 % or less of the population; however, with the advent of MDCT and MRI, some clinicians now believe the true incidence to be higher [22]. Right aortic arch results when the developmental pattern of the fourth branchial arch is reversed. Normally, the left fourth arch forms a portion of the aortic arch, while the right fourth arch forms the right subclavian artery; however, reversal of this pattern results in development of a right aortic arch. Development of right aortic arch may occur in isolation or in association with intracardiac abnormalities, esophageal atresia, or tracheoesophageal fistula. Although frequently asymptomatic, patients may present with a number of symptoms such as dysphagia, dyspnea, hypertension, and heart failure. The molecular etiology of right aortic arch remains poorly understood; however, alterations in embryonic blood flow have been hypothesized to contribute to the condition.

Classification of right aortic arch anomalies has historically been accomplished based on the arrangement of the arch vessels as well as the position of the ligamentum arteriosum [23]. Under this system there are three subgroups of right aortic arch:

1. Right aortic arch with mirror image branching (type I)
2. Right aortic arch with aberrant left subclavian artery (ALSA) (type II)
3. Right aortic arch with isolation of the left subclavian artery (type III)

Within these subgroups, the ligamentum arteriosum is most frequently left sided but may be situated on the right or both sides. If the ligamentum arteriosum is situated on the left opposite the aorta, a complete vascular ring may result in tracheoesophageal compression, a condition known as a "Neuhauser" anomaly.

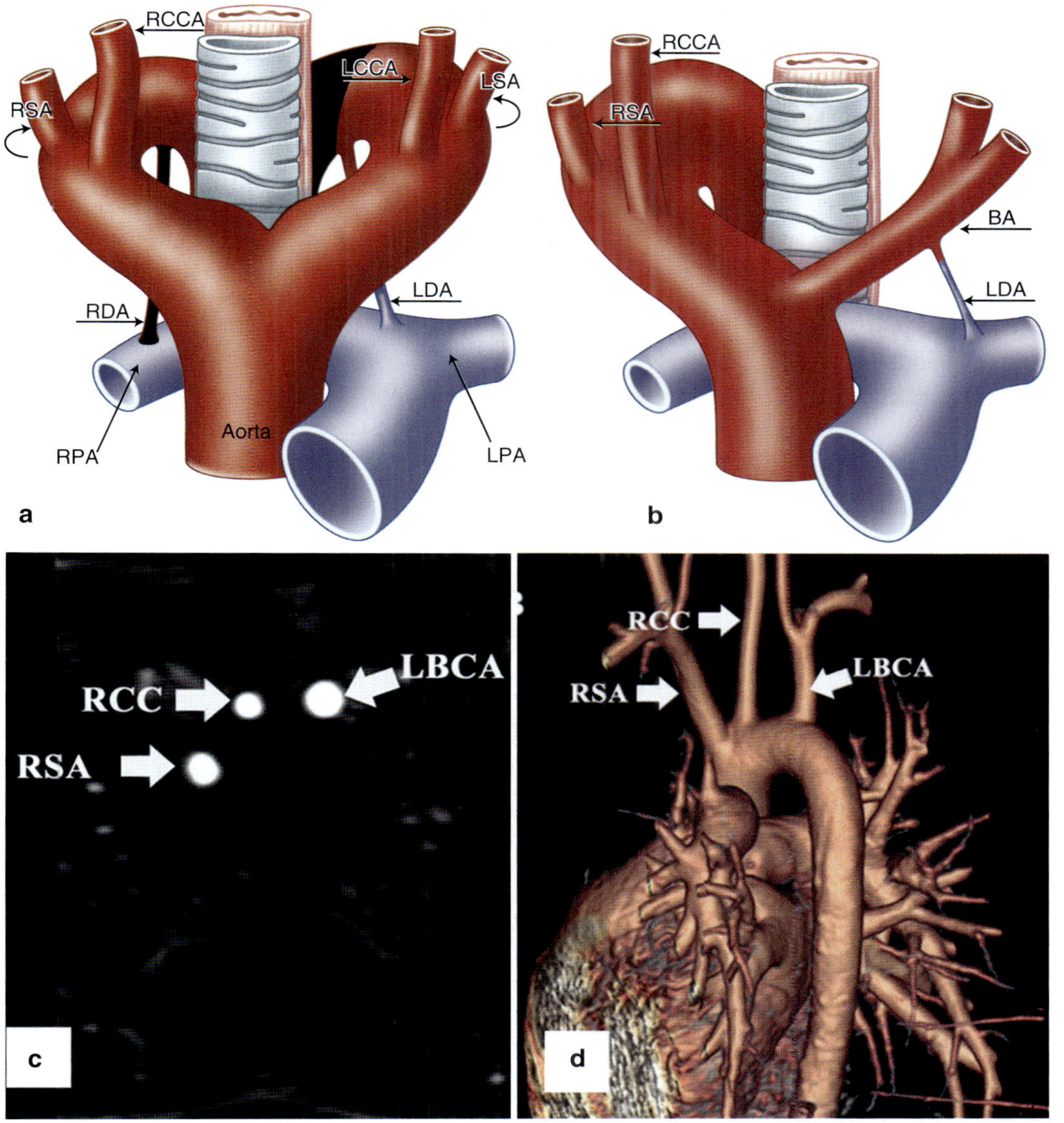

Fig. 24.5 (**a, b**) Schematic illustration of right aortic arch (*RAA*) with mirror image branching pattern. (**a**) The *black-shaded* area represents the break point in the Edwards hypothetical double arch model. (**b**) Schematic of the evolved RAA with mirror image branching. (**c**) Axial reformatted MR angiography and (**d**) 3D volume-rendered image (posterior oblique view) demonstrate RAA with mirror image branching pattern in an 18-year-old young man with history of tetralogy of Fallot status post repair. *LCCA* left common carotid artery, *LSA* left subclavian artery, *LBCA* left brachiocephalic artery, *RCC* and *RCCA* right common carotid artery, *RSA* right subclavian artery, *LDA* left ductus arteriosus, *RDA* right ductus arteriosus, *LPA* left pulmonary artery, *RPA* right pulmonary artery, *BA* brachiocephalic artery

Right Aortic Arch with Mirror Image Branching (Type I)

Pathology and Embryology

Embryologically, this condition results from disruption of the Edwards hypothetical double arch between the descending aorta and the left subclavian artery (Fig. 24.5). Typically, the aorta both originates and descends on the right side of the thorax, eventually crossing over the anterior thoracic vertebrae inferiorly before exiting through the aortic hiatus.

In most cases the ductus arteriosus is left sided, and it is the origin of the ductus that determines whether or not a complete vascular ring is formed [24]. Often a left-sided ductus connects the left pulmonary artery to the left subclavian artery or descending aorta, and there is no complete vascular ring. However, in the rare event that the ductus originates from the posterior aspect of the aorta, a complete vascular ring is formed and may present with tracheoesophageal compression [24]. Occasionally, a patient may present with bilateral ductus arteriosus, in which case a constrictive vascular ring may also be present. Finally, in several instances, a right-sided ductus has been described, in which case there is no vascular ring.

Associations

Based on case reports and case series studies, right aortic arch with mirror image branching is associated with intracardiac malformations in many cases [25, 26]. Most commonly this condition is seen in association with pulmonary atresia with ventricular septal defect (VSD) (46 %), tetralogy of Fallot (32 %), and double-outlet right ventricle with right atrial isomerism (14 %) [27].

Clinical Symptoms

Right aortic arch with mirror image branching is generally asymptomatic, even in cases of left-sided ductus arteriosus and complete vascular ring. In rare cases, infants or young children may present with symptoms of tracheoesophageal compression. Occasionally, patients may become symptomatic late in life due to atherosclerotic hardening of the aortic arch or subsequent compression of mediastinal structures by aneurysmal dilation [28].

Imaging

As most patients with this condition remain asymptomatic, it is often identified incidentally on imaging obtained for unrelated reasons. CXR may demonstrate a right-sided aortic knob with right-sided para-aortic stripe. Occasionally a right-sided aortic arch may mimic a right superior mediastinal mass.

Cross-sectional imaging demonstrates a right-sided aortic arch with a left brachiocephalic trunk emerging as the first arch branch, followed by the right common carotid artery and the right subclavian artery (Fig. 24.5). The brachiocephalic trunk courses anterior to the left pulmonary artery before dividing into the left subclavian and left common carotid arteries. The ductus arteriosus arises from either the posterior aspect of the aortic arch opposite the right subclavian artery or from the origin of the left brachiocephalic artery.

Treatment

In the rare instance that an isolated complete vascular ring is present, treatment may be needed to divide the ligamentum arteriosum. More commonly, treatment of this condition centers on correcting the associated intracardiac defects. Importantly, the surgeon should be made aware of the presence of a right-sided aortic arch prior to intervention requiring a modified Blalock-Taussig shunt as it will be placed on the contralateral side of the arch.

Right Aortic Arch with Aberrant Left Subclavian Artery (Type II)

Pathology and Embryology

Right aortic arch with aberrant left subclavian artery (ALSA) is the most common of the right aortic arch subtypes, and it is the second most common cause of constrictive vascular ring, the first being double aortic arch. In approximately 5–10 % of cases, it may occur in conjunction with intracardiac disease; however, most cases are an isolated phenomenon [26, 29]. Embryologically, interruption of the Edwards hypothetical double arch occurs between the left subclavian and left common carotid arteries (Fig. 24.6). The first major arch vessel to emerge is the left common carotid artery followed by the right common carotid artery, right subclavian artery, and aberrant left subclavian artery. The aberrant left subclavian artery arises at the junction of the right arch and the descending aorta, often from a remnant of the distal left fourth arch.

Most often the ductus arteriosus is left sided and runs from the aortic remnant to the left pulmonary

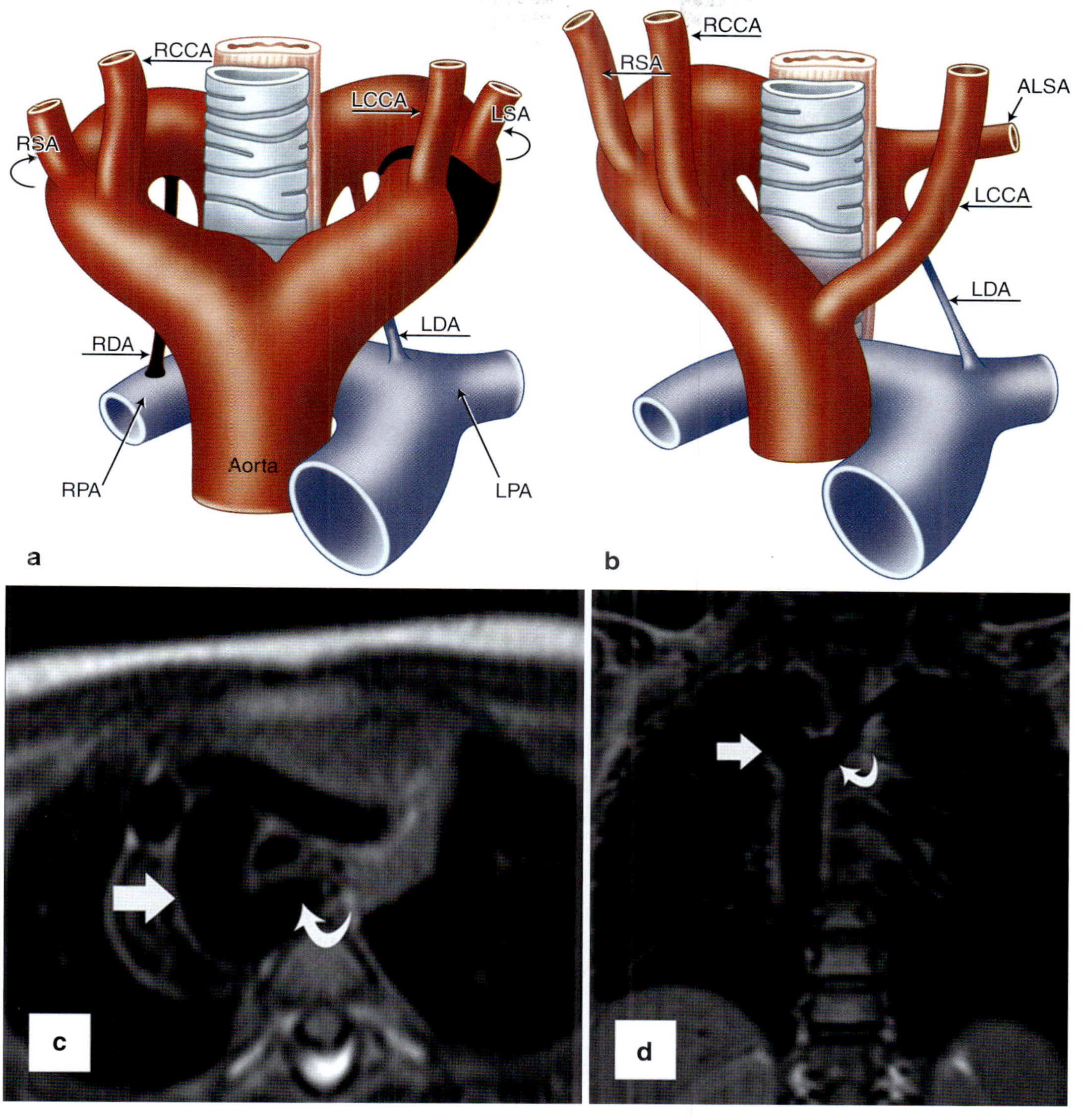

Fig. 24.6 (**a**, **b**) Schematic representation of right aortic arch (*RAA*) with aberrant left subclavian artery (*ALSA*). (**a**) The *black-shaded* area represents the break point in the Edwards hypothetical double arch model. (**b**) Schematic of the evolved *RAA* with *ALSA*. Note the persistent left ductus arteriosus forming a complete vascular ring. (**c**) Axial and (**d**) coronal black-blood MR images demonstrate RAA (*straight arrows*) with ALSA (*curved arrows*). A large diverticulum of Kommerell is seen posterior to the esophagus. The trachea is mildly narrowed. *LCCA* left common carotid artery, *LSA* left subclavian artery, *RCCA* right common carotid artery, *RSA* right subclavian artery, *LDA* left ductus arteriosus, *RDA* right ductus arteriosus, *LPA* left pulmonary artery, *RPA* right pulmonary artery

artery, thus forming a complete vascular ring [29]. In many instances the ring remains relatively loose and is asymptomatic; however, in some patients the ring may be sufficiently tight so as to result in tracheoesophageal compression. This is a much more frequent occurrence in children and young adults, with most adults remaining symptom-free. In rare circumstances, the ductus arteriosus may be right sided, in which case there is no vascular ring and patients remain asymptomatic.

Associations

As stated previously, only approximately 5–10 % of cases of right aortic arch with aberrant left subclavian artery are associated with intracardiac disease. Most often this type of arch branching pattern occurs in isolation and may be detected only incidentally on cross-sectional imaging.

Clinical Symptoms

In general, most patients with this condition are asymptomatic. In the setting of a tight vascular ring formed by the left-sided ductus arteriosus, some patients may experience symptoms of tracheoesophageal compression. This is seen more commonly in infants and young adults, with only rare patients presenting in adulthood due to vessel atherosclerosis (most commonly of the carotid arteries) and/or aneurysmal dilation of Kommerell diverticulum [30]. Some of the more severe symptoms in pediatric patients may include poor feeding tolerance, recurrent aspiration, and failure to thrive.

Imaging

Diagnosis of this condition is best accomplished with cross-sectional imaging via MDCT or MRI. On CXR, a right-sided aortic knob and para-aortic stripe with widening of the right superior mediastinum provides evidence for right aortic arch. When present, an aortic diverticulum (Kommerell diverticulum) may present as a soft-tissue density to the left of the spine and may be mistaken for other mediastinal lesions such as tumors [23]. Occasionally on lateral CXR an area of increased opacity in the retrotracheal space may be present due to the aberrant left subclavian artery [22].

As the last of the major arch vessels to emerge from the aortic arch, the aberrant left subclavian artery is seen originating at the juncture of the aortic arch and descending aorta, possibly from a Kommerell diverticulum. After emerging from the aorta, the vessel courses obliquely upward behind the trachea and esophagus, often visibly indenting the esophagus, before assuming its normal trajectory to supply blood to the left upper extremity (Fig. 24.6). Kommerell diverticulum may contribute to esophageal compression and may make it difficult to distinguish between right aortic arch with aberrant left subclavian and double aortic arch with atresia of the left arch [31]. Importantly, double aortic arch is a more common cause of vascular ring, and any uncertainty about the diagnosis should be communicated preoperatively to the surgeon for appropriate surgical planning.

When performing imaging for this condition, it is important to remember that the ligamentum arteriosum may be poorly visible or not at all visible on cross-sectional imaging [32]. Indentation of the left lateral trachea and/or esophagus in the setting of right aortic arch with aberrant left subclavian artery may suggest the presence of a constrictive ligamentum arteriosum; however, it is frequently difficult to identify this structure with any certainty prior to direct visualization in the operating room.

Treatment

Patients with symptoms of tracheoesophageal compression due to vascular ring are candidates for surgical transection of the ligamentum arteriosum. The Kommerell diverticulum is tacked posteriorly to the prevertebral fascia to prevent impingement on the esophagus. If the diverticulum appears enlarged or frankly aneurysmal, it can be resected. This is generally accomplished through a limited left-sided thoracotomy or minimally invasive approach.

Asymptomatic patients with an aneurysmal Kommerell diverticulum are candidates for surgical resection of the diverticulum with reimplantation of the aberrant left subclavian artery to the aorta as the risk of rupture is relatively high. One study of 32 patients reported a rupture rate of 53 % among those with right aortic arch and aberrant left subclavian artery; however, identification of asymptomatic patients with this condition remains challenging and the true denominator is unknown [33]. However, if identified, surgical resection of the aneurysm is recommended when the maximum diameter reaches 3–5 cm in diameter [33, 34]. All symptomatic patients are candidates for surgical resection. Surgical treatment options include both traditional open approaches and a hybrid approach including both an open component and endovascular component. Often, treatment involves left common carotid to left subclavian bypass with transcatheter occlusion of the origin of the ALSA. An associated Kommerell diverticulum may be treated via open aneurysmorrhaphy, graft interposition, or endovascular stent graft placement in candidates with favorable anatomy [30].

Postoperative imaging may demonstrate occlusion of the ALSA at its origin via an occlusion plug with reconstitution of flow via carotid-subclavian bypass. Alternatively, in patients who underwent an open repair, there may be evidence of graft interposition at the site of the resected Kommerell diverticulum with reimplantation of the ALSA directly to the aortic arch or proximal left common carotid artery [30].

Right Aortic Arch with Isolated Left Subclavian Artery (Type III)

Pathology and Embryology

Isolation of a subclavian artery is a rare malformation, with reports in the literature generally being limited to case studies. This condition results from disruption of the Edwards hypothetical double arch both proximal and distal to the origin of the affected artery, with the isolated artery originating from the ipsilateral pulmonary artery via the ductus arteriosus (Fig. 24.7). Depending on the patency of the ipsilateral ductus arteriosus as well as pulmonary arterial pressure, the affected subclavian artery may perfuse via several different mechanisms.

Associations

Isolation of left subclavian artery is a rare defect and occurs much more commonly with right aortic arch than left. Given that the isolated artery is generally opposite the side of the aortic arch, the lesion is typically found on the left side. In over half of cases, it is associated with intracardiac defects, the most common of which is tetralogy of Fallot [35, 36]. There is also a high incidence of bilateral ductus arteriosus, which may have implications for any surgical correction requiring placement of a modified Blalock-Taussig shunt.

Genetically, this condition is associated with a 22q11 monoallelic microdeletion (DiGeorge syndrome, velocardiofacial syndrome, Catch 22), and the diagnosis of isolated subclavian artery with associated intracardiac defects should prompt a genetic study for 22q11 monoallelic microdeletion [37].

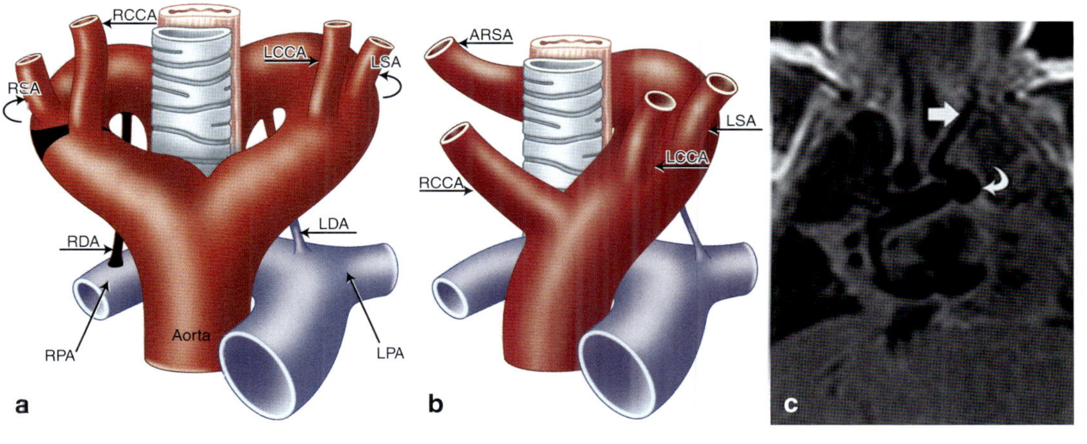

Fig. 24.7 (**a**, **b**) Schematic of right aortic arch (*RAA*) with isolated left subclavian artery (*ILSA*). (**a**) The areas in *black* represent the break points in the Edwards hypothetical double arch model. (**b**) Schematic of the evolved *RAA* with isolation of the left subclavian artery (*LSA*). Note the origin of the *ILSA* from the left pulmonary artery (*LPA*). (**c**) 1-month-old ex-28-week premature boy with double-outlet right ventricle, side-by-side great arteries (aorta to the right), subaortic ventricular septal defect, and *ILSA*. Coronal black-blood image shows the ILSA (*straight arrow*) arising anomalously from the LPA (*curved arrow*). *LCCA* left common carotid artery, *RCCA* right common carotid artery, *RSA* right subclavian artery, *LDA* left ductus arteriosus, *RDA* right ductus arteriosus, *RPA* right pulmonary artery

Clinical Symptoms

Patients with isolation of the subclavian artery may present with a range of symptoms depending on the nature of the connection of the isolated artery to the circulatory system. The great majority of patients with isolated subclavian artery are asymptomatic. In certain circumstances where the artery is completely isolated, it must fill via retrograde flow from the vertebrobasilar system. This can result in a so-called "subclavian steal" syndrome, in which cerebral symptoms occur due to significant shunting of blood away from the brain to supply the subclavian artery. This condition is rare in children since this vascular arrangement is relatively well tolerated in the young. It is more commonly symptomatic in the adult population when it occurs as an acquired condition.

The isolated subclavian artery may also originate from a branch pulmonary artery. When pulmonary vascular resistance is low, blood is shunted away from the subclavian artery into the pulmonary circulation resulting in a "pulmonary steal syndrome." Over time this may result in heart failure due to volume overload from left-to-right shunting. If, due to other associated cardiac malformations, pulmonary vascular resistance remains suprasystemic, the isolated subclavian artery fills via perfusion from the ipsilateral pulmonary artery. Oxygen saturation in the affected limb decreases proportionately with the degree of deoxygenated pulmonary blood "stolen" from the pulmonary circulation, and the patient may have difficulty maintaining oxygen saturation due to decreased pulmonary circulation [38].

Imaging

In general the diagnosis of isolated subclavian artery is accomplished through cross-sectional imaging [39]. Due to the rarity of this condition, it may not be suspected prior to imaging, which is often performed for coexisting congenital heart disease. Imaging will demonstrate a right-sided aortic arch giving rise to the left and right common carotid arteries, followed by the right subclavian artery with the left subclavian artery arising from the proximal pulmonary artery via a ligamentum arteriosus (Fig. 24.7). 3D volume-rendered images may also demonstrate complete isolation of the artery, in which case phase-contrast MRI imaging may be able to demonstrate the direction of blood flow in the isolated vessel [40].

Treatment

Asymptomatic isolated subclavian artery with significant supply from other systemic arteries (e.g., from the vertebrobasilar system without symptoms of "subclavian steal") does not require intervention. For symptomatic patients, or in the case of an origin form the pulmonary artery, treatment for this condition generally involves proximal transcatheter or surgical occlusion of the subclavian artery and reimplantation or bypass grafting (e.g., carotid-subclavian artery) of the isolated artery. Postoperative imaging will demonstrate the reimplanted artery emerging from either the aortic arch or the ipsilateral common carotid artery with preserved flow dynamics.

Circumflex Retroesophageal Aorta

Another uncommon variant of right aortic arch is circumflex retroesophageal aorta. In this condition the aorta may compress the trachea and/or esophagus as the aorta crosses the midline posterior to the esophagus before descending on the contralateral side (left) (Fig. 24.8). This results in the ascending and descending aorta on opposite sides of the thoracic vertebrae, which, in the setting of a left ligamentum arteriosum, may form a complete vascular ring [41]. Treatment of this condition consists of interruption of the vascular ring through surgical division of the ligamentum arteriosum or, in rare cases, total arch replacement.

Double Aortic Arch

Pathology and Embryology

Double aortic arch results from the abnormal persistence of the right and left segments of the Edwards hypothetical double arch (Fig. 24.9a). It is an uncommon vascular anomaly occurring in an estimated 0.05–0.3 % of the population; however, it remains the most frequent cause of symptomatic vascular ring, occurring in 40–50 % of cases [42, 43]. In this condition the ascending aorta arises anterior to the trachea and rapidly bifurcates to form both a left and right arch, both of which

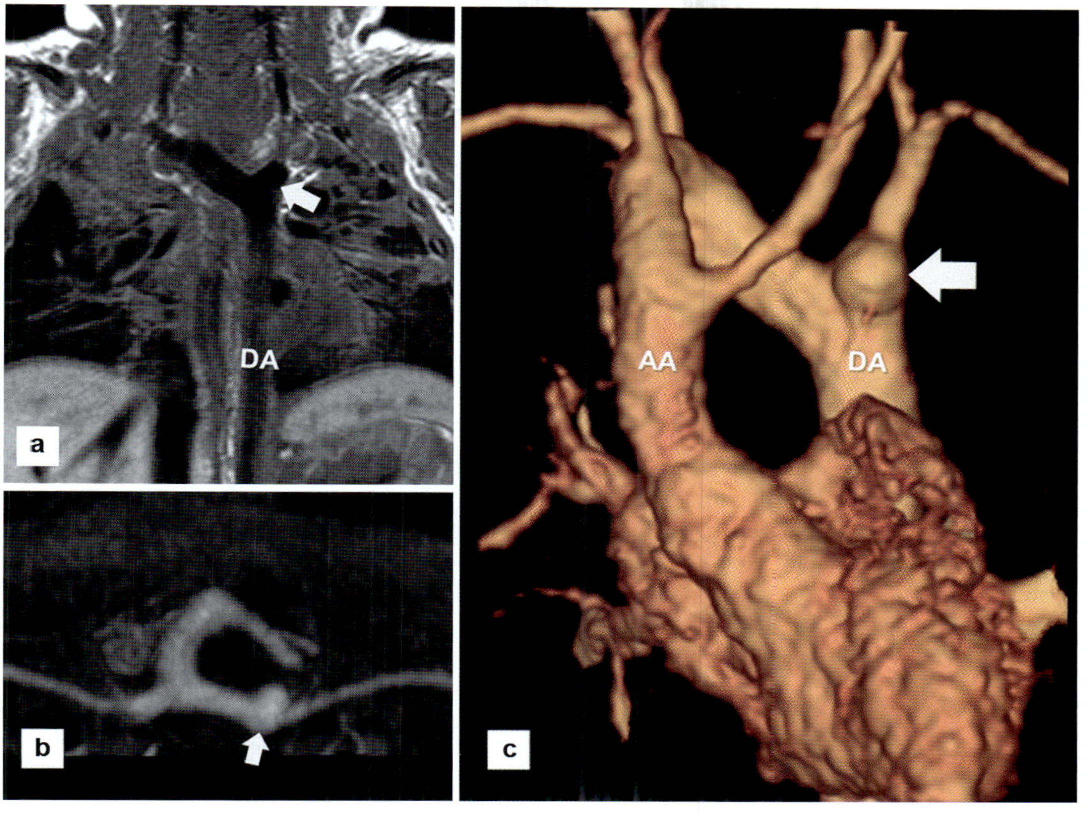

Fig. 24.8 1-year-old boy with right aortic arch and respiratory distress shows anomalous origin of the left subclavian artery (*arrows*). (**a**) Coronal black-blood MR image shows retroesophageal course of the posterior aortic arch and a large diverticulum of Kommerell (*arrow*). (**b**) Axial subvolume maximum intensity projection MR angiography demonstrates a right aortic arch, transverse retroesophageal segment, and left descending thoracic aorta. (**c**) 3D volume-rendered MRA image confirms the diagnosis of a circumflex aortic arch, with the ascending aorta (*AA*) on the right and the descending thoracic aorta (*DA*) on the left. The left subclavian artery has an anomalous origin, arising from the diverticulum of Kommerell (*arrow*). Findings are compatible with a vascular ring

course laterally and superior to the two main bronchi before rejoining posterior to the esophagus to form a single descending aorta. The two arches thus form a complete vascular ring encircling the trachea and esophagus, although the caliber of both arches may vary such that they may be equal in size or one may be hypoplastic [44]. In approximately 75 % of cases, the right arch is larger and more cephalad than the left, which, in a minority of cases, may be completely atretic (forming a fibrous band). This condition, known as incomplete double aortic arch, may be subclassified based on the position and degree of involution of the arch segment, with the most severe cases resembling complete right aortic arch with mirror image branching.

In general, the major arch vessels each arise independently from the ipsilateral arch such that the common carotid arteries originate anterior to the subclavian arteries. The ductus arteriosus, when present, is generally left sided and may contribute to the formation of a complete vascular ring.

Clinical Symptoms

Many patients with double aortic arch begin to display symptoms within the first 3 months of life due to significant tracheoesophageal compression; however, those patients with a relatively loose vascular ring may remain clinically asymptomatic for life. Patients may occasionally develop

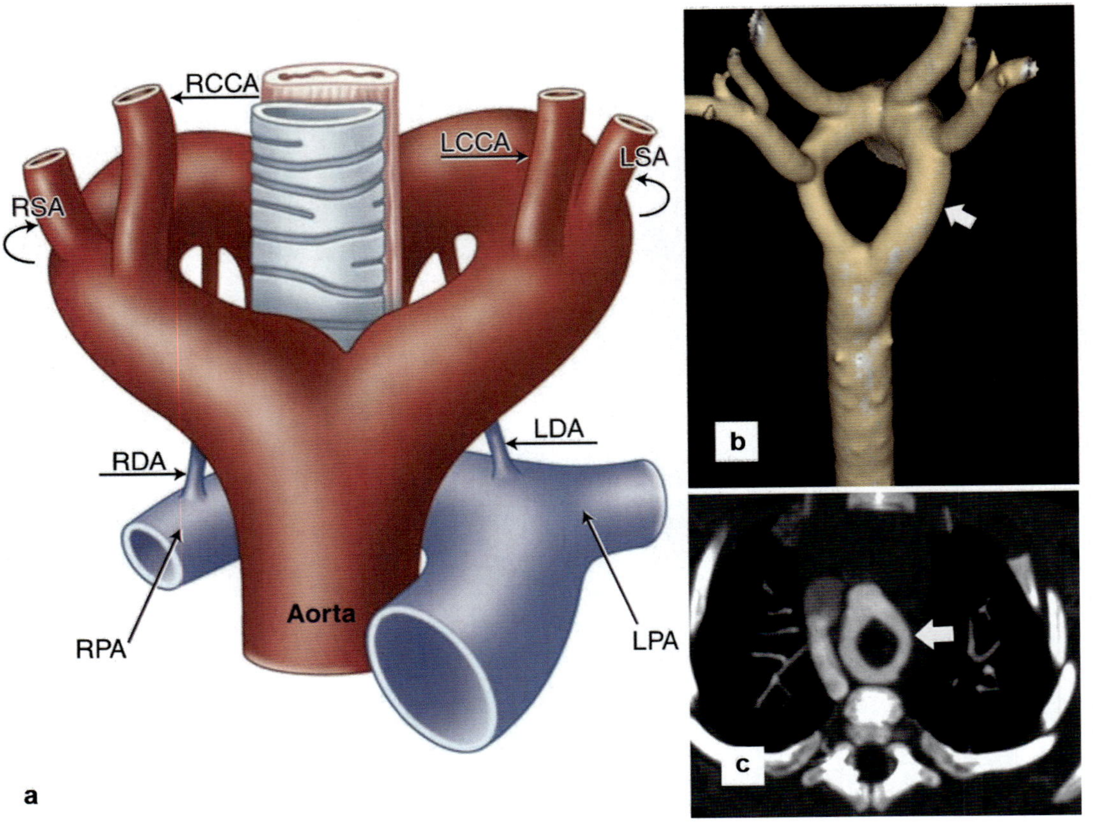

Fig. 24.9 (**a**) Schematic demonstration of the embryology of double aortic arch via the Edwards hypothetical double arch model. Note the absence of a break point in the primitive double arch, thus resulting in the persistence of both left- and right-sided aortae. (**b**) 3D volume-rendered CT angiography and (**c**) axial CT images in an 11-week-old boy with stridor show double aortic arch (*arrows*) with bilateral arches of nearly equal size. The trachea is located in the vascular ring and narrowed. *LCCA* left common carotid artery, *LSA* left subclavian artery, *RCCA* right common carotid artery, *RSA* right subclavian artery, *LDA* left ductus arteriosus, *RDA* right ductus arteriosus, *LPA* left pulmonary artery, *RPA* right pulmonary artery

symptoms in adulthood due to aortic noncompliance or dilation of an existing diverticulum; however, the frequency of this occurrence remains unknown. Typical symptoms in infancy usually include respiratory distress, stridor, and/or chronic lower respiratory tract infections. Older children may also present with dysphagia as their diet transitions to solid food. Delay in diagnosis of a symptomatic vascular ring is common as signs and symptoms can mimic other more common diagnoses, such as asthma, reflux with aspiration, or upper respiratory tract infection. Those patients who present later in life often report subtle symptoms of dysphagia and give a history of respiratory symptoms when closely questioned [22, 25].

Associations

Double aortic arch generally occurs in isolation of cardiac anomalies; however, occasional cases have been reported in association with congenital heart disease such as VSD, tetralogy of Fallot, and truncus arteriosus, among others. Approximately 20 % of cases of double aortic arch are, however, associated with chromosomal abnormalities [24].

Imaging

On CXR the trachea is generally midline with slight bilateral indentations visible from the dual aortic arches. Depending on the degree of tracheal compression, there may be evidence of bilateral pulmonary hyperinflation with constriction of the

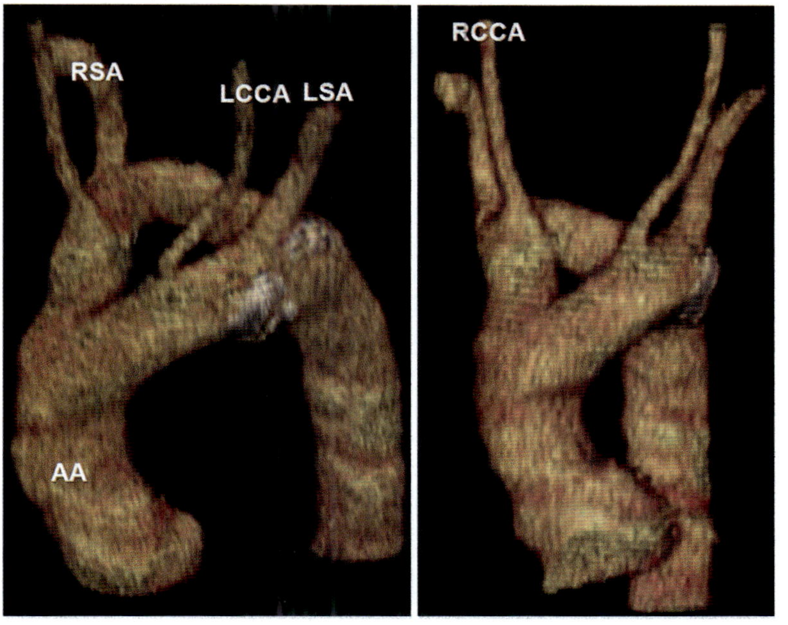

Fig. 24.10 3-dimensional volume-rendered CT angiography images in an asymptomatic 58-year-old male show double aortic arch with bilateral arches of nearly equal size. Not that part of the aortic arch is calcified. *AA* ascending aorta, *LCCA* left common carotid artery, *LSA* left subclavian artery, *RCCA* right common carotid artery, *RSA* right subclavian artery

tracheal lucency and loss of the left-sided aortic knob and para-aortic stripe. The presence of any of these findings should be followed up with cross-sectional imaging to better define the mediastinal vascular anatomy.

MDCT or MRI demonstrates a double aortic arch with four separate vessels emerging independently from their respective ipsilateral arches just above the expected aortic level (Figs. 24.9 and 24.10). On axial imaging the four vessels appear as the points of a square or trapezoid, a finding known as the "four-vessel sign." MDCT or MRI images also allow visualization of the tracheobronchial tree and estimation of the degree of tracheal compression caused by the dual arch segments. Cine-sequence MRI may demonstrate the pulsatile nature of the tracheal compression, and phase-contrast imaging provides information regarding blood flow through both arch segments. This information may also prove useful in preoperative planning as the surgeon may opt for a more invasive approach if there is significant blood flow through the nondominant arch segment. In the event that surgical correction is required, such information will assist in planning the operative approach as well as selecting the appropriate segment of the vascular ring for division.

Differentiation between double aortic arch with atresia of the left segment and right aortic arch with mirror image branching may be difficult as detection of the atretic segment is often challenging. In such cases there are several reported findings that may assist in distinguishing these two conditions. Radiographic findings unique to double aortic arch include symmetric appearance of the subclavian and common carotid arteries originating from the right arch as well as the atretic left side, a more posterior position of the proximal left arch when compared with a more anterior position in right aortic arch with mirror image branching, and the presence of a diverticulum on the descending aorta [45, 46].

Treatment

The treatment for symptomatic double aortic arch involves surgical division of the smaller segment (ideally through an atretric portion) to disrupt the vascular ring and relieve compression on the trachea and/or esophagus. As most cases of double aortic arch are right dominant, the left arch is frequently divided between the left subclavian artery and the descending aorta in order to preserve flow to the major arch vessels. In general, repair is accomplished through a limited left posterolateral thoracotomy, although a right thoracotomy may rarely be needed, particularly if imaging localizes the optimal point of division to the proximal right arch. Median sternotomy is generally reserved for repair of associated cardiac defects.

Cervical Aortic Arch

Pathology

Cervical aortic arch or "Gothic aortic arch" refers to the displacement of the arch from its typical mediastinal position to a level above the clavicle. In general, the condition is not considered pathologic, and most reported cases appear to have been identified incidentally. The condition is thought to result from a disturbance in the normal pattern of growth, regression, and migration in the third and/or fourth pharyngeal arches such that the arch forms abnormally high in the chest or fails to migrate to its typical mediastinal location. Persistence of the third pharyngeal arch, failure of the normal caudal migration of the fourth arch, and/or the abnormal confluence of the third and fourth arches have all been postulated as possible explanations for cervical aortic arch [47].

Associations

Cervical aortic arch is rarely associated with intracardiac malformations such as tetralogy of Fallot, pulmonary atresia with VSD, double-outlet right ventricle, VSD, and a patent ductus arteriosus (PDA) [47–51]. Coarctation of the aorta has also been observed in this condition. Occasionally 22q11 microdeletion has been observed in patients with this condition [52].

Clinical Presentation

In general cervical aortic arch is asymptomatic and identified only incidentally; however a minority of patients may present with symptoms of dysphagia, wheezing, coughing, stridor, or recurrent pneumonia secondary to tracheoesophageal compression [47]. Occasionally, a pulsatile mass may be felt in the left or right neck, corresponding to the position of the cervical arch.

Imaging

Cervical aortic arch may be suggested by the absence of an aortic knob at the typical site, descending aorta on the wrong side, posterior indentation of the trachea, and a large posterior indentation on the mid-third of the back of the esophagus (Fig. 24.11). Definitive diagnosis may be obtained via MDCT or MRI imaging, which will clearly demonstrate the aortic arch ascending above the level of the clavicle. Variations include separate origins of the carotid arteries contralateral to the side of the arch, anomalous origin of the contralateral subclavian artery from the aortic isthmus via a diverticulum, separate internal and external carotid arteries, variations in the position of the ductus/ligamentum arteriosum attachments, the presence of an aortic diverticulum (often at the site of the origin of the contralateral subclavian artery), and a variable relationship between the descending aorta and spine [47].

Treatment

Most patients with an incidentally diagnosed cervical aortic arch require no treatment; however, late in life a small minority of patients may develop aneurysms. These may present as an increasing pulsatile neck mass or symptoms of tracheoesophageal compression [53]. Given the inherent fragility of the aneurysmal tissue, open or endovascular repair is recommended. Repair is most often accomplished via total open arch replacement, rarely, in patients who are poor operative candidates, a two-staged endovascular repair with graft placement, and subsequent axillary-axillary bypass [53]. However, the brachiocephalic vessels and the acute angle of the arch may preclude safe endovascular repair.

As there is significant variability to the branching pattern of major arch vessels, corrective surgery varies considerably for this condition [54]. Depending on the symptomatic vascular anomaly, several different treatment options may be employed on a case-by-case basis. In instances where repair is necessary, treatment generally focuses on correcting major arch vessel anomalies as opposed to altering the arch itself.

Coarctation of the Aorta

Pathology and Embryology

Coarctation of the aorta is defined as a discrete obstructive narrowing in the proximal descending

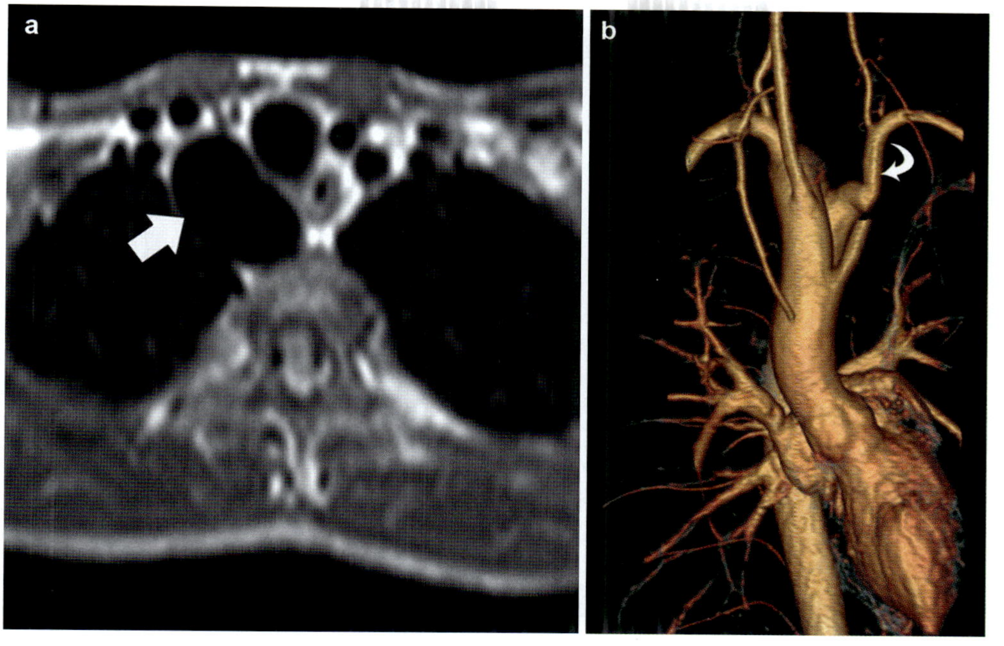

Fig. 24.11 24-year-old asymptomatic man with incidentally detected right cervical aortic arch. (**a**) Axial black-blood MR image shows that the aortic arch (*arrow*) is located near the level of the thoracic inlet, just to the right of the trachea. (**b**) 3D volume-rendered MR angiography image confirms the diagnosis of a right cervical aortic arch. The left subclavian artery (*curved arrow*) is anomalous, arising from a diverticulum of Kommerell. Findings are compatible with a vascular ring

aorta involving or adjacent to the aortic isthmus (between the left subclavian artery and ligamentum arteriosum) (Figs. 24.12 and 24.13). Coarctation can occur in a more tubular fashion in the mid-aortic arch. The condition accounts for approximately one in 3,000–4,000 live births and 5–7 % of all live births with congenital heart disease [55–58]. A slightly higher incidence has been noted in males [59, 60]. Although the cause of aortic coarctation remains unknown, there is considerable evidence that both genetics and alterations in fetal hemodynamics play a role in the development of this condition [61–63]. An abnormal persistence of fetal ductal tissue at the aortic isthmus and decreased fetal antegrade flow through the proximal aorta have both been proposed as possible mechanisms of coarctation. The majority of cases of aortic coarctation are sporadic; however, several studies have identified clear genetic associations between aortic coarctation and other types of congenital heart disease [63–65].

Associations

Aortic coarctation is associated with additional congenital cardiovascular anomalies in 44–84 % of cases, with up to 75 % of patients with aortic coarctation also having a bicuspid aortic valve [60, 66–68] (Fig. 24.13). Conversely, among patients with bicuspid aortic valve, the incidence of aortic coarctation is approximately 25 % [67]. Additional malformations associated with aortic coarctation include PDA, atrial septal defect, VSD, left-sided obstructive lesions, and transposition of the great arteries.

Aortic coarctation is also commonly associated with several genetic syndromes. Several studies have placed the incidence of aortic coarctation at 15–17 % of Turner's syndrome (45XO) patients [69, 70]. Additional genetic syndromes associated with aortic coarctation include Shone complex, PHACE syndrome, Williams syndrome, Noonan syndrome, trisomy 13, and trisomy 18.

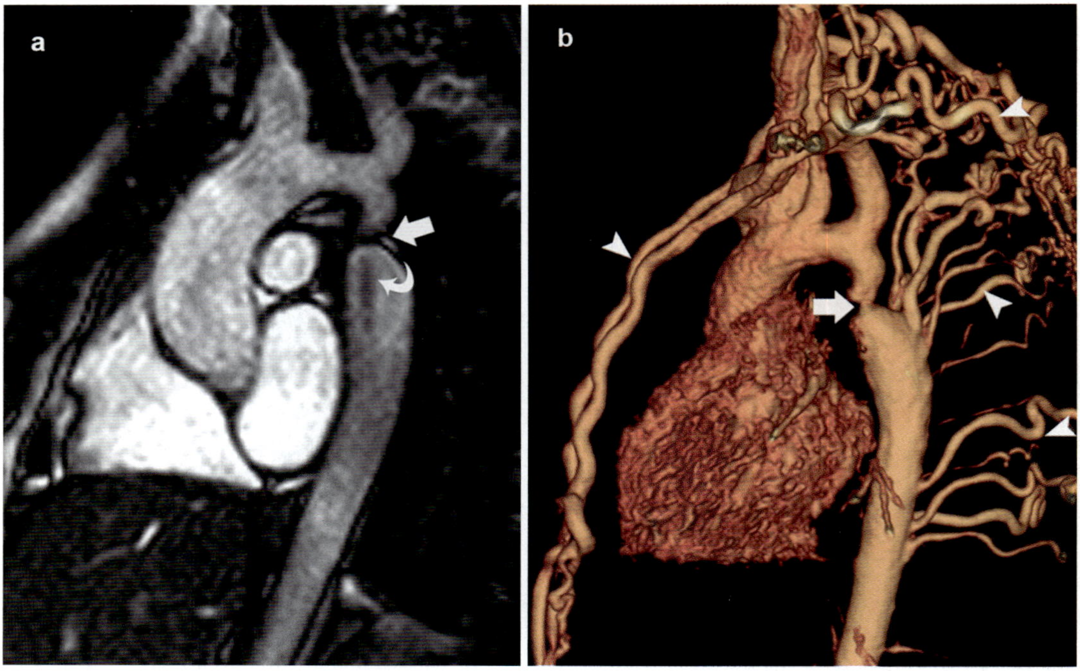

Fig. 24.12 12-year-old boy presented to ED with abdominal pain. Hypertension noted on exam. Renal ultrasound demonstrated evidence of renovascular hypertension with abnormal suprarenal abdominal aortic spectral Doppler waveforms. (**a**) Sagittal-oblique bright-blood (balanced steady-state free precession) MR image shows severe focal narrowing (*arrow*) of the thoracic aorta in the region of the ligamentum arteriosum. A low signal dephasing jet (*curved arrow*) is present within the aorta just distal to the site of coarctation. The ascending aorta is mildly dilated. (**b**) 3D volume-rendered MR angiography image confirms the presence of severe juxtaductal aortic coarctation. Large paraspinal, intercostal, and internal mammary artery collateral vessels (*arrow heads*) are present indicating hemodynamically significant stenosis

Clinical Presentation

Aortic coarctation most frequently presents in infancy shortly after birth; however, milder cases may not be diagnosed until adolescence or later in life. The time of presentation depends on the severity of the stenosis as well as the presence or absence of sufficient collateral circulation. Infants with severe aortic coarctation may be dependent on a PDA to maintain systemic perfusion, and closure of the ductus shortly after birth may precipitate severe left ventricular pressure overload and failure. In untreated aortic coarctation, lower body systemic perfusion will be decreased, resulting in diminished peripheral pulses in the lower body as well as activation of the renin-angiotensin-aldosterone system and upper body hypertension. Severe cases of infantile aortic coarctation may present with kidney failure and metabolic acidosis due to splanchnic organ hypoperfusion if not recognized and treated appropriately.

Common collateral pathways include intercostal, internal thoracic (mammary), cervical, scapular, and thoracodorsal arteries (Fig. 24.12). Rarely such collaterals are unable to provide sufficient flow during periods of exertion, and patients may experience symptoms of lower extremity claudication relieved by rest resulting in varying degrees of lower limb hypoplasia due to chronic hypoperfusion.

Imaging

Findings on CXR may be nonspecific, especially in very young patients who have not developed associated compensatory changes such as cardiomegaly or enlarged collateral vessels. Individuals presenting later in life will

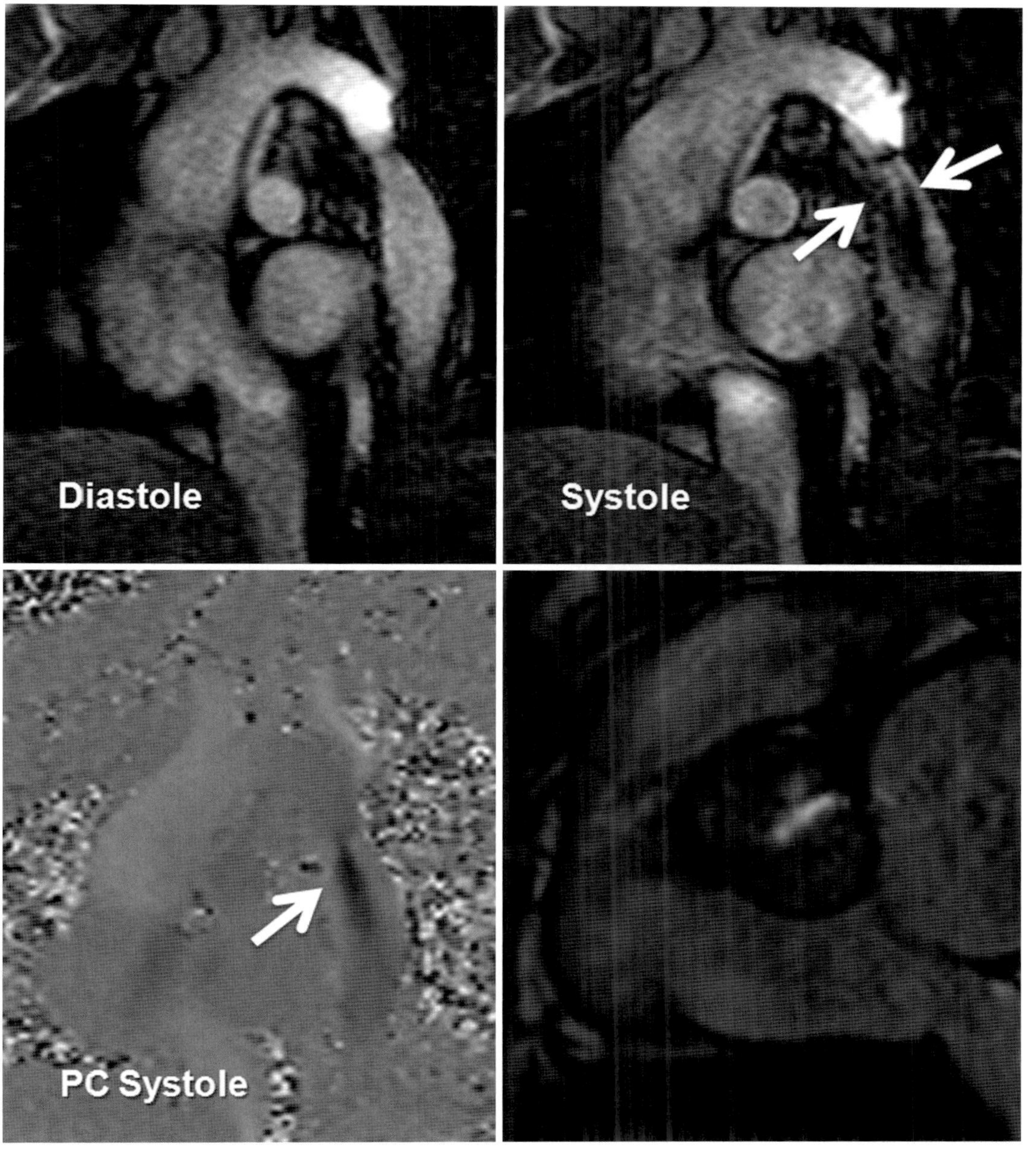

Fig. 24.13 Coarctation of aorta shown by MRI. *Upper row* images are diastolic and systolic frames of cine MR. Signal void from high-velocity flow is seen in systole distal to stenosis. The stenosis size was 1.1 × 0.8 cm at the narrowest point. In plane phase contrast (*PC*) also shows jet of flow with a maximum velocity measured at 200 cm/s with through plane *PC*. A bicuspid aortic valve is seen with evidence of moderate-to-severe stenosis. The peak aortic valve area was 0.9 cm^2 by planimetry. Note dilated ascending aorta (Courtesy of Farhood Saremi MD, USC)

frequently demonstrate a prominent aortic arch with distal indentation (the "3 sign"), inferior rib sclerosis or "notching," and cardiomegaly [71]. In neonates aortic coarctation is most frequently detected via transthoracic echocardiogram, which has a sensitivity of 94–98 % [72]. Older children and adolescents are better suited by evaluation via MRA to more define both anatomical and functional changes in thoracic vasculature (Fig. 24.12). A combination of "black-blood" inversion recovery fast spin echo and balanced steady-state free precession still images in axial and sagittal-oblique planes usually demonstrates the anatomical narrowing. Cine images are very useful to show the jet of blood flow through the stenosis and allow subsequent planning for phase-contrast analysis (Fig. 24.13). Phase-contrast MR may serve as an appropriate complementary study due its ability to measure the pressure gradient across the area of stenosis and quantify the collateral flow. It is important that the phase-contrast image plane is correctly aligned perpendicular to a perceived dephasing "jet" distal to the stenosis so that the maximum velocity and an estimated gradient (using the modified Bernoulli equation) can be accurately determined (Fig. 24.13). A systolic pressure gradient of 20 mmHg or more is an important benchmark for hemodynamically significant aortic stenosis. Presence of collateral flow also indicates hemodynamically significant stenosis. Collateral flow can be directly shown by MRA. Alternatively, a second phase-contrast study in the distal aorta (above the diaphragm) can assess flow recruitment from collateral vessels draining into the descending aorta. The percentage of flow increase in the distal compared with proximal descending aorta helps determine the severity of the stenosis and is proportional to the collateral flow. MRI can predict the need for surgical or transcatheter intervention in patients with coarctation of aorta. Indexed minimum aortic cross-sectional area is shown the strongest predictor of subsequent intervention [73]. It is important to know that flow measurements just distal to stenosis are limited by flow turbulence, aliasing, and stent-related artifacts, and it can be difficult to measure the exact stenosis in severe cases. MRI also allows the evaluation of left ventricular size, function and mass in order to assess the impact of the increased afterload on the heart. Recently three-directional velocity-sensitive, phase-contrast magnetic resonance imaging (four-dimensional phase-contrast MRI) has been use to assess the hemodynamic alterations in coarctation of aorta. It is shown in coarctation patients that aortic wall shear stress is increased and because of systemic nature of the disease alterations in aortic hemodynamics can be found in the entire aorta causing aneurysm formation in the ascending aorta [74]. Four-dimensional flow is also a quick way of evaluating collateral blood flow to establish hemodynamic significance [75].

CT has a special place in diagnosis of the aortic coarctation. Higher spatial resolution and large area of anatomic coverage can accurately show the stenotic segment and the extent of collateral vessels (Fig. 24.14).

Treatment

Diagnosis of a significant aortic coarctation is indication for operation. Historically, severe disease is associated with a high mortality rate in neonates and infants (50 % mortality) [76]. Ideally, repair is accomplished as early as possible after diagnosis, as later treatment is associated with long-term sequelae, such as persistent hypertension [68, 77]. Treatment focuses on relieving the area of stenosis and improving flow dynamics. Currently, optimal management in children consists of open surgical resection of the diseased aortic segment with direct primary anastomosis. Other treatment options, such as subclavian flap angioplasty, synthetic patch repair, or graft interposition, may be considered in select cases as needed. These techniques have led to long-term survival, but late complications are not unusual so these patients require monitoring with imaging. Subclavian flap repair involves dividing the subclavian artery a short distance from its origin and using the proximal-most artery to reconstruct the aorta at the site of coarctation. This provides acceptable long-term outcomes but can affect ipsilateral limb development . Patients undergoing synthetic patch repair have a greater tendency to develop aneurysms than other repair types. Recent advances in endovascular therapy have allowed older patients to be treated effectively with balloon angioplasty and/or stent placement. However, younger children treated with angioplasty alone have a high recurrence rate, and stenting results

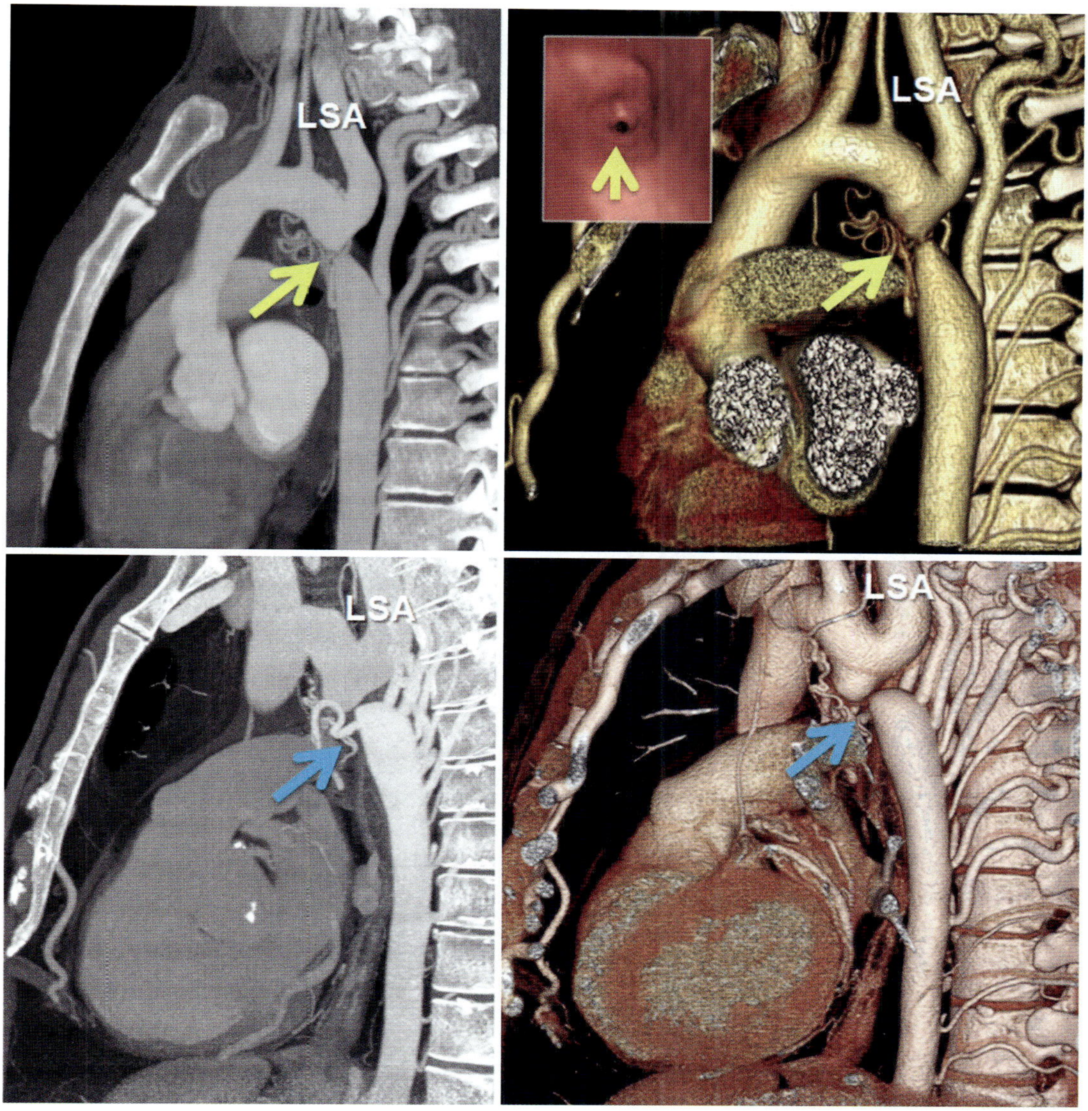

Fig. 24.14 Sagittal two- and three-dimensional volume-rendered CT images in a patient with coarctation of the aorta (*upper row*) and a type A interrupted aortic arch (*lower row*) are presented. Complete luminal discontinuity (*blue arrows*) between the aortic arch and the descending aorta is shown in interrupted aortic arch. The aortic lumen (*yellow arrows*) is not interrupted in coarctation of aorta. Mild poststenotic dilatation, normal caliber of the ascending aorta, and extensive collateral arteries are shown in both cases making differentiation difficult. The left subclavian artery (*LSA*) appears larger in interrupted aortic arch (Courtesy of Farhood Saremi MD, USC)

in the need for multiple reinterventions for redilation of the stent [76, 78]. A recent Cochrane review determined that there is insufficient evidence to determine the best treatment (open vs. endovascular) for coarctation of the thoracic aorta [78–80].

Differential Diagnosis

Pseudocoarctation

(kinking, buckling) of the aorta is an uncommon congenital malformation of the aortic arch characterized by elongation of the aortic arch and acute anterior angulation of the aortic arch at the

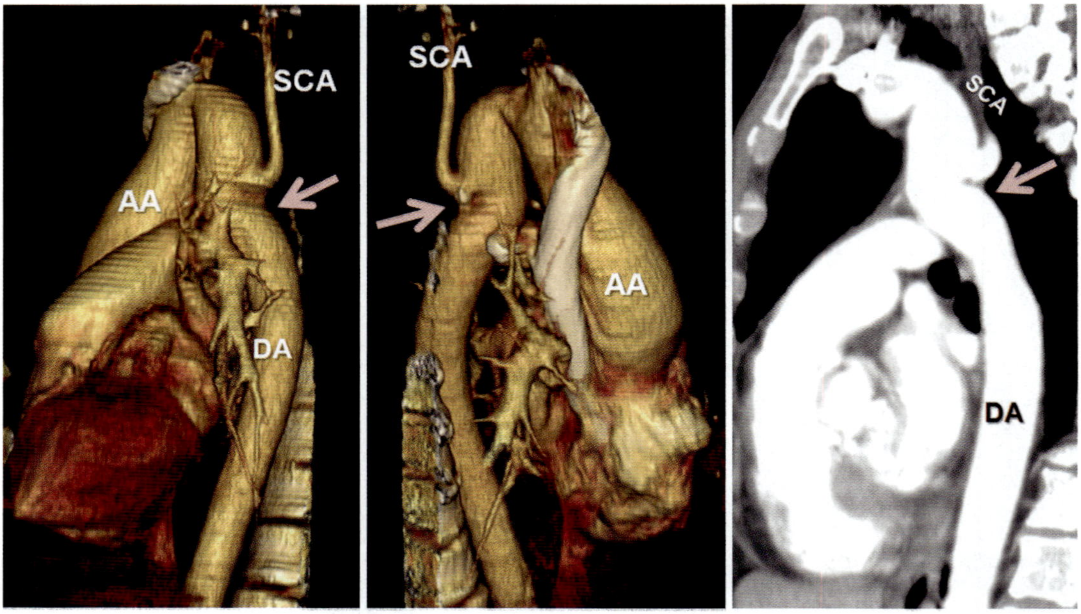

Fig. 24.15 50-year-old female with pseudocoarctation of the aorta. Less than 50 % stenosis is shown at the isthmus (*arrows*). The aortic arch appears elongated and elevates to the thoracic inlet. The left subclavian artery (*SCA*) originates proximal to the stenosis. The ascending aorta (*AA*) appears dilated. A bicuspid aortic valve was seen. *DA* descending aorta (Courtesy of Farhood Saremi, MD, USC)

level of the ligamentum arteriosum with little or no obstruction and absence of increased collateral circulation. Reduction of the isthmic segment cross-sectional diameter may exist, but it is usually less the 50 % of that of the transverse arch. In most cases, pseudocoarctation is an isolated anomaly. Associated abnormalities such as aortic aneurysm, bicuspid aortic valve, and intracardiac shunts are described [81] (Fig. 24.15).

Interrupted Aortic Arch

(IAA) is defined as complete luminal and anatomic discontinuity between the ascending and descending aorta [82]. Three types are described depending on location of the arch interruption and mostly are symptomatic early in infancy. In simple form of IAA, which is more common, bicuspid aortic valve, ventricular septal defect, and persistent ductus arteriosus are common. In complex form, which is less common, other cardiovascular anomalies exist including truncus arteriosus, transposition of the great arteries, double-outlet right ventricle, aortopulmonary window, and functional single ventricle [83].

Simple isolated type A IAA may rarely be discovered late in adulthood (Fig. 24.14). Type A aortic interruption and aortic coarctation or focal atresia have similar anatomic location, at isthmus just distal to the left subclavian artery. In the three situations, hemodynamic effects and clinical manifestations of the aortic arch obstructions are almost identical. The hallmark feature of IAA that is useful to differentiate it from aortic coarctation is the "complete absence" of continuity between both parts of the interrupted segment. In atresia of the isthmus, the lumen is interrupted, but anatomically the aortic wall exists and a fibrous strand extends between the ascending and descending aorta. However with CT or MR it would be difficult to trace the intact aortic wall in a case of atresia. The fact that luminal patency may be lost in severe coarctation of the aorta makes the differential diagnosis more difficult, and the imaging findings are almost identical to those in isolated type A IAA. In IAA, the arch is typically of smaller in caliber than normal, and the branches have a straighter course. Pronounced poststenotic aortic dilatation is more seen in coarctation of the aorta. These distinguishing features may alter or disappear over time especially after development of massive collateral vessels bypassing the interrupted segment (Fig. 24.14). Because of such diagnostic dilemmas, surgical findings may be necessary for the final diagnosis.

Conclusion

Aortic arch anomalies represent a diverse set of malformations with a wide range of clinical symptoms. Successful imaging of arch anomalies relies heavily on the use of cross-sectional imaging such as MRI and/or MDCT in order to delineate the full extent of the vascular anatomy and surrounding mediastinal structures. The most appropriate imaging technique must be decided on a case-by-case basis with particular attention paid to the limitations of each imaging modality. Interpreting the imaging appearance of aortic arch anomalies is best accomplished in the context of an appropriate understanding of the embryological development. Accurate interpretation is particularly important for operative planning when corrective surgery is mandated by symptoms or pathological anatomy.

References

1. Hoffman JI, Kaplan S. The incidence of congenital heart disease. J Am Coll Cardiol. 2002;39(12):1890–900.
2. Raider L, Landry BA, Brogdon BG. The retrotracheal triangle. Radiographics. 1990;10(6):1055–79.
3. Silva F, Godinho C, Carrico A. Prenatal diagnosis of right aortic arch by fetal echocardiography. Rev Port Cardiol. 2011;30(10):803.
4. Hsu KC, Tsung-Che Hsieh C, Chen M, Tsai HD. Right aortic arch with aberrant left subclavian artery–prenatal diagnosis and evaluation of postnatal outcomes report of three cases. Taiwan J Obstet Gynecol. 2011;50(3):353–8.
5. Natsis KI, Tsitouridis IA, Didagelos MV, Fillipidis AA, Vlasis KG, Tsikaras PD. Anatomical variations in the branches of the human aortic arch in 633 angiographies: clinical significance and literature review. Surg Radiol Anat. 2009;31(5):319–23.
6. Jakanani GC, Adair W. Frequency of variations in aortic arch anatomy depicted on multidetector CT. Clin Radiol. 2010;65(6):481–7.
7. Berko NS, Jain VR, Godelman A, Stein EG, Ghosh S, Haramati LB. Variants and anomalies of thoracic vasculature on computed tomographic angiography in adults. J Comput Assist Tomogr. 2009;33(4):523–8.
8. Layton KF, Kallmes DF, Cloft HJ, Lindell EP, Cox VS. Bovine aortic arch variant in humans: clarification of a common misnomer. AJNR Am J Neuroradiol. 2006;27(7):1541–2.
9. Lacout A, Khalil A, Figl A, Liloku R, Marcy PY. Vertebral arteria lusoria: a life-threatening condition for oesophageal surgery. Surg Radiol Anat. 2012;34(4):381–3.
10. Nelson ML, Sparks CD. Unusual aortic arch variation: distal origin of common carotid arteries. Clin Anat. 2001;14(1):62–5.
11. Fawcett SL, Gomez AC, Hughes JA, Set P. Anatomical variation in the position of the brachiocephalic trunk (innominate artery) with respect to the trachea: a computed tomography-based study and literature review of Innominate Artery Compression Syndrome. Clin Anat. 2010;23(1):61–9.
12. Freed K, Low VH. The aberrant subclavian artery. AJR Am J Roentgenol. 1997;168(2):481–4.
13. Branscom JJ, Austin JH. Aberrant right subclavian artery. Findings seen on plain chest roentgenograms. Am J Roentgenol Radium Ther Nucl Med. 1973;119(3):539–42.
14. Kastler B. MRI of cardiovascular malformations. 1st ed. Berlin/Heidelberg: Springer; 2011.
15. Ramaswamy P, Lytrivi ID, Thanjan MT, et al. Frequency of aberrant subclavian artery, arch laterality, and associated intracardiac anomalies detected by echocardiography. Am J Cardiol. 2008;101(5):677–82.
16. Zapata H, Edwards JE, Titus JL. Aberrant right subclavian artery with left aortic arch: associated cardiac anomalies. Pediatr Cardiol. 1993;14(3):159–61.
17. Nakajima Y, Nishibatake M, Ikeda K, Momma K, Takao A, Terai M. Abnormal development of fourth aortic arch derivatives in the pathogenesis of tetralogy of Fallot. Pediatr Cardiol. 1990;11(2):69–71.
18. Bayford D. An account of a singular case of obstructed deglutination. Memoirs Med Soc Lond. 1794;2:11.
19. Proto AV, Cuthbert NW, Raider L. Aberrant right subclavian artery: further observations. AJR Am J Roentgenol. 1987;148(2):253–7.
20. Daniels L, Coveliers HM, Hoksbergen AW, Nederhoed JH, Wisselink W. Hybrid treatment of aberrant right subclavian artery and its aneurysms. Acta Chir Belg. 2010;110(3):346–9.
21. Shennib H, Diethrich EB. Novel approaches for the treatment of the aberrant right subclavian artery and its aneurysms. J Vasc Surg. 2008;47(5):1066–70.
22. Stojanovska J, Cascade PN, Chong S, Quint LE, Sundaram B. Embryology and imaging review of aortic arch anomalies. J Thorac Imaging. 2012;27(2):73–84.
23. Shuford WH, Sybers RG, Edwards FK. The three types of right aortic arch. Am J Roentgenol Radium Ther Nucl Med. 1970;109(1):67–74.
24. McElhinney DB, Hoydu AK, Gaynor JW, Spray TL, Goldmuntz E, Weinberg PM. Patterns of right aortic

arch and mirror-image branching of the brachiocephalic vessels without associated anomalies. Pediatr Cardiol. 2001;22(4):285–91.
25. Kanne JP, Godwin JD. Right aortic arch and its variants. J Cardiovasc Comput Tomogr. 2010;4(5):293–300.
26. Cina CS, Arena GO, Bruin G, Clase CM. Kommerell's diverticulum and aneurysmal right-sided aortic arch: a case report and review of the literature. J Vasc Surg. 2000;32(6):1208–14.
27. Cantinotti M, Hegde S, Bell A, Razavi R. Diagnostic role of magnetic resonance imaging in identifying aortic arch anomalies. Congenit Heart Dis. 2008;3(2):117–23.
28. Higashikuni Y, Nagashima T, Ishizaka N, Kinugawa K, Hirata Y, Nagai R. Right aortic arch with mirror image branching and vascular ring. Int J Cardiol. 2008;130(1):e53–5.
29. Stewart JR, Kincaid OW, Dewards JE. An atlas of vascular rings and related malformations of the aortic arch system. Springfield: Charles C Thomas; 1964.
30. Panduranga P, Al-Delamie T, Ratnam L, Al-Mukhaini M, Zachariah S. Repair of Kommerell's diverticulum with aberrant left subclavian artery in an elderly patient with right aortic arch and dysphagia lusoria. J Card Surg. 2011;26(6):637–40.
31. Kleinman PK, Spevak MR, Nimkin K. Left-sided esophageal indentation in right aortic arch with aberrant left subclavian artery. Radiology. 1994;191(2):565–7.
32. Fries P, Schneider G, Lindinger A, Abdul-Khaliq H, Schafers HJ, Bucker A. MRI and contrast enhanced MR angiography in a patient with right aortic arch and aberrant left subclavian artery. Clin Res Cardiol. 2009;98(9):573–7.
33. Cina CS, Althani H, Pasenau J, Abouzahr L. Kommerell's diverticulum and right-sided aortic arch: a cohort study and review of the literature. J Vasc Surg. 2004;39(1):131–9.
34. Ota T, Okada K, Takanashi S, Yamamoto S, Okita Y. Surgical treatment for Kommerell's diverticulum. J Thorac Cardiovasc Surg. 2006;131(3):574–8.
35. Luetmer PH, Miller GM. Right aortic arch with isolation of the left subclavian artery: case report and review of the literature. Mayo Clin Proc. 1990;65(3):407–13.
36. Nath PH, Castaneda-Zuniga W, Zollikofer C, et al. Isolation of a subclavian artery. AJR Am J Roentgenol. 1981;137(4):683–8.
37. McElhinney DB, Clark 3rd BJ, Weinberg PM, et al. Association of chromosome 22q11 deletion with isolated anomalies of aortic arch laterality and branching. J Am Coll Cardiol. 2001;37(8):2114–9.
38. Carano N, Piazza P, Agnetti A, Squarcia U. Congenital pulmonary steal phenomenon associated with tetralogy of Fallot, right aortic arch, and isolation of the left subclavian artery. Pediatr Cardiol. 1997;18(1):57–60.
39. Sun AM, Alhabshan F, Branson H, Freedom RM, Yoo SJ. MRI diagnosis of isolated origin of the left subclavian artery from the left pulmonary artery. Pediatr Radiol. 2005;35(12):1259–62.
40. Van Grimberge F, Dymarkowski S, Budts W, Bogaert J. Role of magnetic resonance in the diagnosis of subclavian steal syndrome. J Magn Reson Imaging. 2000;12(2):339–42.
41. Philip S, Chen SY, Wu MH, Wang JK, Lue HC. Retroesophageal aortic arch: diagnostic and therapeutic implications of a rare vascular ring. Int J Cardiol. 2001;79(2–3):133–41.
42. Knight L, Edwards JE. Right aortic arch. Types and associated cardiac anomalies. Circulation. 1974;50(5):1047–51.
43. Schlesinger AE, Krishnamurthy R, Sena LM, et al. Incomplete double aortic arch with atresia of the distal left arch: distinctive imaging appearance. AJR Am J Roentgenol. 2005;184(5):1634–9.
44. Lowe GM, Donaldson JS, Backer CL. Vascular rings: 10-year review of imaging. Radiographics. 1991;11(4):637–46.
45. Newman B. MR of right aortic arch. Pediatr Radiol. 1996;26(5):367–9.
46. Dillman JR, Attili AK, Agarwal PP, Dorfman AL, Hernandez RJ, Strouse PJ. Common and uncommon vascular rings and slings: a multi-modality review. Pediatr Radiol. 2011;41(11):1440–54; quiz 1489–90.
47. Felson B, Strife JL. Cervical aortic arch: a commentary. Semin Roentgenol. 1989;24(2):114–20.
48. Haughton VM, Fellows KE, Rosenbaum AE. The cervical aortic arches. Radiology. 1975;114(3):675–81.
49. Cornali M, Reginato E, Azzolina G. Cervical aortic arch and a new type of double aortic arch. Report of a case. Br Heart J. 1976;38(9):993–6.
50. Khoury NJ, Hourani R, Birjawi GA, Hourani MH. Left-sided cervical aortic arch associated with pseudocoarctation, aneurysm formation, and anomalous left brachiocephalic vein: appearance on MDCT and MR angiography. J Thorac Imaging. 2008;23(3):206–9.
51. Moncada R, Shannon M, Miller R, White H, Friedman J, Shuford WH. The cervical aortic arch. Am J Roentgenol Radium Ther Nucl Med. 1975;125(3):591–601.
52. Nagashima M, Shikata F, Higaki T, Kawachi K. Cervical aortic arch and Kommerell's diverticulum associated with the anomalous subaortic left brachiocephalic vein in a patient with chromosome 22q11.2 deletion. Interact Cardiovasc Thorac Surg. 2010;11(2):202–3.
53. Takahashi Y, Tsutsumi Y, Monta O, Ohashi H. Severe tracheal compression due to cervical aortic arch aneurysm. J Card Surg. 2011;26(4):400–2.
54. McElhinney DB, Thompson LD, Weinberg PM, Jue KL, Hanley FL. Surgical approach to complicated cervical aortic arch: anatomic, developmental, and surgical considerations. Cardiol Young. 2000;10(3):212–9.
55. Samanek M, Slavik Z, Zborilova B, Hrobonova V, Voriskova M, Skovranek J. Prevalence, treatment, and outcome of heart disease in live-born children: a prospective analysis of 91,823 live-born children. Pediatr Cardiol. Fall 1989;10(4):205–11.
56. Fixler DE, Pastor P, Chamberlin M, Sigman E, Eifler CW. Trends in congenital heart disease in Dallas County births. 1971–1984. Circulation. 1990;81(1):137–42.
57. Grech V. Diagnostic and surgical trends, and epidemiology of coarctation of the aorta in a population-based study. Int J Cardiol. 1999;68(2):197–202.

58. Mitchell SC, Korones SB, Berendes HW. Congenital heart disease in 56,109 births. Incidence and natural history. Circulation. 1971;43(3):323–32.
59. Miettinen OS, Reiner ML, Nadas AS. Seasonal incidence of coarctation of the aorta. Br Heart J. 1970;32(1):103–7.
60. Tawes Jr RL, Aberdeen E, Waterston DJ, Carter RE. Coarctation of the aorta in infants and children. A review of 333 operative cases, including 179 infants. Circulation. 1969;39(5 Suppl 1):I173–84.
61. Krediet P. An hypothesis of the development of coarctation in man. Acta Morphol Neerl Scand. 1965;6:207–12.
62. Hutchins GM. Coarctation of the aorta explained as a branch-point of the ductus arteriosus. Am J Pathol. 1971;63(2):203–14.
63. Bruneau BG. The developmental genetics of congenital heart disease. Nature. 2008;451(7181):943–8.
64. Beauchesne LM, Connolly HM, Ammash NM, Warnes CA. Coarctation of the aorta: outcome of pregnancy. J Am Coll Cardiol. 2001;38(6):1728–33.
65. Vriend JW, Drenthen W, Pieper PG, et al. Outcome of pregnancy in patients after repair of aortic coarctation. Eur Heart J. 2005;26(20):2173–8.
66. Becker AE, Becker MJ, Edwards JE. Anomalies associated with coarctation of aorta: particular reference to infancy. Circulation. 1970;41(6):1067–75.
67. Smith DE, Matthews MB. Aortic valvular stenosis with coarctation of the aorta, with special reference to the development of aortic stenosis upon congenital bicuspid valves. Br Heart J. 1955;17(2):198–206.
68. Cheatham Jr JE, Williams GR, Thompson WM, Luckstead EF, Razook JD, Elkins RC. Coarctation: a review of 80 children and adolescents. Am J Surg. 1979;138(6):889–93.
69. Ho VB, Bakalov VK, Cooley M, et al. Major vascular anomalies in Turner syndrome: prevalence and magnetic resonance angiographic features. Circulation. 2004;110(12):1694–700.
70. Lopez L, Arheart KL, Colan SD, et al. Turner syndrome is an independent risk factor for aortic dilation in the young. Pediatrics. 2008;121(6):e1622–7.
71. Bjork L, Friedman R. Routine roentgenographic diagnosis of coarctation of the aorta in the child. Am J Roentgenol Radium Ther Nucl Med. 1965;95(3):636–41.
72. Dodge-Khatami A, Ott S, Di Bernardo S, Berger F. Carotid-subclavian artery index: new echocardiographic index to detect coarctation in neonates and infants. Ann Thorac Surg. 2005;80(5):1652–7.
73. Muzzarelli S, Meadows AK, Ordovas KG, Higgins CB, Meadows JJ. Usefulness of cardiovascular magnetic resonance imaging to predict the need for intervention in patients with coarctation of the aorta. Am J Cardiol. 2012;109(6):861–5
74. Frydrychowicz A, Markl M, Hirtler D, et al. Aortic hemodynamics in patients with and without repair of aortic coarctation: in vivo analysis by 4D flow-sensitive magnetic resonance imaging. Invest Radiol. 2011;46(5):317–25.
75. Hope MD, Meadows AK, Hope TA, et al. Clinical evaluation of aortic coarctation with 4D flow MR imaging. J Magn Reson Imaging. 2010;31(3):711–8.
76. Glass IH, Mustard WT, Keith JD. Coarctation of the aorta in infants. A review of twelve years' experience. Pediatrics. 1960;26:109–21.
77. Liberthson RR, Pennington DG, Jacobs ML, Daggett WM. Coarctation of the aorta: review of 234 patients and clarification of management problems. Am J Cardiol. 1979;43(4):835–40.
78. Padua LM, Garcia LC, Rubira CJ, de Oliveira Carvalho PE. Stent placement versus surgery for coarctation of the thoracic aorta. Cochrane Database Syst Rev. 2012;5:CD008204.
79. Carr JA. The results of catheter-based therapy compared with surgical repair of adult aortic coarctation. J Am Coll Cardiol. 2006;47(6):1101–7.
80. Rodes-Cabau J, Miro J, Dancea A, et al. Comparison of surgical and transcatheter treatment for native coarctation of the aorta in patients>or=1 year old. The Quebec Native Coarctation of the Aorta study. Am Heart J. 2007;154(1):186–92.
81. Atalay MK, Kochilas LK. Familial pseudocoarctation of the aorta. Pediatr Cardiol. 2011;32(5):692–5.
82. Varghese A, Gatzoulis M, Mohiaddin RH. Images in cardiovascular medicine: magnetic resonance angiography of a congenitally interrupted aortic arch. Circulation. 2002;106(3):E9–10.
83. Yang DH, Goo HW, Seo DM, et al. Multislice CT angiography of interrupted aortic arch. Pediatr Radiol. 2008;38(1):89–100.

Pulmonary Hypertension in Congenital Heart Disease

25

William M. Bradlow, Sonya V. Babu-Narayan, and Raad H. Mohiaddin

The occurrence of pulmonary hypertension (PH) in patients with congenital heart disease (CHD) is not uncommon and represents an important complication. The chapter sets out the scale of the problem before describing where cross-sectional imaging is used in diagnosis. Prognostication and assessment of therapeutic effect using these techniques is then explored before examining Eisenmenger's syndrome in detail. A discussion on related abnormalities of the pulmonary arteries is included.

Definition

The meaning of the term pulmonary hypertension (PH) depends on the context in which it is used. PH is defined when certain haemodynamic criteria are met during right heart catheterisation (RHC, mean pulmonary artery pressure (mPAP) >25 mmHg) and is also the name given to the collection of conditions which are known to be associated with this haemodynamic state. According to the most recent reclassification (2008) arising from the fourth WHO conference in Dana Point, California, these diseases are divided into six groups (Table 25.1).

Classification of PH in CHD

The majority of PH in congenital heart disease (CHD) comes under the umbrella of pulmonary arterial hypertension (PAH, Group 1 in the WHO Classification) when it is referred to as *PAH associated with CHD* (APAH-CHD) (Table 25.1). Being 'pre-capillary' PH, the pulmonary wedge pressure is ≤15 mmHg with pulmonary vascular resistance >3 Wood units, and the cardiac output is normal or reduced in the absence of an alternative explanation, i.e. lung disease (Group 3), chronic thrombo-embolic PH (Group 4), or PH associated with unclear/multifactorial mechanisms (Group 5) [1].

Shunts are the commonest CHD abnormality associated with PAH, making up approximately 38 % of patients with CHD and PH in one cohort [2]. This group includes Eisenmenger's syndrome, where the development of PH leads to reversal of blood flow through the shunt and cyanosis, but primarily involves patients with systemic-to-pulmonary shunts and to a lesser extent those with small defects and PAH post-corrective surgery (Table 25.2). A helpful five-point framework by which these individual lesions can be characterised has been provided by the most recent guidelines [1] (Table 25.3).

W.M. Bradlow, BMBS, MRCP, PhD
Department of Cardiology, Queen Elizabeth Hospital Birmingham NHS Foundation Trust, Queen Elizabeth Medical Centre, Edgbaston, Birmingham B15 2TH, UK

S.V. Babu-Narayan, MBBS, BSc, MRCP, PhD (✉)
R.H. Mohiaddin, MD, FRCR, FRCP, FESC, PhD
NIHR Cardiovascular Biomedical Research Unit, Royal Brompton Hospital and National Heart and Lung Institute, Imperial College London, Sydney Street, London SW3 6NP, UK
e-mail: s.babu-narayan@imperial.ac.uk; r.mohiaddin@rbht.nhs.uk, r.mohiaddin@imperial.ac.uk

F. Saremi (ed.), *Cardiac CT and MR for Adult Congenital Heart Disease*, DOI 10.1007/978-1-4614-8875-0_25, © Springer Science+Business Media New York 2014

Table 25.1 The Dana Point classification for pulmonary hypertension

1. Pulmonary arterial hypertension (PAH)
1.1. Idiopathic
1.2. Heritable
1.2.1. BMPR2
1.2.2. ALK1, endoglin (with or without hereditary haemorrhagic telangiectasia)
1.2.3. Unknown
1.3. Drugs and toxins induced
1.4. Associated with (APAH)
1.4.1. Connective tissue diseases
1.4.2. HIV infection
1.4.3. Portal hypertension
1.4.4. Congenital heart disease
1.4.5. Schistosomiasis
1.4.6. Chronic haemolytic anaemia
1.5. Persistent pulmonary hypertension of the newborn
1′. Pulmonary veno-occlusive disease and/or pulmonary capillary haemangiomatosis
2. Pulmonary hypertension due to left heart disease
2.1. Systolic dysfunction
2.2. Diastolic dysfunction
2.3. Valvular disease
3. Pulmonary hypertension due to lung diseases and/or hypoxia
3.1. Chronic obstructive pulmonary disease
3.2. Interstitial lung disease
3.3. Other pulmonary diseases with mixed restrictive and obstructive pattern
3.4. Sleep-disordered breathing
3.5. Alveolar hypoventilation disorders
3.6. Chronic exposure to high altitude
3.7. Developmental abnormalities
4. Chronic thromboembolic pulmonary hypertension
5. PH with unclear and/or multifactorial mechanisms
5.1. Haematological disorders: myeloproliferative disorders, splenectomy
5.2. Systemic disorders: sarcoidosis, pulmonary Langerhans cell histiocytosis, lymphangioleiomyomatosis, neurofibromatosis, vasculitis
5.3. Metabolic disorders: glycogen storage disease, Gaucher disease, thyroid disorders
5.4. Others: tumoural obstruction, fibrosing mediastinitis, chronic renal failure on dialysis

From Galie et al. [1], with permission
ALK-1 activin receptor-like kinase 1 gene, *APAH* associated pulmonary arterial hypertension, *BMPR2* bone morphogenetic protein receptor, type 2, *HIV* human immunodeficiency virus, *PAH* pulmonary arterial hypertension

Table 25.2 Classification of shunts in APAH-CHD

(a) *Eisenmenger's syndrome*
Eisenmenger's syndrome includes all systemic-to-pulmonary shunts due to large defects leading to a severe increase in PVR and resulting in a reversed (pulmonary to systemic) or bidirectional shunt. Cyanosis, erythrocytosis and multiple organ involvement are present
(b) *Pulmonary arterial hypertension associated with systemic-to-pulmonary shunts*
In these patients with moderate to large defects, the increase in PVR is mild to moderate, systemic-to-pulmonary shunt is still largely present, and no cyanosis is present at rest
(c) *Pulmonary arterial hypertension with small[a] defects*
In cases with small defects (usually ventricular septal defects <1 cm and atrial septal defects <2 cm of effective diameter assessed by echocardiography), the clinical picture is very similar to idiopathic PAH
(d) *Pulmonary arterial hypertension after corrective cardiac surgery*
In these cases, congenital heart disease has been corrected, but PAH is either still present immediately after surgery or has recurred several months or years after surgery in the absence of significant post-operative residual congenital lesions or defects that originate as a sequela to previous surgery

Reproduced with permission [1]
PAH pulmonary arterial hypertension, *PVR* pulmonary vascular resistance
[a]The size applies to adult patients

The likelihood of developing PAH depends on the shunt itself – in patients with pre-tricuspid defects, it can be rare (i.e. ASD) or up to 15–20 % for sinus venosus defect. For post-tricuspid defects, it is more common (50–70 % for large VSD/PDA) and almost universal in patients with truncus arteriosus [3]. It is important to recognise that not all PH in CHD is due to PAH. Other causes include left heart disease (Group 2) and lung disease (Group 4), including obstructive sleep apnoea.

Pathophysiology and Presentation

In CHD, the pulmonary vasculature is exposed to higher than normal blood flow (i.e. pre-tricuspid shunts) and pressures (in post-tricuspid shunts). This leads to damage of the vascular endothelium which sets into motion a series of deleterious

Table 25.3 5-point framework with which to classify shunts in APAH-CHD

1. Type
1.1. Simple pre-tricuspid shunts
1.1.1. Atrial septal defect (ASD)
1.1.1.1. Ostium secundum
1.1.1.2. Sinus venosus
1.1.1.3. Ostium primum
1.1.2. Total or partial unobstructed anomalous pulmonary venous return
1.2. Simple post-tricuspid shunts
1.2.1. Ventricular septal defect (VSD)
1.2.2. Patent ductus arteriosus
1.3. Combined shunts
Describe combination and define predominant defect
1.4. Complex congenital heart disease
1.4.1. Complete atrioventricular septal defect
1.4.2. Truncus arteriosus
1.4.3. Single ventricle physiology with unobstructed pulmonary blood flow
1.4.4. Transposition of the great arteries with VSD (without pulmonary stenosis) and/or patent ductus arteriosus
1.4.5. Other
2. Dimension (specify for each defect if more than one congenital heart defect exists)
2.1. Haemodynamic (specify Qp:Qs)[a]
2.1.1. Restrictive (pressure gradient across the defect)
2.1.2. Non-restrictive
2.2. Anatomic[b]
2.2.1. Small to moderate (ASD ≤2.0 cm and VSD ≤1.0 cm)
2.2.2. Large (ASD >2.0 cm and VSD >1.0 cm)
3. Direction of shunt
3.1. Predominantly systemic to pulmonary
3.2. Predominantly pulmonary to systemic
3.3. Bidirectional
4. Associated cardiac and extracardiac abnormalities
5. Repair status
5.1. Unoperated
5.2. Palliated [specify type of operation(s), age at surgery]
5.3. Repaired [specify type of operation(s), age at surgery]

From Galie et al. [1], with permission
ASD atrial septal defect, *VSD* ventricular septal defect
[a]Ratio of pulmonary (Qp)-to-systemic (Qs) blood flow
[b]The size applies to adult patients

pathways. These culminate in a pulmonary vasculopathy characterised by medial hypertrophy and plexiform lesions. The end effect is elevated pulmonary vascular resistance corresponding to an attenuation of pulmonary vasculature.

Symptoms of PH tend to be non-specific and include breathlessness, effort intolerance, chest pain and syncope. Presentation is influenced by a number of factors including the severity of PH, the nature of the underlying defect and prior surgery. PH associated with post-tricuspid shunts tends to manifest with symptoms in infancy whilst pre-tricuspid shunts may take a number of decades to become apparent.

Clinical features are dominated by those of PH (i.e. elevated venous pressure, right ventricular heave, loud second heart sound, ascites, peripheral oedema) with diminishment of murmurs associated with post-tricuspid shunts with the onset of the Eisenmenger's syndrome [4].

Epidemiology and Outcomes

Consistent data has emerged from contemporary registries defining the frequency with which PH affects patients with CHD. In the Dutch National Registry, PH (defined as an echocardiographic-derived systolic PA pressure >40 mmHg) affected 5 % of adults with CHD [5] compared to data from Quebec, Canada, where 5.8 % had received a diagnosis of PH [2].

When considered in terms of etiologies underling PAH, CHD is an important contributor (Fig. 25.1). In the REVEAL Registry of consecutively screened PAH patients, the most common individual subset was idiopathic PAH (46.2 %), followed by collagen vascular disease/connective tissue diseases (25.2 %) and then CHD (9.8 %) [6].

It is not felt likely that these figures will remain static in the future [4]. Advances in surgical and medical treatments continue to expand the numbers of patients with CHD surviving to adulthood. This population is likely to comprise increasingly complex disease with higher rates of associated PAH.

As well as defining its prevalence, registry data has proven what was long suspected that PH in CHD confers a worse prognosis. In the Dutch group, patients with PH had a HR of 3.8 (95 % CI 2.7–5.4, $p<0.001$) for all-cause mortality,

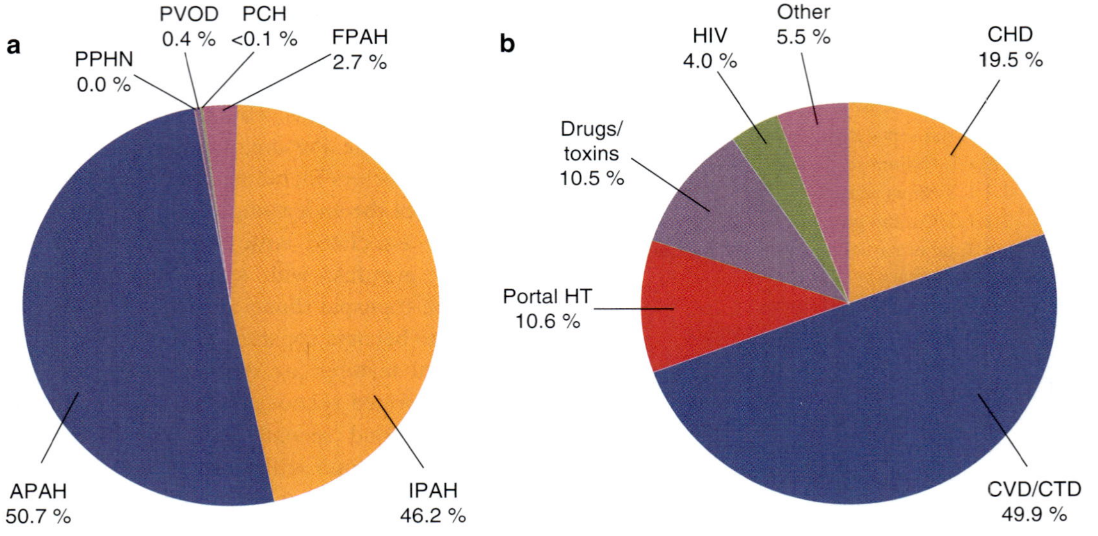

Fig. 25.1 Pie charts demonstrating percentage of patients with WHO Class I (PAH, **a**) and of these the percentage comprising associated PAH in the REVEAL Registry (**b**). Note that CHD is the third most common diagnosis underlying PAH. *APAH* associated PAH, *CHD* congenital heart disease, *CVD/CTD* colleague vascular disease/connective tissue disease, *FPAH* familial PAH, *HT* hypertension, *IPAH* idiopathic PAH, *PAH* pulmonary arterial hypertension, *PCH* pulmonary capillary haemangiomatosis, *PPHN* pulmonary hypertension of the newborn, *PVOD* pulmonary veno-occlusive disease, *REVEAL* Registry to Evaluate Early and Long-Term PAH Disease Management (From Badesch et al. [6], with permission)

adjusted for age and gender. In the Canadian cohort, patients with PH and CHD had a 2-fold higher all-cause mortality and 3-fold higher morbidity [2] than case controls without PH (Fig. 25.2). Finally, the REVEAL Registry has shown that children with APAH-CHD have a similar 5-year survival from RHC (71 ± 13 %) than patients with IPAH (75 ± 7 %) [7]. This argues against the assertion that patients with APAH-CHD fare better than those with IPAH since the RV in CHD has been ‘trained’ to deal with high right-sided pressures over a long period of time.

Treatment

Interventions to the defect itself, when pulmonary blood flow is high but pulmonary vascular disease minimal, represent an important treatment goal in patients with APAH-CHD. The general consensus is that this should be undertaken when the pulmonary vascular resistance is less than 6 Wood units. Management is less clear when the value lies between 6 and 10 Wood units [3]. In Eisenmenger’s syndrome, shunt closure is contraindicated.

For the remainder of patients with APAH-CHD in whom an intervention is not possible, benefit has come in the wake of trials of targeted medical therapies in individuals suffering with idiopathic PAH. Agents include intravenous epoprostenol, endothelin receptor antagonist and phosphodiesterase-5 inhibitors which address deficiencies in prostacyclin (potent vasodilator) and overexpression of endothelin-1 and phosphodiesterase-1 (vasoconstrictors), respectively. Class I support for Bosentan and Class IIa for sildenafil and prostanoids has been given in the most recent recommendations [1].

The Role of Imaging in Management of PH in Congenital Heart Disease

Diagnosis

Given the potential to cure or prevent progression of PH, there is an imperative to identify it promptly in patients with established CHD and, conversely, to diagnose CHD when present in patients with a

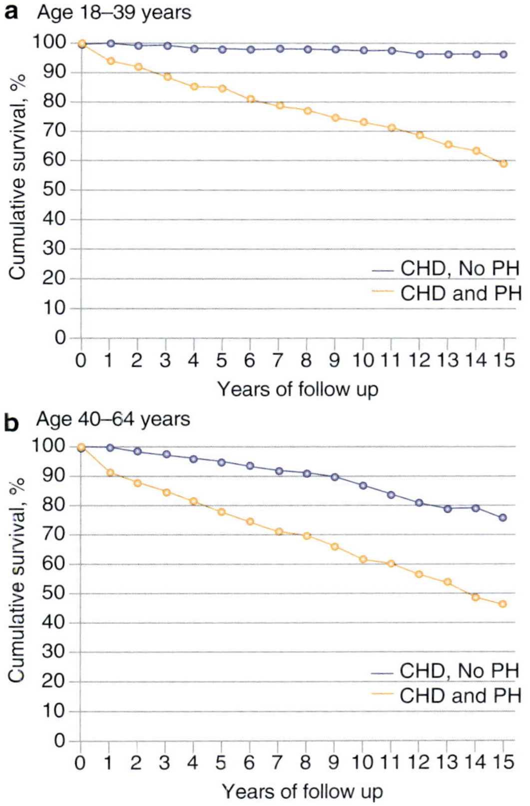

Fig. 25.2 Survival curves for adults with CHD without (triangular data points) and with PH (diamond data points) showing adverse prognosis in both 18–39-year-olds (**a**) and 40–46-year-olds (**b**) (From Lowe et al. [2], with permission)

known diagnosis of PH. The recommended diagnostic algorithm [1] for patients suspected of having PH focuses first on exclusion of common causes of PH in order of likelihood (Groups 2 and 3 and then chronic thromboembolic PH with a VQ scan). If these investigations are non-contributory, a RHC is then recommended before specific tests are undertaken to identify rarer causes of PH including CHD. For patients with established CHD, there is merit in taking the same systematic approach given the potential for there being more than one cause contributing to PH.

The algorithm emphasises the key role of multimodality imaging in patients with APAH-CHD, recognising the strengths and complementary nature of these modalities and the complex nature of the diagnostic questions arising.

Being portable, cheap and available transthoracic echocardiography is used first. It allows assessment of intracardiac shunts (site, size and direction) as well as identifying features which might suggest PH. These include right ventricular remodelling (dilatation, hypertrophy and impaired systolic function), right atrial enlargement, compression of the left ventricle, pulmonary artery dilatation and pericardial effusion. Flattening of the interventricular septum can also be quantified using the eccentricity index [8].

The extent of right ventricular dilatation is best appreciated in the apical four-chamber view. Right ventricular size can be quantified using linear dimensions, fractional area change, M-mode and tissue Doppler. Enlargement of the right atrium can be quantified. Right ventricular hypertrophy is measured in the subcostal view.

Right heart and pulmonary pressures can be non-invasively estimated using Doppler interrogation of the tricuspid regurgitant (TR) jet, right ventricular outflow tract acceleration time, pulmonary regurgitation jet and M-mode measurements of the inferior vena caval size and response to respiration. In day-to-day practice, TR jet velocity (V) is most often used. The right ventricular systolic pressure can be calculated by adding right atrial pressure to $4V$ [2]. This equates to systolic pulmonary artery pressure in the absence of pulmonary stenosis. PH is likely when velocity is >2.8 m/s particularly when a dilatation or dysfunction of the right ventricle coexist.

The ESC guidelines [1] draw attention to the finding of higher than expected pulmonary blood flow in the setting of a small shunt or significant PA dilatation with only moderate PH as these are strongly suggestive of an aberrant pulmonary vein or sinus venosus defect. In these cases, transoesophageal echocardiography can be particularly helpful in imaging the atrial septum, specifically where the superior vena cava enters the right atrium.

Cardiac Computed Tomography

Although disadvantaged by the need for ionising radiation and contrast, computed tomography (CT) has an important part to play in the investigation of

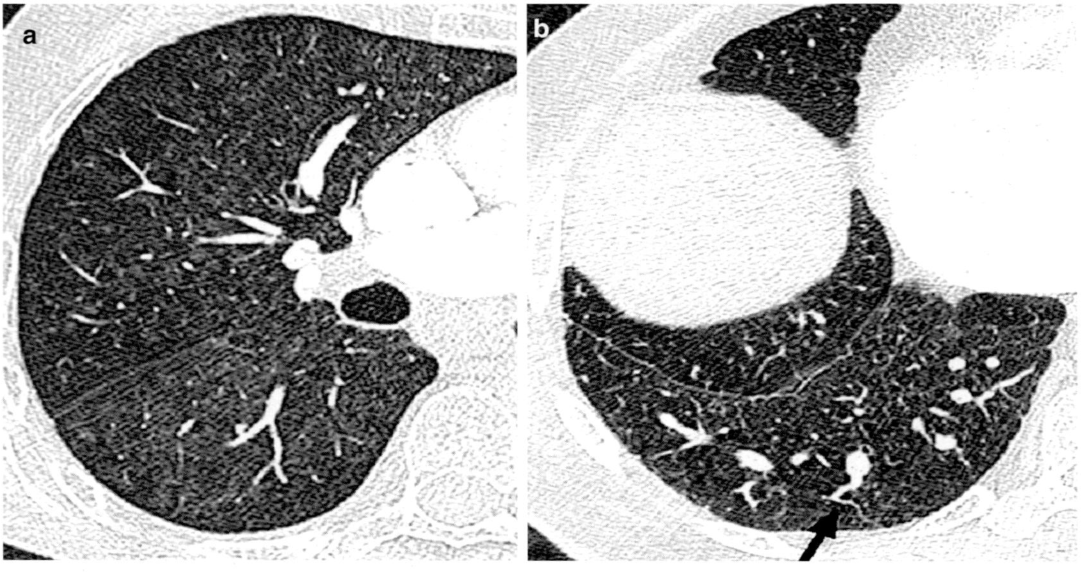

Fig. 25.3 High-resolution CT findings in a patient with pulmonary arterial hypertension. Ground glass changes and small nodular opacities are seen in the lung parenchyma in pulmonary arterial hypertension (**a**) and serpiginous intrapulmonary vessels (**b**), *black arrow* (Courtesy of Dr Michael Rubens, Royal Brompton Hospital, UK)

APAH-CHD where it can provide information on cardiac chambers, great arteries, lung vasculature and parenchyma and mediastinal structures in a single acquisition with high spatial resolution.

This is particularly the case when acoustic windows have been poor (limiting echocardiography), lung disease is present and devices including pacemakers prevent CMR scanning.

The same features of cardiac remodelling associated with PH described previously can also be identified using cardiac CT. Communications between chambers can be visualised and the direction of shunt inferred by the direction of contrast. Although excellent at providing anatomical detail, it is generally not the modality of choice for providing functional data. If necessary, biventricular function can be assessed though this necessitates greater radiation exposure to capture information throughout the cardiac cycle.

The CT pulmonary angiogram is the test of choice to assess the proximal and distal pulmonary arteries non-invasively. In doing so, pulmonary artery dilatation can be identified as well as thrombus, which may form in situ due to sluggish blood flow rather than being embolised from the lower peripheries.

High-resolution CT scan provides valuable information on lung parenchyma which can be abnormal in patients with CHD because of bronchiectasis or hypoplasia. High-resolution CT may also detect parenchymal changes due to pulmonary arterial hypertension, for example, ground glass changes, nodular opacities and serpiginous intrapulmonary small vessels representing plexogenic arteriopathy (Fig. 25.3). In those with chronic thromboembolic PH, it may also identify within the lung tissue haemorrhage, infarction or a mosaic attenuation pattern (due to heterogenous lung perfusion). High-resolution CT has a vital role in identifying those with pulmonary veno-occlusive disease where advanced therapies might be harmful (Fig. 25.4). The key features of this rare entity on CT are interlobular septal thickening, ground glass shadowing and adenopathy.

When contrast enhanced, this technique is particularly adept in the assessment of extracardiac features, particularly native or surgically fashioned systemic-to-pulmonary shunts. Collateral vessels are readily identified. These include dilated bronchial arteries (a commonly seen feature in PH) or bypassing vessels in cases of pulmonary venous occlusion.

Enlarged central pulmonary arteries is a non-specific sign and can be seen in patients with large left-to-right shunt with or without increased pulmonary vascular resistance. A cross-sectional diameter of >3 cm or larger than the aorta for distal main pulmonary artery is suggestive of pulmonary hypertension. Abrupt decrease in the calibre of segmental and subsegmental arteries may indicate increased pulmonary vascular resistance. An analytic technique called fractal analysis was employed to determine whether the degree of branching within the pulmonary arteries of children and young adults with PAH, half of whom had CHD (Fig. 25.5), could be used as a non-invasive measure of PH [9]. This index compared well with conventional markers of disease severity such as functional class, 6-min walk test distance and indexed pulmonary vascular resistance and predicted death amongst the cohort (HR 5.6 (95 % CI 1.2–25; $p = 0.027$)). Associated cardiac findings in CT may include enlarged right ventricle and atrium, bowing of the inter-atrial septum, straightening of the ventricular septum, right ventricle hypertrophy, dilatation and decreased fractional shortening of the right ventricle outflow tract and reflux of contrast into a dilated inferior vena cava, hepatic veins or azygos system.

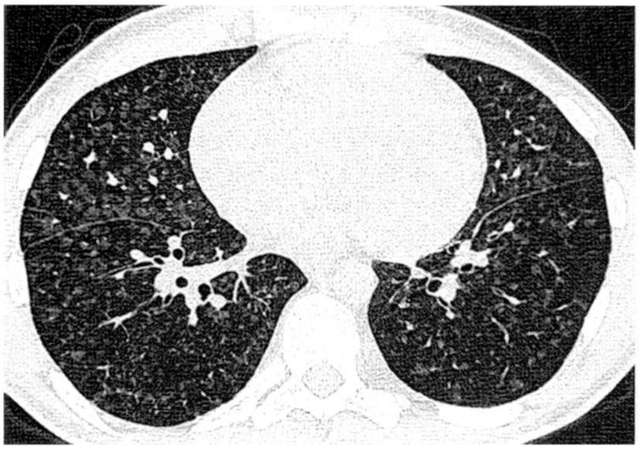

Fig. 25.4 High-resolution CT scan showing classic features of pulmonary veno-occlusive disease. Though this condition is rare, its recognition is important as conventional vasodilator treatment (Courtesy of Dr Michael Rubens, Royal Brompton Hospital, UK)

Cardiovascular Magnetic Resonance

CMR has the strong advantage of being able to image in any plane with high spatial and temporal resolution without ionising radiation. As repeated examinations become commonplace, the latter characteristic is increasingly important.

In order to optimise image quality, breath holding is required which may be problematic in this population of patients. In addition, pacemakers/devices currently represent a contraindication to CMR.

CMR provides the gold standard assessments of right [10] and left ventricular size and function. Especially for the heavily trabeculated right ventricle, analysis remains dependent on the individual undertaking it.

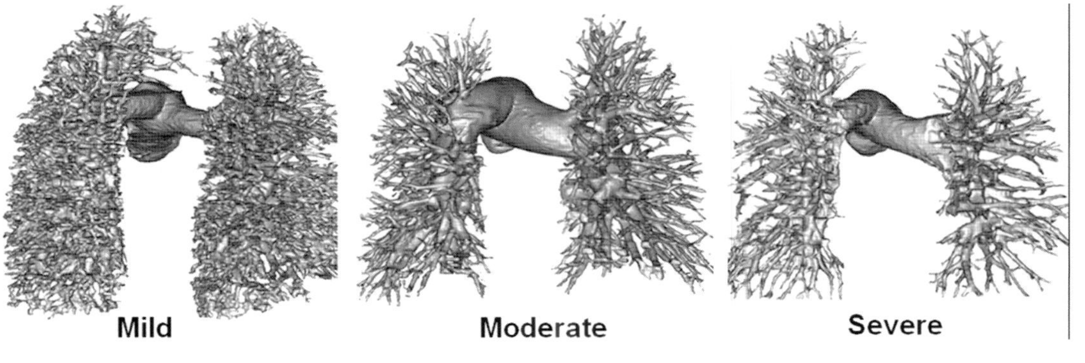

Fig. 25.5 Surface-rendered data taken from patients with increasingly severe PH (*left* to *right*). Note attenuation in branch pulmonary arteries. This is reflected in their fractal dimensions which diminish with reduced branching (1.66, 1.48 and 1.27, respectively) (From Moledina et al. [9] with permission)

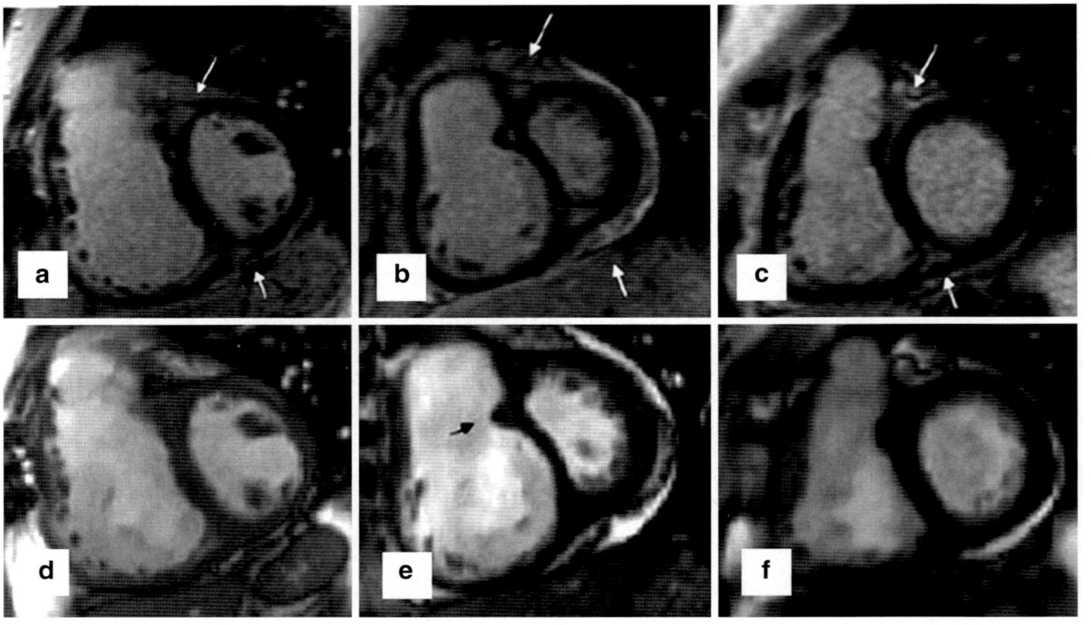

Fig. 25.6 The characteristic late gadolinium enhancement pattern of pulmonary arterial hypertension. The characteristic late gadolinium enhancement pattern of PH. (**a–c**) insertion region enhancement (*arrows*) is triangular in shape with the base at the epicardial surface where both ventricles meet and its apex directed into the interventricular septum. Corresponding short-axis cine slices (**d–f**). The septomarginal trabeculation is *arrowed* (**e**) – enhancement is often seen within this structure (From Bradlow et al. [15] with permission)

Using both cine imaging and in-plane flow mapping, intracardiac shunts can be easily identified. By comparing the ratio of flow through the pulmonary artery to that in the aorta using flow mapping, Qp:QS can be determined and the shunt quantified.

With the addition of contrast, magnetic resonance angiography can delineate extracardiac shunts (especially partial anomalous venous drainage [11]) as well as the pulmonary vasculature.

Late gadolinium enhancement typically demonstrates areas of enhancement at the RV-LV insertion points [12, 13]. Histological data however supports the concept that the myocardial disarray at these sites is a normal feature of insertion region anatomy exaggerated in PH by the hypertrophy of the right ventricle [14] (Figs. 25.6 and 25.7).

Significant efforts have been given over to non-invasively assessing pulmonary pressures using CMR with indices such as right ventricular mass [17], septal deviation [18], pulmonary artery stiffness [19] and, more recently, four-dimensional flow patterns [20]. Of the longer-established measures, none have emerged as a reliable measure in patients with PAH [21]. Moreover, none have been routinely tested in a CHD population where the presence of pre-existing right ventricular hypertrophy, septal defects, shunts and arterial abnormalities is likely to confound many of these measures.

In the setting of a hybrid CMR interventional lab, pulmonary vascular resistance derived from the Fick method has been shown to be inaccurate in conditions of high pulmonary blood flow or increased oxygen concenration [22]. With promising results, the same technique has been used to show that pulmonary vascular resistance can be determined non-invasively in a small cohort with mainly atrial and ventricular septal defects. A pulmonary flow of 6.05 l/min/m^2 or a Qp:QS ratio <2.5/1 had a specificity of 100 % for predicting PVR of ≤3.5 Wood units/m ^{2} on receiver-operator characteristic analysis [23].

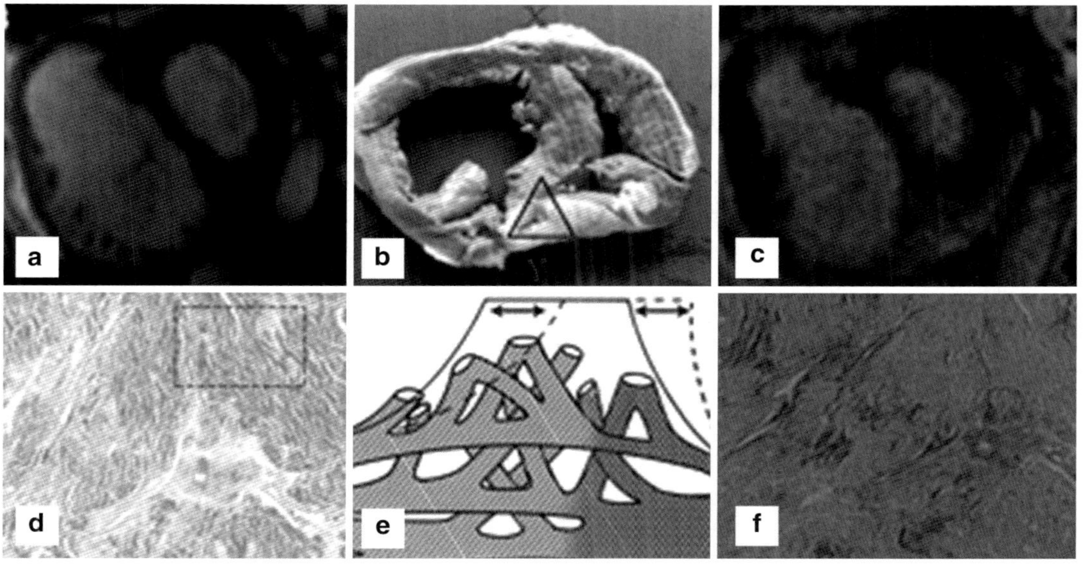

Fig. 25.7 Histological correlations and mechanism for late gadolinium enhancement in RV-LV insertion point regions in pulmonary arterial hypertension. (**a**) Short-axis cine at end diastole. Note straightening of the interventricular septum. (**b**) Corresponding post-mortem section showing a dominant hypertrophied right ventricle with no macroscopic scarring of the insertion regions. Interventricular sulci (*X*, *Y*) and posterior insertion region (*triangle*) are identified. (**c**) Late gadolinium enhancement is apparent in both insertion regions. (**d**) Microscopy findings (picrosirius red stain) typical of the insertion regions. Fibre disarray is shown in the *boxed area*. The pale region immediately below represents increased connective tissue. This territory is illustrated by the broad spaces between crossing fibre bundles from the right (*single lines*) and left (*hatched lines*) ventricle in the sketch (**e**) depicting the posterior insertion region. Abnormal interventricular septum motion is reflected by *arrows* and *dashed lines* (From Fox and Hutchins et al. [16] with permission). (**f**) Plexiform fibrosis; collagen lies between 'disarrayed' myocardial fibres but does not replace them (trichrome staining; and From Bradlow et al. [14] with permission)

Guiding Intervention

Echocardiography (particularly three dimensional), CT and CMR all play an important role in deciding whether a patient would benefit from an intervention. For atrial and ventricular septal defects and patent ductus arteriosus, these modalities are also relied upon in planning whether closure can be undertaken in the catheter laboratory or surgically by defining the exact size, shape and location of the shunt.

Assessment of Treatment and Prognosis

Excluding work arising from the Eisenmenger's syndrome population, there is relatively little data to draw upon when assessing treatment effect and prognosticating in the APAH-CHD population in isolation. The majority of data that are available are derived from PAH patients.

The main measure used in clinical practice and as a trial end point is the 6-min walk test. However, this has faced considerable criticism given its limitations [24] and failure to demonstrate a relationship with clinical end points [25]. This has spurred investigation into alternative surrogates, one of which has been right ventricular mass as assessed by CMR [26, 27]. This measure was employed after medical and surgical therapies have been shown to cause improvements in indices of remodelling [15]. The high interstudy repeatability of CMR makes it an attractive tool for repeated non-invasive measurements, but it is uncertain whether right ventricular mass is the best surrogate to assess as there is no data to say whether reducing it ultimately benefits the patient.

CMR has also been used to prognosticate in patients with PAH. These data suggest that dilatation [28] and impaired systolic function [29] of the right ventricle as well as increased degrees of pulmonary artery stiffness [30] are predictors of a poor outcome. These results cannot be directly extrapolated to the APAH-CHD population, but do serve as a useful starting point for further investigations.

Eisenmenger's Syndrome

Historical Perspective

Eisenmenger's syndrome is severe pulmonary arterial hypertension in conjunction with congenital heart disease and reversal of shunt resulting in cyanosis.

Victor Eisenmenger described ventricular septal defect with reversed shunt in the absence of pulmonary stenosis which was named Eisenmenger's complex in 1897 [31]. He described a 32-year-old man suffering from dyspnoea, cyanosis and in later years heart failure. At post-mortem after he died from massive haemoptysis, he was found to have a large non-restrictive ventricular septal defect and overriding aorta without pulmonary stenosis. The pulmonary arteries were noted to have atheroma, but there was no mention of pulmonary hypertension.

It was Paul Wood that was the first to describe the pathophysiology of Eisenmenger's, specifically the cause of the reversed central shunt being pulmonary vascular resistance at systemic or close to systemic level [32, 33]. He refined his definition of Eisenmenger's syndrome in 1958 as 'pulmonary hypertension due to a high pulmonary vascular resistance with reversed or bidirectional shunt at aorto-pulmonary, ventricular or atrial level' – a definition that remains relevant today.

Clinical Pathophysiology and Course

Eisenmenger's syndrome results from pulmonary hypertension and pulmonary vascular disease induced by the increased pulmonary blood flow consequent to any large congenital heart defect at atrial, ventricular or arterial level with an initially primarily left-to-right shunt. The increased pulmonary blood flow results in the transmission of elevated pressure to the pulmonary circulation. The high pulmonary blood flow results in mechanical stretch, intimal damage and progressive structural abnormalities in the pulmonary vasculature. Medial hypertrophy and smooth muscle proliferation occurs in normally non-muscularised pulmonary arterioles and subsequently concentric laminar intimal fibrosis and plexiform lesions representing irreversible vascular disease. The vascular changes lead to progressive obstruction of small pulmonary arterioles which have the effect of reducing the total cross-sectional area of the pulmonary vascular bed resulting in fixed elevation of resistance and pressure. When the elevated pulmonary resistance exceeds systemic vascular resistance, the initially left-to-right shunt reverses to become a right-to-left (or bidirectional) shunt causing desaturation of systemic arterial blood and clinical cyanosis. Eisenmenger's syndrome patients represent the most severe form of pulmonary arterial hypertension associated with congenital heart disease.

Eisenmenger patients present with multisystem disorders including coagulopathy with both bleeding tendency and predisposition to thrombus formation, haemoptysis, pulmonary haemorrhage, secondary erythrocytosis, cerebral abscess, thromboembolism, renal dysfunction, hypertrophic osteoarthropathy, cholelithiasis, for example, as well as heart failure arrhythmia, sudden death and endocarditis. They are also at risk from pregnancy or noncardiac surgery.

Despite histopathological similarities in adverse pulmonary vascular remodelling, Eisenmenger patients enjoy much better survival with a long asymptomatic period of decades until the 30s [34] compared with idiopathic pulmonary arterial hypertension patients. There is relatively slow disease progression though patients have significant exercise limitation [35] and impaired quality of life. The median survival is probably 40–50 years versus 2.8 years in idiopathic pulmonary arterial hypertension [36–38]. New pharmacological treatments with endothelin receptor antagonists such as Bosentan, phosphodiesterase inhibitors such as sildenafil and prostanoids are recommended for WHO Class ≥ III Eisenmenger patients [1, 39, 40].

Right Ventricular Adaptive Remodelling

The risk and speed at which Eisenmenger's physiology develops depends on the location and size of the systemic-to-pulmonary shunt and the presence of pulmonary stenosis. The nature of the underlying congenital heart defect may be relevant to the adaptive response of the subpulmonary RV. The position and function of semilunar and AV valves, hypertrophy or hypoplasia of any part of the tripartite RV and the effect of surgical incisions and patching from previous palliation or repair all have an effect on myocardial adaptation and function. In Eisenmenger's syndrome versus idiopathic pulmonary arterial hypertension or even APAH-CHD, the RV is considered better adapted to high pulmonary artery pressures having been primed since birth through long-standing exposure to volume and pressure overload. Additionally, regression of the physiological right ventricular hypertrophy present at birth does not occur.

CMR for Underlying Congenital Anatomy and Features of Pulmonary Hypertension

Given that patients tend to volunteer few symptoms and complain of symptoms late in the disease progress [35], functional imaging has a potentially valuable clinical role in Eisenmenger patients.

CMR may occasionally correctly diagnose the precise nature of the underlying congenital heart disease for the first time. CMR can pursue the assessment of each underlying congenital heart lesion appropriately. It is important for CMR to assess both native and operated anatomy and their haemodynamic functional consequences. The location of shunts as pre-tricuspid or post-tricuspid should be determined. The dimension of shunts (ASD >2 cm, VSD >1 cm, arterial shunt >5–7 mm are significant; Table 25.3) and the direction of shunt flow (left to right, right to left or bidirectional) should be measured. In operated patients, CMR can be used to assess the presence and patency of surgical shunts. Contrast-enhanced MR angiography is also useful for extracardiac involvement such as presence of associated PDA or aortopulmonary collaterals.

Both aortic and pulmonary phase-contrast velocity flow mapping data should be acquired to measure shunt ratio. Aortic flow mapping can be used to quantify cardiac output. The presence and degree of tricuspid or pulmonary regurgitation should also be sought

Acquisition of cines for RV and LV ventricular volumes and function should be performed in all patients though accurate and reproducible performance of RV volume measures is not straightforward. For example, it requires accounting for the presence of a VSD where relevant in a consistent fashion, addressing the highly trabeculated boundaries of the RV and the complex RV architecture that can be associated with previous surgery, identifying when systole is a different time frame for the RV than the LV correctly (Fig. 25.8) and correctly identifying enlarged RV the most basal part of which can dilate above the tricuspid valve plane such that part of the RV is present also in systole. Thus, RV volumes and in particular mass measurements remain labour intensive for everyday clinical practice.

Septal flattening in systole and leftward deviation of the ventricular septum when RV systole continues beyond LV systole reflects changing relative pressures and time courses of LV and RV contraction. This can be qualitatively noted on cine imaging just as in echocardiography.

The central pulmonary arteries require imaging. Contrast-enhanced MR angiography is a useful, complementary approach to balanced steady-state free precession cine imaging for assessment of aneurysmal, poorly expansile pulmonary arteries which may demonstrate sluggish flow and in situ pulmonary arterial thrombus [41] (Fig. 25.9). Pulmonary arterial

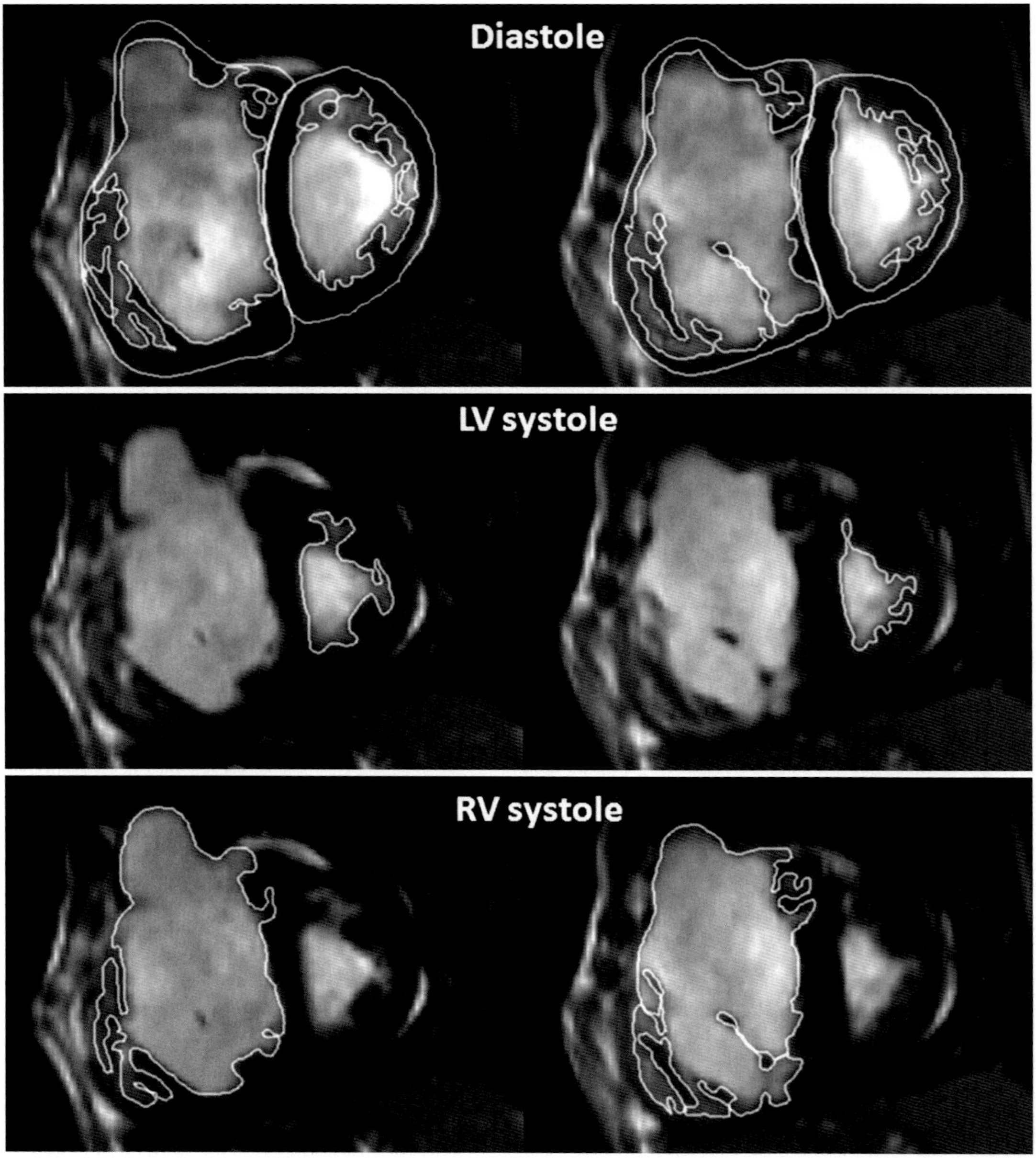

Fig. 25.8 Measurements of right and left ventricular mass, volumes and function in Eisenmenger's syndrome patient. Manual planimetry of short-axis contiguous slices from base to apex of the heart has proven highly reproducible for research in our centre. As right ventricular mass may be prognostically important and given hypertrophy of the trabeculated myocardium, trabeculations have been excluded from the blood pool and included in the ventricular mass. In this example, right ventricular end systole was in a different frame from left ventricular end systole. Whilst reproducible with a single experienced operator, this method is labour intensive and requires about 30 min per patient

thrombosis is well recognised in Eisenmenger's syndrome and is often due to in situ thrombus formation rather than thromboembolic disease. Pulmonary arterial thrombus is predisposed to by slow pulmonary blood flow and biventricular dysfunction [42].

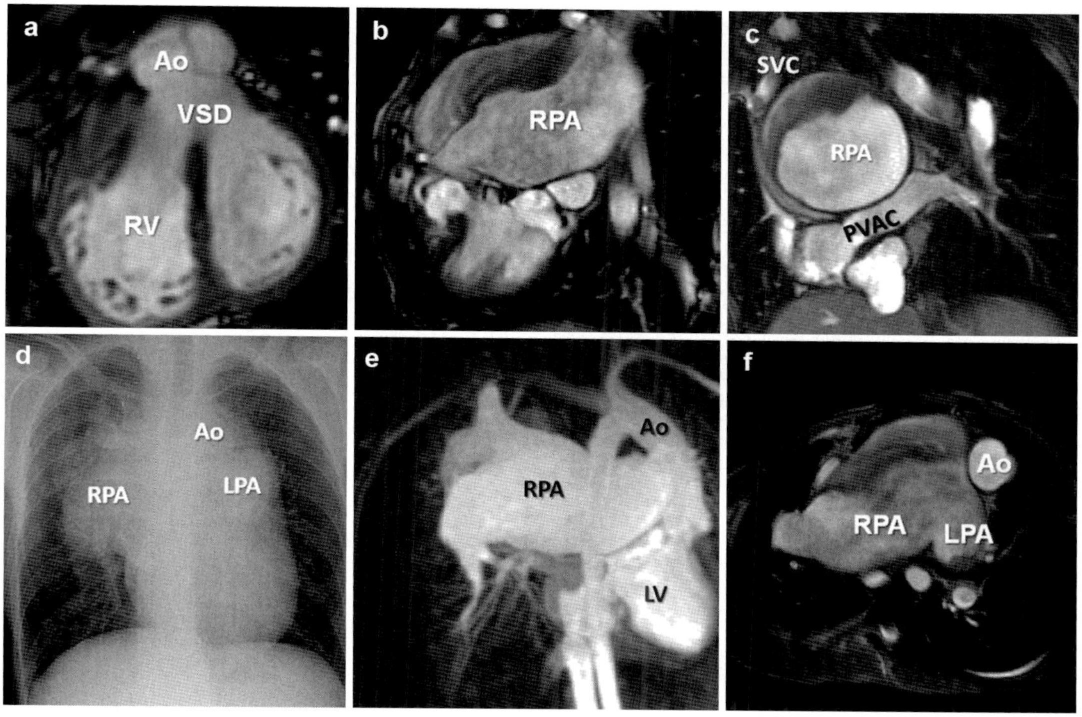

Fig. 25.9 Eisenmenger's physiology in the context of complex underlying congenital heart disease complicated by in situ thrombus. The native anatomy is transposition of the great arteries with subaortic VSD and pulmonary stenosis for which the patient has undergone a palliative Mustard procedure (VSD left open) after early development of increased pulmonary vascular resistance. Image (**a**) shows large, subaortic unrestrictive VSD. Images (**b**–**f**) all show massively enlarged right pulmonary artery (*RPA*) measuring up to 8 cm diameter. In images (**b**, **c**) and (**f**), dark, laminar thrombus is clearly demonstrated in the RPA and also in the LPA on image (**f**). Image (**c**) shows massive dilatation of the RPA and its local effect on the superior vena cava (*SVC*) return to the baffled atrial pathways. Image (**d**) is a plain posteroanterior chest X-ray demonstrating massive pulmonary arterial aneurysmal dilatation correlating with the corresponding contrast-enhanced MR image in (**e**). Cine images from which stills (**b**, **c**) and (**f**) were taken demonstrate sluggish pulmonary blood flow. *Ao* aorta, *LPA* left pulmonary artery, *LV* left ventricle, *PVAC* pulmonary venous atrial compartment, *VSD* ventricular septal defect

Planimetry of the RA and LA from four-chamber cine CMR could be useful as increased RA size and increased RA:LA ratio have been shown to be predictive of mortality in a recent prospective Eisenmenger's study using echocardiography [43].

Ongoing research may define a role for quantitative assessment of pulmonary artery stiffness, the abnormal time course of septal displacement and the degree of septal curvature, late gadolinium enhancement and 4D flow techniques applied to Eisenmenger patients, but outcomes data for these measures is currently limited.

Specific Congenital Heart Defects with Coexisting Pulmonary Arterial Hypertension

Eisenmenger's is associated with a wide variety of underlying heart defects, and as with all pulmonary arterial hypertension associated with congenital heart disease, there is variable rate of pulmonary arterial hypertension disease progression. In order to enable appropriate decision-making, more refined classifications of pulmonary arterial hypertension that coexists with congenital heart disease have been proposed in order to better address an otherwise very heterogenous

Table 25.4 Van Albada and Berger proposed modification: characterisation of pulmonary hypertension associated with congenital cardiac disease

Presence of a systemic-to-pulmonary shunt
Yes/no
Previously (age, duration)
(Note: if such a shunt does not exist – nor has it existed in history – then another form of pulmonary hypertension than that described in the first group of the Venice classification should be considered)
Location of the shunt
Pre-tricuspid level – interatrial communication or abnormal pulmonary venous drainage
Post-tricuspid level – interventricular communications, patent arterial duct, functionally univentricular hearts
Direction of the shunt
Systemic to pulmonary
Pulmonary to systemic
Bidirectional
Size of defect (anatomical and functional, both at present and at early age)
Quantification of the shunt in terms of ratios of pulmonary-to-systemic flows
Restriction: is there a pressure drop over the (post-tricuspid) defect
State of repair
Correction of shunt and age at correction
Pulmonary arterial banding: age at and duration of the banding
Presence, type and duration of surgical shunts (Pott's, Waterston, Blalock-Taussig)
Residual shunting (quantification and location)
Associated cardiac anomalies
Affecting pulmonary haemodynamics, such as pulmonary stenosis
Affecting pulmonary venous outflow, such as divided left atrium, mitral stenosis, or left ventricular dysfunction
Affecting ventricular function and/or cardiac output
Associated extracardiac anomalies
Including syndromes, chromosomal abnormalities, airway anomalies, metabolic disorders, and so on
NB. A full description of pulmonary haemodynamics at the time of examination and, if available, at early age is recommended, as is a full history regarding interventions and timelines, in order fully to establish the impact of the cardiac malformations on the development of pulmonary arteriopathy

group that cannot be assumed to be similar in terms of clinical decision-making and research [44, 45] (Tables 25.4 and 25.5). The differing morphology (even within specific congenital heart subgroups), previous medical history and intervention and associated co-morbidity result in characteristics that differ markedly. For example, children that present with a small, restrictive left-to-right intracardiac shunt with associated pulmonary hypertension may be able to undergo repair with reversibility of the pulmonary hypertension. The time period after which irreversible pulmonary arterial hypertension occurs varies with the precise malformation. Post-tricuspid non-restrictive shunt lesions result in both increased blood flow to the lungs and increased pulmonary arterial pressure and will commonly result in increased pulmonary arterial hypertension in the first years of life and progression to Eisenmenger's syndrome. Examples are large ventricular septal defect, atrioventricular septal defect and functionally univentricular heart. Shunts may also be at arterial level delivering blood flow and systemic pressure to the pulmonary bed continuously through systole and diastole and hence associated with rapidly progressive increase in pulmonary vascular resistance. Examples are aortopulmonary window, patent ductus arteriosus (Fig. 25.10) and truncus arteriosus (Fig. 25.11). Surgical shunts from the aorta such as Waterston (ascending aorta to right pulmonary artery) and Potts (descending aorta to left pulmonary artery) were difficult to size and if non-restrictive result in significant elevation in

Table 25.5 Schulze-Neick and Beghetti new proposed classification of pulmonary arterial hypertension in the setting of congenitally malformed hearts as based on circulatory pathophysiology

Significant shunting lesions	IPAH-like physiology	PAH due to past or present PVH	Eisenmenger physiology	Fontan-like physiology	Unilateral PAH	Hypoplastic PA system
(a) For corrective surgery, PVR is low and presents no problem	(a) Small unoperated lesion (e.g. POF, ASD, VSD, PAD) not haemodynamically related to PAH	(a) After corrective surgery of pulmonary venous stenosis or aortic/mitral valvular disease or coarctation, with normal wedge pressure and left ventricular function	(a) Classical Eisenmenger physiology: no subpulmonary outflow obstruction; predominantly right-to-left shunting at atrial, ventricular or arterial level; no intraventricular mixing	(a) After Fontan operation with the right atrium being incorporated	(a) Due to a *surgical shunt* previously created to increase pulmonary blood flow which has led to significant PAH on that side	(a) After corrective surgery of tetralogy of Fallot without major anatomical obstructions of the pulmonary vascular system and PAH
(b) For corrective surgery, PVR elevated, risk increased but accepted	(b) Small residue after corrective surgery of a shunting lesion, not haemodynamically related to PAH	(b) PAH due to left ventricular dysfunction with abnormal wedge pressure and increased PVR	(b) Functionally univentricular physiology: no subpulmonary outflow obstruction; systemic desaturation is *due to* intraventricular mixing	(b) Fontan with a lateral or extracardiac conduit, right atrium excluded, *no* fenestration	(b) Due to *congenital origin* of one pulmonary artery or of major collateral vessels from the aorta, causing PAH	(b) After corrective surgery of pulmonary atresia without major anatomical obstructions of the pulmonary vascular system and PAH
(c) For corrective surgery, PVR elevated, risk too high, *not operable*				(c) Anatomy as above under (b), *with* fenestration		

Abbreviations: *ASD* interatrial communication, (*i*)*PAH* (idiopathic) pulmonary arterial hypertension, *PVR* pulmonary vascular resistance, *PA system* pulmonary vascular system, *PAD* persistently patent arterial duct, *POF* patent oval foramen, *PVH* pulmonary venous hypertension, *VSD* ventricular septal defect

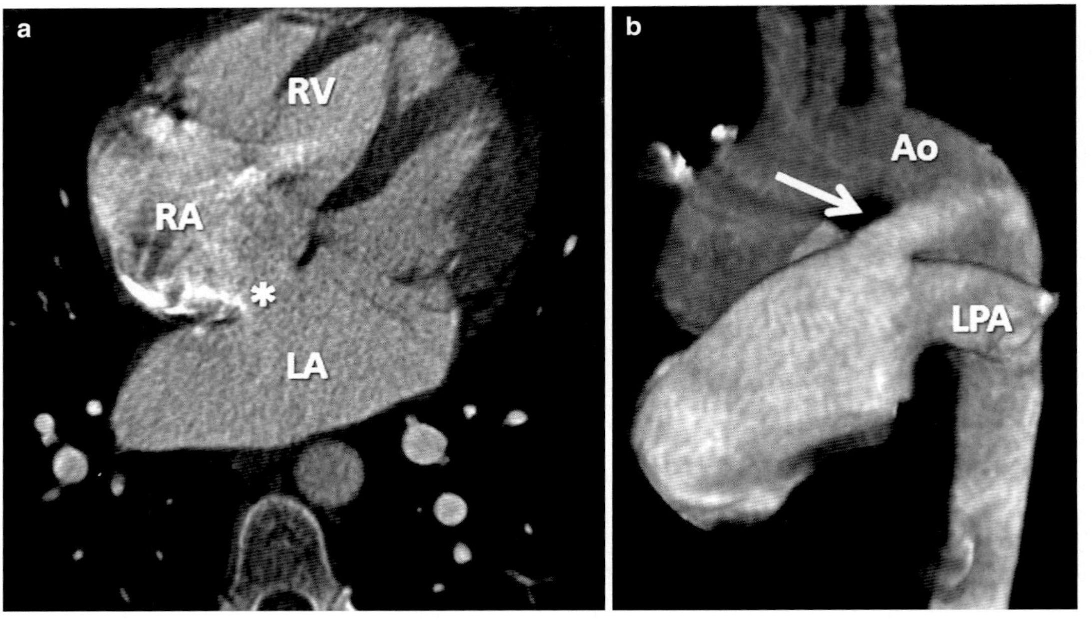

Fig. 25.10 CT demonstration of simple pre-tricuspid or post-tricuspid shunts. The large secundum atrial septal defect (**a**), an example of a simple pre-tricuspid shunt, is marked with an *asterisk*. The right ventricle (*RV*) is enlarged and hypertrophied. A large patent ductus arteriosus (*arrow*), an example of a simple post-tricuspid shunt, is seen between the aorta (*Ao*) and left pulmonary artery (*LPA*) on volume-rendered image (**b**). *LA* left atrium, *RA* right atrium

pulmonary vascular resistance. In contrast, pre-tricuspid lesions result in increased blood flow without increased pulmonary arterial pressure, and pulmonary arterial hypertension develops less frequently and later in the third and fourth decade of life. Examples are anomalous pulmonary venous drainage, sinus venosus defects, secundum atrial septal defects (Fig. 25.10) and common atrium. A late adult presentation of sinus venosus atrial septal defect (Fig. 25.12) or secundum atrial septal defect with associated pulmonary hypertension will likely be suitable to undergo repair with reversibility of any associated pulmonary hypertension.

In combined shunt lesions the combination and the predominant defect should be defined (Fig. 25.13). Further individual variation is explained by the presence of coexisting 'protective' pulmonary stenosis or limited (restrictive) shunt size. Co-morbidity such as the presence of trisomy 21 appears to increase susceptibility to pulmonary arterial hypertension [46]. Schulze-Neick and Beghetti have proposed a cogent classification that allows clear thinking in the assessment of all forms of pulmonary hypertension causing clinical problems in congenital heart disease based on circulatory physiology [45] (Table 25.4). In this classification cyanosis due to intraventricular mixing versus cyanosis due to classical Eisenmenger's physiology with predominant right-to-left shunt at ventricular or arterial level are differentiated.

Fig. 25.12 Known pulmonary hypertension revealed by CMR study to have unexpected congenital heart disease pre-tricuspid cause entirely treatable by surgical repair. Images (**a**, **b**) show *RV* dilatation and hypertrophy. Image (**c**) shows main and right PA dilatation also consistent with pulmonary arterial hypertension. However in addition a RUPV draining to the SVC is notable. In a trans-axial cine (**d**) and sagittal cine (**e**), the underlying sinus venosus ASD is clearly seen (*asterisk*). Image (**f**) is taken from the contrast-enhanced CMR angiogram and demonstrates the RUPV return to the *SVC*. *Ao* aorta, *LA* left atrium, *PA* pulmonary artery, *RA* right atrium, *RUPV* right upper pulmonary vein, *RV* right ventricle, *SVC* superior vena cava

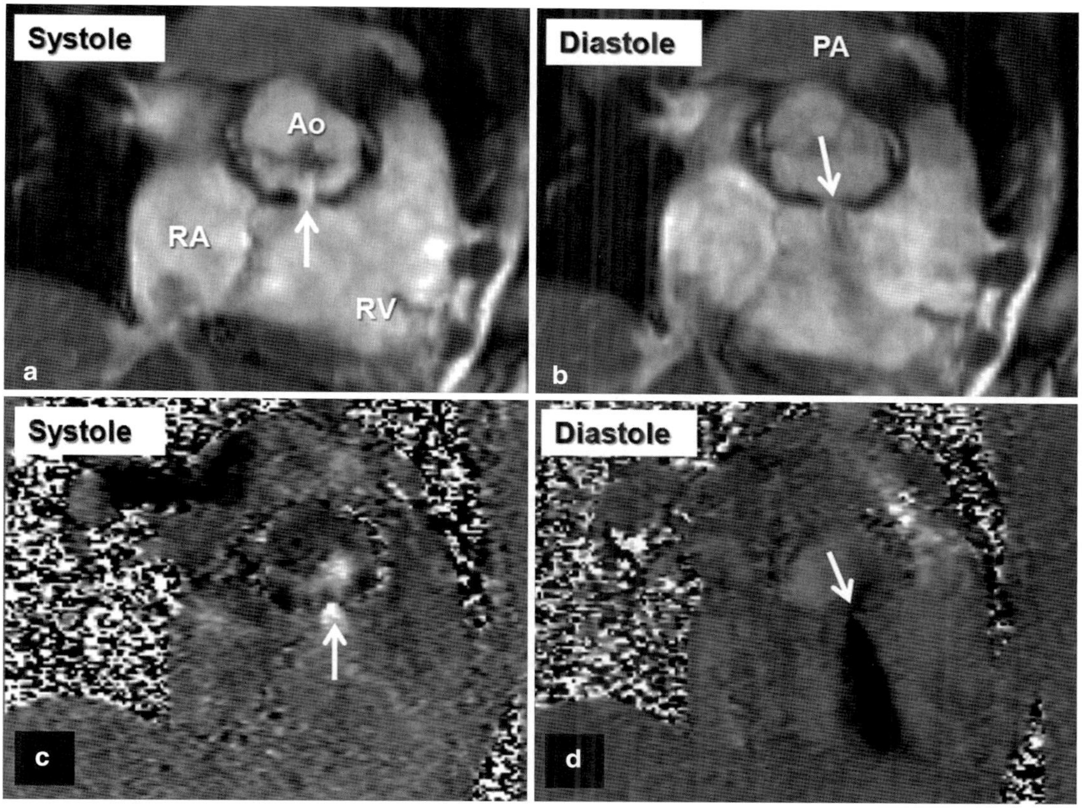

Fig. 25.11 Residual ventricular septal defect (VSD) despite previous truncus arteriosus repair with pulmonary hypertension and bidirectional shunt. Images (**a**, **c**) are in systole and images (**b**, **d**) in diastole. Images (**a**, **b**) are still frames from balanced steady-state free precession cine imaging in a RV oblique view aligned for tricuspid and pulmonary valves and aorta in short axis. Images (**c**, **d**) are corresponding in-plane velocity images. A defect in the VSD patch is *arrowed* highlighting with the direction of the *arrow* that flow is bidirectional, right to left in systole and left to right in diastole. *Ao* aorta, *PA* pulmonary artery, *RA* right atrium, *RV* right ventricle

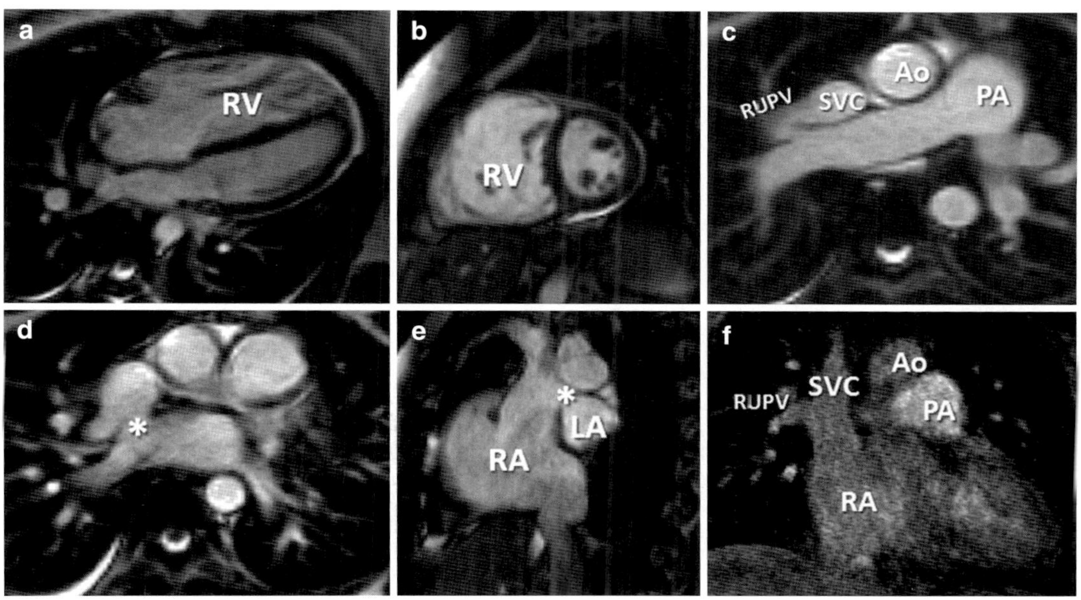

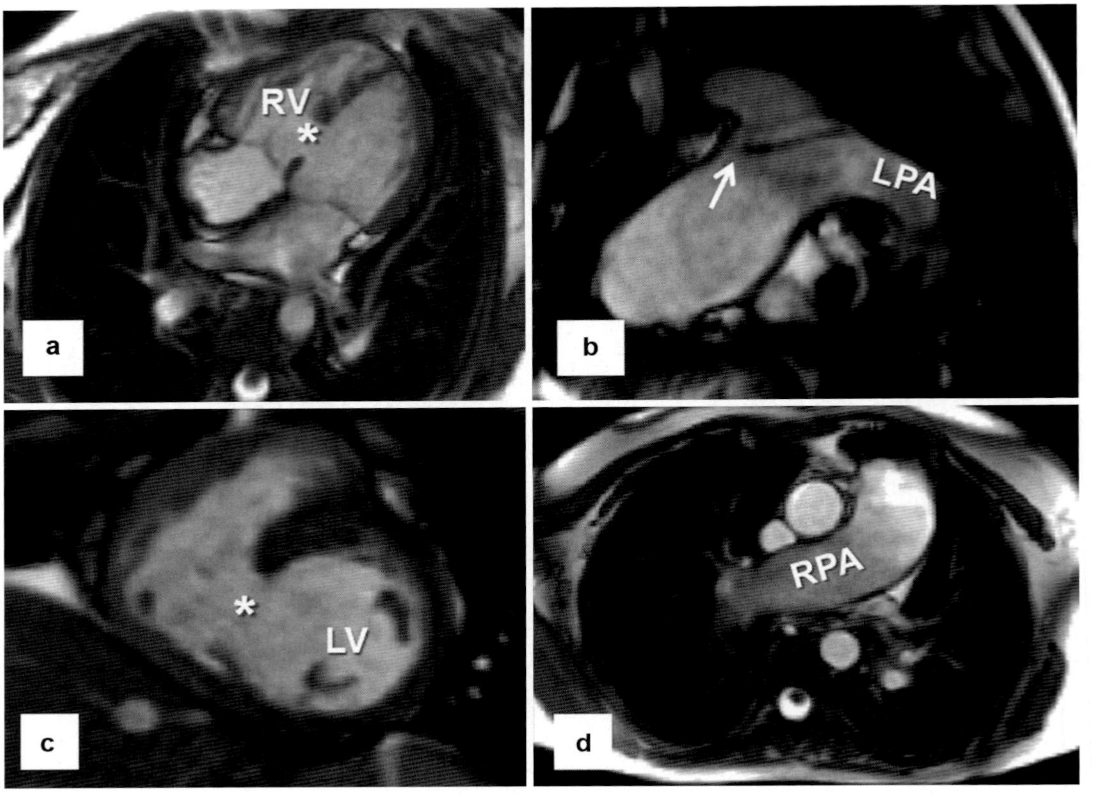

Fig. 25.13 Combined shunt. This patient has a 20 mm unrestrictive muscular VSD with bidirectional predominantly right-to-left shunt which is the predominant lesion (images **a** and **c**, *asterisk*). There is also a PDA measuring 5 mm (**b**, *arrow*). The dilated central pulmonary arteries (**d**) reflect the associated pulmonary arterial hypertension. *LPA* left pulmonary artery, *LV* left ventricle, *RPA* right pulmonary artery, *RV* right ventricle

Acknowledgments William Bradlow and Sonya Babu-Narayan have been or continue to be supported by the British Heart Foundation. This work was supported by the NIHR Cardiovascular Biomedical Research Unit of Royal Brompton & Harefield NHS Foundation Trust and Imperial College London. This report is independent research by the National Institute for Health Research Biomedical Research Unit Funding Scheme. The views expressed in this publication are those of the authors and not necessarily those of the NHS, the National Institute for Health Research or the Department of Health.

References

1. Galie N, Hoeper MM, Humbert M, Torbicki A, Vachiery JL, Barbera JA, Beghetti M, Corris P, Gaine S, Gibbs JS, Gomez-Sanchez MA, Jondeau G, Klepetko W, Opitz C, Peacock A, Rubin L, Zellweger M, Simonneau G. Guidelines for the diagnosis and treatment of pulmonary hypertension: the Task Force for the Diagnosis and Treatment of Pulmonary Hypertension of the European Society of Cardiology (ESC) and the European Respiratory Society (ERS), endorsed by the International Society of Heart and Lung Transplantation (ISHLT). Eur Heart J. 2009;30(20):2493–537.
2. Lowe BS, Therrien J, Ionescu-Ittu R, Pilote L, Martucci G, Marelli AJ. Diagnosis of pulmonary hypertension in the congenital heart disease adult population impact on outcomes. J Am Coll Cardiol. 2011;58(5):538–46.
3. Gatzoulis MA, Alonso-Gonzalez R, Beghetti M. Pulmonary arterial hypertension in paediatric and adult patients with congenital heart disease. Eur Respir Rev. 2009;18(113):154–61.
4. Diller GP, Gatzoulis MA. Pulmonary vascular disease in adults with congenital heart disease. Circulation. 2007;115(8):1039–50.
5. Verheugt CL, Uiterwaal CS, van der Velde ET, Meijboom FJ, Pieper PG, van Dijk AP, Vliegen HW, Grobbee DE, Mulder BJ. Mortality in adult congenital heart disease. Eur Heart J. 2010;31(10):1220–9.
6. Badesch DB, Raskob GE, Elliott CG, Krichman AM, Farber HW, Frost AE, Barst RJ, Benza RL, Liou TG,

Turner M, Giles S, Feldkircher K, Miller DP, McGoon MD. Pulmonary arterial hypertension: baseline characteristics from the REVEAL Registry. Chest. 2010;137(2):376–87.
7. Barst RJ, McGoon MD, Elliott CG, Foreman AJ, Miller DP, Ivy DD. Survival in childhood pulmonary arterial hypertension: insights from the registry to evaluate early and long-term pulmonary arterial hypertension disease management. Circulation. 2012;125(1):113–22.
8. Creager MA, Massie BM, Faxon DP, Friedman SD, Kramer BL, Weiner DA, Ryan TJ, Topic N, Melidossian CD. Acute and long-term effects of enalapril on the cardiovascular response to exercise and exercise tolerance in patients with congestive heart failure. J Am Coll Cardiol. 1985;6(1):163–73.
9. Moledina S, de Bruyn A, Schievano S, Owens CM, Young C, Haworth SG, Taylor AM, Schulze-Neick I, Muthurangu V. Fractal branching quantifies vascular changes and predicts survival in pulmonary hypertension: a proof of principle study. Heart. 2011;97(15):1245–9.
10. Bradlow WM, Hughes ML, Keenan NG, Bucciarelli-Ducci C, Assomull R, Gibbs JS, Mohiaddin RH. Measuring the heart in pulmonary arterial hypertension (PAH): implications for trial study size. J Magn Reson Imaging. 2010;31(1):117–24.
11. Kafka H, Mohiaddin RH. Cardiac MRI and pulmonary MR angiography of sinus venosus defect and partial anomalous pulmonary venous connection in cause of right undiagnosed ventricular enlargement. AJR Am J Roentgenol. 2009;192(1):259–66.
12. McCann GP, Beek AM, Vonk-Noordegraaf A, van Rossum AC. Delayed contrast-enhanced magnetic resonance imaging in pulmonary arterial hypertension. Circulation. 2005;112(16):e268.
13. Blyth KG, Groenning BA, Martin TN, Foster JE, Mark PB, Dargie HJ, Peacock AJ. Contrast enhanced-cardiovascular magnetic resonance imaging in patients with pulmonary hypertension. Eur Heart J. 2005;26(19):1993–9.
14. Bradlow WM, Assomull R, Kilner PJ, Gibbs JS, Sheppard MN, Mohiaddin RH. Understanding late gadolinium enhancement in pulmonary hypertension. Circ Cardiovasc Imaging. 2010;3(4):501–3.
15. Bradlow WM, Gibbs JS, Mohiaddin RH. Cardiovascular magnetic resonance in pulmonary hypertension. J Cardiovasc Magn Reson. 2012;14:6.
16. Fox CC, Hutchins GM. The architecture of the human ventricular myocardium. Johns Hopkins Med J. 1972;130(5):289–99.
17. Saba TS, Foster J, Cockburn M, Cowan M, Peacock AJ. Ventricular mass index using magnetic resonance imaging accurately estimates pulmonary artery pressure. Eur Respir J. 2002;20(6):1519–24.
18. Roeleveld RJ, Marcus JT, Faes TJ, Gan TJ, Boonstra A, Postmus PE, Vonk-Noordegraaf A. Interventricular septal configuration at mr imaging and pulmonary arterial pressure in pulmonary hypertension. Radiology. 2005;234(3):710–7.
19. Bradlow WM, Gatehouse PD, Hughes RL, O'Brien AB, Gibbs JS, Firmin DN, Mohiaddin RH. Assessing normal pulse wave velocity in the proximal pulmonary arteries using transit time: a feasibility, repeatability, and observer reproducibility study by cardiovascular magnetic resonance. J Magn Reson Imaging. 2007;25(5):974–81.
20. Reiter G, Reiter U, Kovacs G, Kainz B, Schmidt K, Maier R, Olschewski H, Rienmueller R. Magnetic resonance-derived 3-dimensional blood flow patterns in the main pulmonary artery as a marker of pulmonary hypertension and a measure of elevated mean pulmonary arterial pressure. Circ Cardiovasc Imaging. 2008;1(1):23–30.
21. Roeleveld RJ, Marcus JT, Boonstra A, Postmus PE, Marques KM, Bronzwaer JG, Vonk-Noordegraaf A. A comparison of noninvasive MRI-based methods of estimating pulmonary artery pressure in pulmonary hypertension. J Magn Reson Imaging. 2005;22(1):67–72.
22. Muthurangu V, Taylor A, Andriantsimiavona R, Hegde S, Miquel ME, Tulloh R, Baker E, Hill DL, Razavi RS. Novel method of quantifying pulmonary vascular resistance by use of simultaneous invasive pressure monitoring and phase-contrast magnetic resonance flow. Circulation. 2004;110(7):826–34.
23. Bell A, Beerbaum P, Greil G, Hegde S, Toschke AM, Schaeffter T, Razavi R. Noninvasive assessment of pulmonary artery flow and resistance by cardiac magnetic resonance in congenital heart diseases with unrestricted left-to-right shunt. JACC Cardiovasc Imaging. 2009;2(11):1285–91.
24. Macchia A, Marchioli R, Marfisi R, Scarano M, Levantesi G, Tavazzi L, Tognoni G. A meta-analysis of trials of pulmonary hypertension: a clinical condition looking for drugs and research methodology. Am Heart J. 2007;153(6):1037–47.
25. Savarese G, Paolillo S, Costanzo P, D'Amore C, Cecere M, Losco T, Musella F, Gargiulo P, Marciano C, Perrone-Filardi P. Do changes of 6-minute walk distance predict clinical events in patients with pulmonary arterial hypertension?: a meta-analysis of 22 randomized trials. J Am Coll Cardiol. 2012;60(13):1192–201.
26. Wilkins MR, Paul GA, Strange JW, Tunariu N, Gin-Sing W, Banya WA, Westwood MA, Stefanidis A, Ng LL, Pennell DJ, Mohiaddin RH, Nihoyannopoulos P, Gibbs JS. Sildenafil versus Endothelin Receptor Antagonist for Pulmonary Hypertension (SERAPH) study. Am J Respir Crit Care Med. 2005;171(11):1292–7.
27. Wilkins MR, Ali O, Bradlow W, Wharton J, Taegtmeyer A, Rhodes CJ, Ghofrani HA, Howard L, Nihoyannopoulos P, Mohiaddin RH, Gibbs JS, The Sipht Study G. Simvastatin as a treatment for pulmonary hypertension trial (SiPHT). Am J Respir Crit Care Med. 2010;181(10):1106–13.
28. van Wolferen SA, Marcus JT, Boonstra A, Marques KM, Bronzwaer JG, Spreeuwenberg MD, Postmus PE, Vonk-Noordegraaf A. Prognostic value of right ventricular mass, volume, and function in idiopathic pulmonary arterial hypertension. Eur Heart J. 2007;28(10):1250–7.

29. van de Veerdonk MC, Kind T, Marcus JT, Mauritz GJ, Heymans MW, Bogaard HJ, Boonstra A, Marques KM, Westerhof N, Vonk-Noordegraaf A. Progressive right ventricular dysfunction in patients with pulmonary arterial hypertension responding to therapy. J Am Coll Cardiol. 2011;58(24):2511–9.
30. Dogan OF, Karcaaltincaba M, Yorgancioglu C, Demircin M, Dogan R, Ersoy U, Celiker A, Alehan D, Haliloglu M, Boke E. Demonstration of coronary arteries and major cardiac vascular structures in congenital heart disease by cardiac multidetector computed tomography angiography. Heart Surg Forum. 2007;10(1):E90–4.
31. Eisenmenger V. Die angeborenen Defecte der Kammerscheidewand des Herzens. Z Klin Med. 1897;32:1–28.
32. Wood P. The Eisenmenger syndrome or pulmonary hypertension with reversed central shunt. I. Br Med J. 1958;2(5098):701–9.
33. Wood P. The Eisenmenger syndrome or pulmonary hypertension with reversed central shunt. Br Med J. 1958;2(5099):755–62.
34. Saha A, Balakrishnan KG, Jaiswal PK, Venkitachalam CG, Tharakan J, Titus T, Kutty R. Prognosis for patients with Eisenmenger syndrome of various aetiology. Int J Cardiol. 1994;45(3):199–207.
35. Diller GP, Dimopoulos K, Okonko D, Li W, Babu-Narayan SV, Broberg CS, Johansson B, Bouzas B, Mullen MJ, Poole-Wilson PA, Francis DP, Gatzoulis MA. Exercise intolerance in adult congenital heart disease: comparative severity, correlates, and prognostic implication. Circulation. 2005;112(6):828–35.
36. Cantor WJ, Harrison DA, Moussadji JS, Connelly MS, Webb GD, Liu P, McLaughlin PR, Siu SC. Determinants of survival and length of survival in adults with Eisenmenger syndrome. Am J Cardiol. 1999;84(6):677–81.
37. Hopkins WE, Ochoa LL, Richardson GW, Trulock EP. Comparison of the hemodynamics and survival of adults with severe primary pulmonary hypertension or Eisenmenger syndrome. J Heart Lung Transplant. 1996;15(1 Pt 1):100–5.
38. Daliento L, Somerville J, Presbitero P, Menti L, Brach-Prever S, Rizzoli G, Stone S. Eisenmenger syndrome. Factors relating to deterioration and death. Eur Heart J. 1998;19(12):1845–55.
39. Gatzoulis MA, Beghetti M, Galie N, Granton J, Berger RM, Lauer A, Chiossi E, Landzberg M. Longer-term bosentan therapy improves functional capacity in Eisenmenger syndrome: results of the BREATHE-5 open-label extension study. Int J Cardiol. 2008;127(1):27–32.
40. Mukhopadhyay S, Sharma M, Ramakrishnan S, Yusuf J, Gupta MD, Bhamri N, Trehan V, Tyagi S. Phosphodiesterase-5 inhibitor in Eisenmenger syndrome: a preliminary observational study. Circulation. 2006;114(17):1807–10.
41. Broberg C, Ujita M, Babu-Narayan S, Rubens M, Prasad SK, Gibbs JS, Gatzoulis MA. Massive pulmonary artery thrombosis with haemoptysis in adults with Eisenmenger's syndrome: a clinical dilemma. Heart. 2004;90(11):e63.
42. Broberg CS, Ujita M, Prasad S, Li W, Rubens M, Bax BE, Davidson SJ, Bouzas B, Gibbs JS, Burman J, Gatzoulis MA. Pulmonary arterial thrombosis in eisenmenger syndrome is associated with biventricular dysfunction and decreased pulmonary flow velocity. J Am Coll Cardiol. 2007;50(7):634–42.
43. Moceri P, Dimopoulos K, Liodakis E, Germanakis I, Kempny A, Diller GP, Swan L, Wort SJ, Marino PS, Gatzoulis MA, Li W. Echocardiographic predictors of outcome in eisenmenger syndrome. Circulation. 2012;126(12):1461–8.
44. van Albada ME, Berger RM. Pulmonary arterial hypertension in congenital cardiac disease–the need for refinement of the Evian-Venice classification. Cardiol Young. 2008;18(1):10–7.
45. Schulze-Neick I, Beghetti M. Classifying pulmonary hypertension in the setting of the congenitally malformed heart–cleaning up a dog's dinner. Cardiol Young. 2008;18(1):22–5.
46. Yamaki S, Horiuchi T, Sekino Y. Quantitative analysis of pulmonary vascular disease in simple cardiac anomalies with the Down syndrome. Am J Cardiol. 1983;51(9):1502–6.

Congenital Thoracic Venous Anomalies

26

Farhood Saremi

Congenital abnormalities of the major mediastinal venous structures occur in less than 2 % of people who have no other abnormalities [1–6]. Although many congenital anomalies have been described, three occur with sufficient frequency that they will be encountered in routine clinical practice: azygos or hemiazygos continuation of an interrupted inferior vena cava (IVC), persistence of a left superior vena cava (SVC) with and without a coexisting right SVC, and partial anomalous pulmonary venous return (PAPVR). Although they may occur in adults who have no other abnormalities, these three abnormalities also may be associated with a wide variety of vascular anomalies and cardiac defects [1–6]. Classifications of systemic and pulmonary venous anomalies are shown in Tables 26.1 and 26.2.

Imaging Techniques

Thoracic venous anomalies may not be diagnosed until adulthood. The decision to perform surgical correction relies on preoperative knowledge of the systemic or pulmonary venous anatomy, associated cardiac anomalies, and the magnitude of the left-to-right or right-to-left shunts. Multiple complementary diagnostic tests are usually necessary in order to obtain complete anatomic and functional data. Although echocardiography has

Table 26.1 Classification of systemic venous anomalies

Anomalies of SVC
Persistent left SVC (connection to coronary sinus)
Persistent left SVC with unroofed coronary sinus
Persistent left SVC connecting to left atrium
Absent right SVC with persistent left SVC
Right SVC connecting to left atrium
Aberrant right atrial insertion
Aneurysm
Absent both SVC with azygos continuation of IVC
Anomalies of IVC
Azygos continuation to SVC
Hemiazygos continuation to left SVC
Connection to left atrium
Connection to coronary sinus
Aberrant right atrial insertion
Situs inversus
Miscellaneous thoracic venous disorders
Absent left brachiocephalic vein with venous return via (LSICV)
Anomalous courses (subaortic) of the left brachiocephalic vein
Anomalous hepatic venous connection to right atrium
Anomalous hepatic venous connection to coronary sinus
Absent azygos vein
Common associated anomalies
Heterotaxy syndrome, TOF

IVC inferior vena cava, *LSICV* left superior intercostal vein, *SVC* superior vena cava, *TOF* tetralogy of Fallot

F. Saremi, MD
Department of Radiology, Cardiothoracic Section,
University of Southern California,
USC Keck Hospital, 1500 San Pablo St.,
Los Angeles, CA 90033, USA
e-mail: fsaremi@usc.edu

F. Saremi (ed.), *Cardiac CT and MR for Adult Congenital Heart Disease*,
DOI 10.1007/978-1-4614-8875-0_26, © Springer Science+Business Media New York 2014

Table 26.2 Classification of pulmonary venous anomalies

Anatomical variant in connection or course: common trunk, supernumerary vein, meandering pulmonary vein
Intrinsic abnormality: stenosis, hypoplasia, atresia, aneurysm (varix)
Partial anomalous pulmonary venous return
Right pulmonary veins: SVC, right atrium, both, IVC (scimitar), azygos vein
Left pulmonary veins: left brachiocephalic vein (left vertical vein), coronary sinus
Partial bilateral
Total anomalous pulmonary venous return
Supracardiac: left brachiocephalic vein, right SVC, azygos vein
Cardiac: coronary sinus, right atrium
Infracardiac: portal vein or tributary, ductus venosus, IVC, left gastric vein
Associated anomalies
Pulmonary: bronchopulmonary sequestration, AVM, congenital cystic adenomatoid malformation
Common cardiac: cor triatriatum

AVM arteriovenous malformation, *IVC* inferior vena cava, *SVC* superior vena cava

a variety of diagnostic strengths especially in the evaluation of many congenital heart disease in children, it can be suboptimal for comprehensive assessment of thoracic venous anomalies. With magnetic resonance imaging (MRI) or computed tomography (CT), detailed anatomic information regarding the number, origin, course, and drainage of all thoracic veins and their relationships to cardiac and extracardiac structures can be easily obtained. They provide volumetric data that are essential for diagnosis and therapeutic planning [7–11]. Associated great vessels and intracardiac anomalies can also be evaluated. Both modalities are useful postoperatively and facilitate the evaluation of patency, anastomotic narrowing, right ventricular systolic function, and residual abnormal communications.

CT provides rapid acquisition of data with high spatial resolution and a wide anatomic coverage. Isotropic multiplanar reformatting and volume rendering reconstruction capabilities both excellently depict anomalous pulmonary venous structures [7]. The primary disadvantage of CT is that it requires the use of ionizing radiation. Using high pitch modes and iterative reconstruction methods radiation dose can significantly be reduced. Major advantages of MRI are the lack of ionizing radiation and the power for dynamic imaging and function analysis with or without contrast. However, when compared with CT angiography, high-quality MRI capabilities are not nearly as widely available and currently do not offer a comparable level of spatial resolution, and susceptibility artifacts can be problematic. In patients with a cardiac pacemaker or claustrophobia, CT may be a better choice.

In both CT and MR angiographies, timing of the intravenous contrast material bolus is critical because a suboptimally timed bolus may limit opacification of targeted venous structures. In a patient with left-sided SVC, a left arm approach may be the preferred route of injection. In postoperative patients with bidirectional cavopulmonary shunts and azygos continuation of IVC, it may be necessary to perform a dual injection method using both arms or one arm and one lower extremity injections simultaneously.

Regarding CT technique, the narrowest allowable beam collimation should be used to produce isotropic reformatted and 3-dimensional volume-rendered images. Most scanners have the capability of 0.5 mm collimation that can easily provide an isotropic resolution of 0.5 mm in a 25-cm field of view. Nonionic low-osmolality (or iso-osmolality) iodinated contrast material (1–1.5 mL/kg, 80–120 mL volume) is typically administered intravenously using a power injector at injection rates of 3–5 mL/s, depending on quality of venous access. In the evaluation of systemic venous anatomy, diluted contrast (30–50 %) without bolus triggering is the preferred method of injection. The scan can be started immediately after contrast injection or with a few seconds delay depending on "scan start delay" timing specific to the machine used. Bolus triggering generally delays scan initiation for an additional 5–7 s. Without triggering this can be reduced to 2–3 s delay. For pulmonary vein anatomy, anomalous pulmonary venous drainage, and cor triatriatum, the timing of imaging after the injection of contrast material may be precisely determined using either a timing bolus or real-time contrast material tracking. In general the CT technique for evaluation of the pulmonary veins is very similar to coronary CT angiography. In our institution we prefer to start scan with contrast arrival in the descending thoracic aorta below the level of tracheal bifurcation using a 180 Hounsfield unit trigger threshold. Generally, cardiac gating is not required for the evaluation of systemic or pulmonary venous structures, although it may prove useful if the patient is being specifically evaluated for cor triatriatum, associated intracardiac lesions, or central pulmonary vein hypoplasia/stenosis.

MRI is the preferred imaging technique for noncontrast imaging of venous system, flow quantification, and functional analysis [11–13]. Not only can MRI detect the extracardiac anomalous vessels, it can also clearly delineate the intracardiac anatomy (i.e., sinus venosus defect). Furthermore, velocity flow mapping allows accurate assessment of the Qp/Qs without the need for or the risk associated with cardiac catheterization. The thoracic venous system can be evaluated using a variety of MRI techniques. Images are ideally acquired using a dedicated phased-array cardiac coil. Both black blood and bright blood images may be obtained without intravenous contrast material. High-resolution double-inversion recovery fast spin-echo (black blood) images are typically acquired in axial, coronal, and sagittal directions to assess anatomy. Fast gradient echo and balanced steady-state free precession (b-SSFP) pulse sequences provide bright blood cine images that are useful for the venous stenosis, thrombosis, or anomalies. These sequences can be applied using 2-dimensional (2D) or 3D modes without and with ECG gating. The use of contrast-enhanced MR angiography in patients with anomalous thoracic veins has been advocated as a way to improve diagnosis and reduce the patient's time in the scanner. However, recent concerns about complications associated with gadolinium contrast agents have led to using other imaging techniques that do not require the administration of gadolinium contrast. Noncontrast respiratory-triggered ECG-gated free-breathing T2-prepped 3D b-SSFP pulse sequences allow the acquisition of a near-isotropic volumetric dataset (1.5 mm^3) that can be reformatted and reviewed in any plane [14]. For respiratory triggering a navigator pulse with a 5-mm acceptance window is placed over the right hemidiaphragm. A large (40 cm) field of view permits imaging of the entire chest. To reduce the sensitivity of SSFP to field inhomogeneities, which can be problematic for large field-of-view imaging, a nonselective radio frequency excitation is used to shorten the repetition time. Unenhanced MR angiography using this technique is shown to be as accurate as contrast-enhanced MR angiography for showing pulmonary veins [14]. The SSFP technique also permits evaluation of the extravascular pathologies.

For contrast-enhanced MR angiography, a non-ECG-gated 3D fast gradient is usually used [15, 16]. Gadolinium-based contrast material may be either injected by hand or power-injected at 3–4 mL/s using a double dose (0.20 mmol/kg). Depending on the desired anatomical coverage, large field-of-view 1.5–2 mm oblique coronal or sagittal images (i.e., imaging slab of 60–80 mm are partitioned into 40 slices) can be acquired using two or three sequential breath holds or during quiet breathing (Fig. 26.1). A delay of 5 s can be used for the systemic vein evaluation and 15–20 s for the pulmonary veins. Newer dynamic, time-resolved 3D MRA sequences using high-performance gradients obviate the need for a timing strategy. Because a complete 3D MRA dataset can be acquired in 4–7 s, several sequential acquisitions can be obtained immediately following contrast injection. Subsequently, the best quality dataset is selected for image analysis. Although reviewing the individual source images is important, these images are typically reformatted in multiple planes as well as reconstructed as either maximum-intensity-projection (MIP) or volume-rendered images [17].

In addition to anatomy, MRI can be used to detect and measure shunts in a patient with anomalous venous return [13, 18, 19]. Classically the oximetry with cardiac catheterization remains the most widely accepted clinical standard for the QP/QS measurement. However, very small shunts, especially at the atrial level, are hardly assessed by the currently used oximetric technique, because of the pO_2 right chamber variability observed even in normal subjects without left-to-right shunt [20]. On the other side the accuracy of MRI QP/QS assessment in vitro and in vivo has

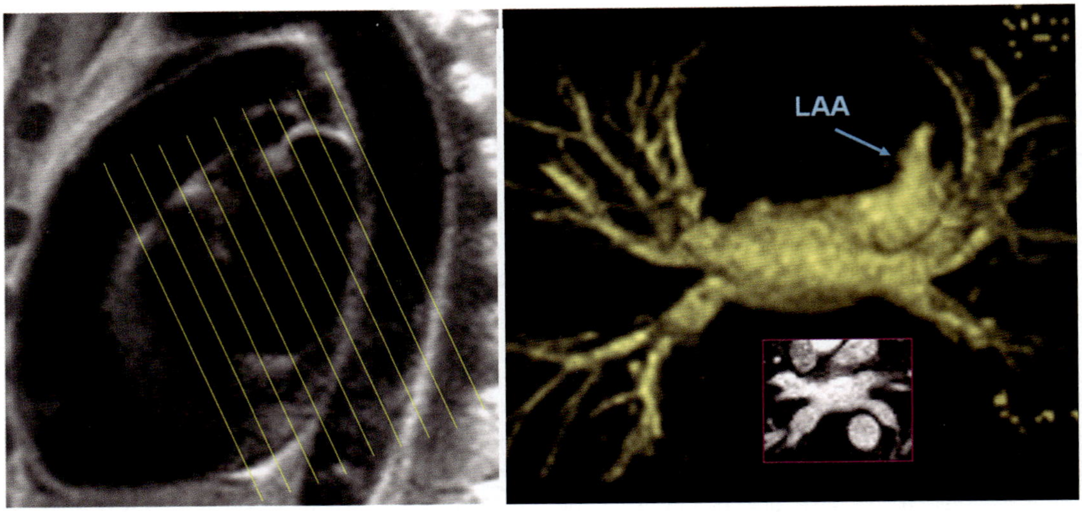

Fig. 26.1 MR angiography technique for the left atrium and pulmonary veins. Using a sagittal reference, oblique coronal partitions will be obtained parallel to the short axis of the heart. An anteroposterior angle (approximately 20°) brings the plane of 3-dimensional dataset parallel to the long axis the pulmonary veins. *LAA* left atrial appendage

already been demonstrated [18]. Phase-contrast MRI flow measurements have been shown more reproducible and tended to correlate better with defect area than oximetry calculations.

Systemic Venous Anomalies

Embryology

Systemic venous anomalies of the thorax are the result of complex variations in the persistence and regression of segments of three pairs of venous channels during the first 4 weeks of fetal development. All these three venous channels drain into the sinus venosus: the omphalomesenteric (vitelline) veins, carrying blood from the yolk sac; the umbilical vein, originating in the chorionic villi and carrying oxygenated blood from placenta; and the common cardinal veins (ducts of Cuvier), draining the body of the embryo.

The right and left common cardinal veins are formed by the confluence of the anterior and posterior cardinal veins [1, 21, 22] (Fig. 26.2). The anterior cardinal vein drains the cephalic portion of the embryo, and the posterior cardinal vein drains the remainder of its body. The left vitelline and cardinal veins regress during embryogenesis. The right vitelline vein forms hepatic segment of the IVC (hepatocardiac channel). The right horn of the sinus venosus and the right common cardinal vein will be developed and eventually form the posterior wall of the right atrium (RA) and the SVC, respectively. The left horn of the sinus venosus, in conjunction with the regressing left common cardinal vein, forms the coronary sinus (CS) and the ligament or vein of the left atrium (Marshall) (Fig. 26.2). A bridging venous plexus forms between the right and left anterior cardinal veins around 24 mm crown-rump embryonic stage and develops to be the left brachiocephalic vein [23]. The left anterior cardinal vein below this connection gradually obliterates. Its upper portion remains as part of the left superior intercostal vein (SICV). The right anterior and common cardinal veins persist and form the SVC.

The right sinus valve persists as the valve of the IVC (eustachian valve) and the valve of the coronary sinus (thebesian valve) [24]. A double SVC is the result of persistence of the left anterior cardinal vein. If, in addition, the normally persistent right cardinal vein regresses, then there is only one SVC on left. In the normal atrial situs, persistence of the left anterior cardinal vein connected to the left atrium (LA) is an infrequent occurrence, this vein usually draining into the

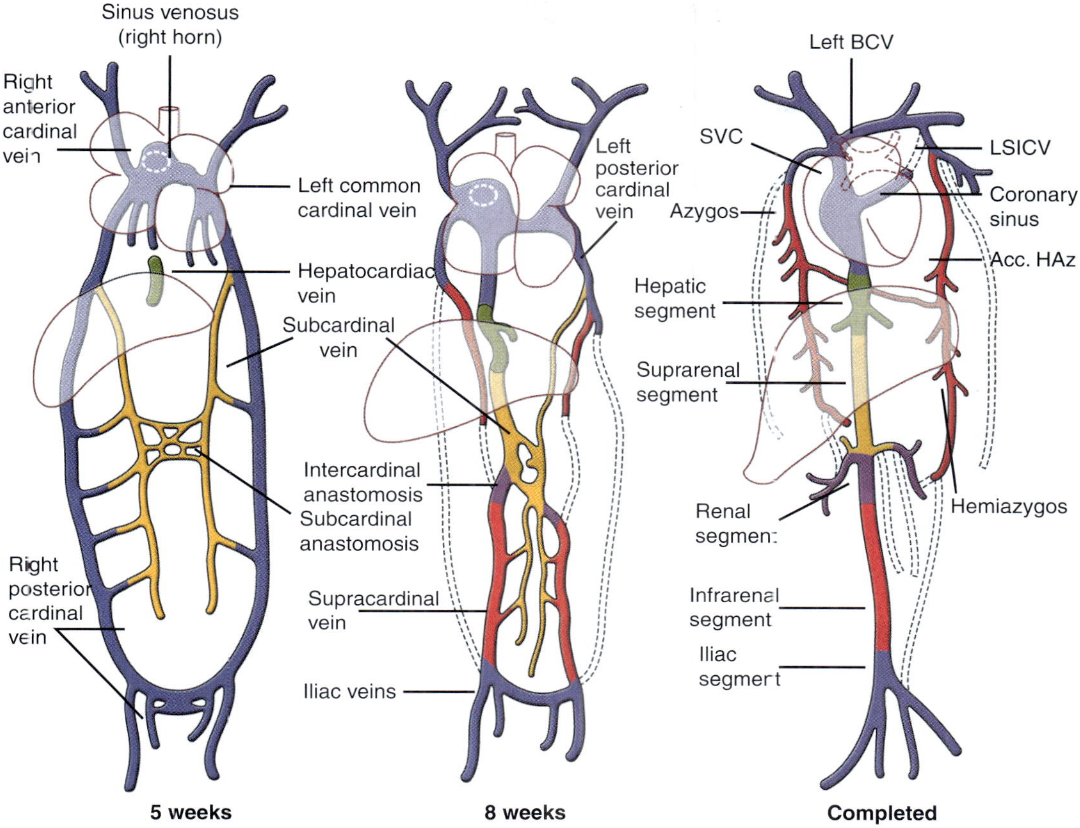

Fig. 26.2 Development of the cardinal veins. The relative relationship and the timing of development of the structures in cartoons are speculative. Anterior views. *Acc* accessory, *BCV* brachiocephalic vein, *HAZ* hemiazygos, *LSICV* left superior intercostal vein, *SVC* superior vena cava

RA via the coronary sinus. In atrial isomerism, conversely, the left anterior cardinal vein usually persists, draining either into the roof of the left-sided atrium (mainly in right atrial isomerism) or into the CS (usually in left atrial isomerism).

Anomalies of the Right SVC

The SVC starts at the confluence of the right and left brachiocephalic veins. It travels 5–7 cm on the right anterior aspect of the upper mediastinum from the level of first sternocostal junction to the superior cavoatrial junction. At the junction with the RA, the SVC is located posterolateral to the ascending aorta, anterior to the right pulmonary artery, and anteromedial to the right superior pulmonary vein (Fig. 26.3). Isolated anomalies of the right SVC are rare [25]. Anomalous low insertion of the right SVC into the right atrium can be seen as an isolated anomaly. Anomalous high insertion of IVC can be seen in congenital heart diseases (CHD). A case of cyanotic CHD with left ventricular hypertrophy described that cardiac catheterization showed a right SVC draining into the left atrium without other cardiovascular abnormality [26]. Congenital aneurysmal dilatation of the SVC may be mistaken with a mass [27] (Fig. 26.4). It may involve the SVC only or multiple veins in the upper mediastinum (Fig. 26.5). This anomaly is usually an incidental finding but has been associated with thrombosis leading to embolization and SVC obstruction [28]. Congenital aneurysmal dilatation can be associated with cystic hygromas [29]. Agenesis of the SVC with two brachiocephalic veins draining separately is also reported without intracardiac malformations [30].

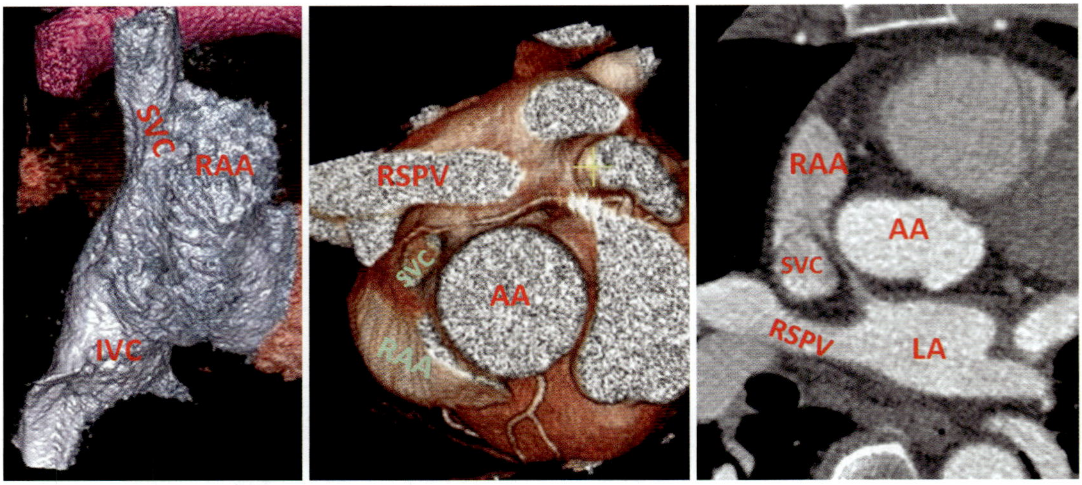

Fig. 26.3 Anatomy of the superior and inferior cavoatrial junctions. Relationship of the superior vena cava (*SVC*) with the right superior pulmonary vein (*RSPV*) and the ascending aorta (*AA*) is shown. Note the SVC connects to posteromedial aspect of the right atrial appendage (*RAA*). *LA* left atrium

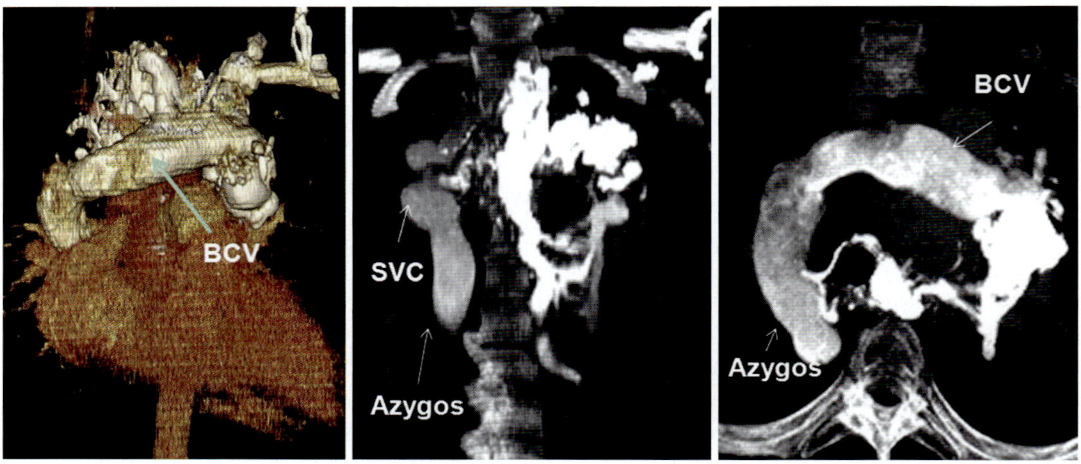

Fig. 26.4 Varicoid veins of upper mediastinum mainly involving the left brachiocephalic vein (*BCV*), azygos system, and superior vena cava (*SVC*) above the confluence with the azygos

Left SVC

The left SVC is the most common anomalous systemic vein drainage in the thorax, incidentally found in one out of 200 (0.5 %) of CT or MRI studies of chest. In patients with congenital heart malformation, it is more common and may be seen in 5–10 % of patients [1, 31–33]. Isolated left SVC is less common than duplicated SVC. Similar to PAVR of the left upper lobe, it results from failure of parts of the left anterior and common cardinal veins to regress. The left SVC drains the tributaries of the left subclavian and jugular veins into the CS via the oblique vein of the left atrium (vein of Marshall). The LSIV becomes a tributary of the left LVC in 20 % of cases and may connect it to the accessory hemiazygos, analogous to the azygos arch on the right that connects the right SVC to the azygos vein (Fig. 26.6). In 80–90 % of patients, the left and right SVCs coexist, although the left is usually smaller especially when the left brachiocephalic vein bridges the two veins (Fig. 26.7). In about 40–60 % of cases, the left brachiocephalic vein connecting the two SVCs is absent [31, 34].

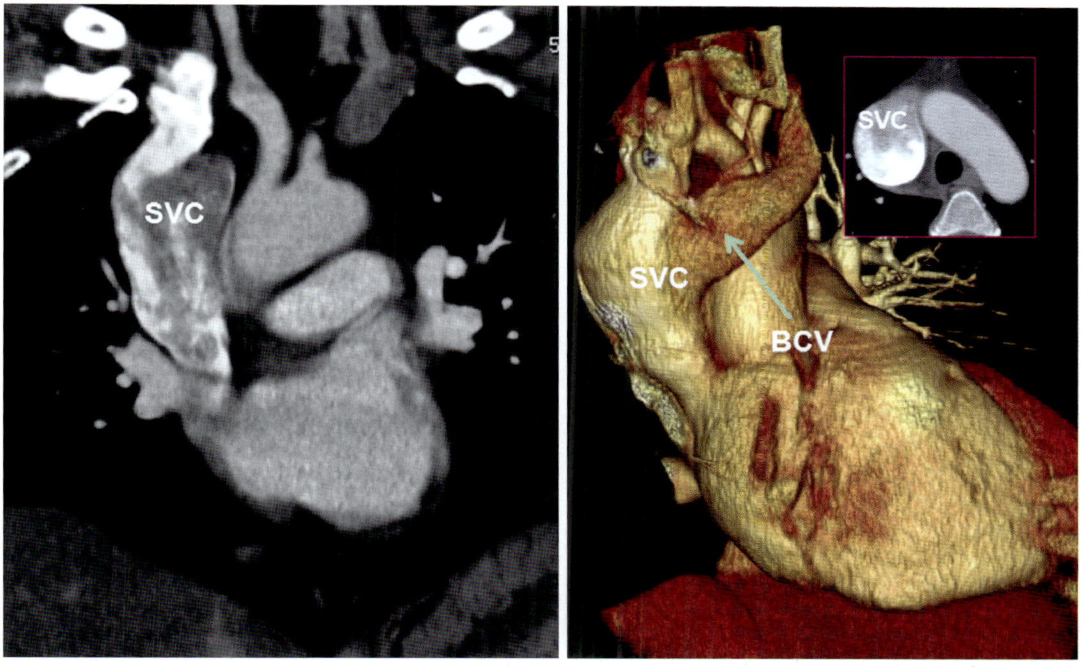

Fig. 26.5 Superior vena cava (*SVC*) aneurysm above the confluence with the azygos vein. The azygos vein was normal sized. The left brachiocephalic vein (*BVC*) is mildly enlarged. The patient referred to CT for possible mass seen on chest X-ray

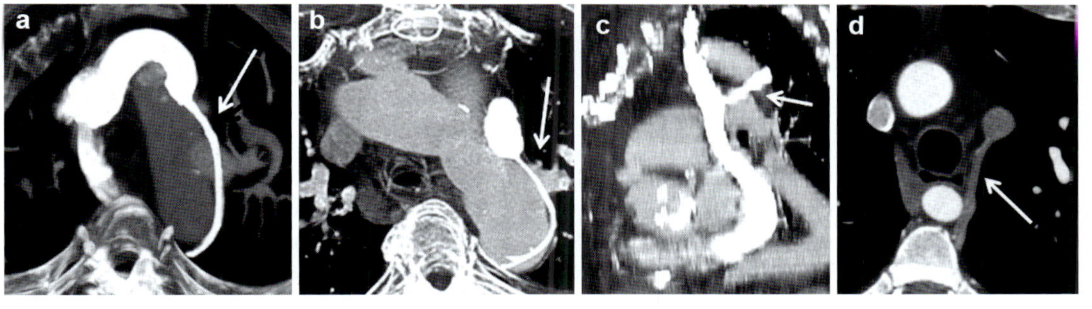

Fig. 26.6 Different patterns of left superior intercostal vein (LSICV) (*arrows*). (**a**) Normal with right superior vena cava (SVC) only. (**b**) Duplicated SVC and small LSICV. (**c**) Left SVC with large LSICV. (**d**) Duplicated SVC with LSICV entering left and the azygos entering right SVC. *SVC* superior vena cava

In this situation the left SVC is larger (Fig. 26.8). In persistent left SVC, especially isolated left SVC, the incidence of CHD increases including atrial septal defect (ASD), tetralogy of Fallot, heterotaxy, coarctation of aorta , pulmonary atresia or stenosis, cor triatriatum, atrioventricular septal defects, double-outlet right ventricle, and anomalous pulmonary venous drainage [1, 35] (Fig. 26.9).

The left SVC descends lateral to the aortic arch and anterior to the hilum, enters the pericardium in the posterior atrioventricular groove, and in almost all cases drains into the CS (90 %) with no significant hemodynamic effects (Figs. 26.8 and 26.10). The CS is large especially when the brachiocephalic vein is absent and will be heavily opacified in CT or MR angiographies when contrast is injected in the left arm. Rarely (8 %), the drainage of the left SVC is not into the CS, but instead into the left atrium or left superior pulmonary vein. In these

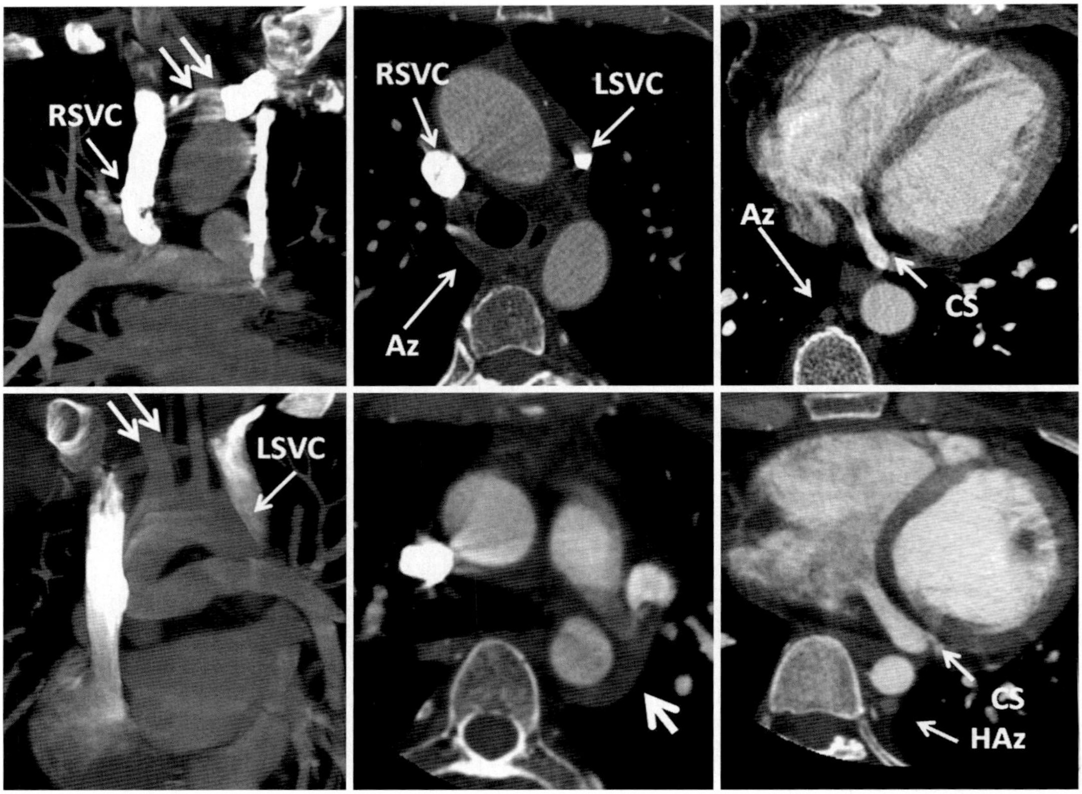

Fig. 26.7 Double superior vena cava (SVC) system connecting through a normal brachiocephalic vein (*double arrow*) in two different patients. The left SVC (*LSVC*) drains into a normal-sized coronary sinus (*CS*) in both cases. In the first case (*upper row*), azygos vein (*Az*) connects to the right SVC (*RSVC*). In the second case (*lower row*), the azygos vein is absent but the hemiazygos (*HAz*) connects to the LSVC by the left superior intercostal vein (*large arrow*)

cases as well, the incidence of CHD increases (Fig. 26.11). Isolated connection of the left SVC to the left atrial roof is very rare [36–38]. Patients with an isolated left SVC draining into the left atrium usually have a right-to-left shunt, unless there is a big bridging vein between the two SVCs, which may allow a left-to-right shunt, instead. Usually, the left SVC draining into the left atrium causes mild cyanosis and polycythemia. Patients are minimally symptomatic or asymptomatic. Cardiac examination, chest X-ray, and electrocardiogram are usually normal. As a result, these rare cases are often an incidental finding during other diagnostic exams [36]. A major complication of this form of hidden right-to-left shunt would be paradoxical embolism with complication such as cryptogenic stroke (Fig. 26.11). Similar situation can occur in cases of left SVC with an unroofed CS especially if the CS ostium to the right atrium is atretic. The anomalies can also interfere with catheterization and may cause difficulty placing a cardiac pacer or defibrillator leads when a left arm approach is used. During the development of the embryo, the left SVC draining into the CS causes an enlargement of this vessel and dissolution of the wall of the CS adjacent to the LA causing either a coronary sinus–left atrium fenestration (unroofing) or an interatrial communication through the mouth of the CS (coronary sinus type ASD) [39]. Therefore, unroofed CS is mostly associated with a left SVC, with or without a connection between both the two SVCs. The diagnosis of this lesion is important to the prognosis of the patient because of the consequences of brain abscess or cerebral emboli that may result from a right-to-left shunt [40, 41]. Injection of contrast in the arm

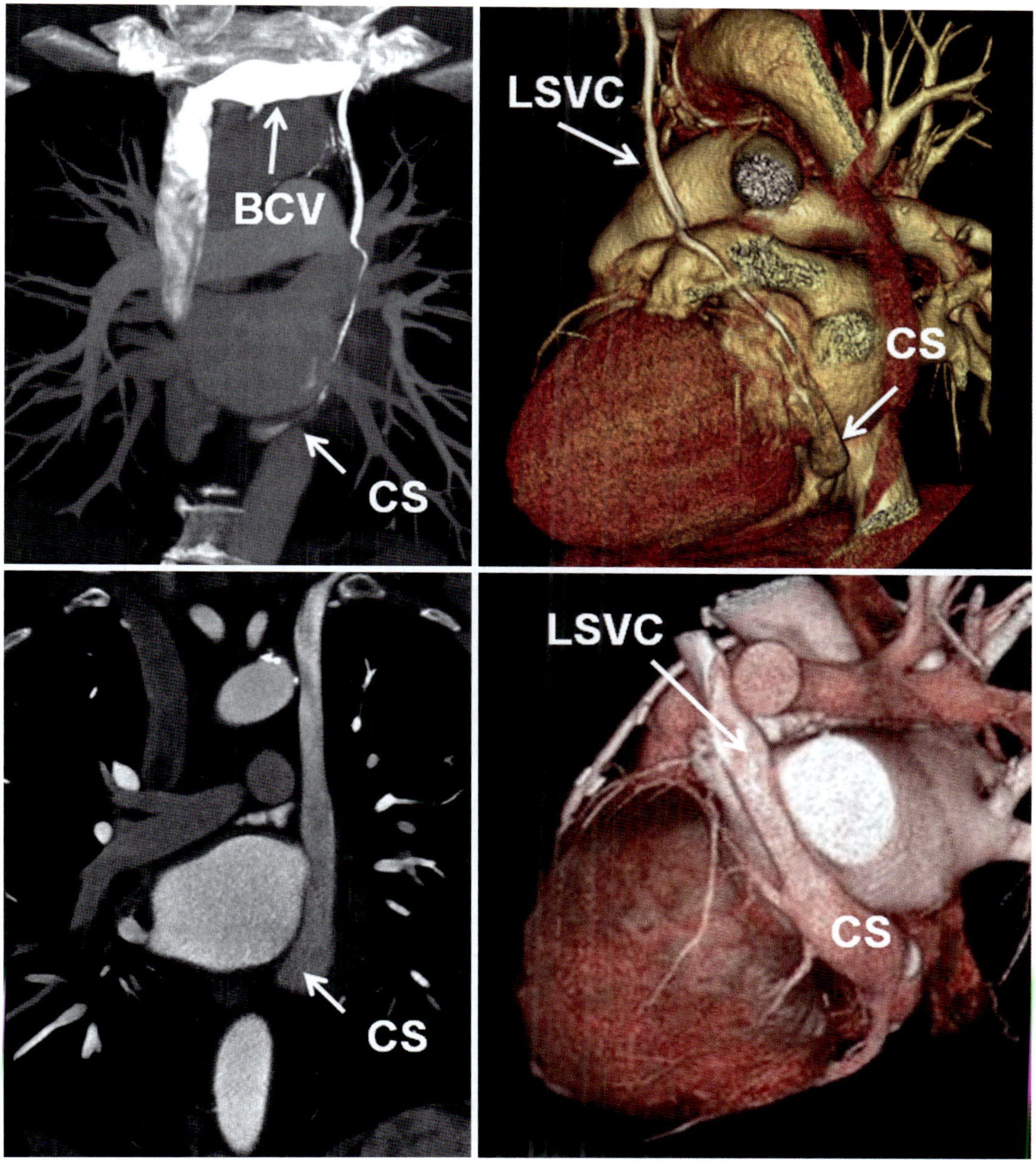

Fig. 26.8 Double superior vena cava (SVC) system with (*upper row*) and without (*lower row*) left brachiocephalic vein (*BCV*). Note the coronary sinus (*CS*) is generally larger in the absence of left brachiocephalic vein. The size of left SVC (*LSVC*) is variable in the presence of left brachiocephalic vein but it is generally smaller than the right SVC

during CT or MR angiography can improve demonstration of this anomaly and associated right-to-left shunting.

Bilateral SVCs are seen in 60–70 % of patients with situs anomalies [35, 42]. In right atrial isomerism, the left SVC drains into the roof of the left-sided atrium. In the hearts with right atrial isomerism, a coronary sinus defect does not exist as there is no orifice of the CS [39]. Whereas in left atrial isomerism, bilateral SVCs are usually present, and both tend to connect low on the atrial wall near the atrioventricular junction [36]. In 50 % of the cases, the left SVC connects to the right-sided atrium through

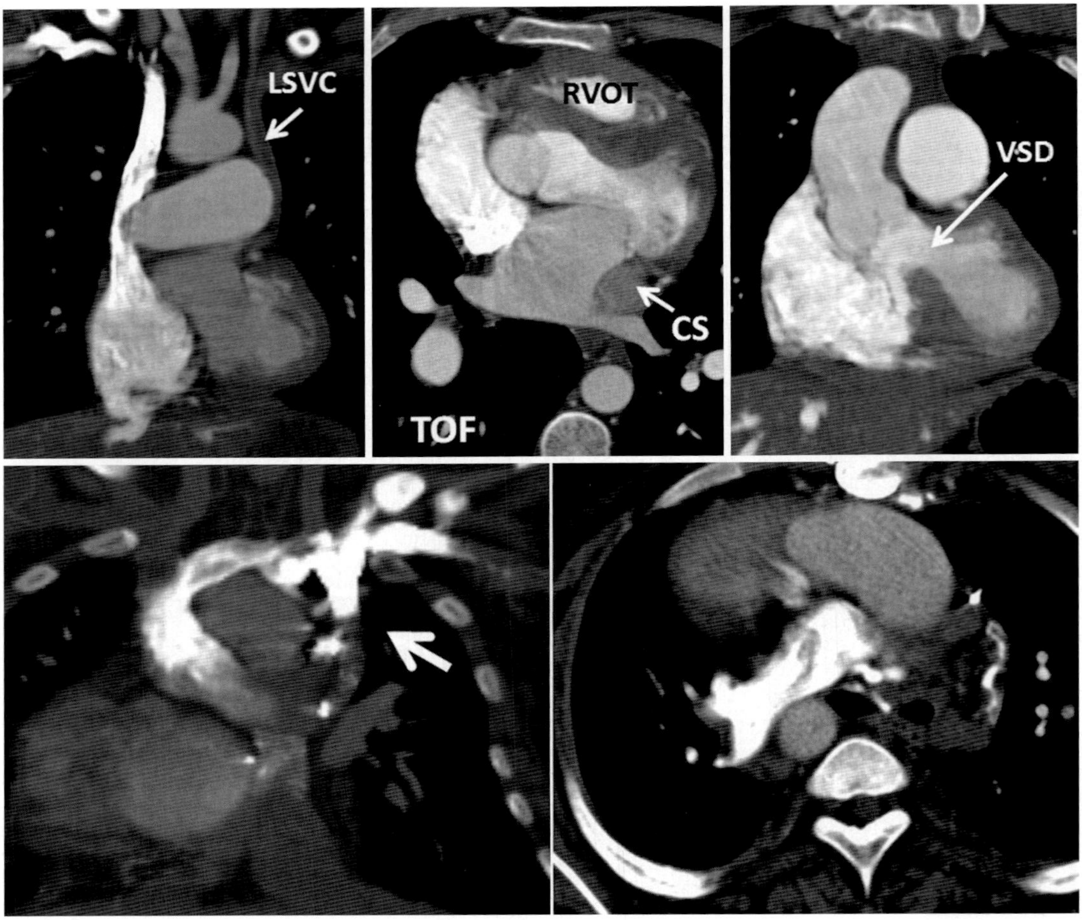

Fig. 26.9 *Upper row*: a 27-year-old male with unrepaired tetralogy of Fallot (*TOF*). Absence of the brachiocephalic vein and a left superior vena cava (*LSVC*) draining into a large coronary sinus is shown. Note the hypertrophied right ventricle outflow tract (*RVOT*) and the ventricular septal defect (*VSD*). The pulmonary arteries are enlarged. *Lower row*: ligated left superior vena cava (SVC) is shown (*arrow*) in a patient with dextrocardia, and double-outlet right ventricle, status post bilateral Glenn shunts and Fontan procedure. Injected contrast has entered into the right pulmonary artery through a right cavopulmonary anastomosis

a CS, but both veins can connect directly into the superior atrial wall.

In situs anomalies, the current trend is to divide and anastomose both SVCs to the pulmonary arteries in a bidirectional cavopulmonary anastomosis, hemi-Fontan, or Fontan procedure [43]. However, a small-caliber left SVC, especially when associated with a large innominate vein, may not be considered worthy of anastomosing and may simply be ligated. In adult repaired CHD the residual of a ligated left SVC can seen in CT or MR (Fig. 26.9). If the left SVC draining the CS is preserved during the Glenn and Fontan-type operations, the ensuing systemic venous hypertension could adversely affect the coronary flow and myocardial perfusion. A persistent left SVC is rarely associated with coronary sinus orifice atresia [44, 45]. Other congenital cardiac lesions associated with coronary sinus orifice atresia with left SVC include ASD, ventricular septal defect, transposition of the great arteries, tricuspid atresia, and mitral atresia [32].

Left Superior Left Intercostal Vein (LSICV) Collateral Pathway

The residuals of an obliterated left anterior cardinal vein are seen as the oblique vein of the left atrium (Marshall) on the cardiac end and as

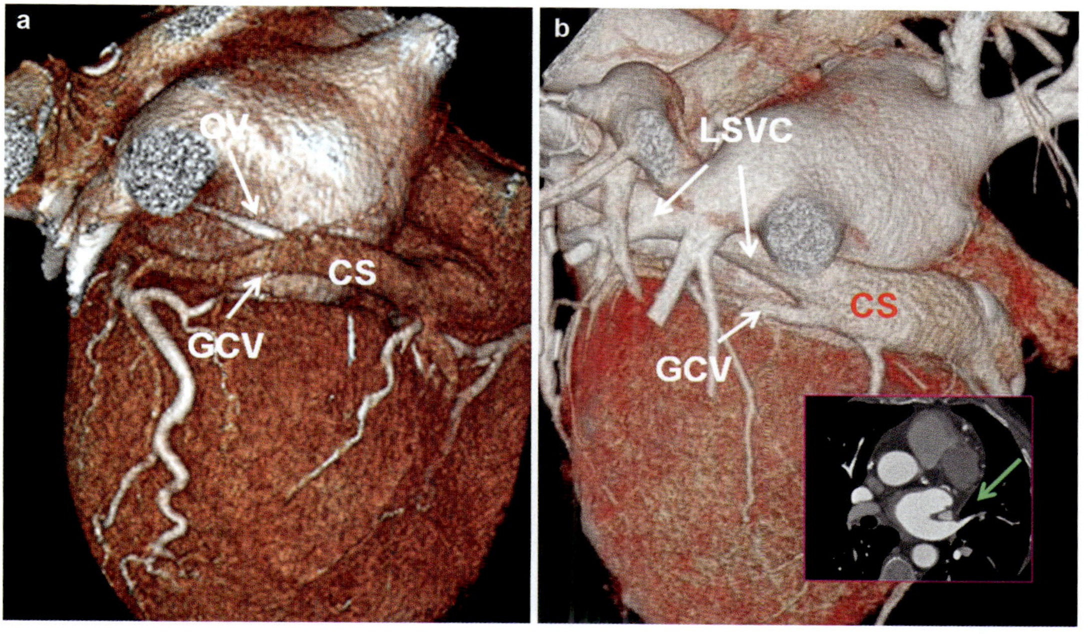

Fig. 26.10 (**a**) Posterolateral view of the heart demonstrates a normal relationship between the coronary sinus (*CS*) and the oblique vein of left atrium (*OV*). The OV is much smaller than the CS and connects to the CS with an angle between 30° t5°. (**b**) In persistent left superior vena cava (*LSVC*), the CS is generally larger than normal. The OV and the LSVC pass along the lateral wall of the left atrium between the left atrial appendage and the left superior pulmonary vein (*green arrow* in **b**). *GCV* great cardiac vein

a small vertical vein on the venous end between the LSICV and the left brachiocephalic vein [22, 31, 46] (Fig. 26.10a). The LSICV is a bridging vessel that links the posteriorly located azygos–hemiazygos systems with the anteriorly located left brachiocephalic vein. The LSICV drains the second, third, and fourth posterior intercostal veins and then passes forward and upward along the aortic arch to drain into the left brachiocephalic vein near the venous angle. In 2/3 the vein connects to the accessory hemiazygos vein which is recognizable in most CT angiographies [47, 48] (Fig. 26.6). The LSICV is described as "aortic nipple" in up to 10 % [47] of chest radiographs. Obviously with CT, it can be seen more frequently (45 %) along the lateral side of aortic arch. This bridging venous pathway has the potential of creating a right-to-left shunt when the SVC or left brachiocephalic vein is narrowed or obstructed. In this situation, venous connections develop between mediastinal veins or tributaries of the LSICV on the systemic side and the superior pulmonary veins (rarely left atrium) on the pulmonary side [49].

Left Brachiocephalic Vein

The brachiocephalic veins are formed by the junction of the internal jugular and subclavian veins behind the sternoclavicular joint. The left brachiocephalic vein passes obliquely from left to right, and the right brachiocephalic vein moves downward behind the manubrium. They join to form the SVC. The left vein is longer than the right; neither has a valve. Anomalous brachiocephalic vein is uncommon, accounting for approximately 1 % of congenital cardiovascular anomalies [23, 50]. The cause of an anomalous brachiocephalic vein remains controversial and is related to abnormal regression of the anterior cardinal anastomosis. The presence of two or more (a plexus) transverse precardinal anastomoses is proposed to explain four patterns of anomalous brachiocephalic vein development: anomalous subaortic left brachiocephalic vein, persistent left SVC with

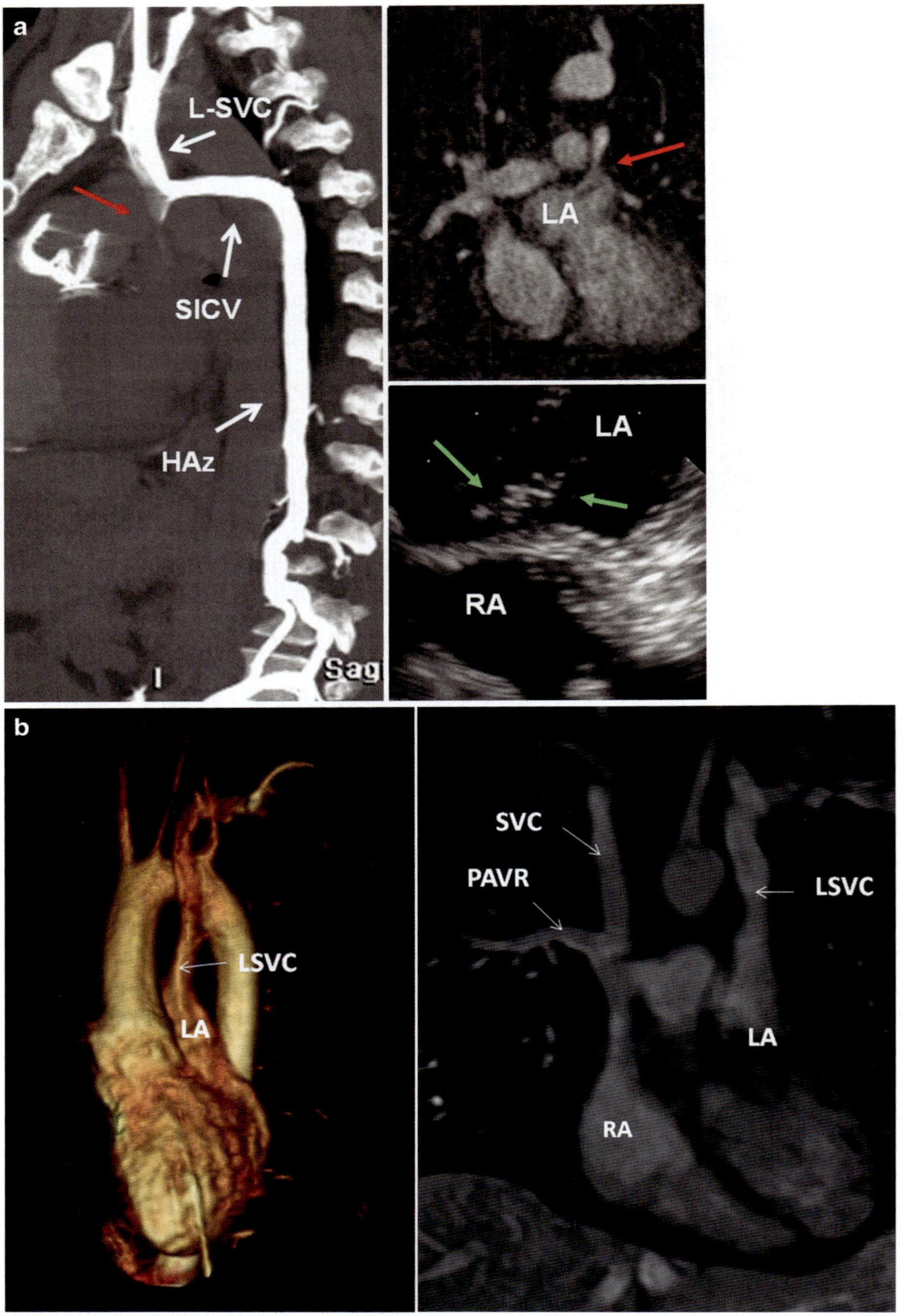

Fig. 26.11 (**a**) Direct communication of the left superior vena cava (*LSVC*) with the left atrium (*LA*) in a patient repaired tetralogy shown by CT and MR angiographies (*red arrows*) using a left arm injection of contrast method. Maximal intensity projection CT in lateral view (*left image*) shows that the LSVC is also connecting with the hemiazygos system (*HAz*) by the superior left intercostal vein (*SICV*). This was confirmed with transesophageal echocardiography after injection of agitated saline in the left arm. Echocardiography image showing bubbles first entered the LA (*green arrows*). The communication was coil embolized as the patient had multiple episodes of paradoxical embolic brain infarctions. (**b**) Volume-rendered left heart MR angiogram from left-sided venous injection in a patient with congenital corrected transposition of the great arteries showing direct communication of the left superior vena cava (*LSVC*) to the left atrium (*LA*). There is no connection between the two SVCs. Note partial anomalous venous return (*PAVR*) of the right upper lobe into the right SVC. *RA* right atrium

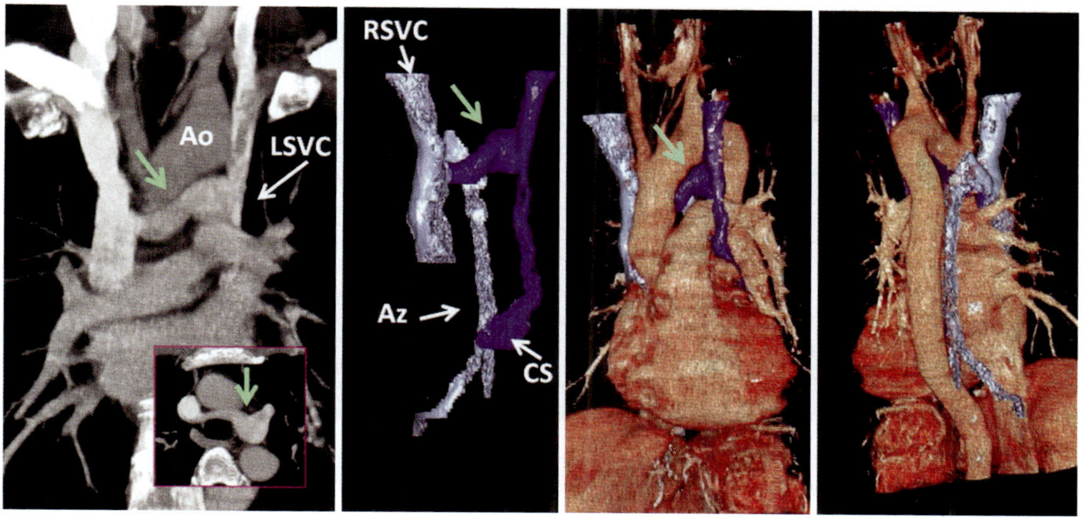

Fig. 26.12 Retroaortic left brachiocephalic vein (*green arrow*) with persistent left superior vena cava (*LSVC*). The azygos vein (*Az*) enters normally into the right SVC (*RSVC*) and the anomalous brachiocephalic vein connects to SVC caudal to the azygos ostium. *Ao* aorta, *CS* coronary sinus

a hypoplastic left brachiocephalic vein connecting to the right SVC, double SVC with agenesis of the left brachiocephalic vein [23], and circumaortic left brachiocephalic vein (Figs. 26.12 and 26.13). An anomalous subaortic left brachiocephalic vein is usually associated with congenital heart disease including right-sided aortic arch and underdeveloped pulmonary artery [23, 51]. This vein, rather than joining the right brachiocephalic vein ventral to the aorta, crosses the midline dorsal to the ascending aorta to join the SVC caudal to the azygos vein (Fig. 26.12). Recognition of the brachiocephalic vein anomalies is important to avoid misdiagnosis and prevent technical difficulty in a left arm approach for the insertion of a central venous catheter and cardiovascular intervention. Congenital aneurysm of the brachiocephalic vein is rare [52]. Most aneurysms are asymptomatic and usually manifest incidentally as mediastinal widening on chest radiographs. There may be a marked difference in the appearance of the aneurysm depending on the patient's posture. A brachiocephalic vein aneurysm can manifest as a mediastinal mass on a supine radiograph but can be barely seen with the patient in the erect position. In this case CT or MR can be diagnostic (Fig. 26.4). A brachiocephalic vein aneurysm, however, can be complicated by a pulmonary embolus, rupture, and venous obstruction, necessitating surgical repair [8].

Azygos System and IVC

In the thorax the azygos system receives blood from the posterior intercostal and mediastinal venous tributaries. The superior intercostal vein drains the second through the fourth intercostal spaces. The right superior intercostal vein communicates with the azygos knob. The left SICV drains into the left brachiocephalic vein along the lateral margin of the aortic arch and may connect to the accessory hemiazygos in 70–80 % of cases. The azygos vein drains into the SVC just cephalad to the right main bronchus. The hemiazygos vein crosses midline at T8–T9 level and behind the descending thoracic aorta to join the azygos vein (Fig. 26.14). From this point, the accessory hemiazygos vein extends further cephalad in a left paravertebral position and may communicate with the azygos vein at different levels.

Embryology

During the fourth to sixth weeks of embryologic development, a pair of posterior cardinal veins drain all but the cephalic portion of the embryo

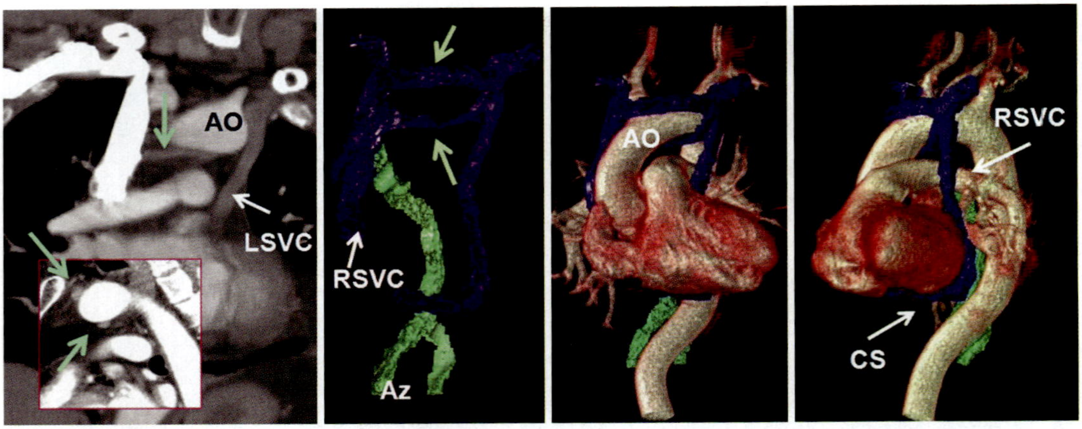

Fig. 26.13 Circumaortic left brachiocephalic vein (*green arrows*) with dual superior vena cava (SVC) system. The azygos system (*Az*) connects with the right SVC (*RSVC*) and the left SVC (*LSVC*) connects with the coronary sinus (*CS*), *Ao* aortic arch

[31, 53, 54]. Later at sixth week, a second new pairs of vein, the subcardinal veins, develop which become dominant at 7 weeks while most of the posterior cardinal veins gradually disappear (Fig. 26.2). Important anastomoses develop between the right and left subcardinal veins anterior to the aorta. The right subcardinal vein further develops to the renal and suprarenal portions of the IVC which connect with the posthepatic segment of IVC (derived from vitelline vein). At 8 weeks, the posterior cardinal veins will be replaced proximally by a third pair of veins, the supracardinal veins, which develop medial and dorsal to the posterior cardinal veins and later anatomose each other behind the aorta. The azygos vein derives mainly from the upper right supracardinal vein but the azygos arch seems to originate from the remaining of the cranial segment of the right posterior cardinal vein. Similarly, upper left supracardinal vein turns into the hemiazygos vein, and the residual of the cranial segment of the left posterior cardinal vein may form the posterior portion of LSICV. The IVC development is complex and five embryological segments contribute to its composition. In caudal–cranial order, these segments include posterior cardinal veins (iliac segment), right supracardinal vein (infrarenal segment), anastomosis between the right supra- and subcardinal veins (renal segment), right subcardinal vein (suprarenal segment), and hepatocardiac canal (hepatic segment).

Anomalies

Azygos and Hemiazygos Continuation of the IVC

Abnormal connection of the hepatic and suprarenal segments of the IVC results in azygos or hemiazygos continuation [53, 54] (Fig. 26.14). Therefore, although a large azygos or hemiazygos vein is the predominant finding in this abnormality, the primary anomaly is the IVC maldevelopment.

These anomalies may be isolated or associated with other anomalies (Figs. 26.15 and 26.16). It can be a part of situs anomalies with left isomerism, in which the liver and stomach are located in the midline, multiple spleens are found along the greater curvature of the stomach (polysplenia syndrome), and the minor fissure of the right lung is absent [55]. Azygos continuation is rare in patients with asplenia (right isomerism). Associated anomalies of the abdominal IVC such as left-sided or duplicated IVC are frequent [55].

The imaging features of azygos continuation of the IVC include dilatation of the azygos vein, azygos arch, and SVC caused by increased flow. The hepatic veins drain into the right atrium via the suprahepatic IVC (Fig. 26.15). The hepatic segment of the IVC is absent or hypoplastic, and this condition must be documented to exclude other causes of an enlarged azygos vein.

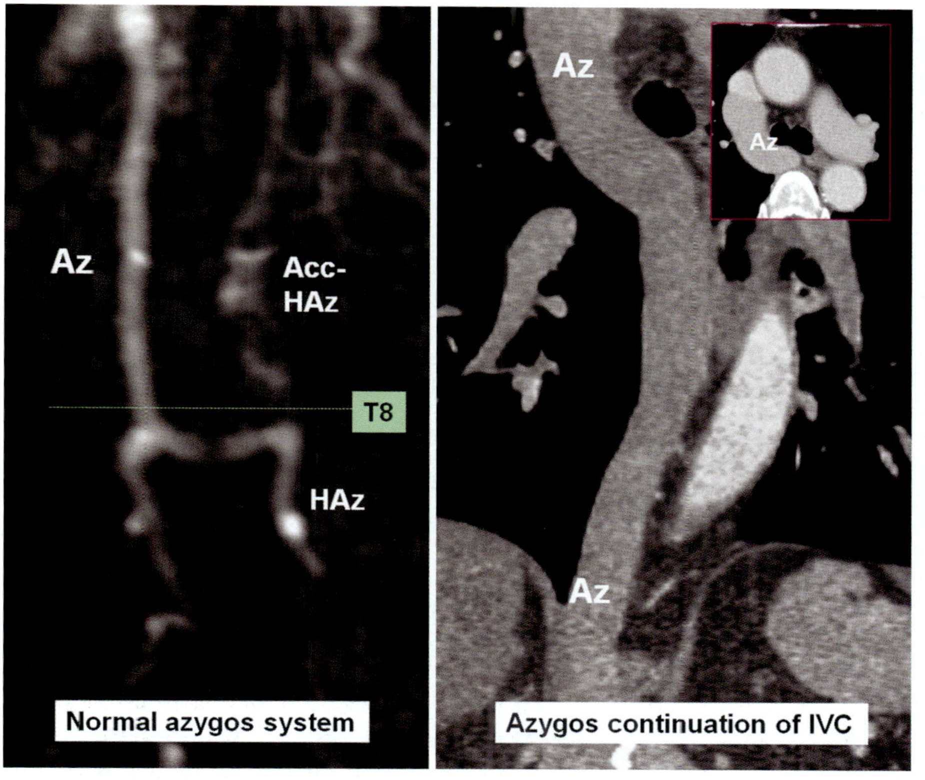

Fig. 26.14 Normal azygos system is shown in MR angiography. The hemiazygos (*HAz*) and accessory (*Acc.*) HAz connect each other approximately at T8 level and cross-link with the azygos (*Az*) at the same level. In azygos continuation of inferior vena cava (*IVC*), the azygos is markedly enlarged and the hemiazygos system is diminutive

Hemiazygos continuation of a left-sided IVC has several variations, including three possible routes for blood in the hemiazygos vein to reach the right atrium [54, 56]. In the first route, the hemiazygos vein drains into the azygos vein at T8–T9. In this case, the findings at more cephalad levels are similar to azygos continuation with enlargement of the distal azygos vein. The hemiazygos vein is also enlarged. The second route involves a persistent left SVC, and blood flows from the hemiazygos vein into the accessory hemiazygos vein and left SVC and then into the CS, all of which are dilated. In the third route, the hemiazygos vein drains to the accessory hemiazygos vein, left SICV, and left brachiocephalic vein into a normal right SVC.

Abnormal Position or Connections or Absence of the Azygos Vein

Azygos lobe of the right lung apex occurs in 1 % of population as a result of malposition of terminal part of the azygos vein [57]. It occurs when the right posterior cardinal vein, one of the precursors of the azygos vein, fails to migrate over the apex of the lung and penetrates it instead, carrying along pleural layers that entrap a portion of the right upper lobe. This is a benign anatomical variant and should not be mistaken with major anomalies. Left azygos lobe is rare and is caused by a malpositioned LSICV draining into the left brachiocephalic vein [58].

In rare occasions, the azygos vein enters the right brachiocephalic vein, right subclavian vein, intrapericardial SVC, or right atrium. Total absence of the azygos vein, a very rare anomaly, arises when the cranial segment of the right supracardinal vein fails to develop [59]. It is usually asymptomatic. Drainage of the right and left intercostal veins will be performed by the hemiazygos and accessory hemiazygos veins as well as through the left brachiocephalic and left superior intercostal veins causing unusual enlargement of these veins.

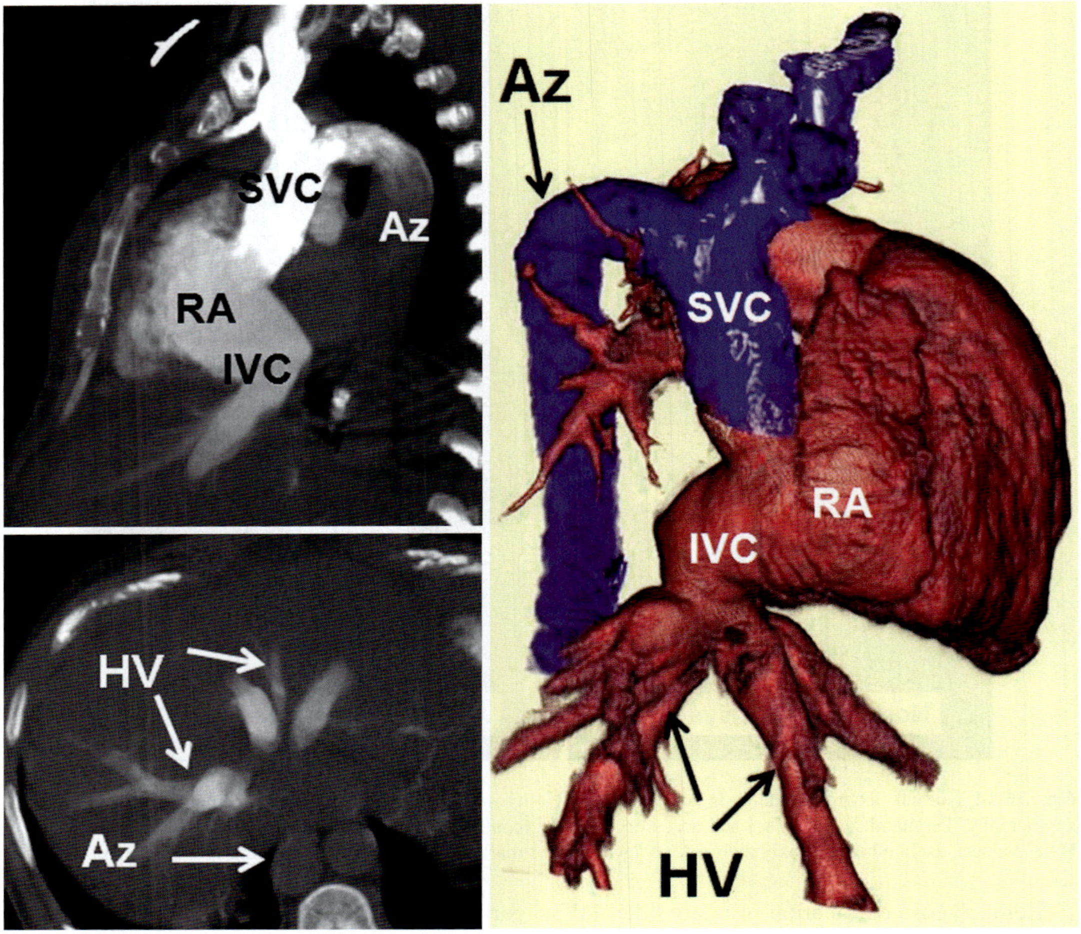

Fig. 26.15 Azygos (*Az*) continuation of inferior vena cava (*IVC*). The azygos is markedly enlarged and enters the posterior aspect of the superior vena cava (*SVC*). The suprahepatic segment of inferior vena cava (*IVC*) persists and connects the hepatic veins (*HV*) with the right atrium (*RA*)

Anomalies of the Pulmonary Veins

Anatomy

Normal pulmonary vein anatomy consists of two right-sided and two left-sided veins with separate ostia. The anatomy and sizes of the LA and pulmonary veins are commonly variable. The pulmonary vein ostia are ellipsoid with a longer superio-inferior dimension. The superior pulmonary veins typically drain the upper and middle lung lobes, whereas the inferior pulmonary veins originate from the lower lobes. The superior pulmonary vein ostia are usually larger than the inferior pulmonary vein ostia.

Embryology

The primary heart tube is formed from fusion of vitelline veins which differentiate into myocardium. Later development of the cardinal and the umbilical venous systems occurs. In those species relying on lungs for the oxygenation of blood, there is also formation of a pulmonary vein [60]. During the first 2 months in utero, the lung buds develop from the foregut. Blood returning from the lung buds initially drains into the splanchnic plexus, which communicates with paired cardinal veins as well as umbilicovitelline veins and drains the systemic veins of the embryo. The right cardinal venous system eventually develops into the right SVC, and the left cardinal venous

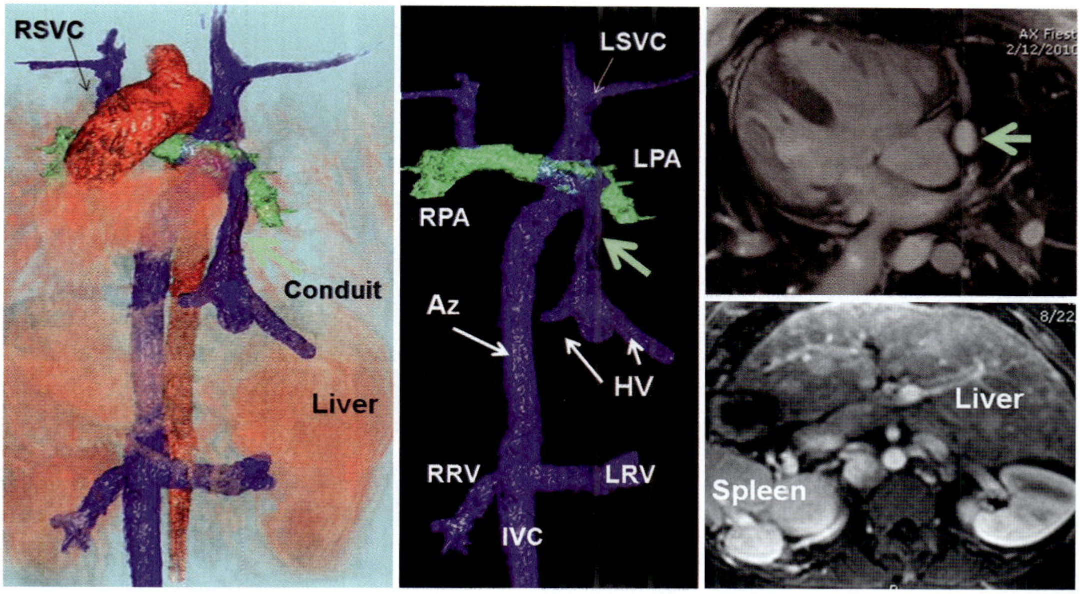

Fig. 26.16 A 21-year-old woman with heterotaxy syndrome, dextrocardia, complex single ventricle, polysplenia, and situs inversus. Status post bilateral bidirectional cavopulmonary shunts (Kawashima procedure). Azygos (*Az*) continuation of inferior vena cava (*IVC*). The hepatic venous (*HV*) flow inclusion into the left pulmonary artery (*LPA*) is performed by an extracardiac conduit (*green arrows*). The left SVC also (*LSVC*) is connected to the LPA. The right SVC (*RSVC*) connected to the right pulmonary artery (*RPA*). *LRV* left renal vein, *RRV* right renal vein

system remains as the oblique vein of the left atrium draining into the coronary sinus. The umbilicovitelline veins develop into the suprahepatic segment of the IVC, portal venous system, and ductus venosus. A primitive common pulmonary vein arises as an outpouching from the dorsal wall of the left atrium and later develops into two and then four separate pulmonary veins. Later, fusion of the common pulmonary vein with the splanchnic venous plexus that drains the lungs occurs, and the pulmonary venous connections to the cardinal and umbilicovitelline veins disappear [61].

Abnormal pulmonary venous connections occur if any of these processes fails to occur properly. If the common pulmonary vein fails to properly incorporate into the dorsal left atrial wall, pulmonary vein stenosis/atresia or cor triatriatum will occur [61]. The sites of anomalous connections are usually divided into (1) direct right atrial; (2) connections through the derivatives of the right-sided common cardinal systems, namely, the SVC and azygos vein; (3) connections through the derivatives of the left common cardinal system, specifically the coronary sinus; and (4) connections through the umbilicovitelline system via the portal vein and venous duct. Direct drainage of the pulmonary veins to the morphologically right atrium, however, is almost always seen in the setting of isomerism of the right atrial appendages and should not necessarily be considered as an error in separation of the splanchnic plexus. Anomalous pulmonary vein return is total if the entire pulmonary vein return is directed to the right atrium and partial if only a portion of the pulmonary vein circulation is affected. The proportion of anomalous pulmonary vein return influences the extent of physiologic compromise and the age of presentation.

Anatomical Variants

Anatomic variations in the course of the pulmonary veins and their connection to the left atrium are common and have attracted attention because of the increasingly use of MRI and CT to depict pulmonary vein anatomy in patients with atrial fibrillation who are treated

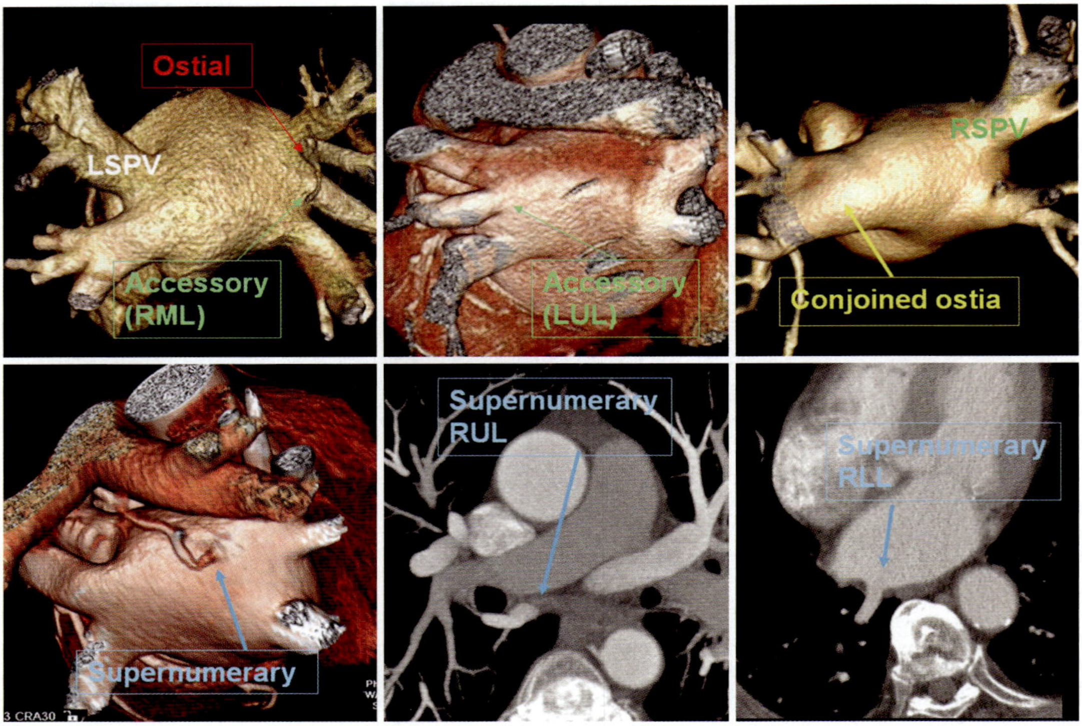

Fig. 26.17 Normal anatomical variations of the pulmonary veins. Accessory right middle lobe (*RML*) and conjoined ostia are relatively common and are seen in one-fourth or one-fifth of studies. Accessory branches on the left side are not common. Supernumerary branch is usually a small branch found in 5–10 % of chest studies. In almost all studies it drains the posterior segment of the right upper lobe (*RUL*) and consistently travels behind the right bronchus before entering the left atrium. Rarely, supernumerary branch arises from the superior segment of the right lower lobe and directly connects to the posteroinferior margin of the left atrium. The significance of these variants is more related to transcatheter ablation of atrial fibrillation arising from the pulmonary vein ostia. *LUL* left upper lobe, *LSPV* left superior pulmonary vein, *RSPV* right superior pulmonary vein

by radiofrequency ablation of arrhythmogenic foci located near the pulmonary vein ostia even in congenital heart malformations. Conjoined (common) pulmonary vein is seen in 30 % of individuals and it is more common on the left side [62]. Supernumerary veins are also frequently seen (Fig. 26.17). The most common is a separate right middle pulmonary vein, which drains the middle lobe of the lung in 25 % of patients [63]. In some patients, the supernumerary pulmonary vein has an aberrant insertion with a perpendicular position in relation to the LA posterior wall (Fig. 26.17). A supernumerary pulmonary vein commonly drains posterior segment of the right upper lobe or superior segment of right lower lobe. Absence of one pulmonary vein requires careful examination of all intrathoracic venous system as it can be associated with partial anomalous venous return. The caliber of the pulmonary veins gradually increased as they approached the left atrium. However, the caliber of the left inferior pulmonary vein may decrease as it enters the LA (Fig. 26.1). This should not be mistaken with a real stenosis. The size of the pulmonary vein ostia is variable during the cardiac cycle. For ablation purposes, any measurement of the pulmonary veins should take place in the same phase of the cardiac cycle during the follow-up studies of patients. Generally, the pulmonary vein ostia enlarge at the end of ventricular systole compared to end ventricular diastole, by the factors of 1.25–1.5 [64].

Anomalies

Stenosis, Atresia, and Aneurysm

Congenital pulmonary vein stenosis and hypoplasia/atresia reflect a spectrum of the same abnormality and may affect individual or multiple pulmonary veins. The abnormality may be focal or may involve a long segment of pulmonary vein and in children can be associated with heart malformations in 50 % of patients [65–67]. Pulmonary vein atresia can be divided into three categories: common, unilateral, and individual pulmonary vein atresia. These categories are based on the extent of involvement, and this depends on the stage in which the normal development of the pulmonary venous drainage is affected. Common and unilateral pulmonary vein atresias are more common in infants and children than in adults. In children recurrent infections, pulmonary edema, and hemoptysis due to the systemic collateral supply to the affected lung can occur [67]. Individual pulmonary vein atresia rarely occurs in adults without specific symptoms or signs [68]. CT findings include a small hemithorax with ipsilateral mediastinal shift, small ipsilateral pulmonary artery, absence of the pulmonary vein connection to the left atrium, and parenchymal abnormalities such as interlobular septal thickening, peribronchovascular thickening, and ground glass opacities. Abnormal vascular structures that represented collaterals can be seen in the involved lung parenchyma. MR imaging may confirm the presence of vascular collaterals and may show retrograde flow in a small pulmonary artery on the affected side. The presence of a small hemithorax without evidence of bronchial obstruction suggests a possible congenital abnormality. These obstructions should be differentiated from acquired form of obstruction secondary to veno-occlusive disease or mediastinitis [66] (Fig. 26.18). Congenital aneurysmal dilatation of the pulmonary vein (varix) can simulate a lung mass [69] (Fig. 26.18).

Partial Anomalous Pulmonary Venous Return

A partial anomalous pulmonary venous return (connection) is a congenital anomaly in which one or more of the pulmonary veins drain into the right atrium or one of its tributaries instead of the left atrium, creating a left-to-right shunt which is usually hemodynamically insignificant [70–73]. Premature atresia of the right or left portion of the primordial pulmonary vein while primitive pulmonary–systemic connections are still present results in a partial anomalous pulmonary venous connection. The overall incidence of partial APVR (PAPVR) is less than 0.5 % in adults [73, 74].

PAPVR can be symptomatic when 50 % or more of the pulmonary blood flow returns abnormally into the systemic side [10]. The ratio of pulmonary to systemic blood flow can be accurately quantified using velocity-encoded phase-contrast MRI [18].

Patients who present with symptoms at an early age tend to have more severe disease and multiple congenital malformations requiring surgical intervention. This explains the frequent detection of right upper lobe PAPVR with associated sinus venosus ASD and other cardiovascular anomalies in the pediatric population. In contrast, in adults PAPVR is an incidental finding in imaging studies of the chest with normal hearts. Sometimes it will be suspected when a usual course of a left-sided central venous catheter is seen on plain chest X-ray [75]. Most reported adult cases involve left upper lobe PAPVR or isolated right upper lobe PAPVR without ASD, and few indications exist for surgical repair (Fig. 26.19). In Haramati et al. series of chest CT scans in adults, the anomalous vein was left sided in 80 % and more common in women without associated ASD [73]. This data was confirmed by another recent report using MDCT [74]. In Ho et al. series [74], PAPVR was observed with 47 % frequency in the left upper lobe, 38 % right upper lobe, 13 % right lower lobe, and 2 % left lower lobe. Among the cases of right upper lobe PAPVR, 42 % were associated with sinus venosus ASD. Other reported anomalies were right-sided volume overload (47 %), isolated upper lobe PAPVR (29 % left and 5 % right), bilateral PAPVR (4 %), and scimitar syndrome (13 %). In another study with cardiac MRI in adult patients with PAPVR and enlarged RV, 75 % were right

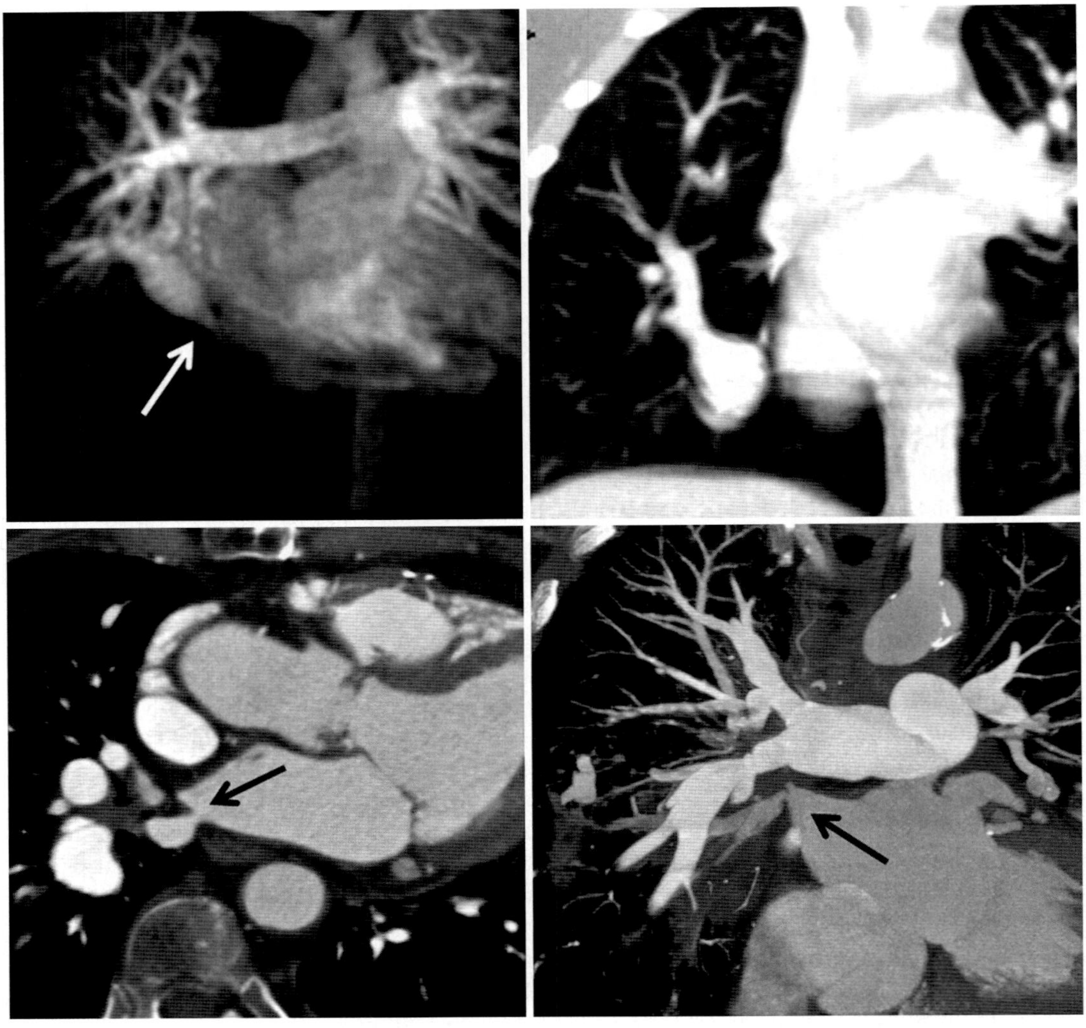

Fig. 26.18 Pulmonary vein stenosis. *Upper row* showing MR angiograms of a congenital stenosis (*arrow*) of the right inferior pulmonary vein and aneurysmal dilatation before entering the left atrium. No pulmonary edema was seen. *Lower row* CT angiograms show stenosis of the right pulmonary vein (*arrows*) and right pulmonary artery due to chronic sarcoid mediastinitis

sided. However, most patients had ASD [76]. Therefore, it seems that isolated PAPVR in adults is more common in the LUL, but it is more common on the right side if complicated by an ASD. In Kafka and Mohiaddin series, 95 % of patients with sinus venosus defect had PAPVR and all were on the right side [76]. In Haramati et al. series, a pulmonary vein in the normal location was seen in 60 % of patients with an anomalous right upper lobe pulmonary vein in contrast to 5 % of patients with an anomalous left upper lobe pulmonary vein (Fig. 26.19). This is possible because of higher incidence of right middle lobe branch of the right side giving the appearance of normal four pulmonary vein patterns in CT or MR studies. In other words, the right upper lobe PAPVR only drains the right upper lobe not the right middle lobe.

Differentiation of the left upper lobe PAPVR with persistent left SVC can be confusing to an inexperienced imager. The origin of both anomalies probably represents a persistent left anterior cardinal vein. In PAPVR of the left upper lobe, the anomalous vein interposed between the

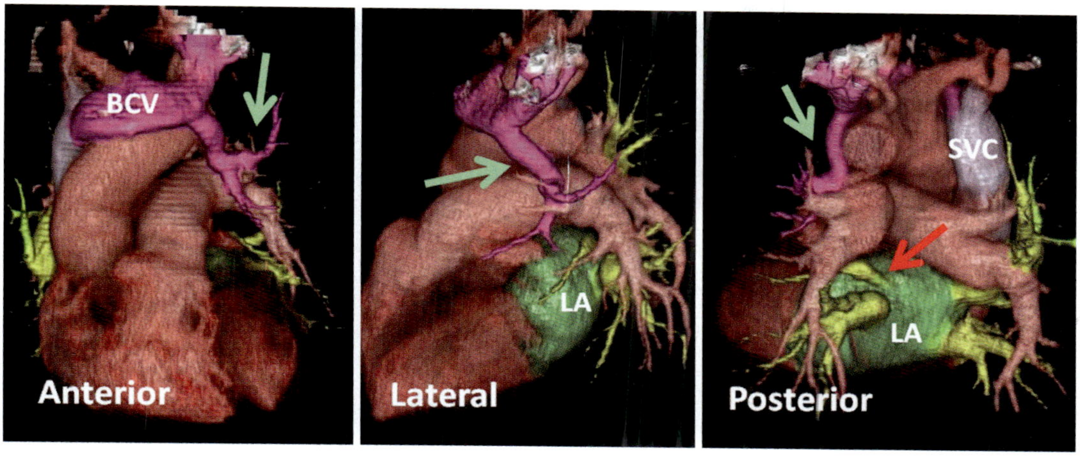

Fig. 26.19 Partial anomalous pulmonary venous return (APVR). Only the anterior segment of the left upper lobe (*green arrows*) drains into the left brachiocephalic vein (*BCV*). Posterior view of the heart shows four pulmonary veins entering the left atrium (*LA*). However, the existing left superior pulmonary vein appears small (*yellow arrow*). *SVC* superior vena cava

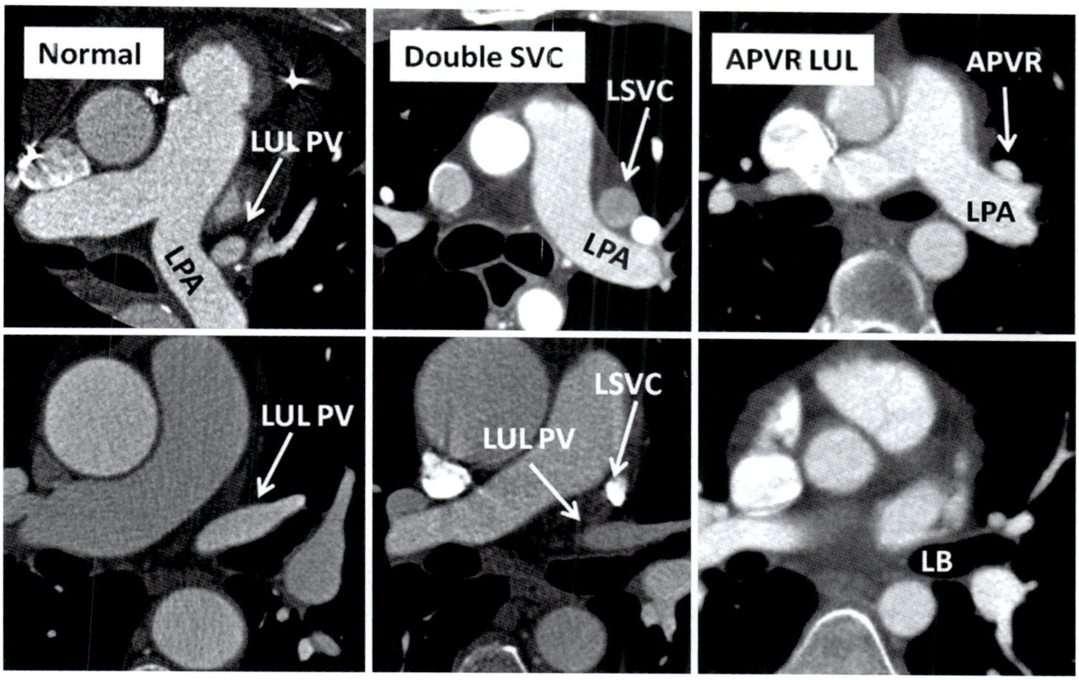

Fig. 26.20 Relationship of veins with left pulmonary artery (*LPA*) and left main bronchus (*LB*) in normal condition, double superior vena cava (*SVC*), anomalous pulmonary venous return of left upper lobe (*APVR LUL*), left upper lobe pulmonary vein (*LUL PV*), and left superior vena cava (*LSVC*)

parenchymal veins of the left upper lobe and the left brachiocephalic vein is described as the "vertical vein" because unlike a persistent left SVC, it does not drain caudally into the coronary sinus. Connection of the left SICV to a persistent left SVC is not uncommon but it is very rare in PAPVR [77]. On axial images, in PAPVR of the left upper lobe, no large vein is seen anterior to the left main bronchus (Fig. 26.20). In the left SVC, two vessels are present anterior to the left

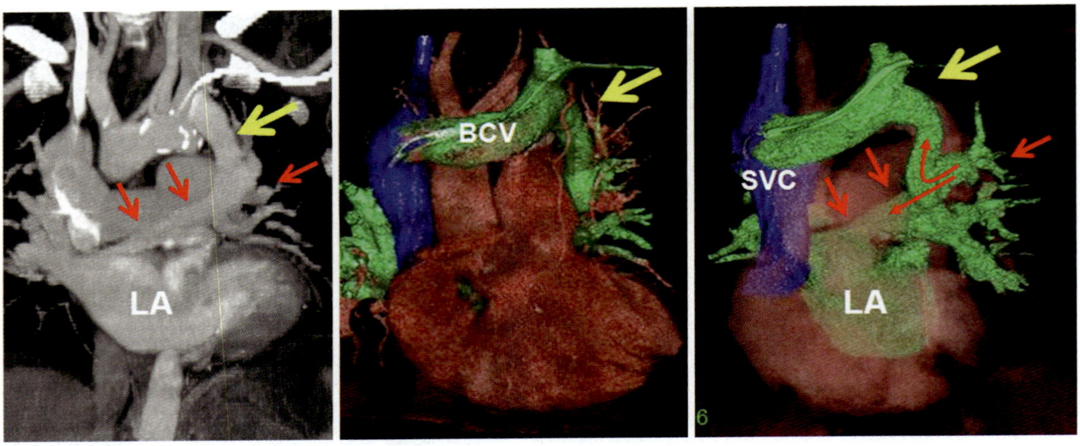

Fig. 26.21 A rare form of anomalous pulmonary venous return (APVR) of left upper lobe into both the vertical vein (*yellow arrows*) and the left atrium (*red arrows*) creating an arcade between the left brachiocephalic vein (*BCV*) and the left atrium (*LA*) with potential for a bidirectional shunt

main bronchus, a left SVC medially and a normal left superior pulmonary vein lateral to it (Fig. 26.20). The left brachiocephalic vein is in the expected position in PAPVR of the left upper lobe but can be absent or small in duplicated SVC. The coronary sinus appears normal in PAPVR but may be enlarged in left SVC. However, if a left innominate vein is present in patients with duplicated SVC, a smaller volume of blood courses through the coronary sinus, and the sinus may be more normal in appearance. In rare occasion, left upper lobe vein can be connected to a vertical vein which interposed between left subclavian vein and left atrium. In this condition, blood flows from the left upper lobe into both the left atrium and the brachiocephalic vein (Fig. 26.21). CT scan of this rare anomaly shows one vein anterior the left bronchus (normal relationship), normal-sized CS, an enlarged brachiocephalic vein, and a vertical vein next to the aortic arch. As a result of bidirectional shunt in this rare anomaly, patient may develop pulmonary hypertension and cyanosis due to reversal of the shunt from a left to right to a right to left.

An asymptomatic left upper lobe PAPVR could become symptomatic if the right lung becomes functionally impaired as a result of lung disease or after pneumonectomy. In that situation, the shunt volume would dramatically increase to approximately 50 % of total pulmonary blood flow, as only the left lower lobe would be contributing to the systemic oxygen supply. A large PAPVR (draining almost entire left lung) with an ASD may also remain asymptomatic due to balanced shunt. If the ASD is surgically closed without repair of the PAPVR, chronic large left-to-right shunt can cause heart failure and pulmonary hypertension (Fig. 26.22) [78]. In PAPVR because the left upper lobe does not drain into the left atrium, the congestion and edema of left-sided heart failure in such patients would spare the left upper lobe. Thrombosis of the left subclavian vein as a result of long-term venous catheterization can cause pulmonary edema limited to the involved lobe.

Anomalous right lung veins usually drain into the SVC, or right atrium, and rarely into the IVC, azygos, coronary sinus, or subdiaphragmatic veins [71, 79–82] (Figs. 26.23 and 26.24). Right upper lobe APVR with sinus venosus ASD may remain asymptomatic. In PAPVR of the right lower lobe, an anomalous pulmonary vein descends from the right lung and drains into the IVC, right atrium, coronary sinus, azygos vein, portal vein, or hepatic vein [83–85]. The anomalous vein usually drains into the subdiaphragmatic IVC and resembles a curved Turkish sword or scimitar. Scimitar (venolobar or hypogenetic lung) syndrome is a collection of findings including dextroposition of the heart, hypoplasia of the right pulmonary artery and right lung, and partial or complete arterial supply to the right lung by

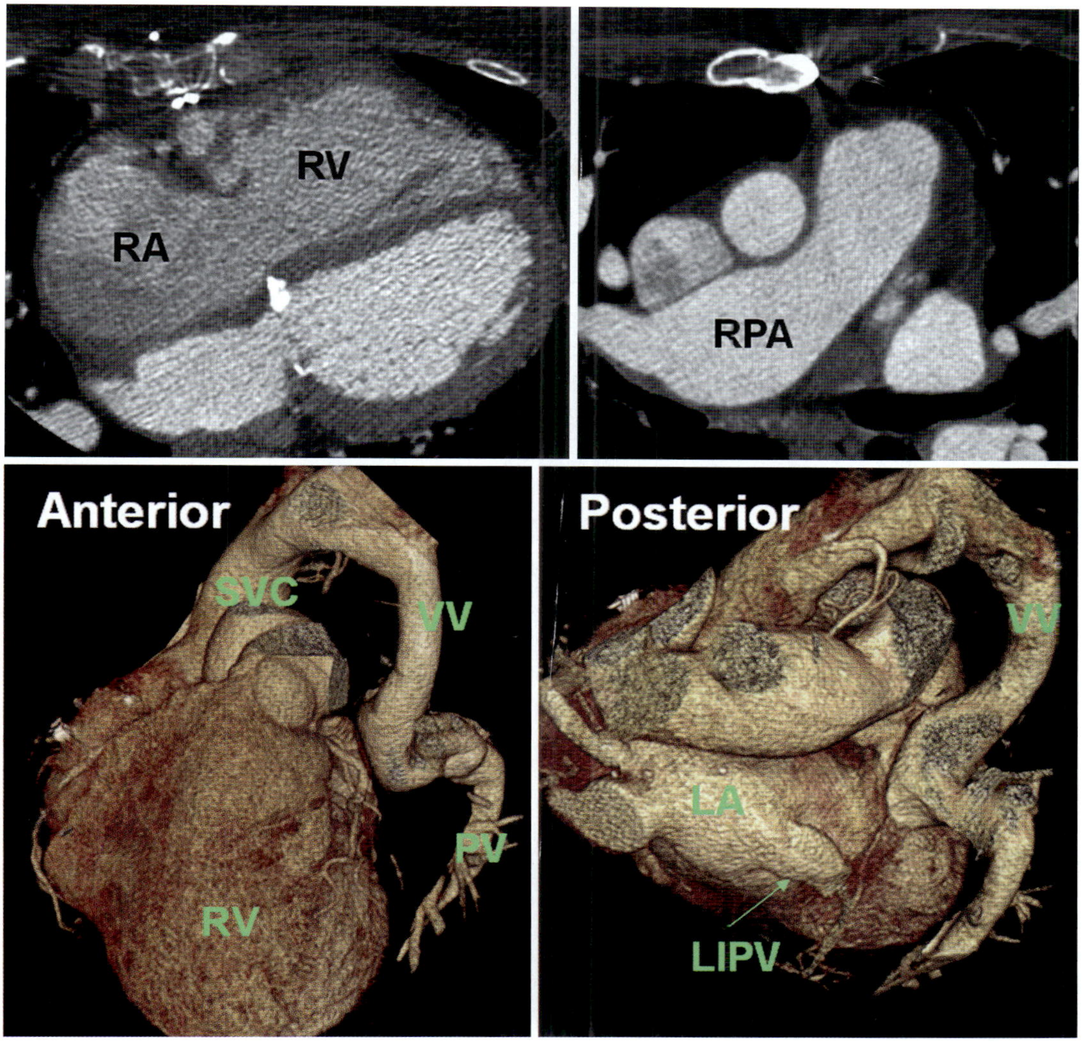

Fig. 26.22 Partial anomalous venous return of the entire left upper lobe in a 46-year-old woman referred for evaluation of right heart enlargement and pulmonary hypertension. Enlarged right atrium (*RA*), right ventricle (*RV*), and right pulmonary artery (*RPA*) are shown. The anomalous pulmonary vein (*PV*) connects to a large vertical vein (*VV*) and the superior vena cava (*SVC*). A 2/1 left-to-right shunt was measured. On posterior view of the left atrium (*LA*), no ostium is seen for left superior pulmonary vein. *LIPV* left inferior pulmonary vein

systemic arteries originating from the descending aorta or abdominal aorta (Fig. 26.24). The spectrum of anomalies and of prognosis in patients with this syndrome is variable. Some patients have severe cardiorespiratory symptoms and large left-to-right shunts requiring surgery, but many others lead a healthy life without surgical correction [83]. Other rare anomalies include ASD, extralobar sequestration, azygos continuation of IVC, and ipsilateral diaphragmatic anomalies [84, 85]. The systemic artery may supply either a segment or a lobe of a normal lung or an abnormal lung with bronchopulmonary sequestration. Isolated scimitar vein (anomalous pulmonary venous connection to the IVC) is another variant and should be differentiated from "meandering" right pulmonary vein [86]. In the latter a relatively large comma-shaped vein with circuitous course exists that drains normally into the left atrium and usually found on the right side.

Patients with PAPVR to the SVC right atrium junction, the right atrium, or both are treated by

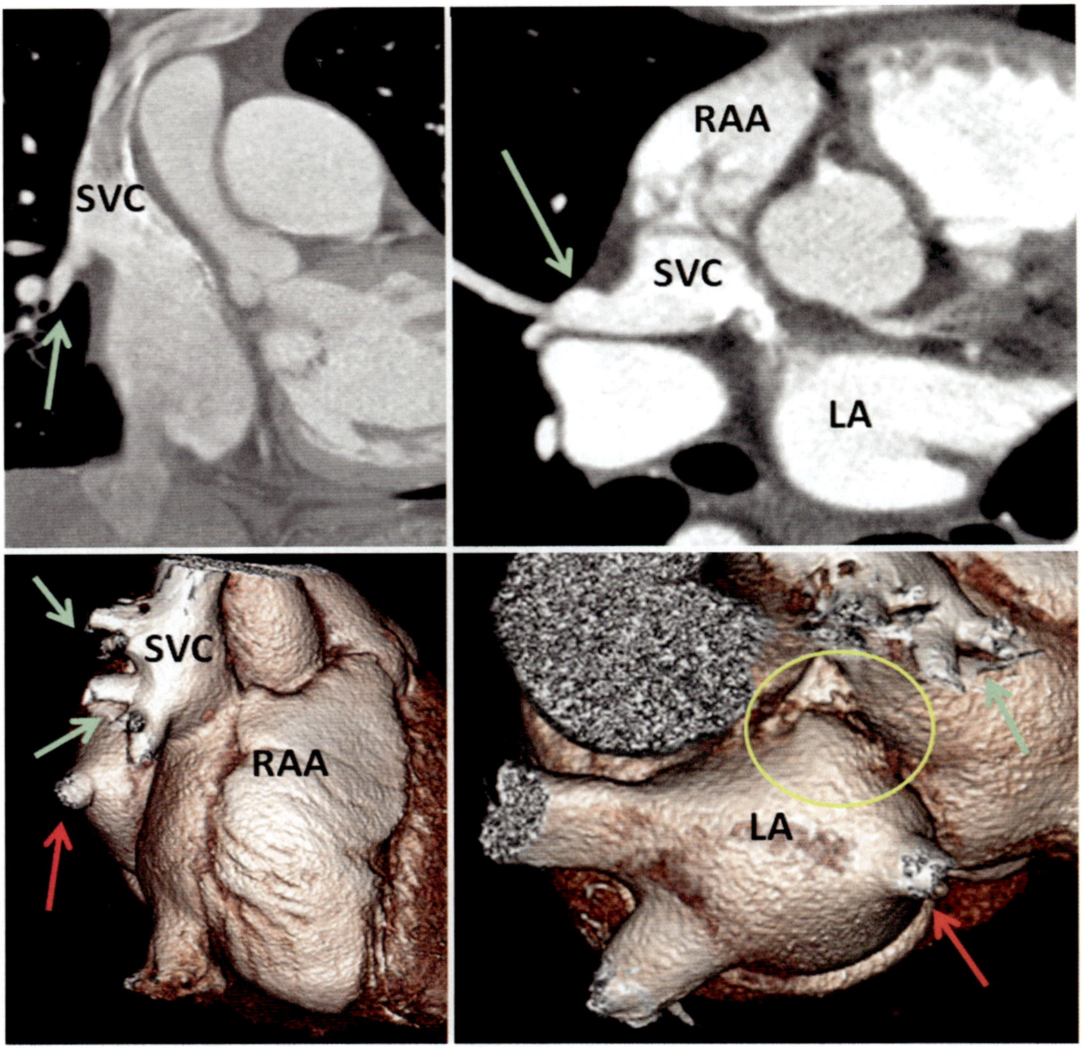

Fig. 26.23 Anomalous pulmonary venous return (APVR) of right upper lobe. Three small anomalous veins (*green arrows*) enter the superior vena cava (*SVC*). The left superior pulmonary vein (*yellow circle*) is absent (*yellow circle*). The left inferior pulmonary vein (*red arrow*) is small. No atrial septal defect was seen. *RAA* right atrial appendage, *LA* left atrium

septal translocation or patch redirection of the anomalous pulmonary venous flow to the left atrium through a native ASD or a surgically created ASD in patients with intact atrial septum [71]. For PAPVR to the high SVC, the SVC is transected and oversewn above the anomalous veins. The anomalous pulmonary venous flow is then redirected through the proximal SVC into the left atrium across a sinus venous atrial septum defect or a surgically created ASD in patients with intact atrial septum [71]. Isolated scimitar vein can be treated with Amplatzer ductal occluder [86].

Total Anomalous Pulmonary Venous Connection or Return (TAPVR)

TAPVR is very rare in adults but accounts for approximately 1–5 % of cardiovascular congenital anomalies in children [87]. This condition is a cause of neonatal cyanosis and the diagnosis is usually made by echocardiography. MR and CT angiography allow detailed and comprehensive evaluation of the anatomy and preoperative assessment of TAPVR [9]. TAPVR is common with asplenia (right isomerism). Four types are described on the basis of the location of pulmonary

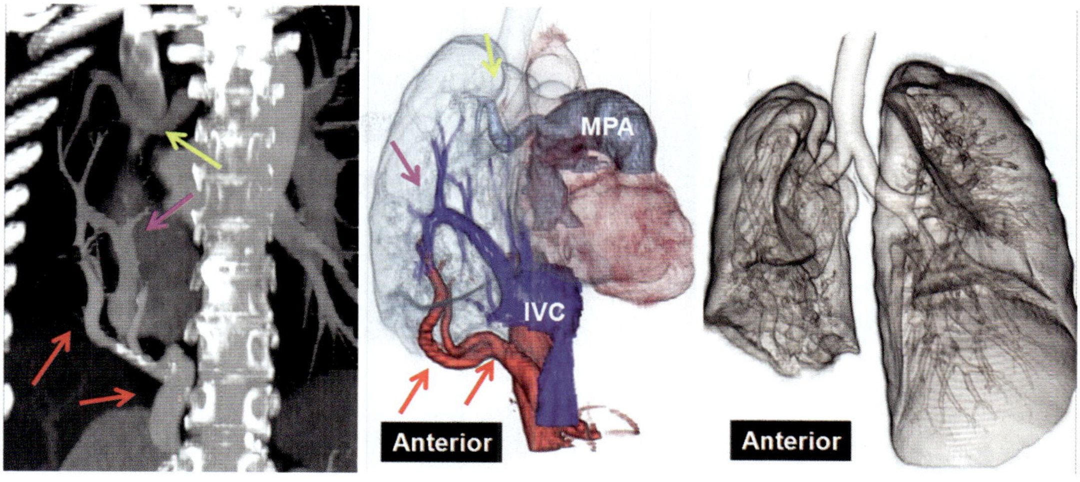

Fig. 26.24 A 51-year-old female with scimitar syndrome shown on CT angiography. Anomalous drainage of the right lower lobe vein (*pink arrows*) into the suprahepatic inferior vena cava (*IVC*) with abnormal arterial supply from celiac to the right lower lobe (*red arrows*). Hypoplastic right lung and a small right pulmonary artery (*yellow arrow*) are seen. *MPA* main pulmonary artery

venous drainage, including supracardiac, cardiac, infracardiac, and mixed forms. Supracardiac drainage is the most common type (45 %) (Fig. 26.25) [86]. In this type, drainage most commonly occurs via an enlarged vertical vein into the left brachiocephalic vein and SVC but rarely may connect to a left SVC or azygos vein. In cardiac type which accounts for 20 % of cases, the pulmonary veins drain into the coronary sinus or the right atrium. The infracardiac type represents 25 % of cases of TAPVR and drains below the diaphragm to the IVC, a hepatic vein, or the portal vein. The draining pulmonary veins in this type of TAPVR may be obstructed when passing through the diaphragm causing neonatal pulmonary edema. In mixed form, the pulmonary veins drain to at least two different locations. Contrast-enhanced MR and CT angiographies are particularly valuable in the characterization of mixed forms of TAPVR; echocardiography may be markedly limited in such cases [88]. Advances in diagnostic imaging and refined surgical techniques have allowed markedly decreased postoperative mortality in TAPVR patients over the last several decades [86].

Cor Triatriatum

Cor triatriatum sinister is a rare anomaly due to incomplete incorporation of the pulmonary vein into the left atrium [89]. In this condition, a membranous diaphragm will divide the left atrium into posterior and anterior chambers [90]. Typically, the membrane lies diagonally in the left atrium and separates the portion containing the pulmonary venous return from the part with the left atrial appendage and mitral valve. The membranous wall between the two chambers typically has one or more openings permitting blood flow from posterior to anterior chamber. A patent foramen ovale is usually present and between the right atrium and either the proximal or distal left atrial chamber. The diagnosis depends on the effective size of the opening in the diaphragm and associated anomalies. In patients with large communications, the diagnosis may present only in adulthood. In children it is associated with other congenital cardiac anomalies in 50 % of cases including ASD, left SVC, and APVR that require surgery during infancy [89]. In adults, it is usually an isolated anomaly incidentally found with imaging. Rarely, a subtotal cor triatriatum is diagnosed when an accessory left atrial chamber receives a portion of pulmonary venous blood flow, whereas the remaining portion of pulmonary venous blood flow drains to the proper left atrium [91]. There are few reports on the role of CT in the evaluation of patients with cor triatriatum in the literature (Fig. 26.26). This rarity is caused by the fact

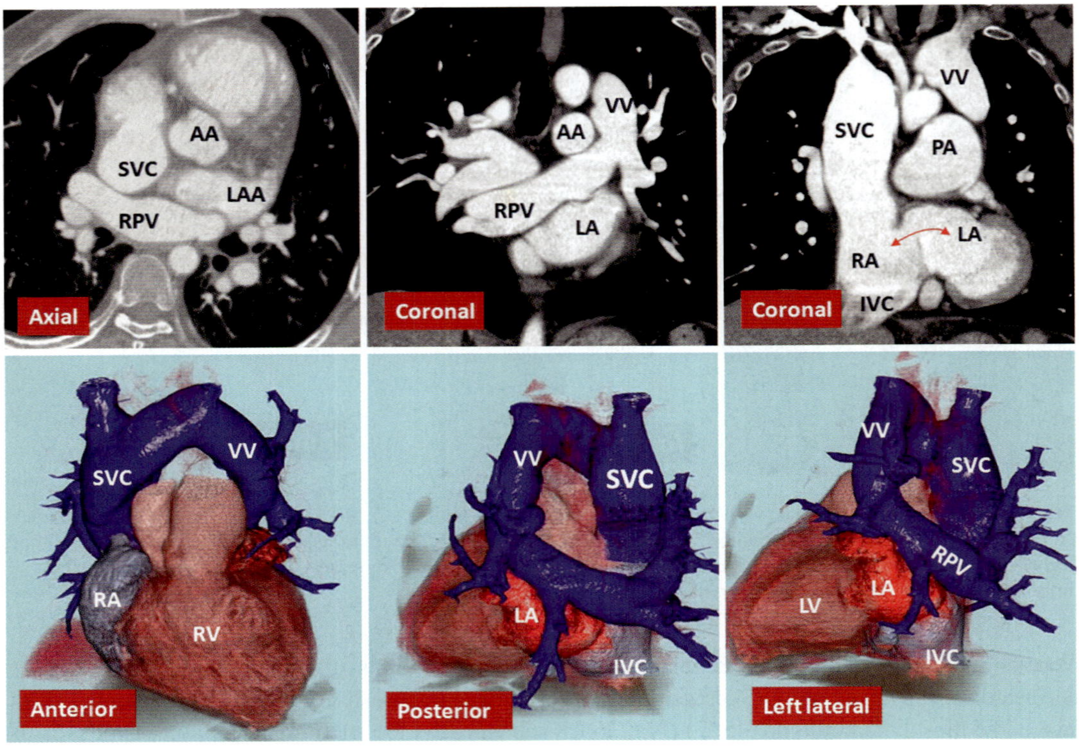

Fig. 26.25 Supracardiac type of total anomalous pulmonary venous return (*TAPVR*) in a 56 year old man presented for evaluation of atrial septal defect (*ASD*) and pulmonary hypertension. CT images shows no pulmonary vein connection to the left atrium. Instead all pulmonary veins connect to a single chamber and drain into a left vertical vein (*VV*). The VV drains into a large right superior vena cava (*SVC*). A large *ASD* (double headed *red arrow*) is shown between the right atrium (*RA*) and the left atrium (*LA*). Inferior vena cava (*IVC*) is normal. The right ventricle (*RV*) is enlarged due to a large left to right shunt but the left ventricle (*LV*) is normal in size. Patient was successfully operated. ASD was closed and the VV was connected to left atrial appendage (*LAA*), *RPV* right pulmonary vein, *AA* ascending aorta

that cor triatriatum is largely diagnosed in children and younger patients by echocardiography. With new-generation scanners, interatrial membrane can be easily shown using ECG gating and proper contrast injection technique. Because the spatial resolution of CT is higher than most routine MR sequences, it seems that CT might be the preferred diagnostic choice of this abnormality [92, 93].

Membranous structures can also be seen in the right atrium. Differential diagnosis are Chiari network, large eustachian valve, and cor triatriatum dexter all representing the remnant of the right valve of sinus venosus (Chap. 13 intracardiac shunts). During the third week of embryonic development, this structure divides the right atrium into two chambers: (1) the smooth sinus portion to which both venae cavae and the coronary sinus are connected and (2) the muscular primitive atrial portion including the right atrial appendage. It normally regresses between the 9th and 15th week of gestation. Dependent on the degree of regression, the patient can keep a complete division of the right atrium (cor triatriatum dexter), a fenestrated membrane, or a network of threads and fibers (Chiari network). Minimal remnants are the eustachian and thebesian valves that guard the orifice of the IVC and the coronary sinus, as well as the crista terminalis.

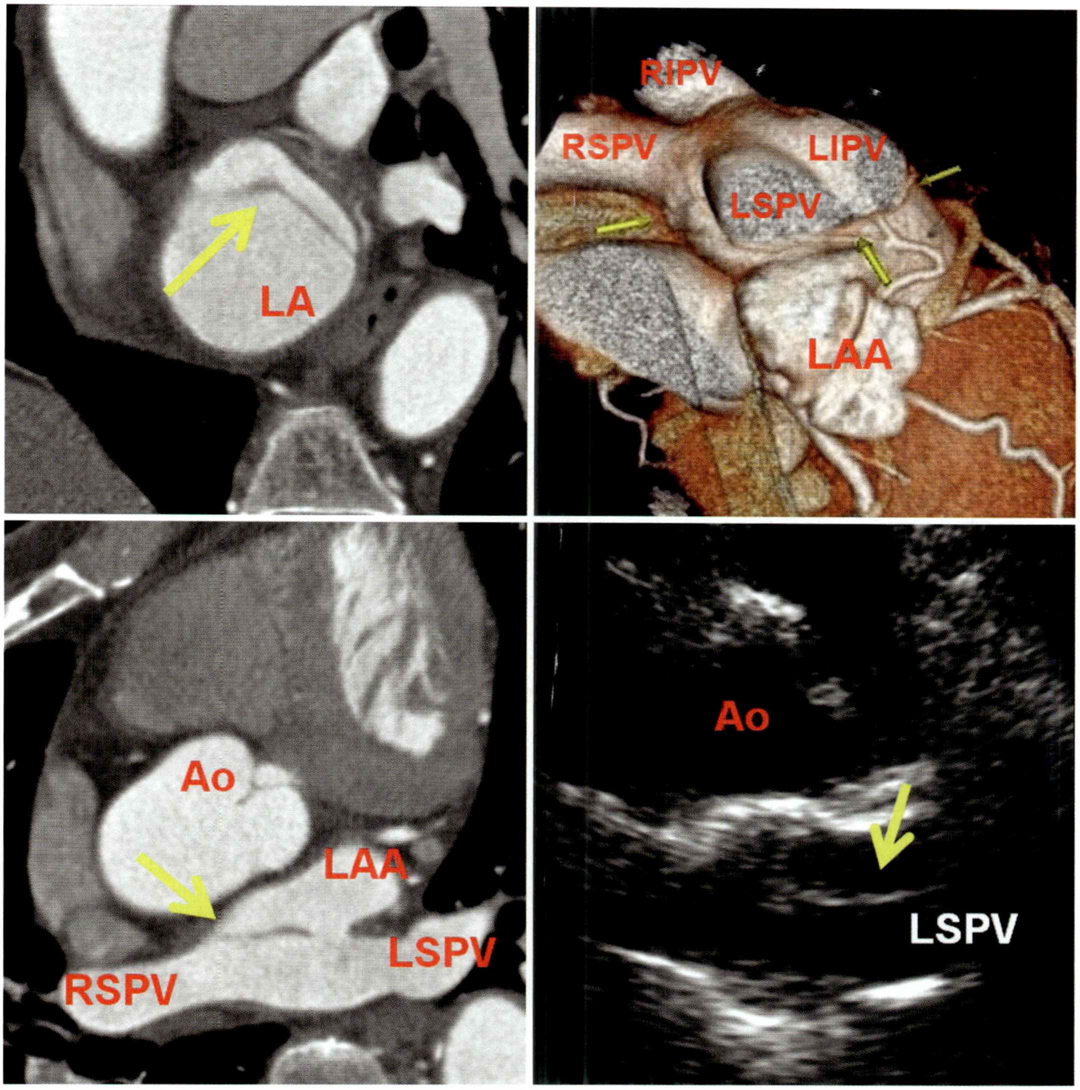

Fig. 26.26 Coronary CT angiography and transthoracic echocardiography in cor triatriatum sinister in a 64-year-old asymptomatic patient referred for screening of the coronary arteries. A membranous diaphragm (*yellow arrows*) in the left atrium (*LA*) parallel to the plane of pulmonary veins is seen separating the pulmonary venous component of the LA from the vestibule and left atrial appendage (*LAA*). Peripheral attachments of the membrane to the LA walls are shown by *yellow arrows* in volume-rendered CT image. *Ao* aorta, *LIPV* left inferior pulmonary vein, *LSPV* left superior pulmonary vein, *RIPV* right inferior pulmonary vein, *RSPV* right superior pulmonary vein

Summary

A wide spectrum of pulmonary venous developmental anomalies exist that can be detected by imaging. Accurate characterization of these abnormalities is important because they all can be associated with significant patient morbidity and mortality. Numerous recent studies have confirmed that both CT and MRI are noninvasive imaging techniques that should play increasingly important roles in the evaluation of these anomalies. CT and MRI are most useful in the evaluation of patients with intrathoracic venous anomalies because these lesions may be difficult to characterize at echocardiography.

References

1. Buirski G, Jordan SC, Joffe HS, Wilde P. Superior vena caval abnormalities: their occurrence rate, associated cardiac abnormalities and angiographic classification in a paediatric population with congenital heart disease. Clin Radiol. 1986;37(2):131–8.
2. Sungur M, Ceyhan M, Baysal K. Partial anomalous pulmonary venous connection of left pulmonary veins to innominate vein evaluated by multislice CT. Heart. 2007;93:1292.
3. Kalke BR, Carlson AG, Ferlic AM, Sellers AD, Lillehei CW. Partial anomalous pulmonary venous connections. Am J Cardiol. 1967;20:91–101.
4. Snellen HA, Dekker A. Anomalous pulmonary venous drainage in relation to left superior vena cava and coronary sinus. Am Heart J. 1963;66:184–96.
5. Pennes DR, Ellis JH. Anomalous pulmonary venous drainage of the left upper lobe shown by CT scans. Radiology. 1986;159:23–4.
6. Demos TC, Posniak HV, Pierce KL, et al. Venous anomalies of the thorax. Am J Roentgenol. 2004;182:1139–50.
7. Kivistö S, Hänninen H, Holmström M. Partial anomalous pulmonary venous return and atrial septal defect in adult patients detected with 128-slice multidetector computed tomography. J Cardiothorac Surg. 2011;6:126.
8. Konen E, Raviv-Zilka L, Cohen RA, et al. Congenital pulmonary venolobar syndrome: spectrum of helical CT findings with emphasis on computerized reformatting. Radiographics. 2003;23:1175–118410.
9. Uçar T, Fitoz S, Tutar E, et al. Diagnostic tools in the preoperative evaluation of children with anomalous pulmonary venous connections. Int J Cardiovasc Imaging. 2008;24(2):229–35.
10. White CS, Baffa JM, Haney PJ, et al. Anomalies of pulmonary veins: usefulness of spin-echo and gradient-echo MR images. AJR Am J Roentgenol. 1998;170:1365–8.
11. Festa P, Ait-Ali L, Cerillo AG, De Marchi D, Murzi B. Magnetic resonance imaging is the diagnostic tool of choice in the preoperative evaluation of patients with partial anomalous pulmonary venous return. Int J Cardiovasc Imaging. 2006;22:685–93.
12. Valsangiacomo ER, Levasseur S, McCrindle BW, MacDonald C, Smallhorn JF, Yoo SJ. Contrast enhanced MR angiography of pulmonary venous abnormalities in children. Pediatr Radiol. 2003;33:92–8.
13. Powell AJ, Geva T. Blood flow measurement by magnetic resonance imaging in congenital heart disease. Pediatr Cardiol. 2000;21:47–58.
14. François CJ, Tuite D, Deshpande V, Jerecic R, Weale P, Carr JC. Pulmonary vein imaging with unenhanced three-dimensional balanced steady-state free precession MR angiography: initial clinical evaluation. Radiology. 2009;250(3):932–9.
15. Prasad SK, Soukias N, Hornung T, et al. Role of magnetic resonance angiography in the diagnosis of major aortopulmonary collateral arteries and partial anomalous pulmonary venous drainage. Circulation. 2004;109(2):207–14.
16. Greil GF, Powell AJ, Gildein HP, Geva T. Gadolinium-enhanced three-dimensional magnetic resonance angiography of pulmonary and systemic venous anomalies. J Am Coll Cardiol. 2002;39(2):335–41.
17. Mohrs OK, Petersen SE, Voigtlaender T, et al. Time-resolved contrast-enhanced MR angiography of the thorax in adults with congenital heart disease. AJR Am J Roentgenol. 2006;187(4):1107–14.
18. Powell AJ, Tsai-Goodman B, Prakash A, Greil GF, Geva T. Comparison between phase-velocity cine magnetic resonance imaging and invasive oximetry for quantification of atrial shunts. Am J Cardiol. 2003;91(12):1523–5.
19. Debl K, Djavidani B, Buchner S, Heinicke N, et al. Quantification of left-to-right shunting in adult congenital heart disease: phase-contrast cine MRI compared with invasive oximetry. Br J Radiol. 2009;82(977):386–91.
20. Hillis LD, Firth BG, Winniford MD. Variability of right sided cardiac oxygen saturations in adults with and without left-to-right intracardiac shunting. Am J Cardiol. 1986;58(1):129–32.
21. Minniti S, Visentini S, Procacci C. Congenital anomalies of the venae cavae: embryological origin, imaging features and report of three new variants. Eur Radiol. 2002;12(8):2040–55.
22. Kellman GM, Alpern MB, Sandler MA, Craig BM. Computed tomography of vena caval anomalies with embryologic correlation. Radiographics. 1988;8:533–56.
23. Chen SJ, Liu KL, Chen HY, et al. Anomalous brachiocephalic vein: CT, embryology, and clinical implications. AJR Am J Roentgenol. 2005;184:1235–40.
24. Steding G, Xu JW, Seidl W, Männer J, Xia H. Developmental aspects of the sinus valves and the sinus venosus septum of the right atrium in human embryos. Anat Embryol (Berl). 1990;181(5):469–75.
25. Takeda K, Matsumura K, Ito T, Nakagawa T, Yamaguchi N. Anomalous insertion of the superior or the inferior vena cava into the right atrium. Pediatr Cardiol. 1998;19(6):474–6.
26. Váquez-Pérez J, Frontera-Izquierdo P. Anomalous drainage of the right superior vena cava into the left atrium as an isolated anomaly. Rare case report. Am Heart J. 1979;97(1):89–91.
27. Moncada R, Demos TC, Marsan RM, Churchill RJ, Reynes C, Love L. CT diagnosis of aneurysms of the thoracic venous system. J Comput Assist Tomogr. 1985;9:305–9.
28. Kalejs M, Kolitis R, Stradins P, Lacis R. Large thrombosed saccular aneurysm of superior vena cava complicated by pulmonary embolism in a young woman. J Invasive Cardiol. 2010;22(8):E159–61.
29. Wong AM, Wa YL, Cheung YC, Ng SH, Lee KF. CT features of mediastinal lymphangiohemangioma asso-

ciated with superior vena cava ectasia: a case report. Acta Radiol. 2000;41:429–31.
30. Quraishi MB, Mufti O, Wase A. Absent left and right superior vena cava and azygos continuation of inferior vena cava: a rare anomaly of systemic venous return. Eur J Cardiothorac Surg. 2012;41(5):e126.
31. Webb W, Gamsu G, Speckman J, Kaiser J, Federle M, Lipton M. Computed tomographic demonstration of mediastinal venous anomalies. AJR Am J Roentgenol. 1982;139:157–61.
32. Mantini E, Grondin CM, Lillehei CW, Edwards JE. Congenital anomalies involving the coronary sinus. Circulation. 1966;33:317–27.
33. Parikh SR, Prasad K, Iyer RN, Desai N, Mohankrishna L. Prospective angiographic study of the abnormalities of systemic venous connections in congenital and acquired heart disease. Cathet Cardiovasc Diagn. 1996;38(4):379–86.
34. Sarodia BD, Stoller JK. Persistent left superior vena cava: case report and literature review. Respir Care. 2000;45:411–6.
35. Rubino M, Van Praagh S, Kadoba K, Pessotto R, Van Praagh R. Systemic and pulmonary venous connections in visceral heterotaxy with asplenia. Diagnostic and surgical considerations based on seventy-two autopsied cases. J Thorac Cardiovasc Surg. 1995;110(3):641–50.
36. Miraldi F, di Gioia CR, Proietti P, De Santis M, d'Amati G, Gallo P. Cardinal vein isomerism: an embryological hypothesis to explain a persistent left superior vena cava draining into the roof of the left atrium in the absence of coronary sinus and atrial septal defect. Cardiovasc Pathol. 2002;11:149–52.
37. Raghib G, Ruttenberg HD, Anderson RC, Amplatz K, Adams P, Edwards JE. Termination of left superior vena cava in left atrium, atrial septal defect, and absence of coronary sinus. A developmental complex. Circulation. 1965;31:906–18.
38. Ezekowitz MD, Alderson PO, Bulkley BH, Dwyer PN, Watkins L, Lappe DL, Greene HL, Becker LC. Isolated drainage of the superior vena cava into the left atrium in a 52-year-old man: a rare congenital malformation in the adult presenting with cyanosis, polycythemia, and an unsuccessful lung scan. Circulation. 1978;58(4):751–6.
39. Knauth A, McCarthy KP, Webb S, Ho SY, Allwork SP, Cook AC, Anderson RH. Interatrial communication through the mouth of the coronary sinus. Cardiol Young. 2002;12(4):364–72.
40. Hahm JK, Park YW, Lee JK, Choi JY, Sul JH, Lee SK, et al. Magnetic resonance imaging of unroofed coronary sinus: three cases. Pediatr Cardiol. 2000;21:382–7.
41. Jian Z, Li J, Xiao Y. Rare association of tetralogy of Fallot with partially unroofed coronary sinus and PLSVC: case report. Thorac Cardiovasc Surg. 2010;58(2):117–9.
42. Macartney FJ, Zuberbuhler JR, Anderson RH. Morphological considerations pertaining to recognition of atrial isomerism. Consequences for sequential chamber localization. Br Heart J. 1980;44(6):657–67.
43. Muster AJ, Naheed ZJ, Backer CL, Mavroudis C. Is surgical ligation of an accessory left superior vena cava always safe? Pediatr Cardiol. 1998;19(4):352–4.
44. Jha NK, Gogna A, Tan TH, Wong KY, Shankar S. Atresia of coronary sinus ostium with retrograde drainage via persistent left superior vena cava. Ann Thorac Surg. 2003;76:2091–2.
45. Gerlis LM, Gibbs JL, Williams GJ, Thomas GDH. Coronary sinus orifice atresia and persistent left superior vena cava. Br Heart J. 1984;52:648–53.
46. Winter FS. Persistent left superior vena cava: survey of world literature and report of thirty additional cases. Angiology. 1954;5:90–132.
47. Ball Jr JB, Proto AV. The variable appearance of the left superior intercostal vein. Radiology. 1982; 144:445–52.
48. McDonald CJ, Castellino RA, Blank N. The aortic "nipple". Radiology. 1970;96:533–6.
49. Gilkeson RC, Nyberg EM, Sachs PB, Wiant AM, Zahka KG, Siwik ES. Systemic to pulmonary venous shunt imaging findings and clinical presentations J Thorac Imaging. 2008;23:170–7.
50. Takada Y, Narimatsu NA, Kohno A, et al. Anomalous left brachiocephalic vein: CT findings. J Comput Assist Tomogr. 1992;16:893–6.
51. Chern MS, Ko JS, Tsai A, Wu MH. Aberrant left brachiocephalic vein: CT imaging findings and embryologic correlation. Eur Radiol. 1999;9:1835–9.
52. Burkill GJ, Burn PR, Padley SP. Aneurysm of the left brachiocephalic vein: an unusual cause of mediastinal widening. Br J Radiol. 1997;70:837–9.
53. Dudiak CM, Olson MC, Posniak HV. Abnormalities of the azygos system: CT evaluation. Semin Roentgenol. 1989;24:47–55.
54. Dudiak CM, Olson MC, Posniak HV. CT evaluation of congenital and acquired abnormalities of the azygos system. Radiographics. 1991;11:233–46.
55. Jelinek JS, Stuart PL, Done SL, Ghaed N, Rudd SA. MRI of polysplenia syndrome. Magn Reson Imaging. 1989;7:681–6.
56. Munechika H, Cohan RH, Baker ME, Cooper CJ, Dunnick NR. Hemiazygos continuation of a left inferior vena cava: CT appearance. J Comput Assist Tomogr. 1988;12:328–30.
57. Mata J, Cáceres J, Alegret X, Coscojuela P, De Marcos JA. Imaging of the azygos lobe: normal anatomy and variations. AJR Am J Roentgenol. 1991;156(5):931–7.
58. Takasugi JE, Godwin JD. Left azygos lobe. Radiology. 1989;171:133–4.
59. Hatfield MK, Vyborny CJ, MacMahon H, Chessare JW. Congenital absence of the azygos vein: a cause for aortic nipple enlargement. AJR Am J Roentgenol. 1987;149:272–4.
60. Anderson RH, Brown NA, Moorman AFM. Development and structures of the venous pole of the heart. Dev Dyn. 2006;235:2–9.
61. Blom NA, Gittenberger-de Groot AC, Jongeneel TH, DeRuiter MC, Poelmann RE, Ottenkamp J. Normal development of the pulmonary veins in

human embryos and formulation of a morphogenetic concept for sinus venosus defects. Am J Cardiol. 2001;87:305–9.
62. Marom EM, Herndon JE, Kim YH, et al. Variations in pulmonary venous drainage to the left atrium: implications for radiofrequency ablation. Radiology. 2004;230:824–9.
63. Tsao HM, Wu MH, Yu WC, et al. Role of right middle pulmonary vein in patients with paroxysmal atrial fibrillation. J Cardiovasc Electrophysiol. 2001;12:1353–7.
64. Choi SI, Seo JB, Choi SH, et al. Variation of the size of pulmonary venous ostia during the cardiac cycle: optimal reconstruction window at ECG-gated multidetector row CT. Eur Radiol. 2005;15(7):1441–5.
65. Heyneman LE, Nolan RL, Harrison JK, McAdams HP. Congenital unilateral pulmonary vein atresia: radiologic findings in three adult patients. AJR Am J Roentgenol. 2001;177(3):681–5.
66. Latson LA, Prieto LR. Congenital and acquired pulmonary vein stenosis. Circulation. 2007;115:103–8.
67. Ou P, Marini D, Celermajer DS, et al. Non-invasive assessment of congenital pulmonary vein stenosis in children using cardiac-non-gated CT with 64-slice technology. Eur J Radiol. 2009;70(3):595–9.
68. Lee HN, Kim YT, Cho SS. Individual pulmonary vein atresia in adults: report of two cases. Korean J Radiol. 2011;12(3):395–9.
69. Vanherreweghe E, Rigauts H, Bogaerts Y, Meeus L. Pulmonary vein varix: diagnosis with multislice helical CT. Eur Radiol. 2000;10:1315–7.
70. Senocak F, Ozme S, Bilgic A, et al. Partial anomalous pulmonary venous return. Evaluation of 51 cases. Jpn Heart J. 1994;35:43–50.
71. Gustafson RA, Warden HE, Murray GF, Hill RC, Rozar GE. Partial anomalous pulmonary venous connection to the right side of the heart. J Thorac Cardiovasc Surg. 1989;98(5 Pt 2):861–8.
72. Dillman JR, Yarram SG, Hernandez RJ. Imaging of pulmonary venous developmental anomalies. AJR Am J Roentgenol. 2009;192(5):1272–85.
73. Haramati LB, Moche IE, Rivera VT, et al. Computed tomography of partial anomalous pulmonary venous connection in adults. J Comput Assist Tomogr. 2003;27:743–9.
74. Ho ML, Bhalla S, Bierhals A, Gutierrez F. MDCT of partial anomalous pulmonary venous return (PAPVR) in adults. J Thorac Imaging. 2009;24(2):89–95.
75. Chintu MR, Chinnappa S, Bhandari S. Aberrant positioning of a central venous dialysis catheter to reveal a left-sided partial anomalous pulmonary venous connection. Vasc Health Risk Manag. 2008;4(5):1141–3.
76. Kafka H, Mohiaddin RH. Cardiac MRI and pulmonary MR angiography of sinus venosus defect and partial anomalous pulmonary venous connection in cause of right undiagnosed ventricular enlargement. AJR Am J Roentgenol. 2009;192(1):259–66.
77. Dillon EH, Camputaro C. Partial anomalous pulmonary venous drainage of the left upper lobe vs duplication of the superior vena cava: distinction based on CT findings. AJR Am J Roentgenol. 1993;160:375–9.
78. Almeda FQ, Barkatullah S, Nathan S, Kavinsky CJ. Partial anomalous pulmonary venous drainage of the superior left pulmonary vein into the innominate vein resulting in right ventricular failure. Am J Med. 2002;113(2):168–9.
79. Otsuka M, Itoh A, Haze K. Sinus venosus type of atrial septal defect with partial anomalous pulmonary venous return evaluated by multislice CT. Heart. 2004;90:901.
80. Toyoshima M, Sato A, Fukumoto Y, et al. Partial anomalous pulmonary venous return showing anomalous venous return to the azygos vein. Intern Med. 1992;31:1112–6.
81. Ibrahim M, Burwash IG, Morton B, Brais M. Direct drainage of the right pulmonary into the coronary sinus with intact interatrial septum: a case report. Can J Cardiol. 2001;17:807–9.
82. Davia JE, Cheitlin MD, Bedynek JL. Sinus venosus atrial septal defect: analysis of fifty cases. Am Heart J. 1973;85:177–85.
83. Dupuis C, Charaf LA, Breviere GM, Abou P, Remy-Jardin M, Helmius G. The "adult" form of the scimitar syndrome. Am J Cardiol. 1992;70:502–7.
84. Woodring JH, Howard TA, Kanga JF. Congenital pulmonary venolobar syndrome revisited. Radiographics. 1994;14:349–69.
85. Celik M, Celik T, Iyisoy A, Ayten O. Scimitar syndrome and azygos continuation of the inferior vena cava Diagnosed in an adult-an unusual association. Congenit Heart Dis. 2012;7(5):E85–8. doi:10.1111/j.1747-0803.2012.00650.x.
86. Lee ML. Isolated and complex scimitar vein anomalies and their differentiation from the meandering right pulmonary vein. Yonsei Med J. 2007;48(6):973–80.
87. Shinozaki H, Shimizu K, Anno H, et al. Total anomalous pulmonary vein drainage in an adult diagnosed by helical computed tomography. Intern Med. 1997;36(12):912–6.
88. Kim TH, Kim YM, Suh CH, et al. Helical CT angiography and three-dimensional reconstruction of total anomalous pulmonary venous connections in neonates and infants. AJR Am J Roentgenol. 2000;175:1381–6.
89. Alphonso N, Norgaard MA, Newcomb A, et al. Cor triatriatum: presentation, diagnosis and long-term surgical results. Ann Thorac Surg. 2005;80:1666–71.
90. Gharagozloo F, Bulkley BH, Hutchins GM. A proposed pathogenesis of cor triatriatum: impingement of the left superior vena cava on the developing left atrium. Am Heart J. 1977;94(5):618–26.
91. Tanaka F, Itoh M, Esaki H, Isobe J, Inoue R. Asymptomatic cor triatriatum incidentally revealed by computed tomography. Chest. 1991;100(1):272–4.
92. Saremi F, Gurudevan SV, Narula J, Abolhoda A. Multidetector computed tomography (MDCT) in diagnosis of "cor triatriatum sinister". J Cardiovasc Comput Tomogr. 2007;1(3):172–4.
93. Sakamoto I, Matsunaga N, Hayashi K, et al. Cinemagnetic resonance imaging of cor triatriatum. Chest. 1994;106:1586–9.

Coronary Artery Anomalies

27

Monvadi B. Srichai and Derek Mason

Isolated congenital coronary artery anomalies have been reported in approximately 1.3 % (range 0.2–5.6 %) of patients undergoing x-ray coronary angiography [1–4] and approximately 0.3 % of patients at autopsy [5]. About 80 % of coronary anomalies are considered benign without significant clinical sequelae, with the remaining 20 % potentially responsible for significant symptoms such as myocardial ischemia and sudden death [1]. The ability to identify coronary artery anomalies and define their anatomic course is important to further evaluate patients in whom a coronary anomaly is suspected. Noninvasive imaging has been the preferred way to evaluate patients with a suspected coronary artery anomaly, and it is important for physicians to recognize and understand the clinical and imaging features of the most commonly encountered coronary artery anomalies.

M.B. Srichai, MD, FAHA, FACC (✉)
Department of Medicine,
Medstar Georgetown University Hospital,
3800 Reservoir Rd NW, 5PHC,
Washington, DC 20007, USA
e-mail: barbarasrichai@yahoo.com,
srichai@alum.mit.edu

D. Mason, MD
Department of Radiology, NYU School of Medicine,
550 First Avenue, New York, NY 10016, USA

Imaging Techniques

Traditional Techniques

Coronary artery anomalies are often not diagnosed or adequately characterized by abnormalities observed on noninvasive tests such as electrocardiography, echocardiography, cardiovascular stress testing, and nuclear cardiac imaging. Identification of high-risk coronary artery anomalies often requires evaluation of coronary artery anatomy, which has traditionally been performed using x-ray coronary angiography. However, there are inherent risks of complications due to the invasive nature of the test and radiation exposure that limit its usefulness as a screening test, particularly for younger patients. Additionally, as only two-dimensional views are obtained, it can be difficult to define the complex three-dimensional course of the anomalous vessels [6], with misdiagnoses occurring in up to 50 % of cases [7, 8], often requiring additional methods such as catheter placement in the pulmonary artery or obtaining comparison angiographic views using a heart model with solder wire positioning in various views to depict the anomalous coronaries in order to determine the course of the coronary anomaly [9].

Noninvasive techniques for evaluation of coronary artery anatomy have included transthoracic echocardiography (TTE), transesophageal echocardiography (TEE), coronary magnetic resonance angiography (MRA), and coronary computed tomography angiography (CTA).

F. Saremi (ed.), *Cardiac CT and MR for Adult Congenital Heart Disease*,
DOI 10.1007/978-1-4614-8875-0_27, © Springer Science+Business Media New York 2014

TTE is a risk-free, noninvasive, widely available technology which has been shown to be an important screening tool for delineation of coronary artery anatomy in children and adolescents [10]. However, TTE imaging in adults is of variable image quality, dependent on many factors including body habitus and presence of underlying pulmonary disease. Visualization of coronary arteries in adults with TTE is difficult due to their small size, mobility, and limits of resolution, and thus is unreliable for excluding the presence of a significant coronary anomaly [11, 12]. TEE has been shown to be superior to TTE for coronary artery imaging [13–15]. However, due to limited tomographic imaging planes on TEE, only short segments of anomalous coronary arteries can be visualized at any one time, requiring meticulous operator technique to follow a vessel from its ostium to the ongoing segments [15].

Coronary MRA and CTA have emerged in recent years as important recommended clinical tests for screening adults for possible anomalous coronary arteries [16]. Both techniques provide 3-dimensional (3D) volumetric image acquisitions to evaluate the (3D) path of anomalous coronary arteries with wide field of view coverage and tissue characterization, allowing for distinguishing an occluded vessel from an anomalous one (e.g., vessel cannot be engaged with conventional angiography catheter) [17]. These newer, noninvasive techniques have been shown to provide better information on the origin and anatomic course of aberrant vessels compared to conventional x-ray angiography [18]. However, there are advantages and disadvantages between the two techniques that may make one more favorable than the other depending on the clinical situation.

Coronary MRA

Coronary MRA is a noninvasive 3-dimensional technique that is useful in the evaluation of congenital anomalous coronary arteries [19, 20] and is recommended as an initial screening method for evaluation of individuals with possible anomalous coronary arteries as part of the differential diagnosis [16, 21]. A major advantage of MRA is the limitless number of imaging planes possible compared with limited angulations in conventional x-ray coronary angiography or TTE and TEE acoustic windows. Moreover, evaluation of the heart and coronary arteries can be performed in a single examination setting (Fig. 27.1).

There have been several different MR methods applied for coronary MRA including both dark-blood and bright-blood techniques. Standard 2D spin-echo MR imaging had been the predominant technique used early on for visualization of the proximal coronary artery segments [22]. However, since 1991, coronary MRA has been mainly performed with "bright blood" gradient-echo techniques. Initial work focused on acquiring multiple thin 2D stacked slices gated to the cardiac cycle and processed with maximum intensity projection (MIP) algorithm to produce a coronary angiogram [23, 24]. Additional 2D methods such as selective arterial tagging with subsequent subtraction, interleaved spiral K-space scanning, and an ultrafast K-space segmented technique have also been described [20].

3D coronary MRA offers several advantages over 2D techniques. With 3D techniques, a volumetric acquisition of thin, truly contiguous partition images that encompass the complete coronary arterial tree can be acquired in 1 acquisition, minimizing the reliance on slice orientation [20]. 3D coronary MRA techniques were developed in the early 1990s, and investigators were able to successfully image volumes up to 64 mm thick across the aortic root with sufficient contrast between blood vessels and surrounding tissues. Further advancements in MRA techniques have led the development of various 3D whole-heart coronary MRA techniques with further improvements in tissue contrast for improved delineation of the coronary arteries [25–30]. Disadvantages over the 2D acquisitions are increased susceptibility to motion artifacts related to phase encoding in two directions [31, 32] and longer acquisition times. Multiple techniques have been applied to overcome the difficulties associated with coronary artery imaging, including suppression of respiratory artifacts with the use of signal averaging, breath-holding or respiratory triggering [33], suppression of cardiac motion with cardiac gating, and ultrafast

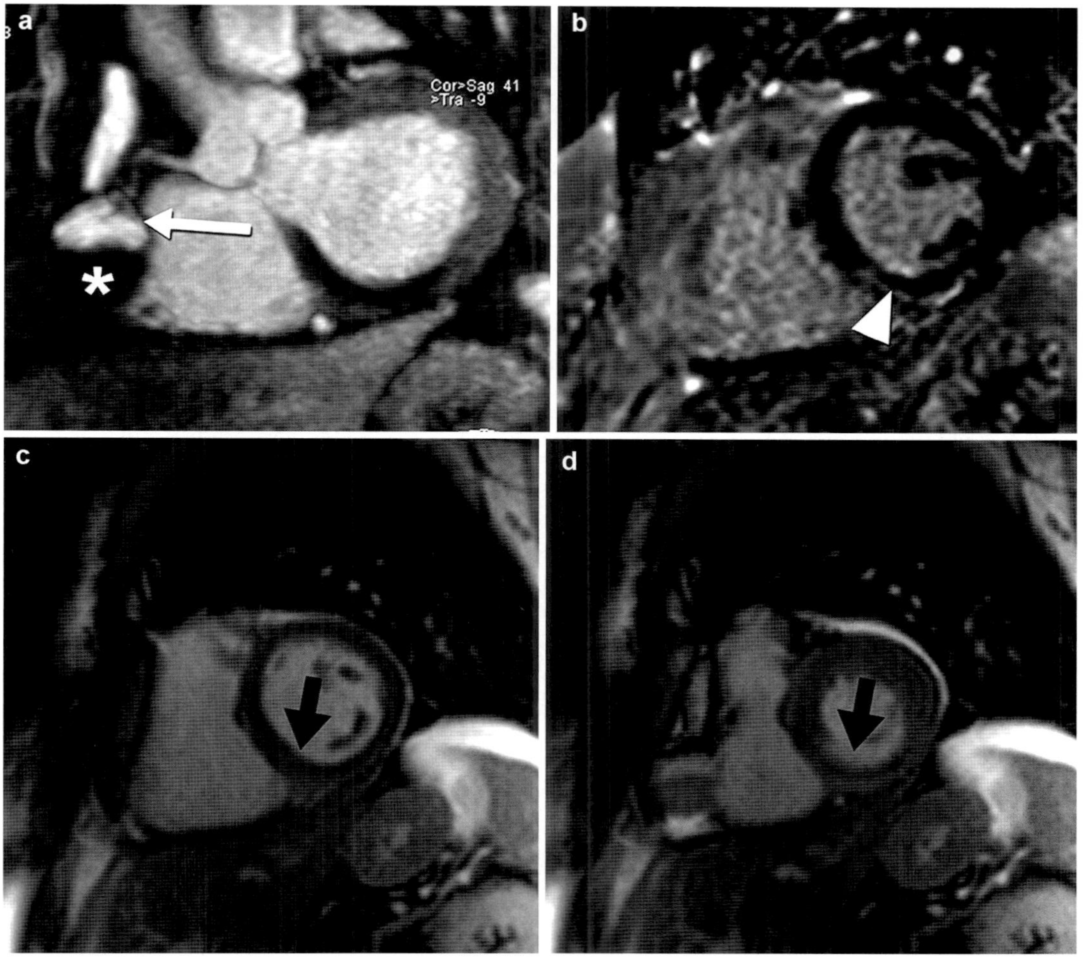

Fig. 27.1 MR techniques in the evaluation of coronary anomalies. Contrast-enhanced 3D coronary MRA (**a**) demonstrates right coronary artery aneurysm (*arrow*) which is partially filled with non-enhancing thrombus (*asterisk*). Late gadolinium enhancement inversion recovery image (**b**) demonstrates segmental infarction involving the basal and mid-inferior and inferoseptal walls (*arrowhead*) within the distribution supplied by the right coronary artery. Cine MR images at end diastole (**c**) and end systole (**d**) demonstrate the associated wall motion abnormality (*black arrows*) involving the basal and mid-inferior and inferoseptal walls

imaging sequences [34] with optimization of coronary artery signal to noise ratio. Other methods to reduce imaging time include limited resolution and coverage for protocols designed for detection of coronary anomalies and not for coronary stenosis detection [35].

The most important advantage of coronary MRA is that it does not require radiation. Another advantage is that it can often be performed free-breathing, often without the need for exogenous contrast agents and beta-blockers, making it useful for diagnostic evaluation in young patients with symptoms of possible anomalous coronary arteries [17] and allowing for repeat acquisitions on the same day in case of artifacts. Additionally, adjunct MR sequences such as velocity-encoded phase-contrast imaging and cine and late gadolinium enhancement imaging can further aid in demonstrating the flow directionality, hemodynamic significance, and structural and functional consequences of anomalous vessels [36]. Limiting factors with coronary MRA include its dependence on regular heart rhythm and respiration pattern for optimizing image quality and shortening image acquisition times. There are contraindications in patients with pacemakers, internal cardiac defibrillations, intracranial surgical clips, hearing aids, or neurostimulators, and MR-compatible metallic implants or clips may lead to problematic susceptibility artifact (i.e., following coronary artery bypass surgery). In addition, because of limited spatial resolution, distal coronary segments are often not well visualized with coronary MRA [37, 38]. Thus, alternative techniques such as coronary CTA are the preferred modality for evaluation of small collateral vessels and arteriovenous fistulas [39].

Coronary CTA

Coronary CTA is a valuable noninvasive 3-dimensional modality for delineating coronary artery anomalies, particularly in patients with equivocal x-ray coronary angiography findings [40], and is recommended as an initial screening method for evaluation of individuals with possible anomalous coronary arteries as part of the differential diagnosis [16, 41]. Recently, numerous studies have confirmed that coronary CTA is superior to conventional x-ray angiography in the detection of coronary artery anomalies [42]. In one study of 1,758 patients who underwent coronary CTA, 28 patients with anomalous coronary arteries were identified. Twenty of these patients subsequently underwent conventional x-ray coronary angiography. The anomalous coronary arteries could be accurately diagnosed with conventional x-ray angiography in only 11 of these patients [42].

There have been significant advances with coronary CTA over the past decade focused on improvement of image quality and reduction of patient radiation exposure. Multi-detector CTA, particularly with newer generation scanners, permits high-speed scanning of large volumes with high in-plane and through-plane resolution with isotropic voxels for evaluation in nearly any imaging plane without loss of spatial resolution. It is important to note that available acquisition and radiation dose reduction modes vary significantly depending on the manufacturer and model of specific CT systems. In depth discussion and comparison of the available technologies will not be covered in this chapter. However, common technical issues including dose reduction features will be mentioned.

ECG gating is an essential requirement for all coronary CTA imaging. Synchronization with the ECG is generally performed with detection of the R wave on the ECG signal. The "R-R interval" represents the time between consecutive R waves. The timing of image acquisition or reconstruction is often expressed as either a percent of the R-R interval or actual delay time (e.g., "400 ms" would be 400 ms after the R wave and "-400 ms" would be 400 ms before the R wave). ECG gating can be performed either in prospective or retrospective modes depending on the type of image acquisition. Retrospective gating is often performed in conjunction with conventional spiral imaging, simultaneous recording of the ECG over several heart beats (usually 6–10 beats), and very low pitch to allow for image reconstruction at any phase of the cardiac cycle. The cardiac phase least affected by cardiac motion artifact can then be chosen for image interpretation. Prospective triggering is commonly performed in conjunction with axial (step and shoot) scanning mode, with data acquisition triggered by a pre-specified time or phase of the cardiac cycle and performed over several heart beats until the entire heart is imaged. Data acquisition can be performed at a single phase of the cardiac cycle (e.g., 70 % of the R-R interval) or across a range of phases (60–80 % of the R-R interval) sometimes denoted as "padding." The advantage with retrospective gating is the ability to obtain ventricular functional information, since image reconstruction can be performed throughout the cardiac cycle. However, this is at the expense of increased patient radiation exposure. The advantage of prospective triggering is the significant reduction in radiation exposure, particularly when little or no padding is used [43–45]. The disadvantage with prospective triggering is the more limited dataset available based on a pre-specified chosen phase (or range of phases if padding is used) of the cardiac cycle with limited ability to compensate for an arrhythmia that may occur during acquisition.

Excellent temporal and spatial resolution is necessary for adequate visualization and interpretation of the small, moving coronary arteries. For CT scanners, temporal resolution is largely dependent on the rotation speed of the gantry, although other parameters may also be important. An estimate of temporal resolution for most scanners is simply the amount of time needed for the gantry to rotate half of a complete rotation (e.g., 150 ms for a scanner with a 300 ms gantry rotation time). Multi-cycle reconstruction techniques can significantly improve the effective temporal resolution by merging the datasets from several different heart beats but at the expense of increased radiation exposure. Dual-source scanners utilize two sets of sources and detector rows positioned at 90° angles to each other within the gantry and allow for simultaneous data acquisition and improved effective temporal resolution of the scanner to one-quarter of the gantry rotation time (e.g., 75 ms for gantry rotation of 300 ms). Given the limitations of temporal resolution with CT, patient heart rates of less than 60–65 beats per minute are often recommended to optimize image quality. Temporary reduction in heart rate is commonly achieved by the administration of beta-adrenergic blocking agents (or calcium channel blockers) which are given to the patient prior to scanning. Beta-blockers and calcium channel blockers have the added advantage of being able to suppress ectopic beats (e.g., premature ventricular contractions) that can adversely affect image quality. However, premedications should be used with caution in patients with low blood pressure or acutely ill. The spatial resolution of most scanners is 0.4–0.5 mm. Current generation CT scanners can acquire images with slice thickness as thin as 0.5 mm and generate nearly isotropic voxels as small as 0.5 mm^3. Field of view of the reconstructions should be generally limited to the smallest diameter possible that includes the cardiac structures and generally no more than 20–25 cm for optimal viewing (assuming a standard 512 × 512 image reconstruction matrix), with axial slice thickness set at the thinnest slices possible. Nitrates are commonly administered prior to scan acquisition for coronary vasodilatation to optimize vessel visualization.

The administration of intravenous iodinated contrast is necessary for optimal evaluation of coronary CTA. Depending on individual manufacturers, models, and protocols, contrast rates range from 4 to 7 mL/s and total contrast volumes usually range from 50 to 120 mL. Dual-head injection pumps allow for injection of saline (40–50 mL) immediately following the contrast injection to maximize contrast enhancement of the coronary arteries. Either "bolus tracking" or the "test bolus" method with tracking of a region of interest (e.g., ascending aorta) may be used to ensure accurate timing of data acquisition with contrast enhancement of the coronary arteries.

The primary disadvantage of coronary CTA is exposure to ionizing radiation, of particular concern in younger patients. Many different strategies have been employed to reduce the radiation exposure associated with coronary CTA, most of which are individualized dependent on patient and scanner-specific qualities. Examples of operator-dependent parameters include choice of scan mode, tube voltage, and tube current dependent on patient size including automated adjustments available on some scanners and scan length. Single-beat whole-heart imaging via wide detector systems (e.g., 320-detector CT system) or using high-pitch helical mode has been shown to provide diagnostic image quality with potential to reduce radiation exposure by over 90 % [46, 47]. Post-processing techniques such as iterative reconstruction algorithms can provide improved image quality and reduced noise, allowing for diagnostic image acquisition at lower tube potential and current compared to standard filtered back projection algorithms [48–50].

Image Interpretation

Visualization of the coronary arteries from different imaging planes is often essential for accurate image interpretation. Isotropic voxels in three-dimensional volumetric datasets (MRA or CTA) allow for MPR with minimal image distortion. Most 3D software packages allow for display of three orthogonal views simultaneously, allowing for manual manipulation of the planes in order to optimize the view for each coronary artery and segment. The use of curved MPR images, often created by an automated or semiautomated algorithm, allows for display of the entire coronary vessel in a single 2-dimentional (2D) image, with the ability to rotate the artery around a focal point. Maximum intensity projections (MIP) are created using thicker sections and can be helpful to reduce image noise and/or visualize a longer vessel segment. Finally, volume-rendered 3D images allow for interpretation of structural relationships such as vessel course in relation to other cardiac or vascular structures with exclusion of surrounding structures such as bones, lung tissue, and extracardiac vessels.

Normal Coronary Artery Anatomy

Embryology

The development of a blood vascular system occurs relatively early during the gestation period, characterized by differentiation of precursor cells into primitive blood cells and endothelial cells. The first endothelial cells appear during formation of the heart tubes and form the endocardial endothelium. As the wall of the heart tube thickens and the cardiac jelly diminishes, the number of myocytes increase in number and the endocardial surface becomes progressively more trabeculated, establishing an endocardial-lined sinusoidal system which minimizes diffusion distances to the myocardium. This sinusoidal system precedes any evidence of vascularization [51].

The initial feature of a developing coronary vasculature occurs around the fourth week of embryogenesis with the appearance of vascular buds or blood islands that arise in the epicardium and consist of a layer of endothelial cells distended by nucleated erythrocytes. These blood islands appear to form from endothelial precursor cells from the liver region which migrate to the epicardium as opposed to endocardial endothelial cells [52]. The gradual disappearance of cardiac jelly and eventual compaction of the myocardium seems to correlate with the appearance of the blood islands. These blood islands initially appear near the ventricular apex in the interventricular sulcus and then eventually over other regions of the ventricles. The blood islands gradually coalesce and form the rudiments of a network of vascular channels, preferentially forming in the sulci or indentations of the epicardial surface [53]. Following early capillarization, the venous vessels appear around the sixth week and arterial vessels during the transition from sixth to seventh week of embryogenesis. Although different concepts have been put forth regarding the development of the coronary arteries from the aorta, current evidence suggests that major coronary arteries form by coalescence of microvessels which grow toward and penetrate the aorta [54], an event that occurs as early as 44 days after gestation [53]. Several studies have shown that the left coronary artery appears to establish a connection earlier than the right [55, 56]. The development of coronary arteries proceeds in orderly sequence, proximal-distal, with smooth muscle alpha actin first expressed at the site of their aortic connection regulated by neural crest [51]. Disruption of the neural crest leads to variability in the site of origin and symmetry of the coronary arteries [51]. Thickening of the media and adventitia, formation of the internal elastic lamina, and increase in collagen content occur between the fourth month and birth [57], with continued increase both medial thickness, length of the arterial segments, and numerical density of arterioles during the first year after birth [58, 59].

Definitions

The basic definition of what constitutes a normal coronary artery and the normal spectrum of coronary artery variation has been the subject of many articles. In general, most experts agree that it is normal to have two coronary arteries, the right and the left. However, some confusion arises with regard to definitions of smaller arteries such as conal (infundibular) branches, particularly when these branches demonstrate independent origin from the aorta. A frequently used definition is that any configuration occurring in >1 % of an unselected general population is considered normal or normal variant [60]. It then follows that coronary anomalies are variants of normal coronary artery anatomy that occur in <1 % of the general population.

Another basic nomenclature principle is that coronary vessels are named for the structures that they supply rather than for their origin. This nomenclature is based on the fundamental embryologic principles, namely, that the coronary vessels arise within the developing epicardium and only later attach to the aorta. Thus, various perturbations in the connections of the coronary vessels to each other and to the aorta occur subsequent to the formation of the coronary vessels in the epicardium. Moreover, three main coronary vessels (left anterior descending, circumflex, and right coronary) are considered arteries and the smaller, more distal vessels are termed coronary branches.

Normal Variants

There are several commonly recognized variations in normal coronary artery anatomy. Some of the more typical coronary artery variants are described below.

Vasculature to the Inferior Wall

The vascular supply to the inferior wall has a spectrum of variants. The origin of the posterior descending artery (PDA) and posterolateral branches that supply the inferior wall can originate from the right coronary artery (RCA) only (right dominant), the left circumflex (LCX) artery only (left dominant), or encompass multiple branches from both arteries (codominant). In most patients the PDA arises from the distal portion of the coronary artery, but some patients have early takeoff of the PDA from the RCA (split RCA), which then courses toward the apex along the diaphragmatic surface of the right ventricle. Others have a left anterior descending (LAD) artery that wraps around the apex to supply some of the apical inferior wall.

Vasculature to the Atrioventricular Node

A better definition of coronary dominance incorporates the arterial supply to the atrioventricular node, an electrically active bundle of tissue that delays conduction of impulses from the atria to the ventricles. Unfortunately, the node is not directly visualized with current coronary artery imaging techniques, but it is closely associated with central fibrous body near the apex of the Koch triangle. This triangle is enclosed by the septal leaflet of the tricuspid valve anteriorly, the coronary sinus ostium inferiorly, and the Eustachian ridge posteriorly. Typically the dominant artery that supplies the PDA and inferior wall also gives rise to small branches at the base of the heart that supply the atrioventricular node.

Vasculature to the Sinoatrial Node

The sinuatrial node is another electrically active tissue bundle that sits near the junction of the right atrium and superior vena cava and serves as the primary pacemaker of the heart. This node is supplied by a single branch from the proximal RCA in 60 % of people. Other variants include sinoatrial node branch from the proximal LCX or distal RCA or LCX artery [61].

Ramus Intermedius

Instead of bifurcating into the LAD and LCX arteries, in some patients the left main trifurcates into an LAD, LCX, and ramus intermedius artery. The ramus intermedius typically supplies the lateral and inferior walls in a territory similar to that supplied by the diagonal or obtuse marginal branches. As a result, the branches that would normally supply these regions are either diminutive or nonexistent and have coalesced into the ramus intermedius.

Right Superior Septal Perforator

The right superior septal perforator is a normal variant seen in approximately 3 % of patients [62]. This branch supplies the anterior septum in a similar territory to other septal perforators but arises from the proximal RCA or right sinus of Valsalva instead of the LAD.

Multiple Coronary Ostia

In addition to the typical LCA and RCA origins from the aorta, some patients have smaller branches that arise directly from the aorta as opposed to from the coronary arteries. Common

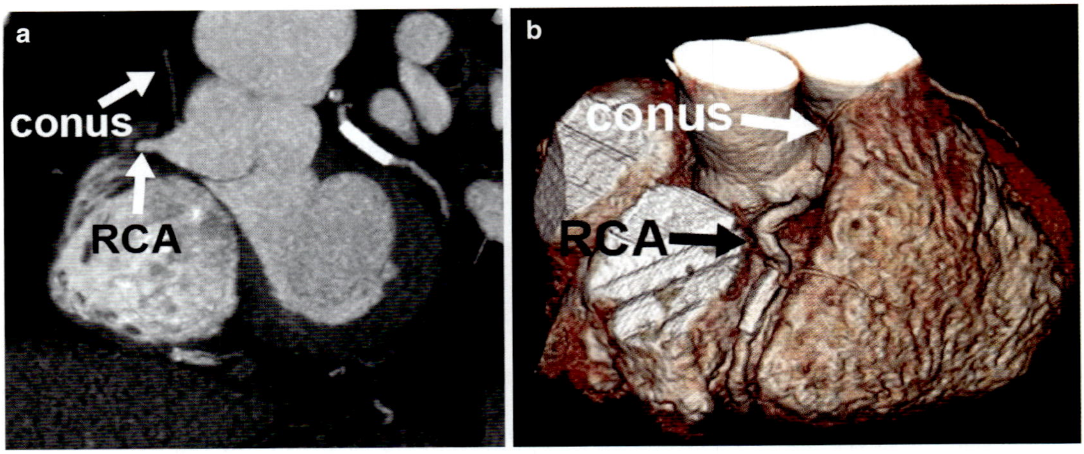

Fig. 27.2 Normal variant of multiple coronary ostia. Coronary CTA 2D thin maximum intensity projection (**a**) and 3D volume-rendered (**b**) images demonstrating a common coronary artery variant of separate origin of the conus branch directly from the aortic root instead of from the right coronary artery (*RCA*)

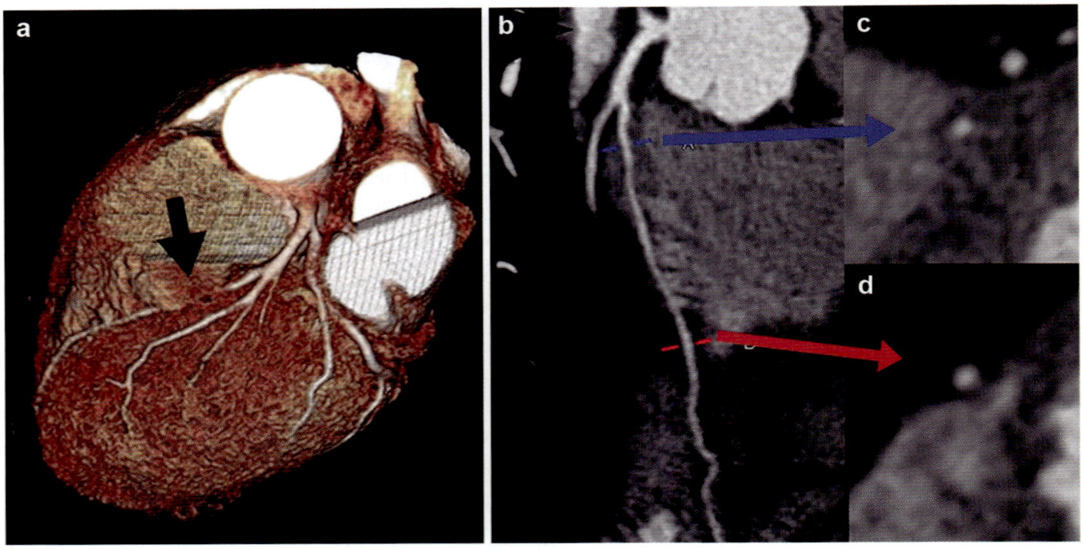

Fig. 27.3 Normal variant of myocardial bridging. Coronary CTA 3D volume-rendered image (**a**) demonstrates that a portion of the left anterior descending artery (LAD) is obscured by overlying myocardium (*black arrow*). Curved multiplanar reformatted images of the LAD (**b**) and corresponding multiplanar reformatted images axial to the vessel (**c**, **d**) demonstrate intramyocardial bridge with the mid-segment of LAD surrounded by myocardium (*blue arrow*, image **c**) and normal epicardial position of the distal LAD surrounded by epicardial fat (*red arrow*, image **d**)

variants of this type include direct origin of the conus or sinoatrial node branch from the aorta (Fig. 27.2). While these variants may have clinical consequences if unrecognized during surgery or coronary catheterization, for the majority of people, these are not clinically significant.

Myocardial Bridging

Myocardial bridging refers to the intramyocardial course of a portion of a normally positioned epicardial coronary artery (Fig. 27.3). The degree in which the coronary artery "dives" into the myocardium is variable in depth and length. With the advent of coronary CTA and MRA, allowing visualization of extra-coronary structures, this variant has been noted to occur much more frequently than previously reported by x-ray coronary angiography. Although typically seen in the mid-LAD segment, myocardial bridges can occur in any coronary artery segment. Although systolic narrowing may be visualized on coronary artery imaging, these findings are rarely clinically significant since most coronary blood flow occurs in diastole.

Coronary Anomalies: Clinical Implications

Incidence

Depending on the series, isolated congenital coronary artery anomalies have been reported in approximately 1.3 % (range 0.2–5.6 %) of patients undergoing x-ray coronary angiography [1–4]. Variations in number are likely related to referral bias in some centers not reflective of the general population and variability in definitions of anomalous versus normal variant coronaries. Although the aortic root is normal in most patients with coronary anomalies, about 26 % of coronary anomalies involve some type of aortic root abnormality, such as asymmetry of the aortic sinuses [63]. In patients with more substantial cardiac defects of the outflow tracts, such as transposition of the great arteries, increased variation of the coronary artery pattern is noted, and it becomes important when describing these patterns to relate them specifically to the aortic and pulmonic valves [64]. The most common coronary anomaly is absent left main with separate origin of the LAD and LCX arteries from the left sinus of Valsalva, with an incidence of 0.41 % followed by the LCX arising from the RCA or directly from the right sinus of Valsalva, with an incidence of 0.37 % [65]. Both of these anomalies are considered benign in clinical significance. The most common potentially serious coronary artery anomaly is anomalous origin of the RCA from the left sinus of Valsalva, with incidence of 0.107 % [65] (Table 27.1).

Table 27.1 Incidence of specific coronary anomalies

	Number	Incidence (%)	Anomalies (%)
Benign			
Absent left main	513	0.41	30.4
LCX from right sinus or RCA	467	0.37	27.7
Coronary artery from noncoronary sinus			
1. LCA from noncoronary sinus	1	0.0008	0.06
2. RCA from noncoronary sinus	4	0.003	0.24
Anomalous origin from above the sinuses			
1. LCA from ascending aorta	16	0.013	0.95
2. RCA from ascending aorta	188	0.15	11.2
Small coronary artery fistulae	163	0.12	9.7
Potentially serious			
Coronary artery from pulmonary artery			
1. LM from pulmonary artery	10	0.008	0.59
2. LAD from pulmonary artery	1	0.0008	0.06
3. RCA from pulmonary artery	2	0.002	0.12
Coronary artery from opposite sinus			
1. LM from right sinus	22	0.017	1.3
2. LAD from right sinus	38	0.03	2.3
3. RCA form left sinus	136	0.107	8.1
Single coronary artery	56	0.044	3.3
1. R-I	1	0.0008	0.06
2. R-II	19	0.015	1.1
3. R-III	5	0.004	0.3
4. L-I	20	0.016	1.2
5. L-II	11	0.009	0.65
Multiple or large-sized fistulae	62	0.06	3.7

Adapted from Yurtdas and Gulen [65] with permission
LM left main, *LAD* left anterior descending, *LCX* left circumflex, *LCA* left coronary artery, *RCA* right coronary artery

Clinical Presentation

Many studies have demonstrated that most coronary artery anomalies are discovered as benign, incidental findings upon angiography studies. Some of these "benign" anomalies include (1) absent left main, (2) ectopic origin of the LCX artery from the right sinus of Valsalva, (3) ectopic coronary origin from the posterior sinus of Valsalva, (4) anomalous coronary origin from the ascending aorta, (5) absent circumflex, (6) intercoronary communications, and (7) small coronary artery fistula. Other anomalies may be associated with potentially more serious sequelae such as angina pectoris, myocardial infarction, syncope, cardiac arrhythmias, congestive heart failure, or even sudden death. Potentially serious anomalies include (1) ectopic coronary origin from the pulmonary artery, (2) ectopic coronary origin from the opposite sinus of Valsalva, (3) single coronary artery, and (4) large coronary fistula [1]. The etiology of myocardial ischemia may be related to disturbed kinetics from oblique origin, ostial stenosis, compression of intramural course, loss of reservoir capacity, and increased myocardial oxygen demand associated with exercise. Physical examination findings depend on the coronary anomaly and are most often entirely normal.

Table 27.2 Clinical significance-based classification of coronary artery anomalies

Class	Coronary artery anomaly
I. Benign	Ectopic origin of LCX from right sinus
	Ectopic origin of LCX from the RCA
	Separate origin of LCX and LAD
	Duplicated LAD
II. Relevant	Coronary artery fistula
Related to myocardial ischemia	Single coronary artery R-L, I-II-III, A-P
	Ectopic origin of LCA from PA
	Coronary artery atresia
	Hypoplastic coronary artery
III. Severe	Ectopic origin of LCA from the right sinus
Potentially related to sudden death	Ectopic origin of RCA from the left sinus
	Ectopic origin of RCA from the PA
	Single coronary artery R-L, I-II-III, B
IV. Critical	Class II and superimposed CAD
Related to sudden death/ myocardial ischemia and associated with superimposed CAD	Class III and superimposed CAD

Adapted from Rigatelli et al. [66] with permission

Classification Schemes

Different classification criteria have been described for coronary artery anomalies. Some investigators prefer to categorize anomalies based solely on clinical significance, such as benign, relevant, severe, or critical [66] (Table 27.2). Other schemes focus on first assessing anatomic variation independent from clinical and hemodynamic sequelae, with judgment about clinical relevance as a secondary clinical classification. Anatomic schemes commonly divide coronary artery anomalies into three general classifications. These include anomalies of origin and course, anomalies of intrinsic coronary arterial anatomy, and anomalies of coronary termination (Table 27.3). Coronary anomalies of origin and course have the highest risk of developing major cardiac events.

Isolated Coronary Anomalies

Anomalies of Origin and Course

The majority of clinically significant coronary artery anomalies are within this group of anomalies. There are three main subcategories within this group including (A) absent left main (LM) artery, (B) anomalous ostium outside the aortic sinuses, and (C) anomalous ostium at an improper sinus.

Absent Left Main

Absent left main, also known as separate origin of LAD and LCX, is typically a benign configuration where the LAD and LCX each have well-defined, separate ostia from the left sinus of Valsalva (Fig. 27.4). Although inability to

Table 27.3 Anatomic classification of coronary artery anomalies

Anomalies of origin and course
Absent left main
Anomalous coronary ostium outside the aortic sinuses
High takeoff
Anomalous origin of coronary artery from pulmonary artery[a]
Anomalous coronary ostium at an improper sinus with anomalous course
Anterior
Interarterial[a]
Intraseptal
Posterior
Single coronary artery
Anomalies of intrinsic anatomy
Congenital ostial stenosis or atresia
Coronary ectasia and aneurysm
Duplicated coronary arteries
Subendocardial coronary course
Coronary crossing
Anomalies of termination
Coronary artery fistulas[a]
Extracardiac terminations
Coronary arcade

[a]Hemodynamically significant anomalies

separately cannulate the LAD and LCX at x-ray angiography may lead to misinterpretation that one of these arteries is completely occluded, with potential failure to perfuse both vessels during cardiopulmonary bypass [67], the wide field of view and tissue characterization possible with coronary CTA and MRA make this diagnostic error uncommon [68]. There is an increased incidence of left coronary artery dominance and myocardial bridging. However, there is no increased association with congenital heart anomalies or coronary artery disease [67, 69].

Anomalous Coronary Ostium Outside the Aortic Sinuses

There is a large subset of coronary anomalies, including origin of the left coronary artery from the pulmonary artery (ALCAPA) (Fig. 27.5), that are part of this subcategory. ALCAPA is also known by the eponym of Bland-White-Garland syndrome with estimated incidence of 0.008 % [65]. This anomaly most often presents as an isolated defect, but in 5 % of cases may be associated with other congenital heart defects,

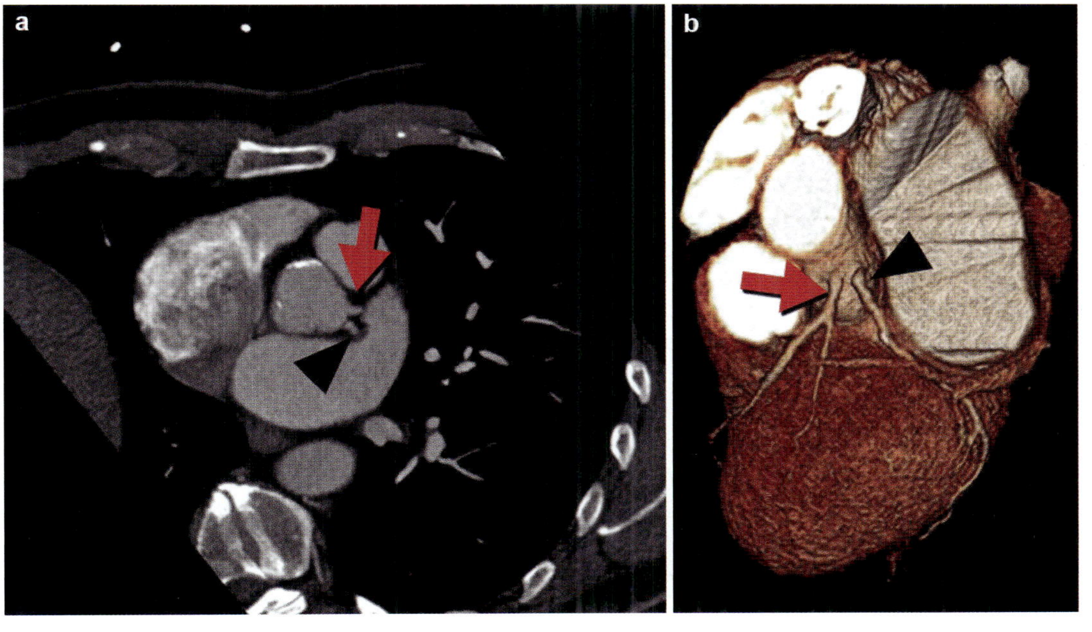

Fig. 27.4 Absent left main or separate origin of the left anterior descending (LAD) and circumflex arteries. Coronary CTA multiplanar reformatted image (**a**) and corresponding 3D volume-rendered image (**b**) demonstrate that the LAD (*red arrow*) and circumflex (*black arrowhead*) arteries arise directly from the left coronary sinus without a common ostium (absent left main)

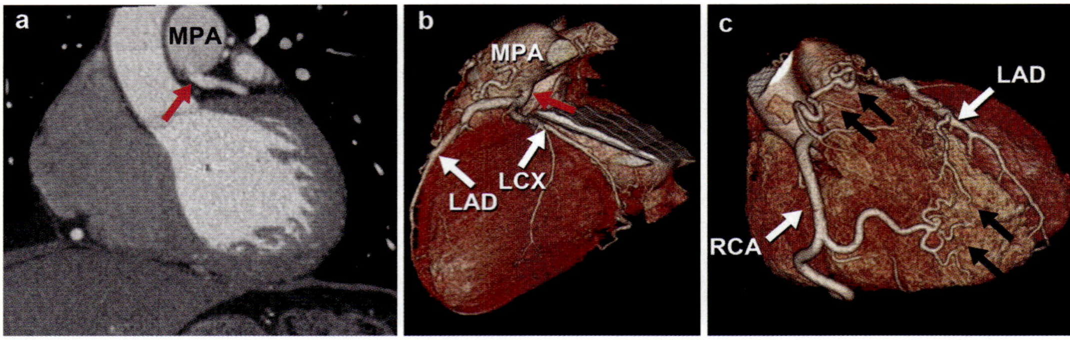

Fig. 27.5 Anomalous left coronary artery from the pulmonary artery (ALCAPA). Coronary CTA multiplanar reformatted images (**a**) and corresponding 3D volume-rendered images (**b**, **c**) demonstrate anomalous origin of the left coronary artery from the main pulmonary artery (*MPA*) (*red arrow*). The right coronary artery (*RCA*) demonstrates normal origin from the right aortic sinus and is significantly dilated due to the inherent left to right shunting present at the coronary artery level with associated large collateral vessels (*black arrows*) between the right and left coronary artery systems. *LAD* left anterior descending artery, *LCX* left circumflex artery

including atrial septal defect, ventricular septal defect, and aortic coarctation. Symptoms usually present in infants or children with symptoms of myocardial ischemia due to coronary steal phenomenon or congestive heart failure. Left to right shunting from the higher pressure left coronary arterial system to the lower pressure arterial system occurs via RCA to left coronary artery (LCA) collateral vessels, with retrograde flow in the left coronary arterial circuit. Thus, blood flows from the aorta --> RCA --> collateral vessels --> LCA --> low pressure pulmonary circuit. The resultant circulatory insufficiency results in left ventricular dysfunction, myocardial infarction, or life-threatening cardiac arrhythmias.

ALCAPA is associated with 90 % mortality if not surgically corrected [70]. Although rare, there have been numerous reports of this anomaly presenting in the adult, with clinical presentations of heart failure from chronic mitral insufficiency or global ischemic cardiomyopathy [71]. There is still ongoing risk of sudden cardiac death due to ischemic malignant ventricular arrhythmias [72]. Survival beyond infancy is attributed to the development of abundant intercoronary collateral arteries, an alteration in hemodynamics that encourages antegrade blood flow in the left coronary arterial tree, and reduction in the size of the left ventricular myocardium supplied by the LCA [70]. Once the diagnosis of ALCAPA is made, early surgical repair is recommended to prevent future potential complications. Surgical repair procedures include aortocoronary saphenous vein or internal mammary artery bypass grafting, aortic root reimplantation with or without a pulmonary flap, or intrapulmonary baffling [72]. Other coronary anomalies arising from the pulmonary artery are even more rare, including anomalous LAD from the pulmonary artery with estimated incidence of 0.0008 % and anomalous RCA from the pulmonary artery (ARCAPA) with estimated incidence of 0.002 % [65] (Fig. 27.6).

Although conventional x-ray coronary angiography can detect and depict the course of ALCAPA and similar variants, diagnosis can be difficult, particularly given the presence of numerous enlarged collateral arteries and high-flow shunting that can make adequate opacification of the coronaries difficult as well as the limited 2-dimensional visualization (Fig. 27.6). CT and MR imaging provide direct visualization of the origin and proximal course of the anomalous coronary artery, including the exact location of the anomalous coronary artery from the pulmonary artery, and visualization of the dilated intercoronary collateral arteries (Fig. 27.5). In addition, dynamically enhanced MR imaging (fast time-resolved MRA or first-pass perfusion MR imaging) may demonstrate the lack of early enhancement of the LCA compared to RCA followed by late enhancement of the LCA in ALCAPA [71]. Finally, phase-contrast MR

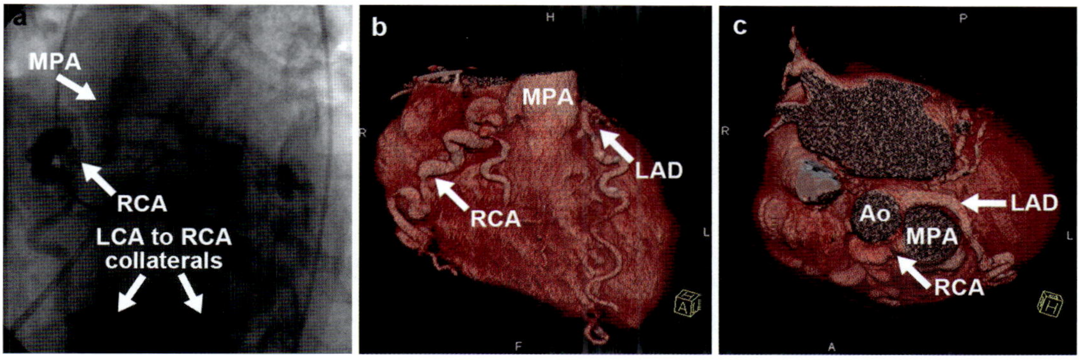

Fig. 27.6 Anomalous right coronary artery from the pulmonary artery (ARCAPA). X-ray coronary angiogram (**a**) and 3D coronary CTA volume-rendered images (**b**, **c**) demonstrating anomalous origin of the right coronary artery (*RCA*) from the main pulmonary artery (*MPA*). The coronary anatomy is more easily appreciated on the 3D coronary CTA images compared to x-ray coronary angiogram. The left coronary artery (*LCA*) system demonstrates normal origin from the left aortic sinus with the presence of large coronary collaterals. *LAD* left anterior descending artery. *Ao* Aorta

imaging can be used to demonstrate the retrograde flow in the anomalous coronary arteries.

Additional sites of anomalous origin of the coronary arteries include origin above or below the aortic sinuses such as the left or right ventricular outflow tracts, the ascending aorta, and the brachiocephalic or subclavian arteries. Although anomalous origin from the ascending aorta is considered a benign anomaly, the clinical sequelae of origins at other sites remain uncertain due to their rarity.

Anomalous Coronary Ostium at an Improper Sinus

Anomalous coronary origin from an improper sinus is probably the most frequent clinically significant coronary anomaly. This type of anomaly is important to recognize, since it is a common cause of sudden cardiac death in young athletes, accounting for approximately 15 % of sudden death causes in young persons [73–75]. The most commonly encountered form of this anomaly is ectopic (aberrant) origin of a coronary artery from the contralateral sinus. Conceptually, there are four potential paths that a coronary may take to its perfusion territory: prepulmonic, anterior to the right ventricular outflow tract (Type 1); interarterial, between the aorta and pulmonary artery (Type 2A); intraseptal, through the proximal interventricular septum similar to a superior septal perforator (Type 2B); or retroaortic, posterior to the aortic root (Type 3) (Figs. 27.7, 27.8, 27.9, and 27.10). Type 2A is considered to be a clinically severe subtype with a high risk of sudden cardiac death. Anomalous LCA from the right sinus of Valsalva is relatively rare with incidence 0.03 %, but with a high association with sudden cardiac death [76–78] (Fig. 27.9). Anomalous RCA form the left sinus of Valsalva is more common (0.1 %) (Fig. 27.10) and is also associated with sudden cardiac death, but at a less frequent rate. In a large retrospective review of sudden cardiac death among military recruits, 33 % of sudden deaths were related to anomalous origin of the LCA from the right sinus and none related to anomalous RCA from left sinus [75]. In other studies, sudden cardiac death was noted with both types of coronary anomalies, although the frequency was significantly less for anomalous RCA from the left sinus [74, 78]. Anatomic features that appear to be associated with risk of sudden death include acute angle takeoff, slit-like coronary orifice, proximal intramural course, double coronary ostia from same sinus, and compression of the anomalous coronary artery between the aorta and pulmonary artery [74, 78]. It is likely that anomalous course between the aorta and right ventricle outflow tract is less harmful than anomalous course of the artery between the aorta and main pulmonary artery.

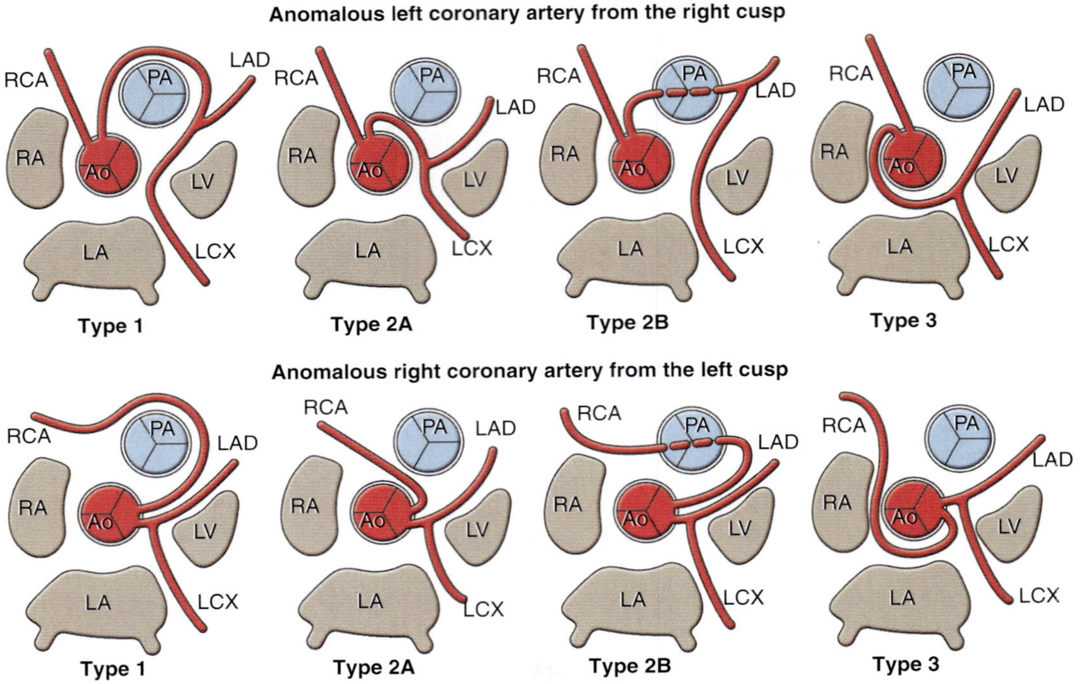

Fig. 27.7 Diagram demonstrating potential paths for anomalous coronary artery from the opposite sinus including prepulmonic (*Type 1*), interarterial (*Type 2A*), intraseptal (*Type 2B*), and retroaortic (*Type 3*). *Ao* aorta, *PA* pulmonary artery, *RA* right atrium, *LA* left atrium, *LV* left ventricle, *RCA* right coronary artery, *LAD* left anterior descending, *LCX* left circumflex

Current AHA guidelines recommend that surgical coronary revascularization be performed for the following indications: (1) anomalous LCA coursing between the aorta and pulmonary artery, (2) documented coronary ischemia due to coronary compression related to anomalous course between the great arteries or an intramural component, and (3) anomalous origin of the RCA coursing between the aorta and pulmonary arteries with evidence of ischemia [79]. Standard surgical revascularization techniques such as bypass grafting, unroofing, and reimplantation and novel techniques such as pulmonary translocation have been performed in these patients. In general, bypass grafting is not a good option for most patients due to potential graft compromise related to competitive flow and possibility of graft thrombosis. Data from surgical series of patients who have undergone intervention for anomalous coronary artery from the opposite sinus have demonstrated good medium-term outcomes at 8–10 years, with elimination of ischemic symptoms, thereby allowing patients to return to normal activities [80].

Single Coronary Artery

Single coronary artery is one of the rarest congenital coronary anomalies occurring in approximately 0.024–0.066 % of the general population undergoing coronary angiography [65]. Single coronary artery is defined as one coronary artery arising from a single coronary ostium from the aortic trunk that supplies the entire myocardium. Although the majority of cases occur in the setting of other congenital cardiovascular disease, isolated single coronary artery anomaly has also been reported, commonly anomalous RCA from the LAD [65]. The modified Lipton classification for describing different types of single coronary artery anomalies uses a coding system defined by the originating sinus and the relationship between the three main coronary arteries. The first letter designates the sinus of Valsalva from which the single coronary ostium is located

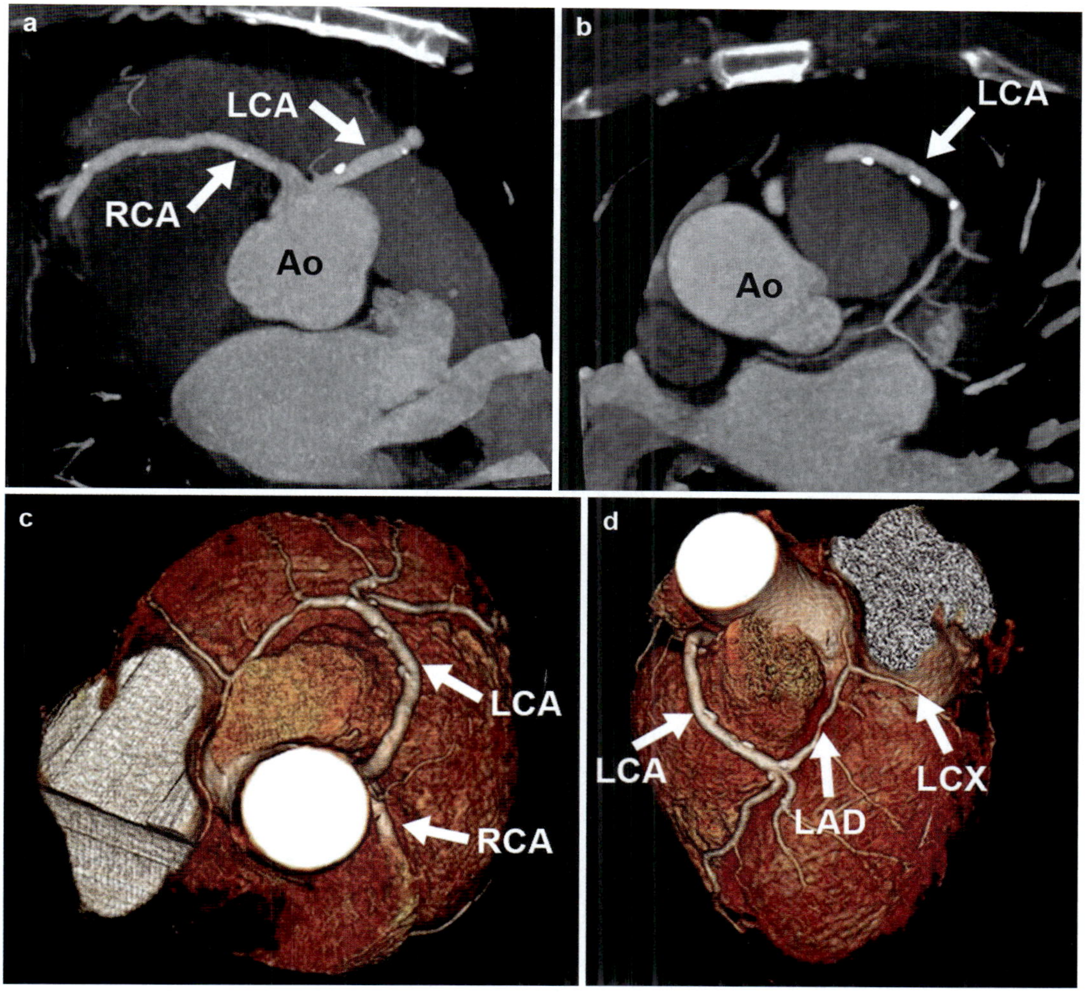

Fig. 27.8 Anomalous left coronary artery from the right aortic sinus, Type I: prepulmonic course. Coronary CTA thin maximum intensity projection images (**a**, **b**) and 3D volume-rendered images. (**c**, **d**) demonstrating anomalous origin of the left coronary artery (*LCA*) from the right sinus adjacent to the right coronary artery (*RCA*) origin. The LCA demonstrates a benign course anterior to the right ventricular outflow tract before giving rise to the normally situated left anterior descending (*LAD*) and left circumflex (*LCX*) arteries. (*Ao*) Aorta

(i.e., left "L" or right "R"). The next position is represented as a Roman numeral (I, II, or III) and describes the anatomic course of the artery. Group I follows the normal anatomic course of either the right or left coronary artery (Fig. 27.11). In Group II, one coronary artery arises from the proximal aspect of the normally located other coronary artery (Fig. 27.12). In group III, the LAD and LCX arise separately (no left main) from the normally positioned RCA (Fig. 27.13). The final letter describes the relationship between the anomalous coronary artery and the aorta and pulmonary artery [i.e., anterior (A), posterior (P), between the great vessels (B), intraseptal (S), and a mixture of types (C)] [1].

The clinical significance and risk of single coronary artery usually depend on the location and course of the abnormal coronary artery origin and the presence and degree of any culprit stenotic or atherosclerotic lesion [65]. Since clinical presentation may vary and there is a risk of sudden death if left untreated, symptomatic patients with demonstrable ischemia need further clinical attention [81].

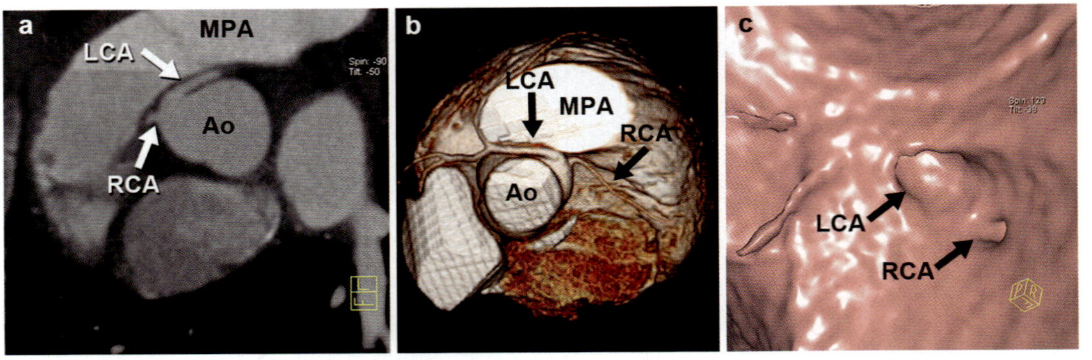

Fig. 27.9 Anomalous left coronary artery from the right aortic sinus, Type 2A: interarterial course. Coronary CTA multiplanar reformatted image (**a**), 3D volume-rendered image (**b**), and corresponding 3D shaded surface endoluminal image (**c**) demonstrating separate origins of the left coronary artery (*LCA*) and right coronary artery (*RCA*) from the right aortic cusp with the LCA coursing between the aorta (*Ao*) and right ventricle outflow tract/main pulmonary artery (*MPA*)

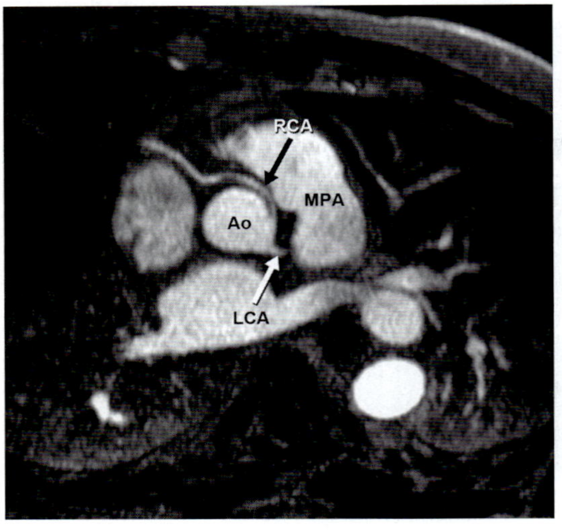

Fig. 27.10 Anomalous right coronary artery from the left aortic sinus, Type 2A: interarterial course. Contrast-enhanced coronary MRA demonstrates separate origins of the left coronary artery (*LCA*) and right coronary artery (*RCA*) from the left aortic cusp with the RCA coursing between the aorta (*Ao*) and main pulmonary artery (*MPA*)/ right ventricle outflow tract

Anomalies of Intrinsic Anatomy

Congenital Ostial Stenosis or Atresia

Ostial atresia is most frequently reported for the left main artery (Fig. 27.14), with subsequent failure of the development of the left main. The LAD and LCX demonstrate retrograde filling via collaterals from the RCA. This anomaly is distinguished from single coronary artery in that the flow is centripetal (from smaller peripheral vessels to larger central vessels) and often from multiple small collaterals in ostial atresia as opposed to centrifugal (from larger to progressively smaller vessels) in single coronary artery [82]. The collateral circulation is usually incapable of providing adequate myocardial perfusion leading to failure to thrive, early myocardial ischemia and infarction, and a poor prognosis without surgical intervention [83].

Coronary Ectasia and Aneurysm

Coronary artery aneurysm is defined as a coronary artery segment that demonstrates a diameter greater than 1.5 times the normal adjacent segment (Fig. 27.1). Coronary artery ectasia is defined as the presence of coronary artery aneurysm that involves more than 50 % of the total length of the coronary artery [84]. Kawasaki's disease accounts for the majority of cases of coronary artery aneurysm worldwide, although atherosclerotic coronary artery disease is frequently implicated for most cases in the United States. Compared with invasive angiography, noninvasive techniques including coronary CTA and MRA allow for more accurate assessment of aneurysm size and presence of associated thrombus [85].

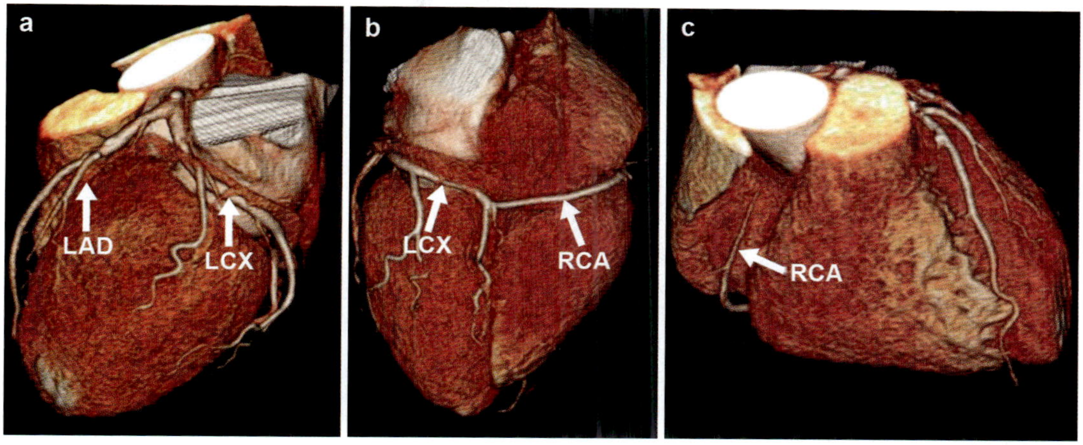

Fig. 27.11 Single coronary artery, Type L-I. Coronary CTA 3D volume-rendered images demonstrate normal origin of the left coronary artery from the left cusp giving rise to normal left anterior descending (*LAD*) and left circumflex (*LCX*) arterial courses (**a**). The LCX runs along the left atrioventricular groove and continues posteriorly along the right atrioventricular groove giving rise to the distal aspect of the right coronary artery (*RCA*) (**b**). The RCA continues along the right atrioventricular groove and is noted to taper in its mid- and proximal segments (**c**)

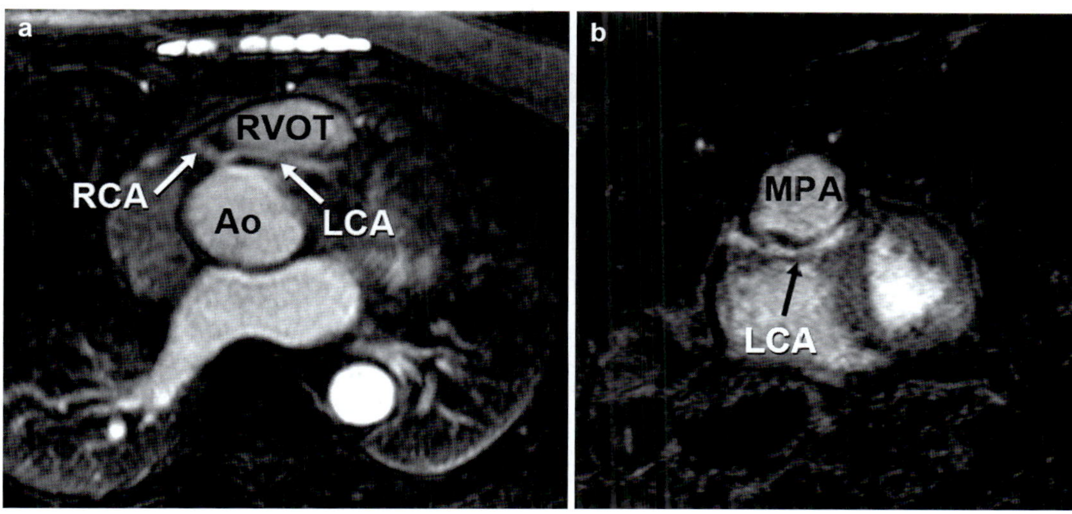

Fig. 27.12 Single coronary artery, Type R-IIS. Coronary MRA multiplanar reformatted image in axial (**a**) and oblique sagittal (**b**) views. The right coronary artery (*RCA*) demonstrates normal origin from the right cusp (**a**). The left coronary artery (*LCA*) arises from the proximal aspect of the RCA with an intraseptal course between the aorta (*Ao*) and right ventricular outflow tract (*RVOT*) (**a**), below the main pulmonary artery (*MPA*) (**b**)

Duplicated Arteries

The LAD, the RCA, or the PDA may appear duplicated. Duplication of the LAD represents the most common type of duplicated artery anomalies and depending on their anatomical course or origins is classified into four to five types. Commonly this anomaly is represented by a short LAD that travels in the proximal two-third of anterior interventricular groove and terminates prior to reaching the apex and running parallel to a longer LAD that continues to supply the apical wall.

Subendocardial Coronary Course

In rare cases, a coronary artery may demonstrate a subendocardial course after penetrating the

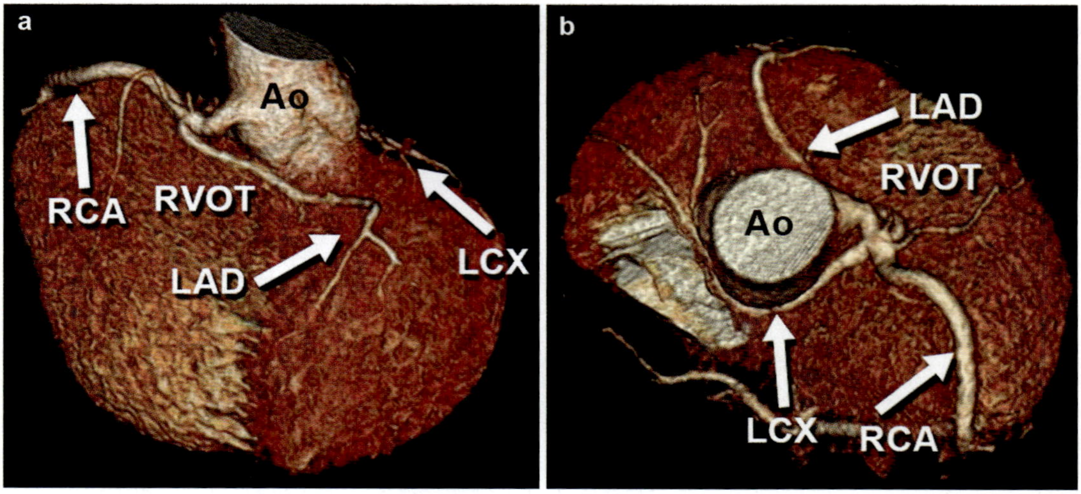

Fig. 27.13 Single coronary artery, Type IIIC. Coronary CTA 3D volume-rendered images (**a**, **b**) demonstrate single coronary ostium from the right cusp with the left anterior descending (*LAD*) coursing between the aorta (*Ao*) and right ventricular outflow tract (*RVOT*) and the left circumflex (*LCX*) coursing posterior to the aorta (*Ao*). The right coronary artery (*RCA*) demonstrates normal course in the right atrioventricular groove. Of note, the main pulmonary artery has been removed from view to demonstrate the course of the LAD

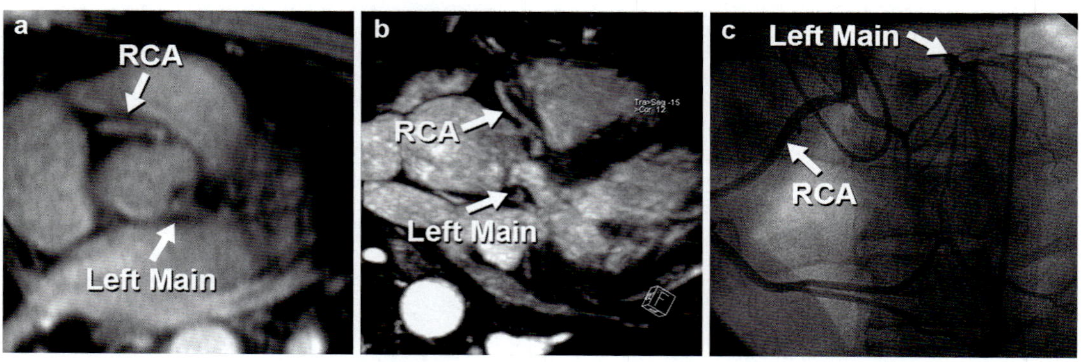

Fig. 27.14 Left main atresia. Coronary MRA 2D multiplanar reformatted (**a**) and thin maximum intensity projection (**b**) views with corresponding x-ray coronary angiogram (**c**). The left main coronary terminates as a blind stump near the left coronary cusp (**a**, **b**). The right coronary artery (*RCA*) demonstrates normal origin from the right cusp and supplies collaterals to the left coronary system (**c**)

myocardium. This anomaly may be seen as an intermediate stage in coronary malposition from intramyocardial to coronary-cameral fistula [63].

Coronary Crossing

Coronary crossing refers to a benign incidental finding where the coronary arteries or their branches demonstrate anomalous crossing over each other as opposed to running parallel to each other (Fig. 27.15).

Anomalies of Termination

Coronary Artery Fistulas

Coronary artery fistulas are abnormal communications between one or more coronary arteries and either a cardiac chamber (coronary-cameral) (Fig. 27.16), the pulmonary artery (Fig. 27.17), or a venous structure. Coronary artery fistulas have an incidence of approximately 0.5 % of patients undergoing angiography [65]. Most coronary artery fistula cases involve the

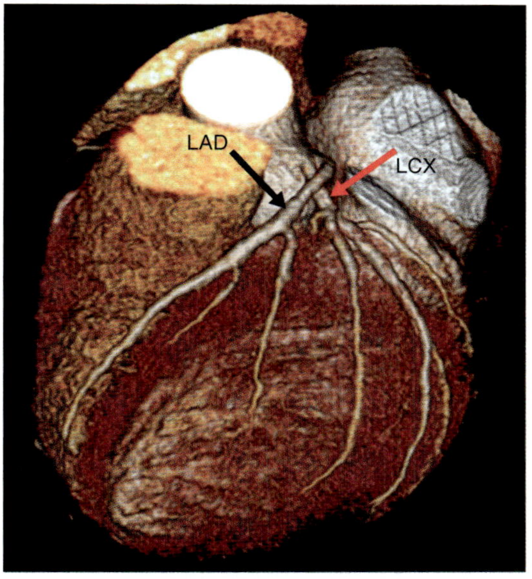

Fig. 27.15 Coronary crossing. Coronary CTA 3D volume-rendered image demonstrates separate origin of the left circumflex (LCX) artery (*red arrow*) and left anterior descending (LAD) artery (*black arrow*) from the left cusp. The LCX demonstrates unusual origin anterior to the LAD origin, and the two vessels cross each other proximally before continuing along their normal anatomic course. *LAD* left anterior descending, *LCX* left circumflex artery

RCA, and the feeding artery is typically dilated and tortuous given that it drains into a lower pressure chamber. Myocardial ischemia may occur due to a hemodynamic steal phenomenon.

Extracardiac Terminations

Connections exist between the coronary arteries and bronchial arteries regardless of patient age or presence of pathology. These connections usually do not become functional unless a pressure gradient exists [86]. Prominent collateral flow from the coronary to bronchial arteries may be seen in patients with any pulmonary disease that decreases perfusion in the bronchial vascular bed (Fig. 27.18). Angina pectoris may result due to "pulmonary steal syndrome" [87].

Coronary Arcade

Coronary arcade is defined as angiographically evident connections between the RCA and LCA in the absence of coronary artery stenosis. While small communications are normal, they are normally not large enough to be visualized on routine angiography. The connections are also distinguished from collaterals by their straight connections in the absence of significant coronary artery disease. Coronary arcade is frequently noted near the crux of the heart [88, 89].

Coronary Artery Anomalies in the Setting of Congenital Heart Disease

Background

There is a higher incidence of coronary artery anomalies in patients with congenital heart disease (CHD) than in the general population, ranging from 3 to 36 % in several studies [90]. In adults with CHD, the origin and course of the coronary arteries, both normal and anomalous, may have implications in surgical reconstruction as the anomalous coronary artery could be inadvertently damaged during surgery. The spatial relationship between the relevant cardiac structure and the coronary arterial system is essential for planning the operation and providing a good outcome. Three-dimensional representation of the data plays an increasingly important role in this regard [54].

Tetralogy of Fallot

The incidence of abnormal coronary artery anatomy is up to 19 % in patients with tetralogy of Fallot (TOF) [91, 92]. Commonly noted anomalies include origin of the LAD from the RCA and single coronary artery [93]. Coronary artery anomalies of greatest concern are those that involve a coronary artery coursing in or anterior to the right ventricular outflow tract (Figs. 27.19, 27.20, and 27.21). Up to 19 % of patients with tetralogy of Fallot are reported to have a conal branch at least as large as the RCA, crossing the right ventricular outflow tract [94, 95]. Although in isolated cases this coronary anomaly is usually considered benign, it is a complicating factor for

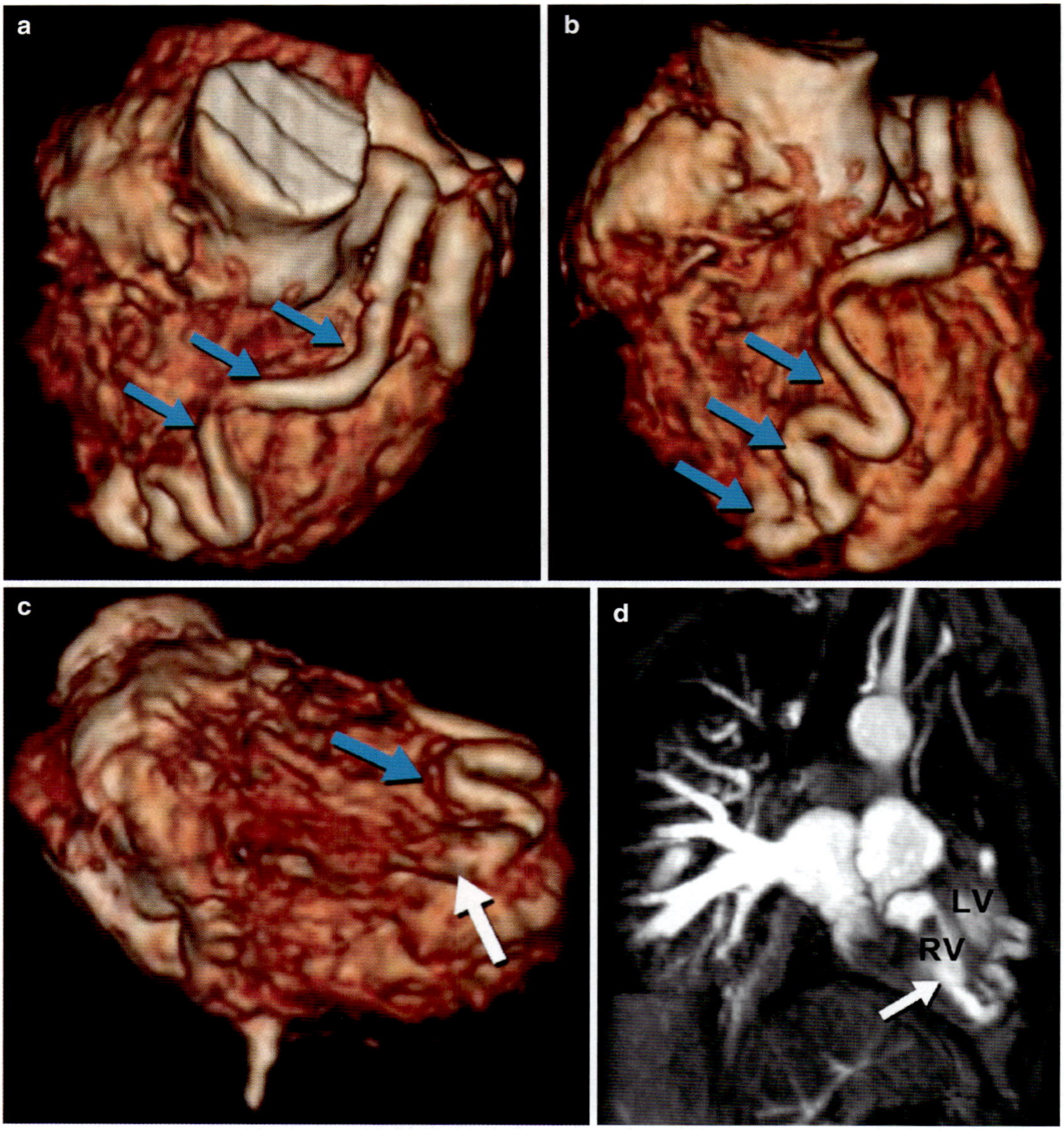

Fig. 27.16 Coronary-cameral fistula. Coronary MRA 3D volume-rendered images (**a–c**) and 2D thin maximum intensity projection image (**d**). The left anterior descending artery (*blue arrows*) is noted to be dilated and tortuous in its course before entering the right ventricle (RV) at its apex (*white arrow*). *LV* left ventricle

surgical correction of patients with TOF, with potential for inadvertent transection at the time of ventriculotomy [94, 96, 97]. Current guidelines recommend determination of coronary artery anatomy prior to any intervention for the right ventricular outflow tract [16] in order to prevent potential complications at the time of intervention [93, 98, 99].

Transposition of the Great Vessels

In congenitally corrected transposition of the great arteries (cc-TGA or Levo-TGA) of the great vessels, the coronary circulation generally demonstrates an "inverted" or "mirror image" of the normal coronary arterial tree pattern, such that the LAD descends to the

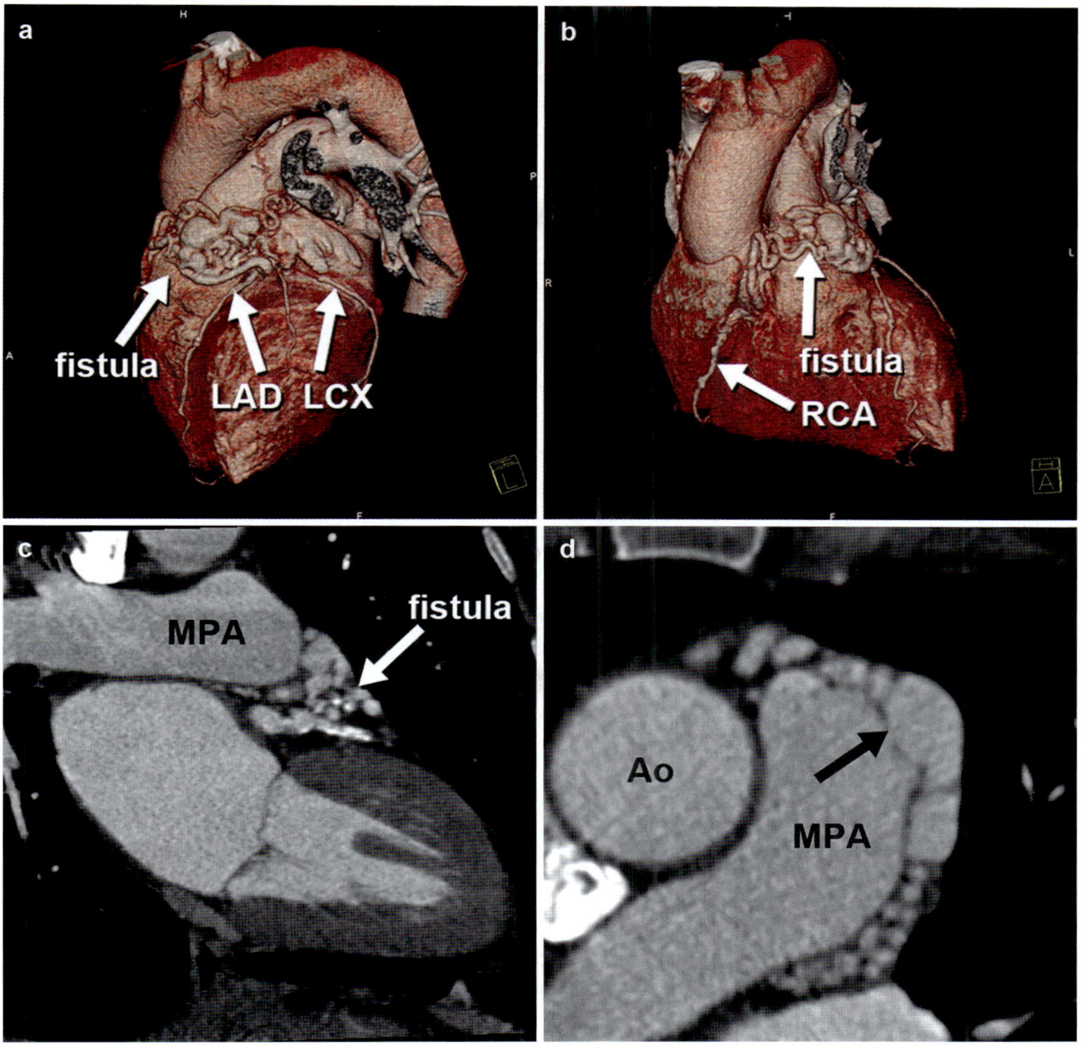

Fig. 27.17 Coronary to pulmonary artery fistula. Coronary CTA 3D volume-rendered images (**a**, **b**) and 2D multiplanar reformatted image (**c**, **d**) demonstrate a mass of dilated tortuous vessels (fistula) arising from the left anterior descending (*LAD*) and right coronary artery (*RCA*) terminating into the main pulmonary artery (**d**, *black arrow*). *Ao* aorta, *LCX* left circumflex

right of the aorta (Fig. 27.22). The terms "morphologically left" and "morphologically right" coronary artery are often used to more accurately describe the coronary arteries and are consistent with the morphologic chamber supplied [100] and segmental terminology used in CHD classification [101]. Reports suggest that deviations from this "inverted" appearance of the coronary arteries are uncommon [102, 103], but others have reported increased number of coronary anomalies comparable to that seen in other forms of congenital heart disease [104]. With the advent of double switch operations (combined atrial and great vessel switch), knowledge of coronary artery anatomy is important prior to surgery, since it may play a role in the course or type of operation or in the decision not to operate at all [104].

Adult patients with complete TGA (Dextro-TGA) also demonstrate considerable variability in the coronary artery anatomy related to

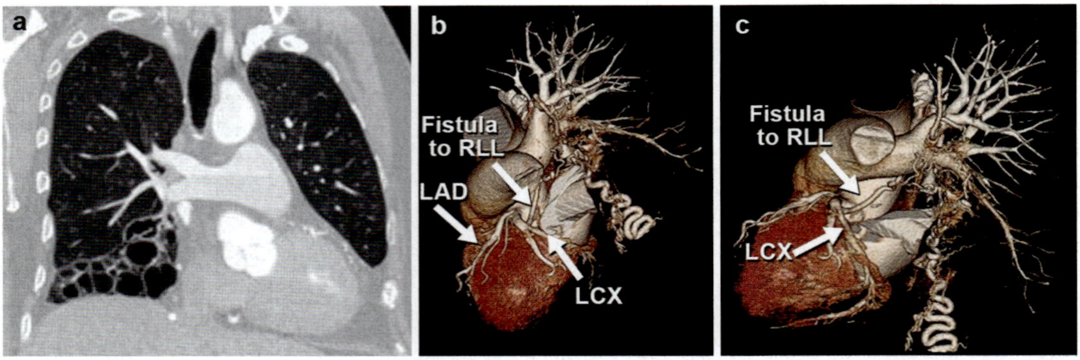

Fig. 27.18 Coronary to bronchial artery collaterals. Chest CTA coronal oblique view (**a**) demonstrates cystic bronchiectasis involving the right lower lobe (*RLL*). Coronary CTA 3D volume-rendered images (**b**, **c**) with coronary artery fistula from left circumflex (*LCX*) to bronchial artery collaterals supplying the RLL. *LAD* left anterior descending artery

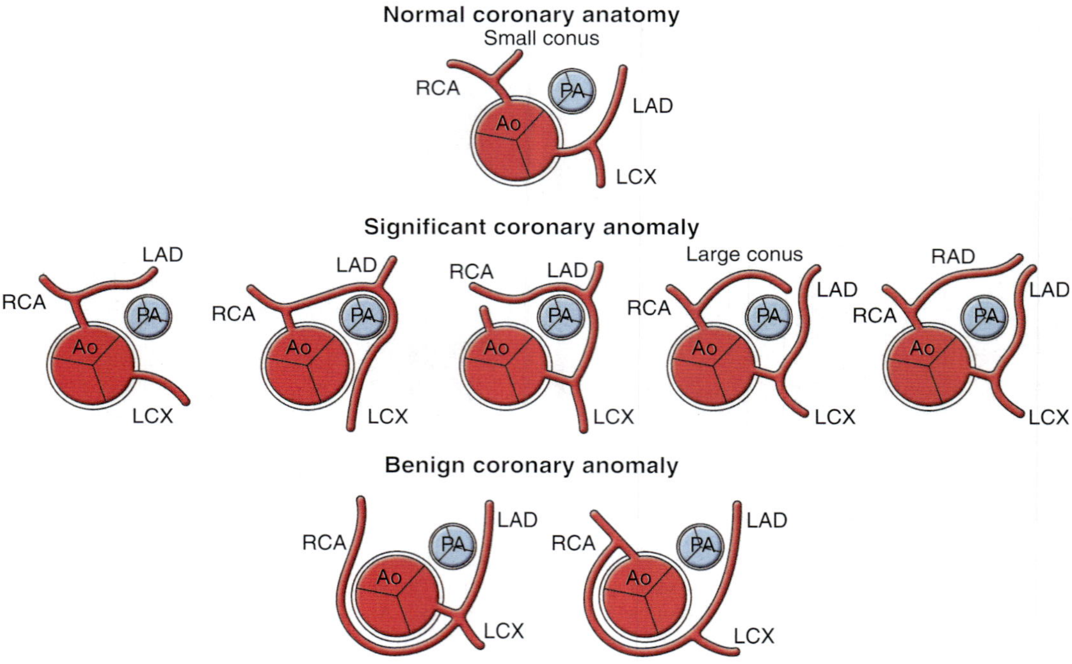

Fig. 27.19 Normal and abnormal coronary artery patterns noted in tetralogy of Fallot. The spatial orientation of the aortic root and relative position of the coronary cusps are kept identical between the normal and abnormal coronary groups to prevent complexity. However, it is important to know the aortic root in tetralogy of Fallot shows variable degrees of clockwise rotation that may move the noncoronary sinus to an anteriorly located position. Anomalies with large vessels or branches crossing the right ventricular outflow tract have the potential for significant complications during surgical repair of tetralogy of Fallot. *Ao* aorta, *PA* pulmonary artery, *RCA* right coronary artery, *LAD* left anterior descending, *LCX* left circumflex

complexity of cardiac anatomy, modification of anatomy by surgery, and potential interference from indwelling devices such as conduits, baffles, stents, and coils. As many as 28 variants of proximal coronary anatomy have been reported [105, 106]. Knowledge of the coronary artery anatomy is important, particularly if a patient is to undergo an arterial switch procedure, since the

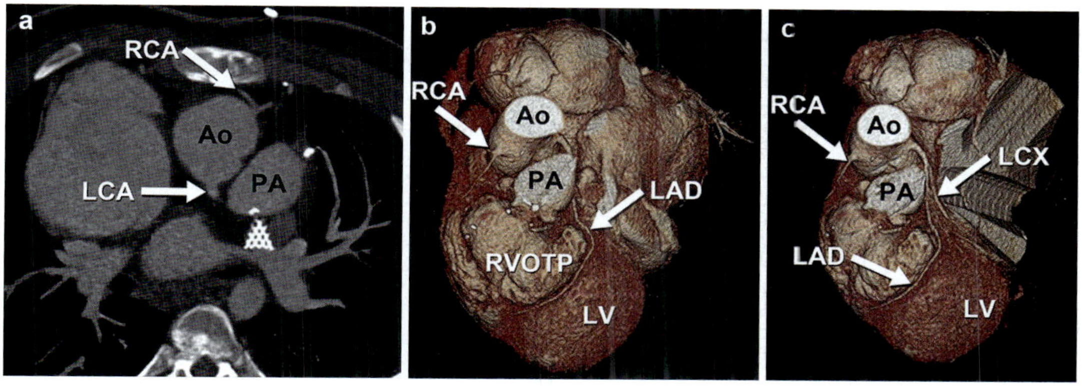

Fig. 27.20 Tetralogy of Fallot, normal coronary anatomy. Coronary CTA 2D multiplanar reformatted image (**a**) and corresponding 3D volume-rendered images (**b**, **c**) demonstrate normal origins of the right coronary artery (*RCA*) and left coronary artery (*LCA*) from their respective cusps. The left anterior descending artery (*LAD*) is noted to course adjacent to the large right ventricular outflow tract surgical patch (*RVOTP*). *Ao* aorta, *PA* pulmonary artery, *LV* left ventricle, *LCX* left circumflex

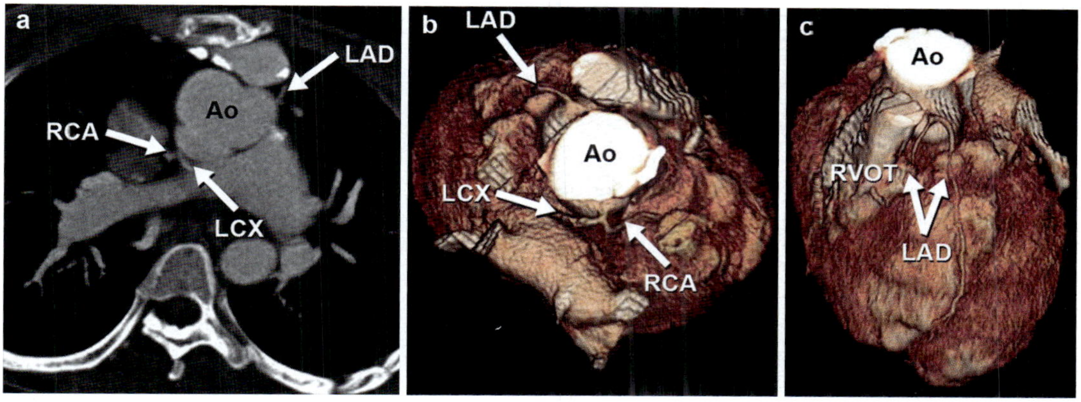

Fig. 27.21 Tetralogy of Fallot with anomalous position of the coronary arteries. Coronary CTA 2D multiplanar reformatted image (**a**) and corresponding 3D volume-rendered images (**b**, **c**) are shown. Assuming clockwise rotation of the aortic root has moved the noncoronary sinus to a right anterior location (**a**), the left anterior descending (*LAD*) is arising from the anterior, right cusp (now located on left side) coursing anterior to the right ventricular outflow tract (*RVOT*) before reaching the anterior interventricular groove. The right coronary artery (*RCA*) and the left circumflex (*LCX*) arteries arise from the left cusp (now located posteriorly). *Ao* aorta, *LCX* left circumflex

coronary arteries also need to be reimplanted, and relatively minor anatomic abnormalities such as high takeoff above the sinotubular junction or non-orthogonal angle from the aortic root can change the clinical course [102]. Several different classification systems have been proposed for describing the different coronary artery variations, but most were complex and not practical for clinical or surgical use [107]. More simplified and practical classification systems focused on origin and/or proximal course of the coronary arteries. The Planche classification system is perhaps the most practical, since it relates directly to anticipated technical difficulties with coronary arterial transfer during the arterial switch operation [108] (Fig. 27.23). Group I is the usual, most common coronary anatomy; Group II refers to coronary arteries originating from and passing through the region between the aorta and pulmonary trunk, often with an associated intramural

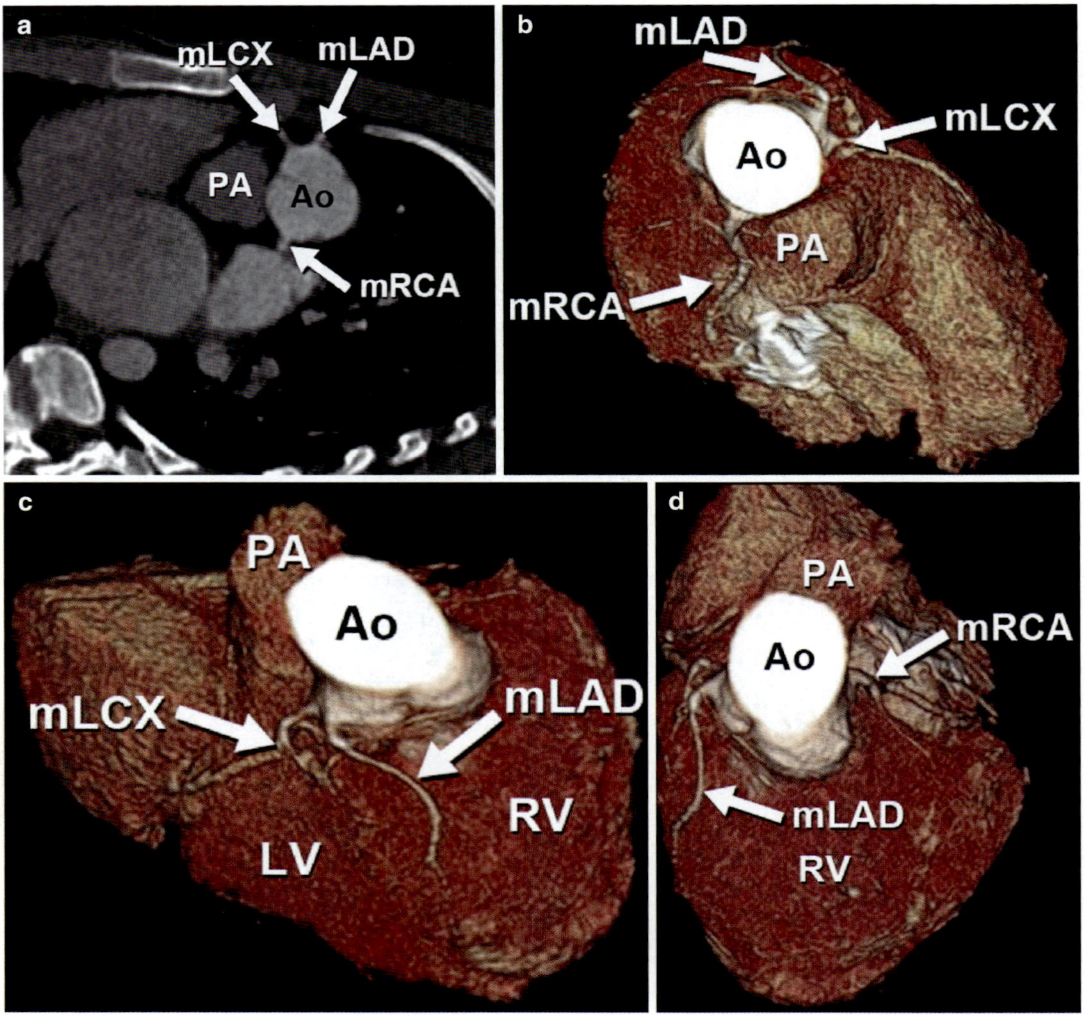

Fig. 27.22 Levo-transposition of the great vessels. Coronary CTA multiplanar reformatted image (**a**) and corresponding 3D volume-rendered images (**b–d**) demonstrate the inverted "mirror" image pattern of the coronary arteries, with the morphologic left anterior descending (*mLAD*) and morphologic left circumflex (*mLCX*) arteries arising from the right facing cusp and course down the right side of the aorta. The morphologic right coronary artery (*mRCA*) arises from the left facing cusp and courses down the left side of the aorta. *Ao* aorta, *PA* pulmonary artery

course; Group III refers to coronary arteries with abnormal looping of one or more coronary arteries either anterior or posterior to the great vessels (Figs. 27.24 and 27.25); and Group IV are miscellaneous other anatomies. Although several studies have been unable to identify a specific relationship between mortality rates and anatomic variants of the coronary arteries [109–111], literature still suggests that certain patterns of origin and coronary artery distribution pose increase surgical risks [107]. The presence of an intramural coronary artery or abnormal coronary looping (either anterior or posterior to the great arteries) with a single coronary ostium is associated with higher mortality risk compared to normal, usual anatomy. This increased risk is related to potential kinking and/or distortion of the transferred segment in the case of posterior looping and stretching or bowstringing of the transferred segment in the case of anterior looping.

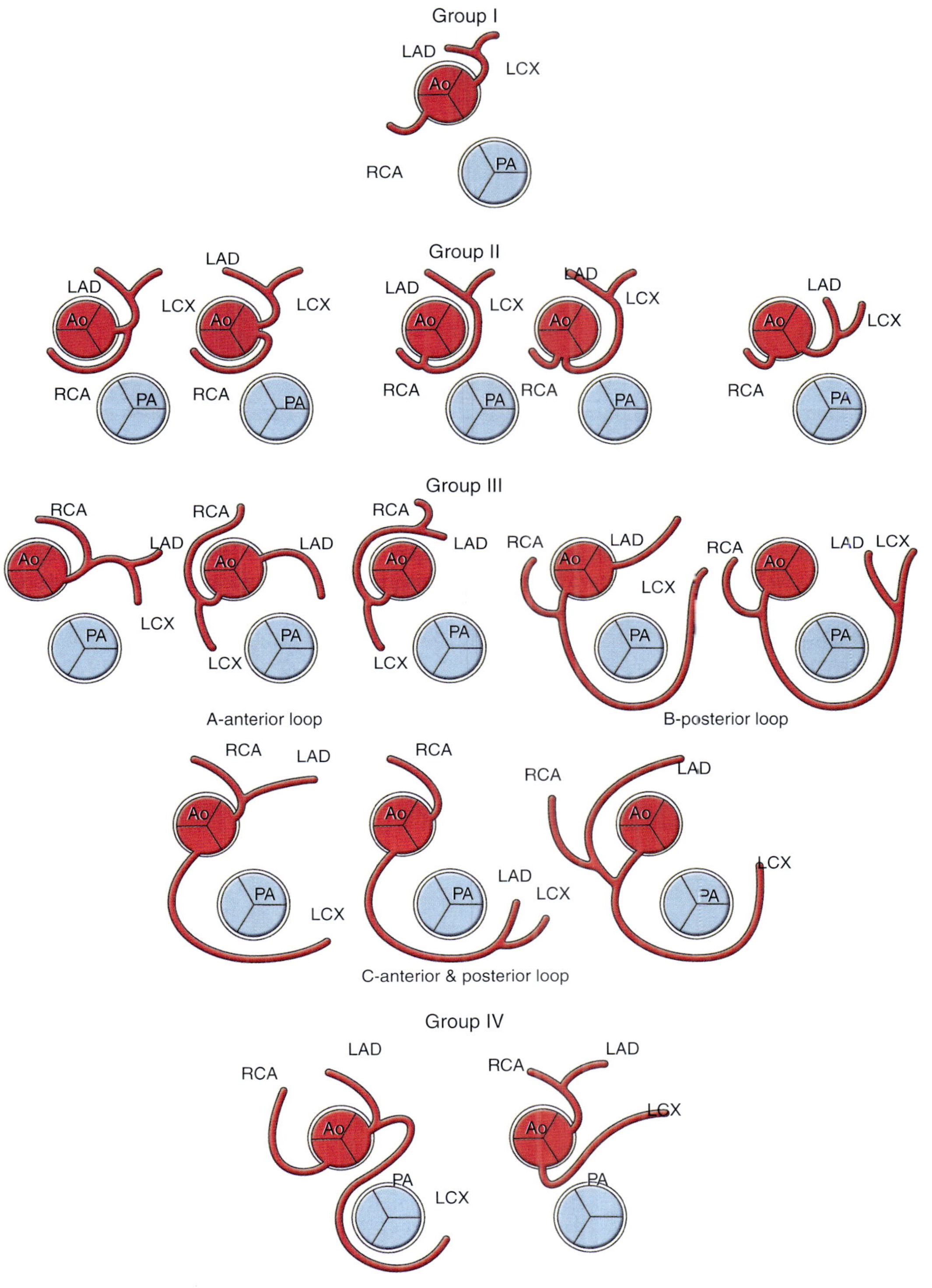

Fig. 27.23 Planche classification system in dextro-transposition of the great vessels. *Ac* aorta, *PA* pulmonary artery, *RCA* right coronary artery, *LAD* left anterior descending, *LCX* left circumflex

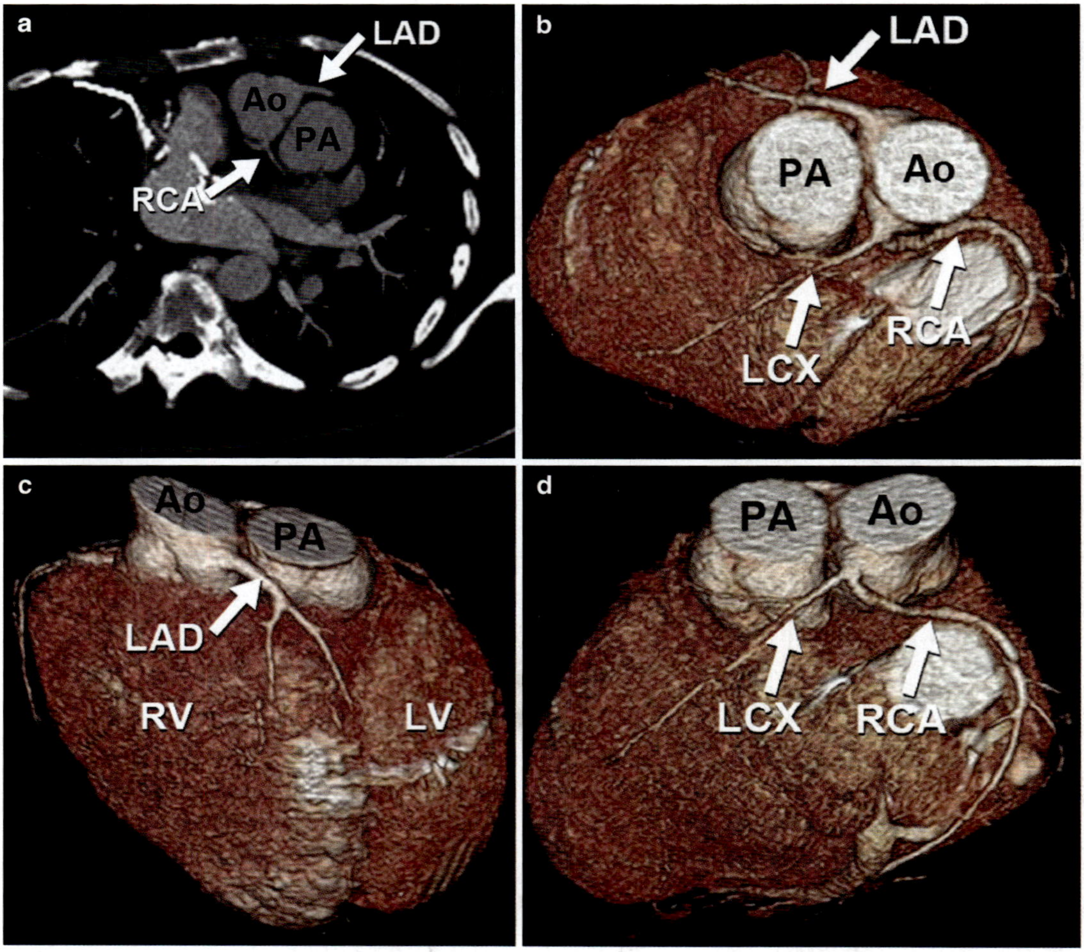

Fig. 27.24 Dextro-transposition of the great vessels post-atrial switch, Planche Group III, Type B: posterior looping. Coronary CTA 2D multiplanar reformatted image (**a**) and corresponding 3D volume-rendered images (**b–d**) demonstrate anterior origin of the left anterior descending (*LAD*) artery and posterior origin of the right coronary artery (*RCA*) and left circumflex (*LCX*) arteries. The RCA and LCX demonstrate posterior looping (Type C) behind the aorta (*Ao*) and pulmonary artery (*PA*)

Adjustments in surgical technique can be made depending on the coronary artery anatomy but, in some cases, may require complete alteration of the surgical technique.

Bicuspid Aortic Valve

Bicuspid aortic valve is the most common congenital heart malformation, present in 1–2 % of the population. Bicuspid aortic valve is highly associated with congenital abnormalities of the aorta and proximal coronary arteries [112], with reported 2 % incidence of associated coronary artery anomalies. Frequently reported anomalies include anomalous origin of the LCX from the RCA or right sinus and absent left main with separate origins of the LAD and LCX from the left sinus [103, 113]. Since many of these patients will require aortic valve surgery, preoperative assessment of coronary artery anatomy for identification of possible anomalies would avoid potential injury to the anomalous coronary artery during surgical aortic repair [114].

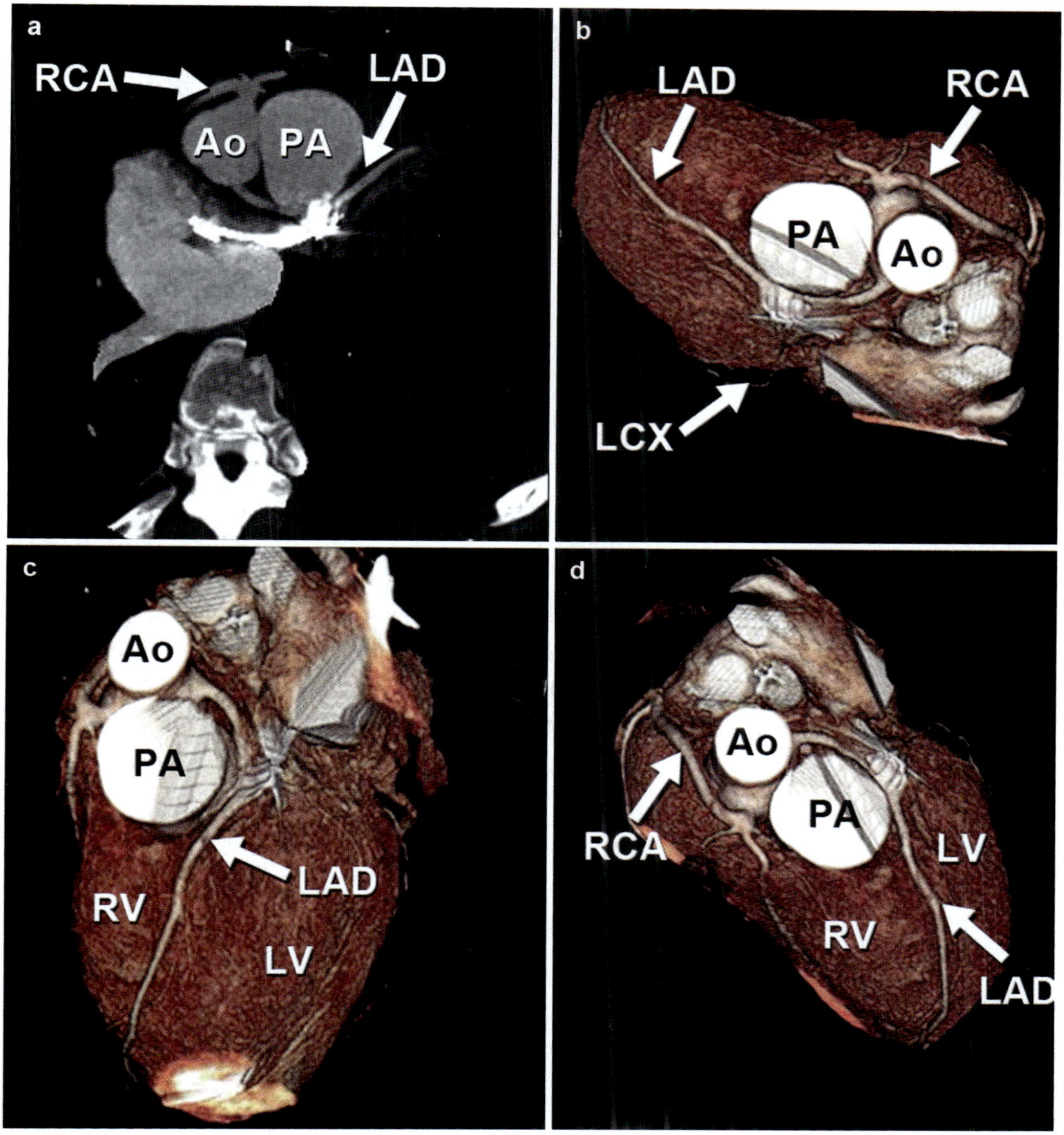

Fig. 27.25 Dextro-transposition of the great vessels post-atrial switch, Planche Group III, Type C: anterior and posterior looping. Coronary CTA 2D multiplanar reformatted image (**a**) and corresponding 3D volume-rendered images (**b–d**) demonstrate anterior origin of the right coronary artery and posterior origin of the left coronary artery. The RCA courses anterior to the pulmonary artery (*PA*) and the left anterior descending (*LAD*) and left circumflex (*LCX*) arteries course posterior to the PA to supply their respective territories. *Ao* aorta, *LV* left ventricle, *RV* right ventricle

Mitral Valve Prolapse

Anomalous coronary arteries demonstrate high association with mitral valve prolapse. In 29 adult patients with mitral valve prolapse, multiple anomalies were described, most involving anomalous origin or the RCA or LCX [115]. Separate origins of the LAD and LCX as well coronary artery fistulae have also been described [116]. Recognition of coronary anomalies is important for patients undergoing surgical valve repair or replacement to avoid inadvertent obstruction of the anomalous coronary ostium and/or compression along its course by a valvular prosthesis.

Acknowledgment We gratefully acknowledge Martha Helmers for her hard work with the preparation of the images and figures for this chapter.

References

1. Yamanaka O, Hobbs RE. Coronary artery anomalies in 126,595 patients undergoing coronary arteriography. Cathet Cardiovasc Diagn. 1990;21:28–40.
2. Click RL, Holmes Jr DR, Vlietstra RE, Kosinski AS, Kronmal RA. Anomalous coronary arteries: location, degree of atherosclerosis and effect on survival – a report from the Coronary Artery Surgery Study. J Am Coll Cardiol. 1989;13:531–7.
3. Baltaxe HA, Wixson D. The incidence of congenital anomalies of the coronary arteries in the adult population. Radiology. 1977;122:47–52.
4. Engel HJ, Torres C, Page Jr HL. Major variations in anatomical origin of the coronary arteries: angiographic observations in 4,250 patients without associated congenital heart disease. Cathet Cardiovasc Diagn. 1975;1:157–69.
5. Alexander RW, Griffith GC. Anomalies of the coronary arteries and their clinical significance. Circulation. 1956;14:800–5.
6. Liberthson RR, Dinsmore RE, Fallon JT. Aberrant coronary artery origin from the aorta. Report of 18 patients, review of literature and delineation of natural history and management. Circulation. 1979;59:748–54.
7. Moodie DS, Gill C, Loop FD, Sheldon WC. Anomalous left main coronary artery originating from the right sinus of Valsalva: pathophysiology, angiographic definition, and surgical approaches. J Thorac Cardiovasc Surg. 1980;80:198–205.
8. Ishikawa T, Brandt PW. Anomalous origin of the left main coronary artery from the right anterior aortic sinus: angiographic definition of anomalous course. Am J Cardiol. 1985;55:770–6.
9. Serota H, Barth 3rd CW, Seuc CA, Vandormael M, Aguirre F, Kern MJ. Rapid identification of the course of anomalous coronary arteries in adults: the "dot and eye" method. Am J Cardiol. 1990;65:891–8.
10. Frommelt PC, Frommelt MA. Congenital coronary artery anomalies. Pediatr Clin North Am. 2004;51:1273–88.
11. Douglas PS, Fiolkoski J, Berko B, Reichek N. Echocardiographic visualization of coronary artery anatomy in the adult. J Am Coll Cardiol. 1988; 11:565–71.
12. Vered Z, Katz M, Rath S, et al. Two-dimensional echocardiographic analysis of proximal left main coronary artery in humans. Am Heart J. 1986;112:972–6.
13. Zwicky P, Daniel WG, Mugge A, Lichtlen PR. Imaging of coronary arteries by color-coded transesophageal Doppler echocardiography. Am J Cardiol. 1988;62:639–40.
14. Mitchell MM, Sutherland GR, Gussenhoven EJ, Taams MA, Roelandt JR. Transesophageal echocardiography. J Am Soc Echocardiogr. 1988;1:362–77.
15. Gaither NS, Rogan KM, Stajduhar K, et al. Anomalous origin and course of coronary arteries in adults: identification and improved imaging utilizing transesophageal echocardiography. Am Heart J. 1991;122:69–75.
16. Warnes CA, Williams RG, Bashore TM, et al. ACC/AHA 2008 Guidelines for the Management of Adults with Congenital Heart Disease: Executive Summary: a report of the American College of Cardiology/American Heart Association Task Force on Practice Guidelines (writing committee to develop guidelines for the management of adults with congenital heart disease). Circulation. 2008;118:2395–451.
17. McConnell MV, Ganz P, Selwyn AP, Li W, Edelman RR, Manning WJ. Identification of anomalous coronary arteries and their anatomic course by magnetic resonance coronary angiography. Circulation. 1995;92:3158–62.
18. Bunce NH, Lorenz CH, Keegan J, et al. Coronary artery anomalies: assessment with free-breathing three-dimensional coronary MR angiography. Radiology. 2003;227:201–8.
19. Duerinckx AJ, Bogaert J, Jiang H, Lewis BS. Anomalous origin of the left coronary artery: diagnosis by coronary MR angiography. AJR Am J Roentgenol. 1995;164:1095–7.
20. Post JC, van Rossum AC, Hofman MB, Valk J, Visser CA. Three-dimensional respiratory-gated MR angiography of coronary arteries: comparison with conventional coronary angiography. AJR Am J Roentgenol. 1996;166:1399–404.
21. Hendel RC, Patel MR, Kramer CM, et al. ACCF/ACR/SCCT/SCMR/ASNC/NASCI/SCAI/SIR 2006 appropriateness criteria for cardiac computed tomography and cardiac magnetic resonance imaging: a report of the American College of Cardiology Foundation Quality Strategic Directions Committee Appropriateness Criteria Working Group, American College of Radiology, Society of Cardiovascular Computed Tomography, Society for Cardiovascular Magnetic Resonance, American Society of Nuclear Cardiology, North American Society for Cardiac Imaging, Society for Cardiovascular Angiography and Interventions, and Society of Interventional Radiology. J Am Coll Cardiol. 2006;48:1475–97.
22. Paulin S, von Schulthess GK, Fossel E, Krayenbuehl HP. MR imaging of the aortic root and proximal coronary arteries. AJR Am J Roentgenol. 1987;148:665–70.
23. Cho ZH, Mun CW, Friedenberg RM. NMR angiography of coronary vessels with 2-D planar image scanning. Magn Reson Med. 1991;20:134–43.
24. Dumoulin CL, Souza SP, Darrow RD, Adams WJ. A method of coronary MR angiography. J Comput Assist Tomogr. 1991;15:705–10.

25. Kim WY, Danias PG, Stuber M, et al. Coronary magnetic resonance angiography for the detection of coronary stenoses. N Engl J Med. 2001;345:1863–9.
26. Weber OM, Martin AJ, Higgins CB. Whole-heart steady-state free precession coronary artery magnetic resonance angiography. Magn Reson Med. 2003;50:1223–8.
27. Prakken NH, Vonken EJ, Velthuis BK, Doevendans PA, Cramer MJ. 3D MR coronary angiography: optimization of the technique and preliminary results. Int J Cardiovasc Imaging. 2006;22:477–87.
28. Shea SM, Deshpande VS, Chung YC, Li D. Three-dimensional true-FISP imaging of the coronary arteries: improved contrast with T2-preparation. J Magn Reson Imaging. 2002;15:597–602.
29. Nezafat R, Stuber M, Ouwerkerk R, Gharib AM, Desai MY, Pettigrew RI. B1-insensitive T2 preparation for improved coronary magnetic resonance angiography at 3 T. Magn Reson Med. 2006;55:858–64.
30. Gharib AM, Abd-Elmoniem KZ, Herzka DA, et al. Optimization of coronary whole-heart MRA free-breathing technique at 3 Tesla. Magn Reson Imaging. 2011;29:1125–30.
31. Li D, Paschal CB, Haacke EM, Adler LP. Coronary arteries: three-dimensional MR imaging with fat saturation and magnetization transfer contrast. Radiology. 1993;187:401–6.
32. Paschal CB, Haacke EM, Adler LP. Three-dimensional MR imaging of the coronary arteries: preliminary clinical experience. J Magn Reson Imaging. 1993;3:491–500.
33. Hofman MB, Paschal CB, Li D, Haacke EM, van Rossum AC, Sprenger M. MRI of coronary arteries: 2D breath-hold vs 3D respiratory-gated acquisition. J Comput Assist Tomogr. 1995;19:56–62.
34. Xu J, Kim D, Otazo R, et al. Initial comparative evaluation of a five-minute comprehensive cardiac MR examination using highly accelerated parallel imaging. Montreal: International Society of Magnetic Resonance in Medicine; 2011.
35. Prakken NH, Cramer MJ, Olimulder MA, Agostoni P, Mali WP, Velthuis BK. Screening for proximal coronary artery anomalies with 3-dimensional MR coronary angiography. Int J Cardiovasc Imaging. 2010;26:701–10.
36. Greer ML, Mondal TK, Yoo SJ. Late presentation of anomalous origin of the left coronary artery from the pulmonary artery: the definitive role of cardiovascular magnetic resonance imaging. Cardiol Young. 2011;21:225–6.
37. McConnell MV, Stuber M, Manning WJ. Clinical role of coronary magnetic resonance angiography in the diagnosis of anomalous coronary arteries. J Cardiovasc Magn Reson. 2000;2:217–24.
38. Hundley WG, Bluemke DA, Finn JP, et al. ACCF/ACR/AHA/NASCI/SCMR 2010 expert consensus document on cardiovascular magnetic resonance: a report of the American College of Cardiology Foundation Task Force on Expert Consensus Documents. Circulation. 2010;121:2462–508.
39. Gowda RM, Vasavada BC, Khan IA. Coronary artery fistulas: clinical and therapeutic considerations. Int J Cardiol. 2006;107:7–10.
40. Datta J, White CS, Gilkeson RC, et al. Anomalous coronary arteries in adults: depiction at multi-detector row CT angiography. Radiology. 2005;235:812–8.
41. Taylor AJ, Cerqueira M, Hodgson JM, et al. ACCF/SCCT/ACR/AHA/ASE/ASNC/NASCI/SCAI/SCMR 2010 appropriate use criteria for cardiac computed tomography. A report of the American College of Cardiology Foundation Appropriate Use Criteria Task Force, the Society of Cardiovascular Computed Tomography, the American College of Radiology, the American Heart Association, the American Society of Echocardiography, the American Society of Nuclear Cardiology, the North American Society for Cardiovascular Imaging, the Society for Cardiovascular Angiography and Interventions, and the Society for Cardiovascular Magnetic Resonance. J Am Coll Cardiol. 2010;56:1864–94.
42. Shriki JE, Shinbane JS, Rashid MA, et al. Identifying, characterizing, and classifying congenital anomalies of the coronary arteries. Radiographics. 2012;32:453–68.
43. Earls JP. How to use a prospective gated technique for cardiac CT. J Cardiovasc Comput Tomogr. 2009;3:45–51.
44. Shuman WP, Branch KR, May JM, et al. Prospective versus retrospective ECG gating for 64-detector CT of the coronary arteries: comparison of image quality and patient radiation dose. Radiology. 2008;248:431–7.
45. Scheffel H, Alkadhi H, Leschka S, et al. Low-dose CT coronary angiography in the step-and-shoot mode: diagnostic performance. Heart. 2008;94:1132–7.
46. Einstein AJ, Elliston CD, Arai AE, et al. Radiation dose from single-heartbeat coronary CT angiography performed with a 320-detector row volume scanner. Radiology. 2010;254:698–706.
47. Achenbach S, Marwan M, Ropers D, et al. Coronary computed tomography angiography with a consistent dose below 1 mSv using prospectively electrocardiogram-triggered high-pitch spiral acquisition. Eur Heart J. 2010;31:340–6.
48. Gosling O, Loader R, Venables P, et al. A comparison of radiation doses between state-of-the-art multislice CT coronary angiography with iterative reconstruction, multislice CT coronary angiography with standard filtered back-projection and invasive diagnostic coronary angiography. Heart. 2010;96:922–6.
49. Leipsic J, Labounty TM, Heilbron B, et al. Estimated radiation dose reduction using adaptive statistical iterative reconstruction in coronary CT angiography: the ERASIR study. AJR Am J Roentgenol. 2010;195:655–60.
50. Leipsic J, Labounty TM, Heilbron B, et al. Adaptive statistical iterative reconstruction: assessment of image noise and image quality in coronary CT angiography. AJR Am J Roentgenol. 2010;195:649–54.
51. Tomanek RJ. Formation of the coronary vasculature: a brief review. Cardiovasc Res. 1996;31 Spec No:E46–51.

52. Mikawa T, Fischman DA. Retroviral analysis of cardiac morphogenesis: discontinuous formation of coronary vessels. Proc Natl Acad Sci U S A. 1992;89:9504–8.
53. Hutchins GM, Kessler-Hanna A, Moore GW. Development of the coronary arteries in the embryonic human heart. Circulation. 1988;77:1250–7.
54. Bogers AJ, Gittenberger-de Groot AC, Poelmann RE, Peault BM, Huysmans HA. Development of the origin of the coronary arteries, a matter of ingrowth or outgrowth? Anat Embryol (Berl). 1989;180:437–41.
55. Hirakow R. Development of the cardiac blood vessels in staged human embryos. Acta Anat (Basel). 1983;115:220–30.
56. Mandarim-de-Lacerda CA. Development of the coronary arteries in staged human embryos (the Paris Embryological Collection revisited). An Acad Bras Cienc. 1990;62:79–84.
57. Matonoha P, Zechmeister A. Structure of the coronary arteries during the prenatal period in man. Funct Dev Morphol. 1992;2:209–12.
58. Kurosawa S, Kurosawa H, Becker AE. The coronary arterioles in newborns, infants and children. A morphometric study of normal hearts and hearts with aortic atresia and complete transposition. Int J Cardiol. 1986;10:43–56.
59. Reinecke P, Hort W. The growth of coronary artery branches in man under physiological conditions. Morphological studies of corrosion casts of the anterior interventricular branch of the coronary artery. Z Kardiol. 1992;81:110–5.
60. Becker AE, Anderson RH. Coronary artery anomalies. In: Becker AE, Anderson RH, editors. Pathology of congenital heart disease. London: Butterworths; 1981. p. 369–78.
61. Kennel AJ, Titus JL. The vasculature of the human sinus node. Mayo Clin Proc. 1972;47:556–61.
62. Bream PR, Souza Jr AS, Elliott LP, Soto B, Curry GC. Right superior septal perforator artery: its angiographic description and clinical significance. AJR Am J Roentgenol. 1979;133:67–73.
63. Angelini P, Villason S, Chan AVJ, Diez JG. Normal and anomalous coronary arteries in humans. In: Angelini P, editor. Coronary artery anomalies: a comprehensive approach. Philadelphia: Lippincott Williams & Wilkins; 1999. p. 27–150.
64. Angelini P, de la Cruz MV, Valencia AM, et al. Coronary arteries in transposition of the great arteries. Am J Cardiol. 1994;74:1037–41.
65. Yurtdas M, Gulen O. Anomalous origin of the right coronary artery from the left anterior descending artery: review of the literature. Cardiol J. 2012;19:122–9.
66. Rigatelli G, Docali G, Rossi P, Bandello A. Validation of a clinical-significance-based classification of coronary artery anomalies. Angiology. 2005;56:25–34.
67. Topaz O, DiSciascio G, Cowley MJ, et al. Absent left main coronary artery: angiographic findings in 83 patients with separate ostia of the left anterior descending and circumflex arteries at the left aortic sinus. Am Heart J. 1991;122:447–52.
68. Hacioglu Y, Budoff M. Is the left anterior descending artery really absent? – a decisive input from coronary CT angiography. Catheter Cardiovasc Interv. 2010;76:117–20.
69. Dicicco BS, McManus BM, Waller BF, Roberts WC. Separate aortic ostium of the left anterior descending and left circumflex coronary arteries from the left aortic sinus of Valsalva (absent left main coronary artery). Am Heart J. 1982;104:153–4.
70. Wesselhoeft H, Fawcett JS, Johnson AL. Anomalous origin of the left coronary artery from the pulmonary trunk. Its clinical spectrum, pathology, and pathophysiology, based on a review of 140 cases with seven further cases. Circulation. 1968;38:403–25.
71. Khanna A, Torigian DA, Ferrari VA, Bross RJ, Rosen MA. Anomalous origin of the left coronary artery from the pulmonary artery in adulthood on CT and MRI. AJR Am J Roentgenol. 2005;185:326–9.
72. Frapier JM, Leclercq F, Bodino M, Chaptal PA. Malignant ventricular arrhythmias revealing anomalous origin of the left coronary artery from the pulmonary artery in two adults. Eur J Cardiothorac Surg. 1999;15:539–41.
73. Maron BJ. Sudden death in young athletes. N Engl J Med. 2003;349:1064–75.
74. Basso C, Maron BJ, Corrado D, Thiene G. Clinical profile of congenital coronary artery anomalies with origin from the wrong aortic sinus leading to sudden death in young competitive athletes. J Am Coll Cardiol. 2000;35:1493–501.
75. Eckart RE, Scoville SL, Campbell CL, et al. Sudden death in young adults: a 25-year review of autopsies in military recruits. Ann Intern Med. 2004;141:829–34.
76. Roberts WC. Major anomalies of coronary arterial origin seen in adulthood. Am Heart J. 1986;111:941–63.
77. Kragel AH, Roberts WC. Anomalous origin of either the right or left main coronary artery from the aorta with subsequent coursing between aorta and pulmonary trunk: analysis of 32 necropsy cases. Am J Cardiol. 1988;62:771–7.
78. Taylor AJ, Rogan KM, Virmani R. Sudden cardiac death associated with isolated congenital coronary artery anomalies. J Am Coll Cardiol. 1992;20:640–7.
79. Warnes CA, Williams RG, Bashore TM, et al. ACC/AHA 2008 guidelines for the management of adults with congenital heart disease: a report of the American College of Cardiology/American Heart Association Task Force on Practice Guidelines (Writing Committee to Develop Guidelines on the Management of Adults With Congenital Heart Disease). Developed in Collaboration With the American Society of Echocardiography, Heart Rhythm Society, International Society for Adult Congenital Heart Disease, Society for Cardiovascular Angiography and Interventions, and Society of Thoracic Surgeons. J Am Coll Cardiol. 2008;52:e143–263.
80. Mainwaring RD, Reddy VM, Reinhartz O, et al. Anomalous aortic origin of a coronary artery: medium-term results after surgical repair in 50 patients. Ann Thorac Surg. 2011;92:691–7.

81. Desmet W, Vanhaecke J, Vrolix M, et al. Isolated single coronary artery: a review of 50,000 consecutive coronary angiographies. Eur Heart J. 1992;13:1637–40.
82. Nishida N, Chiba T, Ohtani M, Yoshioka N. Two adult cases of congenital atresia of the left coronary ostium-comparison of a sudden death case with a long-term survival case. Virchows Arch. 2005;447:742–6.
83. Musiani A, Cernigliaro C, Sansa M, Maselli D, De Gasperis C. Left main coronary artery atresia: literature review and therapeutical considerations. Eur J Cardiothorac Surg. 1997;11:505–14.
84. Pursnani A, Jacobs JE, Saremi F, et al. Coronary CTA assessment of coronary anomalies. J Cardiovasc Comput Tomogr. 2012;6:48–59.
85. Murthy PA, Mohammed TL, Read K, Gilkeson RC, White CS. MDCT of coronary artery aneurysms. AJR Am J Roentgenol. 2005;184:S19–20.
86. Smith SC, Adams DF, Herman MV, Paulin S. Coronary-to-bronchial anastomoses: an in vivo demonstration by selective coronary arteriography. Radiology. 1972;104:289–90.
87. Spindola-Franco H, Weisel A, Delman AJ. Pulmonary steal syndrome: an unusual case of coronary-bronchial pulmonary artery communication. Radiology. 1978;126:25–7.
88. Mahani MG, Agarwal PP. Coronary artery anomalies on CT angiography. Appl Radiol. 2011;40:18–25.
89. Greenberg MA, Fish BG, Spindola-Franco H. Congenital anomalies of the coronary arteries. Classification and significance. Radiol Clin North Am. 1989;27:1127–46.
90. Taylor AM, Thorne SA, Rubens MB, et al. Coronary artery imaging in grown up congenital heart disease: complementary role of magnetic resonance and x-ray coronary angiography. Circulation. 2000;101:1670–8.
91. Shrivastava S, Mohan JC, Mukhopadhyay S, Rajani M, Tandon R. Coronary artery anomalies in tetralogy of Fallot. Cardiovasc Intervent Radiol. 1987;10:215–8.
92. Jureidini SB, Appleton RS, Nouri S. Detection of coronary artery abnormalities in tetralogy of Fallot by two-dimensional echocardiography. J Am Coll Cardiol. 1989;14:960–7.
93. McManus BM, Waller BF, Jones M, Epstein SE, Roberts WC. The case for preoperative coronary angiography in patients with tetralogy of Fallot and other complex congenital heart diseases. Am Heart J. 1982;103:451–6.
94. Berry Jr JM, Einzig S, Krabill KA, Bass JL. Evaluation of coronary artery anatomy in patients with tetralogy of Fallot by two-dimensional echocardiography. Circulation. 1988;78:149–56.
95. Dabizzi RP, Caprioli G, Aiazzi L, et al. Distribution and anomalies of coronary arteries in tetralogy of fallot. Circulation. 1980;61:95–102.
96. Berry BE, McGoon DC. Total correction for tetralogy of Fallot with anomalous coronary artery. Surgery. 1973;74:894–8.
97. Humes RA, Driscoll DJ, Danielson GK, Puga FJ. Tetralogy of Fallot with anomalous origin of left anterior descending coronary artery. Surgical options. J Thorac Cardiovasc Surg. 1987;94:784–7.
98. Heuser RR, Achuff SC, Brinker JA. Inadvertent division of an anomalous left anterior descending coronary artery during complete repair of tetralogy of Fallot: 22-year follow-up. Am Heart J. 1982;103:430–2.
99. Landolt CC, Anderson JE, Zorn-Chelton S, Guyton RA, Hatcher Jr CR, Williams WH. Importance of coronary artery anomalies in operations for congenital heart disease. Ann Thorac Surg. 1986;41:351–5.
100. Shea PM, Lutz JF, Vieweg WV, Corcoran FH, Van Praagh R, Hougen TJ. Selective coronary arteriography in congenitally corrected transposition of the great arteries. Am J Cardiol. 1979;44:1201–6.
101. Van Praagh R. Terminology of congenital heart disease. Glossary and commentary. Circulation. 1977;56:139–43.
102. McKay R, Anderson RH, Smith A. The coronary arteries in hearts with discordant atrioventricular connections. J Thorac Cardiovasc Surg. 1996;111:988–97.
103. Tuzcu EM, Moodie DS, Chambers JL, Keyser P, Hobbs RE. Congenital heart diseases associated with coronary artery anomalies. Cleve Clin J Med. 1990;57:147–52.
104. Ismat FA, Baldwin HS, Karl TR, Weinberg PM. Coronary anatomy in congenitally corrected transposition of the great arteries. Int J Cardiol. 2002;86:207–16.
105. Rowlatt UF. Coronary artery distribution in complete transposition. JAMA. 1962;179:269–78.
106. Pasquini L, Sanders SP, Parness IA, et al. Coronary echocardiography in 406 patients with d-loop transposition of the great arteries. J Am Coll Cardiol. 1994;24:763–8.
107. Suzuki T. Modification of the arterial switch operation for transposition of the great arteries with complex coronary artery patterns. Gen Thorac Cardiovasc Surg. 2009;57:281–92.
108. Planche C, Bruniaux J, Lacour-Gayet F, et al. Switch operation for transposition of the great arteries in neonates. A study of 120 patients. J Thorac Cardiovasc Surg. 1988;96:354–63.
109. Qamar ZA, Goldberg CS, Devaney EJ, Bove EL, Ohye RG. Current risk factors and outcomes for the arterial switch operation. Ann Thorac Surg. 2007;84:871–8; discussion 878–9.
110. Quaegebeur JM, Rohmer J, Ottenkamp J, et al. The arterial switch operation. An eight-year experience. J Thorac Cardiovasc Surg. 1986;92:361–84.
111. Dibardino DJ, Allison AE, Vaughn WK, McKenzie ED, Fraser Jr CD. Current expectations for newborns undergoing the arterial switch operation. Ann Surg. 2004;239:588–96; discussion 596–8.
112. Fedak PW, Verma S, David TE, Leask RL, Weisel RD, Butany J. Clinical and pathophysiological implications of a bicuspid aortic valve. Circulation. 2002;106:900–4.
113. Tajouri TH, Kumar G, Edwards WD, Phillips S, Klarich KW. Coronary artery anomalies in patients with bicuspid aortic valve disease. In: 16th world

congress on Heart Disease Annual Scientific Sessions 2011, Vancouver, 2011.
114. Barriales-Villa R, Penas-Lado M, Moris C. Bicuspid aortic valve and coronary anomalies. Circulation. 2003;107:e105; author reply e105.
115. Topaz O, DeMarchena EJ, Perin E, Sommer LS, Mallon SM, Chahine RA. Anomalous coronary arteries: angiographic findings in 80 patients. Int J Cardiol. 1992;34:129–38.
116. Morimoto K, Taniguchi I, Miyasaka S, Marumoto A. Bicuspid aortic valve stenosis with single coronary artery. Ann Thorac Cardiovasc Surg. 2005; 11:267–9.

28 Coronary Veins

Farhood Saremi, Horia Muresian, and Damián Sánchez-Quintana

Investigation performed on the venous system of the heart is overshadowed by the numerous studies performed on the arterial side of coronary vessels. Recent development in cardiac pacing and transvenous ablations asks for a thorough and a more detailed knowledge of the cardiac venous anatomy and function, concomitantly demonstrating the increasing value of the coronary venous system (CVS) imaging. With increasing longevity of patients with congenital heart disease (CHD), long-term complications including heart failure and arrhythmias have led to increased interest in the roles of cardiac resynchronization therapy (CRT) and radiofrequency ablation in these patients. CT and MR can play an important role in assessment of cardiac morphology and coronary vessel mapping. A detailed review of the anatomical particulars of the CVS represents the major topic of this chapter. The variations, anomalies, and modifications encountered in normal hearts and CHD are subsequently presented. We briefly review clinical applications of this system in CRT. The description of anatomic variants of cardiac veins may also be important for retrograde cardioplegia perfusion (RCP).

F. Saremi, MD (✉)
Department of Radiology, Cardiothoracic Section, University of Southern California, USC Keck Hospital, 1500 San Pablo, St. Los Angeles, CA 90033, USA
e-mail: fsaremi@usc.edu

H. Muresian, MD, PhD
Department of Cardiovascular Surgery, University Hospital of Bucharest, Splaiul Independentei 169, Bucharest, Romania
e-mail: cvsurg@hotmail.com

D. Sánchez-Quintana, MD, PhD
Departamento de Anatomía Humana, Facultad de Medicina de Badajoz, Badajoz 06071, Spain
e-mail: damians@unex.es

Development of the Cardiac Veins

The right and left common cardinal veins (ducts of Cuvier) are formed by the confluence of the anterior and posterior cardinal veins [1, 2]. The right horn of the sinus venosus and the right common cardinal vein will be developed and eventually form the posterior wall of the right atrium (RA) and the superior vena cava, respectively. The left horn of the sinus venosus, in conjunction with the regressing left common cardinal vein, forms the coronary sinus (CS) and the ligament or vein of the left atrium (Marshall) [1, 2] (Fig. 28.1). A vessel connecting the right and left superior cardinal veins enlarges and becomes the left brachiocephalic vein. The right sinus valve persists as the valve of the inferior vena cava and the valve of the coronary sinus (Eustachian and the Thebesian valves, *respectively*) [2].

It was suggested in earlier experiments that coronary vessels arise from the proepicardium, a transitory structure in the embryonic heart that forms epicardium and several internal tissues [3]. Recent histological analysis in mouse and cardiac organ culture has shown that coronary vessels arise from angiogenic sprouts of the sinus

F. Saremi (ed.), *Cardiac CT and MR for Adult Congenital Heart Disease*,
DOI 10.1007/978-1-4614-8875-0_28, © Springer Science+Business Media New York 2014

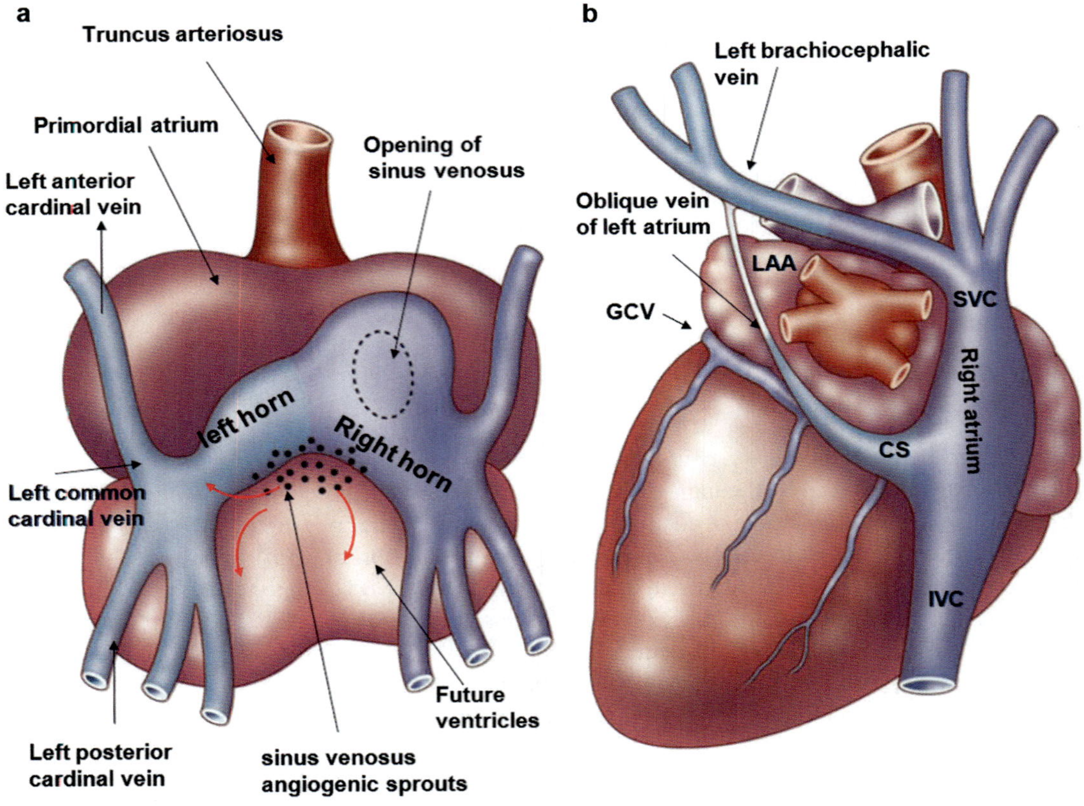

Fig. 28.1 Development of cardiac veins. Posterior drawings of the embryonic heart at 4 weeks (**a**) and well-developed heart (**b**) at 8 weeks. The right and left anterior cardinal veins connect through small anastomotic veins which form the left brachiocephalic vein. The right horn of the sinus venosus and the cardinal veins eventually form the posterior wall of the right atrium (RA) and the vena cava, respectively. The left sinus horn regresses and loses its connection with the left anterior cardinal vein and becomes the coronary sinus (*CS*) and the oblique vein of left atrium (Marshall). Angiogenic sprouts (*small asterisks* in **a**) of the sinus venosus covering the epicardial surfaces (shown by *red curved arrows*) turn into the coronary vessels including veins (colored in *dark green*). *GCV* great cardiac vein, *IVC* inferior vena cava, *SVC* superior vena cava, *LAA* left atrial appendage

venosus, the major vein that returns circulating blood to the embryonic heart [4]. Some sprouting venous endothelial cells dedifferentiate into arteries and capillaries as they invade the myocardium and some remain on the surface and differentiate into veins [4].

Cardiac Vein Classification

A complete, highly efficient and clinically useful classification of the CVS is not as straightforward as in the case of the coronary arteries. The *epicardial* coronary veins depict a very different macroscopic disposition, as compared to the coronary arterial system, and show many more individual variations.

Modern anatomical classification divides the cardiac veins into two main groups including tributaries of the Greater-Cardiac Vascular System (CVS) and tributaries of the Smaller-CVS, consisting of the Thebesian vessels [5–7]. For clarity Greater-CVS is divided into two groups including CS and non-CS tributaries (Fig. 28.2). Branches of the two systems can communicate. The term Compound-CVS has been used to describe

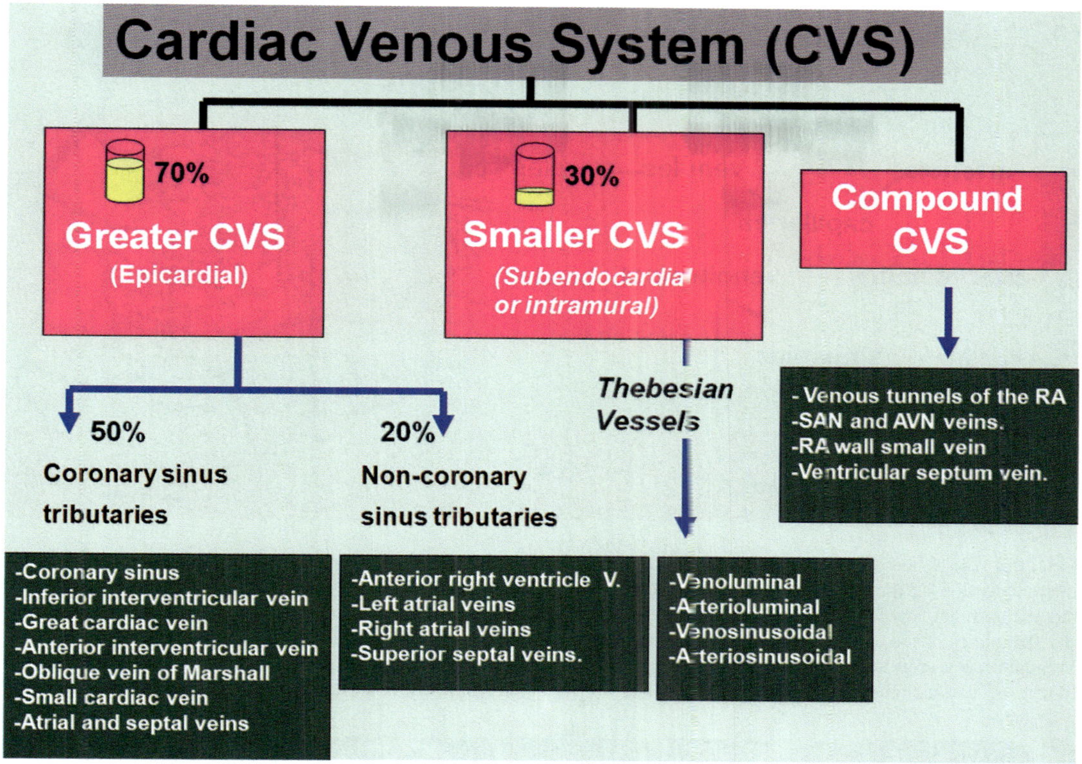

Fig. 28.2 Classification of the cardiac venous system (*CVS*), right atrium (*RA*), sinuatrial node (*SAN*), atrioventricular node (*AVN*), vein (*V*)

structures in which venous drainage is performed equally by both systems (Fig. 28.2) [6].

In ventricular myocardium, the external two thirds are drained by the Greater-CVS, and the internal third is mainly drained by tributaries of the Smaller-CVS [6].

The left ventricle and part of the right ventricle and the left atrium (LA) are drained by the CS tributaries, and the majority of the right ventricle and both atria are drained by the non-CS tributaries. Almost all veins of the Greater-CVS are finally drained into the right atrium. In the right atrium, the wall of sinus venosus is drained by tributaries of the Greater-CVS, and the right atrial appendage is mainly drained by the Smaller-CVS [8].

Smaller-CVS (Thebesian Vessels)

Consisting of sinusoids, channels, and *lacunae*, this subendocardial and intramyocardial bidirectional communicating network runs in every direction conducting blood from epicardial coronary arteries into the cardiac chambers and provides myocardial nourishment (Fig. 28.3). Sinusoids are large capillaries with different morphologies (Figs. 28.4 and 28.5). They are remnant of the primitive cardiac circulation.

The vessels of the Smaller-CVS are collectively called *Thebesian veins*. However, in view of their arterial component, the term "Thebesian vessels" is preferred [6]. Four distinct parts are described (Fig. 28.3b). Their orifices are found in cardiac chambers (mostly RA and right ventricle) and bases of papillary muscles [9, 10] and usually are <0.5 mm in diameter but can be much larger especially in congenital heart disease with abnormal drainage of the CS [11]. Approximately 70–80 % of the left coronary artery blood flow drains through the CS tributaries, and the remainder is drained via the Smaller-CVS [12–15]. The right heart chambers mainly drain thorough the

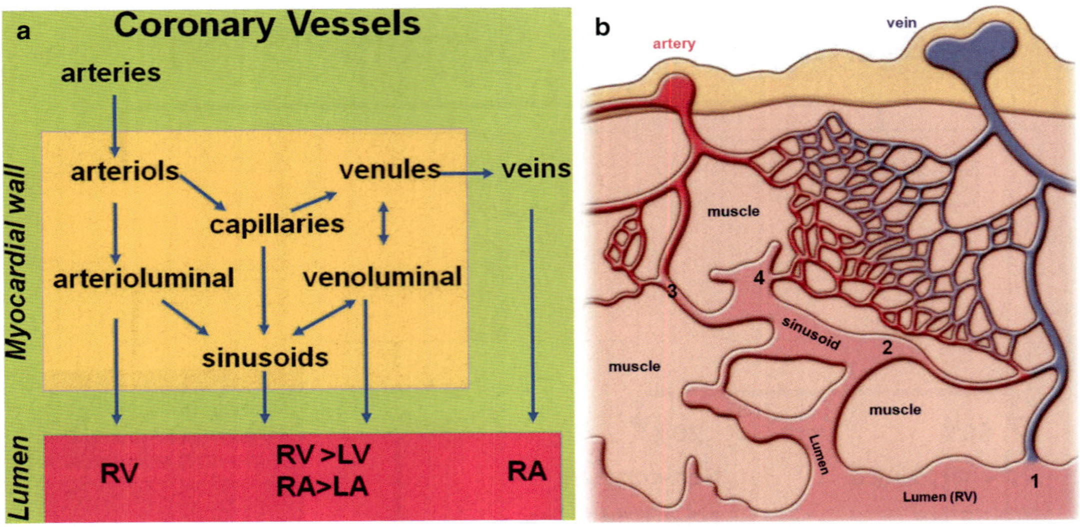

Fig. 28.3 (**a**) Schematic drawing demonstrates extensive interconnection of the epicardial cardiac vessels through the intraluminal Smaller-Cardiac Venous System (CVS). (**b**) Tributaries of the Smaller-CVS (Thebesian vessels): *1*. Venoluminal vessels connect intramural venules with the lumen of cardiac chambers. *2*. Venosinusoidal vessels connect intramural venules with subendocardial sinusoids and then the lumen. *3*. Arterioluminal vessels connect arterioles with the atria or ventricles without traversing capillary beds. Only exist in the right ventricle (RV). *4*. Arteriosinusoidal vessels connect arterioles with sinusoidal spaces. *RA* right atrium, *LV* left ventricle, *LA* left atrium

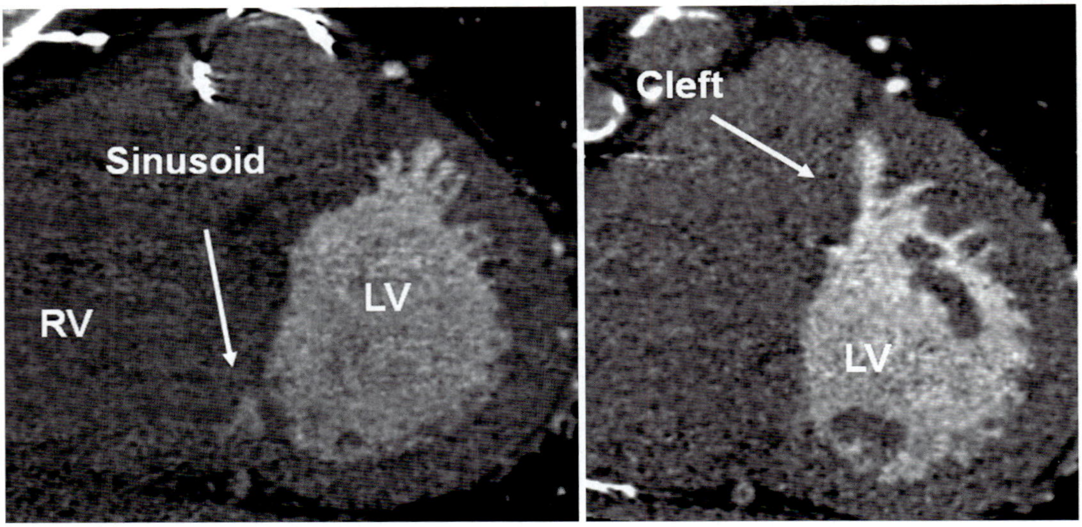

Fig. 28.4 Short-axis CT images of the heart showing large sinusoids in the interventricular septum and an example of myocardial cleft of the interventricular septum. Clefts should not be mistaken with a ventricular septal defect *RV* right ventricle, *LV* left ventricle

Smaller-CVS [6, 8]. In patients with single ventricle and atrial isomerism, this drainage pattern may be different due to rearrangement of the epicardial veins. The Thebesian network can provide reverse flow from ventricles into the epicardial coronary arteries when flow in the latter is compromised [12]. In patients with congestive heart failure, congestion is mainly in large veins not the Thebesian veins [13]. Enlarged Thebesian veins are described in CHD patients.

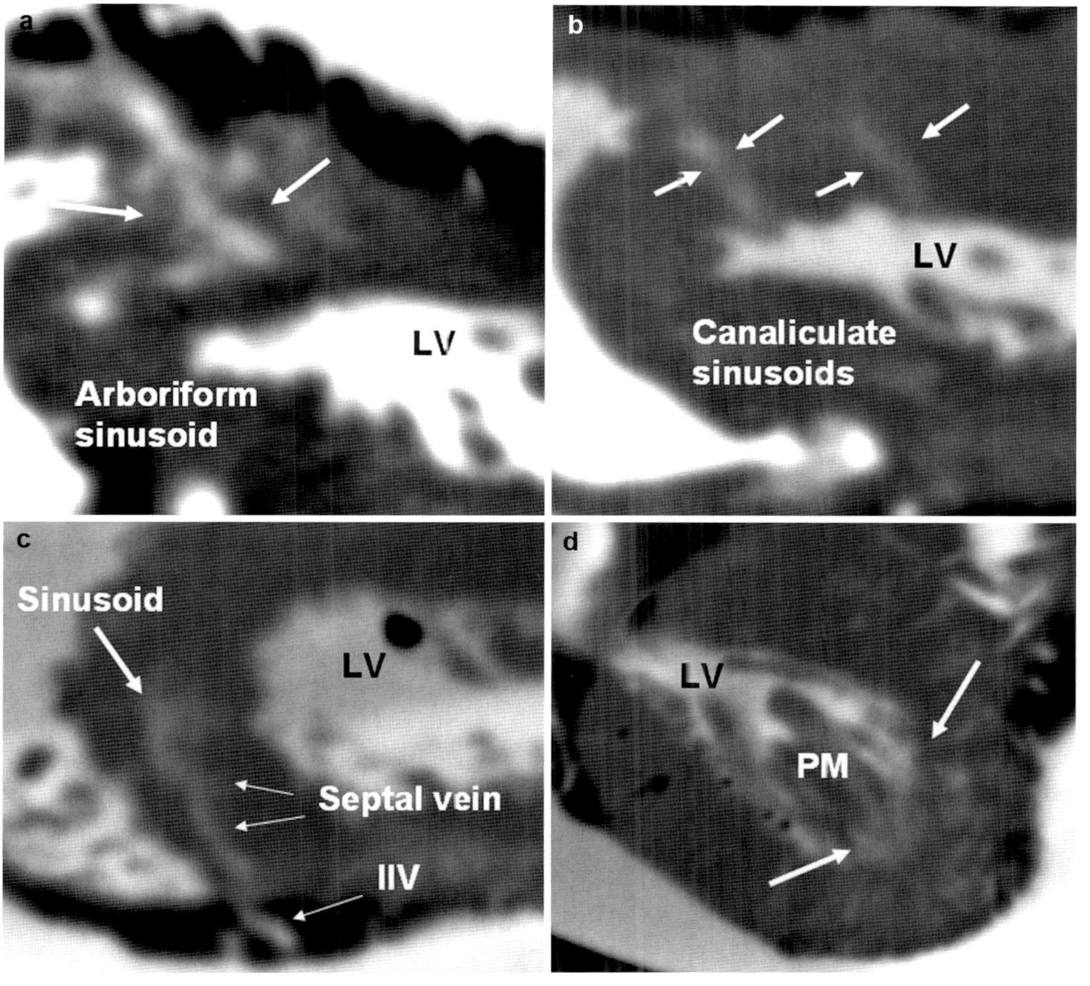

Fig. 28.5 Ex vivo CT of the heart in different specimens. The coronary veins are opacified with 10 % iodinated contrast injected into the coronary sinus. Note numerous contrast-filled intramural Thebesian vessels including sinusoids (*thick white arrows*) some opening into the ventricular lumen. Arboriform (**a**) and canaliculate (**b**) sinusoid morphologies are shown. (**c**) demonstrates a venosinusoidal communication connecting the inferior interventricular vein (*IIV*) with a sinusoid through the septal vein. (**d**) Shows large sinusoids at the base of left ventricle (*LV*) papillary muscle (*PM*). Thebesian vessel foramina are common at the apex of the ventricles and at the base of the papillary muscles

Atrial Venous System

Imaging of these veins is difficult because of small size of vessels. However careful evaluation of cardiac CT images can show these structures in many studies. Different classifications are introduced [6, 8, 16, 17]. The easiest classification is introduced by von Lüdinghausen [8] (Table 28.1).

Veins of the LA Wall

The majority of left atrial veins are tributaries of the Greater-CVS. Three groups are described [6, 8]:

1. Veins of the posterior and lateral walls of the LA empty into the CS and GCV (Fig. 28.6).
2. Septal veins of the LA drain into the RA through the interatrial septum. These veins are commonly seen with CTA. Veins anterosuperior to the fossa ovalis pass through the

Table 28.1 Venous drainage of the left and right atrial walls

Left atrium	Right atrium
1. Posterior and lateral walls (99 %)	1. Small intramural veins (73 %)
Draining into the CS	Draining into the RA, 1 mm diameter
2. Septal walls	2. Venous tunnels of the RA (right atrial CS) (25–60 %)
Draining into the RA (92 %)	1–12 cm in length and 1–4 mm in diameter – emptying into the RA or SCV
Anterosuperior (near SVC) (99 %)	3. SAN region
Posteroinferior (near IVC) (35 %)	Small veins and sinusoids draining into the RA
3. Posterosuperior wall	4. AVN region
Draining into the mediastinal veins (40 %)	Small venous tunnels draining into the RA or CS
Directly draining in the LA (80 %)	
Draining into the pulmonary veins (some)	

Incidence is shown in parenthesis
AVN atrioventricular node, *CS* coronary sinus, *IVC* inferior vena cava, *LA* left atrium, *RA* right atrium, *SVC* superior vena cava, *SAN* sinoatrial node

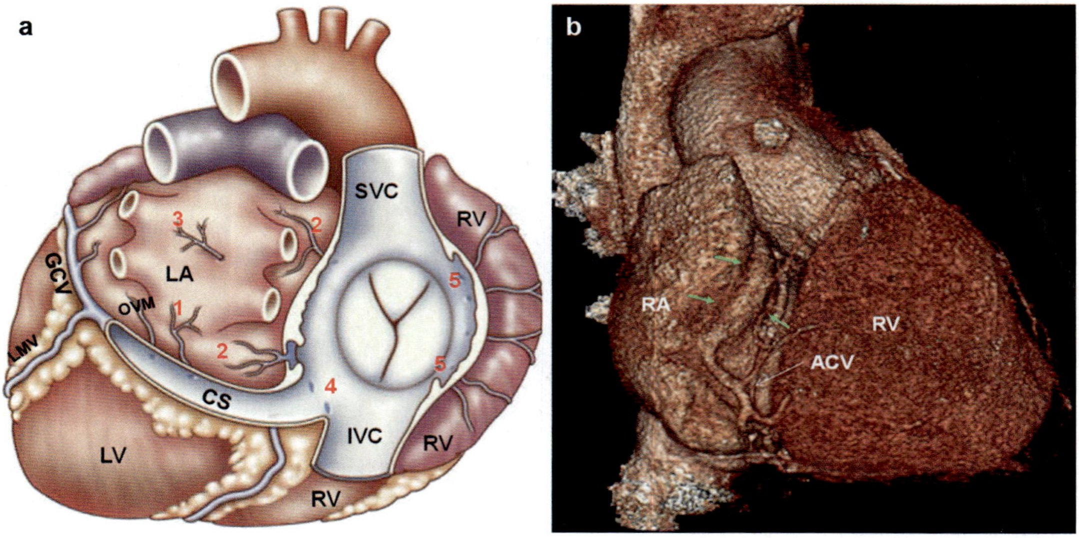

Fig. 28.6 (**a**) Atrial venous system. Posterosuperior view of the heart is depicted. The right atrium is removed. *1*. Veins of the posterior and lateral walls of the left atrium (*LA*) empty into the coronary sinus (*CS*). *2*. Septal veins of the LA drain into the right atrium (*RA*). *3*. Posterosuperior wall of the LA drains into the LA lumen or the superior pulmonary veins. *4*. Atrioventricular node region contains small sinusoids draining into the RA near the CS ostium. *5*. Anterior cardiac veins may drain directly into the RA, small cardiac vein, or into a venous tunnel in the RA wall. (**b**) Drainage of the anterior cardiac vein (*ACV*) into the venous tunnel running (*green arrows*) parallel to the atrioventricular groove. *LV* left ventricle, *RV* right ventricle, *SVC* superior vena cava, *IVC* inferior vena cava, *OVM* oblique vein of Marshall, *LMV* left marginal vein, *GCV* great cardiac vein

interatrial groove and empty in to right atrium near the superior cavoatrial junction (Fig. 28.7). Some (12 %) may pass through superior interatrial muscle connections where Bachmann bundle is located [18] (Fig. 28.8). Enlargement of these veins can rarely occur in arteriovenous malformations of the atrial vessels (Fig. 28.9). Veins inferoposterior to fossa ovalis are less common (Fig. 28.7).

3. Posterosuperior wall of the LA near the left atrial appendage drain into the LA and superior pulmonary veins (Fig. 28.7). They may connect to the mediastinal veins, azygos or hemiazygos venous system, and bronchial

veins [8]. The mediastinal connections can be important alternative route for venous return to the atria incase of occlusion of pulmonary, brachiocephalic, or superior vena cava occlusion (Figs. 28.7 and 28.8). In congenital atresia of the CS, the myocardial venous drainage can be via ectatic atrial veins of the LA [19].

Veins of the RA Wall

The majority of the right atrial wall veins are located intramurally and drain into the RA. The veins draining the wall of the right atrial appendage have no connection with the epicardial veins and therefore are classified as Smaller-CVS. The RA veins are classified into four groups based on anatomical locations (Table 28.1).

1. *Small intramural venous tunnels draining directly into the RA*: They are a few mm in length and 1 mm diameter [6].
2. *Venous tunnels of the RA*: Termination of the anterior cardiac veins of the right ventricle is variable. They may drain directly into the RA, small cardiac vein, or in some into a venous tunnel [6]. When it exists, this venous tunnel runs parallel and 1–2 cm above to the tricuspid orifice along the posterior or posterolateral wall of the RA [20] (Fig. 28.6). In high-quality CTAs, these veins may be partially visible (Fig. 28.6b). This system of drainage was initially described as "the small cardiac vein." This SCV can drain either separately into the right atrium or into the CS.
3. *Sinoatrial node region: The sinoatrial node region* has sinusoids draining into the RA [14] This network of anastomosing blood vessels theoretically can protect the node in case arterial supply is compromised. However, this phenomenon is rare given the common variants of dual or multiple arterial supplies to the node.
4. *Atrioventricular node region*: Venous tunnels are seen at the base of interatrial septum near

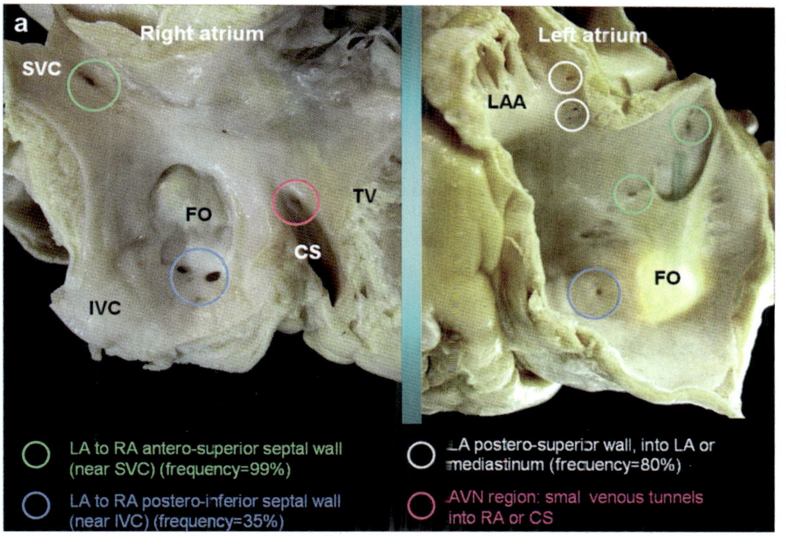

Fig. 28.7 (**a**) Septal views of the right and left atria (*RA*, *LA*) from two different cadaveric specimens are shown. Most of the septal venous drainage occurs from the LA into the RA. Venous drainage of the anterosuperior and posterosuperior of the interatrial septum as well as posterosuperior wall of LA and atrioventricular node (AVN) region is shown by *green*, *blue*, *white*, and *pink circles*, respectively. Most of the septal venous drainage occurs from the LA into the RA. The venous opening can be large enough to be detected by CT scan. (**b**) Short-axis CT images demonstrate the drainage pattern of atrial wall veins matching to the *colored circles* shown in (a) including communication between the two atrial walls near the SVC (*green arrow* in b1) and IVC (*blue arrow* in b3), the superior wall of the LA near confluence with left superior pulmonary vein (*white arrow* in b2), and the medial RA wall near the coronary sinus (CS) ostium (*pink arrow* in b4). Veins of the superior wall of LA may communicate with venous collaterals in the mediastinum (*white arrow* in b2). *LAA* left atrial appendage, *FO* fossa ovalis, *SVC* superior vena cava, *IVC* inferior vena cava, *TV* tricuspid valve

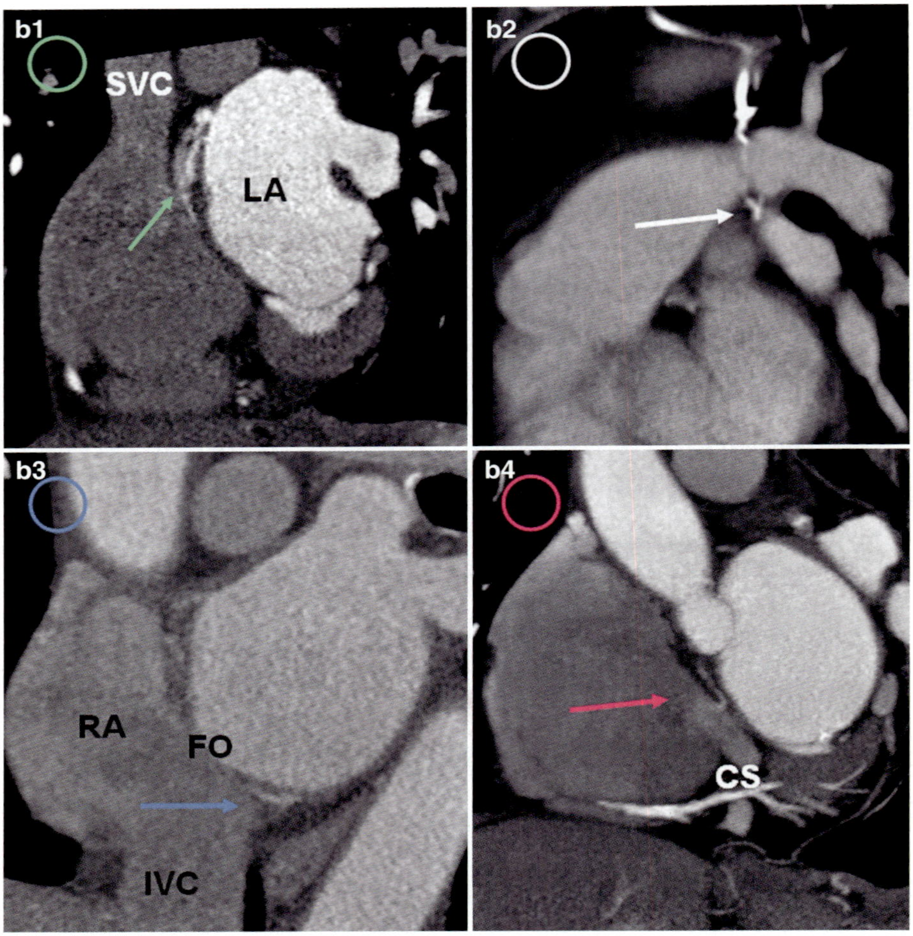

Fig. 28.7 continued)

the atrioventricular node and His bundle and usually open into the RA near the ostium of the CS or directly into the CS (Figs. 28.6 and 28.8). These tunnels can be seen in CTA and should not be confused with anomalous vessels or a patent foramen ovale.

Anterior Right Ventricular Venous System

Including the anterior cardiac, right marginal and conus veins are present in 90 % of cases [6, 20–22] (Table 28.2).

The anterior cardiac veins drain 2/3 of the right ventricle including the anterior and anterolateral walls of the right ventricle. These veins are frequently identified in coronary CTAs (Fig. 28.10). They are variable in sizes and numbers and usually drain into the RA just above the atrioventricular groove [6, 16, 21]. In 5–27 % they merge to form a common trunk before entering the RA [6, 21].

The right marginal vein originates near the right ventricular apex and receives branches from posterior and anterior surfaces of the right ventricle (Fig. 28.10). In one third the vein continues as small cardiac vein into the CS [6]. In the remainder of cases, it drains into the RA or the venous tunnels of the RA.

The conus (infundibular) veins are usually small veins and drain into the RA. However, they

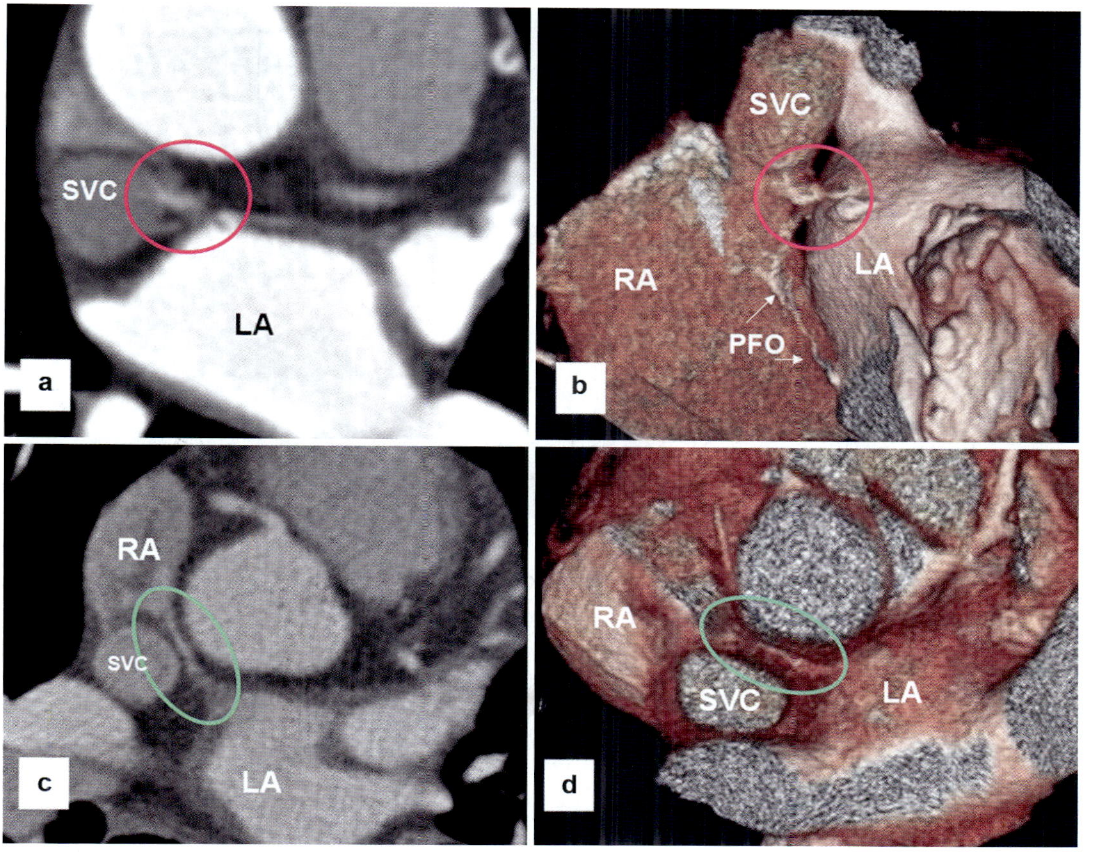

Fig. 28.8 Venous drainage of the anterosuperior septal wall of left atrium (*LA*) into the right atrium (*RA*) through the superior interatrial muscle connection where Bachmann bundle resides. Communications found in two different patients are shown by *pink* (**a**, **b**) and *green* (**c**, **d**) *circles*. This communication is seen in 12 % of CT angiographies. The lumen of a patent foramen ovalis (*PFO*) is incidentally seen (*white arrows*). *SVC* superior vena cava

can be large and varicoid creating diagnostic problems (Fig. 28.11) or causing excessive bleeding during surgery. Veins of Zuckerkandl and Cruveilhier are described in anatomic literature for veins draining the anterior or posterior surfaces of the infundibulum, respectively [20, 21] (Fig. 28.11).

Coronary Sinus Tributaries

The coronary sinus tributaries include the CS, the GCV, the left marginal vein, the posterolateral vein of the LV, and the inferior interventricular vein (IIV) (Fig. 28.12). In 30 % it receives the right marginal vein blood through the small cardiac vein [6] (Table 28.2).

Imaging Methods

The CS is frequently used as a conduit for catheter treatment of arrhythmias as well as left ventricular pacing. These procedures are well known for their potential technical difficulties. As a result different imaging methods are introduced for evaluation of this system. Each technique has its own advantages and limitations [23–29].

Retrograde venography via the CS is currently the standard technique for defining the CS anatomy; however, it is invasive in nature and can be technically challenging. This technique is frequently used to show the anatomy of the CS and target veins for CRT. In this technique using an occlusive balloon contrast in injected into the CS and two orthogonal views including right anterior oblique 45° and left anterior oblique 45° are

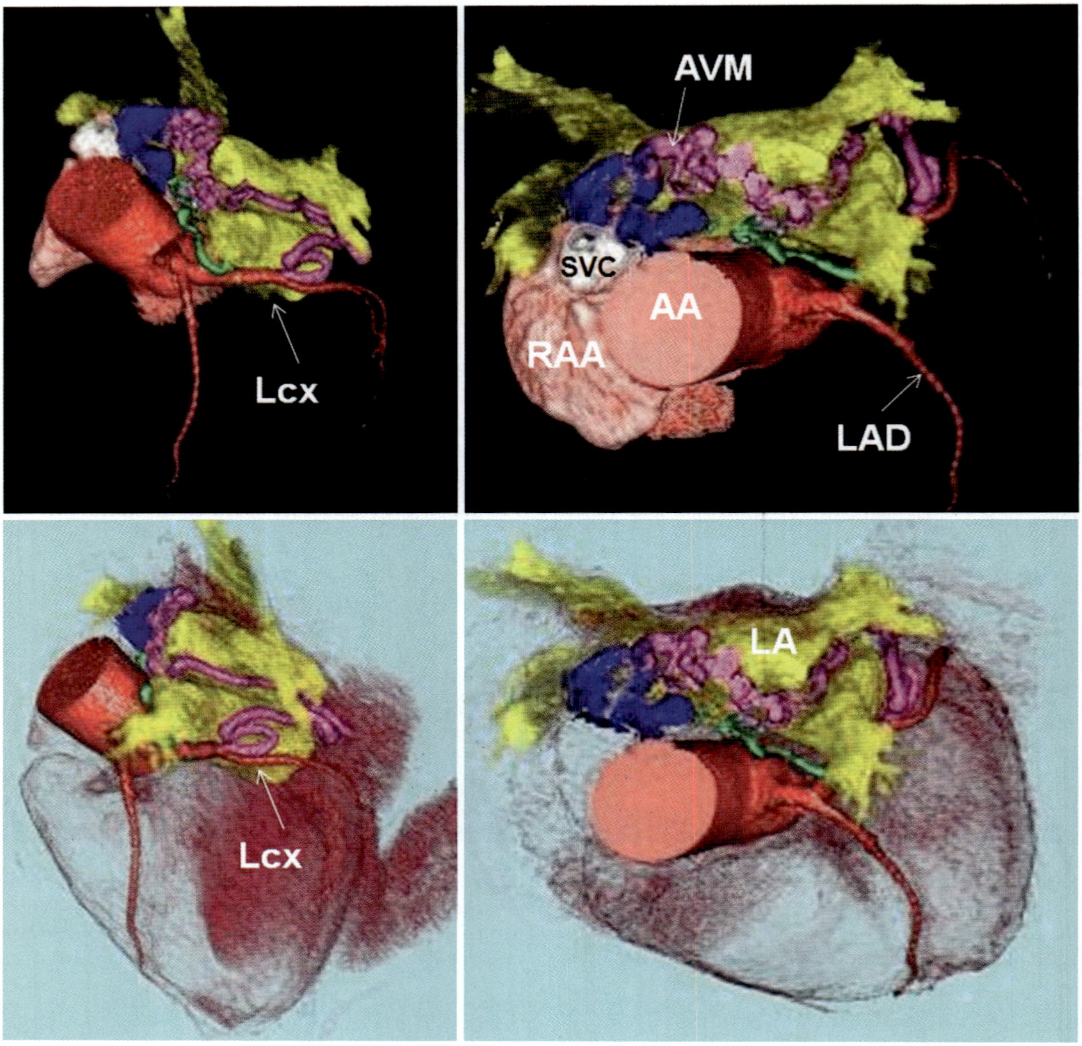

Fig. 28.9 Color-coded CT angiography shows arteriovenous malformation (*AVM*) in the transverse sinus near the superior cavoatrial junction. Arterial supply is provided by an atrial branch (in *green*) and the left sinoatrial node (in *pink*) arteries both arising from the left circumflex (*LCx*) artery. Enlarged draining atrial veins (*blue*) are seen near the junction of the superior vena cava (*SVC*) with the atrium. Left atrium (*LA*) is shown in *yellow*. *AA* ascending aorta, *RAA* right atrial appendage, *LAD* left anterior descending artery

obtained [23]. High-speed rotational coronary venography uses rapid isocentric rotation over a 110° arc in 4 s, acquiring 120 frames/angiogram [23]. With this modification, vessel overlap and foreshortening will be reduced, and target veins including second-degree tributaries can be better defined. Levophase of coronary angiography is preferred by some investigators and claimed to better define the anterior interventricular vein (AIV) and IIV as well as the peripheral branches compared to retrograde venography [24]. However, the sensibility of this method is questionable. The technique takes advantage of the coronary artery angiography procedure commonly indicated in the assessment of candidates for CRT.

MRI and CT have been increasingly used to assess anatomy of the coronary vessels including coronary veins [25–29]. CT has the advantage of

Table 28.2 Characteristics of the epicardial veins of coronary sinus and anterior right ventricle venous system

Veins	Origin	Territory	Ostial diameter (mm)	Frequency %	Drainage	Number	Variant	Ostial valve %
CS	GCV	Left atrioventricular groove	4–14 (10)	99	RA	1, duplication is very rare	Absence (with left SVC), unroofed, atresia (1 %), duplication	80
GCV/AIV	Apex	Anterior septum, anterior of both ventricles, parts of LA and apex	AIV = 09–4.4 (2.7), GCV = 1.2–6.3(3.9)	100	CS (99 %)	1(98 %)	Aberrant course to RA in 1 %, aneurysm, myocardial bridge 2–8 %, duplication 3 %, myocardial belt (6 %)	85
IIV	Apex	Posterior wall of the RV and LV, apex, posterior two third of the interventricular septum	2–5.3 (3.6)	100	CS, rarely RA (2.5 %)	1 (75 %), 2 (24 %)	Aneurysm (8 %), varicoid, duplicated, myocardial cover (2.5 %)	60
LPV	Posterior wall	Lateral and diaphragmatic walls of the LV	1–5.5 (2.4)	95	CS (37–77 %), GCV (13 %)	1 (63 %), 2 (23 %), multiple small (9 %), non (5 %)	Bulbar (5 %), myocardial cover (2 %)	30
LMV	Posterolateral wall of LV	Draining much of LV myocardium	1–3 (2.2)	70–85	GCV (80 %), CS (20 %)	1	Absence common	30
SCV	Right atrioventricular groove	Diaphragmatic surface of RV	<1	30–50	CS (85 %), IIV (12 %)	1	Can receive the right marginal vein in 10 %	–
OVM	Junction of CS and GCV	Posterolateral LA, 2–3 cm length	0.4–1.8	85–95	CS	1	Persistent SVC 0.5 %	–
RMV	Apex	Anterior and posterior RV walls	0.5–3	13–80	SCV (30 %), rest RA or tunnel of RA	1	Large draining into a vertical RA tunnel	–
ACV	Anterior RV	Anterior and anterolateral RV	0.5–1	90	RA (30 %), venous tunnel of RA (66 %), SCV	1 (24–57 %), 2(33–48 %), 3(9–28 %), up to 15 tiny ones	Abnormal course of AIV into SVC, large conus vein	12

Data from von Lüdinghausen [6], Pina [21], Mierzwa and Kozielec [22], Ortale et al. [30], Pejkovic and Bogdanovic [32], von Lüdinghausen [33], Saremi et al. [35], Cendrowska-Pinkosz [41], von Lüdinghausen [5] with permission

Abbreviations: *AV* arteriovenous, *ACV* anterior cardiac vein, *AIV* anterior interventricular vein, *CS* coronary sinus, *LA* left atrium, *LV* left ventricle, *GCV* great cardiac vein, *IIV* inferior interventricular vein, *IVC* inferior vena cava, *OVM* oblique vein of Marshall, *LMV* left marginal vein, *LPV* left posterior vein, *LV* left ventricle, *RV* right ventricle, *RMV* right marginal vein, *RA* right atrium, *SCV* small cardiac vein, *SVC* superior vena cava

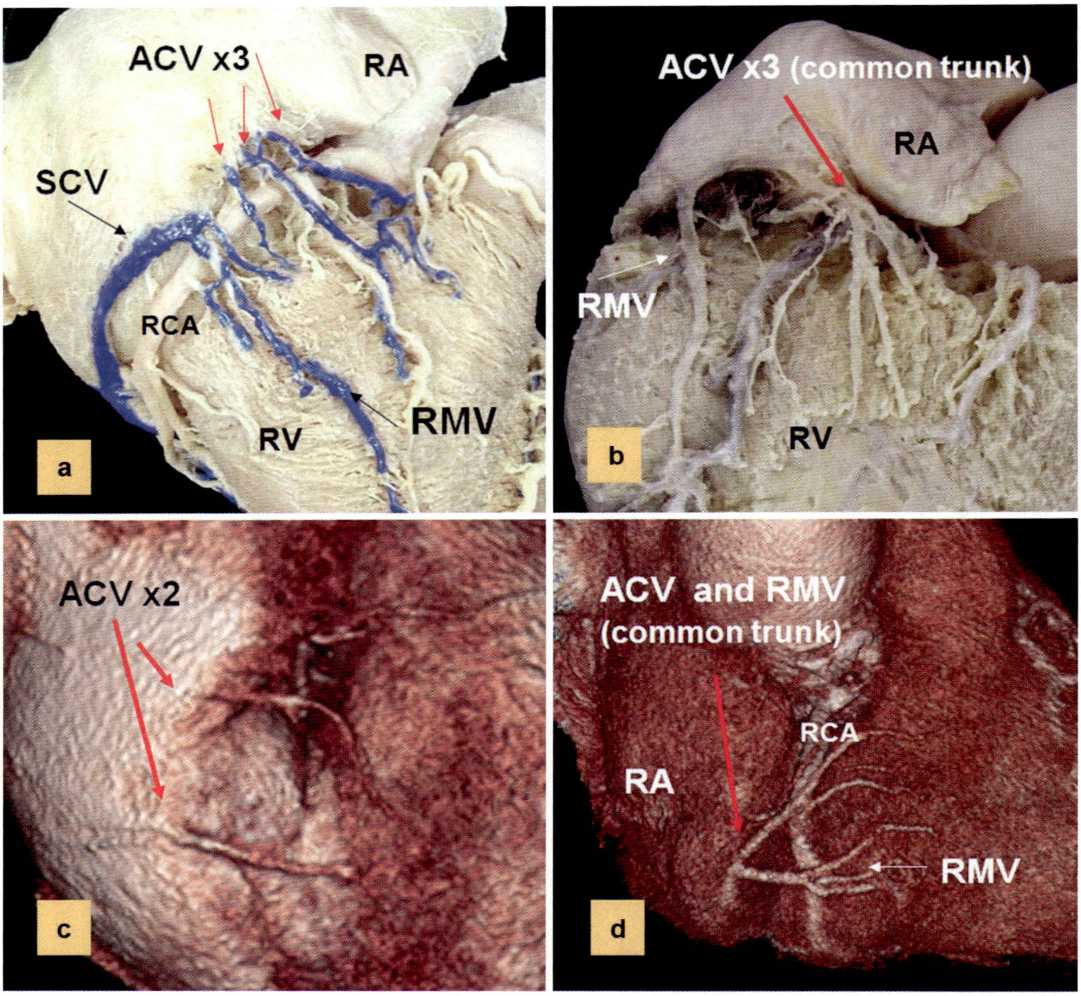

Fig. 28.10 Common variants of the right ventricle (*RV*) venous system are shown: cadaveric specimens (**a**, **b**) and CT angiograms (**c**, **d**). Passing anterior to the right coronary artery (*RCA*), the anterior cardiac veins (*ACV*) commonly enter into right atrium (*RA*) as separate vessels or in some cases form a common trunk (5–27 %). The right marginal vein (*RMV*) is seen in 80 % of cases. It drains in to small cardiac vein (*SCV*) in 30 % or drains directly into the RA in 70 %

Fig. 28.12 Left lateral, posterior, and right lateral views of the cadaveric heart (*upper row*) and CT angiographies of a patient with tetralogy of Fallot (*lower row*). Tributaries of the coronary sinus (*CS*) venous system are displayed in *blue*. The CS tributaries include the CS, the great cardiac vein (*GCV*), the anterior interventricular vein (*AIV*) portion of the GCV, the left marginal vein (*LMV*), the posterior vein (*PV*) of the left ventricle, the inferior interventricular vein (*IIV*), the oblique vein of Marshall (*OVM*), and the small cardiac vein (*SCM*). A very large PV and two small IIVs are shown (*yellow asterisks*) in CT image of patient with tetralogy of Fallot. In cadaveric heart the right marginal vein (*RMV*) drains directly into the right atrium, while in tetralogy case, it is draining into the SCV. That is why SCV is large in this patient; it also drains into the IIV. *MPA* main pulmonary artery

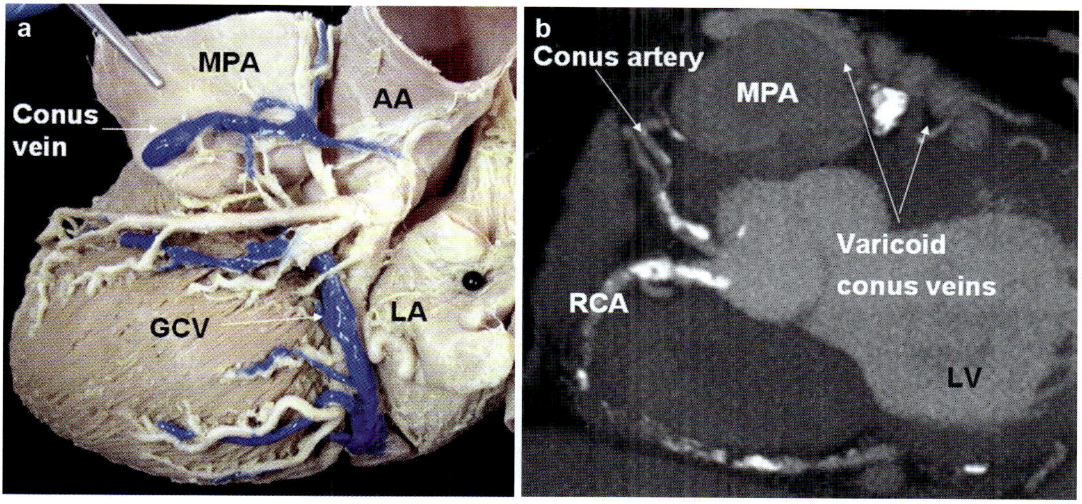

Fig. 28.11 Conus veins. (**a**) In this cadaveric specimen the conus vein is the vein located between the main pulmonary artery (*MPA*) and the ascending aorta (*AA*). Large and varicoid conus veins are seen in coronary artery occlusions, myocardial bridging, and vascular malformations. (**b**) Dilated conus vein is shown in a patient with severe coronary artery disease and right coronary artery (*RCA*) occlusion, (*GCV*) great cardiac vein, (*LA*) left atrium, (*MPA*) main pulmonary artery, (*LV*) left ventricle

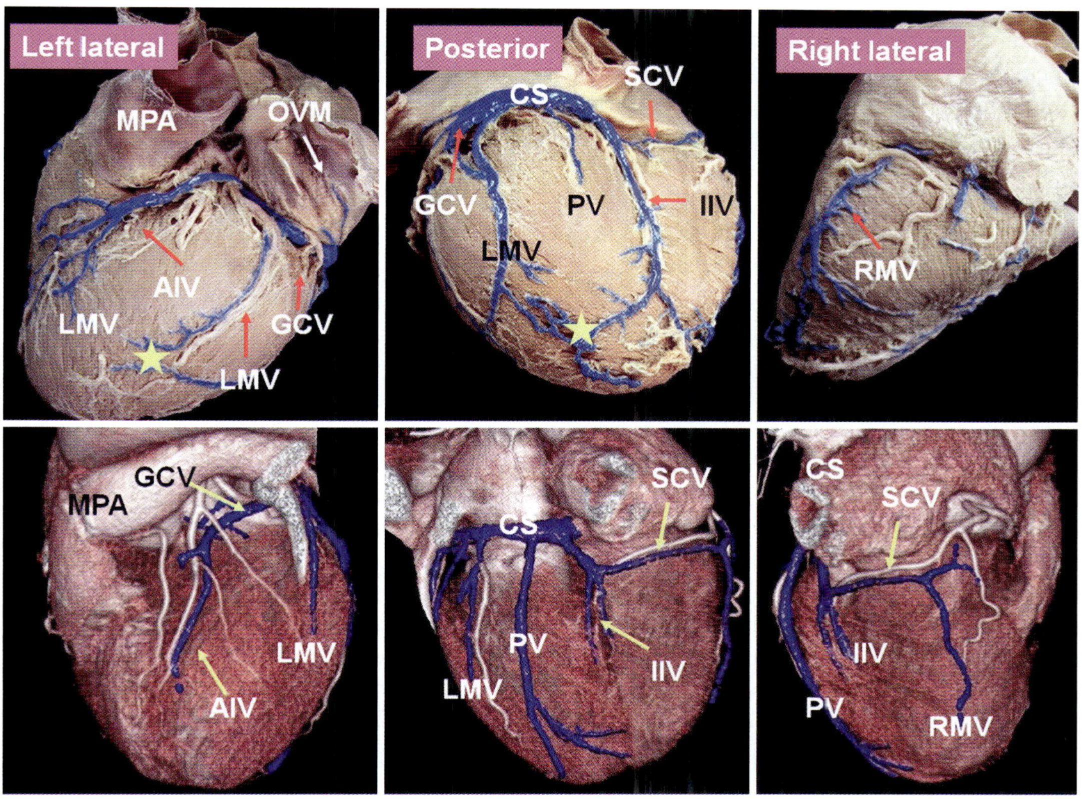

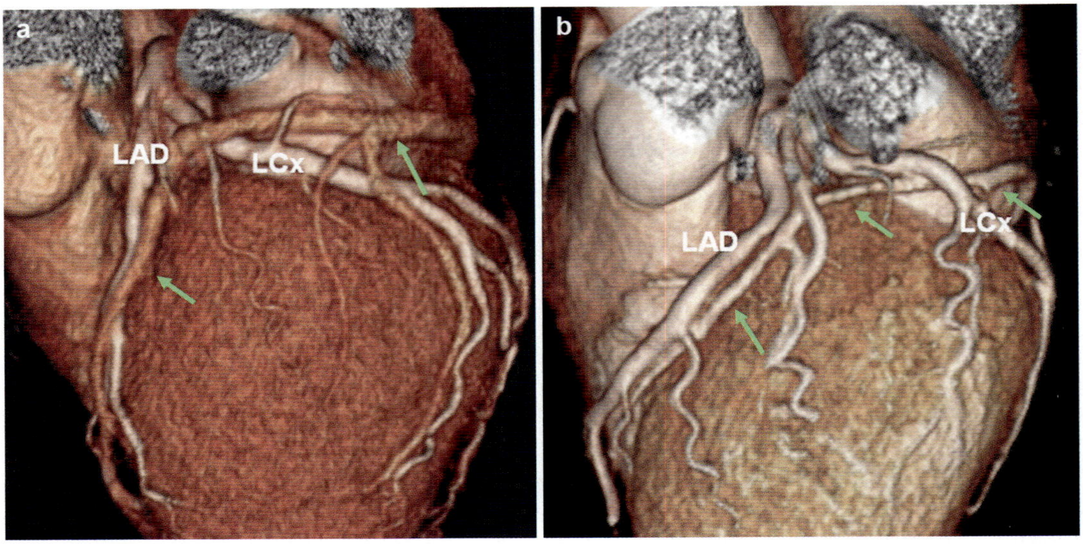

Fig. 28.13 The anterior interventricular vein (*green arrows*) portion of the great cardiac vein crosses the left anterior descending (*LAD*) and the left circumflex (*LCx*) arteries forming a triangle (triangle of Brocq and Mouchet). (**a**) The vein runs superficial to arteries in 60–70 % of population. The relations of the vein and these arteries are highly variable. It passes under both arteries in 20 % (**b**)

showing part of the CS and in some cases *the* confluence of the IIV which may be obscured with balloon in retrograde venography. With CT there is no foreshortening or vessel overlap. CT also demonstrates many ancillary structures such as coronary arteries, old infarctions, interatrial septum anatomy, and variants of the normal anatomy. Higher radiation dose in CT is a limitation [26] which can be modified using dose reduction techniques. CT also may have difficulty showing second-order tributaries of the coronary veins in routine coronary CTAs. Demonstration of the oblique vein of left atrium is also more challenging with CT compared with retrograde venography. However, with some modification of the CT technique, most small branches can be nicely depicted. CT technique for cardiac venous mapping is very similar to routine coronary CTA [18]. For optimal visualization of the coronary venous system, the trigger delay for data acquisition should be delayed 2–3 s to let the coronary venous side fill with contrast. This can easily be achieved with selecting the automated trigger level in the descending aorta approximately 3 cm below the tracheal bifurcation and starting scan 4 s after reaching a threshold of 180 Hounsfield units (HU).

Great Cardiac Vein

The GCV is the longest and the most consistent vessels making up the cardiac venous system almost always enters the CS [30–34]. This vein drains blood from the anterior interventricular septum, the anterior surfaces of both ventricles, part of the LA, and the apical region of the heart [6]. The AIV portion of the vein courses superiorly within the anterior interventricular groove and then enters the left atrioventricular groove where defined as a great cardiac vein (GCV). The GCV may originate at the apex or in the apical or middle third of the anterior interventricular sulcus with a highly variable position with respect to *the left anterior descending artery* ("anterior interventricular artery") which may render very difficult the localization of the latter especially in limited access coronary artery bypass procedures.

The GCV crosses the branches of the left coronary artery system including the anterior descending and the circumflex branches forming a triangle [6, 30] in which the vein is mainly superficial to arteries in 60–70 % [31–34] (Fig. 28.13). The ramus intermedius – when present – traverses this triangle. However, it is important to know that the relations of the vein and

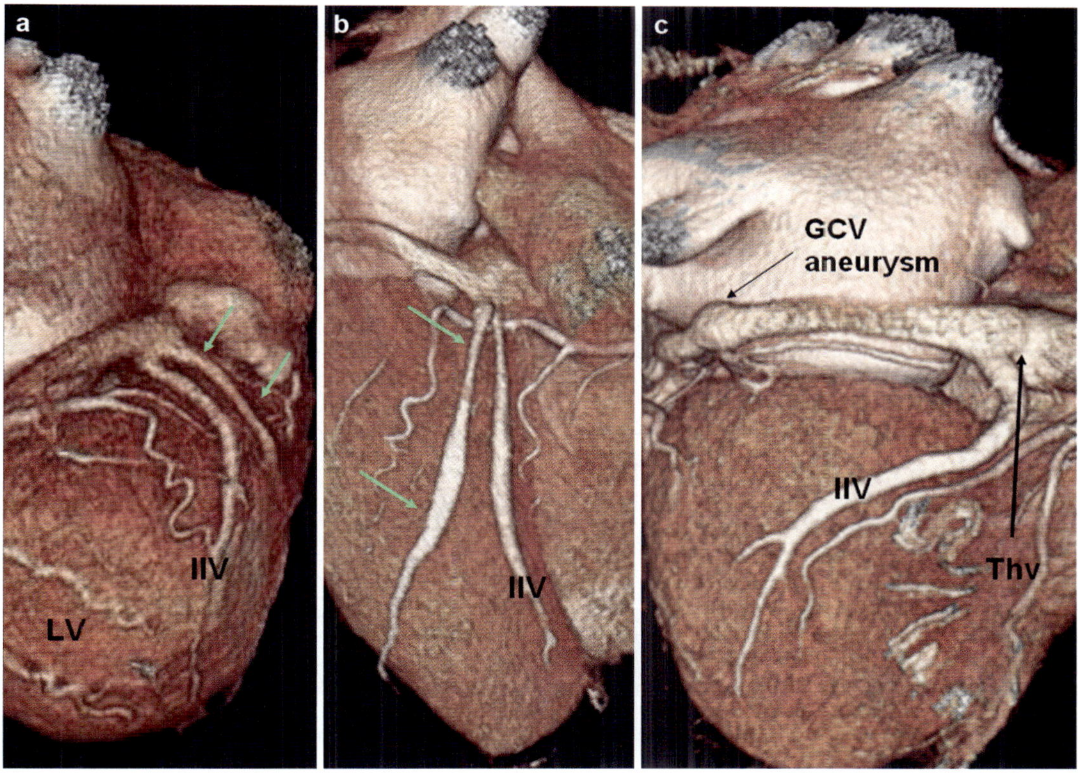

Fig. 28.14 Variants of the inferior interventricular vein (*IIV*). (**a**) Duplicated IIV with one posterior right ventricle (*RV*) vessel (*green arrows*). (**b**) Duplicated IIV with one vessel running along posterior left ventricle (*LV*) wall (*green arrows*). Duplicated IIV can be seen in 3 % of population. (**c**) Rare course of the IIV draining mainly the posterior LV wall. These variants are important as they may remain undetected as a result of their ostial occlusion with balloon at the time of retrograde venography for LV pacing. CT has the advantage of showing all these variants. Note aneurysm of the great cardiac vein (*GCV*) which is seen in 1.5 % of coronary CT angiographies. Also note an outer ring marking the anatomic level of the Thebesian valve (*Thv*)

these arteries are highly variable and practically unpredictable in many cases.

Aberrant drainage of GCV into the RA or superior vena cava is described [33]. In this situation the GCV runs in the transverse sinus and finally joins the azygos vein or the RA. Variation in anatomical course of the AIV is common in CHD, and drainage may occur directly into the right atrium. Knowledge of this anatomy prior to surgery can be important for retrograde cardioplegia perfusion (RCP).

Myocardial bridges are detected above the anterior interventricular vein or its tributaries in 8 % [30]. Aneurysmal dilatation of the distal end of the GCV has been reported and may interfere with coronary artery bypass surgery [34]. It is the second most common location of coronary vein aneurysm seen in 1.5 % of CT examinations [35] (Fig. 28.14).

Inferior Interventricular Vein

The IIV, also known as middle cardiac vein or posterior interventricular, travels along the inferior aspect of the heart (attitudinal orientation) in the interventricular sulcus. The vein is a constant landmark and drains into the CS approximately 1 cm from the CS ostium. Extending from the apex to the CS, it drains the inferior walls of the ventricles as well as the apical area and the posterior 2/3 of the septum [6] (Fig. 28.15). The terminal portion of the vein measures 3–4 mm in diameter and appears angled in 35 % or bulbous

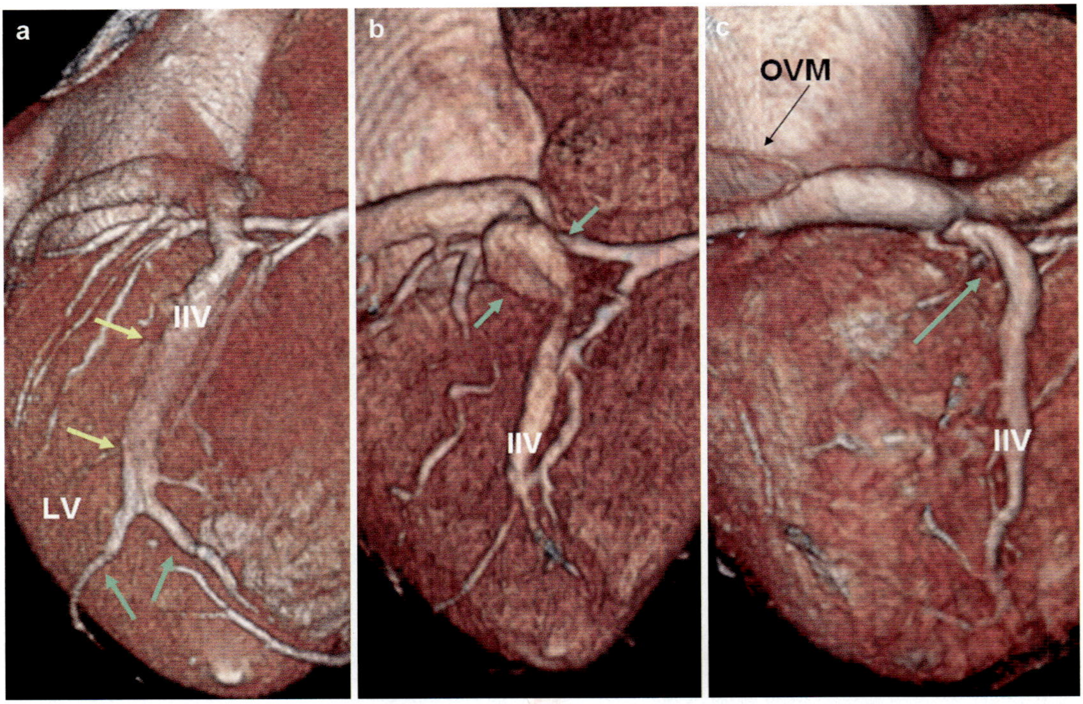

Fig. 28.15 Variants of the inferior interventricular vein (*IIV*) are common. (**a**) The IIV appears bifurcated near the LV apex in 45 % (*green arrows*). This appearance is formed by the confluence of two tributaries with the same caliber. Uncommonly, the entire length may appear varicoid (*yellow arrows*). (**b**) Fusiform aneurysmal dilatation of the venous confluence is seen in 8 % (*green arrows*). It is the most common location for bulbous enlargement of the coronary veins. (**c**) The terminal portion of the vein appears angled in 35 % (*green arrow*). Note the confluence of the oblique vein of Marshall (*OVM*) with the coronary sinus. *LV* left ventricle

in 19 % of population [6]. Fusiform aneurysmal dilatation (focal dilatation of twice the normal diameter) (mean 10.5 ± 1.4 mm) of the venous confluence is reported on CT studies in 8 % (Fig. 28.15). It is the most common location for bulbous enlargement of the coronary veins [35]. Aneurysms, especially the diverticular form, arising from the CS and the confluence of coronary veins with the CS, may be associated with cardiac arrhythmias such as ventricular preexcitation [36, 37].

Left Posterior (Posterolateral) and Left Marginal Veins

Several venous branches drain the myocardial walls located between the IIV and the AIV [30]. Veins draining posterior and lateral walls of the LV are of particular interest for LV pacing in CRT [38] (Fig. 28.16). Imaging techniques permit identification of potential anatomic factors that may pose difficulties to cannulate and advance the LV pacing lead including ostial valves, variceal veins, or absence of posterior or lateral vein.

The left posterior (inferior) veins are 1–3 in numbers and measure 2.5 mm at ostium. While the distal myocardial origin of the left posterior vein is highly variable, it usually terminates in a uniform fashion in the CS (75 %), although it can also drain into the GCV [6, 32, 39]. It is single in 60 %. In absence of the left posterior vein (5 %), it is the left marginal vein which drains most of the left ventricular posterolateral wall [5]. Small diameter of the vein (<2 mm) and acute angulation with the CS may complicate the insertion of the lead for CRT [38]. The left marginal (obtuse marginal) vein is present in 70–95 % of specimens, emptying into the GCV in 80 % of cases and into the CS in the remaining [30]. The frequency of

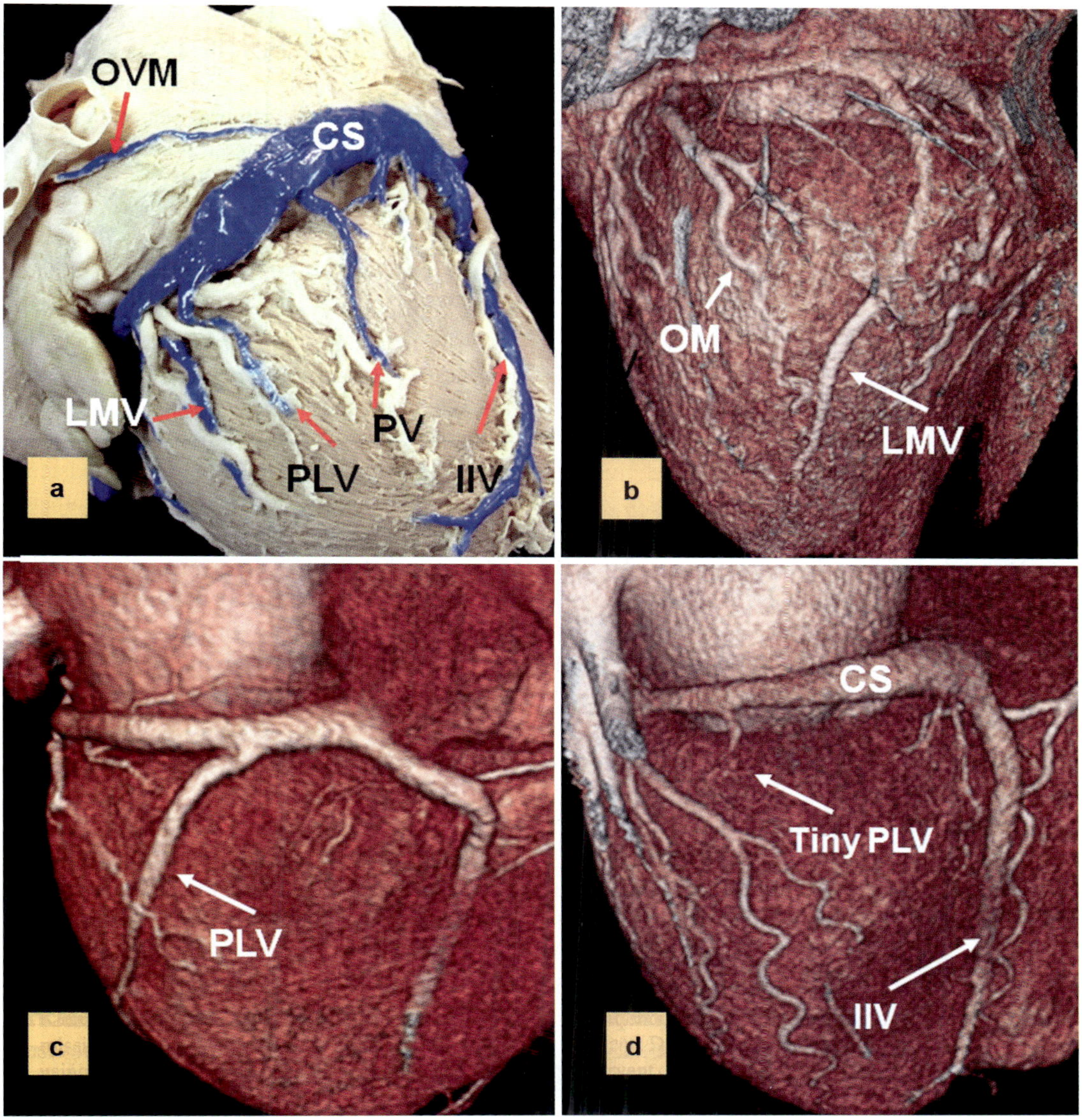

Fig. 28.16 Target veins used for CRT include the posterior, posterolateral, and marginal veins of the left ventricle. (**a**) Posterolateral view of a heart specimen. Veins are colored in *blue*. (**b**) Large left marginal vein (*LMV*) is shown crossing the obtuse marginal (*OM*) branch of the left circumflex artery near the apex. In absence of the left posterior vein (5 %), it is the LMV which drains most of the left ventricular posterolateral wall. The LMV drains into the great cardiac vein in 80 %. (**c**) Single but large posterolateral vein (*PLV*). In 75 % PLV drains into the CS. (**d**) Only a small PLV exists. *PV* posterior vein, *OVM* oblique vein of Marshall, *IIV* inferior interventricular vein

visualization is less with CT or MRI compared with retrograde venography [25–28]. It drains much of the left ventricle myocardium, usually running superficial to the marginal branch of the circumflex artery [32, 40]. Its diameter varies and, like other coronary veins, is enlarged in patients with cardiac failure [40]. Anastomosis of the epicardial veins in the periphery is common. This is especially common between the veins of the left ventricle such as between the GCV and posterolateral vein or between the IIV and posterolateral or marginal veins (Fig. 28.12).

Small Cardiac Vein

With a frequency of 30–50 % and average diameter of 1 mm, the small cardiac vein (right coronary vein) drains the posterolateral wall of the right ventricle into the CS (85 %), the IIV (12 %), or rarely the RA (1 %) [16, 30, 41] (Fig. 28.12). It is seen more frequently in women than in men [41].

Oblique Vein of the Left Atrium (Marshall)

The oblique vein of Marshall, a remnant of the left superior vena cava, descends along the lateral and inferior walls of the left atrium between the left atrial appendage and the left pulmonary veins and joins at the junction of the GCV and the CS approximately 3 cm from the CS ostium [42, 43]. The vein is short (2–3 cm in length) and its superior part obliterated by fibrosis. Complete fibrosis or obliteration in the form of a cord is seen in 5–12 % [6]. The average diameter is 1 mm (0.4–1.8) and the angle with the CS varies between 25 and 50°. It is present in 85–95 % [42] (Fig. 28.12). Balloon-occluded venography of the CS can visualize the oblique vein of Marshall in 73 % of the patients [44]. Demonstration of this vein with CT requires special attention to the detail and quality of the CTA. It is reported in 35–40 % of cases [25, 39] (Figs. 28.15c and 28.16a). The best phase for visualization of the oblique vein of Marshall is ventricular systole, likely due to coronary veins enlargement during this phase [39].

The oblique vein of Marshall is now implicated as a source of activation in atrial tachyarrhythmias [45–49]. This may originate from the muscle sleeve of the vein (Marshall bundle) [50]. This muscle sleeve is connected to musculature surrounding CS or the left pulmonary veins [45–47]. The vein is of greater significance when it persists as a patent left superior vena cava. It is seen in 0.5 % of the normal population and up to 5 % of congenitally malformed hearts [51] draining into the CS.

Ventricular Septal Veins

The right and left aspects of the septum are drained by 20–25 small parallel veins on each side. The anterior septal veins are drained into the AIV and the posterior septal veins into the IIV. Superior (distal) third of IV septum (ventricular outflow tracts) is drained by the left or right superior septal veins. The left superior septal vein, the longest and largest intramural venous channel, can reach 2–3 mm in diameter. It is found in 55 % of the hearts and runs with left superior (first) septal artery [6].

Valves of Coronary Veins

While retrograde coronary venous angiography and CTA reveal gross anatomical features of the coronary venous system, venous valves are not easily viewed using these methods.

Venous valves are common in the human hearts. Knowledge of the venous valves existence can be important before coronary vein catheterization, CRT, or retrograde cardioplegic administration [42, 52]. Valves could hinder advancement of guide wires, catheters, or pacing leads [53]. Venous valves are usually incomplete, unicuspid at ostium of the venous ostium [6]. Larger veins including GCV, IIV, and posterior veins of the left ventricle have an average of 2.5–3 valves per vein, while left marginal veins have an average of 0.8 valves per vein [52].

Coronary Sinus Boundaries

The Thebesian valve demarcates the distal end of CS. It can be seen in 80 % of cadaveric and is highly variable in size and morphology [20, 54–56] (Fig. 28.17). A complete circular valve is seen in 20–30 % of the time, and it is absent in 20 % [20, 55]. In most cases a groove or depression is seen on the outer surface of the CS ostium [56] which can localize the atrial end of CS in the absence of the CS valve (Fig. 28.14c). Since the CS and inferior vena cava valves share the same embryologic origin, both can be affected in congenital heart disease. For example, enlargement of these valves is seen in hypoplastic right heart [57].

Variants of the coronary sinus morphology are shown in Figs. 28.18 and 28.19. The CS length is between 30 and 50 mm in 75 % of the anatomic specimens [21, 25]. A short CS is defined as <2 cm in length [54] (Fig. 28.19).

In order to identify the CS, it is important to localize its origin. Demonstration and localization

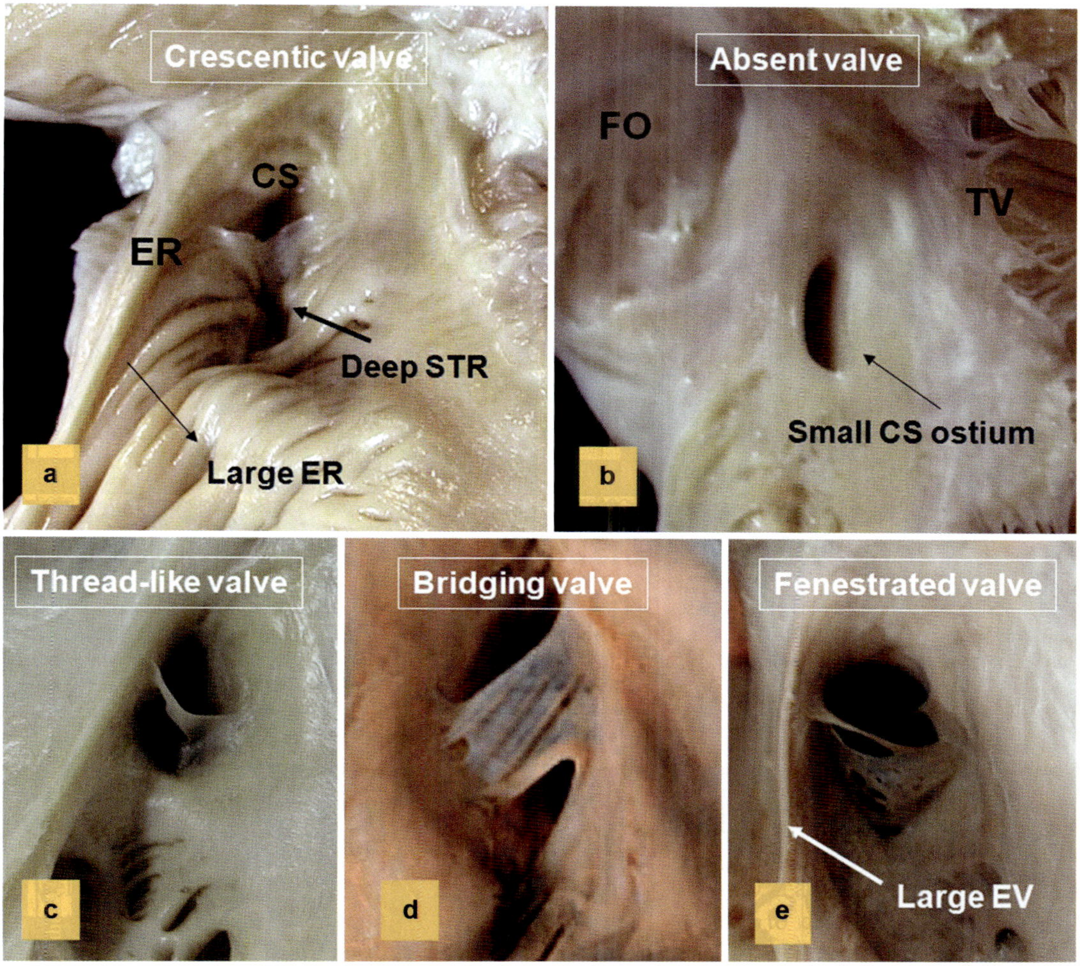

Fig. 28.17 Mechanical barriers to the coronary sinus (*CS*) ostium catheterization and anatomical variations. Mechanical barriers causing difficulty catheterization of the CS include large Eustachian valve/ridge (frequency = 25 %), deep (>5 mm) sub-Thebesian recess (*STR*) (frequency = 45 %) (**a**) hypoplastic CS ostium (**b**) and unusually large Thebesian valve. Anatomic variants of the Thebesian valve are common including circular in 30 %, crescentic in 35 %, absent in 20 %, threadlike in 2 % (**c**) Bridging (**d**) and fenestrated (**e**) in 10 % of population. *ER* Eustachian ridge, *EV* Eustachian valve, *FO* fossa ovalis, *STR* sub-Thebesian recess, *TV* tricuspid valve (From von Lüdinghausen [6], Ortale et al. [30], Silver and Rowley [55], Saremi et al. [69], Cabrera et al. [70] with permission)

of the oblique vein of Marshall and the valve of GCV (Vieussens) are important for ablation approaches and cannulation of the coronary venous system [42, 53]. For example, the valve of Vieussens is a frequent cause of obstruction to passage of a catheter in postmortem and in vivo studies [58, 59], and cannulation of the oblique vein of Marshall can be used to analyze the electrical activity for ablation of paroxysmal AF [50].

Three anatomic landmarks are recognized for localization of the CS-GCV junction including the orifice of the oblique vein of Marshall, the valve of Vieussens, and the left margin of the CS myocardial sleeve with the oblique vein of Marshall as the most constant landmark [6, 30] (Fig. 28.20). These anatomic landmarks are not at the same level and usually are located within a 10 mm interval [30, 42]. Current resolution of

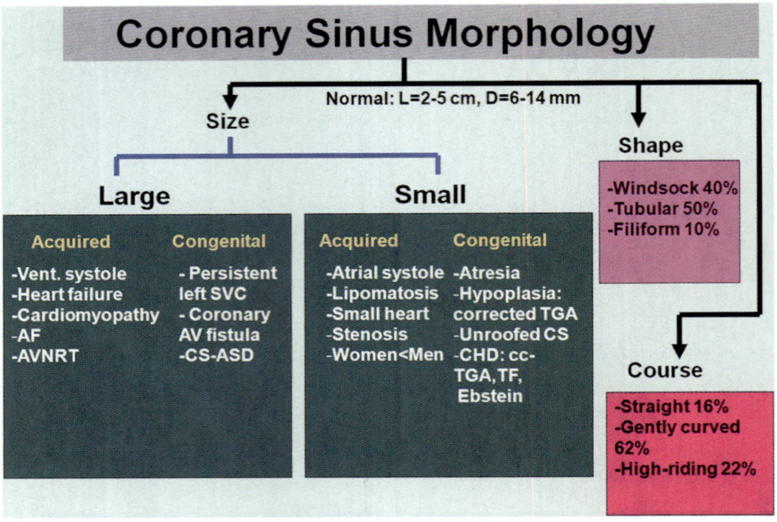

Fig. 28.18 Variants of coronary sinus (CS) morphology. A normal CS is usually 2–5 cm in length (*L*) and 6–14 mm in diameter (*D*). CS is normally larger during ventricular systole and contracts during atrial systole. It is usually tubular or windsock in shape and gently curved toward the left atrium. *AVNRT* atrioventricular node reentrant tachycardia, *AV* arteriovenous, *AF* atrial fibrillation, *SVC* superior vena cava, *ASD* atrial septal defect, *ccTGA* congenitally corrected transposition of great vessels, *TF* tetralogy of Fallot, *CHD* congenital heart disease (From von Lüdinghausen [6], Saremi et al. [35], Miraldi et al. [51], D'Cruz et al. [60], Ong et al. [61] with permission)

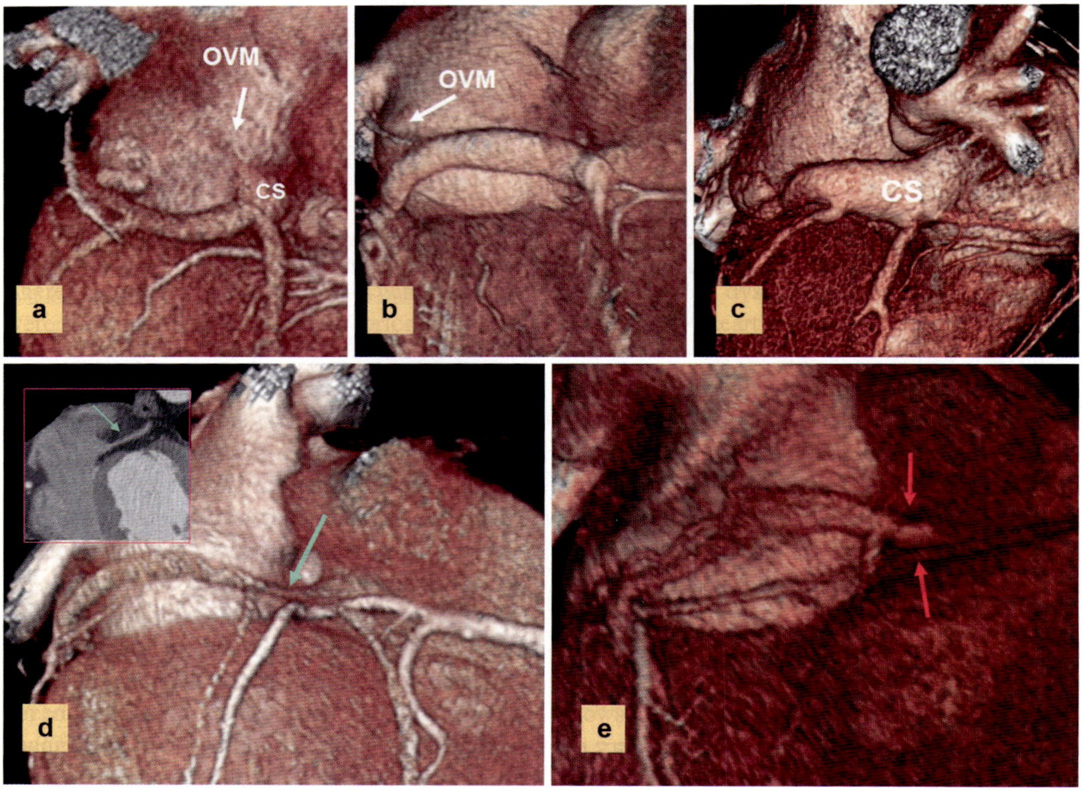

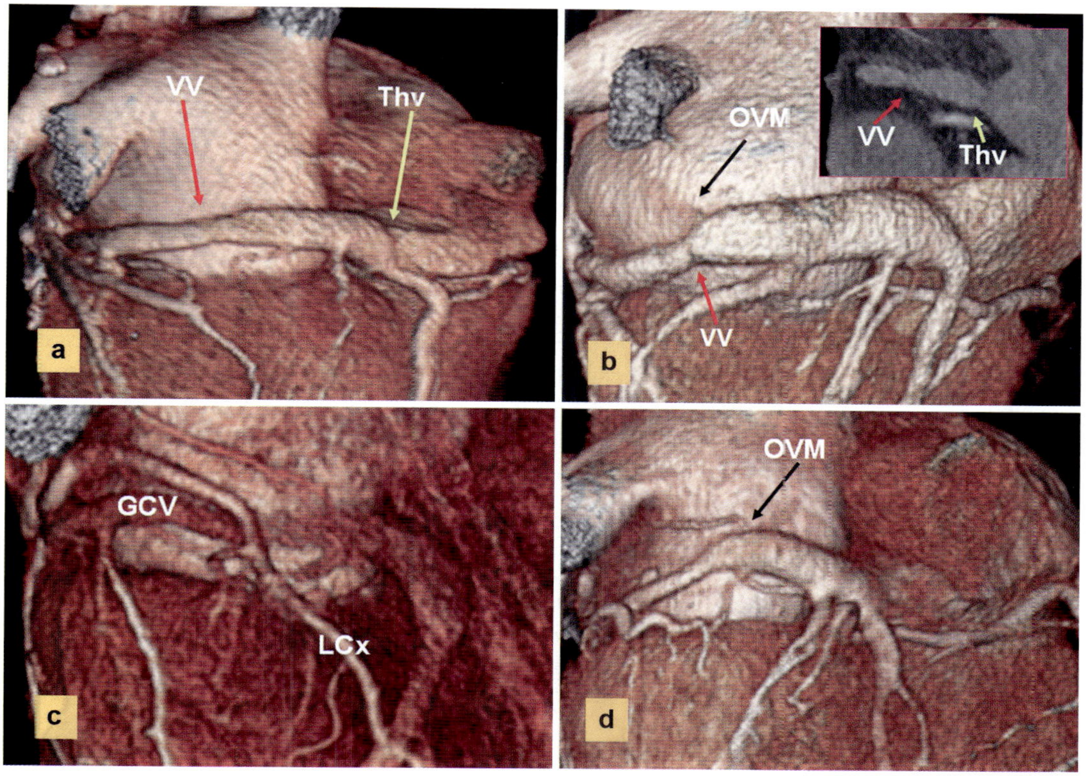

Fig. 28.20 Mechanical barriers for venous intervention: (**a**, **b**) valve of Vieussens (*VV*) and Thebesian valve (*ThV*). (**c**) Arterial compression by overlying left circumflex (*LCx*) artery. (**d**) Oblique vein of Marshall (*OVM*) and CS tortuosity. The VV exists in 80 % and can be seen in 50 % of high-quality CTA images. It is unicuspid (65 %) or bicuspid. The OVM exists in 85 % and can be seen with CT in 35 %. An acute angle with the CS, a small diameter, and a tortuous course are anatomic characteristics that make cannulation of a vein difficult

clinical CT scanners does not permit to directly localize the CS muscle sleeve. The valve of Vieussens is present in 65–85 % of cadaveric heart specimens as a unicuspid or incomplete valve adjacent or proximal to the oblique vein of Marshall [42, 54, 55, 58, 59]. It is located at 32 ± 5 mm from the CS ostium [46]. Utilizing good quality CT images, it is possible to demonstrate the valve of Vieussens in 50 % coronary CTAs [39] (Fig. 28.20). The level of valve of Vieussens at the CS-GCV junction can be localized by an annular narrowing on the external surface in 20 % of cases [3, 30, 53] (Fig. 28.20a, b). This is believed to be secondary to sphincter-like thickening of the CS myocardial sleeve [3].

Phasic Variation of the Coronary Veins

Variation of the coronary vein sizes occurs during the cardiac cycle and in disease [35, 60, 61]. The diameter of the coronary veins is generally greater

◄

Fig. 28.19 Anatomic variants of the length and size of coronary sinus. Oblique vein of Marshall (*OVM*) is best landmark to localize the origin of the CS. The OVM is seen in 40 % of CT studies. (**a**) Short CS (2 cm or shorter) is seen in 10 %. (**b**) Long CS, defined as 5 cm or longer in length, is seen in 15 % of population. In this example the CS appears high riding and more atrialized. (**c**) Shows a large windsock CS in a patient with heart failure. (**d**) Narrowed (filiform) CS secondary to increased epicardial fat (*green arrows*). (**e**) Atretic CS (*red arrows*) in congenitally corrected transposition of the great arteries during late systole compared to mid-diastole. However, the difference between the two phases is not statistically significant [35]. The coronary veins are larger in heart failure and in patients with chronic atrial fibrillation [60]. The CS contracts normally during atrial systole [35] but not in patients with active atrial fibrillation. Windsock CS morphology is more common in patients with atrioventricular nodal reentrant tachycardia [61]. Given the phasic variation of the coronary veins, it is recommended that all images throughout the cardiac cycle be evaluated during pre-procedural planning [39].

Coronary Veins and Congenital Heart Disease

With improved treatment of the congenital heart disease and increasing longevity of these patients, long-term complications including arrhythmias and heart failure are arising as major management issues. These issues have led to increased interest in the roles of CRT and radiofrequency ablation in these patients [11]. CT can play an important role in assessment of cardiac morphology and coronary vessels in adult congenital heart disease (Figs. 28.21 and 28.22).

Device implantation is sometimes required in congenitally corrected transposition of the great arteries (ccTGA) because of morphologic right ventricle dysfunction and complete heart block [11, 62]. However, percutaneous cardiac procedures in these patients can be challenging due to variations in the CS anatomy and venous access, and in some cases, search to identify alternative locations for pacemaker lead placement may be necessary if left ventricular endocardial pacing is not possible. The CS develops with the morphologic atria, and in majority of patients with ccTGA, it drains into the RA. The venous branches, including the GCV and posterior branches, develop with the morphologic ventricles and can be affected in ccTGA.

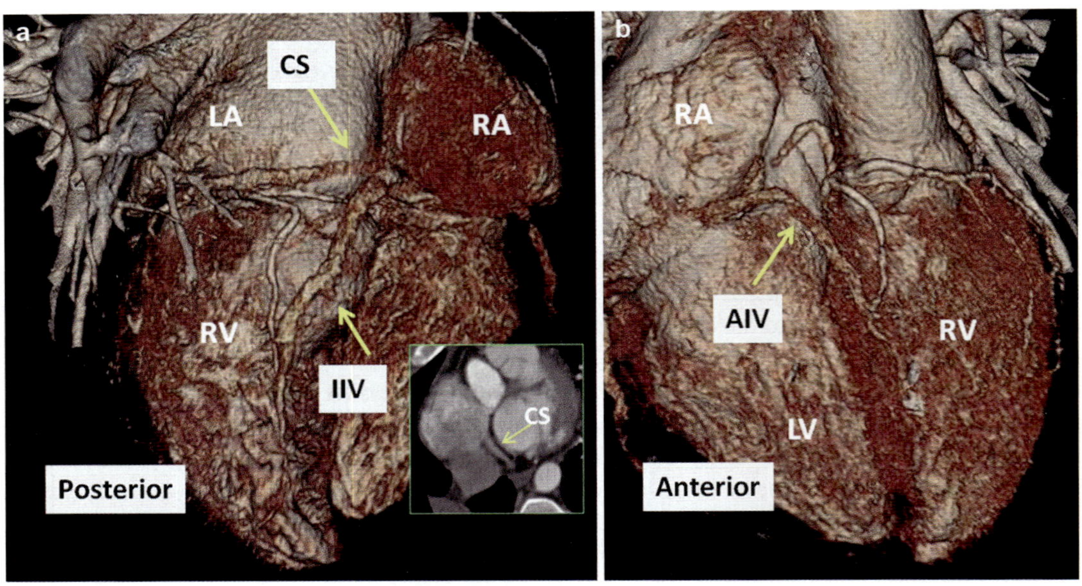

Fig. 28.21 Coronary venous system in congenitally corrected transposition of the great arteries. (**a**) Posterior view of the heart shows the coronary sinus (*CS*) and the inferior interventricular vein (*IIV*) draining into the right atrium (*RA*). Note that the CS appears hypoplastic and connecting high with the RA. High insertion of the CS ostium is not uncommon and may cause difficulty in CS catheterization. (**b**) Anterior view of the heart shows the anterior interventricular vein (*AIV*) draining directly into the RA. Normally it will continue as great cardiac vein. *LV* morphologic left ventricle, *RV* morphologic right ventricle

A comprehensive anatomical data in these patients was provided by Bottega et al. [11]. The location of the CS ostium may be difficult to find as a result of atresia or high ostial location occurring in 15 % of cases [11] (Fig. 28.21). The CS ostium may open above the Eustachian ridge. The absence of AIV is not uncommon; however, the left ventricular marginal vein and IIV are present in most cases (Fig. 28.21). The epicardial veins draining the right ventricle are generally prominent in 75 % of cases [11]. The anterior interventricular vein was shown draining directly into the right atrial appendage in 87 % of the specimens with ccTGA studied by Uemura et al. [62] (Fig. 28.21). The venous drainage of the morphologically left ventricle occurs directly to the right atrium in 20 %, while the morphologically right ventricle veins drain via the coronary sinus in 87 % [61]. When lateral pacing is not possible, the IIV and the AIV can be alternative options for epicardial pacing of the morphologic RV.

Abnormal arrangement of coronary venous return is common in hearts with isomeric atrial appendages (heterotaxy syndrome). Morphologically, the epicardial veins can be divided into circumflex veins (including the CS) in the atrioventricular groove and longitudinal veins over the ventricles (Fig. 28.22). Hearts with isomeric right appendages have absence or hypoplasia of the pulmonary venous component, and the CS is generally absent [62, 63]. The circumflex veins are also absent in nearly all those with isomeric right appendages. Instead, venous drainage of the ventricles occurs through longitudinal veins directly into the atrium. Hearts with isomeric left appendages have hypoplastic systemic venous components. The CS is normal in most patients, and the circumflex venous system is seen in 90 % of the hearts with isomerism of left appendages (Fig. 28.22). A coronary sinus receiving all circumflex veins, as seen in the normal heart, is found in 27 % of cases. The AIV and IIV are highly consistent veins and their anatomical malformations are rare. A rare example of anomalous drainage of the AIV into the superior vena cava is shown in Fig. 28.23.

Anomalies of the Coronary Sinus

A classification of coronary sinus anomalies was suggested by Mantini et al. [64], including (1) enlargement of the coronary sinus with/without a left-to-right shunt, (2) absent coronary sinus, (3) coronary sinus orifice atresia, and (4) hypoplasia of the coronary sinus. In CS atresia or hypoplasia, coronary veins are drained via multiple Thebesian veins into the atria. These enlarged Thebesian veins can be used to directly cannulate the ventricular veins for pacing (Fig. 28.22c, d). The CS orifice atresia can be divided into cases with drainage to a persistent left superior vena cava and those with drainage directly to the cardiac chambers (through fenestrations in the floor of the LA or by emptying of the CS tributaries to into the atria) [51, 64]. Other congenital cardiac lesions associated with CS atresia with left superior vena cava include atrial septal defect, ventricular septal defect, transposition of the great arteries, tricuspid atresia, and mitral atresia [64, 65]. Rarely, anomalous pulmonary venous return can occur via the CS.

Persistent left superior vena cava draining into the CS causes an enlargement of this vessel, and this may interfere with the formation of the posterior wall of the LA causing either a CS-LA fenestration (unroofed coronary sinus) or an interatrial communication through the mouth of the CS (CS-type atrial septal defect) [51, 63, 65]. The diagnosis of this CS anomaly is important to the prognosis of the patient because of the consequences of brain abscess or cerebral emboli that may result from a right-to-left shunt (Figs. 28.24 and 28.25). The CS septal defects may be of particular clinical importance in patients undergoing a modified Fontan procedure as a significant residual right-to-left shunt will result if left unrepaired. Surgical treatment includes closure of the mouth of the coronary sinus, creation of an intra-atrial baffle, or direct repair of the fenestration [66]. Enlargement of the CS is also seen in coronary artery-CS fistula (Fig. 28.26) and rarely in anomalous drainage of left hepatic vein into the CS (Fig. 28.27). Persistence of the left omphalomesenteric vein can cause abnormal communication between the left hepatic vein and the CS.

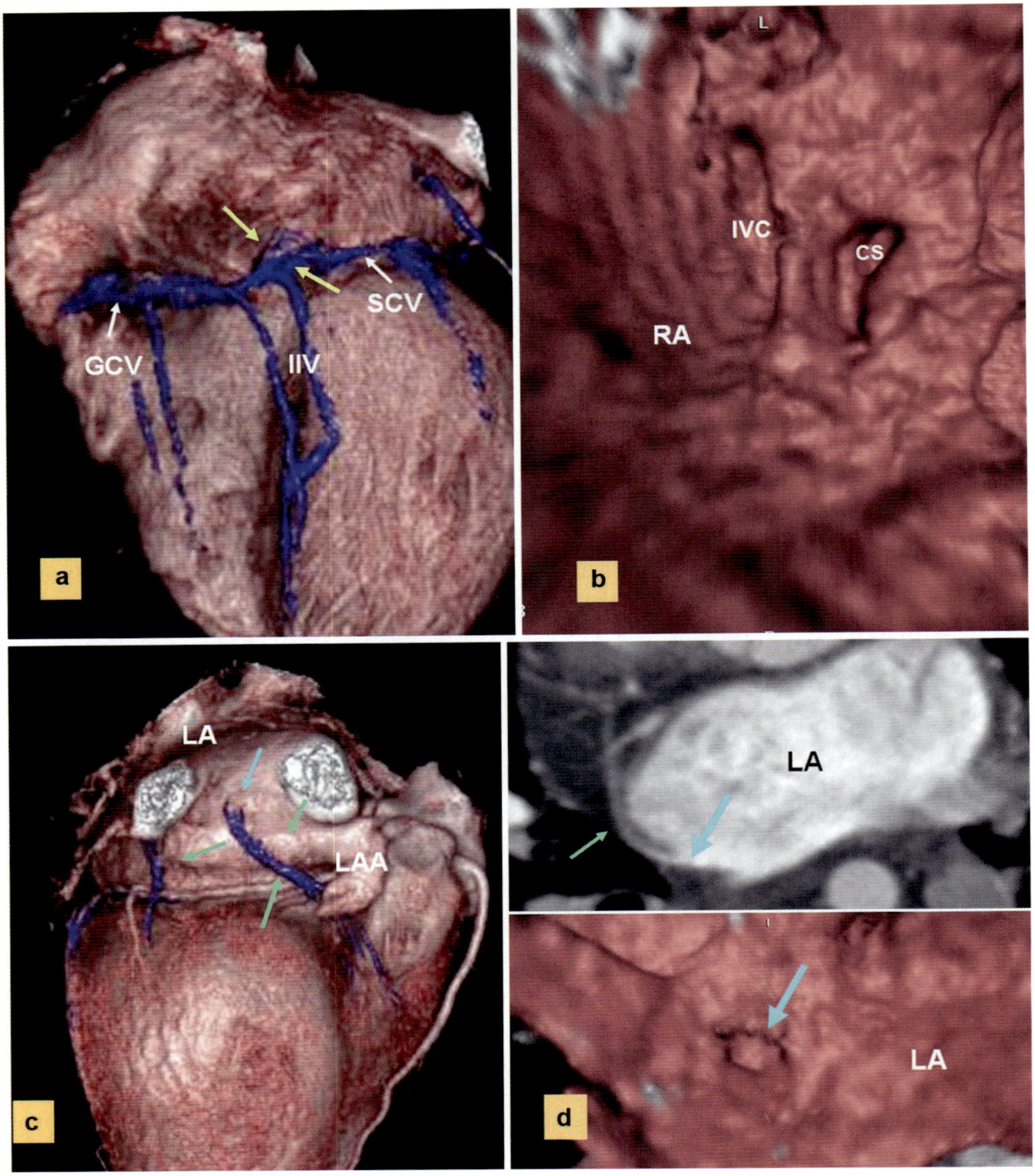

Fig. 28.22 Unusual coronary venous system in a patient with left atrial isomerism, dextrocardia, and azygos continuation of the inferior vena cava. (**a**) Posterior view of the heart shows a hypoplastic coronary sinus (*yellow arrows*) formed by equally sized inferior interventricular vein (*IIV*), great cardiac vein (*GCV*), and small cardiac vein (*SCV*). (**b**) Virtual endoscopy of the right atrium (*RA*) shows small coronary sinus (*CS*) ostium. (**c**, **d**) demonstrate direct drainage of multiple left ventricular veins (*green arrows*) into the left atrium (*LA*). Also shown is the orifice of large Thebesian veins (*blue arrows*) emptying into the LA best seen on endoscopic view (**d**). (*LAA*) left atrial appendage

Cardiac Resynchronization Therapy

CRT has become an acceptable method of treatment in patients with depressed left ventricle systolic function with advanced and symptomatic heart failure (New York Heart Association class III or IV) [67]. Left ventricular lead placement in a suitable coronary vein branch along

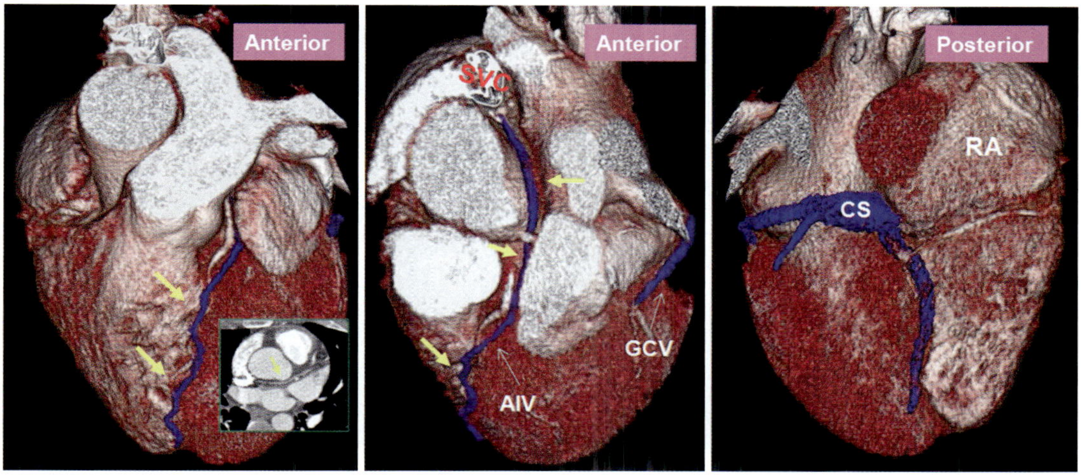

Fig. 28.23 Abnormal drainage of the anterior interventricular vein (*AIV*) into the superior vena cava (SVC) (*yellow arrows*). In this patient the coronary sinus (*CS*) is mainly formed by posterior and marginal veins of the left ventricle (not shown). The great cardiac vein (*GCV*) is not developed and appears short. Although this is a rare anomaly, it may have clinical implications in regard to percutaneous mitral annuloplasty, retrograde cardioplegic perfusion, and myocardial gene transfer. *RA* right atrium

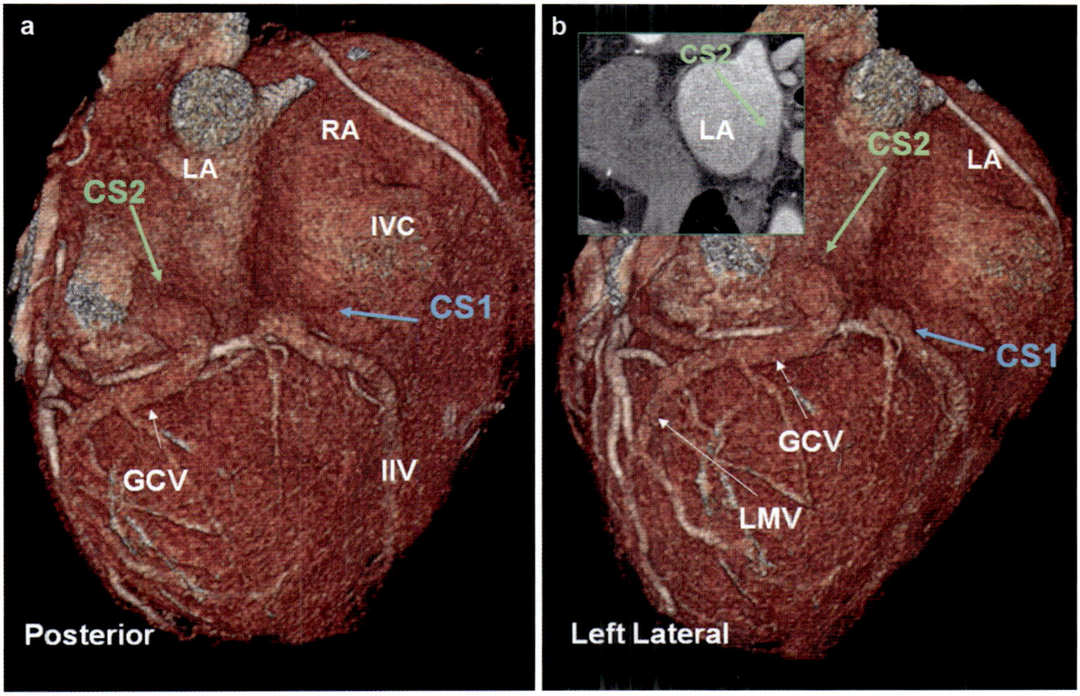

Fig. 28.24 Split coronary sinus (CS) in a patient with repaired tetralogy of Fallot. Status postsurgical correction of tetralogy and ligation of persistent left superior vena fistula to the left atrial roof. Posterior (**a**) and left lateral (**b**) views of the heart are shown. The inferior interventricular vein (*IIV*) and the posterior vein of left ventricle are drained by the CS1 (*blue arrow*) into the right atrium (*RA*), and the great cardiac vein (*GCV*) and the left marginal vein (*LMV*) are drained by the CS2 (*green arrows*) into the left atrium (*LA*). *IVC* inferior vena cava

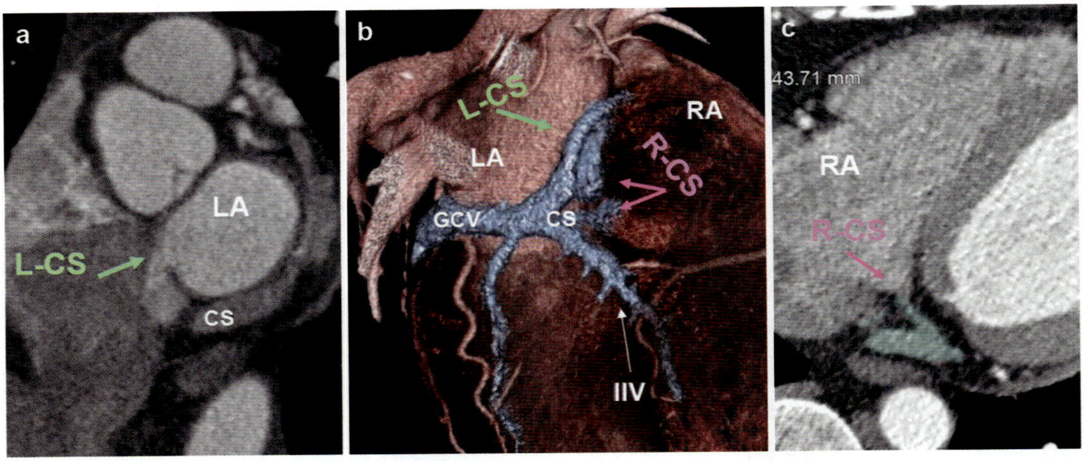

Fig. 28.25 Unroofed coronary sinus (*CS*) in an asymptomatic patient. CS communications with the left atrium (*L-CS*) (**a**, **b**) and the right atrium (*R-CS*) (**b**, **c**) are better shown on two-dimensional images than the volume-rendered posterior view (**b**). *IIV* inferior interventricular vein, *LA* left atrium, *RA* right atrium, *GCV* great cardiac vein, *RV* right ventricle

the dys-synchronous wall of the left ventricle is an important determinant of responsiveness to CRT [38]. Since most patients have cardiomegaly, generally, the CS is larger and anatomic location of a vein can be displaced [23, 26]. Implanting the electrode in a coronary vein can be difficult in up to 20 % of patients, a consequence of unfavorable anatomical factors (Figs. 28.17 and 28.20). In such group accurate anatomic depiction of the vessels can be crucial in success of the left ventricle pacing [23, 68]. Common target vein for placement of the lead is the LMV or posterior veins of the left ventricle (Figs. 28.16). In rare cases the lead is placed in an anterolateral tributary of the GCV (Fig. 28.28).

With the development of newer, smaller caliber pacing leads, the need for an imaging modality to resolve and localize most first- or large second-order tributaries is necessary. Recently a segmental classification of the venous tributaries is introduced using rotational venography [68]. Coronary CTA can easily be used to address the segmental location of the target vein and find anatomic barriers [25, 26, 69, 70]. Information required in radiology report is included in Table 28.3.

Coronary Sinus Retrograde Cardioplegia Perfusion Delivery

RCP is widely used as a method of myocardial protection especially in cases with severe coronary artery disease that can alter the distribution of antegrade cardioplegia [71]. The coronary sinus venous system is not affected by extensive coronary artery disease, and a more uniform venous network remains in the subendocardial zone of both ventricles. RCP is also used in valvar procedures, with normal coronary arteries, as this method allows the surgeon to deliver the maintenance doses only from the CS – facilitating the operation and shortening

Fig. 28.27 Cardiac CT scan shows enlarged coronary sinus (*CS*) with anomalous connection of the left hepatic vein (*L. hepatic V.*) directly into it. No unusual hemodynamic effect is expected in this pattern of connection. The right hepatic vein was connected to the inferior vena cava (*IVC*) with normal drainage into the right atrium (*RA*). The coronary veins were normal. *LA* left atrium, *PLV* posterolateral vein, *RA* right atrium

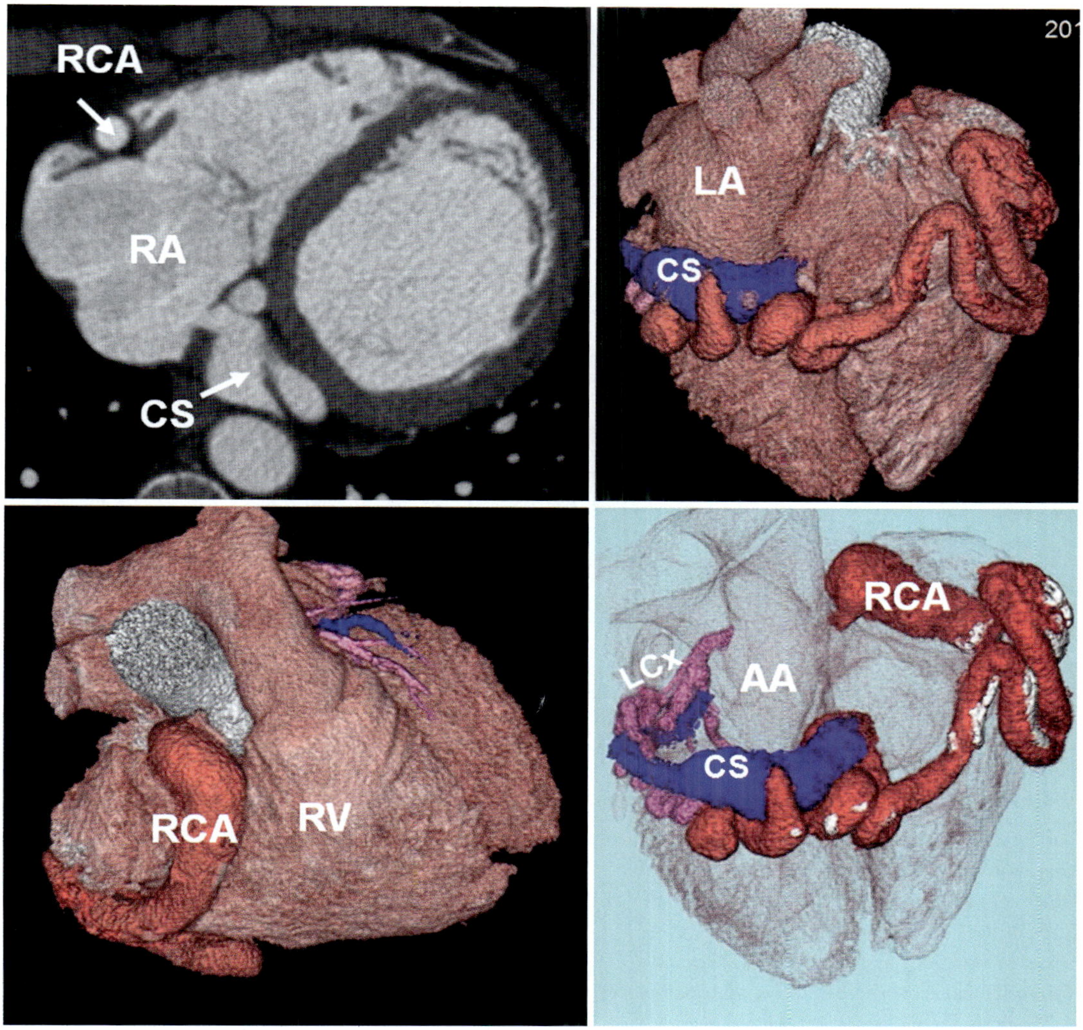

Fig. 28.26 Anomalous fistulous communications between the coronary sinus (*CS*) (*blue colored*) with the right coronary artery (*RCA*) (*red coded*) and the left circumflex (*LCx*) artery (*pink coded*). The RCA and the CS are markedly enlarged. An anomalous tangle of small vessels arising from the LCx is seen connecting to distal end of the CS. RCA calcifications are shown as white plaques on color-coded images. *AA* ascending aorta, *LA* left atrium, *RV* right ventricle, *RA* right atrium

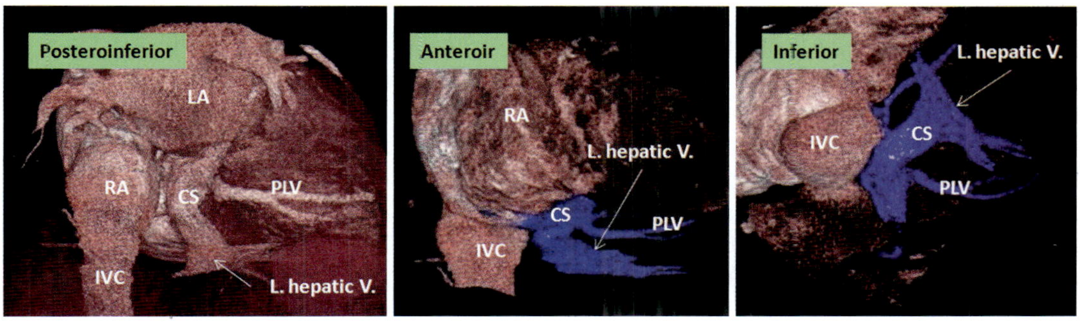

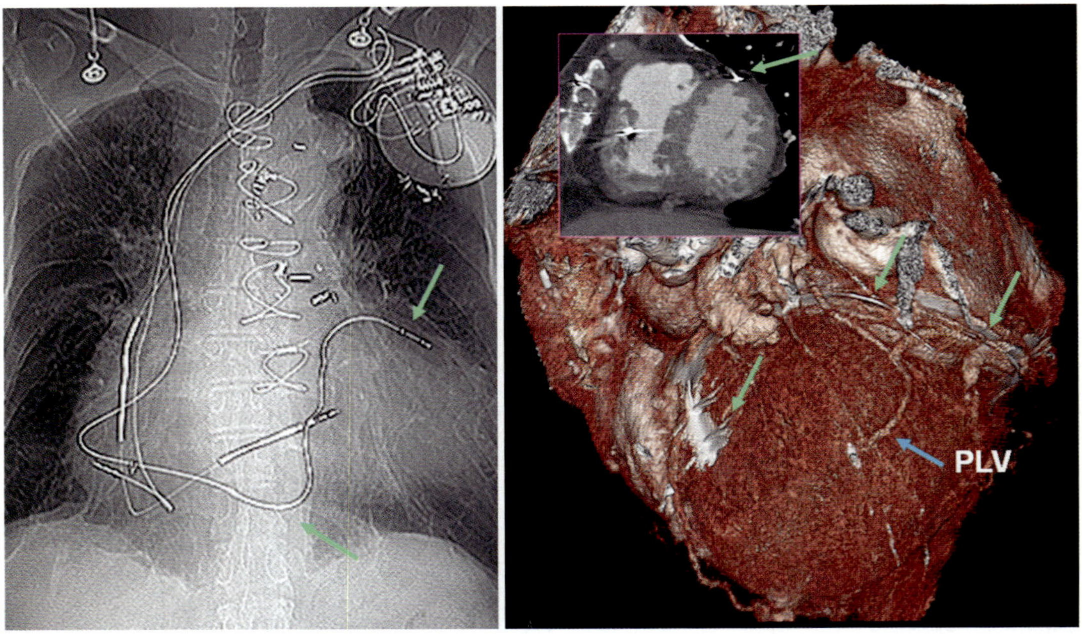

Fig. 28.28 Biventricular pacing in a 49-year-old patient with tetralogy of Fallot. Images show unusual placement of the left ventricle (LV) pacer lead in a branch of the anterior interventricular vein (AIV) (*green arrows*). *PLV* posterolateral vein

Table 28.3 CT angiography: what to look for before CRT

Variants: hypoplasia, absence, duplication, diverticulum
High insertion of the CS (Fig. 28.23)
Other anatomic barriers (Figs. 28.15 and 28.18)
Sizes of the CS for balloon occlusion
Distance of target vein from the Thebesian valve
Tortuosity and acute angle of target vein confluence: The posterior and lateral veins have an acute takeoff in 30 %
First- or large second-order tributaries of the CS. Diameter >1.5 mm (4 F, the current size of the smallest LV pacing lead) allows a lead implant

the aortic cross-clamping times. Knowledge of the anatomic variants of the CS and its tributaries is important as the efficiency and distribution of a RCP may be affected, which leads to partial or poor myocardial protection. It would be difficult to perform RCP in patients with an ostial atresia/stenosis of the CS, large Chiari network, and in congenital heart disease with venous drainage anomalies (Figs. 28.23 and 28.24). With regard to selective retroinfusion of cardiac veins, the GCV/AIV and IIV have highly consistent anatomic course (Fig. 28.29). The distribution of RCP should be assessed by examining the posterior and anterior cardiac veins during perfusion, because RCP may not perfuse all of the right ventricular free wall and septum. Distribution of RCP to the free wall of the right ventricle is often poor, because there is no direct communication between the coronary sinus and anterior cardiac veins. This may cause a problem in some patients especially in hypertrophied hearts in which delivery from the epicardial veins toward the subendocardial plexus is highly impeded. A variant of cardioplegia delivery consists in perfusing the cardioplegic solution into the RA (with the caval veins snared).

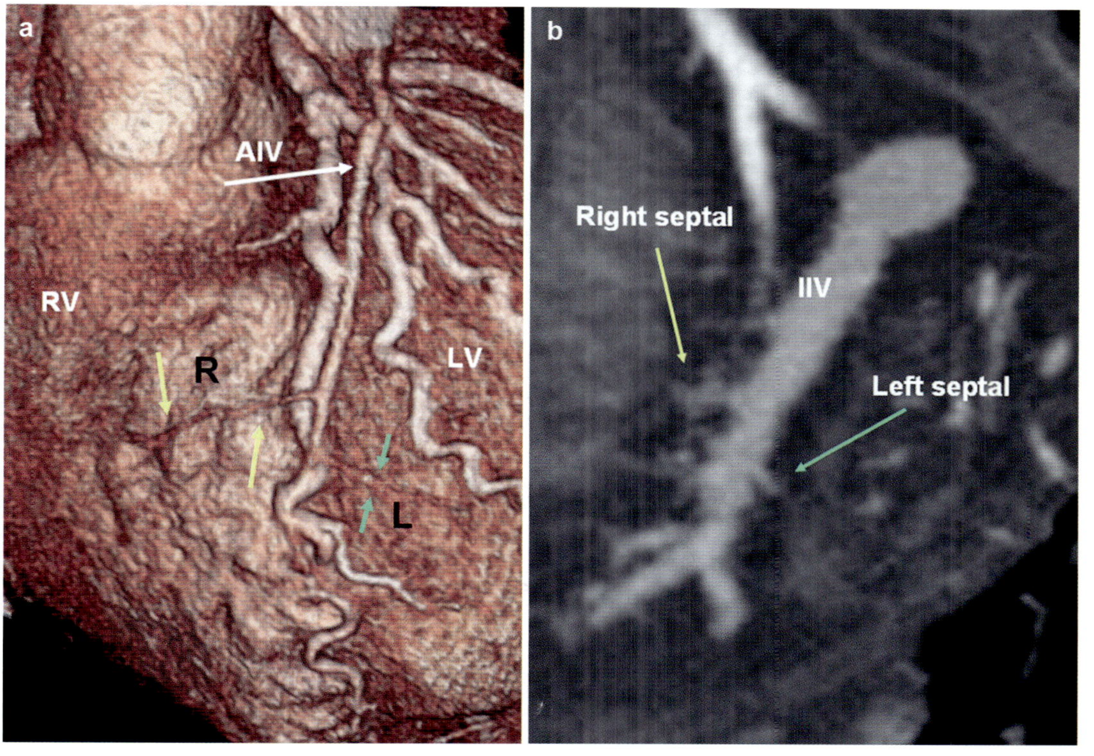

Fig. 28.29 (**a**) Tributaries from both ventricles join the anterior interventricular (*AIV*) portion of the great cardiac vein (*yellow arrows*) right ventricle tributaries, (*green arrows*) left ventricle tributaries. (**b**) Inferior interventricular vein (*IIV*) draining right and left (posterior) septal veins. The AIV and IIV are highly consistent veins. RV branches can drain into these veins. This helps provide distribution of cardioplegic solution in the RV with retrograde CS perfusion

Conclusion

A complete and highly efficient and clinically useful classification of the CVS is not as straightforward as in the case of the coronary arteries. In this chapter we strived to describe the role of coronary CTA in anatomic classification, assessment of anatomic variants, and pathologic changes of the CVS. We also emphasized on the role of CT in transvenous ablation procedure and left ventricular pacing for CRT.

References

1. Anderson RH, Brown NA, Moorman AFM. Development and structures of the venous pole of the heart. Dev Dyn. 2006;235:2–9.
2. Steding G, Xu JW, Seidl W, Männer J, Xia H. Developmental aspects of the sinus valves and the sinus venosus septum of the right atrium in human embryos. Anat Embryol (Berl). 1990;181(5):469–75.
3. Red-Horse K, Ueno H, Weissman IL, Krasnow MA. Coronary arteries form by developmental reprogramming of venous cells. Nature. 2010;464(7288): 549–53.
4. Mark-Paul FM, Peeters V, Gittenberger-de Groot AC, Mentink MMT, Hungerford JE, Little CD, Poelmann RE. Differences in development of coronary arteries and veins. Cardiovasc Res. 1997;36:101–10.
5. von Lüdinghausen M. Clinical anatomy of cardiac veins. Vv. cardiacae. Surg Radiol Anat. 1987;9:159–68.
6. von Lüdinghausen M. The venous drainage of the human myocardium. Adv Anat Embryol Cell Biol. 2003;168:I–VIII. 1–104.
7. Ho SY, Sánchez-Quintana D, Becker AE. A review of the coronary venous system: a road less travelled. Heart Rhythm. 2004;1:107–12.
8. von Lüdinghausen M, Ohmachi N, Besch S, Mettenleiter A. Atrial veins of the human heart. Clin Anat. 1995;8:169–89.
9. Ratajczyk-Pakalska E. Variation of the smallest cardiac veins. Folia Morphol (Warsz). 1978;37(4): 415–8.
10. Ansari A. Anatomy and clinical significance of ventricular Thebesian veins. Clin Anat. 2001;14(2): 102–10.

11. Bottega NA, Kapa S, Edwards WD, et al. The cardiac veins in congenitally corrected transposition of the great arteries: delivery options for cardiac devices. Heart Rhythm. 2009;6(10):1450–6.
12. Ratajczyk-Pakalska E, Fortak W, Gołab B. Sphincters and valves in the walls of the smallest cardiac veins. Folia Morphol (Warsz). 1984;43(2):121–7.
13. Ratajczyk-Pakalska E, Bloch P, Kulig A. Angioarchitectonics of the venous vessels and morphological changes in coronary heart disease. Basic Res Cardiol. 1991;86(6):554–60.
14. Taylor JR, Taylor AJ. The thebesian circulation to developing conducting tissue: a nutrient-nodal hypothesis of cardiogenesis. Can J Cardiol. 1999;15(8):859–66.
15. Taylor JR, Taylor AJ. Thebesian sinusoids: forgotten collaterals to papillary muscles. Can J Cardiol. 2000;16(11):1391–7.
16. Parsonnet V. The anatomy of the veins of the human heart with special reference to normal anastomotic channels. J Med Soc N J. 1953;50:446–52.
17. Huu N, Doutriaux M, Leroy JP, Thuan RH. Small veins of the heart auricle. Bull Assoc Anat (Nancy). 1975;59(167):955–67.
18. Saremi F, Channual S, Krishnan S, et al. Bachmann Bundle and its arterial supply: imaging with multidetector CT-implications for interatrial conduction abnormalities and arrhythmias. Radiology. 2008;248(2):447–57.
19. von Lüdinghausen M, Lechleuthner A. Atresia of the right atrial ostium of the coronary sinus. Acta Anat (Basel). 1988;131(1):81–3.
20. Ortale JR, Marquez CQ. Anatomy of the intramural venous sinuses of the right atrium and their tributaries. Surg Radiol Anat. 1998;20:23–9.
21. Pina JA. Morphological study on the human anterior cardiac veins, venae cordis anteriores. Acta Anat (Basel). 1975;92:145–59.
22. Mierzwa J, Kozielec T. Variation of the anterior cardiac veins and their orifices in the right atrium in man. Folia Morphol (Warsz). 1975;34(2):125–33.
23. Blendea D, Shah RV, Auricchio A, et al. Variability of coronary venous anatomy in patients undergoing cardiac resynchronization therapy: a high-speed rotational venography study. Heart Rhythm. 2007;4(9):1155–62.
24. Arbelo E, García-Quintana A, Caballero E, et al. Usefulness of hyperemic venous return angiography for studying coronary venous anatomy prior to cardiac resynchronization device implantation. Rev Esp Cardiol. 2008;61(9):936–44.
25. Jongbloed MR, Lamb HJ, Bax JJ, et al. Noninvasive visualization of the cardiac venous system using multislice computed tomography. J Am Coll Cardiol. 2005;45(5):749–53.
26. Knackstedt C, Mühlenbruch G, Mischke K, et al. Imaging of the coronary venous system in patients with congestive heart failure: comparison of 16 slice MSCT and retrograde coronary sinus venography: comparative imaging of coronary venous system. Int J Cardiovasc Imaging. 2008;24(8):783–91.
27. Van de Veire NR, Schuijf JD, De Sutter J, et al. Noninvasive visualization of the cardiac venous system in coronary artery disease patients using 64-slice computed tomography. J Am Coll Cardiol. 2006;48(9):1832–8.
28. Younger JF, Plein S, Crean A, Ball SG, Greenwood JP. Visualization of coronary venous anatomy by cardiovascular magnetic resonance. J Cardiovasc Magn Reson. 2009;11:11–26.
29. Chiribiri A, Kelle S, Götze S, et al. Visualization of the cardiac venous system using cardiac magnetic resonance. Am J Cardiol. 2008;101(3):407–12.
30. Ortale JR, Gabriel EA, Iost C, Márquez CQ. The anatomy of the coronary sinus and its tributaries. Surg Radiol Anat. 2001;23(1):15–21.
31. Bales GS. Great cardiac vein variations. Clin Anat. 2004;17:436–43.
32. Pejkovic B, Bogdanovic D. The great cardiac vein. Surg Radiol Anat. 1992;14(1):23–8.
33. von Lüdinghausen M. Aberrant course of the anterior interventricular part of the great cardiac vein in the human heart. Gegenbaurs Morphol Jahrb. 1989;135(3):475–8.
34. Loukas M, Tubbs RS, Jordan R. Aneurysm of the great cardiac vein. Surg Radiol Anat. 2007;29(2):169–72.
35. Saremi F, Channual S, Sarlaty T, Tafti MA, Milliken JC, Narula J. Coronary venous aneurysm in patients without cardiac arrhythmia as detected by MDCT: an anatomic variant or a pathologic entity. JACC Cardiovasc Imaging. 2010;3(3):257–65.
36. Ho SY, Russell G, Rowland E. Coronary venous aneurysms and accessory atrioventricular connections. Br Heart J. 1988;60:348–51.
37. Sun Y, Arruda M, Otomo K, et al. Coronary sinus-ventricular accessory connections producing posteroseptal and left posterior accessory pathways: incidence and electrophysiological identification. Circulation. 2002;106:1362–7.
38. Morgan JM, Delgado V. Lead positioning for cardiac resynchronization therapy: techniques and priorities. Europace. 2009;11 Suppl 5:v22–8.
39. Saremi F, Thonar B, Sarlaty T, et al. Posterior interatrial muscular connection between the coronary sinus and left atrium: an anatomofunctional study of the coronary sinus using multi detector computed tomography. Radiology. 2011;260:671–9.
40. Loukas M, Bilinsky S, Bilinsky E, el-Sedfy A, Anderson RH. Cardiac veins: a review of the literature. Clin Anat. 2009;22(1):129–45.
41. Cendrowska-Pinkosz M. The variability of the small cardiac vein in the adult human heart. Folia Morphol (Warsz). 2004;63(2):159–62.
42. de Oliveira IM, Scanavacca MI, Correia AT, Sosa EA, Aiello VD. Anatomic relations of the Marshall vein: importance for catheterization of the coronary sinus in ablation procedures. Europace. 2007;9(10):915–9.
43. Kim DT, Lai AC, Hwang C, Fan LT, Karagueuzian HS, Chen PS, Fishbein MC. The ligament of Marshall: a structural analysis in human hearts with implications for atrial arrhythmias. J Am Coll Cardiol. 2000;36:1324–7.
44. Kurotobi T, Ito H, Inoue K, et al. Marshall vein as arrhythmogenic source in patients with atrial fibrilla-

tion: correlation between its anatomy and electrophysiological findings. J Cardiovasc Electrophysiol. 2006;17(10):1062–7.
45. Shah D, Haissaguerre M, Jais P, Hocini M. Nonpulmonary vein foci: do they exist? Pacing Clin Electrophysiol. 2003;26(7 Pt 2):1631–5.
46. Chauvin M, Shah DC, Haissaguerre M, Marcellin L, Brechenmacher C. The anatomic basis of connections between the coronary sinus musculature and the left atrium in humans. Circulation. 2000;101:647–52.
47. Cabrera JA, Ho SY, Climent V, Sánchez-Quintana D. The architecture of the left lateral atrial wall: a particular anatomic region with implications for ablation of atrial fibrillation. Eur Heart J. 2008;29:356–62.
48. Tan AY, Chou CC, Zhou S, et al. Electrical connections between the left superior pulmonary vein, left atrium and ligament of Marshall: implications for the mechanisms of atrial fibrillation. Am J Physiol Heart Circ Physiol. 2005;290:H312–22.
49. Hsu LF, Jais P, Keane D, et al. Atrial fibrillation originating from persistent left superior vena cava. Circulation. 2004;109:828–32.
50. Hwang C, Wu TJ, Doshi RN, Peter CT, Chen PS. Vein of Marshall cannulation for the analysis of electrical activity in patients with focal atrial fibrillation. Circulation. 2000;101(13):1503–5.
51. Miraldi F, di Gioia CR, Proietti P, De Santis M, d'Amati G, Gallo P. Cardinal vein isomerism: an embryological hypothesis to explain a persistent left superior vena cava draining into the roof of the left atrium in the absence of coronary sinus and atrial septal defect. Cardiovasc Pathol. 2002;11:149–52.
52. Anderson SE, Quill JL, Iaizzo PA. Venous valves within left ventricular coronary veins. J Interv Card Electrophysiol. 2008;23(2):95–9.
53. Corcoran SJ, Lawrence C, McGuire MA. The valve of Vieussens: an important cause of difficulty in advancing catheters into the cardiac veins. J Cardiovasc Electrophysiol. 1999;10:804–8.
54. Maros TN, Rácz L, Plugor S, Maros TG. Contributions to the morphology of the human coronary sinus. Anat Anz. 1983;154(2):133–44.
55. Silver MA, Rowley NE. The functional anatomy of the human coronary sinus. Am Heart J. 1988;115(5):1080–4.
56. Roberts JT. Arteries, veins, and lymphatic vessels of the heart. In: Luisada AA, editor. Development and structure of the cardiovascular system. New York: McGraw-Hill; 1958. p. 85–118.
57. Schutte DA, Rowland DG, Allen HD, Bharati S. Prominent venous valves in hypoplastic right hearts. Am Heart J. 1997;134(3):527–31.
58. Duda B, Grzybiak M. About variability of Vieussen valve in the adult human heart. Folia Morphol (Warsz). 2000;59(1):43–5.
59. Karaca M, Bilge O, Dinckal MH, Ucerler H. The anatomic barriers in the coronary sinus: implications for clinical procedures. J Interv Card Electrophysiol. 2005;14:89–94.
60. D' Cruz IA, Johns C, Shala MB. Dynamic cyclic changes in coronary sinus caliber in patients with and without congestive heart failure. Am J Cardiol. 1999;83:275–7.
61. Ong MG, Lee PC, Tai CT, et al. Coronary sinus morphology in different types of supraventricular tachycardias. J Interv Card Electrophysiol. 2006;15:21–6.
62. Uemura H, Ho SY, Anderson RH, et al. Surgical anatomy of the coronary circulation in hearts with discordant atrioventricular connections. Eur J Cardiothorac Surg. 1996;10:194–200.
63. Min JY, Kim CY, Oh MH, et al. Arrangement of the systemic and pulmonary venous components of the atrial chambers in hearts with isomeric atrial appendages. Cardiol Young. 2000;10(4):396–404.
64. Mantini E, Grondin CM, Lillehei CW, Edwards JE. Congenital anomalies involving the coronary sinus. Circulation. 1966;33:317–27.
65. Gerlis LM, Gibbs JL, Williams GJ, Thomas GDH. Coronary sinus orifice atresia and persistent left superior vena cava. Br Heart J. 1984;52:648–53.
66. Attenhofer Jost CH, Connolly HM, Danielson GK, Dearani JA, Warnes CA, Jamil Tajik A. Clinical features and surgical outcome in 25 patients with fenestrations of the coronary sinus. Cardiol Young. 2007;17(6):592–600.
67. Kautzner J, Riedlbauchova L, Cihak R, Bytesnik J, Vancura V. Technical aspects of implantation of LV lead for cardiac resynchronization therapy in chronic heart failure. Pacing Clin Electrophysiol. 2004;27:783–90.
68. Singh JP, Houser S, Heist EK, Ruskin JN. The coronary venous anatomy: a segmental approach to aid cardiac resynchronization therapy. J Am Coll Cardiol. 2005;46(1):68–74.
69. Saremi F, Pourzand L, Krishnan S, et al. Right atrial cavotricuspid isthmus: anatomic characterization with multi-detector row CT. Radiology. 2008;247(3):658–68.
70. Cabrera JA, Sánchez-Quintana D, Ho SY, et al. Angiographic anatomy of the inferior right atrial isthmus in patients with and without history of common atrial flutter. Circulation. 1999;99:3017–23.
71. Ruengsakulrach P, Buxton BF. Anatomic and hemodynamic considerations influencing the efficiency of retrograde cardioplegia. Ann Thorac Surg. 2001;71:1389–95.

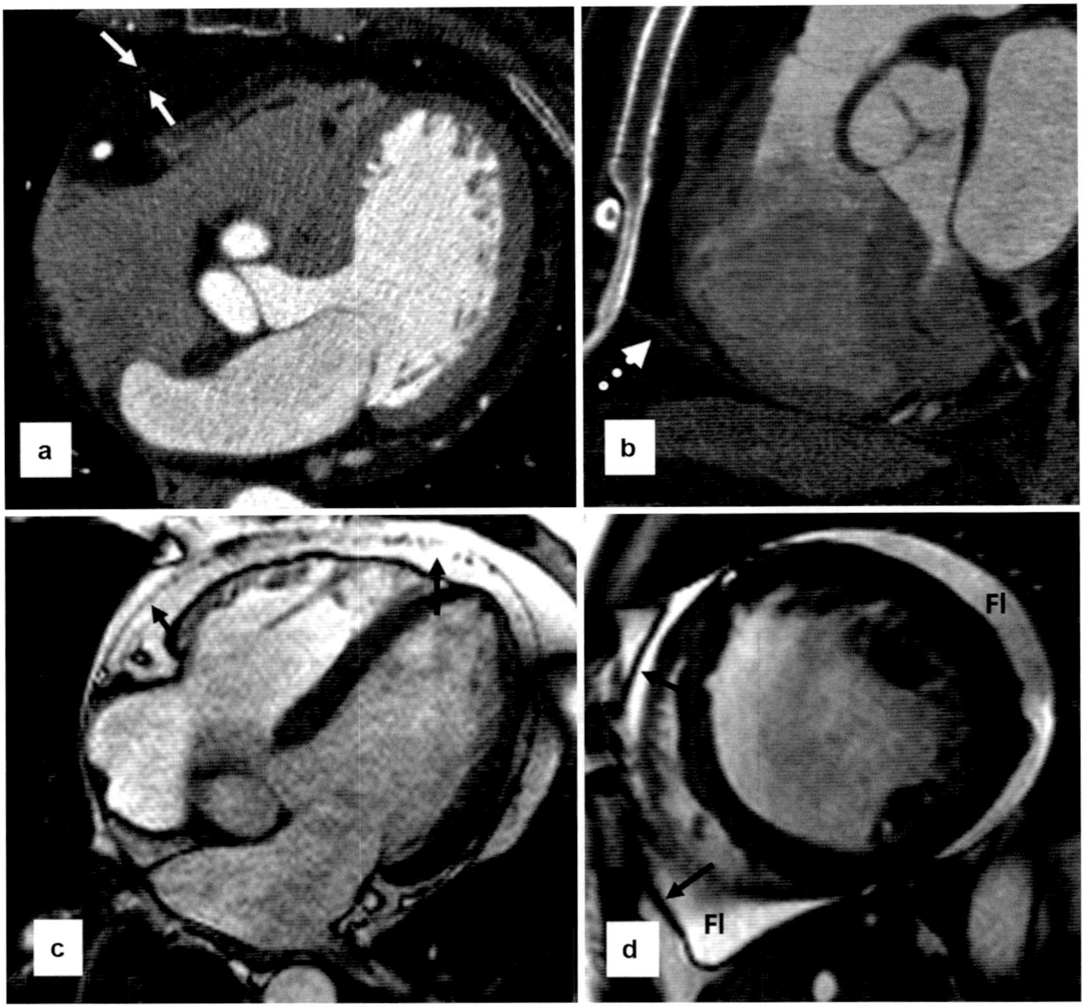

Fig. 29.1 Normal pericardium on CT (**a**, **b**) and MR (**c**, **d**) images. (**b**) Sagittal CT shows attachment of the fibrous pericardium to the central tendon of the diaphragm (*dashed arrow*). (**a**) CT and (**c**) MR axial images of the heart show the epicardial (inside) fat, the mediastinal (outside) fat, and the thin line of pericardial sac (*arrows*) between the two adipose tissue compartments. (**d**) Short-axis cine MR shows accumulation of fluid (*Fl*) in the pericardial sac separating the two fatty compartments. Parietal pericardium is shown by *arrows* in (d). In cine MR sequence (balanced steady-state free precession), it can be difficult to differentiate small amount of pericardial fluid from surrounding fat tissue as both appear high in signal intensity

Imaging

CT and MRI are equally considered the preferred imaging methods for morphological assessment of the pericardial sac and the pericardium. Higher spatial resolution of the CT scan allows improve visualization of the normal pericardium. As a result normal pericardium appears thinner using CT compared with MRI. This is not surprising knowing that most cardiac CT protocols consist of 0.5–1 mm slices, while in cardiac MRI most routine sequences involve 5–8 mm slices. Generally a pericardium thicker than 3 mm is considered abnormal [8]. On the other hand, MRI is the modality of choice for functional evaluation of heart and to differentiate constrictive pericarditis from restrictive cardiomyopathy [9, 10].

tion: correlation between its anatomy and electrophysiological findings. J Cardiovasc Electrophysiol. 2006;17(10):1062–7.
45. Shah D, Haissaguerre M, Jais P, Hocini M. Nonpulmonary vein foci: do they exist? Pacing Clin Electrophysiol. 2003;26(7 Pt 2):1631–5.
46. Chauvin M, Shah DC, Haissaguerre M, Marcellin L, Brechenmacher C. The anatomic basis of connections between the coronary sinus musculature and the left atrium in humans. Circulation. 2000;101:647–52.
47. Cabrera JA, Ho SY, Climent V, Sánchez-Quintana D. The architecture of the left lateral atrial wall: a particular anatomic region with implications for ablation of atrial fibrillation. Eur Heart J. 2008;29:356–62.
48. Tan AY, Chou CC, Zhou S, et al. Electrical connections between the left superior pulmonary vein, left atrium and ligament of Marshall: implications for the mechanisms of atrial fibrillation. Am J Physiol Heart Circ Physiol. 2005;290:H312–22.
49. Hsu LF, Jais P, Keane D, et al. Atrial fibrillation originating from persistent left superior vena cava. Circulation. 2004;109:828–32.
50. Hwang C, Wu TJ, Doshi RN, Peter CT, Chen PS. Vein of Marshall cannulation for the analysis of electrical activity in patients with focal atrial fibrillation. Circulation. 2000;101(13):1503–5.
51. Miraldi F, di Gioia CR, Proietti P, De Santis M, d'Amati G, Gallo P. Cardinal vein isomerism: an embryological hypothesis to explain a persistent left superior vena cava draining into the roof of the left atrium in the absence of coronary sinus and atrial septal defect. Cardiovasc Pathol. 2002;11:149–52.
52. Anderson SE, Quill JL, Iaizzo PA. Venous valves within left ventricular coronary veins. J Interv Card Electrophysiol. 2008;23(2):95–9.
53. Corcoran SJ, Lawrence C, McGuire MA. The valve of Vieussens: an important cause of difficulty in advancing catheters into the cardiac veins. J Cardiovasc Electrophysiol. 1999;10:804–8.
54. Maros TN, Rácz L, Plugor S, Maros TG. Contributions to the morphology of the human coronary sinus. Anat Anz. 1983;154(2):133–44.
55. Silver MA, Rowley NE. The functional anatomy of the human coronary sinus. Am Heart J. 1988;115(5): 1080–4.
56. Roberts JT. Arteries, veins, and lymphatic vessels of the heart. In: Luisada AA, editor. Development and structure of the cardiovascular system. New York: McGraw-Hill; 1958. p. 85–118.
57. Schutte DA, Rowland DG, Allen HD, Bharati S. Prominent venous valves in hypoplastic right hearts. Am Heart J. 1997;134(3):527–31.
58. Duda B, Grzybiak M. About variability of Vieussen valve in the adult human heart. Folia Morphol (Warsz). 2000;59(1):43–5.
59. Karaca M, Bilge O, Dinckal MH, Ucerler H. The anatomic barriers in the coronary sinus: implications for clinical procedures. J Interv Card Electrophysiol. 2005;14:89–94.
60. D' Cruz IA, Johns C, Shala MB. Dynamic cyclic changes in coronary sinus caliber in patients with and without congestive heart failure. Am J Cardiol. 1999;83:275–7.
61. Ong MG, Lee PC, Tai CT, et al. Coronary sinus morphology in different types of supraventricular tachycardias. J Interv Card Electrophysiol. 2006;15:21–6.
62. Uemura H, Ho SY, Anderson RH, et al. Surgical anatomy of the coronary circulation in hearts with discordant atrioventricular connections. Eur J Cardiothorac Surg. 1995;10:194–200.
63. Min JY, Kim CY, Oh MH, et al. Arrangement of the systemic and pulmonary venous components of the atrial chambers in hearts with isomeric atrial appendages. Cardiol Young. 2000;10(4):396–404.
64. Mantini E, Grondin CM, Lillehei CW, Edwards JE. Congenital anomalies involving the coronary sinus. Circulation. 1966;33:317–27.
65. Gerlis LM, Gibbs JL, Williams GJ, Thomas GDH. Coronary sinus orifice atresia and persistent left superior vena cava. Br Heart J. 1984;52:648–53.
66. Attenhofer Jost CH, Connolly HM, Danielson GK, Dearani JA, Warnes CA, Jamil Tajik A. Clinical features and surgical outcome in 25 patients with fenestrations of the coronary sinus. Cardiol Young. 2007;17(6):592–600.
67. Kautzner J, Riedlbauchova L, Cihak R, Bytesnik J, Vancura V. Technical aspects of implantation of LV lead for cardiac resynchronization therapy in chronic heart failure. Pacing Clin Electrophysiol. 2004;27:783–90.
68. Singh JP, Houser S, Heist EK, Ruskin JN. The coronary venous anatomy: a segmental approach to aid cardiac resynchronization therapy. J Am Coll Cardiol. 2005;46(1):68–74.
69. Saremi F, Pourzand L, Krishnan S, et al. Right atrial cavotricuspid isthmus: anatomic characterization with multi-detector row CT. Radiology. 2008;247(3):658–68.
70. Cabrera JA, Sánchez-Quintana D, Ho SY, et al. Angiographic anatomy of the inferior right atrial isthmus in patients with and without history of common atrial flutter. Circulation. 1999;99:3017–23.
71. Ruengsakulrach P, Buxton BF. Anatomic and hemodynamic considerations influencing the efficiency of retrograde cardioplegia. Ann Thorac Surg. 2001;71: 1389–95

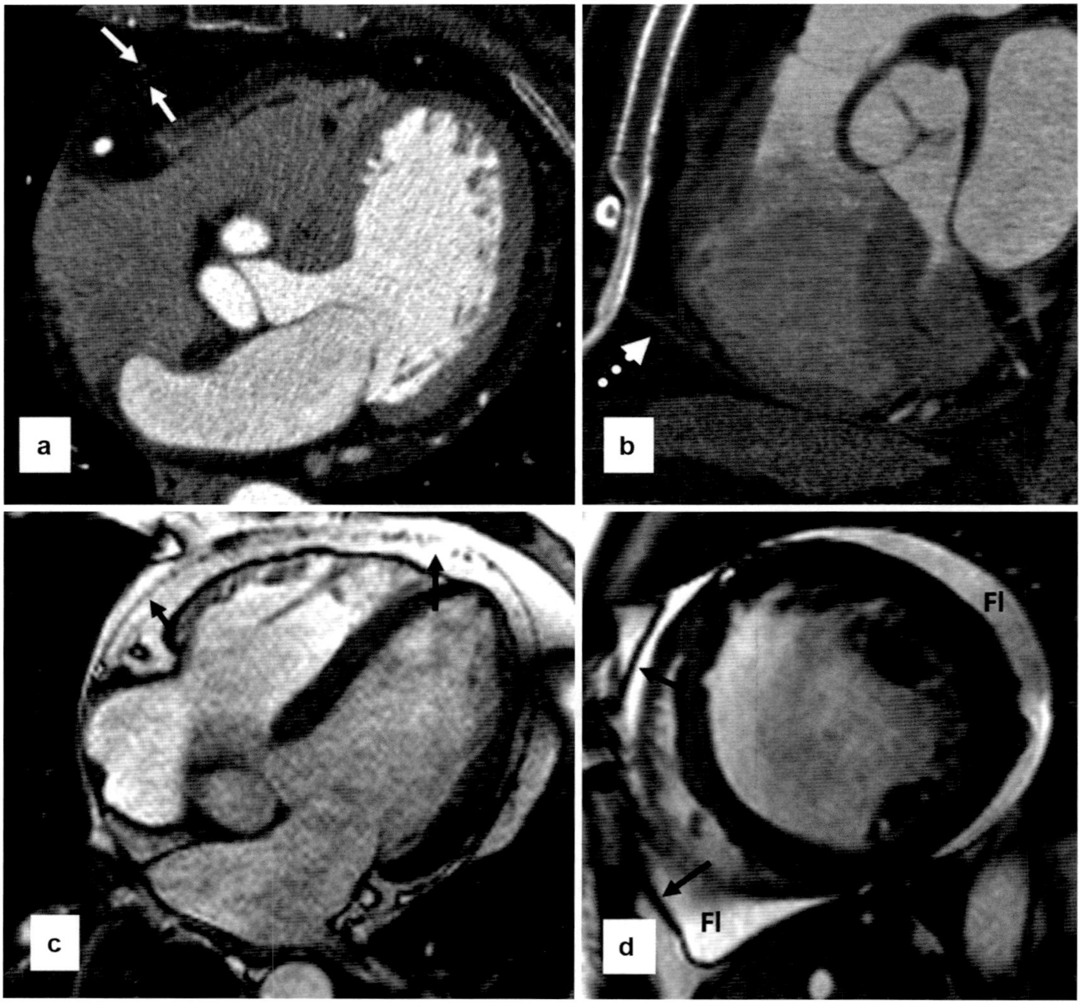

Fig. 29.1 Normal pericardium on CT (**a**, **b**) and MR (**c**, **d**) images. (**b**) Sagittal CT shows attachment of the fibrous pericardium to the central tendon of the diaphragm (*dashed arrow*). (**a**) CT and (**c**) MR axial images of the heart show the epicardial (inside) fat, the mediastinal (outside) fat, and the thin line of pericardial sac (*arrows*) between the two adipose tissue compartments. (**d**) Short-axis cine MR shows accumulation of fluid (*Fl*) in the pericardial sac separating the two fatty compartments. Parietal pericardium is shown by *arrows* in (d). In cine MR sequence (balanced steady-state free precession), it can be difficult to differentiate small amount of pericardial fluid from surrounding fat tissue as both appear high in signal intensity

Imaging

CT and MRI are equally considered the preferred imaging methods for morphological assessment of the pericardial sac and the pericardium. Higher spatial resolution of the CT scan allows improve visualization of the normal pericardium. As a result normal pericardium appears thinner using CT compared with MRI. This is not surprising knowing that most cardiac CT protocols consist of 0.5–1 mm slices, while in cardiac MRI most routine sequences involve 5–8 mm slices. Generally a pericardium thicker than 3 mm is considered abnormal [8]. On the other hand, MRI is the modality of choice for functional evaluation of heart and to differentiate constrictive pericarditis from restrictive cardiomyopathy [9, 10].

tion: correlation between its anatomy and electrophysiological findings. J Cardiovasc Electrophysiol. 2006;17(10):1062–7.
45. Shah D, Haissaguerre M, Jais P, Hocini M. Nonpulmonary vein foci: do they exist? Pacing Clin Electrophysiol. 2003;26(7 Pt 2):1631–5
46. Chauvin M, Shah DC, Haissaguerre M, Marcellin L, Brechenmacher C. The anatomic basis of connections between the coronary sinus musculature and the left atrium in humans. Circulation. 2000;101:647–52.
47. Cabrera JA, Ho SY, Climent V, Sánchez-Quintana D. The architecture of the left lateral atrial wall: a particular anatomic region with implications for ablation of atrial fibrillation. Eur Heart J. 2008;29:356–62.
48. Tan AY, Chou CC, Zhou S, et al. Electrical connections between the left superior pulmonary vein, left atrium and ligament of Marshall: implications for the mechanisms of atrial fibrillation. Am J Physiol Heart Circ Physiol. 2005;290:H312–22.
49. Hsu LF, Jais P, Keane D, et al. Atrial fibrillation originating from persistent left superior vena cava. Circulation. 2004;109:828–32.
50. Hwang C, Wu TJ, Doshi RN, Peter CT, Chen PS. Vein of Marshall cannulation for the analysis of electrical activity in patients with focal atrial fibrillation. Circulation. 2000;101(13):1503–5.
51. Miraldi F, di Gioia CR, Proietti P, De Santis M, d'Amati G, Gallo P. Cardinal vein isomerism: an embryological hypothesis to explain a persistent left superior vena cava draining into the roof of the left atrium in the absence of coronary sinus and atrial septal defect. Cardiovasc Pathol. 2002;11:149–52.
52. Anderson SE, Quill JL, Iaizzo PA. Venous valves within left ventricular coronary veins. J Interv Card Electrophysiol. 2008;23(2):95–9.
53. Corcoran SJ, Lawrence C, McGuire MA. The valve of Vieussens: an important cause of difficulty in advancing catheters into the cardiac veins. J Cardiovasc Electrophysiol. 1999;10:804–8.
54. Maros TN, Rácz L, Plugor S, Maros TG. Contributions to the morphology of the human coronary sinus. Anat Anz. 1983;154(2):133–44.
55. Silver MA, Rowley NE. The functional anatomy of the human coronary sinus. Am Heart J. 1988;115(5):1080–4.
56. Roberts JT. Arteries, veins, and lymphatic vessels of the heart. In: Luisada AA, editor. Development and structure of the cardiovascular system. New York: McGraw-Hill; 1958. p. 85–118.
57. Schutte DA, Rowland DG, Allen HD, Bharati S. Prominent venous valves in hypoplastic right hearts. Am Heart J. 1997;134(3):527–31.
58. Duda B, Grzybiak M. About variability of Vieussen valve in the adult human heart. Folia Morphol (Warsz). 2000;59(1):43–5.
59. Karaca M, Bilge O, Dinckal MH, Ucerler H. The anatomic barriers in the coronary sinus: implications for clinical procedures. J Interv Card Electrophysiol. 2005;14:89–94.
60. D' Cruz IA, Johns C, Shala MB. Dynamic cyclic changes in coronary sinus caliber in patients with and without congestive heart failure. Am J Cardiol. 1999;83:275–7.
61. Ong MG, Lee PC, Tai CT, et al. Coronary sinus morphology in different types of supraventricular tachycardias. J Interv Card Electrophysiol. 2006;15:21–6.
62. Uemura H, Ho SY, Anderson RH, et al. Surgical anatomy of the coronary circulation in hearts with discordant atrioventricular connections. Eur J Cardiothorac Surg. 1996;10:194–200.
63. Min JY, Kim CY, Oh MH, et al. Arrangement of the systemic and pulmonary venous components of the atrial chambers in hearts with isomeric atrial appendages. Cardiol Young. 2000;10(4):396–404.
64. Mantini E, Grondin CM, Lillehei CW, Edwards JE. Congenital anomalies involving the coronary sinus. Circulation. 1966;33:317–27.
65. Gerlis LM, Gibbs JL, Williams GJ, Thomas GDH. Coronary sinus orifice atresia and persistent left superior vena cava. Br Heart J. 1984;52:648–53.
66. Attenhofer Jost CH, Connolly HM, Danielson GK, Dearani JA, Warnes CA, Jamil Tajik A. Clinical features and surgical outcome in 25 patients with fenestrations of the coronary sinus. Cardiol Young. 2007;17(6):592–600.
67. Kautzner J, Riedlbauchova L, Cihak R, Bytesnik J, Vancura V. Technical aspects of implantation of LV lead for cardiac resynchronization therapy in chronic heart failure. Pacing Clin Electrophysiol. 2004;27:783–90.
68. Singh JP, Houser S, Heist EK, Ruskin JN. The coronary venous anatomy: a segmental approach to aid cardiac resynchronization therapy. J Am Coll Cardiol. 2005;46(1):68–74.
69. Saremi F, Pourzand L, Krishnan S, et al. Right atrial cavotricuspid isthmus: anatomic characterization with multi-detector row CT. Radiology. 2008;247(3):658–68.
70. Cabrera JA, Sánchez-Quintana D, Ho SY, et al. Angiographic anatomy of the inferior right atrial isthmus in patients with and without history of common atrial flutter. Circulation. 1999;99:3017–23.
71. Ruengsakulrach P, Buxton BF. Anatomic and hemodynamic considerations influencing the efficiency of retrograde cardioplegia. Ann Thorac Surg. 2001;71:1389–95.

Congenital Pericardial Anomalies

29

Farhood Saremi

Anatomy

The pericardium surrounds the heart and extends superiorly to cover part of the superior vena cava, ascending aorta, and main pulmonary artery. The pericardium consists of an outer fibrous component and an inner double-layered serous sac that surrounds the heart [1, 2]. The outer serous layer which is closely attached to the fibrous layer is the parietal pericardium. The visceral serous pericardium, or epicardium, adheres to the heart and great vessels and forms recesses and sinuses [2]. Normal pericardium can be identified at CT images as a thin smooth line of soft tissue attenuation (isodense to the normal myocardium) outlined by low-attenuation mediastinal and epicardial fat (Fig. 29.1). On MRI the fibrous pericardium appears low in signal intensity on most sequences and is surrounded by high-intensity mediastinal and epicardial fat. Normally, the pericardial sac contains 15–50 mL of fluid allowing visualization of the pericardial recesses on CT or MR imaging studies [3]. The fibrous pericardium is fused with the central tendon of the diaphragm inferiorly and with the tunica adventitia of the great vessels superiorly (Fig. 29.2). Anteriorly, it is attached to the sternum by the superior and inferior sternopericardial ligaments.

The reflections of the serosal layers are arranged around two complex tubes. One tube encloses the aorta and pulmonary trunk. The second tube encloses the superior vena cava, the inferior vena cava, and the four pulmonary veins [2]. The transverse sinus is the passage between these two pericardial tubes and lies posterior to the ascending aorta and main pulmonary artery, above the left atrium (Fig. 29.2). The oblique sinus is the cul-de-sac located posterior and superior to the left atrium and separated from the transverse sinus by two layers of pericardial reflections that extend between the left and right superior pulmonary veins. The superior extent of the transverse sinus along the aortocaval space is the superior aortic recess [2]. Cephalad extension of this recess into the high right paratracheal region (high riding recess) can be mistaken for pathologies or a pericardial diverticulum [4, 5] (Fig. 29.2). Lateral extent of the transverse sinus forms the left and right pulmonic recesses between the pulmonary artery and superior pulmonary vein on each side [6]. Pericardial fat composes of the epicardial fat and the paracardial fat [7] (Fig. 29.1). Paracardial (mediastinal) fat is situated on the external surface of the parietal pericardium within the mediastinum. Epicardial (subepicardial) fat is located between the visceral layer of the pericardium and the myocardium. Epicardial fat is not limited to the surface of the heart but can penetrate deep in the interatrial septum and septal atrioventricular junction.

F. Saremi, MD
Department of Radiology, Cardiothoracic Section,
University of Southern California,
USC Keck Hospital, 1500 San Pablo St.,
Los Angeles, CA 90033, USA
e-mail: fsaremi@usc.edu

F. Saremi (ed.), *Cardiac CT and MR for Adult Congenital Heart Disease*,
DOI 10.1007/978-1-4614-8875-0_29, © Springer Science+Business Media New York 2014

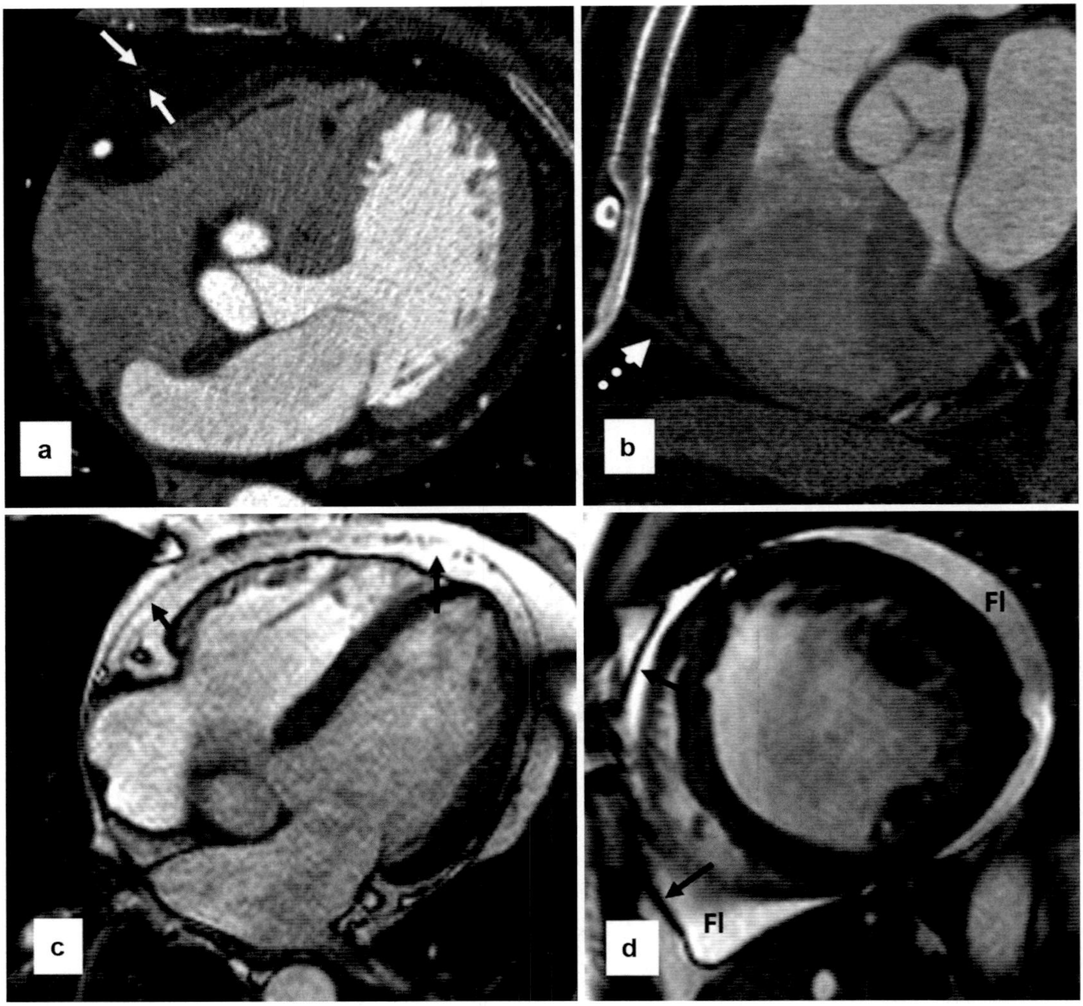

Fig. 29.1 Normal pericardium on CT (**a**, **b**) and MR (**c**, **d**) images. (**b**) Sagittal CT shows attachment of the fibrous pericardium to the central tendon of the diaphragm (*dashed arrow*). (**a**) CT and (**c**) MR axial images of the heart show the epicardial (inside) fat, the mediastinal (outside) fat, and the thin line of pericardial sac (*arrows*) between the two adipose tissue compartments. (**d**) Short-axis cine MR shows accumulation of fluid (*Fl*) in the pericardial sac separating the two fatty compartments. Parietal pericardium is shown by *arrows* in (d). In cine MR sequence (balanced steady-state free precession), it can be difficult to differentiate small amount of pericardial fluid from surrounding fat tissue as both appear high in signal intensity

Imaging

CT and MRI are equally considered the preferred imaging methods for morphological assessment of the pericardial sac and the pericardium. Higher spatial resolution of the CT scan allows improve visualization of the normal pericardium. As a result normal pericardium appears thinner using CT compared with MRI. This is not surprising knowing that most cardiac CT protocols consist of 0.5–1 mm slices, while in cardiac MRI most routine sequences involve 5–8 mm slices. Generally a pericardium thicker than 3 mm is considered abnormal [8]. On the other hand, MRI is the modality of choice for functional evaluation of heart and to differentiate constrictive pericarditis from restrictive cardiomyopathy [9, 10].

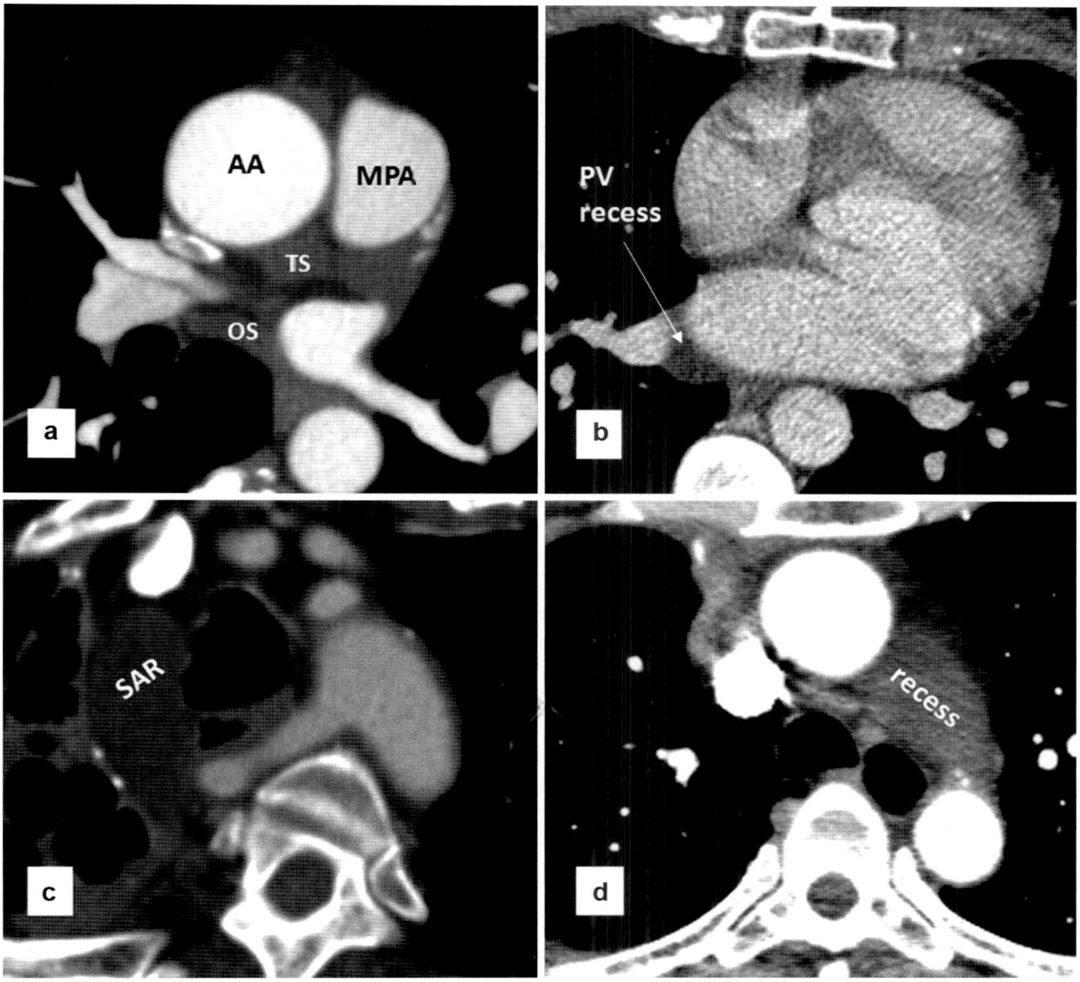

Fig. 29.2 Axial CT images of the heart show pericardial recesses. (**a**) Transverse sinus (*TS*) and oblique sinus (*OS*) are shown. (**b**) A prominent pericardial lateral recess of the pulmonary vein is shown. Lateral recesses are formed between superior and inferior pulmonary veins and commonly seen on the right side. (**c**) High riding aortocaval recess with its superior extent rising to the level of the thoracic inlet. (**d**) Large aortopulmonary pericardial recess. It is due to superior extension of the left pulmonic recess of the transverse sinus. *AA* ascending aorta, *MPA* main pulmonary artery, *SAR* superior aortic recess

Although evaluation of pericardium and pericardial fluid is possible on non-gated CT scans, ECG-gated methods are usually preferred particularly when detailed evaluation of the pathologies is required. For example, pericardial cysts can be characterized in most non-gated CT scans of the heart, while detection of partial absence of pericardium may be optimally performed using gated CT.

Morphological study of the pericardium with MRI can be best obtained with black-blood fast spin-echo (BB-FSA) sequence. Five millimeters axial, coronal, and sagittal images can be obtained to cover the entire pericardium. In this sequence, double inversion recovery (IR) pulses are used to null the blood signal. To remove high signal intensity of fat, a third IR pulse can be included in the pulse sequence, the so-called triple IR. It is important to know that BB-FSE sequence is not designed to be a T1-weighted sequence. As a matter of fact in most applications it is proton

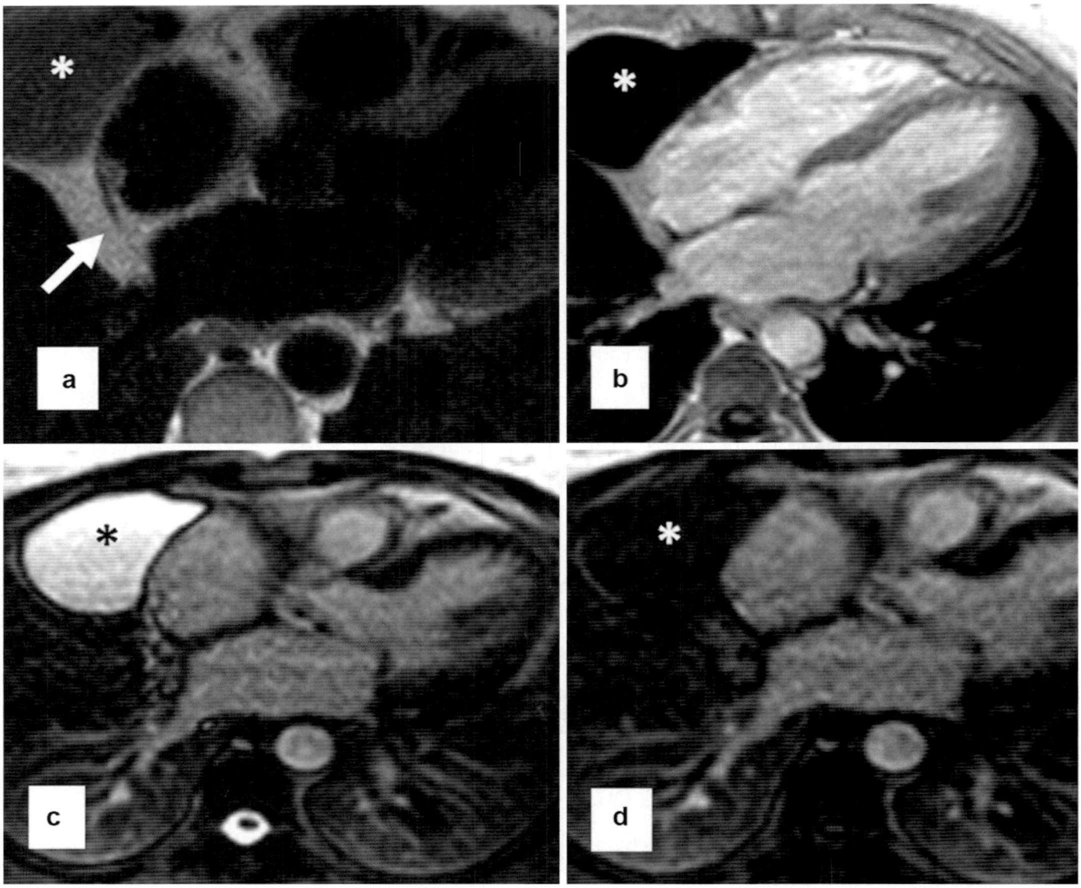

Fig. 29.3 Pericardial cyst (*stars*) in the right anterior cardiophrenic angle shown with MRI. (**a**) Black-blood fast spin echo shows the cyst as a homogeneous medium signal intensity area. This sequence is proton density weighted, and fluid-filled structures may appear isosignal to the myocardium. Note the cyst is separate from the normal pericardium (*arrow*). (**b**) Post-contrast T1-weighted fast gradient-echo sequence shows the cyst as a low-signal area. (**c**, **d**) are T2-weighted single-shot fast spin-echo sequences before (a) and after (b) fluid attenuation inversion pulse

density or T2 weighted; as a result the fluid signal may appear bright not dark (Fig. 29.3). To make it T1 weighted, echo time should be lowered. T2-weighted triple IR sequence has the advantage of demonstration of pericardial edema in cases with inflammatory pericarditis. IR pulse can be adjusted to null pericardial fluid signal (Fig. 29.3). The second most important sequence in the evaluation anatomy as well as regional and global myocardial function with MRI is bright-blood balanced steady-state free precession (b-SSFP). This sequence is mainly T2 weighted and the signal of blood, fat, and pericardial fluid appears bright. Both non-ECG-gated and cine versions of b-SSFP are helpful for evaluation of the pericardium. Although advanced sequences such as tagged MRI and free-breathing real-time SSFP may be better choices for complete analysis of constrictive physiology and to study physiologic events such as ventricular coupling [9], by careful reviewing of routine cine images, it is simply possible to diagnose constrictive pericarditis in most cases (Fig. 29.4). Cine viewing allows better differentiation of motion between the rigid constricted pericardium and the underlying moving myocardium.

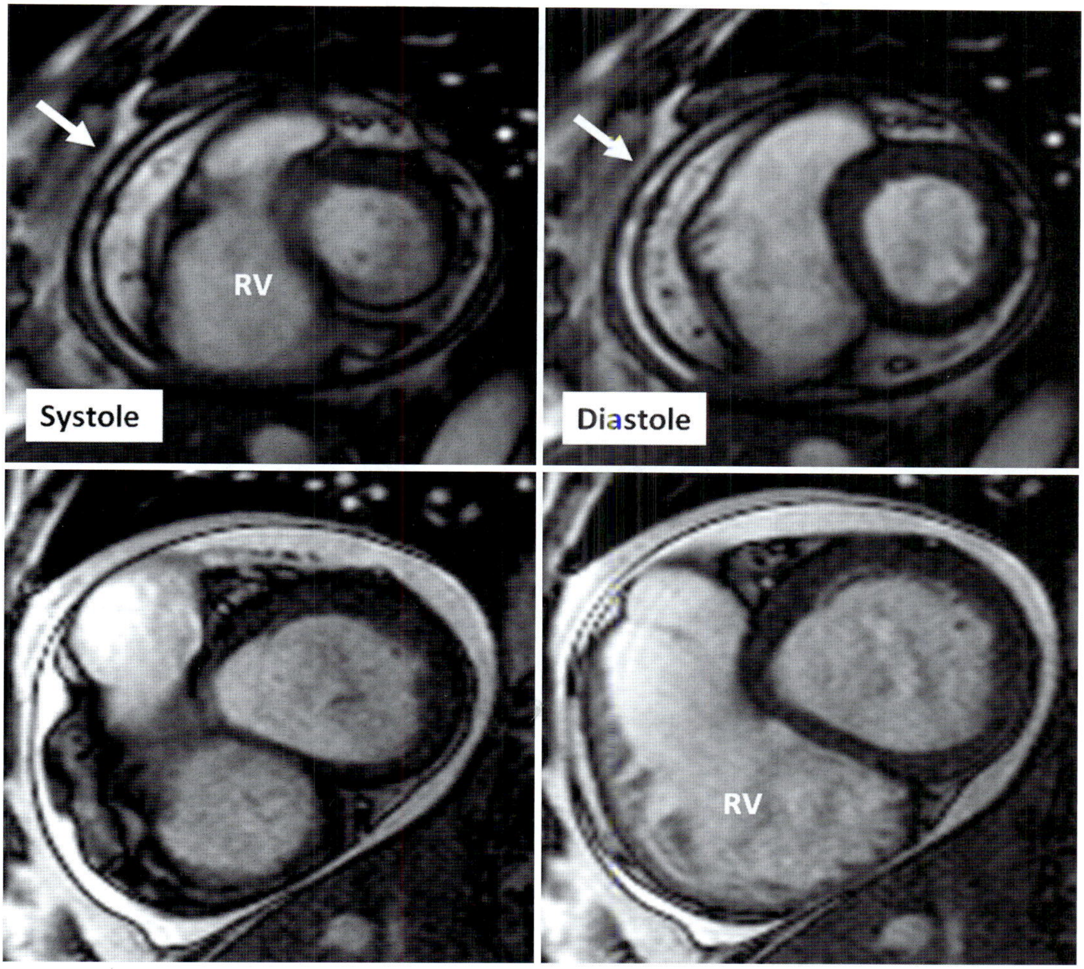

Fig. 29.4 Short-axis cine MR views in systole and diastole in a patient with constrictive pericarditis (*upper row*) and another patient with serous pericardial effusion. Images in constrictive pericarditis patient show thickened rigid pericardium with a fixed pericardial cavity (*arrows*) on both systolic and diastolic images. In contrast, the pericardium appears thin and smooth in pericardial effusion case (*lower images*), and the pericardial cavity (bright in signal intensity) covering the right ventricle (*RV*) appears smaller in diastolic image due to the shift of free fluid in the pericardial sac

Absence of Pericardial Tissue

The pericardial and pleural cavities and diaphragm are so closely related in their development.

The pericardial cavity represents a portion of the original right and left intraembryonic coeloms, and its lining derives from both the parietal (somatic) and the visceral (splanchnic) layers of the mesoderm. Later, the right and left side coeloms fuse, and folds of tissue divide it into separate cavities. The pericardial cavity separates from the peritoneal cavity by the formation of the septum transversum and from the pleura by the growth of the left and right pleuropericardial folds which are linked to the evolution of the incoming cardinal veins of the sinus venosus. Major part of pericardium is derived from the parietal mesoderm which is also primarily the wall of the pericardial cavity. A small dorsal

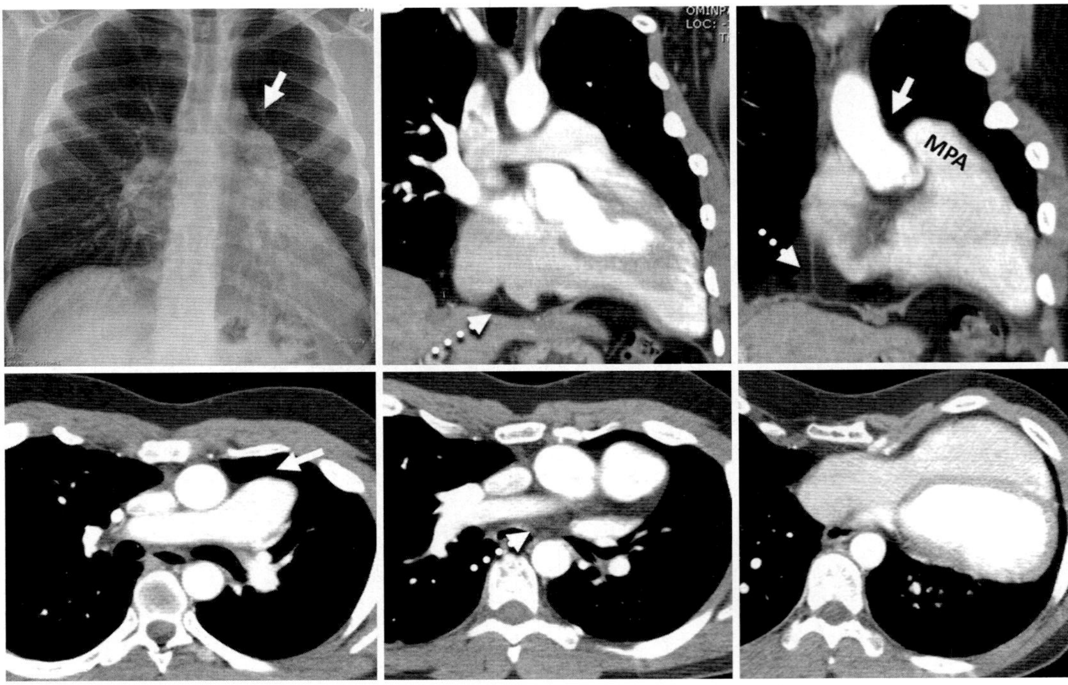

Fig. 29.5 Complete absence of the left pericardium in a 24-year-old male with pectus excavatum. The entire heart is shifted to the left. Plain radiograph and CT images demonstrate a prominent left main pulmonary artery extending beyond the mediastinal margins into the left lung. Because of the absence of left pericardium, a "tongue" of lung tissue interposes between the main pulmonary artery (*MPA*) and aorta (*arrows*), a diagnostic sign for congenital absence of pericardium. Only parts of the right pericardium extending to the diaphragm and left atrial appendage are seen (*dashed arrows*)

portion is probably derived from the mesoderm at the root of the dorsal mesocardium. The septum transversum (a derivative of the visceral layer) forms the caudal wall of the pericardial cavity. Congenital pericardial defects result from incomplete development of either the septum transversum or the pleuropericardial folds. Premature atrophy of the left common cardinal vein (duct of Cuvier) compromises the blood supply to the left pleuropericardial fold and accounts for absence of the left pericardium [11, 12]. If abnormality occurs in early stages of embryonic development, the pleural serosa and diaphragm may also be affected.

Congenital absence of pericardium has been described in literature for more than four centuries and mainly discovered inadvertently during postmortem and thoracotomy procedures [11–14]. Radiologically, it was undiscovered until 1959 when Ellis et al. reported the first case by x-ray [15]. Subsequently, increasing numbers of cases have been reported. Van Son et al. presented the Mayo Clinic experience on congenital absence of the pericardium (15 cases in 34,000 surgeries) [16]. In all, the diagnosis was made in the operating room.

Congenital absence of pericardium occurs on a spectrum from complete absence of the left, right, or both sides of the pericardium to small regional defects. Partial defect may involve part of the left, right, or diaphragmatic pericardium. Approximately 30 % of patients with pericardial agenesis have additional anomalies such as atrial septal defect, bicuspid aortic valve, mitral stenosis, tricuspid insufficiency, patent ductus arteriosus, tetralogy of Fallot, pulmonary sequestration, bronchogenic cyst, and congenital diaphragmatic hernia [14–19]. Pectus excavatum is a common deformity in these patients [14] (Fig. 29.5). Agenesis of the left pericardium is

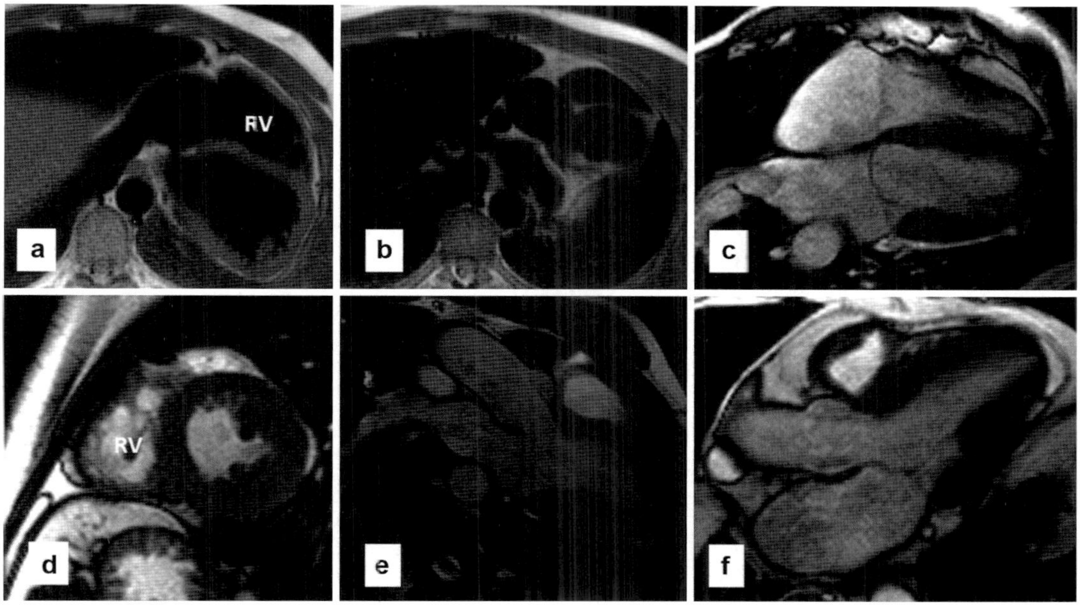

Fig. 29.6 MR images in a patient with complete absence of pericardium. (**a**, **b**) Are axial black-blood images. (**c**–**e**) Are cine images in four-chamber, axial, and three-chamber views, respectively. Normal pericardium cannot be traced. *Dark line* anterior to the right ventricle (*RV*) on short-axis view is related to susceptibility artifact not a real pericardial line. The heart is laterally displaced in the left hemithorax and the apex is rotated posteriorly. (**f**) Three-chamber view of a normal heart is shown for comparison

the most common type accounting for 70 % of cases (Fig. 29.6). It usually involves the entire left side. In Gatzoulis series of ten cases with isolated pericardial defect, 70 % were complete absence of the left side [8]. Partial defects of left pericardium are not uncommon; they are usually located in the upper part of the left pericardium causing herniation of the left atrial appendage or part of the left ventricle (Fig. 29.7). In lower part is involved incarceration of the left ventricle and ischemia by coronary artery compression may ensue [20, 21]. Total aplasia of the pericardium accounts for less than 10 % of the cases identified [8, 16, 17]. It may coexist with an incomplete closure of the anterior chest wall, ectopia of the heart, and omphalocele. In less severe forms, the heart remains intrathoracic but falls over in the left hemithorax and may be associated with diaphragmatic defects. Agenesis of the right pleuropericardial membrane is considered very uncommon (4 %) (Fig. 29.8). Right-sided mediastinal shift of the heart may be observed. In the partial form, the right atrial appendage or ventricle may herniate through the defect or the right lung may herniate in and compress the superior vena cava [22–25]. Defects of the diaphragmatic pericardium are associated with partial diaphragmatic aplasia and intrapericardial herniation of the greater omentum.

In congenital absence of pericardium, patients are generally asymptomatic but 30 % experience recurrent chest pains largely nonexertional, which may be positional, or dyspnea. The etiology of symptoms is speculative but may result from increased heart mobility and distortion of intrathoracic structures (e.g., pleural attachments, great vessels). The shifted apical impulse tends to give the impression of cardiac enlargement. Systolic ejection murmurs can be heard, without clear explanation. Electrocardiography shows right bundle branch block and clockwise rotation of the precordial plane. Palpitations, syncope, or sudden death are features applying to the localized forms. Therefore, it is very important to differentiate partial from complete absence of the pericardium.

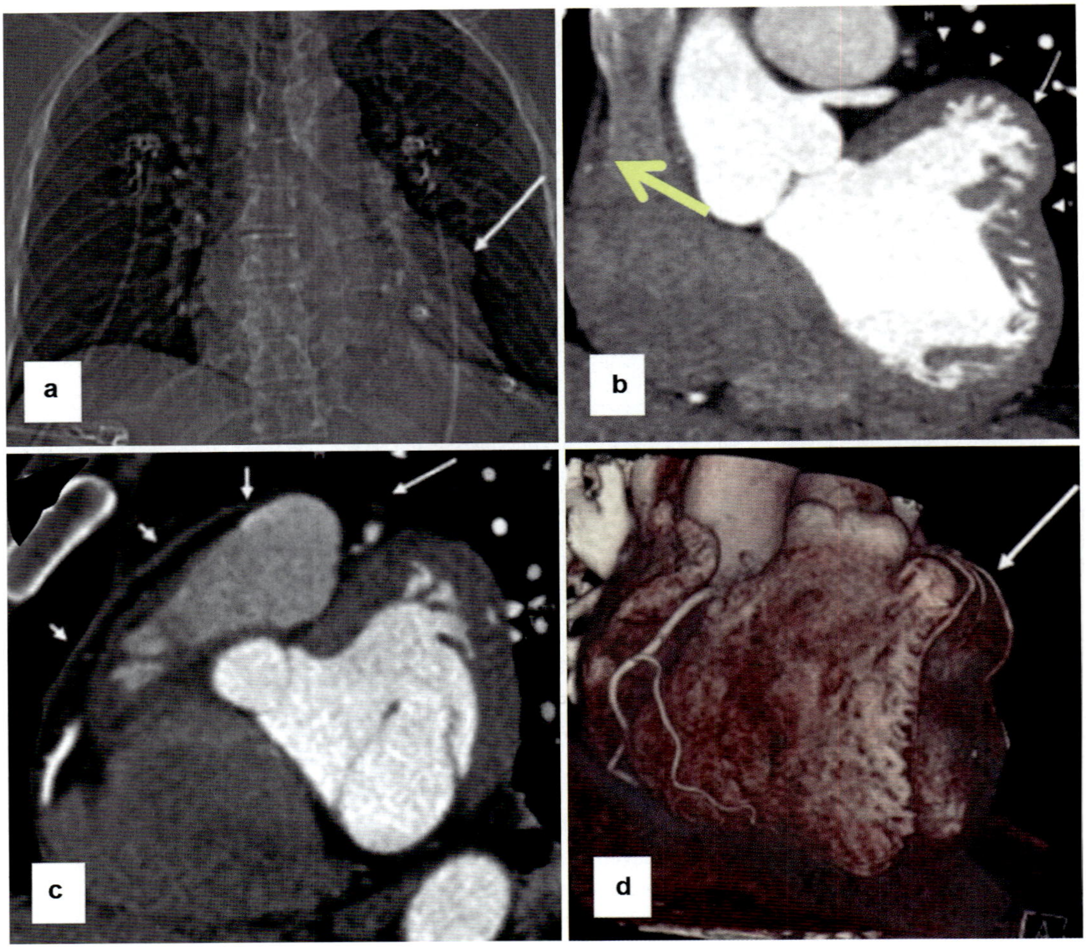

Fig. 29.7 Partial absence of the left pericardium in a 63-year-old man with severe chest pain that worsened with breathing. (**a**) CT topogram shows an abnormal bulge along left cardiac boarder (*arrow*). (**b–d**) CT coronary angiograms show that the focal bulge (*long white arrows*) is due to partially herniated left ventricle. *Arrowheads* in panel **b** show absent left pericardium. Coronal view (**b**) shows intact right pericardium (*yellow arrow*). Sagittal view (**c**) through the base of the heart shows intact anterior pericardium (*short arrows*), free edge of the pericardium at defect (*medium length arrow*), and bare area overlying the left ventricle (*long arrow*) (From Verde et al. [26] with permission)

On left-sided agenesis, prominent pulmonary artery and the lung interposing between the main pulmonary artery and aorta are seen in 90 % of patients establishing this marker as the pathognomonic feature of absent pericardium on plain films [8] (Fig. 29.5). Interposition of lung between heart and diaphragm is seen in 20 %. The heart structure has been described as "teardrop" shaped.

The diagnosis can be confirmed by CT or MR as they more clearly delineate the anatomical relationships with adjacent structures than other modalities. Both delineate the presence of normal pericardium as a thin line of uniform low attenuation/signal intensity against the pericardial fat. Despite high resolution and contrast in CT and MR, it is not always possible to trace the exact margins of the pericardial defect and determine the actual size of pericardial defect (Fig. 29.6). Because of levoposition of the heart, the left inferior pulmonary vein can be compressed between the left atrium and descending aorta/spine [8]. In

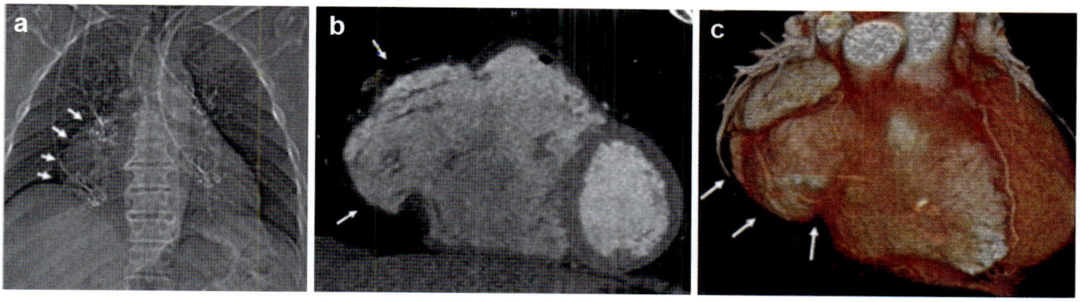

Fig. 29.8 Incomplete absence of the right pericardium in a 42-year-old man with 9-month history of progressive dyspnea. (**a**) CT topogram shows large mass-like opacity in the right hemithorax at the level of the right cardiac boarder (*arrows*). Vessels are seen through the mass. (**b**, **c**) Cardiac CT angiogram shows herniation of the right atrium and ventricle through a large defect in the pericardium (*arrows*) in coronal oblique (**b**) and 3-dimensional volume-rendered imaging (**c**). Note the waist created as the right heart herniates through the incomplete defect (From Verde et al. [25] with permission)

incomplete defects, a rim of residual pericardium may cause compression of the herniated atrial appendage or ventricle that requires urgent attention [26] (Fig. 29.8). MRI and echocardiography also show increased heart mobility and impaired left ventricular torsion. On echocardiography, the right ventricle diameter may falsely appear enlarged due to posterior rotation of the heart. As a result these patients may be referred for MRI for evaluation of right ventricle enlargement and possible atrial septal defect [27]. Symptomatic complete absence of pericardium may benefit from pericardioplasty, but otherwise is not thought to require intervention [28]. Because patients with partial absence of pericardium may be at risk of herniation and strangulation of cardiac structures, closure of the pericardial defect is believed to reduce these risks.

Pericardial Cyst and Diverticulum

Preliminary reports on pericardial cysts and diverticula date back to the middle of the nineteenth century all derived exclusively from autopsy studies [29–32]. Otto Pickhardt accomplished the first resection of a pericardial cyst in 1931 [30]. The appearance of the thin-walled, translucent cysts containing crystal-clear fluid gave rise to the new term "spring water cyst of the mediastinum" by Greenfield and colleagues in 1943 [32].

The pericardial cyst and diverticulum are closely associated, and many believe they have common embryonic origin during development of the pericardium, hence the term "pericardial coelomic cyst or diverticulum" was used. Lillie at al. proposed that both diverticulum and cyst derive from the ventral recess of the pericardial coelom [33]. The authors concluded that persistence of the recess results in formation of a diverticulum, while constriction of the proximal part of the persistent recess accounts for either a diverticulum with a narrow neck or a cyst in communication with the pericardial cavity.

Pericardial cysts are rare congenital encapsulated cysts lined by mesothelium. When the results of a mass radiographic campaign in Edinburgh were published in 1958, Le Roux reported that 3 out of 300,000 subjects were found to have a pericardial cyst [31]. Therefore, 1 in every 100,000 of the population may have such a cyst, constituting 5 % of all mediastinal masses [34].

Pericardial cysts and diverticulum are unilocular and contain clear serous fluid. They usually appear as a solitary encapsulated lesion adjacent to the pericardium, but 20 % may communicate with the pericardium (diverticulum). Pericardial cysts typically occur in the cardiophrenic angle (90 %). Two-thirds are located on the right side (Fig. 29.3). In 10 % they occur in remote locations [35, 36] (Fig. 29.9). Case has been reported that the cyst developed on follow-up studies, while previous CT did not show evidence of any

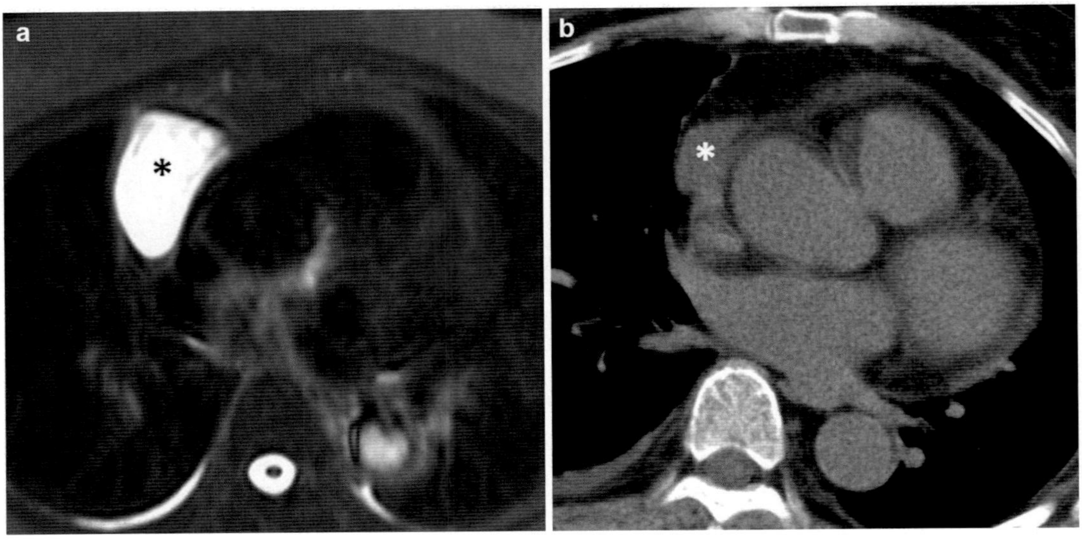

Fig. 29.9 Pericardial cyst (*) located high in right upper paramediastinal area at the superior vena cava level. (**a**) T2-weighted axial fast spin-echo MR. (**b**) Axial CT. Note the cyst appears larger in MR obtained a few weeks later after the CT scan was done. In this unusual location, a pericardial cyst should be differentiated from bronchogenic and thymic cysts

intrathoracic mass [37]. The majority of pericardial cysts are asymptomatic. They can cause nonspecific symptoms including dyspnea, chest pain, and cough in 25 %. Pericardial cysts are usually detected in the third or fourth decade of life with the same frequency in both men and women. In some reports it is more common in women [38].

Pericardial cysts are usually suspected on plain radiographs. However, many cases are incidentally diagnosed on CT or MR studies of the chest or abdomen. The most common radiographic appearance of the pericardial cysts is a well-defined, smooth-walled rounded mass located at right anterior cardiophrenic angle. It may extend into the major fissure. The position in relation to the heart is stable, but the cyst shape may change in different positions and can grow very slowly on follow-up examinations. The attenuation of the cyst fluid is generally similar to transudate fluid (near-water density of 0–20 Hounsfield units). It appears low signal on T1-weighted images and becomes bright on T2-weighted images (Fig. 29.3). Atypical fluid attenuation/signal can occur due to hemorrhage or increased proteinaceous material.

Differential diagnosis includes loculated pericardial effusions and other cystic lesions such as bronchogenic and thymic cysts. For surgical candidates, although thoracotomy was used to treat such lesions in the past, video-assisted thoracic surgery (VATS) is the best option for the treatment of these cysts [38]. Percutaneous aspiration of cyst can be performed as an alternative option to surgical resection in selected cases and may be lifesaving in symptomatic patients [39]. Spontaneous resolution of a pericardial cyst has been reported in few cases managed conservatively, the probable mechanism being cyst rupture [40].

Pericardial diverticulum is rarer than pericardial cyst and corresponds to herniation through a defect in the parietal pericardium that communicates with the pericardial cavity [31].

The distinction between pericardial cysts and diverticula in the historic literature is often quite vague, and the difference between a diverticulum with narrow neck and a cyst that communicates with the pericardial cavity through a pedicle sometimes seems arbitrary [29].

Pericardial diverticulum typically occurs in the cardiophrenic angles and has the tendency to change in size and location overtime [41] (Fig. 29.10). Cysts that disappear on follow-up examination may represent a decompressed diverticulum. Cardiac

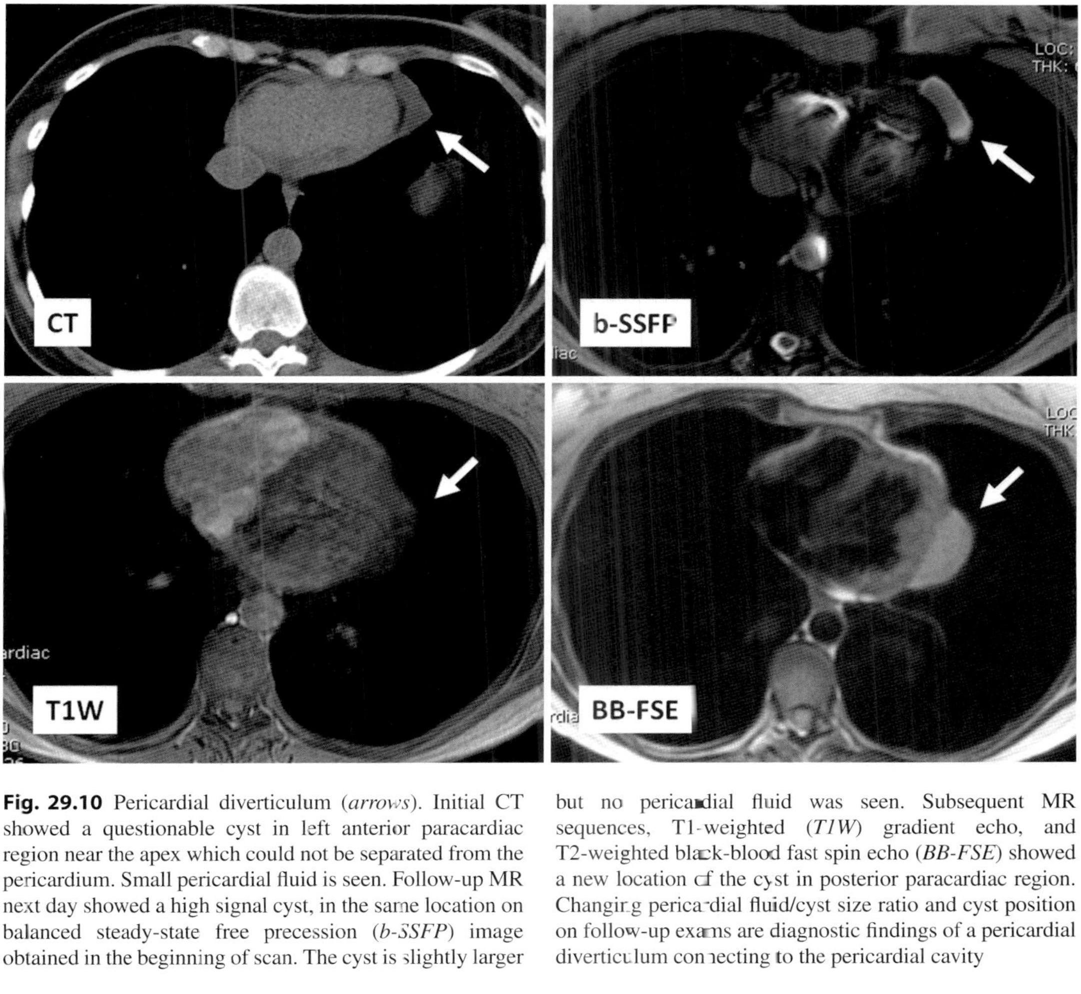

Fig. 29.10 Pericardial diverticulum (*arrows*). Initial CT showed a questionable cyst in left anterior paracardiac region near the apex which could not be separated from the pericardium. Small pericardial fluid is seen. Follow-up MR next day showed a high signal cyst, in the same location on balanced steady-state free precession (*b-SSFP*) image obtained in the beginning of scan. The cyst is slightly larger but no pericardial fluid was seen. Subsequent MR sequences, T1-weighted (*T1W*) gradient echo, and T2-weighted black-blood fast spin echo (*BB-FSE*) showed a new location of the cyst in posterior paracardiac region. Changing pericardial fluid/cyst size ratio and cyst position on follow-up exams are diagnostic findings of a pericardial diverticulum connecting to the pericardial cavity

MR or CT is helpful in reaching a preoperative diagnosis. Although it resembles a pericardial cyst, the diagnosis of a diverticulum should be suspected when a complete wall cannot be identified in all parts of the lesion. Treatment is similar to pericardial cyst [42, 43].

References

1. Vesely TM, Cahill DR. Cross-sectional anatomy of the pericardial sinuses, recesses, and adjacent structures. Surg Radiol Anat. 1986;8:221–7.
2. Levy-Ravetch M, Auh YH, Rubenstein WA, et al. CT of the pericardial recesses. AJR Am J Roentgenol. 1985;144:707–14.
3. Kodama F, Fultz PJ, Wandtke JC. Comparing thin-section and thick-section CT of pericardial sinuses and recesses. AJR Am J Roentgenol. 2003;181: 1101–8.
4. Choi YW, McAdams HP, Jeon SC, et al. The "high-riding" superior pericardial recess: CT findings. AJR Am J Roentgenol. 2000;175:1025–8.
5. Winer-Muram HT, Gold RE. Effusion in the superior pericardial recess simulating a mediastinal mass. AJR Am J Roentgenol. 1990;154:69–71.
6. Protopapas Z, Westcott JL. Left pulmonic recess of the pericardium: findings at CT and MR imaging. Radiology. 1995;196:85–8.
7. Ho E, Shimada Y. Formation of the epicardium studied with the scanning electron microscope. Dev Biol. 1978;66:579–85.
8. Gatzoulis MA, Munk MD, Merchant N, Van Arsdell GS, McCrindle BW, Webb GD. Isolated congenital absence of the pericardium: clinical presentation, diagnosis and management. Ann Thorac Surg. 2000;69:1209–15.
9. Francone M, Dymarkowski S, Kalantzi M, Bogaert J. Real-time cine MRI of ventricular septal motion.

A novel approach to assess ventricular coupling. J Magn Reson Imaging. 2005;21:305–9.
10. Kojima S, Yamada N, Goto Y. Diagnosis of constrictive pericarditis by tagged cine magnetic resonance imaging. N Engl J Med. 1999;341:373–4.
11. Columbus MR. De re anatomica, vol. XV. Edited by N Beurlaquae. Venice; 1559. p. 265.
12. Baille M. On the want of a pericardium in the human body. Trans Soc Improv Med Chir Knowl. 1793;1:91.
13. Southworth H, Stevenson CS. Congenital defects of pericardium. Arch Intern Med. 1938;61:223.
14. Nasser WK, Helmen C, Tavel ME, Feigenbaum H, Fisch C. Congenital absence of the left pericardium. Clinical, electrocardiographic, radiographic, hemodynamic, and angiographic findings in six cases. Circulation. 1970;41:469–78.
15. Ellis K, Leeds NE, Himmelstein A. Congenital deficiencies in the parietal pericardium: a review with 2 new cases including successful diagnosis by plain roentgenography. Am J Roentgenol. 1959;82:125–32.
16. Van Son JA, Danielson GK, Schaff HV, Mullany CJ, Julsrud PR, Breen JF. Congenital partial and complete absence of the pericardium. Mayo Clin Proc. 1993;68:743–7.
17. Saint-Pierre A, Froment R. Total and partial absence of pericardium. Arch Mal Coeur. 1970;63:638–57.
18. Fosburg RG, Jakubiak JV, Delaney TB. Congenital partial absence of the pericardium. Ann Thorac Surg. 1968;5:171–7.
19. Nasser WK. Congenital absence of the left pericardium. Am J Cardiol. 1970;26:466–70.
20. Kogon BE, Butler H, Kanter KR. Partial pericardial defect with left atrial herniation. Pediatr Cardiol. 2006;27(1):180–2.
21. Chassaing S, Bensouda C, Bar O, Barbey C, Blanchard D. A case of partial congenital absence of pericardium revealed by MRI. Circ Cardiovasc Imaging. 2010;3(5):632–4.
22. Karakurt C, Oğuz D, Karademir S, Sungur M, Ocal B. Congenital partial pericardial defect and herniated right atrial appendage: a rare anomaly. Echocardiography. 2006;23(9):784–6.
23. Tamagond SB, Agarwal S, Tomar AS, Satsangi DK. Lung herniation into pericardial cavity: a case of partial congenital absence of right pericardium. Ann Pediatr Cardiol. 2012;5(2):213–4.
24. Minocha GK, Falicov RE, Nijensohn E. Partial right-sided congenital pericardial defect with herniation of right atrium and right ventricle. Chest. 1979;76:484–6.
25. Moene RJ, Dekker A, Van der Harten HJ. Congenital right-sided pericardial defect with herniation of part of the lung into the pericardial cavity. Am J Cardiol. 1973;31:519–22.
26. Verde F, Johnson PT, Jha S, Fishman EK, Zimmerman SL. Congenital absence of the pericardium and its mimics. J Cardiovasc Comput Tomogr. 2013;7(1):11–7.
27. Garnier F, Eicher JC, Philip JL, et al. Congenital complete absence of the left pericardium: a rare cause of chest pain or pseudo-right heart overload. Clin Cardiol. 2010;33(2):E52–7.
28. Drury NE, De Silva RJ, Hall RM, Large SR. Congenital defects of the pericardium. Ann Thorac Surg. 2007;83:1552–3.
29. Schweigert M, Dubecz A, Beron M, Ofner D, Stein HJ. The tale of spring water cysts: a historical outline of surgery for congenital pericardial diverticula and cysts. Tex Heart Inst J. 2012;39(3):330–4.
30. Pickhardt OC. Pleuro-diaphragmatic cyst. In: Transactions of the New York Surgical Society-Stated Meeting held April 12, 1933. Ann Surg. 1934;99(5):814–6.
31. Le Roux BT. Pericardial coelomic cysts. Thorax. 1959;14(1):27–35.
32. Greenfield L, Steinberg L, Touroff ASW. Spring water cyst of the mediastinum. J Thorac Surg. 1943;12: 495–502.
33. Lillie WI, McDonald JR, Clagett OT. Pericardial celomic cysts and pericardial diverticula; a concept of etiology and report of cases. J Thorac Surg. 1950;20(3):494–504.
34. Patel J, Park C, Michaels J, Rosen S, Kort S. Pericardial cyst: case reports and a literature review. Echocardiography. 2004;21:269–72.
35. Raveglia F, Baisi A, Calati AM, Kaiser LR. Bilocular pericardial cyst in an aberrant location. Interact CardioVasc Thorac Surg. 2009;8:160–1.
36. Omeroglu SN, Omeroglu A, Ardal H, Erkilinc A, Bal E, Ipek G, et al. Epicardial mesothelial cyst located over the left anterior descending coronary artery. Tex Heart Inst J. 2004;31(3):313–5.
37. Comoglio C, Sansone F, Delsedime L, Campanella A, Ceresa F, Rinaldi M. Mesothelial cyst of the pericardium, absent on earlier computed tomography. Tex Heart Inst J. 2010;37(3):354–7.
38. Alar T, Bayram AS, Gebitekin C. Pericardial cysts: an analysis of 12 cases. J Laparoendosc Adv Surg Tech A. 2011;21(7):595–8.
39. Okubo K, Chino M, Fuse J, Yo S, Nishimura F. Lifesaving needle aspiration of a cardiac-compressing pericardial cyst. Am J Cardiol. 2000;85:521.
40. Ambalavanan SK, Mehta JB, Taylor RA, Mehta AV. Spontaneous resolution of a large pericardial cyst. Tenn Med. 1997;90:97–8.
41. Guler A, Sahin MA, Kadan M, Erol G, Cingoz F, Tatar H. Incidental diagnosis of asymptomatic pericardial diverticulum. Tex Heart Inst J. 2011;38(2):206–7.
42. Carretta A, Negri G, Pansera M, Melloni G, Zannini P. Thoracoscopic treatment of a pericardial diverticulum. Surg Endosc. 2003;17:158–9.
43. Akiba T, Marushima H, Masubuchi M, Kobayashi S, Morikawa T. Small symptomatic pericardial diverticula treated by video-assisted thoracic surgical resection. Ann Thorac Cardiovasc Surg. 2009;15(2):123–5.

30 Extracardiac Complications

Farhood Saremi

There are approximately one million adult patients with congenital heart disease (CHD) in the United States and the number is increasing. With increasing survival of repaired CHD, it is more common to see both the cardiac and extracardiac complications of surgical repair. Awareness of these common extracardiac findings will aid in making the appropriate diagnosis and may improve clinical management. Utilization of CT and MR can detect early changes in extracardiac organs. This chapter describes common extracardiac manifestations of congenital disease of the heart and reviews the CT and MR findings in this group of patients. Imaging examples of pulmonary, abdominal, neurological, and thromboembolic complications will be presented. Patients with surgical single-ventricle palliative physiology (Fontan circulation) present a unique spectrum of complications including restrictive lung function, plastic bronchitis, liver changes, thromboembolic disease, and protein-losing enteropathy. These complications will be emphasized.

F. Saremi, MD
Department of Radiology, Cardiothoracic Section,
University of Southern California,
USC Keck Hospital, 1500 San Pablo St,
Los Angeles, CA 90033, USA
e-mail: fsaremi@usc.edu

Pulmonary Complications

Pulmonary complications in CHD are common. CHD patients are at greater risk of respiratory tract infections, airway obstruction, pulmonary hypertension, and thromboembolic complications. In these patients the normal interdependent relationship between the functions of the cardiovascular and respiratory systems can be lost. The ability of the heart to increase systemic and/or pulmonary blood flow is often limited, arterial PO_2 may be decreased by shunt lesions, and O_2 delivery cannot meet the needs of the tissues.

Airway Obstruction

Airway obstruction in patients with CHD can be the result of an anomalous relationship between the tracheobronchial tree and vascular structures or the result of extrinsic compression caused by dilated pulmonary arteries, left atrial enlargement, massive cardiomegaly, or intrinsic bronchial obstruction [1, 2]. Intrinsic airway findings include cartilaginous deficiency, bronchial stenosis, or mucus plugs [2].

Cardiac anomalies which predispose to airway compression by markedly dilated pulmonary arteries include ventricular septal defect (VSD), patent ductus arteriosus (PDA), atrial septal defect (ASD), interruption of the aortic arch, and tetralogy of Fallot (TOF) [3]. In unrepaired CHD patients with left-to-right shunting of blood, increased pulmonary blood flow and venous return may result in left ventricular diastolic dysfunction

F. Saremi (ed.), *Cardiac CT and MR for Adult Congenital Heart Disease*,
DOI 10.1007/978-1-4614-8875-0_30, © Springer Science+Business Media New York 2014

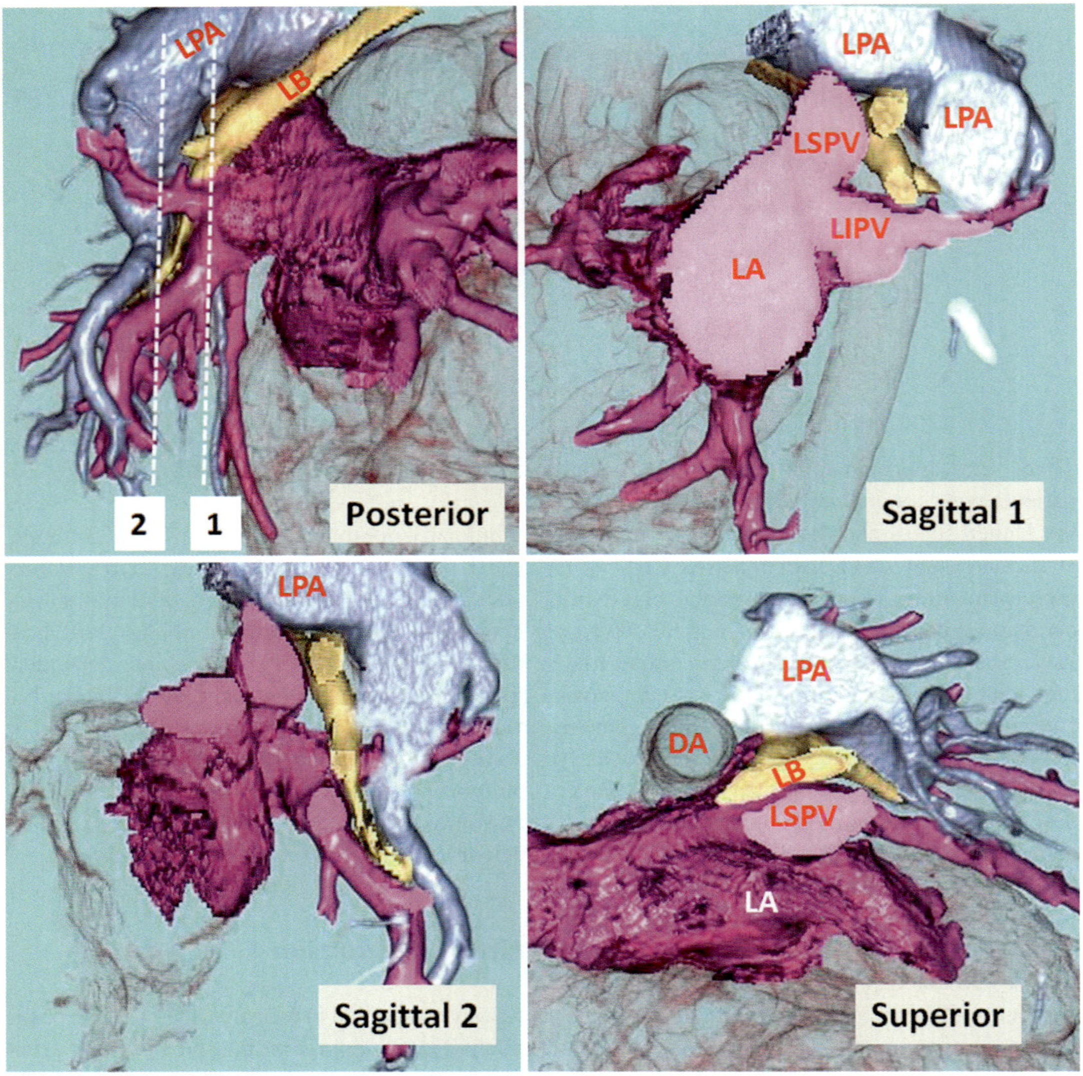

Fig. 30.1 Color-coded CT angiography of chest shows the left main bronchus (*LB*) surrounded by the left pulmonary veins, branches of the left pulmonary artery (*LPA*), and the left atrium (*LA*). The LPA starts superior and immediately turns posterior to the left bronchus, and in the left lower lobe mainly remains posteriorly. The left superior pulmonary vein (*LSPV*) courses anterior to the left bronchus. At left paramedian level (sagittal 1), the left bronchus can easily be squeezed by enlarged vessels causing left lung or left lower lobe atelectasis. An enlarged LA can increase the bronchial compression by elevating the left pulmonary veins. Sagittal 2 image is obtained through left lower lobe branches. *DA* descending aorta, *LIPV* left inferior pulmonary vein

and dilated cardiomyopathy. CHD children with left-to-right shunt often experience respiratory symptoms, which can complicate the management in the preoperative and perioperative periods [2]. An important cause of respiratory insufficiency in such children is external compression by congenital anomalies of the configuration of the great vessels and enlargement of otherwise normal structures [2, 3]. Furthermore, pulmonary venous congestion leads to edema of the bronchiolar mucosa. This in turn leads to bronchiolar spasm and the creation of obstruction [4].

Enlarged left atrium can result in widening of the tracheal bifurcation with or without compression of the main stem bronchi. Enlarged pulmonary arteries and the left atrium together can cause left bronchial compression (Fig. 30.1). Massive cardiomegaly can also compress the left main bronchus and in some cases results in chronic atelectasis and bronchiectasis of the left lower lobe. Malacia and stricture of airway can occur with chronic compression of tracheobronchial tree by anomalous aortic arch and vascular rings [5]. In pulmonary artery slings, the left pulmonary artery arises from the right pulmonary artery and then passes leftward between the trachea and esophagus. This can result in compression of the right main stem bronchus and distal trachea. Complete cartilaginous tracheal ring is common in patients with pulmonary artery slings (ring–sling complex). These cases are generally diagnosed and surgically repaired in newborns and infants. Rare cases can present for the first time during adulthood [6]. Massive enlargement of the pulmonary arteries in Eisenmenger syndrome in association with severe compression of the trachea and main stem bronchi causes lobar atelectasis or emphysema.

Plastic Bronchitis

In this rare, potentially life-threatening condition patients present with recurrent expectoration of branching, mucoid airway casts, which vary in size. It can be found in children with underlying cardiac defects particularly post-shunt procedures with Fontan being the most common [7, 8]. Bronchial casts are acellular noninflammatory composed primarily of mucin and fibrin as compared to the eosinophilic inflammatory casts seen in the other conditions. The pathogenesis of plastic bronchitis includes hypersecretion of airway mucus, abnormalities of pulmonary lymphatic drainage, and poor cardiac output [7, 9]. CT can demonstrate bronchial casts causing partial or complete obstruction of the central airways with associated atelectasis and consolidation. Bronchiectasis and obstructive hyperinflation are usually absent [10]. The airway and lung abnormalities rapidly improve after removal of the bronchial casts.

Parenchymal Changes

Pulmonary edema is a complication of many types of primary cardiovascular diseases [7]. Obstruction of pulmonary venous drainage increases capillary pressure and results in transudation of fluid. Disease states that lead to an increased right atrial pressure impair drainage of pulmonary lymphatics resulting in fluid retention and, often, pleural effusions (right more than left). Left-to-right shunts increase pulmonary blood flow leading to water retention in the lungs.

Pulmonary emphysematous changes in CHD are usually led by airway obstruction. In a recent study by Nabo et al., the frequency of pulmonary emphysema in CHD patients with increased pulmonary blood flow due to left-to-right shunting was assessed using MDCT [11]. The emphysematous change was detected in 44 % of patients. The frequency of segmental emphysematous change in left side was higher than in right side (14.8 % vs. 6.5 %). The left main bronchus is surrounded by the left pulmonary artery, left pulmonary veins, and left atrium (Fig. 30.1). These anatomical features make the left lung vulnerable to develop lobar emphysema. Lobar emphysema due to extrinsic compression by vascular structures is often relieved by correction of the underlying cardiac or vascular defect [12].

Palliative univentricular physiology (so-called Fontan physiology) is associated with passive, non-pulsatile drainage to the pulmonary arteries. Patients typically have congested, small lungs with a restrictive pattern of lung function. The reason why lungs are smaller is unclear but may be related to previous pleurodesis in some cases [7]. Alternatively, there may be an inherent degree of pulmonary hypoplasia due to the lack of pulsatile flow to stimulate lung growth. There is also a high risk of pulmonary embolic disease in this slow-flow state.

Pectus Excavatum

Pectus excavatum is the most common congenital chest wall malformation and is usually seen as an isolated congenital abnormality. However,

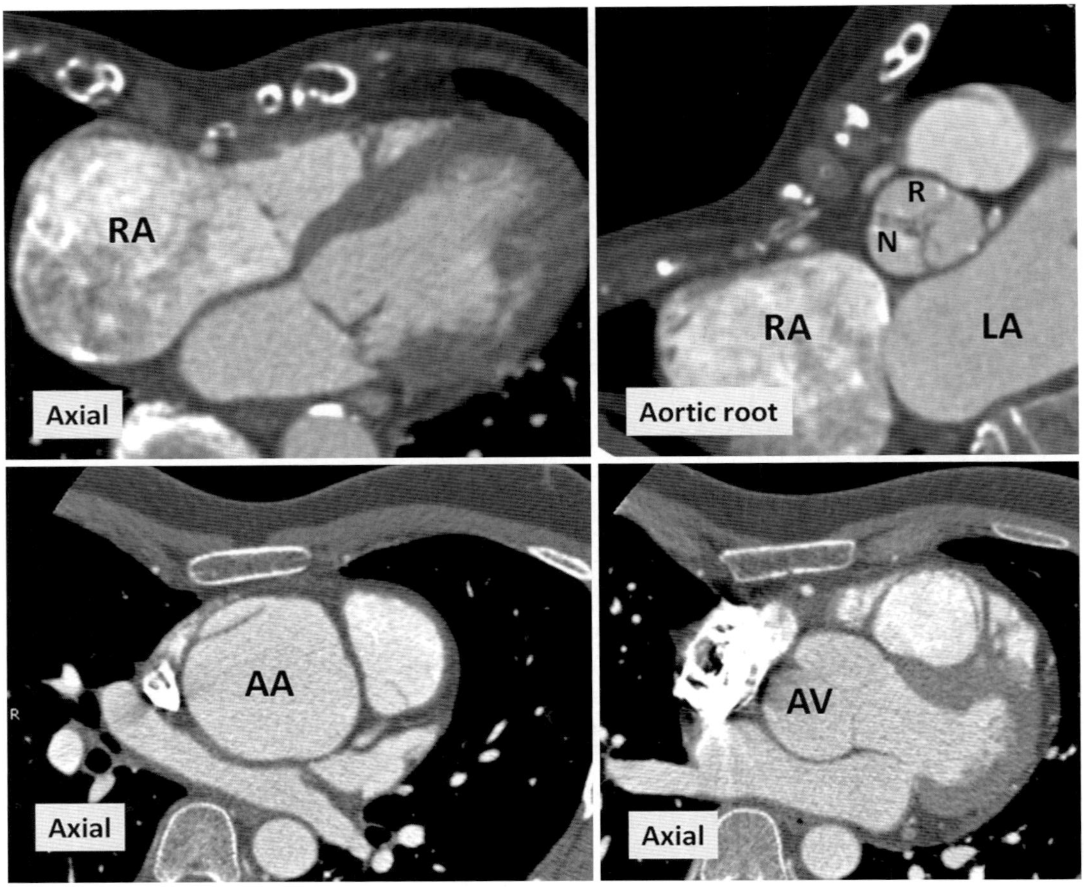

Fig. 30.2 CT images in two different patients with Marfan's syndrome and pectus excavatum. *Upper row* is a 22-year-old male with severe pectus excavatum causing right ventricle outflow tract narrowing and right atrium dilatation (*RA*). Aortic root view shows mild counterclockwise rotation of the aortic valve. *Lower row* demonstrates aortic aneurysm and focal dissection in a 24-year-old male. *AA* ascending aorta, *AV* aortic valve, *N* noncoronary sinus, *R* right coronary sinus

it is occasionally associated with cardiac abnormalities, such as Marfan's syndrome or CHD (5–10 %) [13]. Cardiac or pulmonary compression can result is restrictive lung disease and decreased right ventricle function (Fig. 30.2). Cardiac compression can also contribute to postoperative hemodynamic instability if the pectus deformity is left uncorrected during repair of the CHD. Common CHDs in association with pectus excavatum include VSD, ASD, TOF, double outlet right ventricle, transposition of the great arteries, and aortic coarctation. Aortic aneurysm and dissection are not unusual presentation (Fig. 30.2).

Intrapulmonary Vascular Collaterals and Shunts

Intrapulmonary systemic–pulmonary collaterals (SPC) develop frequently with a bidirectional cavopulmonary connections (BCPC) or Fontan circulation [14]. These systemic to pulmonary shunts usually develop between bronchial and pulmonary vessels causing arterial–arterial or venous–venous communications [15]. Both MR and CT angiography can show the extent of large collaterals. However microscopic communications are difficult to see directly. The mechanism for the development of collateral vessels in

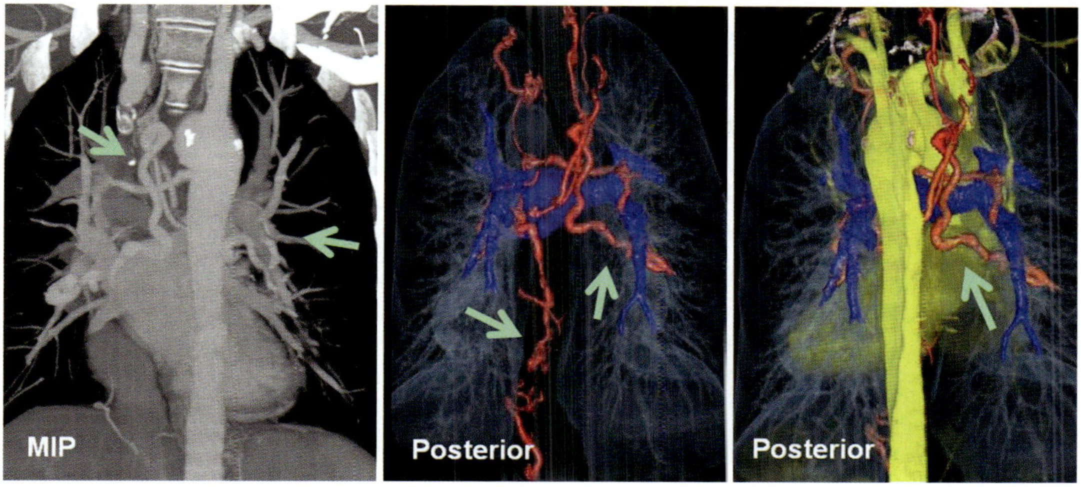

Fig. 30.3 A 35-year-old male with repaired tetralogy of Fallot presented with hemoptysis. Coronal maximum intensity pixel and color-coded multilayer CT angiography images are shown. Enlarged systemic collateral arteries (*green arrows*) arising from the descending thoracic aorta (bronchial), ascending cervical artery, left internal mammary artery, and celiac trunk supplying the lungs (*red vessels*). Pulmonary arteries are relatively small (*dark blue*)

univentricular cases is unknown. Post-Fontan patients typically have passive, non-pulsatile drainage to the pulmonary arteries. This slow-flow state may lead to the development of systemic to pulmonary collateral vessels. Vascular endothelial growth factor and or lack of hepatic venous effluent may also play a role [15–18]. SPC develops more in the lung with less pulmonary arterial flow. Left-to-right shunting via SPCs competes with volume-unloading effect of Fontan. This can contribute to increasing cyanosis, diastolic heart failure, and increased pulmonary artery pressure [19, 20]. Measurement of the magnitude and evaluation of hemodynamic consequences of these shunts are then important. The magnitude of SPC flow can be large and may approach 20–25 % of pulmonary venous return and 18–21 % of aortic output [21]. Evaluation of shunt can be difficult using routine CT or MR angiographic methods, but it can reliably be assessed with phase-contrast MR [19, 20]. It is possible to quantify APC blood flow by subtracting the pulmonary arterial from the pulmonary venous blood flow volume for each lung. For this purpose, Whitehead and colleagues [19] used two-dimensional phase-contrast MR velocity mapping to noninvasively quantify SPC in single-ventricle patients after superior BCPC. Using this method, multiple measurements should be performed at each pulmonary artery and vein levels. For correct quantification of the flow volumes during different phases of cardiac cycle, the phase-contrast sequence should have enough temporal resolution (i.e., 20 or more reconstructed phases per cardiac cycle). Appropriate velocity encoding (VENC) setting is required for correct venous and arterial flow analysis. Due to complex anatomy complete analysis may not be achieved in all patients. Newer 4D velocity mapping technique may be more reliable and even faster than two-dimensional velocity acquisition for quantitative analysis of systemic and pulmonary perfusion including SPC after palliation of single-ventricle physiology [21].

After palliative corrective surgery of TOF with pulmonary atresia, it is not uncommon to find enlarged bronchial arteries and chest wall collaterals (Fig. 30.3). Hemoptysis can result from rupture of these collaterals in to the airways. These enlarged bronchial arteries may be part of major aortopulmonary collaterals (MAPCAs) developing in patients with pulmonary atresia and VSD (i.e., tetralogy of Fallot with pulmonary valve atresia) [22]. Enlarged intercostobronchial

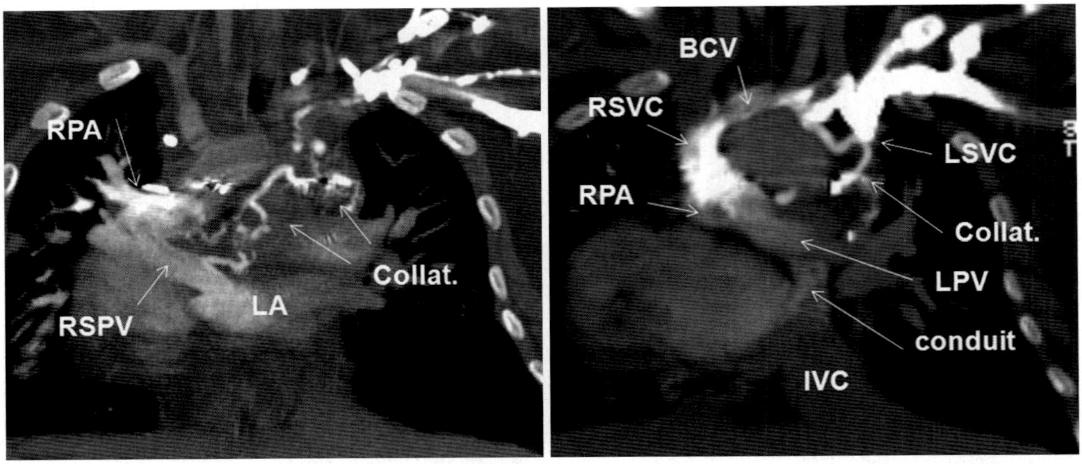

Fig. 30.4 A 17-year-old female with repaired double outlet right ventricle status post-Fontan with hemoptysis and hypoxemia and mild cyanosis. Coronal CT images after injection of contrast into left arm are shown. CT shows partial occlusion of the left brachiocephalic vein (*BCV*) and extensive mediastinal venous collateral (*collat.*) formation. There is a relatively large connection of venous collaterals with the right superior pulmonary vein (*RSPV*) causing early filling of the left atrium (*LA*) indicating a right-to-left shunt. Note the left superior vena cava (*LSVC*) is opacified and appears ligated. The right superior vena cava (*RSVC*) is connected to the right pulmonary artery (*PRA*). The inferior vena cava (*IVC*) flow is directed to the left pulmonary vein (*LPV*) by a conduit. Dextrocardia exists

arteries can be identified in 85 % and subclavian artery chest wall collaterals are seen in 50 % of MAPCAs [23]. For TOF with pulmonary atresia and MAPCAs, a staged surgical approach is usually used. The operative sequence begins with a central aortopulmonary shunt followed by unifocalization of aortopulmonary collateral arteries depending on the source and distribution of pulmonary blood flow. Embolization may be necessary for severe hemoptysis, and stenosis can be corrected with balloon angioplasty and stenting [24, 25]. With CT angiography the extent of bronchial collaterals, stenotic segments, and in selected cases the bleeding site can be detected.

Venovenous collateral vessels can develop between the two cava, the bronchial veins and the caval system, and the upper extremities veins and the pulmonary veins or the left atrium (Fig. 30.4).

Pulmonary Arteriovenous Malformations

Pulmonary arteriovenous malformations (PAVM), also referred to as pulmonary arteriovenous fistulas (PAVF), can occur after superior cavopulmonary anastomosis [26] (Fig. 30.5). Surgical connection of the superior vena cava (SVC) to the right pulmonary artery as classically described by Glenn was initially considered a satisfactory means of palliation for various forms of cyanotic CHD. Substantial morbidity and mortality from the late onset of ipsilateral PAVMs lead to modification of the procedure in which the classic Glenn procedure was replaced by BCPA. Although physiologically similar to the classic Glenn operation, BCPA has been shown to cause bilateral rather than ipsilateral PAVMs under certain conditions, but at a lower incidence [26, 27]. The main reason for the lower incidence may be that the BCPA is usually performed as part of a staged univentricular palliation, with most patients proceeding to incorporation of the inferior vena cava (IVC) and hepatic venous flow into the pulmonary circulation, namely, completion Fontan operation within 1–3 years. An exception to this pattern is the population of patients with polysplenia syndrome and azygos continuation of an interrupted IVC. Such patients commonly develop PAVMs after a Kawashima procedure (BCPA in the setting of azygos continuation of an interrupted IVC to the SVC) [28] (Fig. 30.5). In this procedure most of

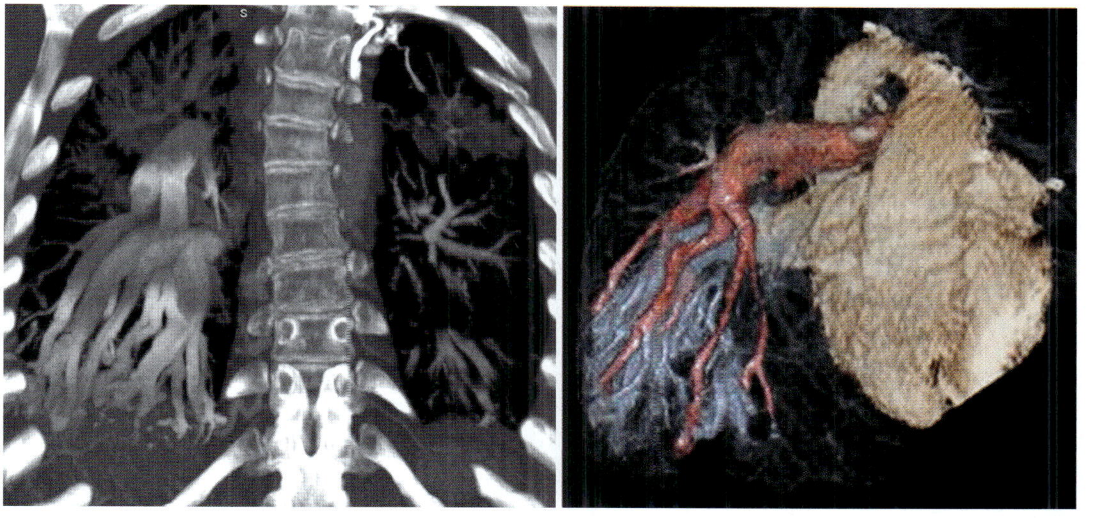

Fig. 30.5 Coronal and color-coded volume-rendered CT images of chest demonstrate extensive arteriovenous malformations (AVM) mainly in the right lower lobe in a patient with bidirectional cavopulmonary connections/Kawashima procedure presented with hypoxemia. Right AVMs did not resolve after hepatic vein inclusion into the left pulmonary circulation. Multiple coil embolizations of the AVMs had been performed before this study. Pulmonary artery branches are colored in *pink*

the systemic venous (85 %) return to the pulmonary circulation, while the hepatic and coronary sinus venous return remains to the right atrium [28]. The PAVMs seen in this population are similar to the hepatopulmonary syndrome seen in children with end-stage liver disease. In other words, exclusion of hepatic blood flow from the pulmonary blood flow contributes to the development of PAVM. In cases of bilateral SVC connections to the left and right pulmonary arteries, the relatively decreased pulmonary circulation on the opposite side to the IVC flow often results in increased AVMs on that side (right side greater than left) [29].

The primary consequence of PAVMs is decreased systemic oxygen saturation due to right-to-left shunting. Resolution of PAVMs after hepatic vein inclusion into the cavopulmonary circulation has been reported [30]. In this procedure, the hepatic veins are taken off of the atrium with a cuff of atrial tissue and anastomosed to the underside of the ipsilateral pulmonary artery with an extracardiac conduit (13–18 mm) or using a lateral caval tunnel constructed with a PTFE (Gore-Tex; W.L. Gore & Associates, Newark, DE) patch [30].

CT findings include the presence of abnormally enlarged pulmonary vessels extending to the periphery of the lung with the PAVM forming a small tangle of vessels (Fig. 30.5). The use of thick-slab (4–20 mm) maximum intensity projections (MIPs) and volume-rendering reconstructions can help detecting and characterizing PAVMs on CT [31].

Palliative Pulmonary Vascular Shunts

Surgical palliation for neonates and children with diminished pulmonary artery blood flow is usually accomplished with systemic–pulmonary artery shunts. TOF is the most common CHD cases who had a palliative shunt procedure in the past (70 %) [32]. In complex CHD, this procedure is performed before cavopulmonary connection. In CT or MR angiographic assessment of this group of adult CHD patients, it is not uncommon to see the remnant of the shunt after surgical closure or embolization or rarely an intact systemic–pulmonary artery shunt (Fig. 30.6). In some cases with history of modified or classic Blalock–Taussig shunts distortion and stenosis (up to 20 %) of the pulmonary artery at the site of the shunt anastomosis can be seen [33, 34].

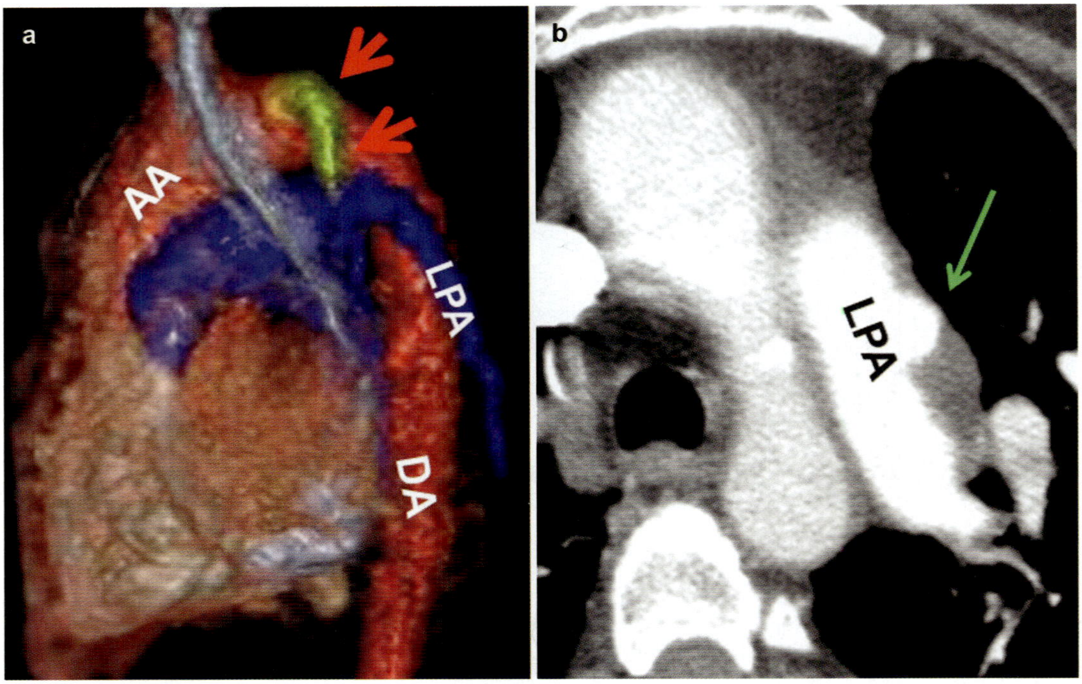

Fig. 30.6 Extracardiac palliative systemic–pulmonary shunts. (**a**) Classic Blalock–Taussig anastomotic shunt is seen between the left subclavian artery (*red arrows*) and left pulmonary artery (*LPA*) in a patient with repaired tetralogy of Fallot. (**b**) Left pulmonary artery (*LPA*) partially thrombosed aneurysm (*green arrow*) possibly at the site of a closed shunt in a patient with repaired tetralogy. *AA* ascending aorta, *DA* descending aorta

Pulmonary Hypertension

Pulmonary hypertension is defined as mean pulmonary artery pressure greater than 25 mmHg at rest, or as pulmonary vascular resistance greater than 3 Wood units. According to the current WHO classification [35], pulmonary hypertension is divided into five classes: (1) pulmonary arterial hypertension (idiopathic, veno-occlusive, etc.), (2) secondary to left heart diseases, (3) associated with lung diseases and/or hypoxemia, (4) secondary to chronic thrombotic and/or embolic disease, and (5) miscellaneous. Pulmonary hypertension associated with CHD is commonly assigned to the first category [36]. The likely mechanism behind the development of pulmonary hypertension in CHD, as in idiopathic pulmonary hypertension, is multifactorial. Vasoconstriction, proliferative and obstructive remodeling of the pulmonary vascular bed, inflammation, and thrombosis all appear to be involved [35, 37]. If pulmonary vascular resistance increases to the point where pulmonary artery pressure exceeds systemic blood pressure, right ventricular diastolic and systolic function decrease acutely and can rapidly progress to right ventricular dilation, dysfunction, and failure [38, 39]. Among Eisenmenger patients, the response of the right ventricle tends to resemble idiopathic pulmonary hypertension in those with pretricuspid defects (ASD) causing atrial and right ventricle dilatation [39]. However, in Eisenmenger patients secondary to a large VSD, the right ventricle is able to sustain an elevated afterload over a much longer period of time and becomes hypertrophied [38]. The rate of progression of pulmonary arterial disease in patients with large VSDs and PDAs is generally faster. A large ASD may also induce an increase in pulmonary arterial pressure but at much slower rate and only rarely result in severe pulmonary hypertension early in life (Fig. 30.7). Eisenmenger syndrome demonstrates pulmonary vascular changes

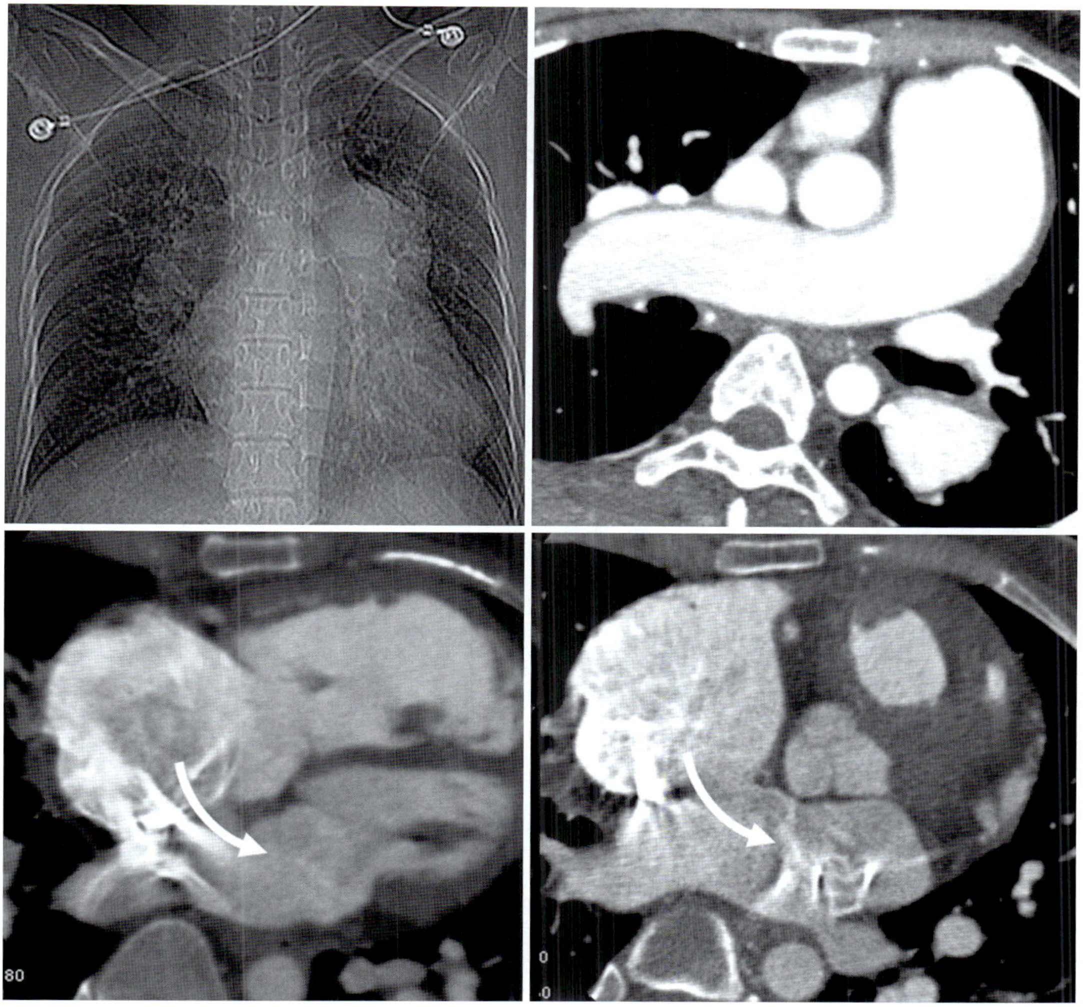

Fig. 30.7 Typical findings of Eisenmenger syndrome in a patient with large atrial septal defect (*arrows*). Enlarged pulmonary arteries, dilated hypertrophic right ventricle, and dilated right atrium are evident. The left atrium is mildly dilated and left ventricle is normal in size

on CT which is similar to idiopathic pulmonary hypertension. These changes include centrilobular ground-glass opacities, mosaicism, and neovascularity [40]. Neovascularity due to enlarged bronchial arteries and intercostal systemic collaterals are more common in patients with Eisenmenger syndrome especially in posttricuspid communications [41] (Fig. 30.8). However, there is no correlation between these findings and severity of pulmonary hypertension [40]. Mosaic attenuation due to pulmonary hypertension can be optimally seen on minimum-intensity projection reconstructions CT angiographies (Fig. 30.9) [42]. In the presence of severe pulmonary hypertension, intrapulmonary hemorrhage can be life-threatening. In mild cases, pulmonary hemorrhage may resolve in a few days.

Thromboembolic Complications

Eisenmenger syndrome typically results in severe dilation of the pulmonary arteries, sluggish flow, and mural thrombus formation of the

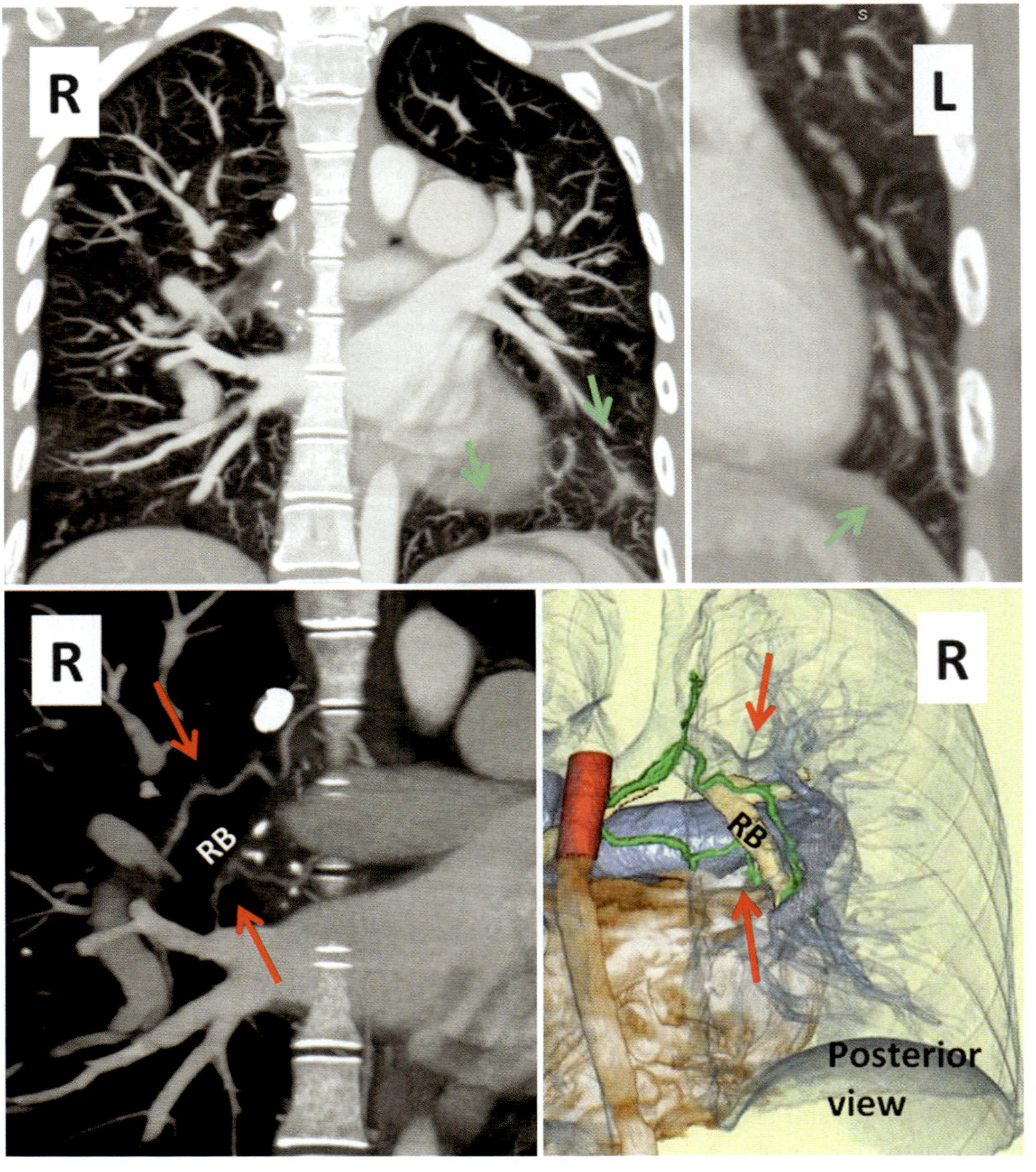

Fig. 30.8 Coronal CT images show systemic to pulmonary collaterals (SPC) in Eisenmenger syndrome. These collaterals develop between bronchial and/or chest wall intercostal arteries on the systemic side and the intraparenchymal pulmonary arteries (*green arrows*). *Upper row* images show multiple tortuous small collateral arteries best shown in the left lower lung extending to the chest wall (*green arrows*). *Lower row* images show enlarged bronchial arteries (*red arrows*) along the right bronchus (*RB*)

central pulmonary arteries affecting 20–30 % of patients [43, 44]. Pulmonary artery calcifications are seen more frequently in patients with pulmonary thrombosis. Women and patients with lower oxygen saturations are at the highest risk of developing thrombosis [44]. Thrombosis of the central pulmonary arteries may be the source for peripheral pulmonary thrombi and

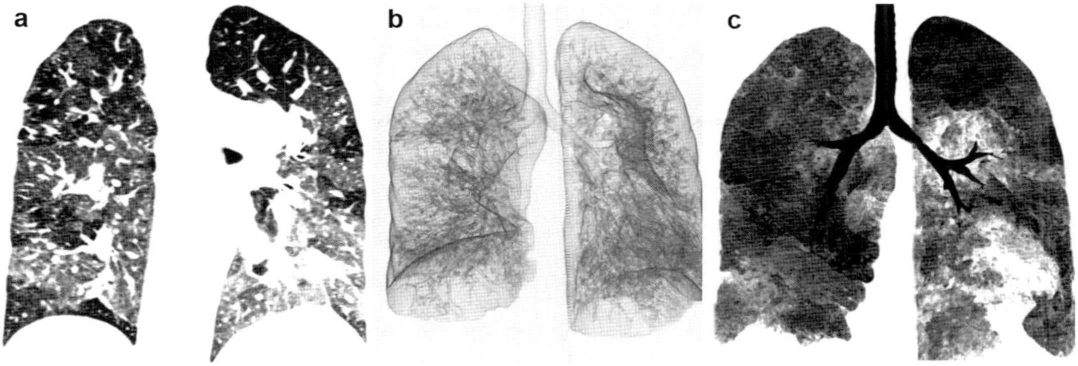

Fig. 30.9 Mosaic attenuation of the lungs in Eisenmenger syndrome. (**a**) Maximum intensity pixel. (**b**) Three-dimensional minimum-intensity pixel. (**c**) Coronal thin slab minimum-intensity pixel. Note improved demonstration of the abnormal perfusion with minimum-intensity pixel technique

pulmonary infarction leading to hemoptysis. CT angiography of chest can provide information about the size of pulmonary arteries and the presence of in situ thrombosis, as well as right ventricular dimensions and function and associated cardiac or extracardiac lesions. It is shown by MRI that pulmonary arterial thrombosis among adults with Eisenmenger syndrome relates to older age, biventricular dysfunction, and slow pulmonary artery blood flow rather than degree of cyanosis or coagulation abnormalities [45].

Thrombosis of the right-sided circulation and chronic pulmonary embolic disease are complications of single-ventricle palliative procedures with an incidence of 5–16 % [46] (Figs. 30.10 and 30.11). The increased risk of thromboembolic complications in this patient population is thought to be multifactorial. Ligation of the pulmonary trunk results in a blind cul-de-sac distal to the pulmonary valve where thrombi can form. The pulmonary blood flow after these procedures is passive and dependent on the transpulmonary gradient between the pulmonary artery and left atrium. The classic Fontan circuit is associated with right atrial dilatation and slow flow, increasing the risk of atrial thrombus [47] (Fig. 30.10). Though the lateral tunnel and extracardiac conduit Fontan modifications result in better streaming of blood flow between the IVC and pulmonary artery, the risk of thromboembolism is still high [48, 49].

Infected systemic to pulmonary shunts (aortopulmonary and ventriculopulmonary) may produce septic pulmonary emboli [50]. The development of right-to-left shunts can lead to systemic embolism from a clot in the systemic vein.

When evaluating for intravascular thrombosis, first-pass imaging with CT or MR angiography is the ideal method to evaluate for intravascular filling defects. However, a high prevalence of variant vascular anatomy in this patient population, such as bilateral SVCs or interrupted IVC with polysplenia, can cause mixing of contrast and unopacified blood resulting in pseudo-filling defects that can limit evaluation for intravascular thrombus (Fig. 30.12). To keep mixing artifacts at a minimum, the site of intravenous contrast injection should be carefully selected based on a patient's known vascular anatomy. Simultaneous injection of contrast agent from more than one site, e.g., simultaneous injection of contrast agent from both an upper and a lower extremity vein to adequately opacify the Glenn and Fontan circuits, can help avoid pitfalls due to mixing artifacts when performing first-pass imaging [51]. Dual-phase imaging, with a second set of images in the equilibrium phase, can also help circumvent this problem. While this is done routinely with MR angiography, a case-by-case decision has to be made with CT angiography to keep the radiation exposure as low as reasonably possible.

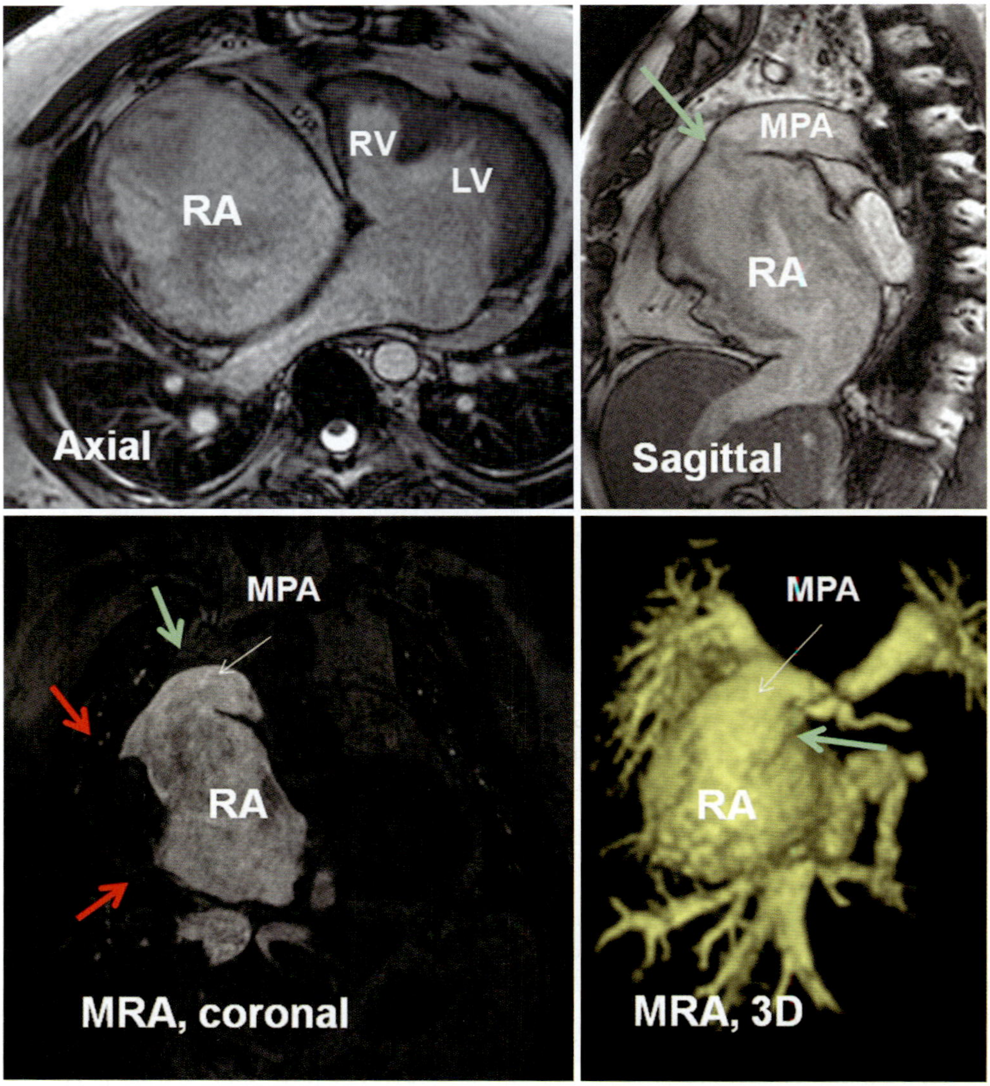

Fig. 30.10 MR images show a large right atrial mural thrombus (*red arrows*) in a 50-year-old male with tricuspid atresia, status post classic atriopulmonary Fontan. The anastomosis between the right atrium (*RA*) and main pulmonary artery (*MPA*) is shown by green arrows. The right atrium (RA) is massively enlarged. A large mural thrombus is shown along the lateral wall of right atrium (*red arrows*). Pulmonary emboli were confirmed on chest CT angiography (not shown). The right ventricle is hypoplastic and a large ventricular septal defect is seen. The tricuspid valve is absent. The MPA was disarticulated distal to the pulmonary valve (not shown). The blind pouch of MPA could also be a hidden location for thrombus formation. It was clear in this patient. Coronal and three-dimensional (*3D*) images of a right heart MR angiography (*MRA*) are presented. *LV* left ventricle, *RV* right ventricle

Paradoxical Embolism

The risk of paradoxical embolism in CHD is high and can be related to intracardiac or extracardiac shunts. Paradoxical embolism can be associated with cerebral infarct, brain abscess, fat embolism after trauma, and limb ischemia [52, 53]. In this regard CT and MR have crucial role in diagnosis of the primary cause and secondary complications of paradoxical embolism. Direct

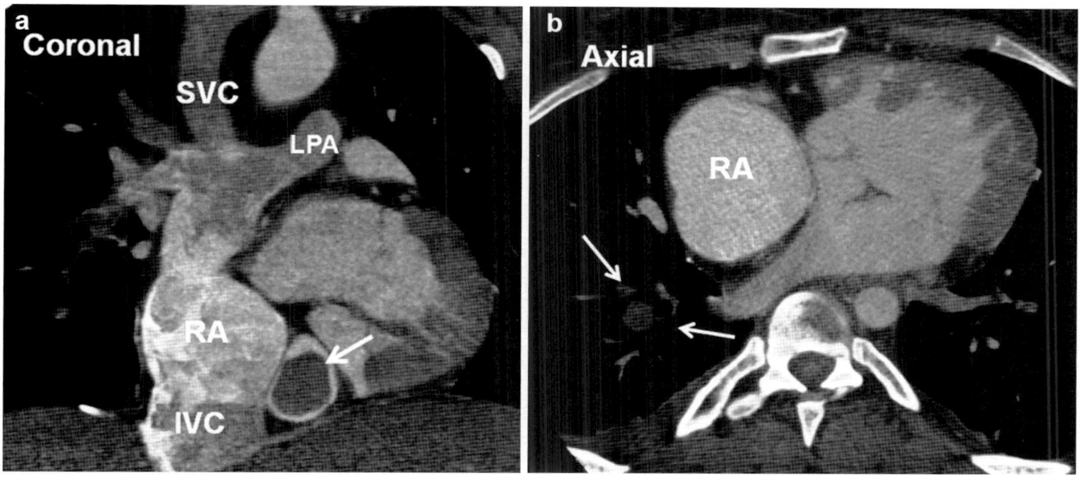

Fig. 30.11 A 22-year-old male with tricuspid atresia, status post bidirectional cavopulmonary connection (BCPC) and intracardiac Fontan presented with shortness of breath. CT angiography showed multiple pulmonary emboli (*arrows* in **b**). A large thrombus is shown in a dilated coronary sinus (*arrow* in **a**). The right atrium (*RA*) is moderately dilated. *IVC* inferior vena cava, *LPA* left pulmonary artery, *SVC* superior vena cava

assessment of an intracardiac shunt is mainly performed by echocardiography and MRI; for extracardiac shunts, CT or MR is commonly performed. However, given the widespread use of cardiac CT for other indications, it has recently gained momentum for the analysis of intracardiac shunts. An indirect diagnosis of an intracardiac shunt can also be performed by transcranial Doppler sonography.

Similar to patients with patent foramen ovale (PFO), non-cyanotic intracardiac shunts including ASD, VSD, and PDA, along with precipitating hemodynamics, can result in paradoxical embolism [52]. In a retrospective study, Bannan et al. demonstrated that 14 % of patients undergoing ASD closure for an indication of significant left-to-right shunt presented with paradoxical embolism [52]. This incidence may be higher than expected, and a diagnosis of paradoxical embolism should be considered more frequently in patients with ASD and cryptogenic stroke [52]. Cyanotic CHDs typically encompass multiple or severe structural abnormalities that allow large volumes of venous blood to shunt directly into the systemic circulation. Paradoxical embolism can complicate the problems in patients with TOF, Eisenmenger syndrome, transposition of the great arteries, and truncus arteriosus [54–57].

In repaired CHD, the presence of residual intracardiac shunts can increase the risk of paradoxical embolism. Patients with transposition of the great arteries and concomitant baffle leaks may have an increased risk of paradoxical embolism [58] (Fig. 30.13). It is important to exclude baffle leak if the patient is scheduled for intracardiac lead placement [59, 60]. A potential site of interatrial communication may be seen by cardiac CT through enlarged Thebesian veins passing along superior interatrial muscle bundle (Bachmann) between the right and left atrial appendages (Fig 30.14).

As explained earlier in this chapter, PAVMs are known complication after some types of cavopulmonary anastomoses due to the diversion of normal hepatic venous flow from the pulmonary circulation that may lead to additional complication including paradoxical embolism [61]. The risk for paradoxical embolism following a Fontan procedure with or without fenestrations has been documented [62]. Paradoxical cerebral embolus can originate on the sutures crossing the fenestration, and it is more common in large (>4 mm) fenestrations [63, 64].

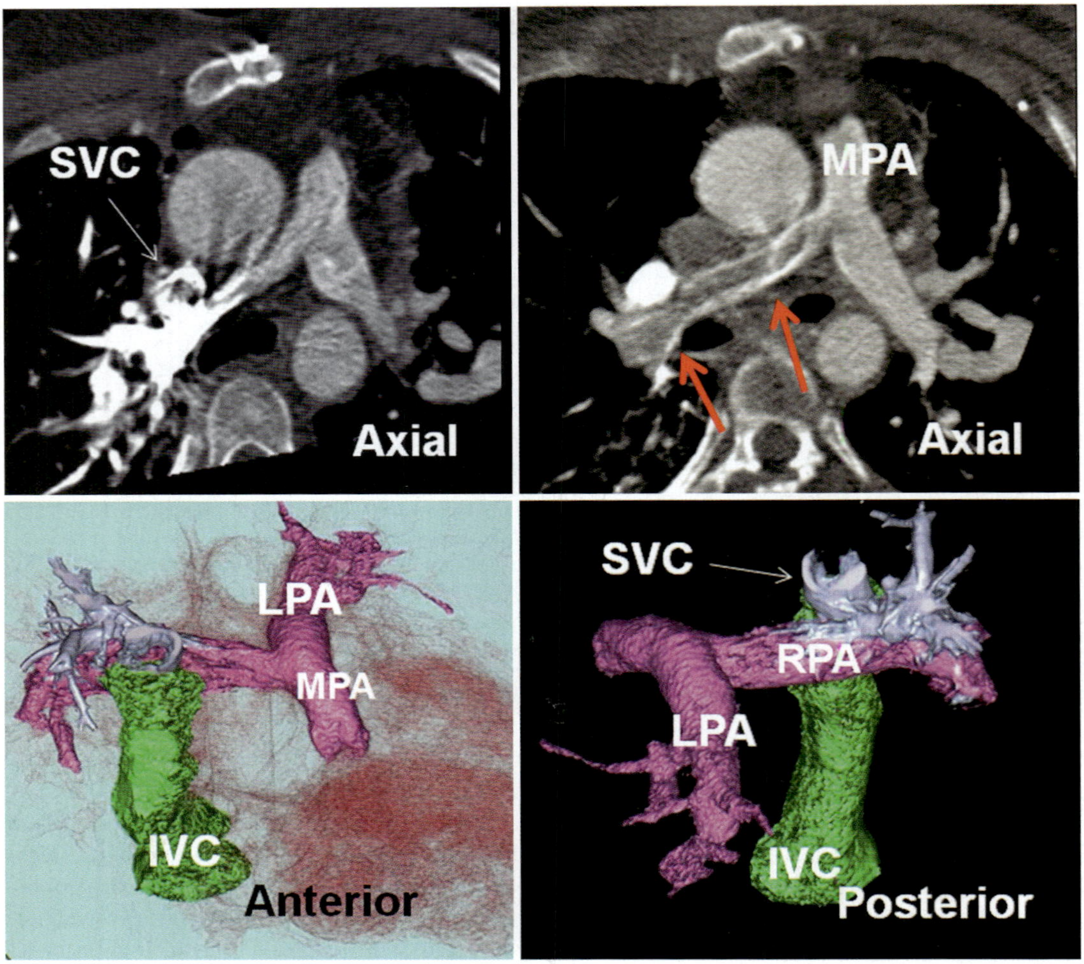

Fig. 30.12 Pseudothrombus of right pulmonary artery (*red arrows*) due to streaming of nonenhanced inferior vena cava (*IVC*) flow. In a patient with bidirectional Glenn and extracardiac Fontan (*green* structure) for pulmonary atresia. Axial CT scans and color-coded images are presented. Injection of contrast is performed in the right arm causing severe enhancement of the superior aspect of right pulmonary artery (shown in *blue* in color images). The inferior margin remained nonopacified (*red arrows*) due to streaming of noncontrast blood of the IVC entering the right pulmonary artery (*RPA*) by extracardiac Fontan tunnel (*green* structure). To avoid this problem simultaneous contrast injection into the upper and lower extremity veins may be necessary. *LPA* left pulmonary artery, *MPA* main pulmonary artery, *SVC* superior vena cava

One important role of CT or MR in the evaluation of paradoxical embolism is to exclude any anomalous venous drainage which may remain undetected in previous imaging studies using echocardiography. Among the list of congenital causes of right-to-left shunting, anomalous drainage of the left SVC into the right atrium and fenestrated coronary sinus should be investigated. A persistent left SVC usually drains into the coronary sinus is usually an incidental finding of no physiological significance. In less than 10 % of cases, however, the persistent left SVC will drain into the left atrium, either directly or through an unroofed coronary sinus, creating a right-to-left shunt [65] (see Fig. 26.11).

Large collateral mediastinal veins causing a visible right-to-left shunt (systemic to pulmonary venous shunt) and paradoxical embolism can

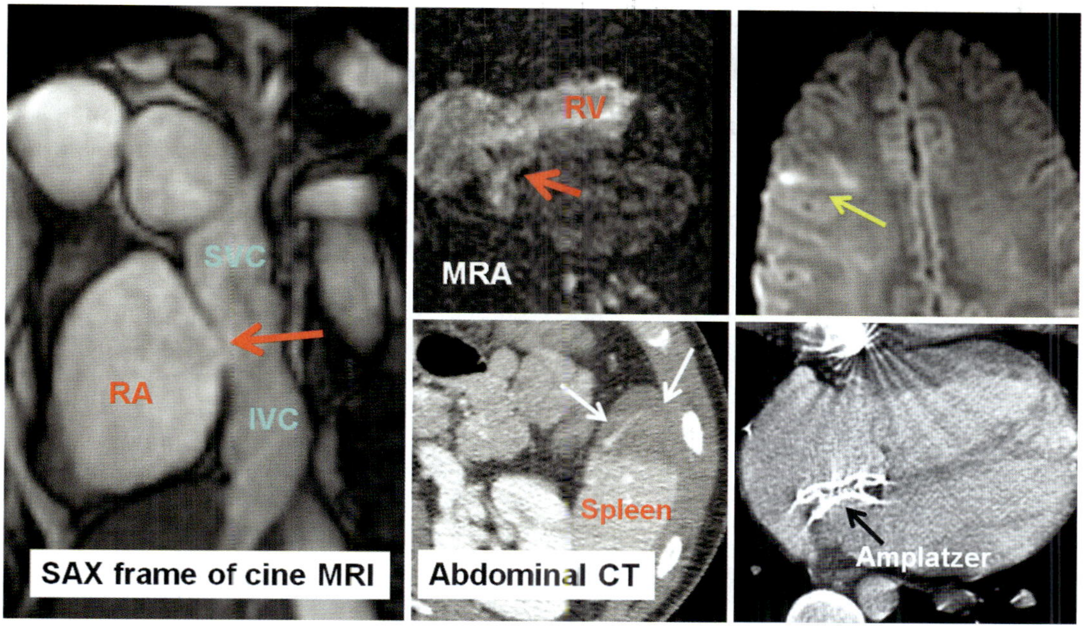

Fig. 30.13 A 24-year-old male with transposition of great arteries status post-Mustard operation evaluated for the cause of brain infarction. MRI of brain showed embolic infarct in the distribution of middle cerebral artery (*yellow arrow*) and CT scan of the abdomen showed anterior splenic infarction (*white arrows*). A large baffle defect was shown by MRI (*red arrows*) which subsequently closed with a transcatheter Amplatzer device (shown in CT of chest). *IVC* inferior vena cava, *MRA* magnetic resonance angiography, *RA* right atrium, *RV* right ventricle, *SAX* short axis, *SVC* superior vena cava

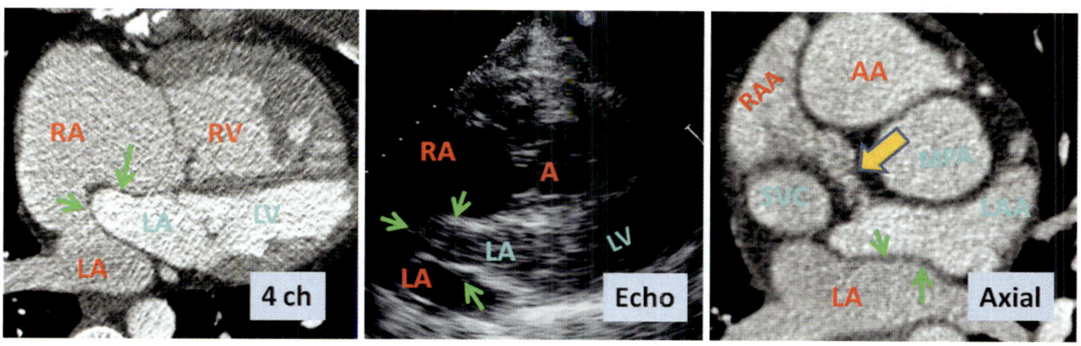

Fig. 30.14 A 32-year-old female status post-Mustard for transposition of great arteries (TGA) showing an intact baffle (*green arrows*) on both four-chamber (*4ch*) CT and left ventricle outflow view of post agitated saline contrast-enhanced echocardiography (*echo*). Echo also showed early entrance of the bubbles into the systemic atrium but could not find the reason. A CT was ordered. CT showed a small shunt between medial wall of the right atrial appendage (*RAA*) and the left atrial appendage (*LAA*) lumen through enlarged Thebesian veins passing along Bachmann bundle (*large arrow*). Thebesian veins are common around the superior cavoatrial junction and within the interatrial muscle bundle. In this patient these small vessels are markedly enlarged possibly due to chronically increased right atrial pressure. *A* aortic valve, *AA* ascending aorta, *LA* left atrium, *LV* left ventricle, *MPA* main pulmonary artery, *RA* right atrium, *RV* right ventricle, *SVC* superior vena cava

develop with stenosis, thrombosis, or absence of the left brachiocephalic vein and severe stenosis or occlusion of the SVC [66]. The collateral venous pathways frequently extend between the left brachiocephalic vein and left atrium through an arcade comprising the left superior intercostal vein or left vertical vein and a pulmonary vein to the left atrium. These collateral pathways can best be shown by CT (Fig. 30.4).

MR and CT have been used for the assessment of ASDs before and after transcatheter closure of the defect and demonstrated some advantages over transesophageal echocardiography [67, 68]. For example, the presence of a short limbus which can be easily shown with CT scan may interfere with appropriate placement of the closure device and can increase complications such as dislodgment of closure device or injury of adjacent structures such the aortic root.

Hepatic Complications

Hepatic complications are common in CHD and usually occur secondary to persistent chronic passive venous congestion or decreased cardiac output due to the underlying cardiac disease [69]. Chronic passive systemic venous congestion in the Fontan circulation results from the absence of normal right ventricular pumping, increased systemic ventricular end diastolic pressure, higher transpulmonary gradient, or stenosis within the Fontan pathway. The spectrum of liver disease includes passive congestion, dilation of hepatic sinusoids, portal and sinusoidal fibrosis, cirrhosis, and rarely hepatocellular carcinoma [70, 71].

In CT or MR imaging hepatic perfusion patterns are generally classified as reticular and zonal enhancement patterns [71–73]. In reticular pattern diffuse patchy enhancement during portal venous phase is seen which can be more pronounced in the periphery of liver. Liver margin can be smooth or irregular. Zonal enhancement is identified by reticular pattern limited to the liver periphery with preservation of normal enhancement in the liver center. Zonal enhancement correlates with lower hepatic vein pressures and a lower likelihood of cardiac cirrhosis, whereas reticular enhancement is commonly associated with extensive hepatic fibrosis [71]. This appearance is similar to the hepatic congestion seen in chronic obstructive venous outflow conditions such as Budd–Chiari syndrome and constrictive pericarditis. Hypervascular nodules occur frequently when there is congestive hepatopathy. This form of regenerative nodules has an imaging appearance similar to that of focal nodular hyperplasia of the liver. Patients with nodules have higher mean right atrial pressures [74]. Single-ventricle patients have higher incidence of nonalcoholic cirrhosis than those without a CHD (4 % vs. 0.3 %) [68]. There have been increasing reports of hepatocellular carcinoma in Fontan hepatopathy and correlates with the duration of the Fontan circuit [74–76]. Regenerative nodules are usually peripherally located and measure less than 2 cm in size

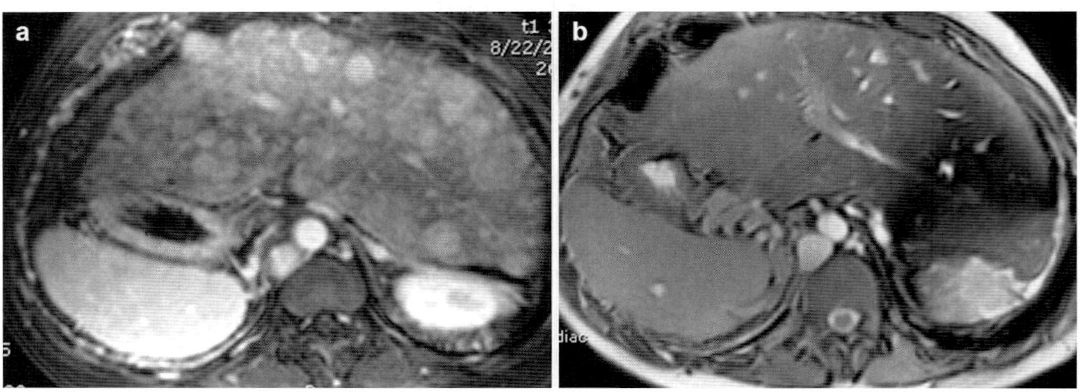

Fig. 30.15 MRI of abdomen in a patient with bidirectional Glenn. Situs inversus is seen. (**a**) Arterial phase MR angiography shows multiple enhancing liver nodules consistent with nodular hyperplasia. Also shown is mild reticular enhancement of the liver. (**b**) T2-weighted MR shows homogenous liver parenchyma. The spleen appears normal. Azygos continuation of inferior vena cava was documented

(Fig. 30.15). The lesions are typically isointense to liver on precontrast images, enhancing on arterial phase with no washout on portal and equilibrium phases and retain contrast on delayed images obtained 1–3 h after injection of gadolinium- BOPTA (Multihance®) or 30 min after injection of gadoxetate disodium (Eovist®). In contrast, hepatocellular carcinoma washes out contrast and becomes hypointense on delayed images [72, 73].

Protein-Losing Enteropathy

Protein-losing enteropathy is a rare but life-threatening complication after the Fontan operation [77]. It is characterized by hypoalbuminemia secondary to the excessive loss of proteins from the intestinal lumen. In a multicenter study of 114 children with protein-losing enteropathy after the Fontan procedure, the median age at diagnosis was 11.7 years [78]. Clinical manifestations include peripheral edema, ascites, pleural/pericardial effusions secondary to hypoalbuminemia, diarrhea secondary to malabsorption, and hypocalcemia.

Neurological Changes in CHD

Recent MR studies have demonstrated a high prevalence of preoperative and postoperative brain injury in neonates with CHD [79–83]. Cerebral lesions occur in 30–50 % of neonates and consist of focal ischemic lesions (stroke), white matter injuries (WMI), and intraventricular hemorrhages; delayed brain maturation also may occur. Multiple factors are likely to contribute to brain injury in patients with CHD [80]. In the past, attention has largely been focused on methods of surgery and perfusion strategies adopted at the time of operation [82–85]. It is now recognized that variation in intraoperative management fails to account for the majority of variability in neurodevelopmental outcomes. More recently the focus has expanded to include preoperative events and prenatal brain development [79].

The predominant preoperative cerebral MR abnormality is WMI, with infarction, hemorrhage, and abnormalities of maturation also seen [81, 82, 86]. MR spectroscopy reveals elevated brain lactate in 50 % [82]. WMI is the most common type of injury after surgery in young infants with CHD and has been associated with hypoxemia and hypotension [76]. WMI has also been described before surgery and is sometimes labeled periventricular leukomalacia [82, 83]. Periventricular leukomalacia is necrosis of the cerebral white matter adjacent to the lateral ventricles in premature infants and may evolve into cystic lesions over time. This type of damage could be different from WMI. The WMI described before and after surgery in term infants with CHD does not appear to undergo the same radiologic and clinical evolution as periventricular leukomalacia in premature infants. Resolution of these lesions is common 4–6 months after surgery. Both conditions, however, relate to the vulnerability of immature oligodendrocytes to ischemic injury during the first few weeks of life [83, 87].

Many brain studies have focused on children with transposition of the great arteries (TGA) because this condition is common, has relatively standard anatomy and surgical repair, and is rarely associated with genetic syndromes. Despite the fact that repair has a low mortality and is usually straightforward, longitudinal follow-up studies have demonstrated neurodevelopmental and learning difficulties in school-aged children who underwent the arterial switch operation in infancy. Approximately one-half have deficits in at least one domain and one-third require remedial academic assistance [79, 80]. McQuillen et al. [88] reported preoperative MRI abnormalities in 40 % of infants with TGA, with the predominant injury—in contrast to other groups with CHD—being arterial ischemic stroke (75 %). In these infants, brain injury was strongly associated with balloon atrial septostomy (BAS). However, a more recent study by Beca et al. showed no association between BAS and brain injury in infants with TGA [89]. Another common pattern in MRI of TGA infants is WMI in 30 % of patients. There seems a trend toward increased brain injury in

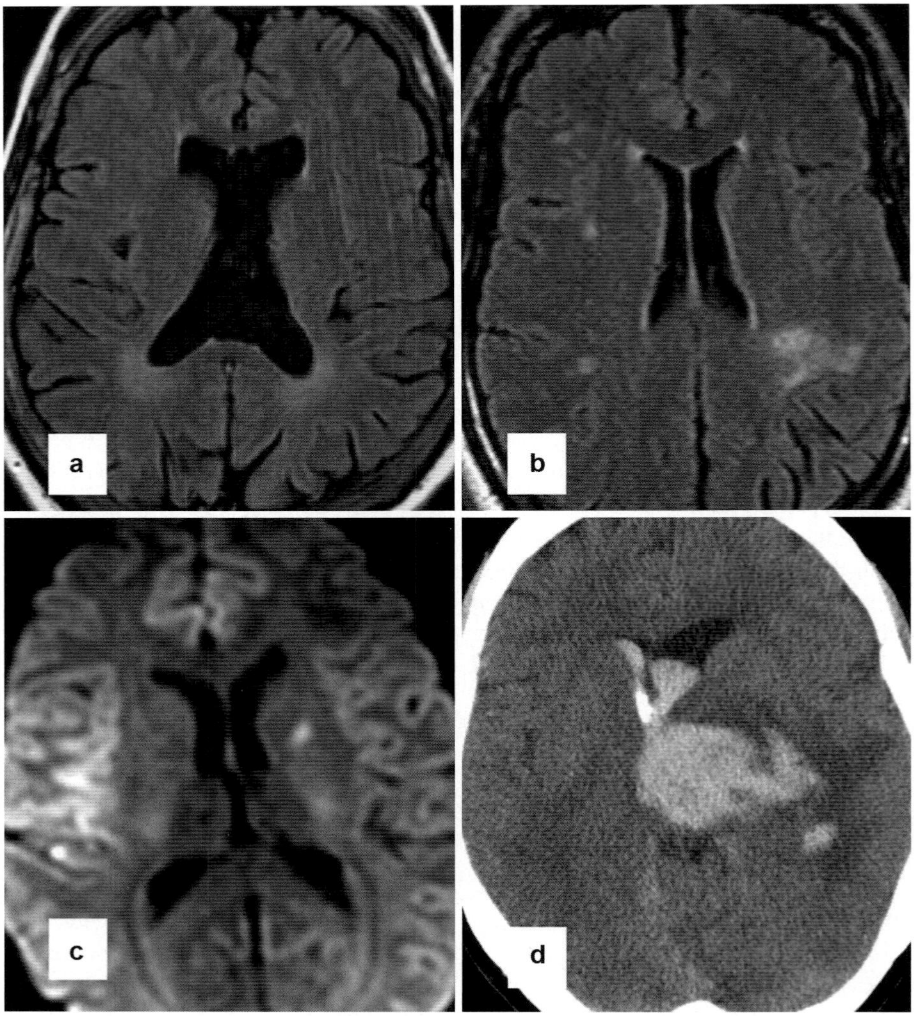

Fig. 30.16 Various neurological complications in adult patients with congenital heart disease. (**a**) T2-weighted MRI shows brain volume loss in a 53-year-old female with unrepaired tetralogy of Fallot (TOF). (**b**) T2-weighted MRI shows multiple white matter degenerative lesions in a 50-year-old male with repaired TOF. (**c**) Diffusion-weighted MRI shows right middle cerebral cortical infarct and left ganglionic lesion due to paradoxical emboli through a baffle defect after atrial switch for transposition of great arteries. (**d**) CT shows extensive intracranial hemorrhage a few days after cardiac catheterization for the assessment of arteriovenous malformation in a 21-year-old post-Fontan patient

TGA with an intact interventricular septum compared with TGA with a ventricular septal defect (38 % vs. 8 %) [89]. Neurologic deficits are common after the Norwood procedure for hypoplastic left heart syndrome and in patients with Fontan operation. Although preoperative MRI usually shows brain lesions in 23 % of patients, postoperative MRI demonstrates new or worsened ischemic and WMI lesions in 73 % of patients (Fig. 30.16). The use of deep hypothermic circulatory arrest (DHCA) seems to play a role in poor neurologic and developmental outcome [90]. The long-term functional impact of these lesions is not clear. Previous studies of patients after the Fontan operation have reported IQ scores lower than population norms. With newer staged approach to Fontan earlier in life, neurodevelopmental outcome appears to be in normal range, although performance remains lower than the general population [91].

Follow-up MR studies have shown cerebral abnormalities in 20 % of adolescents with corrected CHD likely acquired during the neonatal period [92]. On MRI, the majority of findings involve mild white matter changes, such as small patchy T2 hyperintensities in the deep white matter of the corona radiata and at the border of the frontal gray matter and white matter. Diffuse T2 hyperintensity is not common, but varying degrees of white matter atrophy as well as periventricular or cortical volume loss can be seen leading to ventricular enlargement or punctual cystic lesions. Some patients may show poststroke changes involving cortical defects with adjacent enlargement of the subarachnoid space, corresponding to a vascular distribution (Fig. 30.16). Follow-up MR study has shown that the frequency of brain lesions in adults is less than neonates with CHD [92]. It appears that a considerable proportion of the focal changes seen in the neonatal period becomes less visible over time and that the only visible residue of these acute changes could be the white matter volume loss. The lower incidence of brain lesions in MR studies of adolescents with CHD may also be attributed to patients with less severe forms of CHD compared with populations in neonatal MRI studies. Overall, the more common finding in repaired CHD patients in school-age group is brain volume loss not the signal changes.

As explained earlier thromboembolic lesion including those from paradoxical embolism may be the cause of additional brain damage in older patients with CHD (Fig. 30.16). Brain abscesses are reported in cyanotic CHD with the tetralogy of Fallot being the most common. Abscess are usually in frontal and parietal lobes and multiple in one-third of cases [93].

References

1. Kussman BD, Geva T, McGowan FX. Cardiovascular causes of airway compression. Paediatr Anaesth. 2004;14:60–74.
2. Berlinger NT, Long C, Foker J, Lucas Jr RV. Tracheobronchial compression in acyanotic congenital heart disease. Ann Otol Rhinol Laryngol. 1983;92:387–90.
3. Castañer E, Gallardo X, Rimola J, et al. Congenital and acquired pulmonary artery anomalies in the adult: radiologic overview. Radiographics. 2006;26(2):349–71.
4. Nakagawa R, Saijo T, Kagami S. Tracheal compression due to an elongated aortic arch in patients with congenital heart disease: evaluation using multidetector-row CT. Pediatr Radiol. 2009;39:1048–53.
5. Conti VR, Lobe TE. Vascular sling with tracheomalacia: surgical management. Ann Thorac Surg. 1989;47(2):310–1.
6. Lee JC, Kim GS, Lee SJ, et al. An adult case of pulmonary sling with complete tracheal ring. Korean J Intern Med. 1996;11(2):175–7.
7. Healy F, Hanna BD, Zinman R. Pulmonary complications of congenital heart disease. Paediatr Respir Rev. 2012;13(1):10–5.
8. Tzifa A, Robards M, Simpson JM. Plastic bronchitis; a serious complication of the Fontan operation. Int J Cardiol. 2005;101(3):513–4.
9. Watanabe K, Ishida T, Sugawara A, Tachihara M, Munakata M. An adult case of plastic bronchitis. Intern Med. 2008;47(17):1549.
10. Goo HW, Jhang WK, Kim YH, et al. CT findings of plastic bronchitis in children after a Fontan operation. Pediatr Radiol. 2008;38:989–93.
11. Nabo MM, Hayabuchi Y, Sakata M, Ohnishi T, Kagami S. Pulmonary emphysematous changes in patients with congenital heart disease associated with increased pulmonary blood flow: evaluation using multidetector-row computed tomography. Heart Lung Circ. 2011;20(9):587–92.
12. Moideen I, Nair SG, Cherian A, Rao SG. Congenital lobar emphysema associated with congenital heart disease. J Cardiothorac Vasc Anesth. 2006;20(2): 239–41.
13. Willekes CL, Backer CL, Mavroudis C. A 26-year review of pectus deformity repairs, including simultaneous intracardiac repair. Ann Thorac Surg. 1999;67(2):511–8.
14. Triedman JK, Bridges ND, Mayer JE, Lock JE. Prevalence and risk factors for aortopulmonary collateral vessels after Fontan and bidirectional Glenn procedures. J Am Coll Cardiol. 1993;22:207–15.
15. Kanter KR, Vincent RN, Raviele AA. Importance of acquired systemic-to- pulmonary collaterals in the Fontan operation. Ann Thorac Surg. 1999;68:969–74.
16. Ichikawa H, Yagihara T, Kishimoto H, Isobe F, Yamamoto F, Nishigaki K, Matsuki O, Fujita T. Extent of aortopulmonary collateral blood flow as a risk factor for Fontan operations. Ann Thorac Surg. 1995;59:433–7.
17. McElhinney DB, Reddy VM, Tworetzky W, Petrossian E, Hanley FL, Moore P. Incidence and implications of systemic to pulmonary collaterals after bidirectional cavopulmonary anastomosis. Ann Thorac Surg. 2000;69:1222–8.
18. Mori Y, Shoji M, Nakanishi T, Fujii T, Nakazawa M. Elevated vascular endothelial growth factor levels are

associated with aortopulmonary collateral vessels in patients before and after the Fontan procedure. Am Heart J. 2007;153:987–94.
19. Whitehead KK, Gillespie MJ, Harris MA, Fogel MA, Rome JJ. Noninvasive quantification of systemic-to-pulmonary collateral flow: a major source of inefficiency in patients with superior cavopulmonary connections. Circ Cardiovasc Imaging. 2009;2:405–11.
20. Grosse-Wortmann L, Al-Otay A, Yoo SJ. Aortopulmonary collaterals after bidirectional cavopulmonary connection or Fontan completion: quantification with MRI. Circ Cardiovasc Imaging. 2009;2(3):219–25.
21. Valverde I, Nordmeyer S, Uribe S, et al. Systemic-to-pulmonary collateral flow in patients with palliated univentricular heart physiology: measurement using cardiovascular magnetic resonance 4D velocity acquisition. J Cardiovasc Magn Reson. 2012;14(1):25.
22. Duncan BW, Mee RB, Prieto LR, et al. Staged repair of tetralogy of Fallot with pulmonary atresia and major aortopulmonary collateral arteries. J Thorac Cardiovasc Surg. 2003;126(3):694–702.
23. Nørgaard MA, Alphonso N, Cochrane AD, Menahem S, Brizard CP, d'Udekem Y. Major aorto-pulmonary collateral arteries of patients with pulmonary atresia and ventricular septal defect are dilated bronchial arteries. Eur J Cardiothorac Surg. 2006;29(5):653–8.
24. van der Weijden P, Baur LH, Kool LJ, Vliegen HW, van der Wall EE. Embolization as a treatment of life-threatening haemoptysis in an adult with tetralogy of Fallot with pulmonary atresia. Int J Card Imaging. 1998;14(2):123–6.
25. Brown SC, Eyskens B, Mertens L, Dumoulin M, Gewillig M. Percutaneous treatment of stenosed major aortopulmonary collaterals with balloon dilatation and stenting: what can be achieved? Heart. 1998;79(1):24–8.
26. Moore JW, Kirby WC, Madden WA, et al. Development of pulmonary arteriovenous malformations after modified Fontan operations. J Thorac Cardiovasc Surg. 1989;98:1045–50.
27. Dasi LP, Whitehead K, Pekkan K, et al. Pulmonary hepatic flow distribution in total cavopulmonary connections: extracardiac versus intracardiac. J Thorac Cardiovasc Surg. 2011;141(1):207–14.
28. Brown JW, Ruzmetov M, Vijay P, et al. Pulmonary arteriovenous malformations in children after the Kawashima operation. Ann Thorac Surg. 2005;80:1592–6.
29. Kim SJ, Bae EJ, Lee JY, Lim HG, Lee C, Lee CH. Inclusion of hepatic venous drainage in patients with pulmonary arteriovenous fistulas. Ann Thorac Surg. 2009;87:548–54.
30. McElhinney DB, Kreutzer J, Lang P, et al. Incorporation of the hepatic veins into the cavopulmonary circulation in patients with heterotaxy and pulmonary arteriovenous malformations after a Kawashima procedure. Ann Thorac Surg. 2005;80(5):1597–603.
31. Choi YH, Lee W, Cheon JE, et al. CT findings in unilateral hepatopulmonary syndrome after the Fontan operation. Pediatr Radiol. 2009;39:336–42.
32. Williams JA, Bansal AK, Kim BJ, et al. Two thousand Blalock-Taussig shunts: a six-decade experience. Ann Thorac Surg. 2007;84(6):2070–5.
33. Godart F, Qureshi SA, Simha A, et al. Effects of modified and classic Blalock-Taussig shunts on the pulmonary arterial tree. Ann Thorac Surg. 1998;66(2):512–7.
34. Reidy JF, Jones OD, Tynan MJ, Baker EJ, Joseph MC. Embolisation procedures in congenital heart disease. Br Heart J. 1985;54(2):184–92.
35. McLaughlin VV, Archer SL, Badesch DB, et al. ACCF/AHA 2009 expert consensus document on pulmonary hypertension: a report of the American College of Cardiology Foundation Task Force on Expert Consensus Documents and the American Heart Association: developed in collaboration with the American College of Chest Physicians, American Thoracic Society, Inc., and the Pulmonary Hypertension Association. J Am Coll Cardiol. 2009;53(17):1573–619.
36. van Albada ME, Berger RM. Pulmonary arterial hypertension in congenital cardiac disease — the need for refinement of the Evian–Venice classification. Cardiol Young. 2008;18:10–7.
37. Vogel M, Berger F, Kramer A, et al. Incidence of secondary pulmonary hypertension in adults with atrial septal or sinus venosus defects. Heart. 1999;82:30–3.
38. Dimopoulos K, Giannakoulas G, Wort SJ, Gatzoulis MA. Pulmonary arterial hypertension in adults with congenital heart disease: distinct differences from other causes of pulmonary arterial hypertension and management implications. Curr Opin Cardiol. 2008;23:545–54.
39. Van De Bruaene A, De Meester P, Voigt JU, et al. Right ventricular function in patients with Eisenmenger syndrome. Am J Cardiol. 2012;109(8):1206–11.
40. Griffin N, Allen D, Wort J, et al. Eisenmenger syndrome and idiopathic pulmonary arterial hypertension: do parenchymal lung changes reflect aetiology? Clin Radiol. 2007;62:587–95.
41. Sheehan R, Perloff JK, Fishbein MC, et al. Pulmonary neovascularity: a distinctive radiographic finding in Eisenmenger syndrome. Circulation. 2005;112:2778–85.
42. Hayabuchi Y, Inoue M, Watanabe N, Sakata M, Nabo MM, Kagami S. Minimum-intensity projection of multidetector-row computed tomography for assessment of pulmonary hypertension in children with congenital heart disease. Int J Cardiol. 2011;149(2):192–8.
43. Perloff JK, Hart EM, Greaves SM, et al. Proximal pulmonary arterial and intrapulmonary radiologic features of Eisenmenger syndrome and primary pulmonary hypertension. Am J Cardiol. 2003;92:182–7.
44. Silversides CK, Granton JT, Konen E, Hart MA, Webb GD, Therrien J. Pulmonary thrombosis in adults with Eisenmenger syndrome. J Am Coll Cardiol. 2003;42:1982–7.
45. Broberg CS, Ujita M, Prasad S, et al. Pulmonary arterial thrombosis in eisenmenger syndrome is associated with biventricular dysfunction and decreased pulmonary flow velocity. J Am Coll Cardiol. 2007;50(7):634–42.

46. Rosenthal DN, Friedman AH, Kleinman CS, Kopf GS, Rosenfeld LE, Hellenbrand WE. Thromboembolic complications after Fontan operations. Circulation. 1995;92:287–93.
47. Jacobs ML, Pelletier G. Late complications associated with the Fontan circulation. Cardiol Young. 2006;16 Suppl 1:80–4.
48. Lee SY, Baek JS, Kim GB, et al. Clinical significance of thrombosis in an intracardiac blind pouch after a Fontan operation. Pediatr Cardiol. 2012;33(1):42–8.
49. Tsang W, Johansson B, Salehian O, Holm J, Webb G, Gatzoulis MA, Therrien J. Intracardiac thrombus in adults with the Fontan circulation. Cardiol Young. 2007;17:646–51.
50. Mahar T, Katzman P, Alfieris G. A case of fatal septic pulmonary embolus arising from an infected Sano conduit. Pediatr Cardiol. 2009;30:181–3.
51. Greenberg SB, Bhutta ST. A dual contrast injection technique for multidetector computed tomography angiography of Fontan procedures. Int J Cardiovasc Imaging. 2008;24:345–8.
52. Hirsch R, Streifler JY. Stroke in congenital heart disease and patent foramen ovale. Isr Med Assoc J. 2006;8(11):798–802.
53. Bannan A, Shen R, Silvestry FE, Herrmann HC. Characteristics of adult patients with atrial septal defects presenting with paradoxical embolism. Catheter Cardiovasc Interv. 2009;74(7):1066–9.
54. Kurlan R, Griggs RC. Cyanotic congenital heart disease with suspected stroke. Should all patients receive antibiotics? Arch Neurol. 1983;40(4):209–12.
55. Yang SY. Brain abscess associated with congenital heart disease. Surg Neurol. 1989;31(2):129–32.
56. Geva T, Frand M, Benjamin P, Hegesh J. Cerebral embolization from an inferior vena cava thrombus in tetralogy of Fallot. Pediatr Cardiol. 1990;11(1):44–6.
57. Oppenheimer EH. Arterial thrombosis (paradoxical embolism) in association with transposition of the great vessels. Johns Hopkins Med J. 1969;124(4):202–10.
58. Klein AJ, Kim MS, Salcedo E, Fagan T, Kay J. The missing leak: a case report of a baffle-leak closure using real-time 3D transoesophageal guidance. Eur J Echocardiogr. 2009;10(3):464–7.
59. Kuppahally SS, Litwin SE, Green LS, Ishihara SM, Freedman RA, Michaels AD. Utility of intracardiac echocardiography for atrial baffle leak closure in repaired transposition of the great arteries. Echocardiography. 2010;27(8):E90–3.
60. Saremi F, Kang J, Rahmanuddin S, Shavelle D. Assessment of post-atrial switch baffle integrity using a modified dual extremity injection cardiac computed tomography angiography technique. Int J Cardiol. 2013;162(2):e25–7.
61. Srivastava D, Preminger T, Lock JE, et al. Hepatic venous blood and the development of pulmonary arteriovenous malformations in congenital heart disease. Circulation. 1995;92(5):1217–22.
62. Day RW, Boyer RS, Tait VF, Ruttenberg HD. Factors associated with stroke following the Fontan procedure. Pediatr Cardiol. 1995;16(6):270–5.
63. Quinones JA, Deleon SY, Bell TJ, Cetta F, Moffa SM, Freeman JE, Vitullo DA, Fisher EA. Fenestrated fontan procedure: evolution of technique and occurrence of paradoxical embolism. Pediatr Cardiol. 1997;18(3):218–21.
64. Bando K, Turrentine MW, Park HJ, Sharp TG, Scavo V, Brown JW. Evolution of the Fontan procedure in a single center. Ann Thorac Surg. 2000;69(6):1873–9.
65. Ezekowitz MD, Alderson PO, Bulkley BH, et al. Isolated drainage of the superior vena cava into the left atrium in a 52-year-old man: a rare congenital malformation in the adult presenting with cyanosis, polycythemia, and an unsuccessful lung scan. Circulation. 1978;58(4):751–6.
66. Gilkeson RC, Nyberg EM, Sachs PB, Wiant AM, Zahka KG, Siwik ES. Systemic to pulmonary venous shunt imaging findings and clinical presentations. J Thorac Imaging. 2008;23(3):170–7.
67. Rickers C, Jerosch-Herold M, Hu X, et al. Magnetic resonance image-guided transcatheter closure of atrial septal defects. Circulation. 2003;107(1):132–8.
68. Lee T, Tsai IC, Fu YC, Jan SL, Wang CC, Chang Y, Chen MC. MDCT evaluation after closure of atrial septal defect with an Amplatzer septal occluder. AJR Am J Roentgenol. 2007;188(5):W431–9.
69. Asrani SK, Asrani NS, Freese DK, et al. Congenital heart disease and the liver. Hepatology. 2012;56(3):1160–9.
70. Schwartz MC, Sullivan LM, Glatz AC, et al. Portal and sinusoidal fibrosis are common on liver biopsy after Fontan surgery. Pediatr Cardiol. 2013;34(1):135–42.
71. Kiesewetter CH, Sheron N, Vettukattill JJ, et al. Hepatic changes in the failing Fontan circulation. Heart. 2007;93(5):579–84.
72. Fredenburg TB, Johnson TR, Cohen MD. The Fontan procedure: anatomy, complications, and manifestations of failure. Radiographics. 2011;31:453–63.
73. Ginde S, Hohenwalter MD, Foley WD, et al. Noninvasive assessment of liver fibrosis in adult patients following the fontan procedure. Congenit Heart Dis. 2012;7(3):235–42.
74. Bryant T, Ahmad Z, Millward-Sadler H, et al. Arterialised hepatic nodules in the Fontan circulation: hepatico-cardiac interactions. Int J Cardiol. 2011; 151(3):268–72.
75. Krieger EV, Moko LE, Wu F, et al. Single ventricle anatomy is associated with increased frequency of nonalcoholic cirrhosis. Int J Cardiol. 2012.
76. Ghaferi AA, Hutchins GM. Progression of liver pathology in patients undergoing the Fontan procedure: chronic passive congestion, cardiac cirrhosis, hepatic adenoma, and hepatocellular carcinoma. J Thorac Cardiovasc Surg. 2005;129:1348–52.
77. Khanna G, Bhalla S, Krishnamurthy R, Canter C. Extracardiac complications of the Fontan circuit. Pediatr Radiol. 2012;42(2):233–41.
78. Mertens L, Hagler DJ, Sauer U, et al. Protein-losing enteropathy after the Fontan operation: an international multicenter study. PLE study group. J Thorac Cardiovasc Surg. 1998;115:1063–73.

79. Bird GL, Jeffries HE, Licht DJ, Wernovsky G, Weinberg PM, Pizarro C, Stellin G. Neurological complications associated with the treatment of patients with congenital cardiac disease: consensus definitions from the Multi-Societal Database Committee for Pediatric and Congenital Heart Disease. Cardiol Young. 2008;18 Suppl 2: 234–9.
80. Miller SP, McQuillen PS, Hamrick S, et al. Abnormal brain development in newborns with congenital heart disease. N Engl J Med. 2007;357:1928–38.
81. McQuillen PS, Barkovich AJ, Hamrick SE, et al. Temporal and anatomic risk profile of brain injury with neonatal repair of congenital heart defects. Stroke. 2007;38:736–41.
82. Mahle WT, Tavani F, Zimmerman RA, et al. An MRI study of neurological injury before and after congenital heart surgery. Circulation. 2002;106: I109–14.
83. Galli KK, Zimmerman RA, Jarvik GP, et al. Periventricular leukomalacia is common after neonatal cardiac surgery. J Thorac Cardiovasc Surg. 2004; 127:692–704.
84. Hovels-Gurich HH, Seghaye MC, Schnitker R, et al. Long-term neurodevelopmental outcomes in school-aged children after neonatal arterial switch operation. J Thorac Cardiovasc Surg. 2002;124:448–58.
85. Wypij D, Newburger JW, Rappaport LA, et al. The effect of duration of deep hypothermic circulatory arrest in infant heart surgery on late neurodevelopment: the Boston circulatory arrest trial. J Thorac Cardiovasc Surg. 2003;126:1397–403.
86. Miller SP, McQuillen PS, Vigneron DB, et al. Preoperative brain injury in newborns with transposition of the great arteries. Ann Thorac Surg. 2004;77: 1698–706.
87. Miller SP, Ramaswamy V, Michelson D, et al. Patterns of brain injury in term neonatal encephalopathy. J Pediatr. 2005;146:453–60.
88. McQuillen PS, Hamrick SE, Perez MJ, et al. Balloon atrial septostomy is associated with pre-operative stroke in neonates with transposition of the great arteries. Circulation. 2006;113:280–5.
89. Beca J, Gunn J, Coleman L, et al. Pre-operative brain injury in newborn infants with transposition of the great arteries occurs at rates similar to other complex congenital heart disease and is not related to balloon atrial septostomy. J Am Coll Cardiol. 2009;53(19): 1807–11.
90. Dent CL, Spaeth JP, Jones BV, et al. Brain magnetic resonance imaging abnormalities after the Norwood procedure using regional cerebral perfusion. J Thorac Cardiovasc Surg. 2006;131(1):190–7.
91. Forbess JM, Visconti KJ, Bellinger DC, Jonas RA. Neurodevelopmental outcomes in children after the Fontan operation. Circulation. 2001;104(Suppl I): 127–32.
92. von Rhein M, Scheer I, Loenneker T, Huber R, Knirsch W, Latal B. Structural brain lesions in adolescents with congenital heart disease. J Pediatr. 2011; 158(6):984–9.
93. Chakraborty RN, Bidwai PS, Kak VK, et al. Brain abscess in cyanotic congenital heart disease. Indian Heart J. 1989;41(3):190–3.

Cardiac MR in Patients with Implantable Arrhythmia Devices

31

Roy Beinart and Saman Nazarian

Magnetic resonance imaging (MRI) has become an established method of cardiovascular imaging in many clinical situations. In recent years, newer MRI techniques have been developed allowing both morphology assessment and functional evaluation of patients with congenital heart disease (CHD) [1, 2]. Furthermore, it has been shown that MRI is superior to echocardiography for certain anatomic regions due to acoustic window limitations, particularly in the pulmonary artery branches and the aortic arch in adult patients. MRI is currently established as the gold standard for measurements of ventricular volumes as well as for blood flow analysis [3–6]. These advantages coupled with the freedom from ionizing radiation make MRI an attractive noninvasive imaging tool for patients with CHD [7].

The number of patients with CHD who require pacemakers [8–12], implantable cardioverter defibrillators (ICD) [13–15], and biventricular resynchronization pacing [16–23] is constantly increasing. These trends raise a crucial clinical problem because MRI scans are generally contraindicated in patients who have implanted cardiac devices. The concern for performing MRI in the setting of implantable cardiac devices is related to the potential for current induction in leads within the scanner [24, 25], force and torque exerted upon ferromagnetic components [26], and heating and tissue damage at the lead-tissue interface [27, 28]. In addition, MRI electromagnetic inference may result in inappropriate pacing secondary to tracking, inhibition of pacing, inappropriate ICD shocks, and/or programming changes with ultimately unpredictable pacing and antitachycardia behaviors [29]. Nevertheless, some patients with CHD that have undergone device implantation stand to derive significant clinical benefit from MRI in comparison to other imaging alternatives. Therefore, strategies for safe performance of MRI in this population of cardiac device recipients are necessary. Importantly, most of the studies to date addressed the risk of MRI in the setting of implanted cardiac devices in patients without CHD. Their results, however, appear to be relevant to the adult CHD population. At the same time, there are additional unique considerations that must be taken into account when planning an MRI examination for the CHD patient with an implantable device. For example, due to abnormal venous structures and the risk of systemic embolus from residual intracardiac shunting, many CHD patients undergo epicardial rather than endocardial pacing or defibrillator lead/patch implantation. As a result, the studies, which included a limited number of cases with epicardial leads, cannot be generalized to all patients with CHD.

R. Beinart, MD (✉)
Division of Cardiology, Johns Hopkins University School of Medicine, 702 Rutland Avenue, Traylor 903, Baltimore, MD 21287, USA
e-mail: rbeiner1@jhmi.edu

S. Nazarian, MD, PhD
Ventricular Arrhythmia Ablation Service, Cardiac Electrophysiology, Johns Hopkins Hospital, Carnegie 592C, 600 N. Wolfe Street, Baltimore, MD 21287, USA
e-mail: snazarian@jhmi.edu

F. Saremi (ed.), *Cardiac CT and MR for Adult Congenital Heart Disease*,
DOI 10.1007/978-1-4614-8875-0_31, © Springer Science+Business Media New York 2014

The American Heart Association and European guidelines discourage, in general, the use of MRI in patients with implanted devices. However, they do not define the procedure as absolutely contraindicated [30, 31]. Therefore, the decision of performing MRI in patients with cardiac devices, including those with CHD, should be made on an individual basis. Importantly, the MRI must be performed under unique conditions, applying strict safety measures and documenting informed consent. Individualized risk assessment, the presence of specialized personnel with adequate emergency medical equipment and expertise, continuous monitoring during the procedure, and thorough follow-up are essential.

MRI Safety Protocol

Over the past decade, we have developed and tested a protocol for noncardiac and cardiac MR imaging of patients with permanent pacemakers or ICDs. So far, we have safely performed nearly 1,000 MRI examinations using this protocol [32]. It comprises several steps including device selection based on previous in vitro and in vivo studies [26], device programming to minimize inappropriate activation or inhibition of brady- or tachyarrhythmia therapies, and patient monitoring (Fig. 31.1). In general, ferromagnetic devices in a magnetic field are subject to static and gradient magnetic field-induced force and torque. Therefore, we include only patients with leads that were implanted 6 weeks or more prior to referral for MRI to avoid risk of lead or generator movement in magnetic field. To avoid the risk of heating, it would be rational to exclude patients with epicardial and/or abandoned leads. Depending on their length and configuration (i.e., loops), retained segments may be prone to significant temperature rises than leads that are attached to pulse generators and can cause electrical currents and additional susceptibility artifacts. Also, pacemaker-dependent ICD recipients are excluded from MRI scans at our institution. In pacemaker-dependent patients, pacemaker programming is changed to an asynchronous mode (DOO/VOO) in order to avoid electromagnetic interference (EMI)-induced inappropriate inhibition of pacing. In non-pacemaker-dependent patients, we program the device to an inhibited pacing mode (DDI/VVI) to avoid EMI-induced inappropriate tracking. Other pacing functions, including tachyarrhythmia monitoring and therapies, and rate response mode are also disabled. During the examination, we monitor patients continuously using ECG, blood pressure, and pulse oximetry. Additionally, the patient is asked to report any symptoms using the in-room speaker system. At the end of the scan, we interrogate the device and reprogram it to baseline settings. Up to now, the primary clinically significant event attributable to MRI that we have detected is power-on reset, with an incidence of up to 1.5 % [32]. Other minor changes in device parameters including lead sensing and capture thresholds have also been detected. Such lead parameter changes, in our experience, were clinically nonsignificant and did not require any alteration in device programming or need for system revision.

MRI in Patients with CHD and Cardiac Devices

Pulver and colleagues have recently published their experience in MRI scanning of patients with CHD and implanted cardiac devices using a 1.5-T magnet [33]. They performed 11 MRI scans in eight patients who had undergone device placement for sinus node dysfunction, long QT syndrome, and complete heart block. All patients were non-pacemaker dependent, three of them had dual-chamber devices, and most had epicardial leads. Four of these scans were cardiac, and the rest were non-thoracic scans. Inappropriate pacing or significant changes in generator or lead parameters were absent. The authors concluded that MRI could be safely performed in patients with CHD despite having predominantly epicardial leads [33].

Thoracic Scans

An important aspect of MRI imaging in patients with CHD is related to image quality when

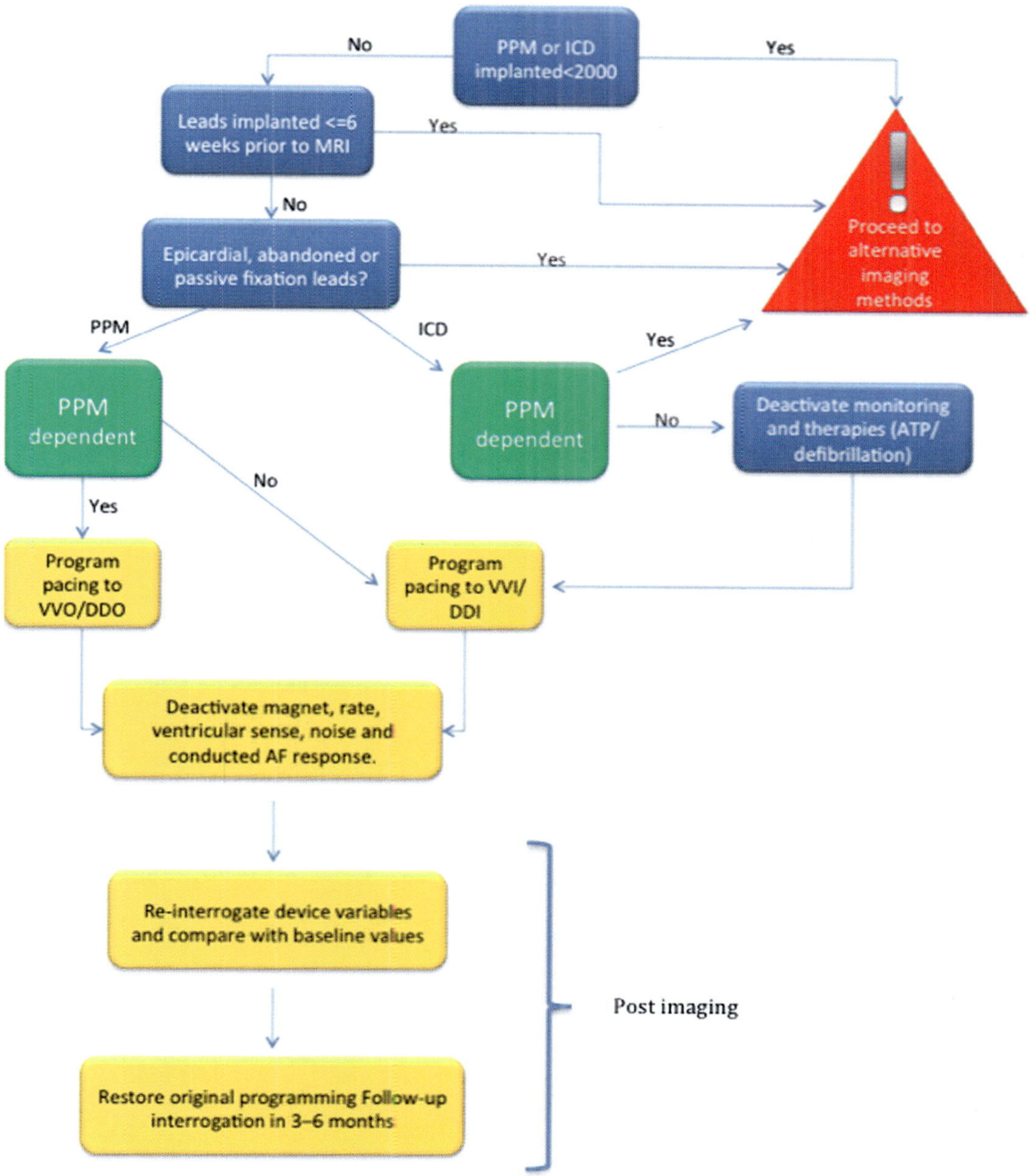

Fig. 31.1 Safety protocol for MRI in patients with implanted cardiac devices. *AF* atrial fibrillation, *ATP* antitachycardia pacing, *DDI* dual-chamber inhibited pacing without atrial tracking, *DOO* dual-chamber asynchronous pacing, *ICD* implantable cardioverter defibrillator, *PPM* pacemaker, *VOO* ventricular asynchronous pacing, *VVI* ventricular inhibited pacing (Adapted from Nazarian et al. [32] with permission)

performing cardiac MR scans. In patients with implantable devices, metal susceptibility artifacts may potentially limit the image quality especially in higher magnetic fields such as 3-T magnets. Metal artifacts due to magnetic susceptibility effect or induction of eddy currents by radio-frequency pulses appear as bands with increased or decreased signal in the vicin-

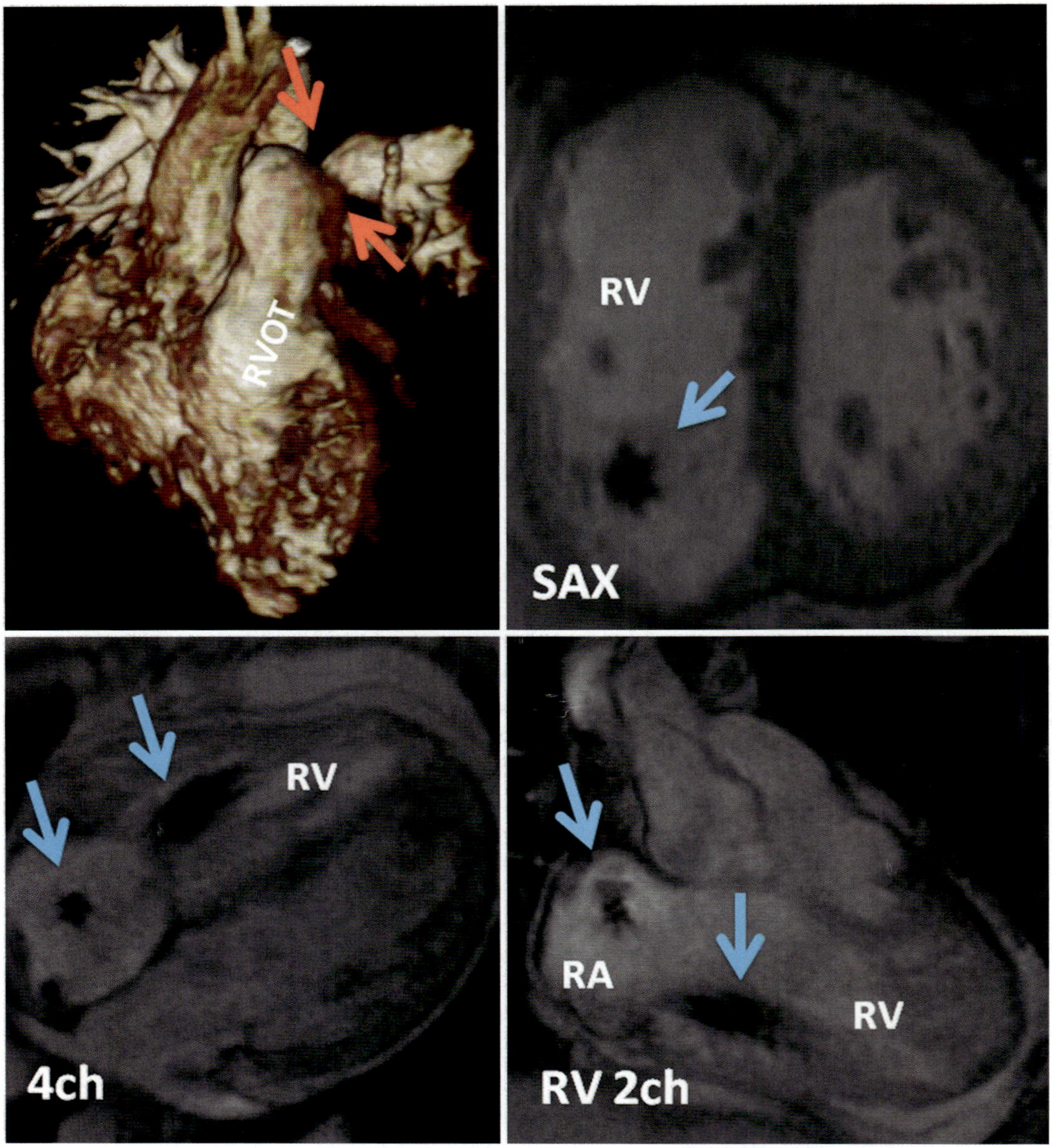

Fig. 31.2 Thoracic MRI of a patient status post complete repair of tetralogy of Fallot and implanted dual-chamber pacemaker. Volume-rendered reconstruction shows left pulmonary artery stenosis (*red arrows*) and the right ventricle outflow tract patch (*RVOT*). Cine MR images in short axis (*SAX*), four chamber (*4ch*), and right ventricle (*RV*) two chamber (*2ch*) showing the lead artifacts in the right atrium(*RA*) and RV (*blue arrows*)

ity of the leads or generators. On delayed post-contrast images, artifactual increased signal may be confused with hyperenhancing myocardial scars [24]. In our experience, these artifacts can be reduced by selecting imaging planes perpendicular to the plane of the device generator, shortening the echo time, and using spin echo and fast spin echo sequences (Fig. 31.2). In general, compared to balanced steady-state free-precession (SSFP) sequence, spoiled fast gradient echo sequence demonstrates fewer artifacts from metallic devices. This is likely related to shorter echo times used in the later sequence. Pulver and colleagues have reported that in their experience, in patients with CHD, all MRIs yielded diagnostic quality images with no evidence of major artifacts despite having predominantly epicardial leads [33]. They used routine MR sequences for their cardiac cases. Mild atrial lead artifact was seen in SSFP cine imaging, but double inversion recovery black blood series were essentially artifact-free. Notably, artifacts from leads and pacemaker generators are minimal in size. Moreover, left-sided ICD generators are the primary cause of image distortion in device recipients [34].

MRI-Conditional Cardiac Devices

Given the increased clinical need for MRI scans in patients with implantable cardiac device, implantable cardiac device manufacturers have developed devices that are specifically designed to be safe in the MRI environment. These "MRI-conditional" devices pose no known hazards when MRI is performed using a specific device programming and detailed monitoring conditions [35]. Recently, the United States Food and Drug Administration (FDA) approved the Revo MRI SureScan Pacing System (Medtronic, Inc., Minneapolis, MN), one of the MRI-conditional pacing systems [36]. Additional MRI-conditional devices are available outside of the United States. These devices include the Accent MRI (St Jude Medical, St. Paul, MN) [37], Evia and Estella (Biotronik, Berlin, Germany) [38], as well as Lumax 740 (Biotronik, Berlin, Germany) [38]. Of note, these devices are approved for MRI only when attached to specific leads (e.g., CapSureFix (Medtronic, Inc., Minneapolis, MN), Tendril MRI (St Jude Medical, St. Paul, MN), and Linoxsmart (Biotronik, Berlin, Germany)) and when the MRI field strength is limited to 1.5 T.

Several modifications were made in these devices in order to make them "MRI conditional." Due to manufacturer proprietary designs, not all changes are disclosed. However, these changes include design features to minimize the use of ferromagnetic materials. Changes in the lead conductor design and filtering are used to alleviate heating. The use of a Hall sensor rather than a reed switch results in more predictable pacemaker performance within the MRI environment [39]. Other changes include modules to simplify MRI safe device programming. For example, in the Revo MRI SureScan Pacing System (Medtronic, Inc., Minneapolis, MN), the MRI mode streamlines the choice between asynchronous and non-stimulation modes, increases pacing output to 5.0 V at 1.0 ms during MRI, and enables MRI mode programming only after system integrity has been checked and approved.

The first feasibility study for such an MRI-conditional device included 107 patients. During this study, patients underwent implantation of the EnRhythm MRI-conditional device or a conventional dual-chamber device. The authors reported no complications during the follow-up period [40]. They observed, however, a trend towards lower successful cephalic vein access when using MRI dedicated leads compared to conventional leads (60.0 % vs. 68.4 %, respectively). Also, subclavian vein access was used more frequently in patients with MRI-conditional leads (40.0 % vs. 31.6 % respectively, p=NS). Finally, there was no difference in fluoroscopy time (6.0 ± 3.6 min vs. 6.6 ± 3.8 min), overall procedure times (71.7 ± 27.6 min vs. 76.9 ± 30.3 min), or duration of hospitalization. This study suggested that the EnRhythm MRI-compatible pacemaker is safe and could be used for cardiac pacing. Following this study, a larger-scale randomized prospective multicenter study was performed. The study included 464 patients and recruited both pacemaker-dependent and non-pacemaker-dependent patients [39]. Twelve weeks following the procedure, 211 patients underwent MRI examination using a 1.5-T scanner. Other technical parameters included a maximum specific absorption rate of 2 W/kg and a maximum gradient slew rate of 200 T/m/s. During these scans, the isocenter was limited to extra-thoracic region (above the superior surface of C1 vertebra and below the inferior surface of the body of T12). Device interrogation was performed before MRI, immediately after MRI, 1 week after MRI, and at 1 month after MRI. No events were reported during MRI examinations, and no device-related adverse events were attributable to MRI. There were no differences between the study groups with regard to pacemaker measurements including capture threshold, sensitivity, and impedances. Importantly, since this study was limited to specific isocenter locations, the results cannot be generalized to assess safety of this MRI-conditional system with MRI isocenter in the thorax (between C1 and T12 vertebra). This study led to the approval of the Revo MRI Pacemaker System with 5086 MRI CapSureFix MRI Pacing Leads (Medtronic) and the SureScan Software (Medtronic) as "MRI conditional" by the United States FDA [41].

Future Directions

The currently approved MRI-conditional devices were assessed and approved for conditional use in 1.5-T MRI scanners. Higher field strengths are increasingly used in the clinical setting and offer improved signal-to-noise ratio (SNR), spatial resolution, image quality, and diagnostic strength. Gimbel and colleagues observed no arrhythmias or significant changes in device parameters with 3.0-T MRI in 14 patients with cardiac devices. Minor observed events did include, however, one patient with a burning sensation in his chest [42] and two cases of inhibition of pacing during the scan related to both EMI-induced output inhibition [43] and possibly the magnetohydrodynamic effect (i.e., the inhibition of pacing due to current induction from the to-and-fro motion of MRI induced charged ions contained in aortic blood) [44]. Future studies to examine the safety of preforming 3.0-T MRI in patients with implanted MRI-conditional cardiac devices are warranted.

The use of currently approved MRI-conditional devices excludes isocenter localization between C1 and T12 vertebra. The thoracic isocenter restriction could potentially decrease the image SNR and resolution. Since high SNRs are required for various thoracic scans, including assessment for myocardial viability, blood vessels, vascular malformation, and existence of shunts, it is highly important to study the safety of MRI-conditional devices with MRI isocenter located in the thorax and to characterize the extent of artifacts related to the implanted device system.

The population of patients that qualify for ICD and/or CRT devices, including those with CHD, is growing. Many such patients will benefit from an MRI scan at some point after the implant procedure. Hence, it is essential to develop MRI-conditional ICD and/or CRT systems. The "MR-pro" (Lumax 740, Biotronik, Germany) was recently approved in Europe. The data regarding these newly approved devices has not yet been published.

MRI-conditional technologies represent innovation that could facilitate the use of MRIs in patients who require pacemaker or ICD systems. The availability of such technology will surely benefit patients with CHD.Hence, additional studies are needed to investigate safety in the setting of higher static magnetic field strengths, serial MRI examinations, image isocenter located between C1 and T12, and abandoned or epicardial leads.

Acknowledgments Dr. Nazarian is on the MRI advisory panel (unpaid) for Medtronic. Dr. Nazarian is a scientific advisor to and is principal investigator for research funding to Johns Hopkins University from Biosense Webster Inc. Dr. Nazarian is funded by the National Institutes of Health Career Development Grant K23HL089333.

References

1. Knauth Meadows A, Ordovas K, Higgins CB, Reddy GP. Magnetic resonance imaging in the adult with congenital heart disease. Semin Roentgenol. 2008;43:246–58.
2. Marcotte F, Poirier N, Pressacco J, et al. Evaluation of adult congenital heart disease by cardiac magnetic resonance imaging. Congenit Heart Dis. 2009;4:216–30.
3. Koskenvuo JW, Karra H, Lehtinen J, et al. Cardiac MRI: accuracy of simultaneous measurement of left and right ventricular parameters using three different sequences. Clin Physiol Funct Imaging. 2007;27:385–93.
4. Maceira AM, Prasad SK, Khan M, Pennell DJ. Reference right ventricular systolic and diastolic function normalized to age, gender and body surface area from steady-state free precession cardiovascular magnetic resonance. Eur Heart J. 2006;27:2879–88.
5. Kilner PJ, Gatehouse PD, Firmin DN. Flow measurement by magnetic resonance: a unique asset worth optimising. J Cardiovasc Magn Reson. 2007;9:723–8.

6. Prakash A, Powell AJ, Krishnamurthy R, Geva T. Magnetic resonance imaging evaluation of myocardial perfusion and viability in congenital and acquired pediatric heart disease. Am J Cardiol. 2004;93:657–61.
7. Rebergen SA, de Roos A. Congenital heart disease. Evaluation of anatomy and function by MRI. Herz. 2000;25:365–83.
8. Anderson RH, Becker AE, Arnold R, Wilkinson JL. The conducting tissues in congenitally corrected transposition. Circulation. 1974;50:911–23.
9. Huhta JC, Maloney JD, Ritter DG, Ilstrup DM, Feldt RH. Complete atrioventricular block in patients with atrioventricular discordance. Circulation. 1983;67:1374–7.
10. Connelly MS, Liu PP, Williams WG, Webb GD, Robertson P, McLaughlin PR. Congenitally corrected transposition of the great arteries in the adult: functional status and complications. J Am Coll Cardiol. 1996;27:1238–43.
11. Thiene G, Wenink AC, Frescura C, et al. Surgical anatomy and pathology of the conduction tissues in atrioventricular defects. J Thorac Cardiovasc Surg. 1981;82:928–37.
12. Manning PB, Mayer Jr JE, Wernovsky G, Fishberger SB, Walsh EP. Staged operation to Fontan increases the incidence of sinoatrial node dysfunction. J Thorac Cardiovasc Surg. 1996;111:833–9; discussion 839–40.
13. Alexander ME, Cecchin F, Walsh EP, Triedman JK, Bevilacqua LM, Berul CI. Implications of implantable cardioverter defibrillator therapy in congenital heart disease and pediatrics. J Cardiovasc Electrophysiol. 2004;15:72–6.
14. Alexander ME, Walsh EP, Saul JP, Epstein MR, Triedman JK. Value of programmed ventricular stimulation in patients with congenital heart disease. J Cardiovasc Electrophysiol. 1999;10:1033–44.
15. Dore A, Santagata P, Dubuc M, Mercier LA. Implantable cardioverter defibrillators in adults with congenital heart disease: a single center experience. Pacing Clin Electrophysiol. 2004;27:47–51.
16. Dubin AM. Resynchronization in pediatrics who needs it? J Am Coll Cardiol. 2005;46:2290–1.
17. Janousek J, Vojtovic P, Hucin B, et al. Resynchronization pacing is a useful adjunct to the management of acute heart failure after surgery for congenital heart defects. Am J Cardiol. 2001; 88:145–52.
18. Zimmerman FJ, Starr JP, Koenig PR, Smith P, Hijazi ZM, Bacha EA. Acute hemodynamic benefit of multisite ventricular pacing after congenital heart surgery. Ann Thorac Surg. 2003;75:1775–80.
19. Bacha EA, Zimmerman FJ, Mor-Avi V, et al. Ventricular resynchronization by multisite pacing improves myocardial performance in the postoperative single-ventricle patient. Ann Thorac Surg. 2004;78:1678–83.
20. Janousek J, Gebauer RA. Cardiac resynchronization therapy in pediatric and congenital heart disease. Pacing Clin Electrophysiol. 2008;31 Suppl 1:S21–3.
21. Khairy P, Fournier A, Thibault B, Dubuc M, Therien J, Vobecky SJ. Cardiac resynchronization therapy in congenital heart disease. Int J Cardiol. 2006;109:160–8.
22. Strieper M, Karpawich P, Frias P, et al. Initial experience with cardiac resynchronization therapy for ventricular dysfunction in young patients with surgically operated congenital heart disease. Am J Cardiol. 2004;94:1352–4.
23. Janousek J, Gebauer RA, Abdul-Khaliq H, et al. Cardiac resynchronisation therapy in paediatric and congenital heart disease: differential effects in various anatomical and functional substrates. Heart. 2009;95:1165–71.
24. Nazarian S, Halperin HR. How to perform magnetic resonance imaging on patients with implantable cardiac arrhythmia devices. Heart Rhythm. 2009;6:138–43.
25. Tandri H, Zviman MM, Wedan SR, Lloyd T, Berger RD, Halperin H. Determinants of gradient field-induced current in a pacemaker lead system in a magnetic resonance imaging environment. Heart Rhythm. 2008;5:462–8.
26. Roguin A, Zviman MM, Meininger GR, et al. Modern pacemaker and implantable cardioverter/defibrillator systems can be magnetic resonance imaging safe: in vitro and in vivo assessment of safety and function at 1.5 T. Circulation. 2004;110:475–82.
27. Sommer T, Naehle CP, Yang A, et al. Strategy for safe performance of extrathoracic magnetic resonance imaging at 1.5 tesla in the presence of cardiac pacemakers in non-pacemaker-dependent patients: a prospective study with 115 examinations. Circulation. 2006;114:1285–92.
28. Vahlhaus C. Heating of pacemaker leads during magnetic resonance imaging. Eur Heart J. 2005;26:1243; author reply 1243–4.
29. Nazarian S, Roguin A, Zviman MM, et al. Clinical utility and safety of a protocol for noncardiac and cardiac magnetic resonance imaging of patients with permanent pacemakers and implantable-cardioverter defibrillators at 1.5 tesla. Circulation. 2006;114:1277–84.
30. Levine GN, Gomes AS, Arai AE, et al. Safety of magnetic resonance imaging in patients with cardiovascular devices: an American Heart Association scientific statement from the Committee on Diagnostic and Interventional Cardiac Catheterization, Council on Clinical Cardiology, and the Council on Cardiovascular Radiology and Intervention: endorsed by the American College of Cardiology Foundation, the North American Society for Cardiac Imaging, and the Society for Cardiovascular Magnetic Resonance. Circulation. 2007;116:2878–91.
31. Roguin A, Schwitter J, Vahlhaus C, et al. Magnetic resonance imaging in individuals with cardiovascular implantable electronic devices. Europace. 2008;10:336–46.
32. Nazarian S, Hansford R, Roguin A, et al. A prospective evaluation of a protocol for magnetic resonance imaging of patients with implanted cardiac devices. Ann Intern Med. 2011;155:415–24.

33. Pulver AF, Puchalski MD, Bradley DJ, et al. Safety and imaging quality of MRI in pediatric and adult congenital heart disease patients with pacemakers. Pacing Clin Electrophysiol. 2009;32:450–6.
34. Sasaki T, Hansford R, Zviman MM, et al. Quantitative assessment of artifacts on cardiac magnetic resonance imaging of patients with pacemakers and implantable cardioverter-defibrillators. Circ Cardiovasc Imaging. 2011;4:662–70.
35. Standard practice for marking medical devices and other items for safety in the magnetic resonance environment. American Society for Testing and Materials (ASTM) International 2008.
36. http://www.fda.gov/MedicalDevices/default.htm.
37. http://www.sjmprofessional.com/Products/index.aspx.
38. http://www.biotronikusa.com/manuals/.
39. Wilkoff BL, Bello D, Taborsky M, et al. Magnetic resonance imaging in patients with a pacemaker system designed for the magnetic resonance environment. Heart Rhythm. 2011;8:65–73.
40. Forleo GB, Santini L, Della Rocca DG, et al. Safety and efficacy of a new magnetic resonance imaging-compatible pacing system: early results of a prospective comparison with conventional dual-chamber implant outcomes. Heart Rhythm. 2010;7:750–4.
41. http://www.medtronic.com/mrisurescan-us/pacing_system_description.html.
42. Gimbel JR. Magnetic resonance imaging of implantable cardiac rhythm devices at 3.0 tesla. Pacing Clin Electrophysiol. 2008;31:795–801.
43. Gimbel JR. Unexpected asystole during 3T magnetic resonance imaging of a pacemaker-dependent patient with a 'modern' pacemaker. Europace. 2009;11:1241–2.
44. Gimbel JR. Unexpected pacing inhibition upon exposure to the 3T static magnetic field prior to imaging acquisition: what is the mechanism? Heart Rhythm. 2011;8:944–5.

Index

F. Saremi (ed.), *Cardiac CT and MR for Adult Congenital Heart Disease*,
DOI 10.1007/978-1-4614-8875-0, © Springer Science+Business Media New York 2014

E

H

I

J

K

T

U

W

Y

Printed in the United States of America